General

— AND —

Applied

Toxicology

GENERAL

—— AND ——

APPLIED

TOXICOLOGY

SECOND EDITION

EDITORS

Bryan Ballantyne
MD, DSc, PhD, FFOM, FACOM, FAACT, FATS, FRCPath, FIBiol, MRCS
Director of Applied Toxicology
Union Carbide Corporation, Danbury, Connecticut, USA
Adjunct Professor of Pharmacology and Toxicology
West Virginia University, USA

Timothy C. Marrs
MD, DSc, MRCP, FRCPath, FIBiol
Senior Medical Officer
Joint Food Safety and Standards Group
London, UK

Tore Syversen
MSc, DrPhil
Professor of Toxicology
Norwegian University of Science and Technology
Trondheim, Norway

VOLUME 1

Published in the United Kingdom by
MACMILLAN REFERENCE LTD., 1999
25 Eccleston Place, London, SW1W 9NF
Basingstoke and Oxford

Companies and representatives throughout the world.

http://www.macmillan-reference.co.uk

Distributed in the UK and Europe by
Macmillan Distribution Ltd.,
Brunel Road, Houndmills,
Basingstoke, Hampshire, RG21 2XS, England

General and Applied Toxicology - 2nd ed.
1. Toxicology
I. Ballantyne, Bryan.   II. Marrs, Timothy C.   III. Syversen, Tore L. M.
615.9
ISBN 0-333-698681

Published in the United States and Canada by
GROVE'S DICTIONARIES INC., 1999
345 Park Avenue South, 10th Floor
New York, NY 10010-1707, USA

ISBN 1-56159-242-0

A catalog record for this book is available from the Library of Congress

Typeset by Kolam Information Services Ltd, India
Printed and bound in the UK by Bath Press, Bath

CONTENTS

VOLUME 1

PART ONE: BASIC SCIENCE

VOLUME 2

PART FOUR: TARGET ORGAN AND TISSUE TOXICITY

PART FIVE: GENETIC TOXICOLOGY, CARCINOGENICITY, REPRODUCTIVE AND DEVELOPMENTAL TOXICOLOGY

PART SIX: ENVIRONMENTAL TOXICOLOGY

VOLUME 3

PREFACE TO SECOND EDITION

It is with sadness that we have to note the death of one of the original editors, Paul Turner, *CBE*, Emeritus Professor of Clinical Pharmacology, University of London. Professor Turner was a remarkable man in many respects. As an internationally renowned clinical pharmacologist, his political and negotiating skills were called on widely by National and International organizations. However, his interests and expertise flowed well beyond the boundaries of medical sciences. He was, for example, well versed in music and an accomplished pianist, and just before his death was ordained into the Church. He was a kind, compassionate, and deeply sincere man. His guiding skills were much missed during the preparation of this second edition.

Since publication of the first edition of this textbook, there have been several major advances in toxicology and its sub-specialties. New horizons have appeared, subjects previously covered by generic considerations have become areas for investigation on their own, and concepts in some established areas have been modified or radically changed. Regulatory approaches continue to be amended, harmonization has become a major issue, and inevitable politics has fashioned some elements of applied toxicology. All these trends have been reflected in the planning of this new edition. Chapters on subjects carried over from the first to this edition have been completely updated and rewritten by the authors, additional co-authors, or replacement authors. New chapters have been added in the areas of molecular toxicology, apoptosis, species variability, toxicogenetics, extrapolation, biological rhythms and toxicity, neurobehavioural toxicology, endocrine disruption, environmental toxicology, mixtures, risk assessment, biomarkers, interactions, and education. In view of recent and unfortunate trends, chapters have been included which are devoted to terrorism and to the toxicologist as an expert witness. A new section has been added dealing with the toxicology of special groups of substances. This is not intended to be an all-inclusive compendium of substance toxicology, but rather to illustrate the wide spectrum of toxicity from substances of differing structure and origin. The section on regulatory toxicology has been totally updated with respect to changes in regulatory activity and attitudes. As in the previous edition, in order to get the best representation of expertise and attitude, contributions have been obtained from a wide geographical area. Authors are from Canada, the Czech Republic, Finland, France, Germany, Jordan, the Netherlands, Norway, South Africa, Sweden, Switzerland, the United Kingdom and the United States.

We continue to have concern about some unfortunate trends in toxicology and its applications. Even though there is some increasing flexibility, regulators generally still maintain a restricted and compartmentalized mindset to testing needs and classifications. One notable example of this has been the guidelines for the classification of substances having a respiratory sensitizing potential, introduced by the EEC and apparently adopted by OECD without question. Based on known political pressures from one country, the criteria include one that states that for the purposes of classification as a respiratory sensitizer it does not have to be demonstrated that the material operates through an immune mechanism. Not only does this qualification mean that some purely irritant substances will be wrongly classified, but the approach flagrantly ignores the definition of a respiratory sensitizer. This is but one of several examples where regulatory activity goes contrary to credible scientific concepts. However, there are some encouraging signs. Thus, since the Uruguay round of the General Agreement on Tariffs and Trade (GATT), codex standards are, in most circumstances, accepted food standards for world trade purposes. This has inevitably raised the profile of the various codex committees and the World Health Organisation/Food and Agricultural Organisation Committees that advise the codex committees. This has placed the Joint Expert Committee on Food Additives (JECFA) and the Joint Meeting on Pesticide Residues (JMPR) in a key position in protection of public health. In a number of areas the EU has continued to harmonise its regulatory requirements, while NAFTA (USA, Canada and Mexico) continues to make progress on harmonisation. In both the USA and UK, there have been major changes since the last edition: the passage of the Food Quality Protection Act in the USA is making major changes on risk assessment of food in that country and possibly elsewhere. In the UK, the Joint Food Safety and Standards Group, in the Department of Health and the Ministry of Agriculture,

Fisheries and Food is intended to be the fore-runner of a Food Standards Agency.

Whilst the majority of full-length publications in respected scientific, medical, and technical journals are of high quality and add to our knowledge and understanding of various facets of toxicology, some publications are less desirable. We still continue to see a few examples of the same, or very marginally altered data, appearing from the same individuals or groups in two different journals at different times. We believe it highly unlikely that this is a desire, on the part of the authors, to ensure that the widest audience have access to the information. More likely the motivation is related to attempted publication proliferation in a competitive or research restricted environment. Those who see such examples of unethical duplication of information, often against the stated objectives of a journal, should make this known to the respective editors. Also, some publications contain data which must clearly have been selective, or manipulated, with the objective of supporting a viewpoint, which could be personal, commercial, or political in motivation. Again, editors and referees should be constantly vigilant to detect such submitted contributions with a potentially unethical and/or unprofessional content. We do not suggest that the referee should significantly impact on the subjective interpretation of the data, unless this is clearly biased or ignores well established facts. Indeed it is reprehensible for a referee to insist that opinion (as opposed to observed fact) be modified to accord with his or her own viewpoint, a situation which we have known to occur. Rather, the editor and referees should ensure, as far as possible, that methodology is appropriate and that the information submitted represents a true and complete record of the measurements and observations. Finally, a not insignificant number of published papers seem to add little to the factual basis of knowledge or an understanding of processes and mechanisms. Editors and referees should be more willing to reject such inadequate contributions, even though this may go contrary to objectives of attracting papers to a particular journal. One way to have more impartial review of papers, although very rarely practiced, would be for editors to send manuscripts to reviewers by an anonymous process. This is to say, referees should be asked to review papers without a knowledge of the authors or the institution of origin. Although, clearly, style and interest may be recognized, this would at least be one way to restrict 'bias' or 'the old boy' attitudes in recommendations on the acceptability or otherwise of papers for publication in recognized reputable scientific journals.

We have some concerns over the increasing use of the 'internet' to distribute information related to health sciences. Whilst much information that can be derived from internet sources has a credible origin, in some instances false or manipulated information is to be found. Pallen and Loman [*Brit. Med. J.*, **317**, 1522 (1998)] have drawn attention to, and illustrated, the way in which appropriate software can easily allow alteration of the true likeness of real individuals, or create fictional images of near-photographic quality which illustrate medical conditions. It is feasible that data distributed through the internet could be 'hacked' and manipulated for unethical reasons. Since the electronic network is being used increasingly for distribution of, and access to, information, the scientific and medical communities need to develop approaches and methodologies in order to ensure the source and credibility of the information, and prevent on-line manipulation of the data.

The production of a work of this size needs the devoted contribution from a number of persons. The individual editors are grateful for the help received at their own respective geographical locations. Bryan Ballantyne is particularly thankful for the consistently devoted help and contribution from Ms. Sandra Morris, and for her continuing support, persistence, and patience. Tim Marrs would like to thank Dr. Jeremy Metters and Dr. Andrew Wadge for their encouragement, and Mrs. Carole Dobson for her help and support. Tore Syversen would like to acknowledge Ms. Janne HjeldeWold for her dedicated attention to work carried out in Trondheim. Once again, it has been the utmost of pleasure to work with the staff of Macmillan. Mrs. Rosemary Foster guided us through the first edition and the initial stages of planning for the second edition. In particular, and for this edition, we wish to thank Dr. Gina Fullerlove, Publishing Director (Science) and Ms. Diana Levy, Senior Production Controller. Their extreme level of devotion and professionalism is reflected in the high quality of production.

Bryan Ballantyne   **Timothy C. Marrs**   **Tore Syversen**
Connecticut, USA   *Edenbridge, UK*   *Trondheim, Norway*

PREFACE TO FIRST EDITION

Some fifty years ago, toxicology was barely recognized as a discipline and had few active participants, although some experimental pathologists at that time would now be regarded as within the sphere of toxicology. Over the past three decades there has been a considerable expansion in our understanding and applications of the various facets associated with exposure to natural and synthetic potentially harmful materials. This has been reflected in an expansion of the population calling themselves professional toxicologists, an increase in the number of units and establishments devoted to toxicological investigations, the formation of many learned societies devoted to general and specialist aspects of toxicology, and a proliferation of publications on toxicology and its subspecializations. Accompanying all these factors has been the appearance of a number of journals devoted to general, special, and applied toxicology. Additionally, the number of textbooks devoted to toxicology has shown a dramatic increase. In general, however, the majority of these texts have been concerned with specialist areas or subdisciplines. General toxicology texts are relatively few in number, particularly those devoted to use in undergraduate and postgraduate courses, and for those working for toxicology certifying examinations. Many general texts are brief, of limited technical scope, and several are directed at an audience more general than toxicologists in training or practice. We therefore saw the need for a textbook of toxicology for both educational and reference use which complements, rather than conflicts with, existing texts.

This textbook is intended to give a comprehensive review of the scientific basis of toxicology and its application, and to be used both as a reference volume and a text for educational purposes. Both general and specialist needs are considered, with particular reference to basic principles, definitions, laboratory aspects, interpretation of data, and practical applications of toxicology. Thus, there are sections devoted to basic concepts, techniques, toxicity by specific routes of exposure and by organ systems, special aspects of toxicology, and the increasingly dominant, though sometimes scientifically suspect, area of regulatory toxicology. Environmental topics are covered in several chapters, notably those dealing with air pollution, toxicology of pesticides, toxicology and disasters, and the section on regulatory toxicology in the second volume. Amongst the many objectives of this book during its planning phase were to inter-relate knowledge gained in the toxicology laboratory to its practical applications, and to present topics not normally, or inadequately, covered by other texts.

Toxicology is primarily concerned with defining the potential of natural and synthetic substances to produce adverse health effects and, if they do so, to determine their nature, incidence, mechanism of production, and reversibility. The implications with respect to human health and the environment are clear. Interpretation and application of knowledge gained in the toxicology laboratory may be overshadowed by political, commercial, regulatory and technological issues and pressures. We thus feel that there is a need to stress a concern about ethical and moral issues being fundamental to the practice of toxicology as a profession with wide-ranging social implications. For this reason reference is made to these issues in several chapters, and a specific chapter is devoted to this consideration.

The practice of toxicology has been the subject of attacks, usually verbally but sometimes physically violent, because of the excessive use of animal models. Therefore, in several areas of this book the use of alternatives, and their validation, is presented.

We hope that this textbook will be of use for those working toward a first or higher degree in toxicology or in courses with a toxicological facet, or for those reading for certification in general or specialist toxicology. Additionally, we believe that the book will serve as a useful reference text for general, clinical, industrial, environmental, forensic, and experimental toxicologists, and to occupational health physicians, industrial hygienists, epidemiologists, experimental and general pathologists, biochemists and pharmacologists.

During the preparation of this book we have received nothing but the utmost help, guidance and courtesy from Mrs. Rosemary Foster, Mr. John Normansell and Ms. Grace Evans. Their professionalism is to the significant credit of Macmillan.

Bryan Ballantyne   **Timothy C. Marrs**   **Paul Turner**
Danbury, Connecticut, USA   *London, UK*   *London, UK*

LIST OF CONTRIBUTORS

Lisbeth Aasmoe, *MSc, PhD*
Department of Clinical Pharmacology, University
Hospital of Tromso, N-9038 Tromso, Norway

Gerald E. Adams, *PhD, DSc, FACR*
Medical Research Council Radiobiology Unit,
Chilton, Didcot, Oxfordshire OX11 0RD, UK
Professor Adams died in 1998

Catrine Ahlen,
Senior Scientist, SINTEF UNIMED, Department
of Extreme Work Environment, N-7489
Trondheim, Norway

Antero Aitio, *MD, PhD*
Programme for Chemical Safety, World Health
Organization, Avenue Appia 20, Geneva 27
CH-1211, Switzerland

Diana Anderson, *BSc, MSc, PhD, Dip Ed,
FRCPath, FIBiol, FIFST, FATS*
Senior Associate, Coordinator External Affairs,
BIBRA International, Woodmansterne Road,
Carshalton, Wallington, Surrey SM5 4DS, UK

Charles M. Auer, *BSc*
Director, Chemical Control Division, Office
of Pollution Prevention and Toxics, US
Environmental Protection Agency (7405), 401 M
Street SW, Washington DC 20460, USA

Ronald C. Backer, *PhD, DABFT*
Universal Toxicology Laboratories, 10210 West
Highway 80, Midland, Texas 79706, USA

Bryan Ballantyne, *MD, DSc, PhD, FFOM,
FACOM, FAACT, FATS, FRCPath, FIBiol, MRCS*
Director of Applied Toxicology, Union Carbide
Corporation, 39 Old Ridgebury Road, Danbury,
Connecticut 06817-0001, USA

Steven I. Baskin, *PharmD, PhD, FCP, FACC,
DABT, FATS*
Team Leader and Principal Investigator, Division
of Pharmacology, U.S. Army Medical Research
Institute of Chemical Defense, 3100 Ricketts
Point Road, Aberdeen Proving Ground, Edgewood
Area, Maryland 21010-5400, USA

D. Nicholas Bateman, *BSc, MD, FRCP*
Director, Scottish Poisons Information Bureau,
Royal Infirmary, 1 Lauriston Place, Edinburgh
EH3 9YW, UK

George S. Behonick, *BS, MS, PhD*
NRC/NAS Research Associate, U.S. Army Medical
Research Institute of Chemical Defense, 3100
Ricketts Point Road, Aberdeen Proving Ground,
Edgewood Area, Maryland 21010-5400, USA

Sir Colin Berry, *DSc, MD, PhD, FRCP, FRCPath,
FFPM, FFOM*
Professor of Morbid Anatomy and Histopathology,
Department of Morbid Anatomy, Institute of
Pathology, Royal London Hospital, Whitechapel,
London E1 1BB, UK

Chantal Bismuth, *MD*
Professor of Medicine, Medical and Toxicological
Intensive Care Unit, Hôpital Lariboisière,
Université Paris VII, 2 rue Ambroise Paré, 75010
Paris, France

Olav Bjørseth, *MSc, PhD*
Associate Professor, Department of Industrial
Economics and Technology Management,
Norwegian University of Science and Technology,
A Getz vl, N-7491 Trondheim, Norway

Stephen W. Borron, *MD, MS*
Associate Clinical Professor of Emergency
Medicine, School of Medicine, George Washington
University, 1215 Seventeenth Street NW,
Washington DC 20036-3008; Visiting Researcher,
Hôpital Lariboisière, Université Paris VII, 2 rue
Ambroise Paré, 75475 Paris, France

Joan M. Braganza, *DSc, MSc, FRCP, FRCPath*
Pancreato-Biliary Service, Manchester Royal
Infirmary, Oxford Road, Manchester M13 9WL,
UK

John Caldwell, *PhD, DSc, FIBiol, HonMRCP*
Section of Molecular Toxicology, Division of
Biomedical Sciences, Imperial College School of
Medicine, South Kensington, London SW7 2AZ,
UK

Flemming R. Cassee, *PhD*
Laboratory for Health Effects Research, National
Institute for Public Health and the Environment,
P.O. Box 1, NL-3720 BA Bilthoven, The
Netherlands

Cheryl E.A. Chaffey, *BSc*
Head, Health Re-evaluation Section, Pest
Management Regulatory Agency, Health Canada,
2250 Riverside Drive, 6606E1 Ottawa, Ontario
K1A 0K9, Canada

John J. Clary, *PhD, FATS*
BioRisk, P.O. Box 2326, 2407 Oakfield Drive,
Midland, Michigan 48641, USA

Mary E. Clinton, *MD*
Clinical Professor, Department of Neurology,
School of Medicine, Vanderbilt University, 2100
Pierce Avenue, Medical Center South, Nashville,
Tennessee 37232, USA

David M. Conning, *OBE, MB, BS, FRCPath,
FIBiol, FIFST*
Blacksmith's Cottage, Totnor, Brockhampton,
Hereford HR1 4TJ, UK

Philip T. Copestake, *BSc, MSc*
Information and Advisory Service, BIBRA
International, Woodmansterne Road, Carshalton,
Surrey SM5 4DS, UK

Ian A. Cotgreave, *PhD*
Associate Professor, Division of Biochemical
Toxicology, Institute of Environmental Medicine,
Karolinska Institute, Box 210, S-17177 Stockholm,
Sweden

P.F. D'Arcy, *OBE, BPharm, PhD, DSc, DSc(Hon),
FRPharmS, CChem, FRSC, FPSNI*
Emeritus Professor, School of Pharmacy, The
Queen's University of Belfast, Medical Biology
Centre, 97 Lisburn Road, Belfast BT9 7BL,
Northern Ireland, UK

Susan Davies, *BPharm, MRPS, MBIRA*
Head of Regulatory Affairs, Schering Health Care
Ltd., The Brow, Burgess Hill, West Sussex RH15
9NE, UK

Rebecca J. Dearman, *BSc, PhD*
Research Toxicology Section, AstraZeneca Central
Toxicology Laboratory, Alderley Park,
Macclesfield, Cheshire SK10 4TJ, UK

Anthony P. DeCaprio, *BS, PhD, DABT*
Associate Professor, School of Public Health,
University at Albany, State University of New
York, One University Place, Rensselaer, New York
12144, USA

Wolf-D. Dettbarn, *MD*
Professor, Departments of Pharmacology and
Neurology, School of Medicine, Vanderbilt
University, 2100 Pierce Avenue, Medical Center
South, Nashville, Tennessee 37232, USA

Ian C. Dewhurst, *BSc, PhD*
Mallard House, Kings Pool, 3 Peasholme Green,
York YO1 7PX, UK

Geoff E. Diggle, *MB, BS, DipPharmMed, FFPM*
97 Bennetts Way, Croydon, Surrey CR0 8AG, UK

Virginia A. Dobozy, *VMD, MPH*
Office of Pesticide Programs, Health Effects
Division (7509C), US Environmental Protection
Agency, 401 M Street SW, Washington DC 20460,
USA

Lennart Dock, *PhD*
National Institute of Environmental Medicine,
Karolinska Institute, Box 210, S-17177 Stockholm,
Sweden

Gareth O. Evans, *BSc, MSc*
Principal Clinical Pathologist, Clinical Pathology,
Astra Safety Assessment, Astra Charnwood,
Bakewell Road, Loughborough LE11 5RH, UK

Steven Fairhurst, *BSc, PhD*
Head of Toxicology, Toxicology Unit, Health and
Safety Executive, Room 156, Magdalen House,
Trinity Road, Bootle, Merseyside L20 3QZ, UK

Victor J. Feron, *PhD*
Emeritus Professor of Biological Toxicology, Toxicology Division, TNO Nutrition and Food Research Institute, P.O. Box 360, NL-3700 AJ Zeist, The Netherlands

Robin J. Fielder, *BSc, PhD, DipToxRCPath*
Department of Health, Skipton House, 80 London Road, London SE1 6LW, UK

Brent L. Finley, *PhD, DABT*
Exponent, 149 Commonwealth Drive, Menlo Park, California 74025, USA

Trond Peder Flaten, *PhD*
Department of Chemistry, Norwegian University of Science and Technology, N-7491 Trondheim, Norway

Frode Fonnum, *BSc, PhD*
VISTA Professor, Forsvarets forskninsinstitutt, Postboks 25, N-2007 Kjeller, Norway

Andrew Forge, *BSc, MSc, PhD*
Institute of Laryngology and Otology, University College London, 330-332 Gray's Inn Road, London WC1X 8EE, UK

John R. Foster, *BSc, PhD, DipRCPath, FRCPath*
Senior Pathologist, AstraZeneca Central Toxicology Laboratory, Alderley Park, Macclesfield, Cheshire SK10 4TJ, UK

Etienne Fournier, *MD*
Professor Emeritus of Clinical Toxicology, Clinique Toxicologique, Hôpital Fernand Widal, 200 rue du Faubourg-St-Denis, 75475 Paris, Cedex 10, France

Arthur Furst, *PhD, ScD*
Institute of Chemical Biology, Harney Science Center, University of San Francisco, San Francisco, California 94117-1080, USA

Shayne C. Gad, *PhD, DABT*
Gad Consulting Services, 1818 White Oak Road, Raleigh, North Carolina 27608, USA

Sharat D. Gangolli, *BSc PhD, MChemA, CChem, FRSC, FRCPath*
157 Old Lodge Lane, Purley, Surrey CR8 4AU, UK

Michael L. Gargas, *PhD*
ChemRisk, The Courtland East Building, 29225 Chagrin Boulevard, Cleveland, Ohio 44122, USA

David G. Gatehouse, *CBiol, BSc, PhD, FIBiol, FRCPath*
Department of Genetic Toxicology, Preclinical Safety Sciences, Glaxo Wellcome Research and Development Ltd., Park Road, Ware, Hertfordshire SG12 ODP, UK

Paul Grasso, *BSc, MD FRCPath, DCP, DTM&H*
Robens Institute, University of Surrey, Guildford, Surrey GU2 5XH, UK

Peter Greaves, *MB, ChB, FRCPath*
Head of Safety of Medicines, Safety of medicines, AstraZeneca, Mereside, Alderley Park, Macclesfield, Cheshire SK10 4TG, UK

John P. Groten
Department of Explanatory Toxicology, TNO Nutrition and Food Research Institute, PO Box 360, 3700 AJ Zeist, The Netherlands

Ramesh C. Gupta, *DVM, PhD, DABT*
Professor and Head of Toxicology, Toxicology Department, Breathitt Veterinary Center, Murray State University, P.O. Box 2000, 715 North Drive, Hopkinsville, Kentucky 42241-2000, USA

Güneyt Güzey, *MD*
Institute of Cancer Research and Molecular Biology, Medical Technical Research Centre, Norwegian University of Science and Technology, N-7005 Trondheim, Norway

Hakam Hadidi, *MD, PhD*
Associate Professor, Department of Pharmacology, Faculty of Medicine, Jordan University of Science and Technology, P.O. Box 3030, Irbid, Jordan

Roy Hamlet, *BSc, PhD, CBiol, MIBiol*
Department of Health, Skipton House, 80 London Road, London SE1 6LW, UK

Ernest S. Harpur, *BSc, PhD, MRPharmS*
Department of Toxicology, Sanofi Research, Alnwick Research Centre, Willowburn Avenue, Alnwick, Northumberland NE66 2JH, UK

Jan G. Hengstler, *MD*
Institute of Toxicology, University of Mainz, Obere
Zahlbacher Strasse 67, D-55131 Mainz, Germany

Steven J. Hermansky, *MS, PharmD, PhD, DABT*
Principal Toxicologist, Schering-Plough
HealthCare Products, 3030 Jackson Avenue,
Memphis, Tennessee 38151, USA

Paul M. Hext, *BSc, PhD*
AstraZeneca Central Toxicology Laboratory,
Alderley Park, Macclesfield, Cheshire SK10 4TJ,
UK

Elwood F. Hill, *BA, PhD*
Wildlife Toxicologist, Adjunct Professor,
University Center for Environmental Sciences and
Engineering, University of Nevada, Reno, Nevada
USA; P.O. Box 1615, Gardnerville, Nevada 89410,
USA

Richard H. Hinton, *BA, PhD, FRCPath*
School of Biological Science, University of Surrey,
Guildford, Surrey GU2 5XH, UK

Bo Holmberg, *PhD*
Professor Emeritus, Department of Toxicology and
Chemistry, National Institute for Working Life,
S-17184 Solna, Sweden

William J.M. Hrushesky, *MD*
Professor of Medicine, Department of Medicine,
Stratton Veterans Affairs Medical Centre and
Albany Medical College, Albany, New York
12208, USA

Deborah J. Hussey, *BSc*
Mallard House, Kings Pool, 3 Peasholme Green,
York YO1 7PX, UK

Jeffrey R. Idle, *PhD, CChem, FRSC*
Professor in Medicine and Molecular Biology,
Institute for Cancer Research and Molecular
Biology, Norwegian University of Science and
Technology, Medisinsk Teknisk Senter, 7005
Trondheim, Norway

H. Paul A. Illing, *PhD, FIBiol, FRSC, FRIPHH,
FIOSH*
Centre for Occupational and Environmental

Health, Medical School, University of Manchester,
Stopford Building, Oxford Road, Manchester
M13 9PT, UK

Imran Imam
Research Service, Stratton Veterans Affairs
Medical Centre, Albany, New York 12208, USA

Bengt Jernström, *PhD*
Associate Professor, Division of Biochemical
Toxicology, Institute of Environmental Medicine,
Karolinska Institute, Box 210, S-17177 Stockholm,
Sweden

Sam Kacew, *PhD, FATS*
Department of Pharmacology, University of
Ottawa, 451 Smyth Road, Ottawa, Ontario K1H
8M5, Canada

James P. Kehrer, *PhD*
Professor and Head, Division of Pharmacology and
Toxicology, College of Pharmacy, The University
of Texas at Austin, Austin, Texas 78712-1074,
USA

Ian Kimber, *BSc, MSc, PhD*
Research Manager, AstraZeneca Central
Toxicology Laboratory, Alderley Park,
Macclesfield, Cheshire SK10 4TJ, UK

Alan B.G. Lansdown, *BSc, PhD, FRCPath,
FIBiol, MIMgt*
Hon.Senior Lecturer and Research Fellow, Skin
Research and Wound Healing Laboratory, Clinical
Chemistry, Division of Investigative Sciences,
Imperial College School of Medicine, London W6
8RP, UK

Peter N. Lee, *MA, FSS, CStat*
P. N. Lee Statistics and Computing Ltd., Hamilton
House, 17 Cedar Road, Sutton, Surrey SM2 5DA,
UK

Hon-Wing Leung, *PhD, DABT, CIH*
Union Carbide Corporation, 39 Old Ridgebury
Road, Danbury, Connecticut 06817-0001, USA

David W. Lincoln II, *PhD*
Research Service, Stratton Veterans Affairs
Medical Centre, Albany, New York 12208, USA

Edward A. Lock, *MIBiol, PhD, FRCPath*
AstraZeneca Central Toxicology Laboratory,
Alderley Park, Macclesfield, Cheshire SK10 4TJ,
UK

Thomas F. Long, *MS*
Senior Health Scientist, ChemRisk, McLaren Hart
Inc., 5900 Landerbrook Drive, Suite 100,
Cleveland, Ohio 44124, USA

David P. Lovell, *BSc, PhD, FSS, CStat, MBiol,
CBiol*
BIBRA International, Woodmansterne Road,
Carshalton, Surrey SM5 4DS, UK

Timothy C. Marrs, *MD, DSc, MRCP, FRCPath,
FIBiol*
Joint Food Safety and Standards Group, Skipton
House, 80 London Road, London SE1 6LH, UK

Robert L. Maynard, *BSc, MB, BCh, MRCP,
FRCPath, FFOM, FIBiol*
Department of Health, Skipton House, 80 London
Road, London SE1 6LH, UK

Patricia R. McElhatton, *MSc, PhD, CBiol, FIBiol*
National Teratology Information Service, Regional
Drug and Therapeutics Centre, Wolfson Unit,
Claremont Place, Newcastle-upon-Tyne NE2 4HH,
UK

Douglas McGregor, *PhD, FIBiol, FRCPath*
International Agency for Research on Cancer, 150
Cours Albert Thomas, 69372 Lyon, Cedex 08,
France

Clive Meredith, *MA, MSc, PhD*
Immunotoxicology Department, British Industrial
Biological Research Association International,
Woodmansterne Road, Carshalton, Surrey SM5
4DS, UK

Klara Miller, *ChemEng, MSc, PhD, FRCPath*
Consultant, Immunotoxicology, Food Science and
Biotechnology, 35D Arteberry Road, Wimbledon,
London SW20 8AG, UK

Jeremy J. Mills, *BSc, PhD*
Section of Molecular Toxicology, Division of
Biomedical Sciences, Imperial College School of
Medicine, South Kensington, London SW7 2AZ,
UK

Neil A. Minton, *BSc, MD, MRCP, MFPM*
Medical Toxicology Unit, Guy's Hospital, London
SE1 9RT, UK

Karl E. Misulis, *PhD, MD*
Clinical Professor, Department of Neurology,
School of Medicine, Vanderbilt University, 2100
Pierce Avenue, Medical Center South, Nashville,
Tennessee 37232, USA

Ralf Morgenstern, *PhD*
Associate Professor, Institute of Environmental
Medicine, Karolinska Institute, Box 210, S-17177
Stockholm, Sweden

Roy C. Myers, *BS, DABT*
Manager, Risk Assessment Information Group,
Union Carbide Corporation, 39 Old Ridgebury
Road, Danbury, Connecticut 06817-0001, USA

B.K. Nelson, *PhD, MSc, BSc*
Research Toxicologist, Division of Biomedical and
behavioral Science (C-24), National Institute for
Occupational Safety and Health, Centers for
Disease Control and Prevention, 4676 Columbia
Parkway, Cincinnati, Ohio 45226, USA

James C. Norris Jr., *PhD, DABT, MS, BS*
Head, Inhalation Toxicology, Covance Laboratories
Ltd., Otley Road, Harrogate, North Yorkshire HG3
1PY, UK

Frederick W. Oehme, *DVM, PhD*
Professor of Toxicology, Pathobiology, Medicine
and Physiology, Comparative Toxicology
Laboratories, Kansas State University, 1800
Denison Avenue, Manhattan, Kansas 66506-5606,
USA

Franz Oesch, *PhD*
Professor, Director, Institute of Toxicology,
University of Mainz, Obere Zahlbacher Strasse 67,
D-55131 Mainz, Germany

Eugene J. Olajos, *BA, MS, PhD*
US Army SBCCOM, Edgewood Chemical
Biological Center, Office of Director, Research and
Technology Directorate, Aberdeen Proving
Ground, Maryland 21010-5424, USA

Sten G. Orrenius, *MD, PhD*
Professor, Institute of Environmental Medicine, Karolinska Institute, Box 210, S-17177 Stockholm, Sweden

Alan J. Paine, *DSc, PhD, FRCPath, FIBiol*
Department of Toxicology, School of Medicine and Dentistry, Queen Mary and Westfield College, University of London, Charterhouse Square, London EC1M 6BQ, UK

Dennis J. Paustenbach, *PhD, DABT*
Group Vice President and Principal, Environmental Group, Exponent, 149 Commonwealth Drive, Menlo Park, California 94025, USA; Adjunct Professor of Toxicology, University of Massachusetts, Amherst, USA

Ellen K. Pedersen, *MSc*
Research Fellow, Department of Pharmacology and Toxicology, School of Medicine, Norwegian University of Science and Technology, N-7489 Trondheim, Norway

Alphonse Poklis, *PhD, DABFT, DABCC-TC*
Professor, Departments of Pathology and Pharmacology/Toxicology, Medical College of Virginia Campus at Virginia Commonwealth University, Richmond, Virginia 23298-0165, USA

Frances D. Pollitt, *MA, DipRCPath*
Department of Health, Skipton House, 80 London Road, London SE1 6LH, UK

Christopher J. Powell, *PhD, DipRCPath(Tox), MSc, BSc, FRCPath*
Vanguard Medica, Chancellor Court, Surrey Research Park, Guildford, Surrey GU2 5SF, UK

B.V. Rama Sastry, *DSc, PhD*
Professor of Pharmacology Emeritus, Adjunct Professor of Anesthesiology, Vanderbilt University Medical Center, 209 Oxford House, Nashville, Tennessee 37232-4245, USA

Jennifer M. Ratcliffe, *PhD, MSc, BSc*
Senior Epidemiologist, Statistics and Public Health Research Division, Analytical Sciences Inc., 2605 Meridian Parkway, Durham, North Carolina 27713, USA

Sidhartha D. Ray, *PhD, FACN*
Associate Professor, Division of Pharmacology, Toxicology and Medicinal Chemistry, Arnold and Marie Schwartz College of Pharmacy and Health Sciences, Long Island University, University Plaza, Brooklyn, New York 11201, USA

Daniel F. Reidy, *PhD, JD*
Attorney at Law, Suite 825, 545 Sansome Street, San Francisco, California 94111, USA

Andrew G. Renwick, *BSc, PhD, DSc*
Professor of Biochemical Pharmacology, Clinical Pharmacology Group, School of Medicine, Biomedical Sciences Building, University of Southampton, Bassett Crescent East, Southampton SO16 7PX, UK

Christopher Rhodes, *BSc, PhD, DABT*
Safety of Medicines Department, AstraZeneca, Mereside, Alderley Park, Macclesfield, Cheshire SK10 4TG, UK

Ian R. Rowland, *BSc, PhD*
Professor of Human Nutrition, Northern Ireland Centre for Diet and Health, School of Biomedical Sciences, University of Ulster, Coleraine BT52 1SA, Northern Ireland, UK

Wilson K. Rumbeiha, *BVM, PhD, DABVT, DABT*
Assistant Professor of Clinical Toxicology, Animal Health Diagnostic Laboratory, Michigan State University, G303 VMC, East Lansing, Michigan 48824-1314, USA

Harry Salem, *BA, BSc, MA, PhD, FNYAS, FCP, FATS, FACT*
Chief Scientist, Research and Technology Directorate, US Army SBCCOM, Edgewood Chemical and Biological Center, 5183 Blackhawk Road, Aberdeen Proving Ground, Maryland 21010-5424, USA

Jeffrey D. Simon, *PhD*
Political Risk Assessment Company, P.O. Box 82, Santa Monica, California 90406-0082, USA

Robert Snyder, *PhD*
Environmental and Occupational Health Sciences Institute, Rutgers University, 170 Frelinghuysen Road, Piscataway, New Jersey 08854-8020, USA

Patricia J. Sparks, *MD, MPH*
Private Consultant, 7683 SE 27th Street, Suite 291, Mercer Island, Washington 98040, USA

Maria A. Stander, *MSc*
SASOL Center for Chemistry, Potchefstroom University, Private Bag X60001, Potchefstroom 2520, Republic of South Africa

Eiliv Steinnes, *DrPhil*
Department of Chemistry, Norwegian University of Science and Technology, N-7491 Trondheim, Norway

Pieter S. Steyn, *MSc, PhD*
Director of Research, Division of Research Technology, University of Stellenbosch, Stellenbosch 7600, Republic of South Africa

Tim R. Stiles, *MBA*
Stiles Quality Associates, 1 Old Farm Close, Needingworth, Huntingdon, Cambridgeshire PE17 3SG, UK.

Michael D. Stonard, *BSc, PhD*
Independent Toxicology Consultant, 4A Somerset Close, Congleton, Cheshire CW12 1SG, UK

Jürgen Sühnel
Biocomputing, Institute of Molecular Biotechnology, Beutenbergstr. 11, D-07745 Jena, Germany

Frank M. Sullivan, *BSc Hons*
National Teratology Information Service, Regional Drug and Therapeutic Centre, Wolfson Unit, Claremont Place, Newcastle-upon-Tyne NE2 4HH, UK

F. William Sunderman, Jr., *MD*
Department of Chemistry and Biochemistry, Bicentennial Hall, Middlebury College, Middlebury, Vermont 05753, USA

Tore Syversen, *MSc, DrPhilos*
Professor of Toxicology, Department of Pharmacology and Toxicology, School of Medicine, Norwegian University of Science and Technology, N-7489 Trondheim, Norway

Hanna S. E. Tahti, *PhD*
Research Director, Medical School, University of Tampere, P.O. Box 607, FIN-33101 Tampere, Finland

John A. Thomas, *PhD, FATS*
Professor Emeritus, Department of Pharmacology, Health Science Center, University of Texas, 219 Wood Shadow, San Antonio, Texas 78216, USA

Michael J. Thomas, *MD, PhD*
Department of Internal Medicine, Division of Endocrinology, School of Medicine, University of North Carolina, Chapel Hill, North Carolina 27599-7170, USA

John A. Timbrell, *BSc, PhD, DSc, MRCPath, FIBiol, FRSC*
Biochemical Toxicology, Pharmacy Department, King's College London, Franklin Wilkins Building, Stamford Street, London SE1 8WA, UK

John A. Tomenson, *BSc, DipStat (Cantab), PhD*
ICI Epidemiology Unit, Brunner House, P.O. Box 7, Winnington, Northwich, Cheshire CW8 4DJ, UK

David J. Tweats, *CBiol, BSc, PhD, FIBiol, FRCPath*
Director, Preclinical Safety Sciences UK, Glaxo Wellcome Research and Development Ltd., Park Road, Ware, Hertfordshire SG12 ODP, UK

Rochelle W. Tyl, *PhD, DABT*
Director, Center for Life Sciences and Toxicology, Chemistry and Life Sciences Division, Research Triangle Institute, 3040 Cornwallis Road, P.O. Box 12194, Research Triangle Park, North Carolina 27709-2194, USA

Tipton R. Tyler, *PhD, DABT*
Associate Director, Corporate Applied Toxicology, Union Carbide Corporation, 39 Old Ridgebury Road, Danbury, Connecticut 06817-0001, USA

Marie Vahter, *PhD*
Professor, National Institute of Environmental Medicine, Karolinska Institute, Box 210, S-17177 Stockholm, Sweden

John P. Van Miller, *PhD, DABT*
Associate Director of Applied Toxicology, Union Carbide Corporation, 39 Old Ridgebury Road, Danbury, Connecticut 06817-0001, USA

Duncan W. Vere, *MD, FRCP, FFPM*
14 Broadfield Way, Buckhurst Hill, Essex IG9
5AG, UK

David Walker, *BVSc, CBiol, FIBiol, FRCVS*
APT Consultancy, Old Hawthorn Farm, Hawthorn
Lane, Four Marks, Alton, Hampshire GU34 5AU,
UK

Robert E. Waller, *BSc*
72 King William Drive, Charlton Park,
Cheltenham, Gloucester GL53 7RP, UK

Simon P.F. Warren, *CBiol, MIBiol, BSc, MSc,
DIBT, DABT, DipRCPath*
Mallard House, Kings Pool, 1-3 Peasholme Green,
York Y01 2PX, UK

Catherine J. Waterfield, *BSc, PhD*
Senior Principal Toxicologist, General and
Reproductive Toxicology, Glaxo Wellcome
Research and Development Ltd., Park Road, Ware,
Hertfordshire SG12 0DP, UK (for all correspon-
dence); Department of Pharmacy, King's College
London, Manresa Road, London SW3 6LX, UK

Mike Watson, *BSc*
Ricerca Inc., 7528 Auburn Road, PO Box 1000,
Painesville, Ohio 44077-1000, USA

Gregory P. Wedin, *PharmD, DABAT*
Hennepin Regional Poison Center, Hennepin
County Medical Center, 701 Park Avenue,
Minneapolis, Minnesota 55415, USA

Bernard Weiss, *PhD*
Professor of Environmental Medicine and
Pediatrics, Department of Environmental
Medicine, School of Medicine and Dentistry,
University of Rochester, Rochester, New York
14642, USA

Peter G. Wells, *BSc, MSc, PhD*
Research Scientist, Coastal Ecosystems,
Environment Canada, Environmental Conservation
Branch, 45 Alderney Drive, Dartmouth, Nova
Scotia B2Y 2N6, Canada; Associate Professor,
School for Resource and Environmental Studies,
Dalhousie University, Halifax, Nova Scotia B3H
3E2, Canada

Randy D. White, *PhD*
Director, Toxicology, Corporate Research and
Technical Services, Baxter HealthCare
Corporation, Round Lake, Illinois 60073, USA

Martin F. Wilks, *MD, PhD*
Zeneca Agrochemicals, Fernhurst, Haslemere,
Surrey GU27 3JE, UK

Angela Wilson, *BSc, PhD*
Medical Research Council Radiobiology Unit,
Chilton, Didcot, Oxfordshire OX11 ORD, UK

Patricia A. Wood, *MD, PhD*
Associate Professor of Medicine, Department of
Medicine and Experimental Pathology, Stratton
Veterans Affairs Medical Centre and Albany
Medical College, Albany, New York 12208, USA

Kevin N. Woodward, *BA, BSc, MSc, PhD,
DipRCPath, EurChem, CChem, FRSC, EurBiol,
CBiol, FIBiol, MBIRA*
Schering-Plough Animal Health, Breakspear Road
South, Harefield, Uxbridge, Middlesex UB9 6LS,
UK

Frequently Used Abbreviations

Most abbreviations, either standard or infrequently used, are defined by authors in individual chapters. For ease of reference, the most frequently used abbreviations are listed below.

ACGIH	American Conference of Governmental Industrial Hygienists
ACh	acetylcholine
AChE	acetylcholinesterase (specific cholinesterase)
ACTH	adenocorticotrophic hormone
ADH	antidiuretic hormone
ADI	acceptable daily intake
ADME	absorption, distribution, metabolism and excretion
ADR	adverse drug reaction
ALAD	δ-aminolevulinic acid dehydratase
ALT	alanine aminotransferase
ANOVA	analysis of variance
ANSI	American National Standards Institute
APase	alkaline phosphatase
APTT	activated partial thromboplastin time
ASR	acoustic startle response
AST	aspartate aminotransferase
ATP	adenosine triphosphate
ATPase	adenosine triphosphatase
ATSDR	Agency for Toxic Substances and Disease Registry (US)
AUC	area under the curve
BAC	blood alcohol concentration
BAL	biological action level
BBB	blood-brain barrier
BCF	bioconcentration factor
BChE	butyryl cholinesterase (non-specific cholinesterase; pseudocholinesterase)
BEI	biological exposure index
BMD	bench mark dose
BOD	biological oxygen demand
BP	blood pressure; boiling point
BrDU	bromodeoxyuridine
BUN	blood urea nitrogen
CA	chromosomal aberration
CalEPA	California Environmental Protection Agency
CAM	chorioallantoic membrane
CAS	Chemical Abstracts Service
cAMP	cyclic adenosine monophosphate
ChE	cholinesterase
CHO	Chinese hamster ovary
CK	creatine kinase
CL	confidence limit(s)
CNS	central nervous system

CO	carbon monoxide
COHb	carboxyhaemoglobin
CPSC	Consumer Product Safety Commission (US)
CSF	cerebrospinal fluid
Ct (or CT)	inhalation exposure dosage (atmospheric concentration x time)
CVS	cardiovascular system
CW	chemical warfare
DHHS	Department of Health and Human Services (US)
DNA	deoxyribonucleic acid
DNase	deoxyribonuclease
DOT	Department of Transportation (US)
EAC	endocrine-active compound
EC	effective concentration [with respect to a particular (specific) end-point]
EC$_{50}$	effective concentration producing (or calculated to produce) a 50% response for the specific end-point
ECG	electrocardiogram
EDSTAC	Endocrine Disrupter Screening and Testing Advisory Committee (US)
EEG	electroencephalogram
EGF	epidermal growth factor
ELISA	enzyme-linked immunosorbent assay
EM	electron microscopy
EMEA	European Medicines Evaluation Agency
EMG	electromyogram
ER	endoplasmic reticulum
ERG	electroretinogram
ESR	erythrocyte sedimentation rate
ETS	environmental tobacco smoke
EU	European Union
FAD	flavine adenine dinucleotide
FAO	Food and Agricultural Organisation of the United Nations
FAS	foetal alcohol syndrome
FDA	Food and Drug Administration (US)
FEV	forced expiratory volume
FEV$_1$	forced expiratory volume in one second
FGF	fibroblast growth factor
FID	flame ionization detector
FIFRA	Federal Insecticide, Fungicide and Rodenticide Act (US)
FMO	flavin-containing monooxygenase
FOB	functional observation battery

FRC	functional residual capacity	**IOP**	intraocular pressure
FSH	follicle stimulating hormone	**ip**	intraperitoneal
FVC	forced vital capacity	**IPCS**	International Programme on Chemical Safety (WHO)
GABA	γ-aminobutyric acid		
GATT	General Agreement on Tariffs and Trade	**IRIS**	Integrated Risk Information System
GC	gas chromatography	**ISO**	International Standards Organization
GC-MS	gas chromatography - mass spectrometry	**iv**	intravenous
GD (gd)	gestational day	**JECFA**	Joint Expert Committee on Food Additives
GFR	glomerular filtration rate		
GGT	γ-glutamyl transferase	**JMPR**	Joint Meeting on Pesticide Residues
GH	growth hormone	K_D	dissociation constant
GI	gastrointestinal	K_M	Michaelis constant
GLC	gas-liquid chromatography	K_{ow}	octanol-water partition coefficient
GLP	good laboratory practice	**LAA**	laboratory animal allergy
GOT	glutamate-oxaloacetate transaminase (now referred to as AST, qv)	**LAP**	leucine aminopeptidase
		LC	lethal concentration (atmosphere or liquid)
GPT	glutamate-pyruvate transaminase (now referred to as AST, qv)		
		LC_{50}	concentration causing (or calculated to cause) 50% mortality in population studied
GRAS	generally recognised as safe		
GSH	glutathione		
GST	glutathione-*S*-transferase	$L(Ct)_{50}$	inhalation dosage causing (or calculated to cause) 50% mortality in population studied
G6P	glucose-6-phosphate		
G6Pase	glucose-6-phosphatase		
G6PD	glucose-6-phosphate dehydrogenase	**LD**	lethal dose
6TG	6-thiogaunine	LD_{50}	dose causing (or calculated to cause) 50% mortality in the population studied
Hb	haemoglobin		
HDLP	high density lipoprotein		
HDN	hyaline droplet nephropathy	**LDH**	lactate dehydrogenase
HGH	human growth hormone	**LDLP**	low-density lipoprotein
HGPRT	hypoxanthine-guanine-phosphoribosyl transferase	**LH**	luetinizing hormone
		LLNA	local lymph node assay
		LOAEL	lowest observed adverse effect level
HIV	human immunodeficiency virus	**LVET**	low volume eye test
HPLC	high performance liquid chromatography	**MAO**	monoamine oxidase
HPV	high production volume	**MAT**	mean absorption time
HSE	Health and Safety Executive (UK)	**MCA**	Medicines Control Agency (UK)
HVAC	heating, ventilation and air control	**MCH**	mean (red blood cell) corpuscular haemoglobin
5-HT	5-hydroxytryptamine (serotonin)		
ia	intra-arterial	**MCHC**	mean (red blood cell) corpuscular haemoglobin concentration
IARC	International Agency for Research on Cancer		
		MCS	multiple chemical sensitivity
ic	intracerebral	**MCV**	mean (red blood cell) corpuscular volume
IC	incapacitating concentration		
ICH	International Conference on Harmonization	**MEST**	mouse ear swelling test
		metHb	methaemoglobin
ICRP	International Commission on Radiological Protection	**MFO**	mixed function oxidase
		MMAD	mass median aerodynamic diameter
ICSH	interstitial cell stimulating hormone	**MN**	micronucleus
IC_{50}	concentration causing (or calculated to cause) 50% incapacitation in the population studied	**MP**	melting point
		MRC	Medical Research Council (UK)
		MRL	maximum residue level
		mRNA	messenger ribonucleic acid
ID	inhibitory dose	**MRT**	mean residue time
ID_{50}	dose causing (or calculated to cause) 50% inhibition in the population studied	**MS**	mass spectometry
		MSDS	material safety data sheet
		MTD	maximum tolerated dose
Ig	immunoglobulin	**MW**	molecular weight
IL	interleukin	**NAD**	nicotine adenine dinucleotide
im	intramuscular		

NADH	reduced nicotine adenine dinucleotide
NAG	N-acetyl-β-D-glucosaminidase
NDA	new drug application
NIEHS	National Institute of Environmental Health and Safety (US)
NIOSH	National Institute of Occupational Safety and Health (US)
NKC	natural killer cell
NLM	National Library of Medicine (US)
NMR	nuclear magnetic resonance
NOAEL	no observed adverse effect level
NOEL	no observed effect level
NRC	National Research Council (US)
NSAID	nonsteroidal anti-inflammatory drug
5NT	5-nucleotidase
NTE	neurotoxic esterase
NTP	National Toxicology Program (US)
OC	organochlorine
OECD	Organization for Economic Cooperation and Development
OEL	occupational exposure limit
OP	organophosphate
OSHA	Occupation Safety and Health Administration (US)
OTC	over-the-counter
PAH	polycyclic aromatic hydrocarbons
PAS	periodic acid-Schiff reaction
PBPK	physiologically based pharmacokinetics
pc	percutaneous
PCB	polychlorinated biphenyls
PCD	programmed cell death
PCV	packed (red blood) cell volume
PEL	permitted exposure level
PMN	premanufacturing (premarketing) notification
PMR	proportionate mortality ratio
PMS	postmarketing surveillance
PND (pnd)	postnatal day
PNS	peripheral nervous system
po	peroral
PSD	Pesticides Safety Directorate (UK)
PSI	peripheral sensory irritation
PTH	parathyroid hormone
QA	quality assurance
QSAR	quantitative structure-activity relationship
RAST	radioallergosorbent test
RBC	red blood cell
RD	depression of respiration
RD_{50}	inspired concentration of material producing (or calculated to produce) a 50% decrease in respiratory rate

REM	rapid eye movement
RER	rough endoplasmic reticulum
RfC	reference concentration
RfD	reference dose
RIA	radioimmunoassay
RR	relative risk
rRNA	ribosomal ribonucleic acid
RTECS	Registry of Toxic Effects of Chemical Substances
RV	residual volume
SAR	structure-activity relationship
SBS	sick building syndrome
sc	subcutaneous
SCE	sister chromatid exchange
SD	standard deviation
SDH	sorbitol dehydrogenase
SE	standard error
SEM	standard error of the mean
SER	smooth endoplasmic reticulum
SG	specific gravity
SIDS	screening information dab set
SMR	standardized mortality ratio
SOP	standard operating procedure
STEL	short-term exposure limit
T_3	3,5,3′-tridothyronine
T_4	3,5,3′,5′-tetraiodothyronine (thyroxine)
TCA	tricarboxylic acid
TGF	transforming growth factor
TK	thymidine kinase
TLC	thin layer chromatography
TLV	threshold limit value
TOS	toxic oil syndrome
TNF	tumour necrosis factor
tRNA	transfer ribonucleic acid
TSCA	Toxic Substances Control Act (US)
TSH	thyroid stimulating hormone
UDP	uridine diphosphate
UDPG	uridine diphosphate glucuronide
UDS	unscheduled DNA synthesis
USDA	United States Department of Agriculture
US EPA (EPA)	United States Environmental Protection Agency
USP	United States Pharmacopiea
VMD	Veterinary Medicines Directorate (UK)
VOC	volatile organic compound
VP	vapour pressure
WBC	white blood cell
WHO	World Health Organization
WTO	World Trade Organization

PART ONE
BASIC SCIENCE

Chapter 1
Fundamentals of Toxicology

Bryan Ballantyne, Timothy C. Marrs and Tore Syversen

C O N T E N T S

INTRODUCTION

Toxicology, essentially concerned with addressing the potentially harmful effects of chemicals, is a recognized scientific and medical discipline encompassing a very large number of basic and applied issues. Although only generally accepted as a specific area of knowledge and investigation during this century, its principles and implications have been appreciated for aeons. Thus, the harmful and lethal effects of certain substances, plants, fruits, insect bites, animal venoms and minerals have been known since prehistoric times. Indeed, the Greek, Roman and subsequent civilizations knowingly used certain substances and extracts for their lethality in hunting, protection, warfare, suicide and homicide. Current activity in toxicology is mainly, although not exclusively, concerned with determining the potential for adverse effects from chemicals, both natural and synthetic, in order to assess hazard and risk to humans and lower animal forms, and thus define appropriate precautionary, protective, restrictive and therapeutic measures. For example, substances used or of potential use in commerce, the home, the environment and medical practice may present variable types of harmful effects, whose nature is determined by the physicochemical characteristics of the material, its potential to interact with biological materials and the pattern of exposure. For man-made and man-used materials, a critical analysis may be necessary in order to determine the risk–benefit ratio for their employment in specific circumstances and to determine what protective and precautionary measures are needed. Indeed, with drugs, pesticides, industrial chemicals, food additives and cosmetic preparations, mandatory toxicology testing and government regulations exist. Substances not occurring naturally are often generically referred to as xenobiotics.

HISTORY OF TOXICOLOGY

Except in a few countries, including the UK, where safety evaluation toxicology has been closely associated with pathology, toxicology as a discipline is a daughter science of pharmacology. Toxicology is therefore, in formal terms, a young science. However, the origins of toxicology are very old and it is likely that man undertook his first experiments in toxicology in a search for an acceptable diet when he moved out of the habitat in which he evolved. Of course, many of these experiments must have had an unfortunate outcome. In Greek and Roman times poisons, generally of plant origin, were used for murder and suicide, while the potential danger of medicinal products and their adulterants has been recognized since Babylonian times. Poisoning for nefarious purposes has remained a problem ever since, and much of the earlier impetus to the development of toxicology has been primarily forensic. Another motive for the development of toxicology has been the careful description of adverse reactions to medicinal products that began to appear in the eighteenth century. Thus, William Withering described digitalis toxicity in 1785 and around 1790 Hahnemann, the founder of homeopathy, carried out toxicological studies on himself and his healthy friends with therapeutic agents of his time, including cinchona, aconite, belladonna, ipececuanha and mercury. The introduction of anaesthesia was followed by formal enquiries into sudden deaths during chloroform anaesthesia in the closing years of the nineteenth century.

In World War I, a variety of poisonous chemicals were used in the battlefields of northern France. This was the stimulus for much work on mechanisms of toxicity as well as medical countermeasures to poisoning. In fact, war or the prospect of war played as great a part in the development of toxicology as of many other sciences. Much of the basic work on organophosphates was stimulated by the discovery of these compounds by the Germans in the 1930s. Although defence considerations stimulated this work, much of it, particularly that related to treatment, is applicable to organophosphorus pesticides. Similarly, chelation therapy, initially studied in relation to organic arsenicals, is now used in the treatment of poisoning by many metals.

Occupational toxicology originated in the nineteenth century as a product of the industrial revolution, with early descriptions of occupational diseases induced by chemicals such as cancer of the scrotum in chimney sweeps. Although, in theory, affected workers have always had some remedies at law, major advances in control of occupational disease of chemical origin came in the period after 1960 with the setting of threshold limit values (TLVs) and occupational exposure limits. Additionally, in western countries the increasing wealth of workers and their unions has enabled them to make use of existing legal remedies. These considerations have caused companies to take greater care of their workers and to devote greater resources to occupational hygiene.

Regulatory toxicology (Chapters 71–77) had its origins in the development of the chemical and pharmaceutical industries in the nineteenth and twentieth centuries. Regulatory toxicology now accounts for the vast majority of toxicological expenditure. However, none of the major national toxicology societies predates World War II. Toxicology has only come of age as a science in the last 20 years as concern for consumer and worker health and for the environment increased. The growth of the science has been fuelled by a succession of disasters such as Serveso, Bhopal and the thalidomide disaster, which have thrown up lacunae in knowledge of the toxic effects of substances, as well as the inadequacy of testing procedures. One of the earliest such disasters resulted in the deaths of 105 people from poisoning by an elixir of sulphanilamide containing the solvent diethylene glycol in 1937 in the USA (Calvery and Klumpp, 1939); this led to legislation forbidding the marketing of new drugs until cleared for safety by the US Food and Drug Administration (FDA). Regulations have been elaborated at national, continental [European Union and North Atlantic Free Trade areas (NAFTA)] and international levels.

The main international organizations for regulating chemicals are the Codex Alimentarius Commission, and its committees, for food standards, and the Organization for Economic Cooperation and Development (OECD) for the standardization of test methods. The International Conference on Harmonization (ICH) and the Veterinary International Conference on Harmonization (VICH) are attempting to harmonize test requirements for pharmaceuticals, both human and veterinary. Because of a tendency for new tests to be required without getting rid of old ones, regulations have inclined to become ever more complex, with the result that the cost of animal toxicity testing has become a significant part of product development. New tests do not always imply added cost; thus the advent of mutagenicity tests *in vitro* may permit the avoidance of large numbers of very expensive and laborious long-term carcinogenicity bioassays. However, the complexity of toxicological regulations may imply not only an effect on the profits of the companies developing the chemical or drug but also a loss to the market of potentially useful substances. In some cases this has given rise to sufficient disquiet for legislative action to be taken. Examples of this are the 'orphan drug' procedure in the USA and the clinical trial exemption procedure in the UK. An interesting phenomenon has been that regulatory requirements have given rise to large departments within chemical and pharmaceutical enterprises whose main role is to satisfy regulatory authorities as to the safety of the company's products. However, for reasons of size or economies, many companies have chosen not to develop their own toxicology facilities.

Organochlorine insecticides probably averted an epidemic of typhus at the end of World War II, but it was the persistence of these compounds in the environment that was probably the greatest stimulus to the evolution of environmental toxicology. A major landmark in the development of this branch of toxicology was the publication of *Silent Spring* by Rachel Carson.

The emphasis in toxicology has moved from its origins in acute, particularly human, toxicology to long term and non-target species toxicology. In parallel, stress has changed from study of natural, usually plant compounds to the products of chemical synthesis. Additionally, a great amount of resources has gone into testing for carcinogenic potential in recent years, while there has been intensive study of *in vitro* alternatives to animals in toxicology studies.

A recent development has been the recognition that differing toxicology requirements may be a barrier to free trade. Within major trading blocks such as the NAFTA and the EC, it has been necessary to elaborate common toxicological requirements for clearance of materials, while the agreement on the application of sanitary and phytosanitary measures ("SPS agreement", WTO, 1994), achieved after tortuous negotiations in 1994, requires that, in most circumstances, Codex Alimentarius Commission (CAC) maximum residue levels (MRLs) for food additives, contaminants and pesticides, be accepted for world trade purposes. This has inevitably raised the profile of the international expert committees such as the Joint Expert Committee on Food Additives (JECFA) and the Joint Meeting on Pesticide Residues (JMPR).

Clinical toxicology, the treatment of acute poisoning, was originally carried out by general physicians in general hospitals; in this respect it is an old branch of toxicology and amyl nitrite, one of the earliest antidotes (for cyanide), had been described in the 1880s. Much of the impetus for the development of clinical toxicology came from defence research establishments. Chelation therapy for heavy metal poisoning was discovered during a search for a method of treatment for organic arsenicals during World War II, while oximes for organophosphate poisoning were developed during the 'cold war' in the 1950s and 1960s. As a distinct specialization, clinical toxicology is fairly new, having arisen out of the fact that clinicians may not have ready access to the information necessary successfully to treat their patients. Furthermore, clinical toxicologists need special skills and analytical expertise. The idea of specialist poisons information services arose in the USA in the 1950s, and the concept has since spread throughout the world. Poisons information services, which have access to information on the many thousands of possible chemicals which people may use to poison themselves, now exist in most developed countries. In some cases units exist not only to back up clinicians with information but also to carry out hands-on treatment of poisoning.

Major, extensive and rapid developments in the scientific basis and practice of toxicology have been obvious since the early part of the 1950s. These developments have resulted for a variety of reasons, principal amongst which are those listed in **Table 1**. Reflecting these developments has been a proliferation in the number of textbooks, monographs and journals devoted to general and special aspects of toxicology; a proliferation of abstracting ser-

Table 1 Major driving forces for the recent expansion and development of the scientific basis and practice of toxicology

- Exponential increase in the number of synthetically produced industrial chemicals
- Major increase in the number and nature of new drugs, pharmaceutical preparations, tissue-implantable materials and medical devices
- Increase in the number and types of pesticides and other substances used in agriculture and the food industry
- Mandatory testing and regulation of chemicals used commercially, domestically and medically.
- Enhanced public awareness of potential adverse effects from xenobiotics (non-naturally occurring) to man, animals and the environment.
- Litigation, principally as a consequence of occupational-related illness, unrecognized or poorly documented product safety concerns (including drugs) and environmental harm

Table 2 Major subspecialities of toxicology

Specialty	Major functional components
Clinical	Causation, diagnosis and management of established poisoning in humans
Veterinary	Causation, diagnosis and management of established poisoning in domestic and wild animals
Forensic	Establishing the cause of death or intoxication in humans, by analytical procedures, and with particular reference to legal processes
Occupational	Assessing the potential of adverse effects from chemicals in the occupational environment and the recommendation of appropriate protective and precautionary measures
Product	Assessing the potential for adverse effects from commercially produced chemicals and formulations and recommendation on use patterns and protective and precautionary procedures.
Pharmacological	Assessing the toxicity of therapeutic agents
Aquatic	Assessing the toxicity to aquatic organisms of chemicals discharged into marine and fresh water
Toxinology	Assessing the toxicity of substances of plant and animal origin and produced by pathogenic bacteria
Environmental	Assessing the effects of toxic pollutants, usually at low concentrations, released from commercial and domestic sites into their immediate environment and subsequently widely distributed by air and water currents and by diffusion through soil
Regulatory	Administrative function concerned with the development and interpretations of mandatory toxicology testing programmes, and with particular reference to controlling the use, distribution, handling and availability of chemicals used commercially, domestically and therapeutically
Laboratory	Design and conduct of *in vivo* and *in vitro* toxicology testing programmes

vices related to toxicology information; the provision of courses at undergraduate and graduate levels dealing with general and specialized areas; and the establishment of a private industry devoted to toxicology testing and consultation. Along with these factors has been an increase in the number of professional organizations and certification boards specifically devoted to toxicology. As a consequence of the markedly expanded scope of toxicology, the number of differing subdisciplines which have emerged, and the need for varying professional activities, the practice of toxicology can be subdivided and described by areas of major involvement and specialization; the principal areas are shown in **Table 2**.

Historical aspects of toxicology have been reviewed in detail by Doull and Bruce (1980) and Decker (1987).

DEFINITION AND SCOPE OF TOXICOLOGY

The essence of toxicology is that it is a discipline concerned with studying the potential of chemicals, or mixtures of them, to produce harmful effects in living organisms and determining the implications of these effects. One overview definition covering the various facets of toxicology (Ballantyne, 1989) is as follows:

Toxicology is a study of the interaction between chemicals and biological systems in order to quantitively determine the potential for chemical(s) to produce injury which results in adverse effects in living organisms, and to investigate the nature, incidence, mechanism of production, factors influencing their development, and reversibility of such adverse effects.

Within the scope of this definition, adverse effects are those which are detrimental to either the survival or the normal functioning of the individual. Inherent in this definition are the following key issues in toxicology:

(a) Chemicals, or their conversion products, require to come into close structural and/or functional contact with tissue(s) or organ(s) for which they have a potential to cause injury.
(b) When possible, the observed toxicity (or an end-point reflecting it) should be quantitatively related to the degree of exposure to the chemical (the exposure dose). Ideally, the influence of differing exposure doses on the magnitude and/or incidence of the toxic effect(s) should be investigated. Such dose–response relationships are of prime importance in confirming a causal relationship between chemical exposure and toxic effect, in assessing relevance of the observed toxicity to practical (in-use) exposure conditions, and to allow hazard evaluations and risk assessment.

(c) The primary aim of most toxicology studies is to determine the potential for harmful effects in the intact living organism, in many cases (and often by extrapolation) to man.
(d) Toxicological investigations should ideally allow the following characteristics of toxicity to be evaluated:
  (i) the basic structural, functional, or biochemical injury produced;
  (ii) dose–response relationships;
  (iii) the mechanism(s) of toxicity, i.e. the fundamental chemical and biological interactions and resultant aberrations that are responsible for the genesis and maintenance of the toxic response;
  (iv) factors that may influence the toxic response, e.g. route of exposure, species, sex, formulation of test chemical and environmental conditions;
  (v) development of approaches for recognition of specific toxic responses;
  (vi) the reversibility of effects, either spontaneously or with treatment.

The word toxicity is used to describe the nature of adverse effects produced and the conditions necessary for their induction, i.e. toxicity is the potential for a material to produce injury in biological systems. For pharmacologically active and therapeutic agents ('drugs'), a description of the non-desired effects is most appropriately undertaken using the following specific terms:

Side-effects: undesirable effects which result from the normal pharmacological actions of the drug.
Overdosage: implies that toxicity will occur.
Intolerance: implies that the threshold dose to produce a pharmacological effect is lowered; this may be a consequence of a genetic abnormality.
Idiosyncrasy: an abnormal reaction to a drug due to an inherent, frequently genetic, anomaly.
Secondary effects: those arising as an indirect consequence of the pharmacological action of a drug.
Adverse drug interactions: adverse effects produced by a combination of drugs, but not seen when the drugs are given separately at the same dose.

Toxicity (i.e. the potential to injure) requires to be clearly differentiated from the process of hazard evaluation, which determines the likelihood that a given material will exhibit its known toxicity under particular conditions of use.

DESCRIPTION AND TERMINOLOGY OF TOXIC EFFECTS

Precision in communication depends on a clear understanding of the definitions of technical and scientific

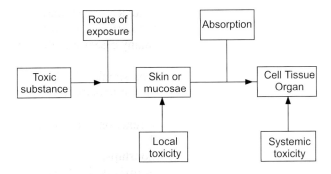

Figure 1 Basis for general classification of toxic effects.

terms in the context of their use. This section discusses the derivation and meanings of frequently used expressions in toxicology.

A schematic representation of the basis for the general classification of toxic effects is given in **Figure 1**. Before toxicity can develop, a substance must come into contact with a body surface such as skin, eye or mucosa of the alimentary or respiratory tract; these are, respectively, the cutaneous, ocular, peroral and inhalation routes of exposure. Other routes of exposure, in experimental or therapeutic situations, are subcutaneous, intravenous, intramuscular and intraperitoneal. Harmful effects that occur at the sites where a substance comes into initial contact with the body are referred to as local effects. If substances are absorbed from the sites of contact, they, or products of their bioconversion, may produce toxic effects in cells, tissues or organs remote from the site of exposure; these remote responses are referred to as systemic effects. Many materials may produce both local and systemic toxicity. Also, since the nature and probability of toxicity depend on the number of exposures, this forms an additional general means for classifying toxic effects into those developing after a single (acute) exposure or multiple (repeated) exposures. Repeated exposure toxicity can cover a wide time span; however, it is descriptively convenient to refer to short-term repeated (not more than 5% of life span), subchronic (5–20% of life span) and chronic (entire life span or the major portion of it). Examples of toxic effects classified according to site and to number of exposures are given in **Table 3**.

Additional descriptions of toxicity are by the time to development and the duration of induced effects. Thus,

Table 3 Examples of toxicity classified according to time-scale and site

Exposure	Site	Effect	Substance
Acute	Local	Skin corrosion	Methylamine
		Lung injury	Hydrogen chloride
	Systemic	Kidney injury	Phenacetin
		Haemolysis	Arsine
	Mixed	Lung injury and methaemoglobinemia	Oxides of nitrogen
Short-term repeated	Local	Skin sensitization	Ethylenediamine
		Lung sensitization	Toluene diisocyanate
		Nasal septal ulceration	Chromates
	Systemic	Neurotoxicity	Acrylamide
		Liver Injury	Arsenic
	Mixed	Respiratory irritation and neurobehavioural	Pyridine
Chronic	Local	Bronchitis	Sulphur dioxide
		I aryngeal carcinoma	Nitrogen mustard
	Systemic	Leukaemia	Benzene
		Angiosarcoma (liver)	Vinyl chloride
	Mixed	Emphysema and kidney injury	Cadmium
		Pneumonitis and neurotoxicity	Manganese

Table 4 Examples of toxicity classified according to time-scale for development or duration

Time-scale	Effect	Substance
Persistent	Testicular injury	Dibromochloropropane
	Scarring (skin/eye)	Corrosives
	Pleural mesothelioma	Asbestos
Transient	Narcosis	Organic solvents
	Sensory irritation	Acetaldehyde
Cumulative	Squamous metaplasia	Irritants (e.g. formaldehyde)
	Liver fibrosis	Ethanol
Latent	Pulmonary oedema	Phosgene
	Peripheral neuropathy	Organophosphates (antiChE)
	Pulmonary fibrosis	Paraquat

they may be described as temporary (reversible or transient) or permanent (persistent). Latent (delayed-onset) toxicity exists when there is a period free from signs following (usually) an acute exposure. Latent toxicity is of particular importance in clinical toxicology since individuals exposed to chemicals of known latency in toxicity should be kept under review in order that any delayed adverse effects may be both promptly recognized and treated. Cumulative toxicity involves progressive injury produced by summation of incremental injury resulting from successive exposures. Examples of toxicity according to the time-scale for development and duration of effect are given in **Table 4**. Effects may also be classified, and described, according to the primary tissue or organ forming the target for toxicity, e.g. hepatotoxic, nephrotoxic, neurotoxic, genotoxic, ototoxic, immunotoxic. A description of toxicity from a material requires inclusion of the following: if effects are local, systemic or mixed; their nature and (if known) mechanism of toxicity; organs and tissues affected; and condition of exposure resulting in toxicity (including species, route and number or magnitude of exposure).

NATURE OF TOXIC EFFECTS

The nature and magnitude of a toxic effect depend on many factors, amongst which are the physicochemical properties of the substance, its bioconversion, the conditions of exposure, and the presence of bioprotective mechanisms. The last factor includes physiological mechanisms such as adaptive enzyme induction, DNA repair mechanisms and phagocytosis. Some of the frequently encountered types of morphological and biochemical injury constituting a toxic response are listed below. They may take the form of tissue pathology, aberrant growth processes, altered or aberrant biochemical pathways or extreme physiological responses.

Inflammation is a frequent local response to irritant chemicals or may be a component of systemic tissue injury. The inflammatory response may be acute with irritant or tissue-damaging materials, or chronic with repetitive exposure to irritants or the presence of insoluble particulate material. Fibrosis may occur as a consequence of the inflammatory process.

Necrosis, used to describe circumscribed death of tissues or cells, may result from a variety of pathological processes induced by chemical injury, e.g. corrosion, severe hypoxia, membrane damage, reactive metabolite binding, inhibition of protein synthesis and chromosome injury. With certain substances, differing patterns of zonal necrosis may be seen. In the liver, for example, galactosamine produces diffuse necrosis of the lobules (Mehendale, 1987), acetaminophen (paracetamol) mainly centrilobular necrosis (Goldfrank *et al.*, 1990) and certain organic arsenicals peripheral lobular necrosis (Ballantyne, 1978).

Enzyme inhibition by chemicals may inhibit biologically vital pathways, producing impairment of normal function. The induction of toxicity may be due to accumulation of substrate or to deficiency of product or function. For example, organophosphate anticholinesterases produce toxicity by accumulation of acetylcholine at cholinergic synapses and neuromuscular junctions (Ellenhorn and Barceloux, 1988). Cyanide inhibits cytochrome oxidase and interferes with mitochondial oxygen transport, producing cytotoxic hypoxia (Ballantyne, 1987).

Biochemical uncoupling agents interfere with the synthesis of high-energy phosphate molecules, but electron transport continues resulting in excess liberation of energy as heat. Thus, uncoupling produces increased oxygen consumption and hyperthermia. Examples of uncoupling agents are dinitrophenol and pentachlorophenol (Williams, 1982; Kurt *et al.*, 1988).

Lethal synthesis occurs when foreign substances of close structural similarity to normal biological substrates become incorporated into biochemical pathways and are then metabolized to a toxic product. A classical example is fluoroacetate, which becomes incorporated in the Kreb's cycle as fluoroacetyl coenzyme A, which combines with oxaloacetate to form fluorocitrate. The latter inhibits aconitase, blocking the tricarboxylic acid cycle and results, particularly, in cardiac and nervous system toxicity (Albert, 1979).

Lipid peroxidation in biological membranes by free radicals starts a chain of events causing cellular dysfunction and death. The complex series of events includes oxidation of fatty acids to lipid hydroperoxides which undergo degradation to various products, including toxic aldehydes. The generation of organic radicals during peroxidation results in a self-propagating reaction (Horton and Fairhurst, 1987). Carbon tetrachloride, for example, is activated by a hepatic cytochrome P450-dependent mono-oxygenase system to the trichloromethyl and trichloromethyl peroxy radicals; the former radical probably covalently binds with macromolecules and the latter initiates the process of lipid peroxidation leading to hepatic centrilobular necrosis. The zonal necrosis is possibly related to high cytochrome P450 activity in centrilobular hepatocytes (Albano *et al.*, 1982).

Covalent binding of electrophilic reactive metabolites to nucleophilic macromolecules may have a role in certain genotoxic, carcinogenic, teratogenic and immunosuppresive events. Important cellular defence mechanisms exist to moderate these reactions, and toxicity may not be initiated until these mechanisms are saturated.

Receptor interaction, at a cellular or macromolecular level, with specific chemical structures may modify the normal biological effect mediated by the receptor; these may be excitatory or inhibitory. An important example is effects on Ca channels (Braunwald, 1982).

Immune-mediated hypersensitivity reactions by antigenic materials are particularly important considerations for skin and lung resulting in allergic contact dermatitis and asthma, respectively (Cronin, 1980; Brooks, 1983; Bardana *et al.*, 1992; see also Chapters 36 and 41).

Immunosuppression by xenobiotics may have important repercussions in increased susceptibility to infective agents and certain aspects of tumorigenesis.

Neoplasia, resulting from aberration of tissue growth and control mechanisms of cell division, and resulting in abnormal proliferation and growth, is a major consideration in repeated exposure to xenobiotics. The terms tumorigenesis and oncogenesis are general words used to describe the development of neoplasms; the word carcinogenesis should be restricted specifically to malignant neoplasms. In experimental and epidemiological situations, oncogenesis may be exhibited as an increase in the total number of neoplasms, an increase in specific types of neoplasm, the occurrence of 'rare' or 'unique' neoplasms or a decreased latency to detection of neoplasm.

Chemical carcinogenesis in many cases is a multistage process. The first, and critical, stage is a genotoxic event followed by other processes leading to the pathological, functional and clinical expression of neoplasia. One multistep model that has received much attention is the initiator–promoter scheme **(Figure 2)**. The first stage, that of initiation, requires a brief exposure to a genotoxically active material which results in binding of the initiator or reactive metabolite to cellular DNA; there is a low, or no, threshold for initiation. The second stage, that of promotion, permits the expression of the carcinogenic potential of the initiated cell. Promoting agents have the following characteristics:

Scheme	Initiator–promoter relations	Neoplasm
A	I	No
B	I P P P P P P P P P	Yes
C	I P P P P P P P P P P	Yes
D	I P P P P P P P P P P	Low/no
E	P P P P P P P P P P P P P P P P	No
F	P P P P P P P P P P P I	No
G	I I I I I I I I I	Yes

Figure 2 Schematic representation of functional interrelationships between initiator and promoter in the two-stage mechanism of carcinogenesis. (A) An initiating dose of a genotoxic carcinogen is not by itself oncogenic. (B) If initiator dose is followed by multiple applications of an epigenetic promoter, neoplasia results (the classical initiator–promoter relationship). (C) If promotion is delayed after initiation a neoplastic response occurs, indicting a persistent initiating process. (D) If promoter dosing is infrequent or doses are small, there may be no neoplasia or a low tumour incidence, indicating a threshold for the promoting effect. (E) Multiple applications of an epigenetic promoter alone do not result in neoplasia. (F) Initiation must precede promotion. (G) A genotoxic carcinogen may act as both initiator and promoter.

■ they need not be genotoxic;
■ repeated exposure is required after initiation;

■ they show some evidence for reversibility;
■ they may have threshold for promoting activity.

Genotoxic initiators may also act in a promotional manner after initiation. Substances causing or enhancing a carcinogenic process may be conveniently described as genotoxic and epigenetic carcinogens; the former are capable of causing DNA injury and the latter exert onocogenic effects by mechanisms other than genotoxicity. Genotoxic materials acting directly with DNA are referred to as primary carcinogens; those requiring to be metabolically activated are procarcinogens, with the metabolically active electrophile being the ultimate carcinogen. Primary carcinogens include alkylene epoxides, sulphate esters and nitrosoureas; procarcinogens include polycyclic aromatic hydrocarbons, aromatic amines, azo dyes and nitrosamines.

Epigenetic carcinogens include the following differing functional classes: promoters, cocarcinogens, hormones, immunosuppresives and solid-state materials. Cocarcinogens, when applied just before or with genotoxic carcinogens, enhance the onocogenic effect. Various mechanisms may cause enhancement, including increased absorption, increased metabolic activation of procarcinogen, decreased detoxification or inhibition of DNA repair. One group of epigenetic carcinogens of current interest are the peroxisome proliferators, which induce liver tumours in experimental rodents. These materials produce hepatomegaly and hepatocyte peroxisome proliferation and induce several liver enzymes, including those of the peroxisomal fatty acid β-oxidation system. Phthlate esters are one class of compound producing peroxisomal proliferation and experimental hepatocarcinogenesis (Rao and Reddy, 1987). For the purposes of risk assessment, it is usually assumed that a threshold for oncogenesis does not exist with genotoxic carcinogens. In contrast, a threshold may exist with epigenetic carcinogens, but there is disagreement about the way in which data from studies with epigenetic carcinogens should be analysed for risk assessment purposes.

Genotoxic chemicals, which interact with DNA and possibly lead to heritable changes, may be conveniently classified as clastogenic or mutagenic.

Clastogenic effects occur at the chromosomal level and are usually visible by light microscopy. They may involve simple breaks, rearrangement of segments or gross destruction of chromosomes. If severe they may be incompatible with normal function, and cell death occurs. The relevance of chemically induced sublethal cytogenetic effects is not clearly understood, but could lead to dysfunction of the reproductive system and tissues with rapid cell turnover rates (see Chapter 49).

Mutagenic effects are focal molecular events in the DNA molecule, which involve either substitution of a base pair or deletion or addition of a base. Base-pair transformations ('point mutations') may occur by direct chemical transformation, incorporation of abnormal base analogues or alkylation. Addition or deletion of a base will result in a disturbance of the triplet code and hence alteration of the codon sequence distal to the addition or deletion ('frameshift mutation'). Intracellular DNA repair enzymes are present, but if the capacity of repair mechanisms is exceeded then abnormal coding will be transcribed into RNA and expressed as altered protein structure and possibly function, depending on the molecular segment affected. The relationship of chemically induced mutation to genetic abnormality is unclear. However, as noted above, it is now generally accepted that in genotoxic carcinogenesis the molecular DNA event of initiation is fundamental to multistage oncogenesis. There is now considerable evidence showing a good correlation (with some test systems) between carcinogenic and mutagenic potential. Thus, the use of certain mutagenicity tests procedures has become widely accepted as a means of screening chemicals for their carcinogenic potential (Krisch-Volders, 1984; Brusick, 1988; see Chapter 48).

Developmental and reproductive toxicity are concerned with, respectively, adverse effects on the ability to conceive and adverse effects on the structural and functional integrity of the conceptus up to and around parturition.

Adverse effects on reproduction may result from a variety of differing effects on reproductive organs and their neural and endocrine control mechanisms (Barlow and Sullivan, 1982). Developmental toxicity deals with adverse effects on the conceptus from the stage of zygote formation, through the stages of implantation, germ layer differentiation, organ formation and growth processes during intrauterine development and the neonatal period. The most extreme toxicity, death, may occur as pre-implantation loss, embryo resorption, foetal death or abortion. Non-lethal foetotoxicity may be expressed as delayed maturation, including decreased body weight and retarded ossification. Structural malformations (morphological teratogenic effects) may be external, skeletal or visceral. The preferential susceptibility of the conceptus to chemical (and other environmental) insults in comparison with the adult state is related to (a) small numbers of cells and rapid proliferation rates; (b) a large number of non-differentiated cells lacking defence capabilities; (c) requirements for precise spatial and temporal interactions of cells; (d) limited metabolic capacity; and (e) immaturity of the immunosurveillance system (Tyl, 1988). There is now considerable awareness that functional, in addition to structural, malformations of development may occur. Malformation from chemical exposure may result from, amongst other mechanisms, (a) genotoxic injury; (b) interference with nucleic acid replication, transcription or translation; (c) essential nutrient deficiency; and (d) enzyme inhibition. The most sensitive period for induction of structural malformations is during organogenesis; functional teratogenic effects may be induced at later stages, particularly neuro-behavioural malformations (Rodier, 1980).

Pharmacological effects may be induced by drugs and chemicals and these may be significant as causes of temporary incapacitation or inconvenience in the occupational environment, as well as side-effects of medication. For example, narcosis from acute overexposure to an organic solvent may clearly be of relevance in safe workplace considerations; such a reversible narcosis needs to be differentiated from central nervous system injury resulting from long-term, low-concentration solvent exposure (World Health Organization, 1985). Another important pharmacological effort, particularly from airborne materials in the workplace, is peripheral sensory irritation. Materials having such effects interact with sensory nerve receptors in skin or mucosae, producing local discomfort and related reflex effects. For example, with the eye there is pain or discomfort, excess lachrymation and blepharospasm. Although such effects are warning and protective in nature, they are also distracting and thus likely to predispose to accidents. For this reason, peripheral sensory irritant effects are widely used in defining, along with other considerations, exposure guidelines for workplace environments (Ballantyne, 1984; see Chapter 32).

DOSAGE–RESPONSE RELATIONSHIPS

A fundamental concept in biology is that of variability. Individual members of the same species and strain differ to variable degrees with respect to their biochemical, cellular, tissue, organ and overall characteristics. Additionally, within a given individual there is a spectrum of variability in certain features, e.g. cell size and biochemical function within a particular cell series. The differences between individuals are usually a consequence of genetic factors and age. Since toxic effects are due to adverse effects on biological systems, or modifications of defence mechanisms, it is not unexpected that the majority of toxic responses will also show variability between individuals of a given strain; also, because of genetic and biochemical variability, even larger discrepancies in response will be observed between species. It is axiomatic to the toxicologist that, within certain limits and under controlled conditions, there is a positive relationship between the amount of material to which given groups of animals are exposed and the toxic response, and that the response of a given animal may differ quantitatively from that of other animals in the same dosage group. As the amount of material given to a group of animals increases, so does the magnitude of the effect and/or the number who are affected. For example, a specific amount of a potentially lethal material given to a group of animals may not kill all of them; however, as the amount of material is increased, so the proportion dying increases. This reflects the variability in the susceptibility of the population studied to the lethal toxicity of the test substance. Likewise, if an irritant material is applied to the skin, as the amount is increased over a given area this is associated with (a) an increase in the number of the population affected and (b) an increase in the severity of the inflammation. For the two examples given above, death is an 'all-or-none' response (a quantal response), whereas inflammation may be considered from a dose–response viewpoint as having two elements, i.e. its presence or otherwise, and the degree of inflammation which represents a continuous (or graded) response. The above considerations, which reflect variability in biological systems, form the basis for the fundamental concept of dose–response relationships in both pharmacology and toxicology, there usually being a positive relationship between dose and response *in vivo* and in many *in vitro* test systems.

It follows from the above discussion that the amount of material to which an organism is exposed is one prime determinant of toxicity. The dose–response relationships for differing toxic effects produced by a given material in a particular species may vary. Thus, as discussed later, dose–response relationships have to be carefully interpreted in the context of the effect of interest and the particular conditions under which the information was obtained.

The word 'dose' is most frequently used to denote the total amount of material to which an organism or test system is exposed; 'dosage' defines the amount of material given in relation to a recipient characteristic (e.g. weight). Dosage allows a more meaningful and comparative indicator of exposure. For example, 500 mg of a material given as a peroral dose to a 250 g rat or a 2000 g rabbit will result in dosages of 2 and 0.25 mg (kg body weight)$^{-1}$, respectively. It follows that comparative dosing should be expressed in dosage units. Dose in most reports usually implies the exposure dose, i.e. the total amount of material which is given to an organism by the particular route of exposure, or the amount incorporated into a test system. Another expression of dose is absorbed dose, which is the amount of material penetrating into the organism through the route of exposure. Absorbed dose may show a closer quantitative relationship with systemic toxicity than exposure dose since it represents the amount of material directly available for metabolic interactions and systemic toxicity. A further expression of dose is target organ dose, which is the amount of material (parent or metabolite) received at the organ or tissue exhibiting a specific toxic effect. This should be expressed (if possible) in terms of the mechanistically causative molecule (parent chemical or reactive metabolite).

Clearly, target organ dose is a more precise quantitative indication of toxicity than exposure dose, since it is a measure of the amount of material at the site of toxicity, whereas exposure dose is total dose to the organism and only a proportion of this (or metabolize) will ultimately gain access to the target site(s) for the toxic response. However, the estimation of target organ or tissue dose requires a detailed knowledge of the pharmacokinetics and metabolism of the material. For this reason, most information relates to the exposure dose.

The exposure dose is of practical importance since it reflects the amount of material to which the organism is actually exposed and the likelihood of the development of a particular toxic end-point, and therefore is of particular use for hazard evaluation purposes. Absolute target organ doses allow a more detailed scientific evaluation of toxicity in relation to bioavailable chemical, and when related to exposure dose may be used for rational risk assessment procedures.

If a material is capable of inducing several differing types of toxicity, the dose (or dosage) of material required to cause the individual effects may differ, with the more sensitive toxic effect appearing at the lower dosages. The first distinct toxicity, at lower dosages, may not necessarily be the most logically significant effect. For example, with epicutaneously applied materials, local inflammation may appear before more sinister systemic toxicity. Conversely, if the most significant toxicity occurs at lower dosages, then other toxicity at higher dosages may be overlooked.

Nature of the Dosage–Response Relationship

As discussed above, with a given population there is a quantitative variability in susceptibility to a chemical by individual members of that population. Thus, with a genetically homogeneous population of animals of the same species and strain, the proportion exhibiting a particular toxic effect will increase as the dosage increases. This is shown schematically in **Figure 3** as a cumulative frequency distribution curve, where the number of animals responding (as a proportion of the total in the group) is plotted as a function of the dosage given (as a $\log_{10}$ function). In many instances there is a sigmoid curve, with a log-normal distribution and being symmetrical about the mid-point. This is a typical dosage–response relationship, often loosely referred to as a dose–response relationship. There are several important elements to this curve that require consideration when interpreting its toxicological significance:

- The majority of those individuals responding do so symmetrically about the mid-point (i.e. the 50% response value). The position of the major portion of the dosage–response curve around its mid-point is sometimes referred to as the potency.
- The mid-point of the curve (50% response point) is a convenient description of the average response, and is referred to as the median effective dose for the

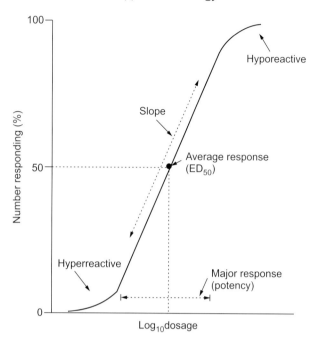

Figure 3 Typical sigmoid cumulative dosage–response curve for a toxic effect, which is symmetrical about the average (50% response) point. The major response (potency) occurs around the average response. The slope of the curve is determined by the increase in response as a function of incremental increases in dosage. Hyperreactive and hyporeactive individuals are found at the extreme left and right sides of the curve, respectively.

effect being considered (ED_{50}). If mortality is the end-point, then this is specifically referred to as the median lethal dose (LD_{50}). The median effective dosage is used for the following reasons: (a) it is at the mid-point of a log-normally distributed cur-veand (b) the 95% confidence limits are narrowest at this point.

- A small proportion of the population, at the left-hand-side of the dosage–response curve, respond to low dosages; they constitute a hypersusceptible or hyperreactive group.
- Another small proportion of the population, at the right-hand-side of the curve, do not respond until higher dosages are given; they constitute a hyposusceptible or hyporeactive group.
- The slope of the dosage–response curve, particularly around the median value, gives an indication of the range of doses producing an effect. It indicates how greatly the response will be changed when the dosage is altered. A steep slope indicates that a majority of the population will respond over a narrow dosage range, and a flatter slope indicates a much wider range of dosages is required to affect the majority of the population.

The shape of the dosage–response curve, and its extreme portions, depend on a variety of endogenous (as well as exogenous) factors, which may include cellular defence mechanisms and reserves of biochemical func-

tion. Thus, toxicity may not be initiated until cellular defence mechanisms are exhausted, or a biochemical detoxification path is near saturation. Also, saturation of a biochemical process which produces toxic metabolites may result in a plateau for toxicity.

An important variant of the sigmoid dosage–response curve may be seen with genetically heterogeneous populations, where the presence of an usually high incidence in the hypersusceptible area could indicate the existence of a special subpopulation that have a genetically determined hypersusceptibility to the substance being tested **(Figure 4)**.

Data plotted on a dosage–response basis may be quantal or continuous. The quantal response is 'all-or-none', e.g. death. The graded, or variable, response is one involving a continual change in effect with increasing dosage, e.g. enzyme inhibition, degree of inflammation or physiological function such as heart rate. The dosage–response curve is often linearly transformed into a log-probit plot (log_{10} dose versus probit response) because it permits the examination of data over a wide range of dosages, and allows certain mathematical procedures (e.g. calculation of confidence limits and slope of response) **(Figure 5)**. Quantal data can also be plotted as a frequency histogram or frequency distribution curve; this is done by plotting the percentage response

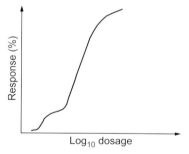

Figure 4 Variant of the sigmoid cumulative dosage–response curve due to enhanced hyperreactive response; this may represent a genetic variant in a proportion of the population causing enhanced sensitivity to the toxic effect.

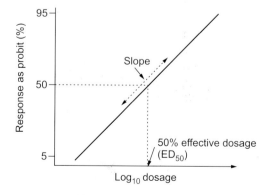

Figure 5 Linear transformation of dosage–response data by log–probit plot.

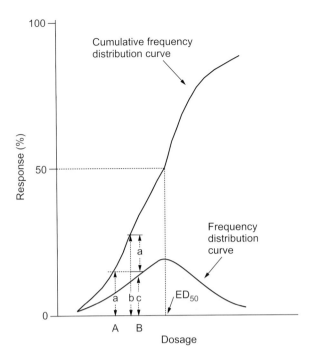

Figure 6 Relationship between cumulative frequency distribution curve and normal frequency distribution curve for quantal data. The cumulative frequency distribution curve shows the proportion responding for each dosage, and hence the expected total response for any given dosage. The frequency distribution curve shows the response specific for that dosage compared with lower dosages. For the frequency distribution curve, the response (c) at any dosage (e.g. B) is obtained by taking the total response at that dosage (b) and subtracting the response (a) at the immediate lower dosage (A).

at a given dose minus the percentage response at the immediate lower dose (i.e. response specific for the dosage). This procedure usually results in a gaussian distribution **(Figure 6)**, reflecting the differential biological susceptibility of the test organism to the treatment. In such a normal frequency distribution curve the mean ± 1 standard deviation (SD) represents 68.3% of the population, the mean ± 2 SD represents 95.5% and the mean ± 3 SD is 99.7% of the population.

It is important to stress that not only will the incidence of the effect of interest vary with dose, and determine the dosage–response relationship, but also the severity or magnitude of the effect will change with varying dosage. Thus, for any given dosage producing a particular response incidence, those responding may show a difference in the magnitude of the effect.

The absence of a clear dosage–response relationship in a controlled experiment may indicate a non-toxic or non-pharmacological action of the material. For example, an aminoalkyltrialkoxydisilane given by gavage to rats resulted in the following mortalities [expressed as (number dying/number dosed)]: 16 g (kg body weight)$^{-1}$ (4/5), 8 g (kg body weight)$^{-1}$ (0/5), 4 g (kg body weight)$^{-1}$ (3/5) and 2 g (kg body weight)$^{-1}$ (0/5). Clearly, there was no dosage–response relationship in this study. Necropsy of

dying rats showed that polymerization of the material had occurred in the stomach, producing a hard, opalescent, solid mass completely occluding the stomach. Hence, the cause of death was a consequence of mechanical obstruction and nutritional deprivation, rather than intrinsic toxicity.

For drugs, one convenient indication of 'safety' often used is the ratio of the median effective dose causing death to that producing the desired therapeutic response (i.e. LD_{50}/ED_{50}); this is frequently referred to as the therapeutic index (TI_{50}). In general, the higher this ratio, the greater is the degree of safety with respect to lethality. However, very considerable caution is needed in applying this information. For example, if the slopes of the dosage–response curves for drug effectiveness and lethality are parallel then the assumption of an equal therapeutic ratio over a range of dosages and to a majority of the population is justified **(Figure 7)**. If, however, the dosage–response curve for lethality is shallower than that for the therapeutic response **(Figure 8)**, then there will be a decreasing therapeutic index at the lower dosages, and the hyperreactive groups may be at greater risk. One approach which can be used to take into account differences in slopes is to calculate the ratio between that dosage causing a 1% mortality (LD_1) and that producing near maximum therapeutic efficacy (ED_{99}). This ratio, LD_1/ED_{99} is referred to as the margin of safety **(Figure 8)**. A complete appraisal of safety-in-use, of course, also requires considerations on sublethal and long-term toxicity, and at therapeutic dosages the likelihood of side-effects and idiosyncratic reactions.

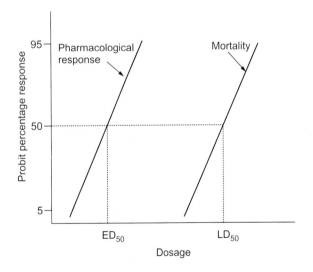

Figure 7 One simplistic method for assessing 'safety ratios' for drugs is by comparing the ratio of the therapeutically effective dose (e.g. ED_{50}) and that causing mortality (LD_{50}); this ratio LD_{50}/ED_{50} is referred to as the therapeutic index (TI). For parallel pharmacological effect and lethality dosage–response lines, the therapeutic index will be similar over a wide range of doses. However, non-parallel lines may give misleading conclusions if the TI_{50} is calculated (see **Figure 8**).

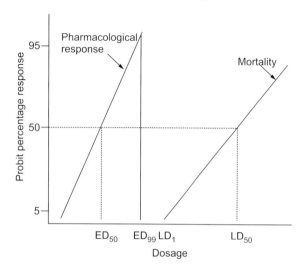

Figure 8 The TI$_{50}$ may give a misleading index of drug safety if the dosage–response lines for pharmacological and lethal effects are not parallel. In the example shown here, there may be a reasonable margin based on LD$_{50}$ and ED$_{50}$. However, owing to the shallow slope of the mortality dosage–response line, the therapeutic index will be significantly lower at the 1 and 5% levels, and thus the hyperreactive group may be at greater risk. In this case a better index of safety will be the ratio LD$_1$ / ED$_{99}$, which is referred to as the 'margin of safety'.

The slope of the dosage–response relationship, particularly around the mid-point, can be of value for more precisely assessing hazard or potential for overdose situations. Thus, for example, in considering lethality a steep slope indicates that a large proportion of the population will be at risk over a small range of doses. Likewise, with a material producing central nervous system depression, a steep slope implies that a small incremental increase of dosage may result in coma rather than sedation.

In most cases of acute lethal toxicity, the dosage–response curve is a log-normal cumulative frequency distribution or gaussian frequency distribution. In a few cases there may be two definite peaks in the frequency distribution curve, and which is distinct from an increase in hyperreactive groups at the left-hand-side of the dosage–response curve. Such a bimodal distribution may reflect different modes of lethality toxicity possibly with differing latency. Earlier deaths at the lower dosages, producing the first phase of the bimodal distribution, represent a quantitatively more potent toxicity; those surviving the first phase toxicity may succumb to the higher dosage latent toxicity. For example, with anticholinesterase organophosphates, the first deaths are due to the cholinergic crisis resulting from acetylcholinesterase inhibition, and late toxicity may result from delayed onset peripheral neuropathy. In some cases, log–probit plots will allow the determination of ED$_{50}$ values for each subgroup in the bimodal distribution.

For many toxic effects, except genotoxic carcinogenesis, there is a dose below which no effect or response can

be elicited; this corresponds to the extreme left-hand-side of the dosage–response curve. This dosage, below which no effect occurs, is referred to as the 'threshold dosage'. The threshold concept, a corollary of the dosage–response relationship, is important in that it implies that it is possible to determine a 'no-observable effect level' (NOEL), which can be used as a basis for assigning 'safe levels' for exposure.

Use of Dosage–Response Information

It is important to reiterate that conclusions drawn from dosage–response studies are valid only for the specific conditions under which the information was collected. Within this constraint, dosage–response information allows at least the following:

(1) Confirmation that the effect being considered is a toxic (or pharmacological) response to the chemical or therapeutic agent. Thus, a positive dosage–response relationship is good evidence for a causal relationship between exposure and the development of toxicity or pharmacological effects.

(2) Quantitative dose–response information allows the determination of an average (median) response, gives the range of susceptibility in the population studied and indicates where the dosage for hyper-susceptible groups is expected.

(3) The slope of the dosage–response curve gives information on the range of effective dosages and the differential proportion of the population affected for incremental increases in dosage. With a shallow slope the range of effective doses is widespread; the proportion of the population additionally affected by incremental increases in dosage is small. In contrast, a steep slope implies that the effective dose for the majority of the population is over a narrow range, and there will be a significant increase in the proportion of the population affected for small incremental increases in dosage.

(4) The shape of the left-hand-side of the dosage–response curve may indicate the existence of an unusually high hypersusceptible proportion of the population. This may, for example, indicate a genetically determined increased susceptibility to the chemical or pharmacologically active substance studied.

(5) The data may allow conclusions on 'threshold' or 'no-effect' dosages for the response.

(6) Quantitative comparison for a specific end-point may be made between different materials with respect to average and range of response, particularly if the information has been collected under similar conditions.

The above considerations are briefly illustrated in the following section.

Dosage–Response Considerations for Acute Lethal Toxicity

Death, a quantal response, is an end-point incorporated in many acute toxicity studies, and often used for the calculation of LD_{50} values.

Acute lethal toxicity studies involve giving differing dosages of the test material to groups of laboratory animals of the same strain by a specific route of exposure and under controlled experimental conditions, e.g. diet, caging, temperature, relative humidity and time of dosing. Mortalities at each dosage are recorded over a specified period of time, usually 14 days. By epicutaneous or respiratory exposure, the exposure time should be stated, since the degree of local injury and the potential for systemic toxicity are a function of this time. For routes other than inhalation, the exposure dosage is usually expressed as mass (or volume) of test material given per unit of body weight, e.g. ml (kg body weight)$^{-1}$ or mg (kg body weight)$^{-1}$. For inhalation, the exposure dose is expressed as the amount of test material present per unit volume of exposure atmosphere: mg m^{-3} or ppm. Dose–response information collected for differing concentrations of an atmospherically disposed material should be over similar periods of time in order to allow the most meaningful comparisons to be made. Alternatively, the effect of differing inhalation exposure doses can be made by exposing different groups to the same concentration of test substance for various exposure periods; this may allow the calculation of a median time to death (50% response rate) for the population exposed to a specific atmospheric concentration of test material (LT_{50}). By using both of these approaches it is possible to reach conclusions on the differential sensitivity of a population to varying concentrations for a specified period of time, or to differing exposure periods for a given concentration.

Dosage–mortality data usually conforms to the sigmoid cumulative frequency distribution curve (**Figure 9A**), which may be converted to a linear form using a log–probit plot (**Figure 9B**). Lethal toxicity is usually initially calculated and compared at a specific mortality level; most frequently used is that causing 50% mortality in the population studied, since this represents the midpoint of the dosage range about which the majority of deaths occur and usually with a symmetrical distribution. This is the median lethal dose for 50% of the population studied (LD_{50}), i.e. that dose, calculated from the dosage–mortality data, which causes death of half of the population dosed under the specific conditions of the test. This concept of the LD_{50} was introduced by Trevan (1927). By inhalation, the reference is the (lethal concentration)$_{50}$ (LC_{50}) for a specified period of time (i.e. X h LC_{50}).

Other values calculated may be the LD_5 and LD_{95}, which give statistical indications of near-threshold and

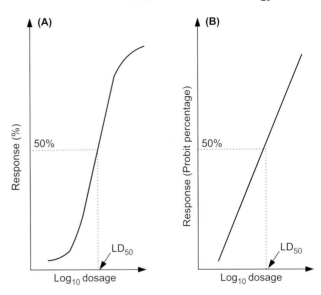

Figure 9 Dosage–mortality data **(A)** plotted as a cumulative frequency distribution curve (% response versus $\log_{10}$ dosage) and **(B)** linearly transformed by log–probit plot.

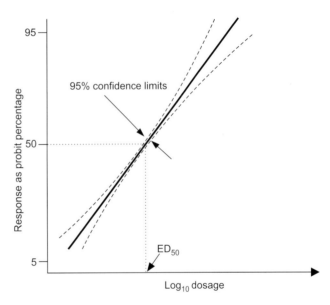

Figure 10 Dosage–mortality curve with 95% confidence limits. The limits are closest at the ED_{50} and diverge as the extremes of the dosage response are reached.

near-maximum lethal toxicity, respectively, and the range of doses over which a lethal response may occur.

Since the LD_{50}, for economical and ethical reasons, is usually conducted with only small numbers of animals, there is an uncertainty factor associated with the calculation of the LD_{50} (or LC_{50} or LT_{50}). This is estimated from the 95% confidence limits, i.e. the dosage range for which there is only a 5% chance that the LD_{50} (or other LD value) lies outside. The 95% confidence limits are narrowest at the LD_{50} (**Figure 10**), which is another reason why this is an appropriate point for the comparison of acute lethal toxicity.

The LD$_{50}$, by itself, is an insufficient index of lethal toxicity, particularly if comparisons are to be made between different materials. The whole of the dosage–response information should be examined, including slope of the dosage–response line and 95% confidence limits. For example, two materials with differing LD$_{50}$ values but overlapping 95% confidence limits are not regarded as being of significantly different lethal toxicity, since there is a statistical probability that the LD$_{50}$ of one material will be within the 95% confidence limits of the other. However, when there is no overlap of 95% confidence limits then the materials are considered to have significantly different lethal toxicity at the LD$_{50}$ level **(Figure 11)**. A particularly important consideration is that of the slope of the dosage–response curve **(Figure 12)**. For example, if two materials have similar LD$_{50}$ values with overlapping 95% confidence limits and identical slopes on the dosage–response lines (and therefore statistically similar LD$_{10}$ and LD$_{90}$ values), they are lethally equitoxic over a wide dosage range (A and B, **Figure 12**). However, materials having similar LD$_{50}$ values but differing slopes (and hence significantly different LD$_{10}$ and LD$_{90}$ values) may not be considered to be lethally equitoxic over a wide dosage range (A or B versus C, **Figure 12**). Thus, materials having a steep slope (A or B, **Figure 12**) may affect a much larger proportion of the population by incremental increases in dosages than is the case with materials having a shallow slope; thus, acute overdose may be a more serious problem affecting the majority population for materials with steeper slopes. In contrast, materials having a shallower slope (C, **Figure 12**) may present problems for the hyper-reactive groups at the left-hand-side of the dosage–response curve, and may occur at significantly lower dosages than for hyperreactive individuals associated with the steep slope group. It follows from the above that a proper interpretation of acute lethal toxicity information should include examination of LD$_{50}$, 95% confidence limits, slope and extremes of the dosage–response curve.

It needs to be stressed that dosage–response information requires to be interpreted in terms of the conditions by which it was obtained; the following few examples are used to illustrate the care necessary:

(a)   The numerical precision of the LD$_{50}$ lies only in the statistical procedures by which it is calculated. If an experiment to determine LD$_{50}$ is repeated at a later time, slightly different dosage–response data may be obtained because of biological and environmental variability, resulting in a different numerical value for the LD$_{50}$. Therefore, LD$_{50}$ values should be regarded as representing an order of lethal toxicity under the specific circumstances by which the information was collected.

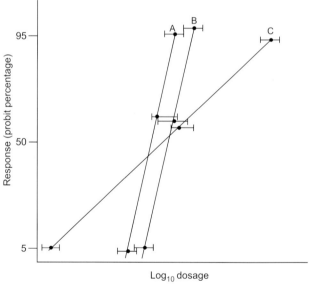

Figure 12 Influence of slopes of dosage–mortality plots on the interpretation of LD$_{50}$ data. All three materials (A, B and C) have overlapping 95% confidence limits at the 50% response level, and are therefore of comparable LD$_{50}$. Materials A and B have parallel dosage–response lines and overlapping confidence limits at 5 and 95%; therefore, these two materials are of comparable lethal toxicity over a wide range of doses. Material C, with a shallower slope, has significantly different LD$_5$ and LD$_{95}$ values, and therefore over a wide range of doses has a differing lethal toxicity to materials A and B. With materials A and B, owing to the steep slope of the dosage–response line, a much larger proportion of the population will be affected by small incremental increases in dosage. With material C, there may be a greater hazard for the hyperreactive groups since the LD$_5$ lies at a much lower dosage than for A and B.

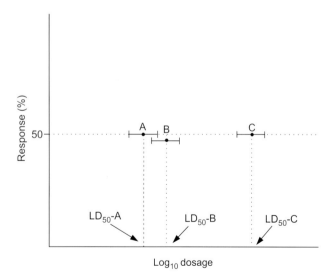

Figure 11 Comparison of the acute lethal toxicity of three compounds using LD$_{50}$ data alone. Compounds A and B have overlapping 95% confidence limits, and therefore have comparable acute lethal toxicities. Compound C, the 95% confidence limits of which are separate from those of A and B, is significantly less toxic (higher LD$_{50}$ dosage) than either A or B, based on LD$_{50}$ values.

(b) An important consideration in interpreting the acute hazard from a chemical is the time to toxic effect. Thus, materials of similar LD_{50}, but differing times to death may present different hazards. For example, with substances having similar LD_{50} and slope values, those having more rapid times to death can be considered as presenting a greater acute hazard. However, those substances with longer latency to effect may have a potential to produce cumulative toxicity by repeated exposure. For example, the acute peroral LD_{50} of 2,4-pentanedione in the rat is 0.58 g (kg body weight)$^{-1}$ and that of 2,2-bis(4-aminophenoxyphenyl)propane (BAPP) is 0.31 g (kg body weight)$^{-1}$, with respective times to death of 2–5 h and 13–14 days; on this basis, 2,4-pentanedione would be regarded as presenting a greater acute potential hazard than BAPP (Tyler and Ballantyne, 1988).

(c) A more complete interpretation of the significance of LD_{50} data may require consideration of the cause of death. If differing potentially lethal toxic effects are produced, it is important to know if this can lead to a multimodal dosage–response curve, and thus to differing hazards by immediate or latent mortality or morbidity. Clearly, latency is of importance in clinical toxicology for decisions on immediate medical management and observations and treatment for latent toxicity. For example, *tert*-butyl nitrite given by acute intraperitoneal injection to mice has a 30 min LD_{50} of 613 mg (kg body weight)$^{-1}$ and a 7 day LD_{50} of 187 mg (kg body weight)$^{-1}$. The earlier deaths were probably related to cardiovascular collapse and methaemoglobin formation, whereas later deaths were due to liver injury (Maickel and McFadden, 1979).

(d) Acute LD_{50} data may not be a direct guide to defining lethal toxicity by multiple exposures. Thus, with a material producing significant cumulative toxicity, the acute lethal dose (and dosage) may be significantly higher than that producing death by multiple smaller exposures. For example, the 4 h LC_{50} for trimethoxysilane is 47 ppm (rat); however, for rats given 20 exposures, each of 7 h over 4 weeks, the LC_{50} was 5.5 ppm for that time period (Ballantyne *et al.*, 1988). Thus, the potentially lethal vapour concentration of trimethoxysilane for repeated exposure is significantly less than that for acute exposure.

Any investigation into lethal toxicity should attempt to allow the maximum amount of usable information to be obtained. For this reason, acute toxicity studies should be designed not only to determine lethal toxicity but also to monitor for sublethal and target organ toxicity; this is possible by incorporating into the protocol observations for signs, body weight, haematology, clinical chemistry, urinalysis, gross and microscopic pathology and other specialized procedures as considered appropriate for the material under test. In this way a significantly greater amount of relevant information can be obtained, and the most useful and meaningful information collected to allow a comparative evaluation of acute toxicity and potential hazards and the potential for cumulative toxicity (Zbinden and Flury-Roversi, 1981).

Detailed discussions on dosage–response relationships and their toxicological and pharmacological relevance have been written by Sperling (1984), Tallarida and Jacob (1979), and Timbrell (1982).

FACTORS INFLUENCING TOXICITY

With both animal studies and human poisoning, the nature, severity, incidence and probable induction of toxicity depends on a large number of exogenous and endogenous factors. Some of the more important are as follows.

Species and Strain

Species and strain differences in susceptibility to chemical-induced toxicity may be due, to variable extents, to differences in rates of absorption, metabolic conversions, detoxification mechanisms and excretion. In some cases animal studies may give underestimates, and in other instances overestimates, for acute peroral toxicity to humans. For example, the acute peroral LD_{50} of ethylene glycol has been determined in several laboratory mammals to range from 4.7 to 7.5 g (kg body weight)$^{-1}$ (Sweet, 1985–1986a) and that for methanol to range from 5.63 to 7.50 g (kg body weight)$^{-1}$ (Sweet, 1985–1986b); both of these chemicals are more toxic to humans with a minimal lethal dosage around 0.5–1.0 ml (kg body weight)$^{-1}$.

Age

With some substances age may significantly affect toxicity, probably mainly due to relative metabolizing and excretory capacities. In one extensive compilation of LD_{50} values for drugs to neonatal and adult mammals (Goldenthal, 1971), the ratio (LD_{50}-adult) (LD_{50}-neonate) varied from < 0.02 (for amidephrine) to 750 (for digitoxin).

Nutritional Status

Nutritional status may significantly influence the level of cofactors and biotransformation mechanisms important for the expression of toxicity. Thus diet can affect toxicity

(Rao and Knapka, 1998). Moreover, diet may markedly influence the natural tumour incidence in animals and modulate carcinogen-induced tumour incidence (Grasso, 1988). Khanna *et al.* (1988) studied the effect of protein deficiency on the neurobehavioural effects of acrylamide in rat pups exposed during the intrauterine and early postnatal stages. They found acrylamide to be more toxic in protein-deficient hosts owing to a significant decrease in dopamine and benzodiazepine receptor binding. Feeding is an important factor in the design and interpretation of acute peroral toxicity studies. For example, Kast and Nishikawa (1981) compared the acute peroral toxicity of several anti-gastric ulcer drugs and β-adrenoceptor agonists and blockers; the ratio (LD_{50} fed)/(LD_{50} fasted) for rats and mice ranged from 1.3 to 1.47, indicating a higher toxicity in the starved animals. The authors concluded that the greater acute toxicity in the starved animals was due to accelerated gastric emptying and intestinal absorption. The importance of dietary factors in toxicity has been reviewed by Angeli-Greaves and McLean (1981) and Grasso (1988).

Time of Dosing

Diurnal and seasonal variations in toxicity may relate to similar variations in biochemical, physiological and hormonal profiles. Examples of temporal variations in biological activity include circadian dependence of metabolic adverse effects of cyclosporin (Malmary *et al.*, 1988), toxicity of methotrexate (Marks *et al.*, 1985) and seasonal variations in gentamicin nephrotoxicity (Pariat *et al.*, 1988).

Environmental Factors

A variety of environmental factors are known to influence the development of toxicity, including temperature, relative humidity and photoperiod. The influence of temperature may vary between differing chemicals and the effects investigated. For example, colchicine and digitalis are more toxic the higher is the temperature (Lu, 1985); in contrast, studies on the behavioural toxicity of the anticholinesterase soman suggest that the lower the temperature, the greater is the susceptibility (Wheeler, 1987). The influence of temperature on toxicity is clearly an important consideration for materials used in arctic and tropical areas.

Exposure (Dosing) Characteristics

The nature, severity and likelihood of inducing toxicity is influenced by the magnitude, number, frequency and profiling of dosing. Thus, local or systemic toxicity produced by acute exposure may also occur by a cumulative process with repeated lower dosage exposures; also, additional toxicity may be seen with the repeated exposure situations. For example, acute exposure to formaldehyde vapour causes peripheral sensory irritant effects and (with sufficiently high concentrations) injury and inflammatory change in the respiratory tract; short-term repeated vapour exposure may result in the development of respiratory sensitization; longer-term vapour exposure may cause squamous metaplasia and nasal tumours (Wartew, 1983). The relationships for cumulative toxicity by repetitive exposure compared with acute exposure toxicity may be complex, and the potential for repeated exposure cumulative toxicity from acutely sub-threshold doses may not be quantitatively predictable. For example, the LC_{50} for a 4 h exposure to trimethoxysilane vapour is 47 ppm; by repeated exposure over a 4 week period (7 h day^{-1}, 5 days a week) the LC_{50} is 5.5 ppm (Ballantyne *et al.*, 1988). In contrast, acute exposure to benzene vapour for 26 h (95 ppm) or 96 h (21 ppm) produced severe bone marrow cytotoxicity, whilst a similar exposure dose given over a longer period of time (95 ppm for 2 h day^{-1} for 2 weeks) produced little toxicity (Toft *et al.*, 1982).

For repeated exposure toxicity, the precise profiling of doses may significantly influence toxicity. For example, with formaldehyde in a 4 week vapour inhalation study, it was determined that exposure of rats to 10 or 20 ppm by interrupted exposure over eight exposure periods produced more nasal mucosal cytotoxicity than did continual exposures (Wilmer *et al.*, 1987). In a 4 week inhalation study with carbon tetrachloride, it was found that interruption of a daily 6 h exposure by 1–5 h periods of non-exposure caused more severe hepatotoxicity than with continuous exposures, but 5 min peak loads superimposed on a steady background only slightly aggravated the hepatotoxic effect of carbon tetrachloride vapour (Bogers *et al.*, 1977).

Formulation and Presentation

For chemicals given perorally or applied to the skin, toxicity may be modified by the presence of materials in formulations which facilitate or retard the absorption of the chemicals. With respiratory exposure to aerosols, particle size significantly determines the depth of penetration and deposition in the respiratory tract (Chapter 30).

Miscellaneous

A variety of other factors may effect the nature and exhibition of toxicity, depending on the conditions of the study, e.g. housing conditions, handling and dosing volume. Variability in test conditions and procedures may result in significant interlaboratory variability in results of otherwise standard procedures (e.g. LD_{50} determination; Griffith, 1964; Hunter *et al.*, 1979).

BIOHANDLING AS A DETERMINANT OF SYSTEMIC TOXICITY

The induction of systemic toxicity results from a complex interrelationship between absorbed parent material and conversion products formed in tissues, their distribution in body fluids and tissues, binding and storage characteristics, and their excretion. Some of these factors are considered below (see also **Figure 13**).

Absorption

The absorption of a substance from the site of exposure may result from passive diffusion, facilitated diffusion, active transport, or the formation of transport vesicles (pinocytosis and phagocytosis). The process of absorption may be facilitated or retarded by a variety of factors, e.g. elevated temperature increases percutaneous absorption by cutaneous vasodilation and surface-active materials facilitate penetration. The integrity of the absorbing surface is important, e.g. the acute percutaneous LD_{50} for HCN (solution) is 6.89 mg (kg body weight)$^{-1}$ for rabbits with intact skin, and 2.34 mg (kg body weight)$^{-1}$ if the skin is abraided (Ballantyne, 1987).

Biodistribution

After absorption, materials circulate either free or bound to plasma protein or blood cells; the degree of binding, and factors influencing the equilibrium with the free form, may influence availability for metabolism, storage or excretion. Within tissues there may be binding, storage, metabolic activation or detoxification; binding may produce a high tissue/plasma partition and be a source for slow titration into the circulation following the cessation of environmental exposure. Examples of storage sites include fat for lipophilic materials (e.g. chlorinated pesticides) and bone for fluoride, lead and strontium. The relationship between exposure dose and release rate may be complex; for example, volatile lipophilic materials are generally more rapidly desorbed than non-volatile lipophilic substances. Tissue permeability may be modified by tissue-specific barriers, e.g. the blood–brain barrier and placenta. This may affect differential toxicity within classes of compounds, e.g. neurobehavioural effects produced by organomercurials but to a lesser degree with inorganic mercury compounds (Lu, 1985).

Biotransformation

Metabolism of substances is conveniently classified under the following two major headings (Williams, 1959):

Phase I reactions A functional group is introduced into the molecule by oxidation, reduction or hydrolysis.
Phase II reactions There is conjugation of an absorbed material or its metabolite with an endogenous substrate.

For many materials there is an initial Phase I reaction to produce materials which are conjugated by Phase II processes. In other instances only a Phase II process may be utilized. Reactions of a Phase I type include oxidation,

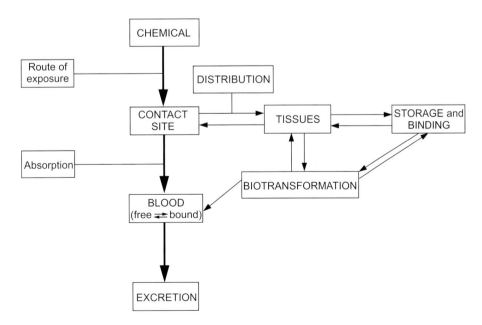

Figure 13 Possible fate of a chemical absorbed from the route of exposure.

Table 5 Examples of metabolic transformations of chemicals

Biotransformation	Chemical	Conversion
Detoxification	Cyanide	Enzymic conversion to less toxic thiocyanate
	Benzoic acid	Conjugation with glycine to produce hippuric acid
	Bromobenzene	3,4-Epoxide reactive matabolite is enzymically hydrated to the 3,4-dihydrodiol or conjugated with glutathione
Activation	Carbon tetrachloride	Microsomal enzyme metabolic activation to hepatotoxic trichloromethylperoxy radicals
	2-Acetylaminofluorene	*N*-Hydroxylation to the more potent carcinogen *N*-hydroxyacetyaminofluorene
	Parathion	Oxidative desulphuration to the potent cholinesterase inhibitor paraoxon

reduction and enzymic hydrolysis; Phase II reactions include conjugation with glucuronic acid, sulphate, glycine and glutathione and acetylation and methylation. Phase I reactions, particularly, may result in the formation of toxic metabolites from relatively innocuous precursors, i.e. metabolic activation. Phase II conjugates are generally more water soluble than the parent compound or Phase I metabolites and hence usually more readily excreted. With toxic parent compounds, or toxic metabolites, there may be conversion to less toxic products, i.e. detoxification has occurred. Examples of metabolic activation and detoxification are given in **Table 5**. Many activation reactions are catalysed by a cytochrome P450-dependent mono-oxygenase system, which is particularly active in the liver. Clearly, a major determinant of the likelihood of toxicity developing, and its severity, is the overall balance between absorption rate of a chemical, its metabolic activation and detoxification and the excretion of toxic species (see Chapter 6).

Excretion

Substances may be excreted as parent compound, metabolites and/or Phase II conjugates. A major route of excretion is by the kidney, and in some cases the urinary elimination of parent compound, metabolite or conjugate, may be used as a means for assessing absorbed dose. Some materials may be excreted in bile and thence in faeces; in such cases there may also be enterohepatic cycling. Certain volatile materials and metabolites may be eliminated in expired air. The excretion of materials in sweat, hair, nails and saliva is usually quantitatively insignificant, but these routes may be of importance for a forensic or industrial diagnosis of intoxication (Paschal et al., 1989; Randall and Gibson, 1989). Materials excreted in milk may be transferred to the neonate.

General Considerations

The probability of adverse effects developing in response to chemical exposure depends particularly on the magnitude, duration, frequency and route of exposure. These will determine the amount of material to which an organism is exposed (the exposure dose), and hence to the amount of material which can be absorbed (the absorbed dose). The latter determines the amount of material available for distribution and toxic metabolite formation, and hence the likelihood of inducing a toxic effect. Opposing absorption and metabolite accumulation is elimination. Hence, for a given environmental exposure situation, the probability of inducing toxicity, and its magnitude, depend on the relationship between rate of absorption, metabolism (activation and detoxification) and elimination of parent material and metabolites.

The amount of a material in contact with the absorbing surface is one of the principal determinants of absorbed dose. In general, the higher the concentration, the greater is the absorbed dose. However, if mechanisms other than simple diffusion across a concentration gradient are operating, a simple proportionate relationship between concentration and absorbed dose may not exist. In such instances, a rate-limiting factor could result in proportionately smaller increases in absorbed dose for incremental increases in concentration at the absorption site. Also, and in particular when there is absorption by active transport, there may be saturation of the absorption process and a ceiling value.

When there is repeated exposure, the relative amounts of biotransformation products, and the distribution and elimination of metabolites and parent compound, may be different from that following an acute exposure. For example, repeated exposure may induce and enhance mechanisms responsible for the biotransformation of the absorbed material and thus alter the relative proportions of parent molecules and metabolites (activation and detoxification), and hence the probability for target organ toxicity. Also, if there is slow detoxification, storage and/or slow excretion, repeated exposures may lead to the accumulation of toxic species and hence a potential for cumulative toxicity.

ROUTES OF EXPOSURE

The primary tissue or system by which a material comes into contact with the body, and from where it may be absorbed in order to exert systemic toxicity, is the route of exposure. The usual circumstances of environmental exposure are by ingestion (peroral), inhalation and skin or eye contact. Also, for investigational, therapeutic and certain forensic purposes, intramuscular, intravenous and subcutaneous injections may be routes of exposure.

The relationship between route of exposure, biotransformation and potential for toxicity may be complex and also influenced by the magnitude and duration of dosing. Materials that undergo hepatic activation are likely to exhibit greater toxicity when given perorally than if absorbed across the lung or skin, owing to the high proportion of material passing directly via the portal vein following peroral dosing. In contrast, materials that undergo hepatic detoxification are likely to be less toxic perorally than when absorbed percutaneously or across the respiratory tract. However, in determining the relevance of route to biotransformation and toxicity, both the magnitude and time-scale for dosing should be considered. Thus, when a single, large dose (bolus) of a metabolically activated material is given perorally, its rapid metabolism may result in the immediate development of a severe acute toxicity. However, if the same material is given perorally at much lower rates (e.g. by dietary inclusion), then there will be slow and sustained absorption, and in such circumstances the rate of generation of the toxic species may approach that resulting from continuous exposure by other routes. With materials that are detoxified by the liver, a slow, continuous alimentary absorption will result in an anticipated low toxicity, compared with other routes of exposure. However, a peroral bolus my result in the detoxifying capacity of the liver being overwhelmed, and unmetabolized material may enter the circulation to initiate toxicity. A few comments on specific routes of exposure follow.

Peroral

If a material is sufficiently irritant or corrosive, it will cause local inflammatory or corrosive effects on the upper alimentary tract. This may lead to, for example, fibrosis, dysphasia and perforation with mediastinitis and/or peritonitis and the complications thereof. Additionally, carcinogenic materials may induce tumour formation in the alimentary tract. The gastro-intestinal tract is an important route by which systemically toxic materials may be absorbed (see Chapter 27).

Cutaneous Contact and Percutaneous Absorption

Skin contact is an important route of exposure in the occupational and domestic environment. Local effects may include acute inflammation and corrosion, chronic inflammatory responses, immune-mediated reactions and neoplasia. The percutaneous absorption of materials can be a significant route for the absorption of systemically toxic materials (Billingham, 1977; Bronough and Maibach, 1985; see Chapter 29), and indeed is now a means for the systemic titration of pharmacologically active materials (Woodford and Barry, 1986). Factors influencing the percutaneous absorption of substances include skin site, integrity of skin, temperature, formulation and physicochemical characteristics, including charge, molecular weight and hydrophilic and lipophilic characteristics (Billingham, 1977; Dugard, 1977; Stuttgen et al., 1982; Kemppainen and Reifenrath, 1990).

Although it is well appreciated that percutaneous absorption of materials may occur when they contaminate the skin as liquid or solid, it has been shown that percutaneous absorption may also result from exposure to the skin to vapour. In the majority of situations, absorption by the inhalation route is generally regarded as being significantly greater than by percutaneous absorption from the vapour phase (McDougal et al., 1986; Jacobs and Phanprasik, 1993). When controlled studies are conducted in humans, difference of opinion may exist, particularly with the need for artifact-free techniques. For example, Johanson and Boman (1991) conducted a comparative study on human volunteers who were exposed for 2 h mouth-only to 50 ppm 2-butoxyethanol, followed by 1 h of no exposure, followed by a further 2 h of skin-only exposure to 50 ppm 2-butoxyethanol. Using areas under the curve for concentrations of 2-butoxyethanol in finger-prick blood samples, they calculated that approximately 75% of the total uptake of 2-butoxyethanol vapour was absorbed through the skin. Subsequently, Corley et al. (1997) criticized this approach, mainly on the basis that the finger-prick sampling was compounded by locally high concentrations of 2-butoxyethanol at the site of absorption. They conducted a study involving exposure of one arm of human volunteers subjected to 50 ppm $[^{13}C_2]$-2-butoxyethanol vapour (50 ppm) for 2 h. Blood samples were taken by finger-prick from the exposed arm and by catheter from the unexposed arm, and analysed for 2-butoxyethanol and its major haemolytic metabolite, butoxyacetic acid. They found the concentration of 2-butoxyethanol in the finger-prick blood samples to be almost 1500 times those taken by catheter from the unexposed contralateral arm. Blood butoxyacetic acid concentrations were found to be within a factor of 4 of each other for the two sampling techniques, and it was considered that the metabolite was a better indicator of absorption into the systemic circulation. In a physiologically based pharmacokinetic model of a 'worst case' scenario (100% body exposure) of an 8 h exposure to 25 ppm vapour, they calculated that only 15–27% of the total uptake of 2-butoxyethanol would be by percutaneous absorption. In contrast, with styrene, measurement of urinary metabolites in workers showed no significant percutaneous absorption of styrene (Limasset *et al.*, 1999).

Inhalation

The likelihood of toxicity from atmospherically dispersed materials depends on a number of factors, the most important of which include physical state and properties, concentration and time and frequency of exposure. The water solubility of a gas or vapour influences the depth of penetration of a material into the respiratory tract. As water solubility decreases, and lipid solubility increases, there is more effective penetration towards the alveoli. Water-soluble molecules, such as formaldehyde, are more effectively scavenged by the upper respiratory tract.

The penetration and distribution of fibres and particulates in the respiratory tract are determined principally by their size. Thus, in general, particles having a mass medium aerodynamic diameter greater than 50 μm do not enter the respiratory tract; those of diameter $> 10\mu$m are deposited in the upper respiratory tract; those having a range of 10–2 μm are deposited in the trachea, bronchi, and bronchioles; and only particles whose diameter is $< 1.2\mu$m reach the alveoli. Thus, larger insoluble particles are more likely to cause local reactions in the upper respiratory tract, and the potential for alveolar injury is greater with smaller diameter particles. Fibres have aerodynamic characteristics such that those having diameters $> 3\mu$m are unlikely to penetrate the lung. In general, fibres having a diameter $< 3\mu$m and length $< 200\mu$m will enter the lung. Fibres of diameter $> 10\mu$m may not be removed by normal clearance mechanisms. Several studies have indicated that fibres of diameter $> 1.5\mu$m and length $< 8\mu$m have maximum biological activity (Asher and McGrath, 1976; Stanton *et al.*, 1981). Dust may be a significant cause of lung disease (Conference, 1990).

The likelihood that inhaled substances will produce local effects in the respiratory tract depends on their physical and chemical characteristics (particularly volatility), reactivity with lining fluids, reactivity with tissue components and site of deposition. Depending on the nature of the material, conditions of exposure and biological reactivity, the types of response produced include acute inflammation and injury, chronic inflammation, immune-mediated hypersensitivity reactions, and neoplasia. The degree to which inhaled gases, vapours and particulates are absorbed and, hence, their potential to produce systemic toxicity, depend on molecular weight, solubility in tissue fluids, metabolism by lung tissue, diffusion rate and equilibrium state (see Chapter 30).

Eye

Local and systemic adverse effects may be produced by contamination with liquids, solids and atmospherically dispersed materials. Local effects include transient inflammation, permanent injury and hypersensitivity reactions. Penetration may lead to iritis, glaucoma and cataract. Systemically active amounts of material may be absorbed from periocular blood vessels and/or nasal mucosa following passage down the nasolachrymal duct (Shell, 1982; Ballantyne, 1983; see Chapter 38).

EXPOSURE TO MIXTURES OF CHEMICALS

Circumstances involving exposure to several xenobiotics can result in prior, coincidental or successive exposure to these chemicals, and the nature of the toxicity may vary considerably depending on the conditions of exposure. Thus, an evaluation of the hazards from exposure to multiple chemicals can be much more demanding than is the case for a single chemical. In assessing toxicity from mixtures it is important to consider (a) chemical and/or physical interactions of the individual materials, (b) the effect that one chemical may have on the absorption, metabolism and pharmacokinetic characteristics of another and (c) the possibility of interaction between parent compound and metabolites (Ballantyne, 1985). A convenient descriptive classification for effects produced by binary mixtures of chemicals is as follows:

Independent effects Substances qualitatively and quantitatively exert their own toxicity independent of each other.

Additive effects Materials with similar qualitative toxicity produce a response which is quantitatively equal to the sum of the effects produced by the individual constituents.

Antagonistic effects Materials oppose each other's toxicity, or one interferes with the toxicity of another; a particular example is that of antidotal action.

Potentiating effects One material, usually of low toxicity, enhances the expression of toxicity by another; the result is more severe injury than that produced by the toxic species alone.

Synergistic effects Two materials, given simultaneously, produce toxicity significantly greater than anticipated from that of either material alone; the effect differs from potentiation in that each substance contributes to toxicity, and the net effect is always greater than additive.

In assessing the toxicity of mixtures, the following need to be taken into consideration:

■   Possible physical and chemical interactions—which may result in the formation of new substances or groupings, or influence bioavailability.
■   Time relationships of the exposure for the various components.

- Route and conditions of exposure.
- Physical and physiological factors affecting absorption.
- Mutual influence of materials and metabolites on biotransformation, pharmacokinetic characteristics and target organ doses of toxic species.
- Relative affinities of the target sites.
- Potential for independent, additive, antagonistic and interactive processes between the various chemical species.

Mixtures may be complex and contain unreacted parent materials, major reaction and degradation products and contaminants and trace additives. It is important to be aware that small quantities of high-toxicity materials may have equal, or greater, significance with respect to adverse health effects than major components. For example, serious consideration needs to be given to repeated exposure toxicity from small quantities of monomer residuals in polymeric materials, e.g. ethylene oxide, propylene oxide, vinyl chloride and formaldehyde (Ballantyne, 1989). The contribution to toxicity by trace materials is well illustrated by, for example, the presence of trialkyl phosphorothioate or phosphorothionate impurities in organophosphate anticholinesterases (Hollingshaus et al., 1981) such as malathion (JMPR, 1998), and the presence of 2,3,7,8-tetrachlorodibenzodioxin in chlorophenols (Kimbrough et al., 1984).

Many instances of enhancement of toxicity by specific routes are known. Thus, on the skin the systemic toxicity of a material may be enhanced by other materials which facilitate percutaneous absorption. For example, the presence of a surface-active material may result in a carrier function, and the presence of a primary irritant may produce local erythema resulting in increased skin blood flow. If the viscosity of a material is increased, this may enhance local or systemic toxicity due to persistence on the skin.

The inhalation exposure dosage of chemicals may be modified by, for example, the presence of sensory irritants or HCN, which can alter the rate and depth of breathing. Some substances may cause anosmia and hence remove an olfactory warning for other inhaled materials. Particulates may absorb other materials which, if inhaled, cause an increased local burden. When trace quantities of highly volatile and toxic materials are present in a substance, they may, depending on the condition of air movement, have a significant influence on toxicity and hazard. For example, if materials containing trace amounts of acrolein are handled in stagnant air conditions, then potentially toxic vapour concentrations of acrolein may develop; in contrast, when there is free airflow the acrolein vapour concentration may be low (Ballantyne et al., 1989). Thus, the degree of ventilation of an area may significantly influence the toxicity of the atmosphere resulting from vaporization of the individual constituents of a liquid mixture.

The endogenous determinants of overall toxicity resulting from exposure to a mixture of chemicals can be very complex. For example, toxicity may be modulated by prior or simultaneous exposure, resulting in enhancement or suppression of metabolic activation or detoxification pathways. The potential for toxicity may depend on the equilibrium state, although this may be continually fluctuating. Modification of toxicity may also result from modulation of pharmacokinetic characteristics, variation in the biodistribution of absorbed materials and metabolites, modifying elimination of the toxic species, and competition for binding sites or receptors. All the above factors will influence the relative and absolute concentration of toxic species at target sites for toxicity. Detailed discussions on the toxicity and hazard evaluation of mixtures of substances have been presented by the World Health Organization (1981), Murphy (1983), Ballantyne (1985) and the National Research Council (1988); see also Chapters 14 and 31.

DRUG TOXICITY

Adverse drug reactions can be classified in several ways. They may be divided into reactions due to overdosage, intolerance, side-effects, secondary effects, idiosyncrasy and hypersensitivity (see pp. 4). Some of these terms are difficult to define, however, and particular reactions are difficult to classify into one of them. Another system divides them into two types: Type A, which are the results of an exaggerated but otherwise normal pharmacological action of a drug, such as uncontrolled bleeding from an anticoagulant drug, and Type B which are totally aberrant effects not expected from the known pharmacological actions of a drug, such as deafness from streptomycin. A third system divides them into three groups: dose dependent, as in Type A above, dose independent, which are of an allergic nature involving antigen–antibody reactions, and pseudoallergic reactions, where allergic reactions are mimicked by mediator release due to direct action of the drug or its metabolite on mast cells.

Factors influencing dose-dependent drug toxicity include formulation, route of administration, pregnancy, age, genetic polymorphism of metabolism, environmental influences on metabolism, renal and hepatic excretion, disease, drug interactions and patient compliance. Nutritional status can affect both dosing efficacy and toxicity (Thomas et al., 1998). Additionally, certain common foods or drinks may interact with drugs or metabolites or modify their metabolism. One well known example is the interaction of monoamine oxidase inhibitors with food rich in tyramine, causing systemic accumulation of amines and hypertensive crises (Lloyd, 1991). A more recently, and not as widely appreciated, finding is drug interactions with grapefruit juice (Fuhr, 1998). A major factor in this interaction is suppression of the cytochrome P450 enzyme CYP3A4 in the wall of the small intestine, resulting in diminished first-pass metabolism with higher bioavailability and increased maximum plasma concentrations of the drug substrates. This, apparently, was first noted in an interaction study of felodipine with ethanol, where grapefruit juice was used to 'blind' for the administration of ethanol (Bailey *et al.*, 1989). It was noted that felodipine concentrations were considerably higher than those previously reported for the dose used. In addition to increasing the bioavailability of drugs, grapefruit juice may prolong the metabolic elimination of some drugs (Fuhr *et al.*, 1993; Bailey *et al.*, 1994). The interaction between drugs and grapefruit juice is marked for felodipine, nimodipine and saquinavir, for which there are marked increases in the area under the curve (AUC) and/or maximum plasma concentrations greater than 70% of controls (Fuhr, 1998). Major drugs implicated in grapefruit interactions include dihydropyridine calcium antagonists, verapamil, terfenadine, cyclosporin, ethinyloestradiol, 17β-oestradiol, prednisone, midazolam, triazolam, quinidine and saguinavir; all these materials share the property of having significant first-pass metabolism by cytochrome P450AL/5, predominantly in the gut wall, resulting in Phase I metabolites (Fuhr, 1998). It has been suggested that psoralens, principally 6′,7′-dihydrobergamottin, are major inhibitors, with a possible contribution from naringenin (Edwards *et al.*, 1996; Runkel *et al.*, 1997). It is proposed that patients be advised to refrain from drinking grapefruit juice when taking a drug that is extensively metabolized, unless a lack of interaction has been demonstrated (Fuhr, 1998).

In many countries, evidence of adverse drug reactions is now sought in normal volunteers and patients in all phases of clinical trial leading up to licensing and marketing of a new product. Post-marketing surveillance (PMS) is then carried out to assess long-term safety in thousands of patients in order to detect low-frequency reactions which were not recognized in the relatively small number of patients studied in pre-marketing trials. There are a variety of post-marketing surveillance schemes, including voluntary reporting of possible cases of drug reaction, while standard epidemiological techniques such as retrospective studies, prospective cohort studies and case-control studies may be useful.

NATURE, DESIGN AND CONDUCT OF TOXICOLOGY STUDIES

Toxicology studies should permit, within the constraints of the time period studied, a quantitative determination of the potential for a chemical, or mixture of chemicals, to produce local and systemic adverse effects and allow a determination of factors that may influence the nature, severity and possible reversibility of effects. Specific features that any toxicology testing programme should allow, are as follows:

- The nature of the adverse effects;
- Relationship of the adverse effects to in-use and practical situations;
- Dose-response relationships (average, range, hyperreactive groups, no-effects and minimum-effects doses);
- Modifying factors;
- Effects of gross acute overexposure;
- Effects of repeated exposure (short and long term);
- Definition of allowable and non-allowable exposures;
- Definition of monitoring procedures;
- Guidance on protective and restrictive procedures;
- Guidance on first-aid and medical management;
- Definition of 'at-risk' populations (e.g. by sex, pre-existing disease or genetic susceptibility).

Information necessary for the above purposes can be obtained only from carefully designed and conducted studies. In some cases, it may not be economically possible to undertake a complete range of toxicology studies, and in such circumstances it is necessary to consider carefully the most appropriate investigational approaches based on known physiochemical properties, existing and suspect toxicology, and anticipated conditions of use. The relevance and credibility of a toxicology study can be no better than its design and conduct permit. For the purposes of hazard evaluation, there is a need to emphasize exposure conditions that may exist under practical conditions of use.

Toxicology testing programmes generally begin with single-exposure *in vivo* or *in vitro* studies and progress to evaluating the effects of long-term repeated exposures. Studies having specific end-points, such as teratology and reproductive effects, are conducted as the emerging toxicology profile and end-use exposure patterns dictate. Toxicology testing procedures can be conveniently subdivided into general and specific. General toxicology studies are those in which animals are exposed to a test material under appropriate conditions, and they are examined for all types of toxicity that the monitoring procedures permit. Specific toxicologicy studies are those in which exposed animals, or *in vitro* test systems, are monitored for a defined end-point (see Chapter 15).

General Toxicology Studies

These are usually conducted as a programme in the sequence of acute, short-term repeated, subchronic and chronic. Ideally, the protocol for general studies should include provision for some animals to be kept for a period after the end of dosing in order to determine a latency and reversibility, or otherwise, of toxic effects. Acute studies give information on toxicity produced by a single exposure, including the effects of massive overexposure; they also give information of use for setting exposure conditions for short-term repeated exposure studies. The type of monitoring employed in general toxicology studies will depend on various considerations, including the chemistry of the test material, its known or suspect toxicology, degree of exposure and the rationale for conducting the test. In general, since multiple exposure studies are most likely to produce the widest range of toxicity, it is usual to employ the most extensive monitoring in these studies. The monitoring employed to detect functional toxicity in the living animal, and for the detection of toxic injury in dead animals, may include the following:

- Inspection, on a regular basis, for signs of toxic and/or pharmacological effects;
- Body weight before dosing and at appropriate intervals during the dosing phase;
- Food and water consumption;
- Haematology for assessment of peripheral blood and haematopoietic tissues;
- Clinical (serum) chemistry of various substances and of specific enzyme activities, and appropriate urinalysis;
- Gross and microscopic pathology with organ weight measurement;
- Special pathological or functional tests may be required on a case-by-case basis.

Specific Toxicology Studies

Many of these procedures are directed at determining a particular toxic effect for hazard evaluation purposes, but others are employed as 'screening' or 'short-term' tests to assess the potential of a substance to induce chronic effects or toxicity with a long latency. Some of the most frequently employed special toxicology methods are listed below.

Primary Irritation

These studies are designed to determine the potential of substances to cause local inflammatory effects, notably in skin and eye (see Chapters 38 and 41). In order to reduce the use of animals for eye irritancy testing, a variety of alternative procedures have been proposed, which include the use of enucleated eyes, various *in vitro* cell or tissue cultures and the measurement of corneal thickness (Nardone and Bradlaw, 1983; Shopsis and Sathe, 1984; Ballantyne, 1986; Borenfreund and Borrero, 1984).

Peripheral Sensory Irritation

Methods to assess the potential to cause eye or respiratory tract discomfort with associated reflexes are particularly useful in occupational toxicology (Owens and

Punte, 1963; Ballantyne *et al.*, 1977; Ballantyne, 1984; see Chapter 32).

Immune-mediated Hypersensitivity

Allergenic materials may produce hypersensitivity reactions by skin contact or inhalation, and several methods are available to determine the potential for chemicals to produce allergic contact dermatitis or asthmatic reactions (Goodwin *et al.*, 1981; Maurer *et al.*, 1984; Karol *et al.*, 1985).

Neurological and Behavioural Toxicity

To confirm the existence, nature, site and mechanism of toxic injury to the central and/or peripheral nervous system, a variety of approaches with varying degrees of sophistication are available (see Chapters 33 and 34). These include observational test batteries (Gad, 1982), light and electron microscopy (Spencer *et al.*, 1980), selective biochemical procedures (Abou-Donia *et al.*, 1987), electrophysiological, pharmacological, tissue culture and metabolism techniques (Dewar, 1981; Mitchell, 1982). The potential to produce delayed polyneuropathy, carried out in hens and sometimes in rodents, and used in the toxicological assessment of organophosphates and some other neurotoxic substances, has been increasingly refined (Veronesi, 1992; OECD, 1995).

Teratology

Most studies are currently directed at assessing the potential for chemicals to induce structural defects of development, and essentially involve administering the test material to the pregnant animal during the period of maximum organogenesis (Tuchmann-Duplessis, 1980; Beckman and Brent, 1984; Tyl, 1988). There has been increasing interest in the development of test methods to assess possible adverse functional effects resulting from exposure of the foetus both during gestation and in the early neonatal period (Zbinden, 1981; Vorhees, 1983; see Chapter 53).

Reproductive Toxicity

Reproductive studies are conducted to assess the potential for adverse structural and functional effects on gonads, fertility, gestation, foetuses, lactation and general reproductive performance. Exposure to the chemical may be over one or several generations. In view of the necessarily comparatively low doses used during these long-term studies, they may not be sufficiently sensitive to detect most potentially teratogenic materials. The basis for these tests has been reviewed (Mattison, 1983; Baeder *et al.*, 1985; Rao *et al.*, 1987; see Chapter 52).

Metabolism and Pharmacokinetics

These studies may be of very considerable importance in the interpretation of conventional toxicology studies, in helping determine the mechanism of toxicity, in assessing the relationship between environmental exposure concentration and target organ toxicity and in the design of additional studies to elucidate mechanisms of toxicity. Metabolic studies should yield information on the biotransformation of a material, the sites at which this occurs and the mechanism of biotransformation. Pharmacokinetic studies should allow a quantitative measurement of the rate of uptake, the absorbed dose, the biodistribution, tissue binding and storage, and the routes and rates of excretion of test material and metabolites (Oehme, 1980; Gibaldi and Perrier, 1982).

Genotoxicity

A number of tests, both *in vitro* and *in vivo*, are available to assess the mutagenic or clastogenic potential of chemicals (see Chapters 48 and 49). A positive genotoxic result is not necessarily a directly usable end-point *per se*, but may assist in defining a potential for adverse health effects or be used in screening for potential longer term toxicity. Thus, materials with clear mutagenic activity may be suspected of being genotoxic carcinogens, and appropriate further studies may be required; clastogenic materials may be suspect of reproductive or haematological toxicity.

The most widely used *in vitro* mutagenicity test has probably been that described by Ames (1982) and which utilizes histidine-dependent mutants of *Salmonella typhimurium*. The bacteria are incubated in a medium deficient in histidine; if the added test chemical is genotoxic it causes a reverse mutation to the histidine-independent state, which permits bacterial growth.

Various mammalian cell culture preparations have been used to assess mutagenic potential. A commonly used test system is a forward gene mutation assay in Chinese hamster ovary (CHO) cells with a strain which is deficient in the enzyme hypoxanthine–guanine phosphoribosyl transferase (HGPRT), and which confers resistance to toxic purine analogues such as 6-thioguanine and permits growth of the cells in a medium containing such substrates. The presence of a mutant chemical will restore sensitivity to the presence of purine analogues, and this may be used to assess mutagenic potential quantitatively. Clastogenic potential can be assessed *in vitro* by exposing cultured cells and subsequently examining them by light microscopy for chromosome damage. It is usual to conduct *in vitro* genotoxicity studies in the pre-

sence and absence of a metabolic activation system in order to assess the possible influence of metabolism on the mutagenic potential of the test chemical. Frequently employed is a homogenate of liver from animals given the polychlorinated biphenyl Arochlor, which induces a broad range of hepatic P450-metabolizing enzymes.

In vivo genotoxicity studies can be conducted in a variety of ways. For example, the specific locus test in mice involves exposure of non-mutant mice to the test substance and subsequently mating them with multiple-recessive stock. Mutant offspring have altered phenotypes such as hair or eye colour, ear length or hair structure. Clastogenic potential can be assessed *in vivo* by exposure to the test chemical and subsequently examining mitotically active tissue, such as bone marrow, for chromosome injury.

Combustion Toxicology

It has been estimated that 50–75% of deaths occurring within a few hours of being exposed to a fire are the result of inhalation injuries and systemic toxicity (Ballantyne, 1981). The primary aim of combustion toxicology is to determine the adverse effects produced as a result of being exposed to heated or burning materials. Although considerable emphasis has been placed on acute effects, there is increasing concern about the long-term consequences of repeated exposure to the products of combustion in occupationally exposed individuals, such as firemen. The design and interpretation of appropriate studies may be difficult because of the large number of variables that may affect the nature, concentration and temporal characteristics of products of combustion. The major, though not exclusive, factors which influence the toxicity and hazard from a fire atmosphere include the nature of the materials available for heating or burning, the phase of the combustion process, temperature, air flow and oxygen availability and potential for interaction between the combustion materials generated. All of these factors may be required to be investigated and considered in evaluating the continually changing hazard from a fire. Principal lines of investigation and sources of information about toxicity and hazards from fire atmospheres are as follows:

(i)   Physicochemical studies to determine the nature of the products of combustion generated under differing conditions of temperature and oxygen availability;
(ii) Animal exposure studies;
(iii) Clinical and forensic observations on fire casualties to determine the nature and cause of morbidity and mortality from exposure to a fire atmosphere.

Although investigations designed to investigate the nature and determinants for materials producing local respiratory or systemic toxicity are of clear importance, it is also necessary to be aware of the presence of materials which may produce sensory irritant or central nervous system depressant effects. Clearly, irritant effects on the eye or narcosis may impede escape from a potentially hazardous situation. Polymers, which constitute a major component of commercial and domestic buildings, provide good examples of the generation of toxic, irritant and neurobehavioural chemical species on combustion (Ballantyne, 1989) (see Chapter 88).

Antidotal Studies

In addition to being aware of the likelihood of spontaneous reversibility of toxic injury (i.e. biochemical and morphological healing), it is of clear practical importance to investigate the induction of reversibility of toxicity by antidotal procedures (Marrs, 1988; see Chapter 20). Indications for such studies include high acute toxicity (including dose and time to onset of effects); serious (but potentially reversible) repeated exposure toxicity; where there are indications that early treatment may reduce or abolish latent toxicity; suspicions of a potential for antidotal effectiveness based on considerations of mechanism of toxicity; and confirmation that antidotal treatment is effective for a new member of a chemical series for which a generic antidote has been established. Examples of chemicals for which specific antidotal treatment has been investigated include cyanides (Marrs, 1987; Meredith *et al.*, 1993), ethylene glycol (Baud *et al.*, 1988; Brent *et al.*, 1999) and organophosphate anticholinesterases (Arena and Drew, 1986; Ellenhorn and Barceloux, 1988; Bismuth *et al.*, 1992).

In addition to investigating specific antidotal therapy, it may also be necessary to confirm, or otherwise, if standard methods of management and support are appropriate for particular substances or groups of materials. This may include, for example, potential for aspiration hazards, influence of dilution (by giving fluid to drink), and potential for adverse interaction with drugs used to maintain cardiovascular or respiratory homeostasis.

Human Studies

Data generated from human exposure may be available for certain chemicals. Such data may be divided into:

(1) those generated experimentally, including clinical trials or drugs;
(2) those resulting from exposed populations using epidemiological techniques.

Exposures of human subjects have been carried out with certain pesticides (JMPR, 1999) and also chemical warfare agents (Marrs *et al.*, 1996). When such data are

available on agrochemicals, it is widely considered that the 100-fold safety factor used on animal extrapolation can be replaced by a factor of 10. The reason for this is that the uncertainty in extrapolation from one group of humans to the world-wide population is less than that involved in extrapolating from laboratory animals. However, some of these studies, especially on older chemicals, have used small numbers of subjects and often of only one sex. The degree to which conclusions drawn from them should overthrow those from well conducted animal studies is debatable. On the other hand, well conducted studies on human subjects can elucidate interesting and relevant aspects of toxicology, such as differential metabolism in humans, as well as different toxicodynamics.

REVIEW OF TOXICOLOGY STUDIES

A critical review of toxicology studies requires detailed case-by-case considerations, but attention should be generally directed to the following:

■ That the laboratory or institution reporting the studies has the necessary scientific and/or medical credibility, capabilities, experience and expertise in the areas being investigated.
■ The objectives of the investigation should be precisely stated, and the study protocol should reflect this in detail.
■ The work should be reported in a clear and unambiguous manner, with all the necessary detail to allow the reader to undertake his/her own assessment and conclusions about the study.
■ There should have been adequate quality control procedures, and standards appropriate to good laboratory practices should have been followed.
■ The material tested should be precisely specified, including stability and the nature and amounts of any impurities, conversion products or additives.
■ It should be confirmed that the methodology which is used for exposure and to monitor the *in vivo* or *in vitro* studies is sufficiently specific and sensitive to allow the various objectives and end-points to be determined.
■ Studies should be designed to allow the determination of the significance of the results and permit hazard and risk assessment procedures. For example, the number of test and control animals should be sufficient to allow for the detection of biological variability in response to exposure, to allow trends to be appreciated and to permit statistical analyses. There should be sufficient dose–response information to allow decisions on causal relationships and the magnitude of doses which produce definite and threshold effects and those not producing toxicity.

■ Monitoring should allow the determination of whether any injury produced is a direct consequence of toxicity or an effect which is secondary to toxicity at another site. A primary effect is one produced as a result of a direct toxic effect of a chemical, or metabolite(s), on a target organ or tissue. Secondary effects are those occurring, often at another non-target site, as a consequence of toxicity in the primary tissue or organ. For example, primary pulmonary injury produced by inhaled potent irritant materials may result in significant hypoxaemia and secondary hypoxic injury to other organs, including liver, kidney or brain. Ideally the study should be carefully assessed to allow a conclusion as to whether the toxicity induced is a consequence of the action of parent material or metabolite, e.g. comparison of routes involving and not involving first-pass effects.

■ Detailed assessment is required to determine if the numerical data have been appropriately and correctly evaluated. Thus, although there may be a statistically significant difference between a test group and the controls, this may not be of biological or toxicological significance. Conversely, changes or trends, not of statistical significance, may be of biological and toxicological relevance. Quantitative information should be viewed against the study as a whole, normal biological variability, quantitative changes which imply pathological processes, and the magnitude of any changes as they may relate to an adverse effect.

The above considerations demand the careful design of toxicology studies, taking into account all factors which are inherent in the defined and inferred objectives of the investigation.

To illustrate the care required in the interpretation of toxicology studies, a few examples are given below of different specific factors that need attention in particular studies:

■ The acute peroral LD_{50} of the undiluted diethylamine is < 0.25 ml (kg body weight)$^{-1}$, whereas with a 10% aqueous solution the acute peroral LD_{50} is 1.41 ml (kg body weight)$^{-1}$, illustrating the influence of dilution of the test material on toxicity. A reciprocal relationship has been demonstrated with glutaraldehyde **(Figure 14)**; in this case, acute peroral toxicity (as mg active material per kg body weight) increases with dilution within the confines of the study.

■ Materials with similar LD_{50} values may have differences in acute toxicity shown by other monitors of their toxicity. For example, 2,4-pentanedione has an acute peroral LD_{50} (rat) of 0.58 g (kg body weight)$^{-1}$, similar to that of 2,2-bis(4-aminophenoxyphenyl) propane (BAPP) at 0.31 g (kg body weight)$^{-1}$; however, times to death were 2–5 h with 2,4-pentanedione and 3–4 days with BAPP, indicating a more serious potential hazard with the former.

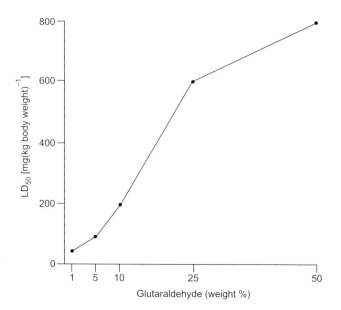

Figure 14 Influence of aqueous dilution on the acute peroral lethal toxicity (as LD_{50}) of glutaraldehyde to rats. As dilution increases the LD_{50} becomes smaller (i.e. greater toxicity).

■ With inhalation studies, the method of generation of the test material in the atmosphere may be highly important, as indicated by the following three illustrative examples:

(1) For acute vapour inhalation studies, and in tests concerned with defining the effects of saturated vapour atmospheres, the vapour may be generated by static or dynamic methods. Static methods involve placing a sample of the test material in the exposure chamber and allowing the atmosphere to equilibrate for an appropriate period of time; thus, all volatile components accumulate to vapour saturation in the chamber. Dynamically generated atmospheres are produced by passing air through the test material and transferring the atmosphere so generated into and through the chamber in a continuous manner; this results in components of the test material being present in the atmosphere in proportion to both their concentration in the test material and volatility. Thus, trace contaminants of highly volatile toxic materials will be present in much higher concentrations with static as opposed to dynamic conditions. For example, methoxydihydropyran (MDP), containing 0.037% acrolein, when generated dynamically did not produce mortalities with rats for a 4 h exposure period (MDP vapour, 7748 ppm; acrolein, trace). However, when the same material was used in a static exposure there were mortalities due to the accumulation of acrolein vapour in the atmosphere (MDP, 8044 ppm; acrolein, 240 ppm); acrolein has a 4 h LC_{50} of 8.3 ppm (Ballantyne et al., 1989a).

(2) The relative humidity of the chamber atmosphere may influence inhalation toxicity with hydrolysable materials. For example, when tris(dimethylamino) silane

(TDMAS) was generated as a vapour with moistened air, a 4 h LC_{50} of 734 ppm was determined (female rat), which accords stoichiometrically with toxicity due to dimethylamine formed by hydrolysis of TDMAS. However, when the vapour was generated under dry air conditions, a 4 h LC_{50} of 38 ppm was calculated from the exposure–mortality data, indicating a highly significantly greater intrinsic toxicity for the TDMAS molecule (Ballantyne *et al.*, 1989b).

(3) A marked difference in toxicity may be obtained for the same material generated in different modes of exposure or different physical states. For example, short-term repeated exposure to vapour from 2-methacryloxypropyltrimethoxysilane does not produce any respiratory tract injury. However, when generated as an aqueous respirable aerosol it produces laryngeal granulomas (Klonne *et al.*, 1987).

■ The use conditions of the test material may influence toxicity, with toxicity being modified by use pattern. Thus, the potential for cutting oil to induce cutaneous neoplasms is significantly enhanced after its industrial use, possibly owing to the generation of polycyclic aromatic hydrocarbons (Agarwal *et al.*, 1986).

HAZARD EVALUATION AND RISK ASSESSMENT

Toxicology is concerned with defining the potential for a material to produce adverse effects, whereas hazard evaluation is a process to determine if any of the known potential adverse effects will develop under specific conditions of use. Thus, toxicology is but one of the many considerations to be taken into account in the hazard evaluation process. The following are some of the other factors that need to be taken into account in defining whether a defined use of a material will be hazardous, and are discussed in detail by Tyler and Ballantyne (1988):

■ Physicochemical properties of the material;
■ Use pattern;
■ Characteristics of the handling procedure;
■ Source of exposure and route of exposure, both normal and possible misuse;
■ Control measures;
■ Magnitude, duration and frequency of exposure;
■ Physical nature of exposure conditions (e.g. solid, liquid, vapour, gas, aerosol);
■ Variability in exposure conditions;
■ Population exposed (e.g. number, sex, age, health status);
■ Any experience and information derived from exposed human populations.

The general approach used to assess hazards is as follows:

(1) Search for all available health-related information on the substance and, if appropriate, substances of close chemical structure. This may include information on physicochemical properties, *in vivo* and *in vitro* toxicology, epidemiology, known occupational and domestic incidents, case reports, monitoring and use patterns.

(2) Detailed impartial review of information accessed, emphasizing those studies conducted by credible scientific standards and by relevant routes of exposure.

(3) Interpretation of the credible and relevant literature in order to define toxicity and, if possible, mechanism, dose–response relationships and factors influencing toxicity (endogenous and exogenous).

(4) Conclusions regarding potential adverse effects from the substance under specific conditions of use.

(5) Determination of acceptable handling or use conditions and acceptable exposure to the substance with respect to immediate and long-term conditions of use.

(6) Determination of the management of overexposure situations.

The process and understanding of hazard evaluation, and its scientific basis, are now at a level where reliable interpretation and prediction can be made. A less reliable and scientifically limited evaluation process is that of risk assessment, which is currently an important developing component of regulatory and occupational toxicology. It is the objective of risk assessment processes to assess the probability that adverse health effects will develop from known, or suspect, xenobiotics in the environment (e.g. drinking water or air) or workplace. Such quantitative risk assessments are most frequently conducted for worktime or lifetime exposure to low concentrations of xenobiotic. They are based on extrapolating dose–response relationships from animal studies, or occasionally human epidemiological data, (a) to determine risk at known or anticipated ranges of occupational or environmental exposure dosages or (b) to assess 'risk-free' dosages. The approaches that are currently most frequently employed are to assess risk from carcinogens, teratogens, reproductively active substances and genotoxic materials.

Currently, with most materials there is insufficient information on mechanisms of toxicity for particular materials to allow scientifically valid, appropriate mathematical models to be developed for a specific toxic effect. The current method of extrapolation makes many, often biologically unreasonable, assumptions which include (a) the existence (or otherwise) of thresholds for specific toxic end-points, (b) linearity of dose–response relationships, (c) comparability of metabolism and pharmacokinetic parameters between species, (d) the interaction between xenobiotics and biological systems at low concentrations and (e) the statistical reliability and biological variability resulting from the relatively small numbers of animals that may technically and ethically be incorporated into animal studies. Thus, with current mathematical approaches of data extrapolation, quantitative risk assessments should be regarded as 'best guesses' for environmentally safe exposure dosages. The findings from quantitative risk assessment may result in risk management measures being undertaken (Hallenbeck and Cunningham, 1986). This involves the development and implementation of regulatory action, taking into account additional factors such as available control measures, cost–benefit analyses and 'acceptable' levels of risk and taking note of various policy, social and political issues. To be encouraged is the developing science of 'biological risk assessment', which allows a more rational risk analysis based upon incorporation of metabolism and pharmacokinetics, including interspecies differences, mechanisms of toxicity and influence of physiological variables (Clayson, 1987; National Research Council, 1987).

SPECIAL CONSIDERATIONS IN HUMAN HAZARD EVALUATION

By the very nature their intended design, laboratory toxicology studies are conducted under highly controlled conditions using healthy animals often of a particular weight range. The extrapolation of such information to a heterogeneous human population, with differing life styles and variable states of health, needs to be undertaken with considerable caution, taking into account all possible known and predictable variables.

The possible interactions of multiple exposures to a variety of chemicals or drugs has been discussed earlier in this chapter. Other illustrative examples are presented below.

Personal Habits

Many personal habits, including diet and the taking of medicinal products, may influence the response to a toxic chemical. Two factors that have received special attention are cigarette smoking and excessive alcohol consumption. Cigarette smoking may lead to increased body burdens of many of the combustion products found in smoke, in particular carbon monoxide. Owing to the significantly increased carboxyhaemoglobin concentrations in smokers, they may be at greater risk in the occupational environment from carbon monoxide and carbon monoxide-generating materials, such as methylene chloride. Other materials in cigarette smoke which

may increase the exposure burden include hydrogen cyanide, hydrogen sulphide, acrolein and polycyclic aromatic hydrocarbons. In some instances, there are clear indications of significantly enhanced toxicity, e.g. synergism between cigarette smoking and asbestos (Hammond and Selikoff, 1973) or radon (Archer et al., 1972). Heavy alcohol consumption may lead to chronic progressive liver injury and fibrosis, and thus increase susceptibility to hepatotoxic substances and impair detoxification pathways.

Co-existing Disease

Individuals with certain illnesses may be at greater risk from particular drugs or industrial chemicals. For example, those with established cardiovascular disease may be at increased risk from exposure to carbon monoxide or methaemoglobin-generating substances, since both may compromise the available oxygen supply to the myocardium. Inhalation of irritant materials may aggravate chronic progressive pulmonary disease.

Genetically Susceptible Subpopulations

Individuals with genetically determined biochemical variants may be at greater risk from certain drugs and chemicals than those with normal biochemical features. Some examples are as follows:

- Individuals with hereditary methaemoglobinemia may generate significant amounts of methaemoglobin at exposure doses of nitrites or aromatic amines which cause only minor methaemoglobin concentrations in the normal population.
- It is well known that slow acetylators are significantly more susceptible to the neurotoxic potential of isoniazid, whereas fast acetylators seem to be more likely to develop liver injury since hepatotoxicity is caused by the metabolite acetylhydrazine (Breckenridge and Orme, 1987). Another aspect of acetylator status relates to the potential of arylamines to induce bladder cancer. Slow acetylators may be more susceptible to arylamine-induced bladder cancer (Cartwright et al., 1987), possibly related to a higher urinary excretion of free arylamine (Derwan et al., 1986).
- Individuals with glucose-6-phosphate dehydrogenase-deficient erythroeytes may be at increased risk from haemolytic effects of oxidants because of the inability of the erythrocyte to generate sufficient NADPH and maintain an adequate concentration of reduced glutathione, resulting in haemolysis (Calabrese et al., 1987). However, animal studies suggest that haemolytic effects occur only on exposure to otherwise toxic concentrations (Amoruso et al., 1986).

■ Exposure of persons with inherited uroporphyrinogen decarboxylase deficiency to dioxin can cause latent chronic hepatic porphyria to develop into porphyria cutanea tarda (Doss and Columbi, 1987).

Other genetically determined variants which have been implicated as increasing susceptibility to chemicals are include α_1-antitrypsin deficiency (emphysema), aryl hydrocarbon hydroxylase deficiency (lung cancer), pseudocholinestese variants (anticholinesterase toxicity) and thalassaemia (lead). An interaction between environmental factors and specific genotypes has been suggested as being involved in the aetiology of a number of diseases, including Parkinsonism (Menegon *et al.*, 1998; Cummings, 1999).

REFERENCES

Abou-Donia, M. B., Lapadula, D. M. and Carrington, C. D. (1987). Biochemical methods for the assessment of neurotoxicity. In Ballantyne, B. (Ed.), *Perspectives in Basic and Applied Toxicology*. Wright, London, pp. 1–30.

Agarwal, R., Gupta, K. P., Sushil, K. P. and Mehrotra, N. K. (1986). Assessment of some tumorigenic risks associated with fresh and used cutting oil. *Indian J. Exp. Biol.*, **24**, 508–510.

Albano, E., Lott, K. A. K., Slater, T. F., *et al.* (1982). Spin-trapping studies on the free-radical products formed by metabolic activation of carbon tetrachloride in rat liver microsomal fractions. *Biochem. J.*, **204**, 593–603.

Albert, A. L. (1979). *Selective Toxicity*. Chapman and Hall, London, p. 469.

Ames, B. N. (1982). The detection of environmental mutagens and potential carcinogens. *Cancer*, **53**, 2034–2040.

Amoruso, M. A., Ryer, J., Easton, D., *et al.* (1986). Estimation of risk of glucose-6-phosphate dehydrogenase-deficient red cells to ozone and nitrogen dioxide. *J. Occup. Med.*, **28**, 473–479.

Angeli-Greaves, M. and McLean, A. E. M. (1981). Effect of diet on the toxicity of drugs. In Gorrod, A. W. (Ed.), *Drug Toxicity*. Taylor and Francis, London, pp. 91–100.

Archer, V. E., Wagner, J. R. and Lurdin, F. E., Jr (1972). Uranium mining and cigarette smoking effects in man. *J. Occup. Med.*, **15**, 204–211.

Arena, J. M. and Drew, R. H. (1986). *Poisoning*. Charles C. Thomas, Springfield, IL, pp. 146–188.

Asher, I. M. and McGrath, P. V. (1976). *Symposium on Electron Microscopy of Microfibers*. Stock No. 017-012-002244-7. Superintendent of Documents, United States Government Printing Office, Washington, DC.

Baeder, C., Wickramarante, G. A. S. and Hummler, H. (1985). Identification and assessment of the effects of chemicals on reproduction and development (reproductive toxicology). *Food Chem. Toxicol.*, **23**, 377–388.

Bailey, D. G., Spence, J. D., Edgar, B., *et al.* (1989). Ethanol enhances the hemodynamic effects of felodipine. *Clin. Invest. Med.*, **12**, 357–362.

Bailey, D. G., Arnold, J. M. and Spence, J. D. (1994). Grapefruit juice and drugs. How significant is the intimation is the intimation. *Clin. Pharmacokinet.*, **26**, 91–98.

Ballantyne, B. (1978). The comparative short-term mammalian toxicology of phenarsazine oxide and phenoxarsine oxide. *Toxicology*, **10**, 341–361.

Ballantyne, B. (1981). Inhalation hazards of fire. In Ballantyne, B. and Schwabe, P. H. (Eds), *Respiratory Protection*. Chapman and Hall, London, pp. 351–372.

Ballantyne, B. (1983). Acute systemic toxicity of cyanides by topical application to the eye. *J. Toxicol. Cut. Ocular Toxicol.*, **2**, 119–129.

Ballantyne, B. (1984). Peripheral sensory irritation as a factor in the establishment of workplace exposure guidelines. In Oxford, R. R., Cowell, J. W., Jamieson, G. G. and Love, E. J. *Occupational Health in the Chemical Industry*. (Eds), Medichem, Calgary. pp. 119–149.

Ballantyne, B. (1985). Evaluation of hazards from mixtures of chemicals in the occupational environment. *J. Occup. Med.*, **27**, 85–94.

Ballantyne, B. (1986). Applanation tonometry and corneal pachymetry for prediction of eye irritating potential. *Pharmacologist*, **28**, 173.

Ballantyne, B. (1987). Toxicology of cyanides. In Ballantyne, B. and Marrs, T. C. (Eds), *Clinical and Experimental Toxicology of Cyanides*. Butterworths, London, pp. 41–126.

Ballantyne, B. (1989). Toxicology. In *Encyclopedia of Polymer Science and Engineering*, Vol. 16. Wiley, New York, pp. 879–930.

Ballantyne, B., Gazzard, M. F. and Swanston, D. W. (1977). Irritation testing by respiratory exposure. In Ballantyne, B. (Ed.), *Current Approaches in Toxicology*, Wright, Bristol, pp. 129–138.

Ballantyne, B., Myers, R. C., Dodd, D. E. and Fowler, E. H. (1988). The acute toxicity of trimethoxysilane (TMS). *Vet. Hum. Toxicol.*, **30**, 343–344.

Ballantyne, B., Dodd, D. E., Pritts, I. M., Nachreiner, D. S. and Fowler, E. M. (1989a). Acute vapor inhalation toxicity of acrolein and its influence as a trace contaminant of 2-methyoxydihydro-2*H*-pyran. *Hum. Toxicol.*, **8**, 229–235.

Ballantyne, B., Dodd, D. E., Myers, R. C., *et al.* (1989b). The acute toxicity of tris(dimethylamino)silane. *Toxicol. Ind. Health*, **5**, 45–56.

Bardana, E. J., Montanara A. and O'Hollaren, M. T. (1992). *Occupational Asthma*. Hanley and Belfus, Philadelphia.

Barlow, S. M. and Sullivan, F. M. (1982). *Reproductive Hazards of Industrial Chemicals*. Academic Press, London.

Baud, F. J., Galliot, M., Astier, A., *et al.* (1988). Treatment of ethylene glycol poisoning with 4-methylpyrolazone. *N. Engl. J. Med.*, **319**, 97–100.

Beckman, D. A. and Brent, R. L. (1984). Mechanisms of teratogenesis. *Annu. Rev. Pharmacol.*, **24**, 483–500.

Billingham, D. J. (1977). Cutaneous absorption and systemic toxicity. In Drill, V. A. and Laza, P. (Eds), *Cutaneous Toxicity*. Academic Press, New York, pp. 53–62.

Bismuth, C., Inns, R. H. and Marrs, T. C. (1992). Efficacy, toxicity and clinical use of oximes in anticholinesterase poisoning. In Ballantyne, B. and Marrs, T. C. (Eds), *Clinical and Experimental Toxicology of Organophosphates and Carbamates*. Butterworths-Heinemann, Oxford, pp. 555–577.

Bogers, M., Appelman, L. M., Feron, V. J., *et al.* (1977). Effects of the exposures profile on the inhalation toxicity of carbon tetrachloride in male rats. *J. Appl. Toxicol.*, **7**, 185–191.

Borenfraund, E. and Borrero, O. (1984). *In vitro* cytotoxicity assays. Potential alternatives to the Draize ocular allergy test. *Cell Biol. Toxicol.*, **1**, 55–65.

Braunwald, E. (1982). Mechanism of action of calcium-channel-blocking agents. *N. Engl. J. Med.*, **307**, 1618–1627.

Breckenridge, A. and Orme, M. L. E. (1987). Principles of clinical pharmacology and therapeutics. In Wetherall, D. J., Ledington, J. G. S. and Warrell, D. A. (Eds), *Oxford Textbook of Medicine*, 2nd edn, Vol. 1. Oxford University Press, Oxford, p. 77.

Brent, J., McMartin, K., Phillips, S., Burkhart, K., Donovan, J. W., Wells, M. and Kulig, K. (1999). Fomepizole for the treatment of ethylene glycol poisoning. *New Eng. J. Med.*, **340**, 832–838.

Bronough, R. L. and Maibach, H. (1985). *Percutaneous Absorption*. Marcel Dekker, New York.

Brusick, D. (1988). *Principles of Genetic Toxicology*. Plenum Press, New York.

Brooks, S. M. (1983). Bronchial asthma of occupational origin. In Rom, W. M. (Ed.), *Environmental and Occupational Medicine*. Little, Brown, Boston, pp. 223–250.

Calabrese, E. J., Moore, G. S. and Williams, P. (1987). The effect of methyl oleate ozonide, a possible oxone intermediate, on normal and G-6-PD deficient erythrocytes. *Bull. Environ. Contam. Toxicol.*, **29**, 498–504.

Calvery, H. O. and Klumpp, T. G. (1939). The toxicity for human beings of diethylene glycol with sulfanilamide. *Southern Med. J.*, **32**, 1105–1109.

Cartwright, R. A., Rodgers, M. J., Barham-Had, D., *et al.* (1987). Role of *N*-acetyltransferase phenotypes in bladder carcinogenesis: a pharmacogenetic epidemiological approach to bladder cancer. *Lancet*, **ii**, 842–846.

Clayson, D. B. (1987). The need for biological risk assessment in reaching decisions about carcinogens. *Mutat. Res.*, **185**, 243–269.

Conference (1990). Organic dust and lung disease. *Amer. J. Ind. Med.*, **17**, 1–148.

Corley, R. A., Markham, D. A., Banks, C., Delorme, P., Masterman, A. and Houle, J. M. (1997). Physiologically based pharmacokinetics and dermal absorption of 2-butoxyethanol vapor by humans. *Fundam. Appl. Toxicol.*, **39**, 120–130.

Cronin, E. (1980). *Contact Dermatitis*. Churchill Livingstone, Edinburgh.

Cummings, J. L. (1999). Understanding Parkinson disease. *J. Amer. Med. Assoc.*, **281**, 376–378.

Decker, W. J. (1987). Introduction and history. In Maley, T. J. and Berndt, W. O. (Eds), *Handbook of Toxicology*. Hemisphere, Washington, DC, pp. 1–9.

Derwan, A., Jani, J. P., Shah, K. S., *et al.* (1986). Urinary excretion of benzidine in relation to acetylator status of occupationally exposed subjects. *Hum. Toxicol.*, **5**, 95–97.

Dewar, A. J. (1981). Neurotoxicity testing. In Gorrod, J. W. (Ed.) *Testing for Toxicity*. Taylor and Francis, London, pp. 199–218.

Doss, M. O. and Columbi, A. M. (1987). Chronic hepatic porphyria induced by chemicals: the example of dioxin. In Foa, V., Emmett, E. A., Maroni, M. and Columbus, A. (Eds), *Occupational and Environmental Chemical Hazards*. Ellis Horwood, Chichester, pp. 231–240.

Doull, J. and Bruce, M. C. (1980). Orgin and scope of toxicology. In Klaassen, C. D., Amdur, M. O. and Doull, J. *Casarett and Doull's Toxicology. The Basic Science of Poisons*, 3rd edn. Macmillan, New York, pp. 3–10.

Dugard, P. H. (1977). Chapter 22. In Marzulli, F. N. and Maibach, H. I. (Eds), *Dermatotoxicology and Pharmacology*. Hemisphere, Washington, DC, pp. 525–550.

Edwards, D. J., Bellevue, F. H. and Wostee, P. M. (1996). Identification of 6',7'-dihydroxybergamottin, a cytochrome P450 inhibitor, in grapefruit juice. *Drug Metab. Dispos.*, **24**, 1287–1290.

Ellenhorn, M. J. and Barceloux, D. G. (1988). *Medical Toxicology*. Elsevier, New York, pp. 1070–1103.

Fuhr, V. (1998). Drug Interactions with grapefruit juice. *Drug Saf.*, **18**, 251–272.

Fuhr, V., Klittich, K. and Staib, A. H. (1993). Inhibiting effect of grapefruit juice and its bitter principal, naringemin, on CYP1A2-dependent metabolism of caffeine in man. *Br. J. Clin. Pharmacol.*, **35**, 431–436.

Gad, S. C. (1982). A neuromuscular screen for use in industrial toxicology. *J. Toxicol. Environ. Health*, **9**, 691–704.

Gibaldi, M. and Perrier, D. (1982). *Pharmacokinetics*. Marcel Dekker, New York.

Goldenthal, E. I. (1971). A compilation of LD_{50} values in newborn and adult animals. *Toxicol. Appl. Pharmacol.*, **18**, 185–207.

Goldfrank, L. R., Flomenbaum, N. E., Lewin, N. A., Weisman, R. S. and Howland, M. A. (1990). Goldfrank's Toxicologic Emergenices, 4th edn. Appleton and Lange, Norwalk, Connecticut, pp. 183.

Goodwin, R. F. J., Crevel, W. R. W. and Johnson, A. W. (1981). A comparison of three guinea-pig sensitization procedures for the detection of 19 reported human contact sensitizers. *Contact Dermatitis*, **7**, 248–258.

Grasso, P. (1988). Carcinogenicity tests in animals: some pitfalls that could be avoided. In Ballantyne, B. (Ed), *Perspectives in Basic and Applied Toxicology*. Wright, London, pp. 268–284.

Griffith, J. F. (1964). Interlaboratory variations in the determination of acute oral LD_{50}. *Toxicol. Appl. Pharmacol.*, **6**, 726–730.

Hallenbeck, W. H. and Cunningham, K. M. (1986). *Quantitative Risk Assessment for Occupational and Environmental Health*. Lewis, Chelsea, MI.

Hammond, E. L. and Selikoff, J. J. (1973). Relation of cigarette smoking to risk of death of asbestos associated disease among insulation workers in the United States. In Bogorski, D., Timbrell, J. C., Wagner, J. C. and Davis, W. (Eds), *Biological Effects of Asbestos*. IARC Scientific Publications, No. 8. IARC, Lyon, pp. 312–317.

Hollingshaus, J. G., Armstrong, D. and Toia, R. F. (1981). Delayed toxicity and delayed neurotoxicity of phosphorothionate and phosphonothionate esters. *J. Toxicol. Environ. Health*, **8**, 619–627.

Horton, A. A. and Fairhurst, S. (1987). Lipid peroxidation and mechanism of toxicity. *CRC Crit. Rev. Toxicol.*, **18**, 27–79.

Hunter, W. J., Lingk, W. and Recht, P. (1979). Intercomparison study on the determination of single administration toxicity in rats. *J. Assoc. Off. Anal. Chem.*, **62**, 864–873.

Jacobs, R. R. and Phanprasik, W. (1993). An *in vitro* comparison of the permeation of chemicals in vapor and liquid phase through pig skin. *Am. Ind. Hyg. Assoc. J.*, **54**, 560–575.

JMPR (1998). *Pesticide Residues in Food—1997. Toxicological and Environmental Evaluations*. Joint Meeting of the FAO Panel of Experts and the WHO Core Assessment Group, 22 September–1 October 1997, Lyon.

JMPR (1999). *Report*. Joint Meeting of the FAO Panel of Experts and the WHO Core Assessment Group, 23 September–3 October, 1998, Rome.

Johanson, G. and Boman, A. (1991). Percutaneous absorption of 2-butoxyethanol vapor in human subjects. *Br. J. Ind. Med.*, **48**, 788–792.

Karol, M. H., Stadler, J. and Magreni, C. (1985). Immunotoxicologic evaluation of the respiratory system: animal models for immediate and delayed-onset pulmonary hypersensitivity. *Fundam. Appl. Toxicol.*, **5**, 459–472.

Kast, A. and Nishikawa, J. (1981). The effect of fasting on oral acute toxicity of drugs in rats and mice. *Lab. Anim.*, **15**, 359–364.

Kemppainen, B. W. and Reifenrath, W. G. (1990). *Methods for Skin Absorption*. CRC Press, Boca Raton, FL.

Khanna, V. K., Husain, R. and Seth, P. R. (1988). Low protein diet modifies acrylamide neurotoxicity. *Toxicology*, **49**, 395–401.

Kimbrough, R. D., Falk, H., Stehr, P., *et al.* (1984). Health implications of 2,3,7,8-tetrachlorodibenzodioxin (TCDD) contamination of industrial soil. *J. Toxicol. Environ. Health*, **14**, 47–93.

Klonne, D. R., Garman, R. H., Snellings, W. M. and Ballantyne, B. (1987). The larynx as a potential target organ in aerosol studies in rats. In *Abstracts, 1987 International Symposium on Inhalation Toxicity*. Karger, Basle, p. 86.

Krisch-Volders, M. (1984). *Mutagenicity, Carcinogenicity and Teratogenicity of Industrial Pollutants*. Plenum Press, New York.

Kurt, T. L., Anderson, R., Petty, C., *et al.* (1988). Dintrophenol in weight loss: the poison center and public health safety. *Vet. Hum. Toxicol.*, **28**, 574–575.

Limasset, J. C., Simon, P., Poirot, P., Subre, I. and Grzeby K. M. (1999). Estimation of the percutaneous absorption of styrene in an industrial situation. *Int. Arch. Occup. Environ. Health*, **72**, 46–51.

Lloyd, G. (1991). Psychiatry. In Edwards, C. R. W. and Bouchier, I. A. D. (Eds), *Davidson's Principles and Practice of Medicine*. Churchill Livingstone, Edinburgh, p. 937.

Lu, F. C. (1985). *Basic Toxicology*. Hemisphere, Washington, DC.

Maickel, R. P. and McFadden, D. P. (1979). Acute toxicology of butyl nitriles and butyl alcohols. *Res. Commun. Chem. Pathol. Pharmacol.*, **26**, 75–83.

Malmary, M.-F., Kabbaj, K. and Oustrin, J. (1988). Circadian dosing stage dependence in metabolic effects of cicyclosporine in the rat. *Annu. Rev. Chromopharmacol.*, **5**, 35–38.

Marks, V., English, J., Aherne, W. and Arendt, J. (1985). Chronopharmacology. *Clin. Biochem.*, **18**, 154–157.

Marrs, T. C. (1987). The choice of cyanide antidotes. In Ballantyne, B. and Marrs, T. C. (Eds), *Clinical and Experimental Toxicology of Cyanides*. Butterworths-Heinemann, Oxford, pp. 383–401.

Marrs, T. C. (1988). Experimental approaches to the design and assessment of antidotal procedures. In Ballantyne, B. (Ed.), *Perspectives in Basic and Applied Toxicology*. Wright, London. pp. 285–308.

Marrs, T. C., Maynard, R. L. and Sidell, F. R. (1996). *Chemical Warfare Agents. Toxicology and Treatment*. Wiley, Chichester, pp. 115–137.

Mattison, D. R. (1983). *Reproductive Toxicology*. Alan R. Liss, New York.

Maurer, T., Weirich, E. G. and Hess, R. (1984). Predictive contact allergenicity influence of the animal strain used. *Toxicology*, **31**, 217–222.

McDougal, J. N., Jepson, G. W., Clewell, H. J., MacNaughton, M. G. and Anderson, M. E. (1986). A physiologically-based pharmacokinetic modal for dermal absorption of vapors in the rat. *Toxicol. Appl. Pharmacol.*, **83**, 286–294.

Mehendale, H. M. (1987). Hepatotoxicity. In Haley, T. J. and Berndt, W. O. (Eds), *Handbook of Toxicology*. Hemisphere, Washington, DC, pp. 74–111.

Menegon, A., Board, P. G., Blackburn, A. C., Mellick, G. D. and LeCouteur, D. G. (1998). Parkinson's disease, pesticides, and glutathione transferase polymorphisms. *Lancet*, **352**, 1344–1346.

Meredith, T. J., Jacobsen, D., Haines, J. A., Berger, J.-C. and van Heist, A. N. P. (1993). *IPCS/CEC Evaluation of Antidote Series, Vol. 2. Antidotes for Poisoning by Cyanide*. Cambridge University Press, Cambridge.

Mitchell, C. L. (1982). *Nervous System Toxicology*. Raven Press, New York.

Murphy, S. D. (1983). General principles in the assessment of toxicity of chemical mixtures. *Environ. Health Perspect.*, **48**, 141–144.

Nardone, R. M. and Bradlaw, J. A. (1983). Toxicity testing with *in vitro* systems: I. Ocular tissue culture. *J. Toxicol. Ocular Cut. Toxicol.*, **2**, 81–8.

National Research Council (1987). *Pharmacokinetics in Risk Assessment*. National Academy Press, Washington, DC.

National Research Council (1988). *Principles of Toxicological Interactions Associated with Multiple Chemical Exposures*. National Academy Press, Washington, DC.

OECD (1995). *OECD Guidelines for Testing of Chemicals. Delayed Neurotoxicity of Organophosphorus Substances Following Acute Exposure*. OECD Guideline 418. Organization for Economic Cooperation and Development, Paris.

Oehme, F. W. (1980). Absorption, biotransformation, and excretion of environmental chemicals. *Clin. Toxicol.*, **17**, 147–158.

Owens, E. J. and Punte, C. L. (1963). Human respiratory ocular irritation studies utilizing *o*-chlorobenzylidenemalononitrile aerosols. *Am. Ind. Hyg. Assoc. J.*, **24**, 262–264.

Pariat, C., Courtois, P., Cambar, J., *et al.* (1988). Seasonal variations in gentamicin nephrotoxicity in rats. *Annu. Rev. Chronopharmacol.*, **5**, 461–463.

Paschal, D. C., DiPietro, E. S., Phillips, D. L. and Gunter, E. W. (1989). Age dependence of metals in hair in selected U. S. population. *Environ. Res.*, **48**, 17–28.

Randall, J. A. and Gibson, R. S. (1989). Hair chromium as an index of chromium exposure of tannery workers. *Br. J. Ind. Med.*, **46**, 171–175.

Rao, G. N. and Knapka, J. J. (1998). Animal diets in safety evaluation studies. In Ioanides, C. (Ed.), *Nutrition and Chemical Toxicity*. Wiley, Chichester, pp. 345–374.

Rao, M. S. and Reddy, J. K. (1987). Peroxisome proliferation and hepatocarcinogenesis. *Carcinogenesis*, **8**, 631–636.

Rao, K. S., Schwetz, B. A. and Park, C. N. (1987). Reproductive risk assessment of chemicals. *Vet. Hum. Toxicol.*, **23**, 167–175.

Rodier, P. M. (1980). Chronology of neuron development: animal studies and their clinical implications. *Childh. Neurol.*, **22**, 525–545.

Runkell, M., Bourian, M., Teglmeier, M., *et al.* (1997). The role of naringin in the interaction of drugs with juices of grapefruit juice. *Arch. Pharmacol.*, **355**, Suppl. 4, R123.

Shell, J. W. (1982). Pharmacokinetics of topically applied ophthalmic drugs. *Surv. Ophthalmol.*, **26**, 207–218.

Shopsis, C. and Sathe, S. (1984). Uridine uptake inhibition as a cytotoxicity test: correlations with the Draize test. *Toxicology*, **29**, 195–206.

Spencer, P. S., Bischoff, M. C. and Schaumburg, H. H. (1980). Neuropathological methods for the detection of neurotoxic diseases. In Spencer, P. S. and Schaumburg, H. H. (Eds), *Experimental and Clinical Neurotoxicology*. Williams and Wilkins, Baltimore, pp. 743–757.

Sperling, F. (1984). Quantitation of toxicology—the dose–response relationship. In Sperling, F. (Ed.), *Toxicology: Principles and Practice*, Vol. 2. Wiley, New York, pp. 199–218.

Stanton, M. F., Layard, M., Tegeris, A., *et al.* (1981). Relation of particle dimension to carcinogenicity in amphobile asbestosis and other fibrous minerals. *J. Natl. Cancer Inst.*, **67**, 965–975.

Stuttgen, G., Siebel, Th. and Aggerbeck, B. (1982). Absorption of boric acid through human skin depending on the type of vehicle. *Arch. Dermatol. Res.*, **272**, 21–29.

Sweet, D. V. (Ed.) (1985–1986a). *Registry of Toxic Effects of Chemical Substances*, Vol. 3. US Department of Health and Human Services, Centers for Disease Control, NIOSH, Washington, DC, p. 2360.

Sweet, D. V. (Ed.) (1985–1986b). *Registry of Toxic Effects of Chemical Substances*, Vol 3. US Department of Health and Human Services, Centers for Disease Control, NIOSH, Washington, DC, p. 3060.

Tallarida, R. J. and Jacob, L. S. (1979). *The Dose–Response Relation in Pharmacology*. Springer, New York.

Thomas, J. A., Stargel, W. W. and Tschanz, C. (1998). Interactions between drugs and diet. In Ioannides, C. (Ed.), *Nutrition and Chemical Toxicity*. Wiley, Chichester, pp. 161–182.

Timbrell, J. A. (1982). *Principles of Biochemical Toxicology*. Taylor and Francis, London, Ch. 2.

Trevan, J. W. (1927). The error of determination of toxicity. *Proc. R. Soc. London, Ser. B*, **101**, 483–514.

Toft, R., Olofason, T., Tuneck, A., *et al.* (1982). Toxic effects on mouse bone marrow caused by inhalation of benzene. *Arch. Toxicol.*, **51**, 295–302.

Tuchmann-Duplessis, M. (1980). The experimental approach to teratogenicity. *Ecotoxicol. Environ. Saf.*, **4**, 422–433.

Tyl, R. W. (1988). Developmental toxicity in toxicologic research and testing. In Ballantyne, B. (Ed.), *Perspectives in Basic and Applied Toxicology*. Wright, London, pp. 206–241.

Tyler, T. R. and Ballantyne, B. (1988). Practical assessment and communication of hazards in the workplace. In Ballantyne, B. (Ed.), *Perspectives in Basic and Applied Toxicology*. Wright, London, pp. 330–378.

Veronesi, B. (1992). Validation of a rodent model of organophosphorus induced delayed neuropathy. In Ballantyne, B. and Marrs, T. C. (Eds), *Clinical and Experimental Toxicology of Organophosphates and Carbamates*. Butterworth-Heinemann, Oxford.

Vorhees, C. V. (1983). Behavioural teratogenicity testing as a method of screening for hazards to human health: a methodological proposal. *Neurobehav. Toxicol. Teratol.*, **5**, 469–474.

Wartew, G. A. (1983). The health hazards of formaldehyde. *J. Appl. Toxicol.*, **3**, 121–126.

Wheeler, T. G. (1987). The behavioural effects of anticholinesterase insult following exposure to different environmental temperatures. *Aviat. Space Environ. Med.*, **58**, 54–59.

Williams, P. L. (1982). Pentachlorophenol, an assessment of the occupational hazard. *Am. Ind. Hyg. Assoc. J.*, **43**, 799–810.

Williams, R. T. (1959). *Detoxification Mechanisms*, 2nd edn. Chapman and Hall, London.

Wilmer, J. W. G. M., Wouterson, R. A., Appleman, L. M., *et al.* (1987). Subacute (4-week) inhalation toxicity study of formaldehyde in male rats: 8-hour intermittent versus 8-hour continuous exposures. *J. Appl. Toxicol.*, **71**, 25–26.

Woodford, R. and Barry, B. W. (1986). Penetration enhancers and the percutaneous absorption of drugs: an update. *J. Toxicol. Cut. Ocular Toxicol.*, **5**, 167–177.

World Health Organization (1981). *Health Effects of Combined Exposures in the Workplace*. Technical Report Series, No. 647. WHO, Geneva.

World Health Organization (1985). *Chronic Effects of Solvents on the Central Nervous System and Diagnostic Criteria*. Environmental Health Criteria Series, No. 5. WHO, Copenhagen.

WTO (1994). *Agreement on the Application of Sanitary and Phytosanitary Measures*. Uruguay Round of the General Agreement on Tariffs and Trade. World Trade Organization, Geneva, 15th April 1994. Also obtainable from the Stationery Office, London, CM2562.

Zbinden, G. (1981). Experimental methods in behavioural teratology. *Arch. Toxicol.*, **48**, 69–88.

Zbinden, G. and Flury-Roversi, M. (1981). Significance of LD_{50} test for the toxicological evaluation of chemical substances. *Arch. Toxicol.*, **47**, 77–99.

ADDITIONAL READING AND REFERENCES

Ballantyne, B. (Ed.) (1988). *Perspectives in Basic and Applied Toxicology*. Wright, London.

Calabrese, E. J. (1991). *Principles of Animal Extrapolation*. Lewis Publishers, Michigan.

Hayes, A. W. (Ed.) (1994). *Principles and Methods of Toxicology*, 3rd edn. Raven Press, New York.

Fan, A. M. and Chang, L. W. (Eds.) (1996). *Toxicology and Risk Assessment. Principles, Methods and Applications*. Marcel Dekker, Inc., New York.

Hodgson, E., Mailman, R. B. and Chambers, J. E. (Eds.) (1998). *Dictionary of Toxicology*, 2nd edn. Macmillan Reference Ltd., London.

Manahan, S. E. (1992). *Toxicological Chemistry*, 2nd edn. Lewis Publishers, Boca Raton, Fl.

Massaro, E. J. (Ed.) (1997). *Handbook of Human Toxicology*. CRC Press, Boca Raton, Fl.

Niesink, R. J. M., de Vries, J. and Hollinger, M. A. (1996). *Toxicology. Principles and Applications*. CRC Press, Boca Raton, Fl.

Svendsen, P. and Hau, J. (Eds.) (1994). *Handbook of Laboratory Animal Science*, Volumes 1 and 2. CRC Press, Boca Raton, Fl.

Chapter 2
Principles of Testing for Acute Toxic Effects

Christopher Rhodes

C O N T E N T S

Toxicology, like medicine, is both a science and an art . . . when we fail to distinguish the science from the art, we confuse facts with predictions and argue they have equal validity, which they clearly do not. In toxicology as in all science, theories have a higher level of certainty than hypotheses which in turn have a higher level of certainty than speculation, opinions, conjectures and guesses.

Michael A. Gallo, History and scope of toxicology. *In* Casarett and Doull's Toxicology: The Basic Science of Poisons, *5th edn., 1996.*

One of the most important tasks in toxicology is to identify early interactions which result in changes which are part of a chain of events leading to toxicity (a biological cascade). The identification of early changes may provide the basis of rational bio-monitoring of human populations. The definition of such early changes, their dose–response relationships and the identification of longer-term consequences require a rather profound understanding of the biology involved.

W. Norman Aldridge, Mechanisms and Concepts in Toxicology, *1996.*

INTRODUCTION

From the quotations above, it is clear that modern toxicology has progressed from simply asking the question 'Is this substance or mixture of substances toxic?' and 'What types of toxicity does this substance produce?' to a more mechanism-based world in which questions such as 'How does this substance produce its toxicity?', 'How can the toxicity of this substance be modulated?', 'How safe is this substance for its intended use?' and 'In which species does this substance exhibit toxicity?'. As in the previous edition of this book (Rhodes *et al.*, 1993), this chapter tries to focus on the principles for testing for acute toxic effects. Several new editions of text books with chapters containing references to acute toxicity testing are listed under References and Further Reading, e.g. Lu (1991).

Data on the acute toxic effects of substances have for many years been collected in academic, industrial, contract and government research laboratories, common both to elective research and non-elective regulatory compliance work, involving a large number of substances of natural origin to chemicals synthesized by man and a wide range of species from both the plant and animal kingdoms. To evaluate the safety of use in each of the more than 30 million species that exist on the earth today is an impossible and unnecessary objective. Instead, selective acute systemic toxicity assessment across a broad range of different animal types does allow some level of prediction of the likely impact of a substance on the environment. Nevertheless, the primary focus of this chapter will be on the assessment of the safety in use of substances for human beings. Other chapters in this book cover the assessment of the impact of acute systemic intoxication of other species in the environment.

Investigation of acute toxicity has led to the identification of selective toxic action and the beneficial use of substances as pesticides in controlling the environment and as drugs for therapeutic use in domesticated animals and man. Natural agonists are selective molecules which contribute to the functioning of cells. Antagonists are inhibitors of natural agonists and are inevitably toxic at certain concentrations. This can be their most valuable property for use by man. Earlier in this century a bacterial infection was frequently fatal. The German scientist Gerhard Domagk tested various newly made chemicals containing a sulphonamide group to determine if any of them would kill bacteria. A red–brown material synthesized in the laboratory containing a sulphonamide grouping, Prontosil, cured mice with an otherwise fatal bacterial infection and subsequently a similarly bacterially infected incurably ill child. However, most people perceive more inherent potential for harm from chemical antagonists with specific and potent toxicity that are synthesized by man than those produced in nature. This is a popular misconception, for several of the most acutely potent intoxicants are a product of mother nature and the guiding hand of evolution. An inquiry into any general toxicology text book will throw up a list of potent natural toxins: tetrodotoxin from puffer fish; α-amanatin from the mushroom *amanita phalloides*; fluoroacetate from the plant *Dichapetalum cymosum*; pyrethin from the plant *Pyrethrum cinariaefolium*; aconite from monks hood, *Aconitum napellus*; conicine from hemlock, *Conium maculatum* L., Umbelliferae; (+)-tubocurarine from curare, an extract from the bark of *Chondodendron*; digitalis from the dried leaves of *Digitalis purpurea* L., Scrophulariaceae; carbon monoxide; hydrogen sulfide; hydrogen cyanide; and arsenic—a list of poisons present in the natural world which can be extended easily. Those who wish to focus negatively rather than positively on the impact of synthetic chemicals can produce a list of acutely poisonous synthetic chemicals, examples of which are paraquat, an extremely effective herbicide; barbiturates, often used sedatives; and organophosphorus agents, the nerve gases of chemical warfare fame. Many synthetic chemical poisons are chemical mimics of natural toxins, often having additional beneficial attributes of specificity, selectivity, potency and 'manufacturability' over those produced in nature.

Definitions of Acute Toxicity

Several definitions of acute toxicity have been formulated: (a) 'the adverse change(s) occurring immediately or a short time following a single or short period of exposure to a substance or substances'; (b) 'adverse effects occurring within a short time of administration of a single dose of a substance or multiple doses given within 24 h; in terms of human exposure it refers to life-threatening events following accidental overdosage, intentional, suicidal and homicidal attempts'. An adverse effect (toxicity) can be defined as any effect that results in functional impairment and/or pathological and/or physiological and/or biochemical lesions that may affect the performance of the whole organism or that reduce the organisms ability to respond to an additional challenge. Pharmacodynamics, the study of the dose and time response to the beneficial biochemical and physiological effects of chemicals and their mechanisms of action, is analogous to what can be considered as toxicodynamics, the study of the dose and time response to the adverse effects of chemicals—natural or synthetic.

Toxicity can be considered to be the 'capacity to cause injury', *hazard* the 'probability for injury to occur' and *safety* the 'improbability of injury'. For a substance to exert a toxic action, the toxicant must reach a sufficient concentration to overcome the inherent reserve capacity within biological systems (threshold level) before it can elicit an adverse change. The inherent reserve capacity which underpins the threshold assumption has as its premise a physiological reserve within the organism which requires depletion or significant alteration or disruption of cellular homeostasis for a toxic response to occur. Consequently, it is a general consensus of toxicologists that toxic events exhibit a threshold dose–response. For a toxic event to occur, a critical receptor of some kind or key endogenous molecule in the organism has to come into contact with the toxicant. These toxic targets can be membrane proteins, transport proteins, receptor proteins, enzyme proteins, nucleic acids and lipids or oxygen. The former is illustrated by the interaction of cyanide, a very small molecule, and cytochrome *c* oxidase, a large enzyme–protein complex. The latter is illustrated by paraquat, an organic dipyridyl molecule, and its interaction with oxygen to form a reactive oxygen species by one-electron donation through a redox recycling. Interestingly, to the author's knowledge, there are few data that indicate carbohydrate molecules as a target of chemical toxicity and yet many inborn errors of metabolism of carbohydrates manifest themselves in severe health effects. As the basic chemical laws apply to these chemical–receptor interactions, they can be and are examined by standard methods of chemistry and biochemistry. This concept of receptor–chemical interaction was the basis for drugs and was further developed as the drug–receptor theory of drug action (toxicant action) which has analogy in enzyme–substrate and ligand–protein theory. Often these types of interaction lead to a cascade of additional change(s), amplifying the initial toxicant–receptor, sometimes leading to the toxicity manifesting itself in a distant tissue or organ from where the initial toxicant–receptor interaction occurred.

Hazard is a function of both toxicity, exposure (external dose) and internal dose, the amount of chemical reaching the biological target. Exposure (external dose) is a measure of the contact between the intoxicant and the outer or inner surface of the human body (e.g. skin, alveolar surface of lung or mucosal surface of gut). It is usually expressed in terms of concentrations of the intoxicant in the medium interfacing with the body surfaces. Once absorbed through body surfaces, the intoxicant gives rise to levels in various organs or tissues. Internal dose is measured in terms of concentrations in the tissues. Exposure and dose should include an indication of the time and frequency at which an individual is subjected to them. Acute exposure to toxins may result in lethality or sub-lethal responses, and the signs and symptoms may be overt or subtle. Consequences of acute exposure to toxins may be *non-specific*, reflecting a mass action effect, *specific*, inhibition of vital cellular receptors (antagonists) and enzymes (inhibitors), mimicking endogenous receptors (agonists), or *reactive*, reflecting chemical modification of cellular chemistry. Responses may occur as a consequence of the formation of reactive intermediates following biotransformation of the parent molecule and consequent modification of physiological processes.

Drugs must have their therapeutic efficacy (benefits) balanced with safety (risk). The margin of safety between the therapeutic and toxic effects of a drug will determine how often physicians will see signs and symptoms of intoxication in their clinic.

Safety Assessment

The assessment of chemical toxicity and the demonstration of safety have been an integral part of pharmaceutical, agricultural and industrial research for many years, with acute systemic toxicity screening being an important aspect of this assessment. In 1944 the preliminary data required to describe the oral, dermal and inhalation toxicity of a chemical were published. Since those early days, the terms 'acute lethality testing' and 'acute toxicity screening', previously synonymous in many people's minds, are now distinct in modern toxicology and pharmacology. Both regulatory bodies and industry expect more than lethality data to be generated from acute systemic toxicity studies. The study of acute toxic effects can be extremely broad. Objectives include the characterization of the acute biological effects of a chemical, defining clinical signs, identifying target organs and describing a chemical's acute toxic syndrome so that intoxicated patients can be diagnosed and treated. Various regulatory guidelines combine under the general heading of acute toxicity studies, evaluations of localized effects on skin and ocular tissues. These topics, which relate to the assessment of irritancy and contact sensitization, will not be dealt with in this chapter and the reader is referred to chapters 38 and 41.

The following section elaborates the principles of acute systemic toxicity assessment as it pertains to the evaluation of acute systemic effects leading to adverse changes in target organs which result in acute ill health and death of a biological organism. Individual chapters which follow in this book cover parenteral, peroral, percutaneous, inhalation, ophthalmic and dermal toxicology in addition to environmental toxicology. The latter is a reflection of the increasing awareness that the maintenance of an ecological balance requires greater attention being given to the effects of chemicals on species other than man and domesticated animals.

DEVELOPMENT OF ACUTE TOXICITY ASSESSMENT

Classification

Many of the principles generally applied to acute (and chronic) toxicity evaluation were established in antiquity. Primitive man undoubtedly observed previously healthy animals becoming ill and occasionally dying following their ingestion or contact with various natural materials. The manuscripts of the ancient Egyptian societies (*Ebers Papyrus*, ca 1500 BC) and the Chinese-speaking peoples (*Yun Chi Ch'i Ch'ien*, ca 1023 BC); the Sanskrit hymns and verses of the Indo-European Hindus (*Vedas*, ca 1500–1200 BC) are considered to be the earliest written records which contain references to poisonous substances and materials. The early Greek philosophers Hippocrates (ca 400 BC), Aristotle (ca 350 BC) and Theophrastus (ca 300 BC) described the use of poisons and Pedanius Dioscorides (ca AD 50), a physician to Nero, introduced, into his *De Materia Medica*, the classification of poisons into plant, animal and mineral. Galen (ca AD 150) and the Persian physician Avicenna (ca AD 1000) further refined this classification, with the latter distinguishing oral from parenteral poisons, concepts which remain extant today.

Dose–Response and Animal Experimentation

Before the twentieth century the art of poisoning of man was the predecessor of acute toxicology testing in animals. In early Greek and Roman times, the prevalence of assassination initiated efforts to discover antidotes. Zopyrus, physician to Mithridates VI, King of Pontus (ca 200 BC), adhering to the adage that 'the best model for man is man', is believed to have used prisoners to identify materials which acted as antidotes against ingested poisons. Eventually a guide to the treatment of accidental or intentional poisoning, *Poisons and Antidotes*, was published by the Judaic philosopher and physician, Moses Maimonides (ca 1198). During the Renaissance period poisoning was seen as a way to advance one's fortune; the Borgias in Italy (ca 1500) and Madame Mon Voisin in France (ca 1680), are reputed to have developed the poisoner's art of assassination. The Marquise de Brinvilliers (ca 1650) is claimed to have administered preparations of toxins to the sick and needy to evaluate potency, speed of onset, specificity, site of action, clinical signs and symptoms prior to their use in assassinations. A handbook of poisons, *De Venenis*, published in the fifteenth century by Peter of Albanos, went to 14 editions, so much was the interest in poisons. From such empirical observations, fundamental principles of toxicity assessment became apparent.

Paracelsus (Philippus Aureolus Theophrastus Bombastus von Hohenheim, ca 1500) is considered by many to have introduced the role of chemistry in medicine. Challenging the establishment views by ritualistically burning the books of Avicenna and Galen in front of his students, he emphasized in his teaching the concept of experimentation. His insight into the relationship of dose and effect resulted in his often paraphrased quotation that 'the dose or amount of a chemical determines whether a substance is a remedy or a poison'. Orfila published his *Traité de Toxicologie* in which he attempted a systematic correlation of chemically induced biological responses based on his observations of the effects of poisons on dogs. Following in the steps of Joseph Plenck (1781), who published *Elementa Medicinae et Chirurgiae Forensis*, describing the role of chemistry in the detection of poisons, Orfila used chemical analysis of autopsy material for detecting and confirming accidental or intentional poisonings. The further advances in the application of experimentation to elucidate toxicity were made by the physiologists Claude Bernard (1813–78) and Magendie (1783–1855). Bernard replaced Magendie's empirical method of experimentation with one of confirmation or refutation of a predefined hypothesis.

Anti-vivisection and Safety Evaluation

It was during this period that the view was held that animals were considered 'machines without consciousness' (Rene Descartes, 1644, *Discourse. The Principles of Philosophy*), a view which was challenged as being morally wrong. Anti-vivisection lobbies arose against using animals in medical experimentation. In 1876 the UK introduced pivotal legislation inappropriately called 'The Cruelty to Animals Act', which required medical experimentation to be conducted only by licensed practitioners and under specified conditions. During the twentieth century legislation to protect the well being of animals has been introduced by the governments of many countries. For example, 110 years after the first legislation of 1876, the UK introduced further legislation, 'The Animal (Scientific Procedures) Act', (1986). The USA likewise has updated 'The Animal Welfare Act' (1987). It is probable that international harmonization of animal welfare legislation will follow the harmonization of study protocols and all mammalian species will be the subject of equivalent animal welfare provisions to ensure their humane treatment, the minimizing of pain and discomfort and the consideration of alternative approaches. This last aspect forms the basis of chapter 19. The increasing legislation for animal welfare has been paralleled by the increase in legislation for chemical safety, which in turn reflects the rapid development of the chemical industry in this century.

International Hazard Labelling and Toxicity Ranking

In 1901, a diphtheria epidemic in the USA resulted in the US Congress passing the virus act of 1902 regulating all biological products sold for the prevention of disease in man with the purpose of achieving consistent potency and requiring batch to batch certification prior to release. In 1906, the US Congress passed the Pure Food and Drug act, which led to the establishment of the Food and Drug Administration in the USA. In these early years the chief of the Bureau of Chemistry of the US Department of Agriculture did pioneering work on the tolerance of various additives to food using human volunteers, the chemicals not having been previously evaluated in animals. Quinine and digitalis were first tested in man before being given to animals. Since these early days, the use of surrogate species prior to exposure of man to chemicals has become the norm rather than the exception from both an ethical and liability point of view.

Descriptions of lethality studies were published in the early 1900s. During the 1920s, several experimentalists evaluated methods to describe the lethality of various biological materials such as insulin and digitalis extracts. Trevan in 1927 proposed an experimental design to define more accurately the lethal concentration or dose for biologically prepared therapeutic materials which were of a variable and inconsistent potency, and introduced the median lethal dose (LD_{50} and LC_{50}), terms consistent with the median effective dose (ED_{50}) used in pharmacology.

Deaths in children following the use of the antibiotic sulphanilamide, which had been formulated in ethylene glycol in 1937, led to the US Congress passing the Federal Food Drug and Cosmetic Act (1938), requiring the obligatory testing of drugs for safety using experimental animals. Advisory guidelines prepared by the staff of the US Food and Drug Administration have subsequently become standardized in International and National regulatory guidelines such as those prepared by the Organization for Economic Cooperation and Development (OECD).

The various legal acts and health and safety regulations of various countries place duties on persons who manufacture, import or supply chemical substances with regard to placing on the label some form of classification of the systemic toxicity potential of the substances, the terminology and classification based on the lethal dose varying slightly from country to country. Generally, if a substance has the potential for lethality at an oral dose of less than 50 mg kg^{-1}, it is described as either 'very' or 'highly' or 'extremely' toxic or hazardous; above 50 mg kg^{-1} but less than 2000 mg kg^{-1} a substance is generally described as 'moderately' or 'slightly' hazardous or harmful, and if there is little potential for lethality at a dose of 2000 mg kg^{-1} and above a substance is not required to be labelled. Consequently, industry conducts acute systemic toxicity assessments as part of a programme to establish the safety of products and to meet obligations under legislation for:

(i) the classification, packaging labelling requirements for transportation; (ii) occupational control of safety and health; (iii) the registration or re-registration of a new drug, food additive or pesticide for sale and use; (iv) new formulations of known products; and (v) re-assessment of a previously developed products safety to maintain its continued sale and use.

The OECD in 1984 identified 'information which should accompany chemicals when they are marketed, especially when traded internationally' as an important aspect of information exchange regarding chemicals when they reviewed international practices of labelling chemicals. The recommendations of the United Nations Committee of Experts on the Transport of Dangerous Goods covering transport by land, sea and air were formulated into guidelines which are generally referred to as the 'Orange Book'. The International Air Transport Association (IATA) Restricted Articles Regulations (established in 1950) was adopted by 57 countries. The International Civil Aviation Organization (ICAO) and its 150 contracting States has adopted as of 1984 Annex 18 to the Chicago convention 'The Safe Transport of Goods by Air' and the 'Technical Instructions for the Safe Transport of Goods by Air'. The World Health Organization's (WHO) 'Classification of Pesticides by Hazard', published in 1975, classifies pesticides into four toxicity groups primarily on acute oral and dermal toxicity in the laboratory rat.

In Japan, labelling requirements are specified under several laws, the primary ones being the Chemical Substances Control Law, the Drugs, Cosmetic and Medical Instruments Law, the Toxic and Deleterious Regulation Law and the Agricultural Chemicals Regulation Law. In Europe, the 'Dangerous Chemical Substances and Proposals Concerning Their Labeling', first published by the Council of Europe in 1962 with a final edition in 1978, was commonly referred to as the 'Yellow Book'. In 1981 the 6th Amendment to the EEC Dangerous Substances Directive made it mandatory for every importer of a new substance to provide to the competent authorities of the Community a set of toxicological, ecotoxicological and physicochemical data before placing a new substance on the market.

Under the 6th Amendment Pre-Marketing Notification of New Chemicals Act, the EEC require acute systemic toxicity assessment by at least two different routes of exposure (oral, dermal and inhalation being the most common) as well as assessment of eye and skin irritation. The Notification of New Substances Regulations of 1982 identify the tests as those defined by the 1984 Annex VI to the Council Directive 67/548/EEC, and these were based on those recommended in 1981 by the OECD Guidelines for Testing of Chemicals.

In the USA, four federal agencies, the Food and Drug Administration (FDA), the Environmental Protection Agency (US EPA), the Occupational Safety and Health (OSHA) and the Consumer Product Safety Commission (CPSC), administer numerous laws, the key ones being the Food, Drug and Cosmetics Act (FDCA) (1938), the Federal Insecticide, Fungicide and Rodenticide Act (FIFRA) (1972), the Occupational Safety and Health Act (1970), the Toxic Substance Control Act (TSCA) (1976), the Consumer Product Safety Act (1972), the Federal Hazardous Substances Act (1960) and all their respective amendments. The last Act stipulates labelling requirements for hazardous substances (toxic, corrosive, irritant, strong sensitizer) for use in the household. Unlike the corresponding European regulation, TSCA does not have a mandatory requirement for a 'base set' of toxicological and ecotoxicological data prior to manufacture or marketing of a new substance but the provisions under Section 8(e) of TSCA do require that adverse effects observed in toxicological studies and in man be notified to the US EPA. The US EPA under Section 4(a) of TSCA can require testing to be conducted to develop data with respect to health and environmental effects for which there is an insufficiency of data and experience. The FDCA and FIFRA specify health and environmental testing requirements in animals for food additives, cosmetics, drugs and pesticides. The transport of hazardous materials in the USA is subject to regulations covered by the Hazardous Materials Transportation Act administered by the Department of Transportation, which it also has provisions for labelling of toxic materials.

In the UK, the Control of Substances Hazardous to Health (COSHH) and OSHA in the USA introduced statutory duties on employers to implement occupational hygiene measures appropriate to the type of hazard and the level of risk. Manufacturers of hazardous substances have two basic devices to impart the necessary information in the material safety data sheet (MSDS) or bulletin (OSHA Hazard Communication Standard) and the labels that they put on their containers. Acute systemic toxicity tests define the appropriate symbols and phrases to be used in MSDS documents and on labels.

The data from acute systemic toxicity studies in laboratory animals are used to indicate the quantitative and qualitative differences between the toxicity of various substances, but as yet there is not complete harmonization between countries or regulations. The lay person needs to understand that the ingestion of no more than a taste of a *very toxic* material, a mouthful of a *toxic* material or a pint of a *harmful* material would be expected to cause death. Ingestion of smaller amounts could well result not in death but in substantial ill-health effects.

Acute Poisoning in Man

The expanding use of synthetically and naturally produced chemicals has led to detrimental effects related to abuse of addictive substances and accidental, incidental and sometimes intentional poisoning of domesticated and wild animals, human adults and most distressingly children. The accidental release of chlorophenols at Seveso resulted in the deaths of many animals; the accidental release of methyl isocyanate at an industrial manufacturing site at Bophal and the natural but catastrophic release of carbon dioxide from a lake in the Cameroons resulted in the death of many adults and children; the 'Spanish toxic oil syndrome', through the use of tainted oil for food preparation, caused illness in thousands of victims in 1981 and still remains inadequately explained; more recently, the 'Gulf war syndrome' has been aligned with exposure to chemicals. The use of chemicals in warfare, for homicidal and suicidal purposes, typify for many the consequences of chemical-induced intoxication. In non-developed countries, accidents due to uncontrolled and incorrect use of synthetic chemicals have led to acute poisoning being a common cause of death and acute illness between 2 and 30 years of age. The American Association of Poisons Control Centers National Data Collection System estimated that 2 million people voluntarily notified them in 1992 as having been exposed to poisonous substances, approximately 90% of exposures occurring at home, 80% being oral ingestion and 60% being children under 5 years of age. In recent years there has been a decline in deaths arising from unintentional ingestion of toxins by children under the age of 5. Of the 2 million reports of exposure to toxins, just under half a million related to therapeutic agents. Therapeutic agents accounted for 600 of the 700 reported deaths from poisoning in 1992. These deaths from acute chemical poisoning need to be seen in the context of the many hundreds who die each year as a consequence of the bacterial contamination of food and from being bitten by poisonous snakes and stung by insects.

Even from such traumatic situations of human poisoning from exposure to chemicals, toxicologists need to look for data regarding human toxicology and dose–response relationships. Suicidal and homicidal sources of knowledge need analysis and comparison with experimental data from animal studies. Adverse effects to drugs in man provide opportunity for examining the process of hazard assessment by the retrospective analysis of clinical symptoms alongside experimental data from animals. Conventional toxicity testing using experiments with laboratory animals aims to detect and characterize the inherent potential for toxicity—hazard assessment—whereas risk assessment aims to extrapolate these data and predict the potential consequences for man at the exposure concentrations which are likely to prevail in a variety of circumstances.

There is a need to extrapolate both qualitatively, *hazard assessment*, and quantitatively, *risk assessment*, using dose–response relationships obtained in animal studies to predict at what exposure level such responses may occur in man. Most toxicologists would agree that animal toxicity testing can reveal a chemical's potential toxicity for man, and that adverse consequences will not be seen in the majority of cases at exposure conditions which are without effect in animals. However, because of the many different drugs available and polymorphism in the human drug metabolism gene pool, several new drugs have produced previously undetected toxicity as a consequence of drug interactions. A recent example is that of cardiac toxicity in patients receiving terfenadine (a non-sedating antihistamine, used for the treatment of allergy) arising from the inhibition of the metabolism of terfenadine following co-administration of ketoconazole, an antifungal. The study of potential drug interactions is becoming an increasingly important focus of the clinical research into a new drug.

Pharmacology and clinical toxicology textbooks are a good source of information on the clinical signs and treatment of poisoning by drugs and acute poisoning by commercial products.

PRINCIPLES AND PROCEDURES

Acute Toxicity Studies

Until the early 1980s, for most of the chemicals in widespread use, there was a paucity of information on their potential to cause harm to mammalian organisms. Most of what was published in the literature was data from a set of short-term studies in the rat. Initial evaluation of the potential of a substance to cause harm to man is often based on an acute systemic toxicity assessment in a laboratory animal, typically the rat or mouse. Many acute systemic toxicity studies are also performed in a whole range of invertebrate species and fish to determine the toxicity potential of substances to the environment. This is not dealt with in this chapter. Acute toxicity assessment studies are a small proportion of the overall experimental studies in mammalian laboratory species. In 1985, of the just over 3.2 million studies in animals reported to the UK Home Office, 6.4% were for the study of the acute medicinal products and 4.7% for the study of acute toxicity in non-medicinal products. In 1995, of the 2.7 million studies in animals, 5.9% were for the study of acute toxicity in medicinal products and only 0.6% for the study of acute toxicity in non-medicinal products.

Assessment of the acute toxicity of substances is of primary importance in the overall evaluation of potential human health hazards. Whilst a principle objective is the detection of adverse effects, it is often overlooked that an equally important objective is to establish the absence of adverse effects, i.e. the demonstration of safety. A second misconception is that the majority of chemicals represent serious acute toxicity hazards. The purpose of acute toxicity tests is more often to confirm the absence of toxic responses. This view is supported by the relatively small proportion of marked effects in acute toxicity studies.

Computer-based systems have been developed for the capture of raw data, subsequent analysis and reporting. One such database comprises of over 3000 acute systemic studies. Using standard classification systems to rank the responses the following prevalence of toxic responses in each study type was obtained. In systemic toxicity studies, 65% of oral and 66% of dermal studies were of low toxicity (> 2000 mg kg^{-1}), 29% and 24% were in the harmful category, respectively, 5% and 9% in the toxic category, respectively, and only 0.8% and 0.9% in the very toxic category.

Such reviews of the outcome of acute systemic toxicity studies completed against a broad spectrum of chemical types (pesticides, intermediates, dyes, pharmaceuticals, cutting oils, biocides, chlorinated solvents, surfactants, formulations) confirms that a majority of the outcomes of these studies did not produce evidence of significant toxicity or lethality at amounts which would be expected to be encountered by human beings.

However, before we are able to begin to understand toxicity, it is necessary to detect toxicity. Acute toxicity testing in whole organisms is one mechanism for achieving this. Traditionally, the emphasis in these types of studies was on determining the LD$_{50}$, time to death, slope of the lethality curve and the prominent clinical signs. Acute lethality testing designed to determine the amount of a chemical that causes death, with death as the only end point, came under extensive criticism in 1990 by the US Society of Toxicology. Acute toxicity studies have achieved a level of notoriety in the public domain owing to the efforts of animal welfare groups. A primary focus has been the LD$_{50}$ test. Regrettably, a considerable amount of rhetoric has been used in the description of these tests, overshadowing more reasoned debate.

The primary goals of acute systemic toxicity studies depend principally on the circumstances in which the study data will be used. At the present time, acute toxicity assessment involves the controlled exposure of various laboratory sentient animal species to a known chemical substance or preparation for a short period of time, following which the clinical signs are monitored for a period of time, whereas acute toxicity generally deals with the adverse effects of single doses. Delayed effects may occur due to accumulation of the chemical in tissues or other mechanisms and it is important to identify any potential for these by repeated dose testing. Dosing periods lying between the single dose and 10% of life-span dosage are often called sub-acute. The OECD considered that this term was semantically incorrect and therefore, to distinguish such dosing periods from the classical sub-chronic, they may be described as 'short-term repeated dose studies'; this applies to 14, 21 and 28 day studies. The term 'para-acute' to describe dosing periods of 1 week or less, with 'sub-acute' for single doses below acute dose levels has been recommended but has not to the author's knowledge, achieved popular usage. The main repeat dose study protocols have usually employed durations of 14, 28 and 90 days, respectively. Other study durations have been used in toxicology but the selection of these three durations is considered to represent a reasonable standardized approach. The term 'sub-chronic' has been used to embrace the toxic effects associated with repeated doses of a chemical greater than a 10% part of an average life-span of experimental animals.

Parameters Studied in Acute Systemic Toxicity Assessments

Establishing a dose–response relationship for exposures at which the probability of a known fraction of a population of a species under study will show lethality is not the only objective of acute systemic toxicity studies. In summary acute studies establish the following:

- Dose ranges for subsequent studies.
- Potency, ranking from extreme to non-toxic.
- Identifying probable physiological systems/target organs being affected.
- Extent or degree of effect, e.g. subdued behaviour, coma death.
- Minimal regulatory guideline requirements.

The following illustrates the additional data that can be obtained with appropriate protocol design:

Clinical signs	Time of onset, duration and recovery
Morbidity	Agonal changes; reflexes; pharmacological effects; dose–response curves (ED$_{50}$).
Lethality	Dose–response (LD$_{50}$ with confidence limits); shape and slope of dose–response curve; estimation of median lethal dose (LD$_{50}$); estimation of minimum lethal dose (LD$_{01}$); estimation of certain lethal dose (LD$_{100}$).
Body weight	Decreased body weight gain; body weight loss; reduced food consumption.
Target organ identification	Necropsy and gross tissue examinations; histological examinations; blood clinical chemistry; hematology.
Physiological function	Immunology; neuromuscular reflexes; behavioral screening; electrocardiogram; electroencephalogram.
Pharmacokinetic	Therapeutic index; bioavailability (AUC, volume of distribution, half-life).
Pharmacodynamics	Relationship between plasma and tissue levels and occurrence of clinical signs.

Identification of the probable physiological systems and target organs involved in acute systemic toxicity is an important objective when conducting these types of assessments.

Protocol Design

For valid conclusions to be reached, application of the scientific method requires the objective of the study to be defined, the use of homogeneous populations of experimental subjects, sensitive and selective indices of effects and analysis of data by appropriate statistical approaches. Whilst some protocols have been defined to meet various international regulations, for other regulations the exact protocols depend on the type of chemical substance and the country in which it will be registered for use. There is a considerable amount of harmony in the requirements for acute oral, dermal, inhalation and parenteral toxicity. The US FDA, for instance, published in the Federal Register in August 1996 a 'Guidance for Industry' on 'Single Dose Acute Toxicity Testing for Pharmaceuticals' as part of a proposed implementation of the 'International Conference on Harmonisation (ICH) Safety Working Group Con-

sensus Regarding New Drug Applications'. Often both sexes of two species are involved, a route of exposure which is anticipated to be the most probable route of exposure for man, and an intravenous dose is necessary for regulatory purposes. Laboratory mice and rats are the species typically selected. Additional species are required by some regulations and in these cases probe studies are often used to select an appropriate dose range and species. The experimental design for acute systemic toxicity assessment has for many years been a modification of the Trevan approach of interval dose levels applied to groups of experimental animals such that an incidence of response can be achieved varying from zero incidence to 100% response and the median lethal dose derived (LD_{50}). The number of replicates and size of sample population will dictate whether the experimentally derived curve reflects the actual response.

In systemic toxicity testing, experimental design should allow broad group classifications of extremely toxic, very toxic, toxic and practically non-toxic and perhaps move away from the need to define the LD_{50}. Lethality should not be the only dose-related systemic effect that would justify a classification and more use would and could be made of the induced clinical signs (**Table 1 and 2**), i.e. the use of qualitative

Table 1 Physiological systems of mammalian organisms, potential targets and clinical signs observed in acute toxicity studies

Main body system	Organs	Examination	Clinical signs
Integumentary	Skin, fur, claws	External observations	Piloerection, oedema, erythema, eruptions, colour, alopecia, irritation, necrosis
Musculature/ skeletal	Muscles, tendons, bones, cartilage	Reflexes	Fasciculation, catalepsy, hyper-hypotonia
Nervous system	CNS—brain, spinal cord Peripheral—nerves and ganglia	Home-cage, external and in-hand passive observations, reflexes, provocation	Ataxia, convulsions, (clonic and tonic) tremor, righting reflex, gait, prostration
	Autonomic	Reflexes	Lachrymation, miosis, mydriasis, ptosis, exophthalmos, chromodacryorrhea,
	Sensory—eye, ear, olfactory	External observations, reflexes	Anaesthesia, parathaesia, corneal/lens opacity, iritis, chemosis, conjunctivitis, nystagmus
Endocrine	Pancreas, adrenal, thymus, parathyroid, pituitary, pineal, testis, ovaries		
Cardiovascular	Heart[a], blood vessels, spleen	Palpitation, heart rate	Arrhythmia, bradycardia, tachycardia, vasodilation, vasoconstriction, hyperthermia, hypothermia
Respiratory	Lungs[a], nasal cavity, pharynx, larynx, bronchus	Breathing rate, external observation	Apnoea, bradypnoea, dyspnoea, tachypnoea, cyanosis, nasal discharge, Cheyne–Stokes, Kussmaul, hypopnoea
Digestive system	Oral cavity, stomach, salivary glands, small/large intestine, rectum, colon, liver[a]	Excreta, external observation	Emesis, flatulence, constipation, diarrhoea, stained faeces, absence of faeces
Urinogenital	Kidney[a], bladder, ovary, testes, placenta, foetus, perineal region	External observations, excreta	Diuresis, rhinorrhoea, anuria, polyuria
Lymphatic	Lymph nodes, thymus, spleen		

[a] Typical organs removed at necropsy for additional histological evaluation if gross observation shows evidence of adverse change

Table 2 Clinical signs of systemic toxicity

Agonal
  Signs of death
Alopecia
  Deficiency of hair
Anaesthesia
  Absence of or reduced response to external stimulus
Analgesia
  Decrease in reaction to pain
Anuria
  Absence of or reduction in urine excretion
Apnoea
  Transient cessation of breathing following a forced respiration
Arrhythmia
  Abnormal cardiac output
Asphyxia
  Suspended animation due to lack of oxygen in blood, suffocation
Ataxia
  Incoordination of muscle action, loss of coordination and steady gait
Blepharospasm
  Rapid or spasmodic eyelid movement
Bradycardia
  Decreased heart rate
Cardiac rhythm
  Response of the heart muscle
Catalepsy
  Animal tends to remain in position it is placed
Chemosis
  Swelling/oedema of the conjunctival tissue
Cheyne—Stokes
  Rhythmic waxing and waning of respiration
Chromodacryorrhea
  Red lachrymation/reddish conjuctival exudate/absence of erthrocytes
Conjuctivitis
  Inflammation of the mucous membranes of the eyelids and junction with the cornea
Convulsion, asphyxial
  Gasping and cyanosis accompanying clonic convulsions
Convulsion, clonic
  Alternating contraction and relaxation of muscles, observed as a cycling of the forelimbs
Convulsion, tonic
  Persistent contraction of muscles with rigid extension of hind limbs
Corneal opacity
  Translucent and opaque to transmission of light
Corneal reflex
  Touching of the cornea causing eyelid to close
Cyanosis
  Bluish appearance of tail, mouth, footpads, due to lack of oxygenation of the blood
Diaphoresis
  Production of perspiration
Diarrhoea
  Frequent defaecation of fluid stools
Discharge
  Excretion/secretion

Diuresis
  Involuntary urination
Dyspnoea
  Difficult or laboured breathing, gasping for air, slow respiratory rate
Emaciation
  Lean wasting muscle mass
Emesis
  Vomiting and retching
Erythema
  Redness of skin due to irritation and inflammation
Exophthalmos
  Protrusion of the eyeball from the orbit
Exudates
  Oozing secretion or discharge
Fasciculation
  Rapid continuous contraction (twitching) involving movements of skeletal muscle on the back, shoulders, hindlimbs and digits
Gait
  Locomotory movement of the limbs during walking, normal carriage of the body
Gasping
  Strain for air with open mouth, convulsive catching of breath often accompanied by a wheezing sound
Grip strength
  Ability to retain hold with digits
Hyperactivity
  Increased level of motor activity
Hyperpnoea
  Deep and rapid breathing
Hypersensitivity
  Excessive reaction to external stimuli such as light, noise or touch
Hypertonia
  Increase in muscle tension
Hypoactivity
  Low level of motor activity
Hypotonia
  Generalized decrease in muscle tension and tone
Iritis
  Inflammation of the iris
Jaundice
  Yellow coloration of mucous membranes due to deposition of bile pigments
Kyphosis
  Curvature of the vertebral column creating a hump back
Lachrymation
  The secretion of tears
Lethargy
  Inability to be aroused from stupor without relapse
Miosis
  Constriction of the pupil irrespective of the presence or absence of light
Motor activity
  Changes in frequency and nature of movements
Mydriasis
  Excessive dilation of pupil

(Continued)

Table 2 *(Contd)*

Myotactic reflex
   Ability to retract when extended over edge of a surface
Necrosis
   Death of tissue
Nictitating membrane
   Inner eyelid of many animals
Nystagmus
   Involuntary rotational, horizontal or vertical movement of
      eyes
Oedema
   Swelling of tissue filling with fluid
Opacity, cornea
   A loss of transparency of the cornea
Opisthotonos
   Tetanic spasm in which the head is pulled towards the dorsal
      position and the back is arched
Paralysis
   Loss of motor function in all or part of the body
Piloerection
   Raising of the hair or fur
Pinna reflex
   Twitch of the outer ear elicited by light stroking of inside
      surface of ear
Polyuria
   Increase above normal in the amount of urine excreted
Preyer's reflex
   Involuntary movement of the ears caused by noise
Prolapsus
   Slipping forward or down of part of an organ, usually uterus or
      rectum
Prostration
   Immobile, resting on ventral surface
Ptosis
   Dropping of the upper eyelid associated with impaired
      conduction in the third cranial nerve and not reversed by
      stimulation

Pupillary reflex
   Contraction of the pupil in response to light
Respiration irregular
   Abnormal breathing
Respiration laboured
   Breathing strained and difficult
Righting reflex
   Ability to regain normal stance on to all four limbs
Salivation
   Excessive salivary secretion
Somnolence
   Drowsiness which can be aroused by external stimulation and
      with resumption of normal activities
Spasticity
   Uncontrolled involuntary movement of limbs
Startle reflex
   Response to external stimuli such as light, touch and noise
Straub tail
   The carriage of the tail in an erect/vertical position (associated
      with interaction with opiate receptor)
Stupor
   Torbidity, dazed state
Tachycardia
   Increased heart rate
Tachypnoea
   Rapid and unusually shallow respiration
Torsion
   Postural incoordination or rolling often associated with the
      vestibular system (ear canal)
Tremor
   Trembling and quivering of the limbs or entire body
Vasoconstriction
   Blanching of the skin or mucous membranes, body
      feels cold
Vasodilation
   Redness of skin and mucous membranes, body feels warm

judgments based on semi-quantitative rather than quantitative dose response data.

A wide variety of intrinsic and extrinsic factors can influence the outcome of a test. In order to establish a dose–response relationship, animals of the same species/strain, sex and age should be divided randomly into equivalent size groups with the different groups treated at the same time of day with different dosages by the same route and observed for a set and consistent period of time. For a single exposure study a mis-delivered dose would have a greater effect on the conclusions than for chronic exposure studies. Toxicity that is clearly the result of accidental events should not be considered in the final conclusion. All protocols should state the ceiling or limit dosage. Small differences in protocols are probably the major cause of the considerable laboratory-to-laboratory variations in results achieved. There is some question concerning the utility of extensive pathological assessments as part of an acute study. Gross necropsies are the minimum requested by most regulatory bodies.

Protocols include necropsies on all animals found dead and those killed following the 2-week post-dosing observation period. Body weights are determined on day 1 (prior to dosing), day 7 and day 14 as required by most regulatory guidelines. Animals should not differ in age by more than 15%; for example, the ratios of the LD_{50}s obtained in adult animals to those in neonates vary from 0.002 to 160.

Clinical Signs

Acute systemic studies are concerned with the detection of adverse changes to the body systems which are likely to be life threatening following single exposure to chemicals. However, they are also concerned with non-life-threatening responses that occur in external tissue which may lead to loss of function, ill health and reduction in quality of life. The assessment of acute systemic toxicity is the assessment of the potential for severe health effects which result from the major systems of the body, cardiovascular, respiratory, central nervous, excretory and locomotory systems being compromised by adverse change. The aim of qualitative extrapolation of toxicity data from animals would be to predict potential signs of toxicity in man and the symptoms that are likely to be described by someone who has been intoxicated, i.e. 'feeling drowsy', 'feeling nauseated'. Animals will not describe such symptoms—they have to be deduced from the clinical signs of toxicity and pharmacological responses expressed in the animal studies and observed and recorded by the toxicologist as cage side observations. It should be remembered that when dealing with animals we are observing clinical signs; animals are not describing their symptoms. Clinical symptoms are the verbal descriptions of feelings provided by a human patient. The term clinical symptoms is often misused when describing animal observations. Signs are overt and observable. Symptoms are apparent only to the subject of intoxication (e.g. headache) and cannot be described or reported by animals. Clinical signs can be reversible or irreversible. Reversible signs are those that dissipate as the chemical is cleared from the body. Irreversible signs are those that do not disappear and are accompanied by organic damage. Signs also represent pharmacological response which may be adverse. The reliability and accuracy of prediction from animal studies can be judged only when a chemical is assessed in both animals and man and any adverse reactions observed are compared. Substantial gross macroscopic findings are rare in minimal acute studies and seldom suggestive of a specific effect. It is difficult to separate the chemical associated effect from agonal and/or autolytic changes in animals found dead. It is difficult to come to a conclusion about the nature of a gross lesion without histological assessment. Confirmation of gross lesions is seldom done because of the autolytic nature of many of the lesions. Pathological examinations in general and histological assessments in particular are most meaningful when the same organs are collected and examined from all animals regardless of the circumstances of death. The kidney and liver are the most frequent target organs of acute toxicity. The clinical laboratory package should be sufficient to detect possible damage to these organs. Serum parameters should include urea, glucose and total protein concentrations and the activities of alanine aminotransferase, aspartate aminotransferase and alkaline phosphatase.

Liver

Liver structure and function are more often altered by acute exposures to chemicals as a consequence of the extensive role of the liver in biotransformation of absorbed exogenous substances. The most sensitive tests for hepatotoxicity are those that monitor elevation in the levels of serum transaminases (asparate amino-

transferase, ASP; alanine aminotransferase, ALT; gamma-glutamyl transpeptidase, γGPT); and serum bile acids. Serum bile acid levels are specific for liver injury and reasonably sensitive and often observable by direct observation of yellowing of external surfaces (jaundice). Signs of hepatotoxicity are not often apparent from cage side observation.

Kidney

As the kidneys receive one quarter of the cardiac output and are the site of concentration and excretion of water-soluble exogenous materials, they are often a target for acute toxic responses. Signs of renal intoxication, however, are rarely prominent in the acute phase. Polyuria and oliguria, proteinuria or haematuria and elevated serum creatinine or blood urea are often not seen until much of the kidneys' capacity to filter, concentrate and re-absorb has been compromised.

Lung

Toxic pulmonary injury is most likely to occur in association with inhaled chemical agents, often by direct irritation, e.g. chlorine gas. However, severe acute toxicity to the lung had been observed following systemic absorption of certain compounds, e.g. methylfurans and some dipyridyl herbicides.

Nervous System

Functional and morphological disturbances of central, peripheral and autonomic systems often occur with acute intoxication, e.g. carbon disulphide and organophosphorus insecticides. The cerebral cortex, cerebellum, peripheral nerves, synapses and spinal cord are often the target for injury. Clinical signs of acute intoxication are often associated with the antagonism of CNS and PNS functions.

Cardiovascular System

Typical chemical-induced cardiac disorders consist of effects on heart rate (chronotropic), contractility (ionotropic), conductivity (dromotropic) and excitability (bathmotropic). A rapid heart beat is referred to as tachycardia and a slow heart rate as bradycardia. Abnormality in rhythm is termed an arrhythmia and can be a consequence of an atrial flutter, atrial fibrillation, ventricular fibrillation or heart block. Cardiac myopathies are characterized by any type of damage to the heart muscle. An elevated level of lactase dehydrogenase (LDH) in the blood is often a signal of damage to the heart.

Haematopoietic System

Whilst the haematopoietic system and immune system may be target tissues following acute exposure, evidence of toxicity from clinical signs is limited. With regard to the blood, the most common acute lesion is induced haemolysis. Haematological assessment of blood, monitoring red and white cell counts, haematocrit, white cell differentials and blood coagulation factors such as clotting time are necessary to diagnose these tissues correctly as targets of acute toxicity.

External Organs

The skin can show evidence of irritation and the eyes opacity of the cornea and/or lens following dermal application, whole body inhalation or systemic exposure. To establish evident toxicity more than a single exposure is often required. Direct contact of external tissues with toxicants often elicits an immediate response within a relatively short period of time following exposure.

Mortality

Mortality in each group is calculated on the basis of the number of animals that die (or are humanely killed because of morbidity) during the observation period, and is normally presented in percentage terms: (number dead/number dosed) × 100. Delayed deaths (those occurring more than 24 h after dosing) are relatively rare and generally restricted to the 72 h period following dosing. The different laboratory practices of including or excluding animals killed because of morbidity may reflect some of the interlaboratory assessments of acute toxicity of equivalent chemicals.

In Vivo Studies

'Fixed-Dose', 'Set-Dose' and 'Sequential Dosing' Procedures

A small number of animals per dose are administered at fixed dose levels approximating to current limits used for labelling. The top dose approximates to the limit dose specified by regulatory guidelines. The set dose method works best if the doses are separated by constant multiples. If there are no effects, the protocol defaults to a limit test. In a limit test, a single dose of the test article is given to one group animals. Additional animals may be required to confirm the limit. One such protocol design consists of three animals per dose at 10, 100 and 1000 mg kg^{-1}. Animals were observed for 14 days post-dosing. Interestingly, one animal per group gave reliable results with 93% of chemicals tested. One method estimated an LD$_{50}$ using six animals by analysing the responses of individual animals. The dose range was defined as 1.5 times a multiplication factor. The approximate lethal dose was the highest dose that did not cause death.

A fixed dose design has been proposed for classification or labelling purposes. Five rats per sex receive 50 mg

kg^{-1} and, if survival is less than 90%, a second group of animals is given 5 mg kg^{-1}. If survival is again less than 90%, the substance is classified as 'very toxic'. If survival is greater than 90%, it is classified as 'toxic'. If survival is 90% but there is evident toxicity after the 50 mg kg^{-1} dose, the substance is classified as 'harmful'. If there is no toxicity at 50 mg kg^{-1}, another group of animals are dosed at 500 mg kg^{-1}. With 90% survival and no evident toxicity, the substance is 'unclassified'. Evident toxicity refers to cage side observations of clinical signs which are likely to be life threatening. This protocol, which has been evaluated and validated, has been introduced into Annex V of Directive 79/83/1/EEC as an alternative to the LD$_{50}$ for toxicity classification for labelling purposes.

Sequential Up-and-Down Dosing

The format for this type of procedure requires single animals to be exposed with subsequent doses adjusted up or down by some constant factor depending on the outcome of the previous dose. In this method, an individual animal is given a randomly selected dose. If the animal dies, the dose is decreased by a constant factor (suggested 1.3) and another animal is dosed at this level. If the animal dose not respond, the dose is elevated by a equivalent constant factor until five animals have been dosed or the limit dose is reached. The data are analysed with the maximum likelihood method or the use of the tables developed by Dixon (1965). In general, only 6–9 animals are required. The up- and-down procedure compares favourably with the fixed-dose procedure.

Rising Dose Procedures

A single group of animals (usually two) receive repeated exposure to the chemical throughout the study (often on alternate days) with the dose increasing at each administration using some constant factor such as doubling until toxicity, morbidity or lethality is observed in one or both animals or the limit dose is achieved. In one such rising dose tolerance design, animals were exposed for 4 days to the initial dosage followed by 3 days of recovery before the next 4 day dosing period at a raised dose level, the sequence being repeated for the three dosing cycles.

Non-Rodent Acute Toxicity Studies

For non-rodents, rising dose procedures are sufficient to support most regulatory submissions. Delayed effects, bioaccumulation due to incomplete clearance between administrations, pharmacological accommodation, induction and inhibition of metabolism may all complicate the interpretation of this type of study. Under some international animal welfare regulations, but not all, non-rodents can be re-used following a wash-out period.

The FDA and the Canadian authorities require acute toxicity testing in at least one non-rodent species, although it has been suggested that is unnecessary to achieve lethal doses in non-rodent species. Animals often used are the dog, monkey and ferret. Agricultural chemicals may have to be tested in domesticated farm animals. The rabbit is the species of choice for a variety of tests, such as dermal toxicity. The use of larger animals permits more extensive observation such as complete physical examinations, palpation, behavioural checks, spinal reflex check, papillary light responses, respiration rate, ECG recording and rectal temperature measurement. Blood samples can also be more easily collected to determine standard clinical chemistry and haematology profiles. The bioanalysis of plasma levels of the parent compound and any significant metabolites would assist in interpretation, but such analytical procedures are often unlikely to be available at the early evaluation stages of a chemical. Such rising multi-dose study designs can replace conventional 2 week studies conducted at a range of fixed dose levels. Gross necropsy examinations, measurement of major organ weights (both absolute and relative) and a battery of serum enzyme assays should all be part of the protocol.

Quality Control Screen

Lethality screening is used in the quality control (QC) monitoring for the standardization of biologically derived materials for potency and the test for gross contamination or adulteration. QC tests for potency generally use a minimum number of groups of few animals dosed at the expected LD_{50}. Such quality assurance limit tests are almost exclusively conducted on mice. If mortality falls within the standardized range of expected responses then the batch would be acceptable. Tests for contamination are often limit tests where only few animals are tested at a set limit dose (MLD, the minimum lethal dose, LD_{01}) with the anticipated outcome of 100% survival. An occasional death may occur because the MLD is in the range of the LD_{01}. There is cause for concern if the repeat response is again not 100% survival and the material should not be released until the cause of enhanced lethality is understood, e.g. possible infection in stock animals.

Rodenticide testing

It should be remembered that the determination of the minimum dose to ensure lethality (LD_{100}) is still an objective in establishing the potency of rodenticides (FIFRA).

Other Species

The US EPA require tests in aquatic non-vertebrates and vertebrates (fish, avian and feral species) for chemicals that may be released into the environment. These areas of acute toxicology assessment are more appropriately covered under ecotoxicology (see Chapter 61).

Factors Affecting Acute Systemic Toxicity Studies

The various factors that influence the outcome of acute systemic toxicity studies are in many respects equivalent to those that modulate all biological studies. In assessing the extent of a toxic hazard there are several important considerations related to route, severity, speed and duration of onset of effect:

Factor	*Type*
Route of exposure	Ingestion, inhalation, dermal, parenteral.
Severity of effect	Harmless, harmful, toxic, very toxic, extremely toxic.
Speed of onset	Immediate, delayed.
Duration of effect	Acute, persistent, reversible, irreversible.
Duration of exposure	Single short duration (acute), Multiple short duration (sub-acute), multiple long duration (sub-chronic), continuous over significant portion of life span (chronic).

As in any biological experiment in which a small sample is taken to estimate the population response, there are many factors that can act as variables:

(1) Interspecies differences relating to heterogeneity of populations, specific physiology, basal metabolic rate and size.
(2) Intraspecies variation regarding strain, sex and age.
(3) Environmental, which includes route of exposure, amount, physical form, formulation exposure intervals and observation intervals.
(4) Statistical, including experimental bias, group size and size of population.

All the above contribute to the difficulties in achieving reproducible, accurate and precise data. However, the route of exposure, the most common being gastrointestinal, inhalation, dermal and parenteral, has a major influence on the toxicity because of the effect of the route of exposure on the rate and extent of absorption (bioavailability) of the chemical. The maximum plasma (tissue level) achieved, the time to maximum plasma levels and the duration of effect are affected by the clearance of the chemical from the system and the extent of distribution within the system. In turn, clearance can be modulated by the physiological changes induced by the chemical itself and the age and disease state of the organism under study.

Acute Inhalation Toxicity

Gases, vapours, smokes, dusts and aerosols when inhaled reach the absorptive surfaces of the lungs and the nasopharyngeal regions. This represents a major route of occupational and incidental exposure to toxins and a significant route of intentional exposure for drugs. In the lungs, inhaled intoxicants have ready access to the systemic circulation because of the extensive surface area and extensive vascularization. The close proximity of the gaseous phase with the vasculature allows toxicant exchange between inspired air and the blood and lymph. A number of factors affect the inhalation of aerosols: characteristics of the aerosols, architecture of the respiratory tract, breathing rate, tidal volume and residual capacity. The anatomy of nasal, buccal and pharyngeal regions, mucous distribution and the geometry of the air passages from nasal turbinates to the alveoli influence the extent and amount of toxicant entering the lungs. The respiratory rate (breaths min^{-1}) and tidal volume (ml) vary between species relative to their size—man has a breathing rate of 12–18 breaths min^{-1} and a tidal volume of 750 ml, dog 20 breaths min^{-1} and 200 ml, guinea pig 90 breaths min^{-1} and 2 ml, rat 160 breaths min^{-1} and 1.4 ml and mouse 180 breaths min^{-1} and 0.25 ml. The disposition of particles is not identical between species. The disposition in the respiratory tract depends on the size of the particle or aerosol: < 1 μm diameter reach the alveolar zone, < 5 μm diameter are deposited in the trachea and bronchi and > 5 μm diameter are deposited in the nose and pharynx. It should be remembered that unlike man, the rodent is an obligatory nose breather and the presence of a toxin may significantly change breathing rates.

Inhalation procedures are more complex and difficult to perform than acute oral, dermal or parenteral procedures, requiring more sophisticated techniques of analysis, formulation preparation and exposure. Acute inhalation toxicity is expressed as a function of concentration in the atmosphere and time of exposure, with 4 h being arbitrarily accepted as the maximum exposure for definition as acute. The practice of using many groups and numbers of animals to define an LC$_{50}$ has been replaced by designs which determine the approximate lowest lethal concentration. Exposure can be whole body in an inhalation chamber or head only, in which the animal is restrained with its head in an inhalation hood. There are limits to the amount of toxicants that can be presented as an atmosphere and common sense should prevail for the concentration used for a limit test. Details of inhalation procedures are given in subsequent chapters.

Acute Dermal Toxicity

Contamination of the skin is considered by many to be the primary route of intentional, adventitious incidental and accidental exposure to toxins. The several mechanisms of percutaneous diffusion of exogenous chemicals into and across the epidermis and into the vascular circulation are as follows:

(1) diffusion through the cells of the stratum corneum;
(2) diffusion between the cells of the stratum corneum;
(3) diffusion down the skin appendages—hair follicles, sweat and sebaceous glands.

The rate and amount of transfer of toxin are influenced by the physical state of the toxicant, the physical state of the skin and the mode of presentation to the skin.

Factors which are considered to make important contributions to the rate and extent of absorption and important during the design of acute dermal toxicity study are the following:

(1) the nature of the vehicle;
(2) the concentration of toxicant in the vehicle;
(3) the state of hydration of the skin;
(4) occluded or un-occluded exposure;
(5) skin abrasion;
(6) viscosity of the formulation;
(7) ionization state of the toxicant, i.e. pK of toxicant and pH of formulation;
(8) the ambient temperature.

Fick's law of diffusion is considered to approximate the percutaneous absorption kinetics of molecules:

$$F = Q_\mathrm{m} = K_\mathrm{p} C A t$$

where Q_m = amount of toxicant that penetrates the skin (mol), A = area of skin (cm^2), t = time (min), F = flux, i.e. moles transferred per unit area in unit time (mol cm^{-2} min^{-1}), K_p = permeability constant (cm min^{-1}) and C = difference between external and internal concentrations (mol cm^{-1}).

The general experimental design and principles are similar for dermal and oral acute toxicity studies. In acute dermal toxicity studies the rabbit has been the recommended species, presumably because of its preferred use in irritancy assessment. The rat, mouse and guinea pig are adequate alternative species which are considerably easier to handle than the rabbit.

The hair is removed in a manner which does not abrade the skin (abrasion increases the extent and rate of absorption of many chemicals) from an area of the dorsal surface (back, shoulder). The area is approximately 10% of the body surface (rat 4 × 5 cm, rabbit 12 × 14 cm, guinea pig 7 × 10 cm). There is a practical limit to the amount of a material than can be sensibly applied to the back of an animal and most regulatory authorities accept a limit dose experiment at approximately 2000–5000 mg kg^{-1}.

Acute Parenteral Toxicity

Several parenteral routes of acute exposure are possible: intravenous, subcutaneous, intraperitoneal, intramuscular, intracerebral. Because of the toxicity which can be elicited by infectious organisms, it is essential for formulations for parenteral acute toxicity to be sterile and for procedures to be aseptic. The intravenous route initially bypasses gut and liver first-pass effects but may demonstrate lung first-pass extraction. The principles and procedures for acute toxicity assessment by the parenteral route of administration are common with those described for oral administration.

STATISTICAL CONSIDERATIONS

Dose–Response/Effect Relationships

It is not the intention of this chapter to give a detailed appraisal of statistical approaches and the reader should consult Chang and Hayes (1989) and Gad and Chengelis (1988) for in-depth analysis. One important way of expressing the severity of response is to establish the **dose–effect** relationship, the relationship between the dose and the magnitude of a defined biological effect either in an individual or in a population sample, or the **dose–response** relationship, the relationship between the dose and the proportion of a population sample showing a defined effect. For solids and liquids the dose is often expressed as mg or ml per kg body weight or as a concentration term expressed as parts per million (ppm) required to cause an effect or an increased incidence of effect. For gaseous or volatile materials concentration is expressed as $mg\,l^{-1}\,h^{-1}$ or $ppm\,h^{-1}$ to combine dose and length of exposure.

Paracelsus (1492–41) in his work *The Third Principle* eloquently defined the dose–response concept: 'What is there that is not a poison? All things are poison and nothing (is) without poison. Solely the dose determines that a thing is not a poison', and the concept of a no-effect level or threshold dose: 'that while a thing may be a poison it may not cause poisoning'. In an individual an effect may be graded from zero to a maximum value. A response may be not graded but either be present or absent, i.e. a quantal response. Occasionally a response may have more than two possible outcomes and is referred to as a polychotomous response. Fundamental to acute toxicology is the relationship of response to log-normal distribution which is commonly expressed in terms related to the principles of population statistics. The first chapter of this book provides an additional discussion of the nature of the dose–response relationship and contains several examples of typical curves to which the reader is referred.

Most often acute responses are expressed as percentage incidence occurring in an exposed population. Groups of experimental subjects are given various doses of a substance and observations are made, the percentage responding being plotted on the y-axis and the logarithm of the dose on the x-axis. The observed cumulative curve is often sigmoidal in shape **(Figure 1–3**; see also Chapter 16).

In a population of subjects there is a range of sensitivity and for any given population a frequency of response curve will form a bell-shaped curve which when plotted as a cumulative frequency will show a sigmoidal relationship. The shape of the dose–response curve in the low-dose region often suggests that a safe level of exposure exists. The general shape and relationship of this dose–response curve can be modelled by sampling over the range of response. How accurately and precisely this

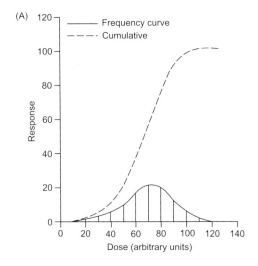
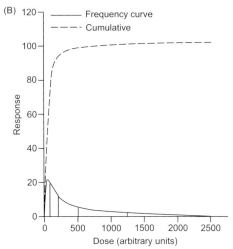

Figure 1 (A) Illustrative normal distribution response–frequency curve and cumulative response–frequency curve plotted against the dose. (B) Skewed distribution response–frequency curve and cumulative response–frequency curve plotted against the dose.

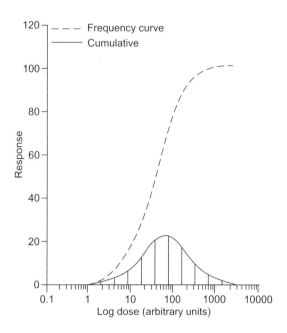

Figure 2 Plot of logarithmic transformation of skewed dose response.

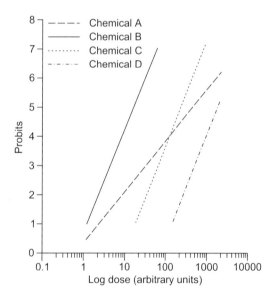

Figure 3 Comparison of probit lines for chemicals with equivalent LD_{50} and different slopes (A and C) and different LD_{50} and equivalent slopes (B and D).

curve will model the true population response will depend upon the number of samples and the size of each sample chosen. Various mathematical transforms convert a sigmoidal curve into a straight-line function. A log transform of a skewed distribution will often normalize the data.

Converting the percentile cumulative response into normal equivalent deviant ranges or probits will often transform a sigmoid response into a linear function. This is expressed mathematically as

$$dP = \frac{1}{\sigma\sqrt{2\pi}} \ \exp\left[\frac{-(x - \mu)^2}{2\sigma^2}\right] dx$$

where $\sigma^2 = $ variance, $\mu = $ mean, $x = $ value at each dose and $dP = $ probability of response. Then,

$$P = \int_{-\infty}^{x} \frac{1}{\sigma\sqrt{2\pi}} \ \exp\left[\frac{-(x - \mu)^2}{2\sigma^2}\right]$$

A linear equation allows more accurate statistical analysis and derivation of the median value, the slope and the confidence intervals. Caution must be exercized as mathematically derived values may well suggest a level of exactitude and credibility which is not justified by the database being used. For many purposes these quantitative values are often no better than a qualitative judgment.

The concept of dose–response and the ranking of substances based on the amount required to produce an effect is generally appreciated. What is not often appreciated is the reason for selecting the median effect dose or concentration (ED_{50}, LD_{50}, EC_{50}, LC_{50}). One could select a dose which would be insufficient to affect any animal in a group, or the dose required which is large enough to affect all the animals in a group. The former would be referred to as the minimum effect dose level and the latter as the certain effect dose. Depending on the data required, the minimum effect dose level (ED_{01}) and the certain effect dose level (ED_{100}) can be derived. The estimated variance associated with these determinations will be greater than the variance for the median value and often with small numbers of animals and dose groups the variances may be very large. For shallow slopes these values may differ significantly; for steep response slopes they may be indistinguishable from each other. There may be little difference between the ED_{01}, ED_{50} or ED_{100}. For another substance, the slope may be shallow with an order of magnitude difference or more between the ED_{01}, ED_{50} and ED_{100}. Although the slopes vary between these two substances, as reflected by dissimilar minimum lethal effect level and certain effect doses, their median effect dose could be equivalent. The question remains of whether it is better to rank substances based on their minimum effect dose, median effect dose or maximum/certain effect dose. The least variability for a derived value from a dose–response curve is the median effect dose. Consequently, this parameter has been selected as the reference point for comparing substances. Unfortunately, whilst the median effect dose is often quoted, the confidence and the slopes are often not reported. All parameters are important in defining the response curve, although it is important to stress that it is questionable whether for lethality data these parameters need to be excessively precise.

Determination of the Median Lethal Dose (LD_{50}/LC_{50})

The LD_{50} value is the median lethal dose and is a statistically derived dose which, when administered in an acute toxicity test, is expected to cause death in 50% of the treated animals in a given period. The LD_{50} is derived from a quantal dose–response curve where the specific response is death. When the route of exposure is inhalation, the term LC_{50} (median lethal concentration) is used. This is also used in aquatic toxicity testing. The LD_{50} / LC_{50} value is commonly misapplied when it is used to describe the acute toxicity of a chemical. The requirement to estimate the LD_{50} value with 95% confidence limits has been subject of criticism. Precise LD_{50} values are not required for the majority of applications. It is the statistical result of a single experiment, and is affected by many parameters such as age, weight, health, food deprivation, route of administration, temperature, caging conditions, seasonal variation, genetic influence and strain of animal. A published source of LD_{50} values [Registry of Toxic Effects of Chemical Substances (RTECS)] was found to cite 62 sources for 87 LD_{50} measurements. Unfortunately, there is a lack of detail in the published sources of LD_{50} values with regard to experimental conditions, strain of animal and method of statistical analysis. It has been proposed that interlaboratory estimates could be better correlated if such information were published.

If mortality at each dosage is plotted against dosages, a sigmoidal dose–response curve is obtained. The LD_{50} is simply the dose, either observed or calculated, that yields 50% mortality. The LD_{50} is difficult to read off a sigmoidal curve and the small number of doses normally used makes drawing an accurate lethal dose curve difficult. The precision with which the curves are described will depend on the number of groups, dose and the number of animals in each group.

In general, all methods of calculation and computation are more readily applied if the doses are evenly spaced and the group sizes are equal. The probit method first developed by Bliss (1935) and later refined by Finney (1971) requires at least two groups of partial responses (i.e. mortality greater than 0% but less than 100%). It also does not deal effectively with groups that have either 0% or 100% lethality. The most common correction for these is to substitute 0.1% for 0% and 99.9% for 100%. The probit method is considered the standard and is required by certain regulatory authorities. The probit method uses the linear relationship resulting from plotting as ordinate values the transformed proportional response in probability units against the logarithmic transformation of the dose plotted as the abscissa values. Probits are based on a theoretical normal population distribution and converted into positive values by the arbitrary addition of the integer five.

Although graphical methods (Litchfield and Wilcoxon, 1949) and tables for easy computation are available, computer techniques are now more often used for the analysis. Alternative approaches have been the use of the logistic function, Logits, and RIDIT analysis, which is based on an empirical distribution rather the theoretical distribution used in probit analysis. The moving average method does not require partial responses and deals effectively with complete responses and can produce an estimate of an LD_{50} with as few as three groups of 3–5 animals in each. This method requires that the doses be separated by a constant geometric factor and groups to be of equal size. Tables allow for the easy calculation of the LD_{50}. An estimate of the LD_{50} and slope can be obtained from as few as three groups of five animals per group provided the data set has responses between 0% and 100% with two of these being less than and greater than 50%, respectively.

The normit chi-squared-squared does not require equally spaced doses or equal group sizes, but does require at least one partial response. Inclusion of complete response is better than for probit analysis, but the procedure is difficult. In general, the best pattern of response will definitely produce close to 100% effect, a minimal effect and a partial effect close to the median effect. If this pattern is obtained, adding more groups does not generally change the results. There is seldom a substantial difference in the LD_{50} determination if sexes are pooled, which perhaps suggests that mixed sex groups should be introduced as a standard procedure. An alternative approach, not generally used, converts the median lethal molar concentration (T) into positive values similar to the pH scale using $pT = -\log(T)$, values greater than unity demonstrating increasing orders of magnitude of toxicity.

Assessing the Acute Effects of Mixtures of Chemicals

This topic is discussed in more detail in another section of this book (see Chapter 14); however, some brief comments on this important aspect of acute toxicity assessment follow.

Toxicology has traditionally concerned itself with the effect of a single substance administered alone or formulated as a single primary substance in an inert vehicle. With the sulphonamide drugs formulated in ethylene glycol, this vehicle was considered inert at the time, but unfortunately it proved to have inherent toxicity. An acute toxicity assessment of this vehicle would have detected the toxic potential. Now vehicles and excipients for use in formulations of drugs have been evaluated for their toxicity potential in order to be on an approved list for pharmaceutical use. More critically, the poly-pharmaceutical approach required to control disease is uncovering initially undetected toxicity due to drug–drug interactions. Terfenadine, introduced in 1985 as the first non-sedating antihistamine, was found in the 1990s to cause cardiac arrhythmia and cardiac arrest when administered with P450 3a inhibitors such as ketoconazole.

Many chemicals which are not drugs are formulated into mixtures with others, varying in their composition and concentration. Many of these formulations before marketing are evaluated in the laboratory using acute toxicity test procedures. Chemicals which are released to the environment become mixtures with chemicals or with their own degradation products. Industrial and municipal effluents either as gases, liquids or solids are usually complex mixtures of chemicals. Again, these can be tested in laboratory acute toxicity procedures.

It is impossible to test every combination of possible mixtures in laboratory tests but it is possible to make an approximate assessment of many of them from the intrinsic toxicity of their components. One approach is to determine the composition of the mixture and estimate approximate total toxicity by adding the toxicity of the individual components. However, the following can make this a too simplistic approach.

Type (1) Additive Effects

If two chemicals produce the same effect by simple independent action (e.g. cholinesterase inhibition by organophosphorus pesticides and inhibition of cytochrome oxidase by sodium cyanide) then the probability of effect (lethality) after administration of a mixture of the two chemicals would be

$$P(d_1, d_2)^* = P_1(d_1) + P_2(d_2) + P_1(d_1)P_2(d_2)$$

where $P_1(d_1)$ represent the probability of the incidence of effect after an administration of dose d_1 of the organophosphorus agent, $P_2(d_2)$ the probability of incidence of effect after administration of dose d_2 of the sodium cyanide and $P(d_1, d_2)$ the probability of the incidence of effect of the combined chemicals.

Type (2) Additive Effects

When two chemicals (C and D) have similar mechanism toxicities, e.g. two different organophosphorus agents, they will probably show parallel regression lines of their probit log dose responses and their cumulative toxicity is the ratio of equally effective doses.

Greater than Additive Effects

When the response from a mixture of two or more components is quantitatively greater or qualitatively different than any which the individual components could elicit when given at an equivalent combined dose, then the response can be described in several ways.

Potentiation is the case when the components of the mixture exhibit toxicity by different mechanisms of action and a quantitatively greater effect is obtained than could be obtained from any of the individual components when given at an equivalent combined dose.

Synergism is the case when the toxicity of the components is elicited by the same or equivalent mechanisms of action and a quantitatively greater response is achieved from the mixture than from the individual components if given at an equivalent combined dose level.

Coalitive effects occur when the response to a mixture of toxicants is qualitatively different to any of the effects elicited by the individual components of the mixture.

Antagonistic Effects

Effects that are quantitatively less than expected from the combined effects of the individual components of a mixture are referred to as antagonistic effects. A chemical which specifically acts an antagonist of toxicity is referred to as an antidote.

Antidotes

Antidotes are discussed elsewhere in this book (see Chapter 20) in more detail but a few remarks are given here for completeness of this chapter. In general, stabilization of the cardiovascular and respiratory function, i.e. the maintenance of vital functions through supportive clinical intervention and symptomatic care, are the first important steps in treating suspected poisoning. Antidotes reduce toxicity by antagonizing the effects of an intoxicant. Specific antidotes are available for relatively few toxins. Antidotes reduce or prevent the absorption and/or distribution of a toxicant to its site of action. They may prevent the action of the toxicant at its site of action by modifying in some way the receptor or the toxicant's interaction with receptors. Antidotes themselves may produce toxicity and therefore the benefits of administration need to be balanced against the potential for additional harm. It must be noted that the antagonism of toxicity by an antidote will be modulated by the pharmacokinetics of both the toxicant and the antidote. Delays in administration or maintenance of antidote therapy to achieve effective controlling concentrations can result in an ineffective antidote. The discovery and evaluation of antidotes are an often overlooked component of acute toxicity assessment

INTER- AND INTRASPECIES SIMILARITIES AND DIFFERENCES

Toxic effects depend on the concentration and duration of exposure of the toxicant to specific target sites. Species differences in response are largely due to differences in pharmacokinetics and biotransformation. The extent of absorption is remarkably consistent between different animal species for a large variety of substances. The amount of the different metabolites reaching the systemic blood circulation and the well perfused and poorly perfused tissues may differ markedly between species owing to variations the rate of biotransformation by the gastrointestinal tract, lung, skin and liver. With large concentrations following acute exposure, often the rates of biotransformation are saturated and variability between species is reduced. Distribution and elimination characteristics of substances tend to be more variable between species; in particular, elimination half-life and serum protein binding have shown marked differences between species. Consequently, interspecies variations in pharmacokinetic parameters such as absolute bioavailability, clearance and elimination half-life are often attributed to quantitative differences in disposition and quantitative rather than qualitative differences in biotransformation.

Allometric Scaling: an Aid to Species Extrapolation

Of the 30 million species on earth today, there are approximately 4000 different species of living mammals. Mammals are clearly of very variable size and appearance, ranging from the tiny shrew (< 10 g), through the rodent (5×10^2 g), rabbit (4×10^3 g), dog (10^4 g), man (10^5 g) and elephant (3×10^7 g) to the largest mammal known to have lived, the blue whale (15×10^7 g)—a 10^7-fold difference in size. However, mammals, including primates, have similar anatomy, physiology, biochemistry and cellular structure and organ sizes and physiological functions have been shown to be correlated with body weight. This relationship is the basis of allometric scaling, which has been used in various areas of the biological sciences. The general relationship which exists between various physiological parameters and the body weight is expressed as

$$X = aw^b$$

where X is the physiological parameter, w is the body weight and a and b are constants. The relative weights of internal organs, pulse and breathing rates, consumption of oxygen, food and water intakes, microsomal enzyme activities, duration of pregnancy, latent periods of tumors, nerve and muscle cell dimensions, maturation time of bone marrow elements and duration of erythrocyte life can all be related to body weight and surface area. Using such relationships, attempts have been made to extrapolate the acute toxicity across animal species to man.

Extrapolation of Acute Toxic Effects

The relationship between body weight and LD_{50} within a single species was established for groups of female mice of different weights. A straight-line relationship existed between log (body weight) and log (LD_{50}). The coefficients of regression differed for different chemicals, sexes and routes of administration. Krasovskii (1975, 1976) reviewed 278 chemicals and between six and ten species of mammals and demonstrated that a linear relationship existed for log (body weight) of different mammalian species against the log (oral LD_{50}) for individual chemicals. Leblic et al. (1984) also found a linear relationship between the log (LD_{50}) of three organophosphorus compounds (esterine, VX and paraoxon) and the log (body weight) of six species (mouse, hamster, rat, rabbit, dog and guinea pig) for three routes of exposure, intravenous (iv), subcutaneous (sc) and intraperitoneal (ip). Book (1982) used the 'body weight' rule to calculate the acute median lethal concentration (LC_{50}) for the inhalation of nitrogen dioxide (NO_2) for a 70 kg man. Extrapolation from the LC_{50} of NO_2 in 1 min obtained in mouse, rat, guinea pig, rabbit and dog predicted 174 ppm as the LC_{50} for a 1 min exposure in man. A published report of a fatality which occurred after acute exposure to 150 ppm NO_2 gives some credence to this extrapolation. Funaki (1974) showed that the familiar straight-line relationship held for three non-steroidal anti-inflammatory drugs when log (body surface area) or log (specific surface area), i.e. surface area/body weight, was plotted against LD_{50}. Onyon (1986) evaluated the relationship between log(LD_{50}) and log(body weight) for seven chemicals, selected from substances most frequently reported as intoxicants in human poisonings in the UK and demonstrated that an accurate prediction of the human lethal dose was obtained for paraquat (data on 12 mammalian species) and phenobarbitone (six mammalian species), the correct order of magnitude of lethal dose for ethanol (four mammalian species), aspirin (six species), an inadequate prediction for paracetamol (three species), amitriptyline (two species) and prediction was not possible for sodium chlorate, which had only one literature LD_{50} value in the rat of 1200 mg kg^{-1}. A prerequisite needed to define the straight-line relationship properly appears to be a relatively large database including three or four animal species.

Physiologically Based Pharmacokinetic Scaling

Alternative approaches to extrapolation include physiologically based pharmacokinetic models (PBPK) which attempt to describe quantitatively the pharmacokinetic processes affecting the disposition of a chemical and its biotransformation from the time it is absorbed to the interaction with different and various body tissues. Such models are used to quantify the magnitude and time course of exposure to the chemical at the critical target tissue sites. The application of such pharmacokinetic simulations to allow extrapolation of acute toxicity data obtained from animals and/or *in vitro* experiments to man is a future possibility which would enhance current allometric scaling approaches and integrate the subsequently obtained pharmacokinetic data on a substance with its acute and sub-acute data.

ALTERNATIVE APPROACHES

Alternative Approaches to Animal Experimentation

Current methodology for acute systemic toxicity assessment is undergoing evaluation and reform because of increasing societal demand for the development and use of *ex vivo, in vitro* and computer-aided quantitative structure–activity response (QSAR) models to replace, reduce and refine procedures (especially acute toxicity procedures) which employ animal experimentation.

Replacement. With the dramatic advances of information management, computer-based expert systems and molecular biology and the comprehensive understanding of the genomic map of human beings and animals, detection and characterization of all the potential individual changes to the underlying biochemical and physiological mechanisms involved in toxicological change are becoming increasingly a possibility.

Quantitative structure–toxicity relationship (QSAR) prediction based upon associating structural elements or groups of molecules to toxicity has been introduced on a commercial basis for general screening of new synthetic molecules. The rapid increase in the development of QSAR may be attributed to the need to evaluate the potential toxicity of the large number of existing chemicals for which there are inadequate or an absence of experimental data from studies in whole organisms. Prediction of biological activity from easily measurable physical and chemical properties of molecules is seen by many as an attractive alternative to whole organism studies.

Considerable effort has gone into the development of *in vitro* and *ex vivo* procedures for the assessment of adverse effects of chemicals. Bacteria, yeast, protista and preparations of higher organisms have been used for *in vitro* testing. The study of single cells rather than organs, tissue cultures or micromass preparations can provide usable information related to the problems of medical, veterinary or environmental safety. The development of such tests is based on a series of assumptions, a principle one being that the manifestation of toxicity observed *in vitro* is relevant when extrapolated to conditions *in vivo*. The majority of us are aware that animals are complex biological entities, consisting of numerous organs and tissues, thousands of enzymes, tens of thousands of proteins and peptides, hundreds of thousands of different molecules and millions of cells. The diversity of animal species is built on an increasing level of organization from molecules through macromolecules, from cells to tissues, from organs to organisms. It is now well established that all animal cells have the same common features of a cell membrane enclosing subcellular organelles for cellular reproduction and energy generation as well as other more specialized cellular functions. A fundamental assumption in the *in vitro* assessment of systemic toxicity is that the disturbance of any part of the basic cellular system by toxins should lead to a common response such as general cytotoxicity. Many different cell types have been used in cytotoxicity investigations and a large number of end points for detecting cytotoxicity have been used: cell viability, cell morphology, cell proliferation, membrane damage, uptake or incorporation of precursors, and metabolic activity. Hundreds of chemicals have now been studied in *in vitro* systems to determine their cytotoxicity to cells at various doses.

It is possible to perceive the development of a classification scheme for transforming the cytotoxicity ID_{50} values into categories of potential hazard statements comparable to those for LD_{50} values. For some industrial chemicals which are not to be manufactured in large amounts and are not for intentional exposure to man, the ability to label the potential hazard from a cytotoxicity index may well be all that is required. For example:

Potentially very toxic	cytotoxicity $ID_{50} < 10\,\mu g\,ml^{-1}$ (million cells ml^{-1}).
Potentially toxic	cytotoxicity $ID_{50} > 10\,\mu g\,ml^{-1}$ and $< 100\,\mu g\,ml^{-1}$ (million cells ml^{-1}).
Potentially harmful	cytotoxicity $ID_{50} > 100\,\mu g\,ml^{-1}$ and $< 1000\,\mu g\,ml^{-1}$ (million cells ml^{-1}).
Potentially non-toxic	cytotoxicity $ID_{50} > 1000\,\mu g\,ml^{-1}$ (million cells ml^{-1}).

The use of molar units rather than concentration units may be more appropriate, to allow comparison across chemicals of a wide diversity of molecular size. Clearly there are many assumptions being made in this extrapolation of cytotoxicity in cells to the complex integrated organism. Many would not be able to recognize the limitation of a potential hazard label derived from a cytotoxicity test compared with a hazard label derived from an *in vivo* study using another animal as a surrogate for man.

What separates the ranking of chemicals by a cytotoxicity *in vitro* screen from those ranked by observing the response of a whole organism is the special functions of selected cells and tissues within the whole organism. It is these special cells and tissues which maintain homeostasis and govern how much and at what rate a chemical is absorbed, transformed, distributed to the tissue, and eventually excreted. The determination of the median lethal dose (LD_{50}) in a laboratory rat provides data which can rank chemicals with regard to their potential to cause lethality in other species but it may not necessarily predict the human toxic dose. Similarly, *in vitro* cytotoxicity ED_{50} data allow some ranking of the potential for chemicals to cause toxicity but cannot predict whether the effect will occur at all or at what dose the effect will be evident in the whole organism. The qualitative and quantitative pharmacokinetics and metabolic dissimilarities between species which compromise intraspecies extrapolation clearly compromise extrapolation from cellular systems to man even when human tissues and cells are used. Whilst possible routes of biotransformation are being predicted from chemical structures using computer-aided analysis, the prediction of internal dose (tissue level) will require very sophisticated modelling indeed (see physiological-based pharmacokinetic modelling, this chapter and Chapter 7).

Mechanism of Cell Injury

An understanding of mechanism of cell injury offers a more rational basis for the design of reliable *in vitro* methods for toxicity screening than simple empiricism. Elucidation of molecular change consequent of chemically induced injury is fundamental to developing an understanding of organ-selective toxicity. The study of isolated cells has the potential to aid in the identification of both the primary molecular mechanism and the cascade of consequent degenerative change. Differentiation of the primary pathological and physiological events from secondary peripheral degenerative processes is required to elucidate the molecular mechanism of cell injury. Often very few cells are adversely affected.

However, multicellular organisms are a complex integration of proliferating and differentiated cells with each cell phenotypically expressing both a set of common sustenance genes and a set of specific genes. From such a perspective, the elimination of *in vivo* animal experimentation to understand toxicological events is a daunting and not to be underestimated goal. With our present knowledge of toxic mechanisms, pharmacokinetics and pharmacodynamics, one cannot envisage *in vitro* cell cytotoxicity screens completely replacing *in vitro* studies. They may, as our knowledge develops and in combination with well designed computer models, eventually predict a chemical's toxic potential to a multicellular organism. Their current application is limited to well defined circumstances, e.g. pyrogenic evaluation using the *Limulus* amoebocyte lysate test. There are *in vitro* techniques other than cytotoxicity assays which can contribute to the *in vivo* assessment of systemic toxicity such as the monitoring of the absorption of chemicals and the study of xenobiotic biotransformation.

Reduction. Reduction in the use of *in vivo* studies in animals for experimental purposes is being achieved. Between 1980 and 1988 the Swiss pharmaceutical companies Ciba-Geigy, Hoffman La Roche and Sandoz reported a reduction in their use of animals in research by 50%. Reports to the UK Home Office of laboratory animal studies indicates a reduction from 4.6 million in 1980 to 3.2 million in 1985 and 2.7 million in 1995. Whilst the use of *in vitro*, *ex vivo* and computer-aided modelling can contribute to savings in resources, it should also be noted that alternative approaches can take considerably more time and resources than the use of *in vivo* studies with the laboratory-bred mouse and rat.

Refinement. Physiological based pharmacokinetic (PBPK) modelling currently combines data from *in vivo*, *in vitro* and *ex vivo* studies to assist in the extrapolation of data generated in laboratory animals in its application to assessing safety to man. PBPK modelling has been introduced into the regulatory environment for the evaluation of chronic toxicity but its use in acute toxicity is not yet apparent. Quantitative and semi-quantitative approaches, many of them using sophisticated computerized treatments of biological data and chemical structure, have been applied with varying degrees of success to predict acute lethal toxicity. They require extensive databases of known dose–effect or dose–response relationships and are limited when the database contains only a few negative results.

DATABASE FOR THE REVIEW OF ACUTE TOXICITY STUDIES

Notable books of reference when searching for acute toxic effects of a chemical are *Sax's Dangerous Properties of Industrial Materials* (Lewis, 1996), *Martindale: The Extra Pharmacopoeia* (Reynolds, 1996), *The Merck Index* (Budavani, 1996), *Registry of Toxic Effects of Chemical Substances* (RTECS), US National Institute for Occupational Safety and Health, *The Physicians Desk Reference and Drug Interactions and Side Effects Index*. Of course, the Internet provides an increasing opportunity for searching any topic. Information searching is covered in a separate chapter of this book (see Chapter 24) and will not be developed further here.

CONCLUDING REMARKS

The detection and characterization of adverse changes following acute exposure to a chemical, the determination of the probable dose at which a chemical will be a poison rather than a remedy, is a large component in safety assessment. The principles for estimating this probable dose have for many years been based on the use of whole animal experimental procedures. Advances in knowledge have established an increasing awareness and desire to minimize the use of whole animal studies, establish humane approaches and introduce alternative approaches to meet these objectives. Such advances are most welcome, but whole animal *in vivo* experiments, especially those conducted to allow studies in the human species, have intrinsic value for studying acute effects which should not be overlooked.

REFERENCES AND FURTHER READING

Aldridge, W. N. (1996). *Mechanisms and Concepts in Toxicology*. Taylor and Francis, London.

Auletta, C. S. (1995). Acute, subchronic and chronic toxicology. In Derlanko, M. J. and Hollinger, M. A. (Eds), *CRC Handbook of Toxicology*. CRC Press, New York, pp. 52–104.

Bliss, C. I. (1935). The calculation of the dosage mortality curve. *Anal. Appl. Biol.*, **22**, 134–167.

Book, S. (1982). Scaling toxicity from laboratory animals to people: an example with nitrogen dioxide. *J. Toxicol. Environ. Health*, **9**, 719–729.

Brown, V. K. (1980). Acute toxicity in theory and practice. In Bridges, J. W. and Grasso, P. (Eds), *Monographs in Toxicology: Environmental and Safety Aspects*. Wiley, New York.

Budavani, S. (Ed.) (1996). *The Merck Index*. Merck, Whitehouse Station, NJ.

Chang, P. K. and Hayes, A. W. (1989). Principles and methods of acute toxicity and eye irritancy. In Hayes, A. W. (Ed.), *Principles and Methods of Toxicology*, 2nd edn. Raven Press, New York, pp. 169–220.

Chappell, W. R. and Mordenti, J. (1991). Extrapolation of toxicological and pharmacological data from animals to humans. *Adv. Drug Res.*, **20**, 1–117.

De Peyster, A. and Sullivan, M. A. (1996). Acute, subchronic and chronic toxicity testing. In Fan, A. M. and Chang, L. W (Eds), *Toxicology and Risk Assessment, Principles, Methods and Applications*. Marcel Dekker, New York.

Dixon, W. J. (1965). The up- and-down method for small samples. *J. Am. Stat. Assoc.*, **43**, 109–126.

ECETOC (1985). Acute toxicity tests, LD$_{50}$ (LC$_{50}$) determination and alternatives. In Oliver, G. J. A., Bomhard, E. M., Carmichael, N., Potokar, M. and Schultz, E. (Eds), *ECETOC Monograph No. 6*. European Chemical Industry Ecology and Technology Center, Brussels.

Ellenhorn, M. J. and Barceloux, D. G. (1988). *Medical Toxicology Diagnosis and Treatment of Human Toxicology*. Elsevier, New York.

Finney, D. J. (1971). *Probit Analysis*, 3rd edn. Cambridge University Press, Cambridge.

Funaki, H. (1974). Drug toxicity (LD$_{50}$) and 'dosis medicamentosa' for children in terms of body surface area and body weight. J. Kyoto Pref. Univ. Med., **83**, 467–477.

Gad, S. and Chengelis, C. P. (1988). *Acute Toxicology Testing Perspectives and Horizons*. Telford Press, Caldwell, NJ.

Gad, S. and Weil, C. (1982). Statistics for toxicologists. In Hayes, A. (Ed.), *Principles and Methods of Toxicology*. Raven Press, New York, pp. 273–320.

Gad, S. and Weil, C. (1986). *Statistics and Experimental Design for Toxicologists*. Telford Press, Caldwell, NJ.

Gallo, M. A. (1996). History and scope of toxicology. In Klaassen, C. D., Amdur, M. O. and Doull, J. (Eds), *Casarett and Doull's Toxicology: The Basic Science of Poisons*, 5th edn. McGraw-Hill, New York, pp. 3–12.

Hayes, A. W. (Ed.) (1989). *Principles and Methods of Toxicology*, 2nd edn. Raven Press, New York.

Klaassen, C. D., Amdur, M. O. and Doull, J. (Eds) (1996). *Casarett and Doull's Toxicology: The Basic Science of Poisons*, 5th edn. McGraw-Hill, New York.

Klaassen, C. D. (1997). Principles of toxicology and treatment of poisoning. In Hardman, J. G., Limbird, L. E., Molinoff, P. B. and Ruddon, R. W. Gilman (Eds), *Goodman and Gilman's The Pharmacological Basis of Therapeutics*, 9th edn. McGraw-Hill, New York.

Krasovskii, G. N. (1975). Species differences in sensitivity to toxic substances. In *Methods Used in the USSR for Establishing Biologically Safe Levels of Toxic Substances*. World Health Organization, Geneva, pp. 109–125.

Krasovskii, G. N. (1976). Extrapolation of experimental data from animals to man. *Environ. Health Perspect.*, **13**, 51–58.

Leblic, C., Coq, H. M. and Le Moan, G. (1984). Etude de la toxicité aigüe de l'Eserine, VX et le Paraoxon pour établir un modèle mathématique de l'être humain. *Arch. Belg. Med. Soc.*, 226–242.

Lewis, R. J. (Ed.) (1996). *Sax's Dangerous Properties of Industrial Materials*, 9th edn. Van Nostrand Reinhold, New York.

Litchfield, J. and Wilcoxon, F. (1949). A simplified method of evaluating dose–effect experiments. *J. Pharmacol. Exp. Ther.*, **96**, 99–113.

Lu, F. C. (1991). *Basic Toxicology: Fundamentals, Target Organs and Risk Assessment*, 2nd edn. Hemisphere Publishing.

Onyon, L. J. (1986). *The Qualitative Extrapolation of Acute Toxicity Data from Animals to Man*. MSc Thesis, University of Surrey, Guildford.

Reynolds, J. E. F. (Ed.) (1996). *Martindale: The Extra Pharmacopoeia*, 31st edn. Pharmaceutical Press, London.

Rhodes, C., Thomas, M. and Athis, J. (1993). Principles of testing for acute toxic effects. In Ballantyne, B., Marrs, T. C. and Turner, P. (Eds), *General and Applied Toxicology*. Macmillan, London.

Chapter 3
Repeated Exposure Toxicity

Bryan Ballantyne

CONTENTS

INTRODUCTION

The amount of detail and usable information on potential adverse health effects that can be obtained from general toxicology studies depends on a multiplicity of factors including, although not limited to, route of exposure, species, total dosage, formulation and purity of test material, the general and specific monitors employed, and the time-scale for exposure. Single (acute) exposures are carried out by giving the dose either perorally by bolus gavage or divided doses over 24 h, percutaneously by skin contact (usually occluded) for a specified period (often 4 or 24 h), or respiratory exposure for a specified period (to various atmospheric concentrations) or for variable periods of time to a specific concentration. Other routes of dosing, such as intravenous, intraperitoneal and intramuscular, usually employ bolus dosing. Observations are often conducted over a 14-day post-dosing period. The majority of acute studies include provision for observation for signs of toxic and/or pharmacological effects. A major end-point is often for mortality, with subsequent calculation of LD_{50} or timed LC_{50} values. Most studies also incorporate observations for non-lethal signs, body weights, and gross pathology by necropsy of animals that die and survivors sacrificed at the end of the 14-day post-dosing observation period (Chapter 15). Many acute studies are conducted as screens for toxicity, to obtain information on potential overexposure situations and/or to satisfy regulatory requirements. Because of this, and sometimes for reasons of economy, most acute studies do not include provision for physiological, biochemical, or histological monitoring. Although adding cost, in selected cases much more information related to potential adverse health effects could be obtained by the use of limited haematology, clinical chemistry and histology. Within the constraints of the limited monitoring usually conducted, acute toxicology studies are useful with respect to the following:

- Give information on potential local and systemic toxicity (and thus hazard) by acute overexposure to the material tested.
- Give information which may be important in determining the acute lethal toxicity, or lack thereof, of the material. In the absence of other information, this is often used as a basis for assuming lethal toxicity in humans, in spite of the difficulties associated with the extrapolation of such data. In a number of cases, acute mortality data obtained from small laboratory animals may be significantly misleading, because of species differences in absorption, pharmacokinetics and metabolism. A notable case is with ethylene glycol: the rat acute peroral LD_{50} is 8.54 ml (kg body weight)$^{-1}$, whereas estimates from human lethal poisoning cases suggests a lethal dose around 1.0 ml (kg body weight)$^{-1}$ (Tyler and Ballantyne, 1988).
- Permits a comparative evaluation, often based on LD_{50}/LC_{50} data, of the toxicity of materials. However, as discussed in Chapter 1, comparison of such data should not be based solely on the LD_{50} or LC_{50} values, since they may result in misleading conclusions with respect to population hazards. An evaluation of all data, including 95% confidence limits, slope on the dose–mortality regression lines and times to death, is required.
- Some acute studies, if adequately monitored, may give information on the potential for long-term adverse health effects; e.g. delayed-onset peripheral neuropathy from overexposure to organophosphates (Johnson, 1992).

■ Give information needed to meet the requirements of regulatory authorities with respect to classification into categories for use in various activities such as handling, transportation and labelling. Although there are geographical differences in the definition of the various classification bands, there is much activity to attempt to reach harmonization of classification standards on an international basis.

Additionally, and when the available information is sufficient, acute exposure studies may give an indication of some of the potential for local and/or systemic toxicity by repeated exposure. For example, local cutaneous or respiratory tract irritant (inflammatory) effects caused by acute exposure may be anticipated to occur also by repeated exposure to lower concentrations. However, the potential for materials to produce systemic toxicity by acute exposure must be carefully interpreted, as must also the extrapolation of such findings to repeated exposure conditions. For example, a dose–response relationship for liver injury when the test substance is given perorally may strongly suggest a potential for cumulative hepatotoxicity by lower dose repeated exposure, e.g. with organic arsenicals (Ballantyne, 1978). In other instances, specific acute organ injury may be a secondary effect; for example, renal tubular necrosis in acute inhalation studies with irritant materials may be a consequence of hypoxaemia secondary to lung injury (Ballantyne and Callaway, 1972). A proper evaluation of the potential for toxicity by repeated exposure requires that repeated exposure studies be conducted. Only in this way can reliable no observed effect levels (NOELs) and no observed adverse effect levels (NOAELs) be established.

DETERMINANTS FOR REPEATED EXPOSURE TOXICITY

As noted previously, acute studies may show a potential for cumulative local and systemic toxicity, if the effects are not secondary to some marked disturbance of physiology and if they are dose-related. However, in most acute studies the test material is given by bolus dosing, resulting in the rapid development of high circulating parent material and metabolites, if the dosed material is readily absorbed by the route of exposure. In these circumstances, the threshold to induce toxicity may be exceeded. With repeated exposure conditions, the individual doses given are usually much smaller than those employed in acute studies, and probably subthreshold for the induction of toxicity by acute dosing. In these circumstances there may be an incremental increase in body load of the material (and/or metabolite) with increasing sequential exposures, and there may be a latency to the onset of toxicity by repeated dose

procedures (Ballantyne, 1989). Many factors are associated with the likelihood for repeated exposure toxicity, and its nature, the most important of these being as follows:

(1) *Repeated exposure duration.* As noted above, there may be a latency to the development of body loading with parent material (or metabolite) which is sufficient to initiate the toxic effect. Clearly the number of exposures will be a determinant of the likelihood of reaching threshold body loads of toxic material and thus for the development of toxicity, as well as the absolute individual dosages.

(2) *Dosing characterisitics.* The precise profiling of exposure doses may have a significant influence on the development of toxicity, which may not be predictable from acute toxicity information. For example, with benzene vapour a 24 h exposure to 95 ppm or a 96 h exposure to 21 ppm produced severe bone marrow toxicity, but in a repeated exposure study involving exposure to 95 ppm vapour for 2 h day^{-1} for 2 weeks there was little toxicity (Toft *et al.*, 1982). The precise influence of profiling of dosing may vary depending on chemical nature. For example, in a 4 week inhalation study with formaldehyde, 8 h continuous exposures were compared with 8 h intermittent exposures (Wilmer *et al.*, 1987). The findings suggested that concentration rather than total dose was the major determinant of toxicity. Thus, interrupted exposures of rats to 10 or 20 ppm formaldehyde vapour induced more cytotoxicity in the nasal mucosa than did continuous exposure to 5 or 10 ppm. In a 4 week inhalation study with carbon tetrachloride, interruption of a daily 6 h exposure by 1–5 h periods free of carbon tetrachloride produced a slightly more severe hepatotoxicity, whereas 5 min peak loads superimposed on a fixed background exposure only slightly enhanced the hepatotoxicity of carbon tetrachloride (Bogers *et al.*, 1987).

(3) *Pharmacokinetics and metabolism.* Given by repeated exposure, the time available for compensatory biological responses is longer, in particular the induction of biotransformation mechanisms, including metabolic activation and detoxification. Depending on the route of exposure (including any first-pass involvement), the development of toxicity and its severity will depend on the relative balance of the induction of activation and detoxification processes.

DURATION OF REPEATED EXPOSURE STUDIES

Repeated exposure studies are usually conducted for a variable combination of the following reasons:

- Determine the potential for non-oncogenic cumulative or long-term toxic effects.
- Determine the *in vivo* oncogenic potential of a material.
- Determine threshold or no-observed adverse effect dosages, particularly when the results are to be used to protect populations, e.g. establishment of workplace exposure guidelines or acceptable daily intakes.
- To meet the requirements of regulatory authorities for activities such as product registration.

Depending on the reason(s) for conducting the investigations, and the stage of assessment of toxicity, repeated exposure studies vary in length from a few days to a lifetime of exposure. It is convenient to subdivide these into short-term, subchronic and chronic studies.

Short-term Repeated Studies

These vary in length from a few days (7–9 days) to 28 days. The shorter studies, around 7 days, have sometimes been referred to as subacute studies. Although the daily dosages employed may be less than the acute doses, the total duration of exposures is much longer [and not below (sub)] than for the acute exposures. The term 'subacute' is not a preferred descriptor. The choice for the duration of a short-term repeated exposure study will depend on a number of factors, including the reason for conducting the study.

Subchronic Studies

These studies involve exposing the test species for 15–20% of their lifespan. Thus, for most laboratory species used in subchronic tests (e.g. rats and mice), exposures will extend over a period of about 90 days. These studies are usually conducted in order to determine the potential for non-oncogenic adverse effects, and their threshold (lowest observed adverse effect level; LOAEL) and no observable adverse effect level (NOAEL). Additionally, and to ensure an appropriate choice of dosing, they are conducted in advance of chronic toxicology studies.

Chronic Studies

Such studies involve exposing the test species to the test material for their lifespan, or the greater part thereof. Although a primary aim of many chronic studies is to investigate the *in vivo* potential for oncogenicity, the majority are usually conducted as combined chronic toxicity/oncogenicity studies. Because of the high cost of such studies, in the region of, or more, than a million dollars depending on the route of exposure, decisions on the need for, and design of, such studies requires very careful consideration.

It is clear that repeated exposure studies of varying duration should be carried out in sequence, with the shorter studies being conducted initially to give guidance on the types of adverse effects to be anticipated (and monitors for), and also to allow the choice of appropriate dosing for the longer studies.

GENERAL DESIGN FEATURES

Details concerning animal use and care, statistical considerations, and design aspects for toxicological studies are given in detail in Chapters 24, 13 and 15, respectively. The following comments give an overview of the major considerations in the development of protocols for repeated exposure studies.

Generic Issues in Experimental Design

During the design of any repeated exposure toxicity study, a multiplicity of differing factors need to be taken into account in developing a protocol. Failure to give adequate thought with respect to all, including minor, details may result in the conduct of an unsatisfactory study, or cause the introduction of artifacts, which complicates interpretation of the findings. Some of the more important relevant considerations are briefly discussed below.

Animals

In order to ensure comparability of groups, and to avoid complications from outlier animals, those which are used in a study are often selected to be of closely comparable age at the start of the study and within a restricted weight range, usually within two standard deviations of the batch mean weight for each sex. To ensure that the animals to be used in a particular repeated exposure toxicity study are healthy, a randomly selected subgroup from the test batch of animals should be checked for health status before the start of the study; this procedure involves, at least, examination by a clinical veterinarian, blood sampling for limited clinical chemistry and viral antibodies, examination for faecal parasites, necropsy for gross pathology, and histology of selected tissues and organs (to include respiratory tract, gastro-intestinal tract, liver, kidney, lymph node and spleen).

Environmental Conditions

To minimize the possible effect of environmental influences on both animal welfare and induced toxicity, factors such as environmental temperature and relative humidity should be maintained within accepted optimum conditions. Significant variations from the recommended range of animal house temperatures can increase susceptibility to infection, impair general health and cause a variation in response to toxic chemicals (WHO, 1978). Changes in temperature may elicit homeostatic changes in various physiological and biochemical systems, and alter rate-determining physiological processes for the absorption and action of toxic chemicals. Also, because of the influence of circadian factors on toxicity (Chapter 11), a constant photoperiod should be used.

The positioning of animals in holding rooms can influence certain physiological and pathological processes, and hence the requirement for randomization and periodic rotation of the position of individual cages at least weekly. It has also been advised (Ecobichon, 1992) that 'sentinel' animals be included in the longer term studies. These animals are not part of the definitive study, but placed in the same room as the test and control animals and periodically monitored for the appearance of bacterial or viral infections, test agent-induced toxic changes due to contamination of the facility or changes in environmental conditions. These animals should be subjected to periodic haematology, clinical chemistry and bacteriology/virology.

Caging

Toxicity can be influenced by a number of factors related to the manner of caging, including type of caging, grouping, and bedding material. For example, the toxicity of isoproterenol was greater in rats caged singly for more than 3 weeks than in rats caged in groups (Hatch *et al.*, 1965). In a study of the influence of housing conditions in skin oncogenicity bioassays, DePass *et al.* (1986) showed that difference in housing conditions can influence both the latency and incidence of local neoplasms resulting from chronic cutaneous application of a carcinogen. Multiple caging can result in unique identification problems and trauma from bites. Additionally, with multiple housing, the susceptibility to transmissible diseases is increased, and if mortalities occur there may be cannibalism. Also, multiple caging does not permit individual animal food consumption values to be obtained, and thus does not allow any correlations between individual weight changes and food consumption to be established. When dosing is by incorporation of test material into the diet, multiple caging does not permit the calculation of individual animal test agent consumption. For these reasons, it is generally recommended that for repeated dose toxicity studies animals should be caged singly (Wilson and Hayes, 1994).

The type of cage employed, metal or plastic, solid floor or suspended, requires careful consideration during protocol design (Stevens and Mylecraine, 1994). For example, solid floor caging requires bedding which may create dust, and certain sawdusts and chips may induce hepatic mixed function oxidase activity. Suspended wire cages, on the other hand, may result in trauma, especially to the feet and legs. Shoebox-type cages may cause problems associated with stasis of the air in the cage.

Most repeated exposure studies with rodents are generally conducted using suspended wire cages with the animals housed singly. This permits ease of clinical examinations and allows information to be obtained on food and water consumption.

Diet

It is well appreciated that both the degree and type of nutrition may affect laboratory animal lifespan, expression of toxicity, and the pattern of carcinogenicity in control and test-agent animals (Allaben and Hart, 1998; Haseman, 1998; Leakey *et al.*, 1998; Turturro *et al.*, 1998). Of particular importance in chronic studies is the marked influence that diet may have on natural tumour incidences, and also on modifying carcinogen-induced tumour incidence (Grasso, 1988). For example, Tucker (1979) demonstrated that Charles River mice on a 20% dietary restriction developed fewer liver tumours than mice fed diet *ad libitum*. Conybeare (1980) found that the incidence of liver tumours in mice was reduced from 47% to 12% by restricting food intake to 75% of the normal amount. Benson *et al.* (1956) found that a higher incidence of spontaneous mammary adenocarinomas developed in rats when olive oil was added to the diet, and Chan and Dao (1981) noted a higher incidence of mammary tumours in rats on a semi-synthetic diet containing 16% corn oil. Both the protein and fat content of diets may influence the induction of tumours by carcinogens. High fat diets enhance mammary tumour incidence caused by dimethylbenzanthracene in rats (Carroll and Khor, 1975), hepatocellular carcinomas in rats by *p*-dimethylaminoazobenzene (Miller and Miller, 1953), colon cancer by 1,2-dimethylhydrazine (Reddy *et al.*, 1976) and pancreatic adenocarcinomas by azaserine (Roebuck *et al.*, 1981). In the rat a high protein diet enhanced hepatocellular carcinoma development from aflotoxin (Madhavan and Gopalan, 1968), and colon carcinoma from 1,2-dimethylhydrazine (Reddy *et al.*, 1976).

Diet should ideally be kept constant over the study period and be of known composition and nutritional status. Diets should be used that have been assayed for contaminants such as pesticides, heavy metals and mycotoxins. They should not be used beyond expiratory dates and stored to prevent contamination.

Test Material

The material to be tested should be of known purity and its chemical identity confirmed. Test material purity, and possible degradation products, should be measured before the start and at the end of the study to ensure stability. With the longer repeated exposure studies, interim analyses may be required. If a dosing matrix, such as drinking water or diet, is used, then stability of the test material and homogeneity of distribution in the matrix are required. Ideally a single batch (lot) of the test material should be used over the study period to ensure an absence of effects due to possible changes and inconsistencies from batch to batch. This, of course, may not be possible with chronic studies, where there should be detailed attention to analyses and to documentation. Also, with materials to be used commercially, the test material should be as close as possible to that intended to be used or marketed.

Choice of Species

Most repeated exposure studies are conducted using rats or mice, with some regulatory agencies also requiring the (additional) use of a larger species (e.g. dog), particularly for subchronic studies. The choice of test species is an important consideration, particularly where there is reason to suspect that species variation in the toxic response may occur, qualitatively or quantitatively. An example is that of butadiene, where the toxic (carcinogenic) potential is greater in the mouse than the rat (Melnick *et al.*, 1990). Since it has been demonstrated that the metabolism of butadiene in the rat is more like that in the human than in the mouse, the rat appears to be a more appropriate model for repeated exposure studies (Bond *et al.*, 1995; Himmelstein *et al.*, 1997; Anderson, 1998).

Criteria for the selection of a species include:

(1) The requirements of regulatory agencies.
(2) The material should have similar pharmacokinetic and metabolic features in both the test species and humans. For the majority of substances, with the possible exception of therapeutic agents, this information is either sparse or not available. Therefore, from a practical viewpoint, this criterion can seldomly be applied.
(3) Use of the most sensitive species (and strain) to the known or suspect toxicity of the test material, on the basis that this represents the most conservative approach in extrapolating toxicity in the test species to humans. Again, such information may not be available at the start of repeated exposure testing, and acute toxicity information may not be a reliable guide to cumulative or long-term toxicity.
(4) Experience of the laboratory and the existence of a good historical control database. Although concurrent control animals should be used in repeated exposure studies, in some instances comparison with the treatment groups may yield equivocal results, and in such cases reference to the historical database may be of use.

In view of the fact that there are species variabilities in the response to toxic chemicals, and since no one species is a perfect surrogate for the human, several regulatory agencies require the use of two species, often citing a rodent and a non-rodent. Often the choice of a species is based on considerations which included experience, animal size, ease of handling, databases, accommodation and economics. However, and if it exists, these should be secondary to information on the pharmacokinetics and metabolism of the test material, its known toxicity, and physicochemical characteristics.

Dosing Procedures

The route of exposure will be determined principally by the intended use of the test material and the likely route by which the user will be exposed. In some instances there could be a need for study by more than one route of exposure. For example, with pesticides the applicator may be exposed cutaneously or by inhalation, whereas the consumers of treated crops will be exposed through the peroral route. In most cases the appropriate route can be used in repeated exposure studies, but in a very few instances because of physical or technical problems an alternative route may be required. An example is provided by ethylenediamine (EDA) for which the respiratory tract is a potential route of exposure. However, generation of the vapour for a long-term study presents difficulties, as do the sampling and analyses of the chamber atmosphere; also, EDA reacts with water and carbon dioxide. These problems hamper the conduct of a chronic inhalation study with EDA. In a comparative pharmacokinetic and metabolism study, EDA was given by oral, intravenous and endotracheal dosing. The equivalency of the fate of EDA by the peroral and endotrachal routes was demonstrated (Yang and Tallant, 1982). Based on these findings, a chronic toxicity/carcinogenicity study was successfully completed in the rat by incorporation of EDA into the diet (Hermansky *et al.*, 1999).

By the peroral route, a multiplicity of dosing procedures are available, the choice of which will depend on the intended use of the test material, physical and chemical characteristics, likely exposure patterns in the user, stability of test material, and the test species. In some instances the material may be given by gavage. This procedure ensures that relatively precise daily pulses of chemical are given, but carries the disadvantage that intubation trauma and dose misplacement may occur. Many peroral repeated dosage studies are conducted by incorporating the test material into diet or drinking water, resulting in a slower titration of the material into the gastrointestinal tract. There may well be differences, therefore, between the absorption pharmacokinetics of test material depending on whether it is given by gavage or dietary/drinking water incorporation. This factor needs consideration in the design and interpretation of studies. When given by inclusion in the diet, it is essential to conduct studies to ensure homogeneity of distribution and stability in the diet, and also to conduct extraction procedures to preclude binding to the diet which will significantly reduce bioavailability. When test material is incorporated into the diet for dosing, it is common practice to adjust the dietary concentration of test material periodically (usually weekly) to achieve constancy of the target daily doses against a progressively changing body weight. Mean projected dietary concentration is calculated from the preceding body weight gain, and the dietary test material concentration is adjusted to achieve constancy of dosing. Feeding at a constant concentration during a study has also been conducted, but this results in loss of control of constant dosage and may modify toxic response and interpretation of the findings from the study (Wilson and Hayes, 1994). As with dietary incorporation studies, when test material is dissolved in drinking water, homogeneity of distribution and stability needs to be confirmed. Also, the test material should not be so unpalatable as to reduce food or water consumption significantly. In special circumstances the test material may require to be dosed using capsules or by an encapsulation procedure; this is particularly useful for highly volatile materials or to mask objectionable taste. Microencapsulation involves uniformly coating the test material with a degradable but impervious material (Melnik *et al.*, 1987; Yuan *et al.*, 1991).

By inhalation, the study design will depend on whether exposure is to gas, vapour or aerosol. The principles of ensuring constancy of exposure dose and avoiding artifacts are similar to those by other routes of exposure. The details of generation, distribution, sampling and analysis of the atmosphere should follow the guidance given in Chapter 30. If whole body exposures are undertaken then the possibility for some percutaneous absorption and, more significantly, swallowing of material due to grooming should be kept in mind, particularly during interpretation of the findings. This can be avoided by the extra precaution of nose-only exposures. Additionally, measures should be in place to avoid exposure of the laboratory worker or contamination of the animal facility after the end of an exposure period. This will include keeping the animals in a stream of fresh air for a period after the exposure has been completed.

Repeated exposure skin contact studies are labour intensive. Again, prevention of secondary route of exposure by licking the test site should be avoided by choosing an appropriate remote application site and/or covering the application site. Based on screening or prior definitive studies, care should be taken to avoid the development of cumulative local skin irritation or injury that could lead to a premature termination of the study.

Repeated exposure studies have been conducted using parenteral routes such as intravenous, intramuscular, intraperitoneal and subcutaneous. Such labour-intensive studies require special careful attention to the dosing techniques in order to avoid trauma associated with the injection process. Alternative parenteral dosing procedures for continuous dosing by slow release procedures have included the use of implanted material or implantable osmotic minipumps (Dey *et al.*, 1982; Ray and Theeuwes, 1987; see also Chapter 26).

Exposure Groups

A prime consideration in the design of repeated exposure studies is the number of groups of animals to be used. A minimum of three groups should be used for exposure to differing concentrations or dosages of the test material. This allows the demonstration of a dose–response relationship, essential for confirmation of a toxic process. Also, and by careful choice of dosages, by using three groups this should allow for one which exhibits toxicity (top dose), one showing a marginal or lowest observable effect level (LOAEL), which should be with the intermediate dose, and a NOAEL or NOEL at the lowest dose. This information is used principally in two ways: first, in using the dose–response information for the purposes of defining safety margins in hazard evaluations and assigning permissible exposures (e.g. TLV or ADI), and second, in setting exposure concentrations or doses for longer term repeated exposure studies. In the latter case, and particularly when using information derived from a subchronic study conducted prior to a chronic study, one prime determinant is the establishment of a maximum tolerated dose (MTD). This is a dose which is usually defined as causing no more than a 10% decrease in body weight, does not produce mortality, and produces effects that will not shorten the lifespan and jeopardize the study, but nevertheless produce some toxicity (Sontag *et al*, 1976; Haseman, 1985). The MTD is mostly used as a basis for assigning the highest dose for a chronic study.

The numbers of animals used per treatment group requires careful planning. There should be sufficient to allow for valid statistical analyses, but not in excess of the numbers dictated by good animal welfare practices. Depending on the length of the study, basic group size (from start to end of dosing) often range from 5 to 20 animals per sex. For subchronic and chronic studies, 20 per sex per group is a reasonable basic group size. Additional animals may be included if 'recovery' groups are required to assess reversibility, or otherwise, of induced toxicity after the end of the dosing period. This is a useful group to have for interpretive purposes, particularly with subchronic studies. The use of 'recovery' animals in the shorter term repeated exposure studies should also be considered. These 'recovery' animals are most frequently added to the high-dose and control groups. Additionally, and in order to study the onset and progression of induced toxicity, many studies also add extra animals for interim sacrifice at predetermined times during the exposure period. These groups also may yield valuable information useful in assessing dose-response relationships.

An untreated control group, equal in size to a dosing group (including interim sacrifice and 'recovery' animals), is of course necessary for primary comparative purposes against the treatment groups. Such a concurrent control group not only serves for the comparison of statistical and dose–response relationships of induced lesions, but may also indicate the presence of any non-treatment and environmental effects. Where the test material has to dosed in a vehicle (solvent or suspending agent), some investigators suggest the need to confirm an absence of effects by the vehicle by inclusion of a vehicle control group. It will have been previously confirmed that the inert vehicle dose not react with the test agent and the preparation has stability. The requirement for a vehicle control group will depend on the length of the study, physicochemical properties of the vehicle and the extent to which it has been investigated toxicologically.

An important consideration in planning and protocol development is the development of criteria for decisions on when, and how, to euthanize animals that become moribund during the dosing period. These criteria should be in accord with Good Laboratory Practice procedures, conducting laboratory practices, and state and/or federal animal welfare regulations (Ecobichon, 1992).

Monitoring for Toxicity

Repeated exposure toxicity studies are costly, in part because of their labour-intensive nature. It therefore follows that the maximum amount of toxicological and usable information should be obtained from them by appropriate extensive monitoring for toxic and other possible treatment related effects. In this way, a repeat of the study can be avoided because of unexpected secondary findings indicating a primary toxicity not detected *per se*. Extensive monitoring is employed in the longer term (subchronic and chronic) studies in order to define, as far as possible, evidence for structural and functional injury to tissues and organs. Whilst the shorter term (7–9 days) studies are often conducted as screening (preliminary) for the longer term studies, and used to set dosages for such longer duration studies, it is wise to undertake some specialized monitoring to assess potential target organs and tissues by short-term repeated exposure, and also aid in the planning of detailed monitoring in the longer term study. The 28 day studies should certainly be well monitored, as for a subchronic study, particularly if they are to be submitted to a regulatory agency.

 For the longer term studies (subchronic and chronic), very detailed monitoring should be planned to include, as a basis, well recognized monitors for the general detec-

tion of potentially adverse effects, and also specific techniques to assess sites of toxic response in particular organs and tissues.

Routinely, and discussed in more detail in the Sub-chronic Studies section, the major overall monitors should include at least the following:

- Clinical observations for signs of toxic and/or pharmacological effects.
- Periodic measurement of body weight.
- Food and water consumption.
- Peripheral blood haematology.
- Blood biochemistry (clinical chemistry).
- Urinalysis.
- Necropsy for signs of gross pathology.
- Organ weights.
- Processing of tissues and organs for histological examination.

It is important to compare clinical pathology findings from treatment groups to those of the concurrent control groups, for which blood has been collected under identical conditions. For example, Walter (1999) compared clinical pathology values for blood collected from the orbital sinus of rats anaesthetized with either pure (100%) carbon dioxide or an oxygen/carbon dioxide mixture (34%, 66%) with the values for blood from un-anaesthetized rats. Small, but statistically significant, differences were found for several values; thus, for the carbon dioxide groups there were smaller values for calcium, and higher values for leukocyte counts, lymphocyte counts, and glucose. A larger proportionate difference was found for creatine kinase and aspartate aminotransferase activities, with values being highest in the unanaesthetized group. This was attributed to the physical activity in this group of animals. When it is necessary to review study findings by comparing with laboratory historical control values, as for example in studies where the chemical pathology findings are borderline, equivocal, or inexplicable, then the comparisons should be made with great care because of the influence of various factors on measured values; e.g. mode and site of collection of blood samples, whether they are taken from anaesthetized, unanaesthetized or sacrificed animals, and the analytical methods employed.

For haematology, clinical chemistry and urinalysis, the choice of individual measurements may vary from laboratory to laboratory, often based on their experience, but certain core measurements are necessary in all studies (see Chapters 17 and 18). In some studies, viewed on a case-by-case basis, additional specialized monitoring may be considered necessary based on information already available or suspect toxicology resulting, for example, from structure–activity considerations. Thus, in the planning of the protocol, there is a clear need to consider the requirement for additional ('non-standard') monitors. For example, with 5-ethylidene-2-norbornene

(ENB), and based on older studies (Kinkead *et al.*, 1971), there was some evidence to suggest a possible effect of ENB on the thyroid gland. Thus, in more recently conducted studies on the repeated exposure toxicity of ENB, provision was made for measurement of thyroid hormones and TSH in serum, and for detailed histology of the thyroid gland including morphometry (Ballantyne *et al.*, 1997). In an NTP study on the subchronic inhalation toxicology of glutaraldehyde, additional monitors included sperm morphology, vaginal cytology and histo-autoradiographic evaluation of respiratory tract cell replication rates in the nasal mucosal epithelium (NTP, 1993). These are but two examples, of many, in which additional monitoring was added to clarify any suspect toxicity. It is becoming more common for additional monitoring to be added to repeated exposure studies to detect effects, some not anticipated, in order to take advantage of the exposure conditions. For example, some regulatory agencies now advise adding monitors for male fertility to repeated exposure studies (e.g. sperm morphology, counts, motility). Thought should be given to the use of histochemical, ultrastructural, neurotoxic, respiratory function and genetic toxicology methods in repeated exposure studies when considered appropriate based on known or suspect toxicology.

Non-invasive procedures (e.g. observations for clinical signs, body weights, food and water consumption) should be conducted before exposure and then sequentially during the treatment and recovery periods. This allows for the detection of any general factors which may indicate the onset of toxicity, or effects secondary to factors not related to test material dosing. Haematology, clinical chemistry and urinalysis, need to be conducted as a minimum at the end of the dosing period. Where there are provisions for interim sacrifices, then chemical pathology should be undertaken at these times in order to detect any early changes. It may also be possible to collect blood and urine samples at interim periods during the dosing phase even if interim sacrifices are not planned. Decisions on whether to conduct chemical pathology on 'recovery' animals in the post-treatment survival groups may depend on whether there are definitive or equivocal changes in the immediate post-treatment sacrificed animals. Because of the automated nature of most chemical pathology investigations, it is recommended that measurements be undertaken on all control and treatment groups, and at the same period of time, to allow valid statistical comparisons. Observations for gross pathology at necropsy and removal of organs for weighing should be conducted on all animals. Organs and tissues showing gross pathological changes, together with those from a predetermined list, should be removed and processed for histological examination. The number of tissues removed will be determined, in part, by the reason for conducting the study and regulatory requirements, but in most cases it is advisable to remove as many as possible and, at least, keep those not to be examined in fixative in case of the need for examination of them in the future. It is usual in both subchronic and chronic studies to undertake light microscopic examination of all removed tissues from the high-dose and control groups. Decisions on whether to examine tissues from the lower dose and recovery groups will depend on the findings from the control and high-dose groups.

SHORT-TERM REPEATED EXPOSURE STUDIES

As noted previously, these studies extend over a period of 7–28 days. They are conducted to obtain an initial indication of the potential for adverse effects by recurrent exposure to the test material, and also as a preliminary to obtain guidance on appropriate doses for a subchronic study. For the latter purpose, it is common to use studies of 7–9 days duration. Since there is a greater likelihood for toxicity to be manifested with increasing time of exposure, 28 day studies may be accepted by some regulatory agencies as meeting the requirements for assessing non-oncogenic toxicity by repeated exposure. Detailed monitoring, equivalent to that for a subchronic study, should be incorporated into the 28 day protocol. However, even with the shorter periods, monitoring should ideally be more than signs, body weight, food and water consumption, and gross pathology. There should, at least, be some limited haematology, clinical chemistry and histology. In this way a better indication of potential toxicity will be obtained, and permit a more reliable guidance for the design of subchronic studies.

SUBCHRONIC STUDIES

These are usually carried out by exposure for 15–20% of the lifespan of the test species. Thus for most common laboratory animals they will be of about 3 months duration with respect to the dosing period. Such studies allow a determination of the potential non-oncogenic toxicity of the test material, allow the determination of definitive, threshold and no-effects dosages, including an MTD, and are essential for the successful planning of a chronic study. Many aspects of the design of these studies (species, housing conditions, mode of dosing, etc.) have been discussed earlier in this chapter and also in Chapter 15.

All subchronic studies should have at least three test chemical treatment groups, together with untreated controls and, if necessary, vehicle controls. It is always advisable to add a recovery group of animals to determine the reversibility, or otherwise, of induced toxicity. The need for interim sacrifice or monitoring groups will be determined by the nature of the test agent and its known toxicology.

It is necessary to incorporate into the study design procedures which may permit the detection of unsuspected toxicity, latency to onset and reversibility. Monitoring procedures should allow for the sensitive detection of early indications of toxicity, latency to toxicity and reversibility of induced toxicity. They should allow for the detection of structural and functional indications of general toxic effects and specific organ or tissue lesions. Standard lists of recommended procedures for monitoring are available in published texts and regulatory guidelines. However, investigators should add, as routine, methods usually conducted in follow-up tests to confirm specific toxic effects, e.g. the inclusion of α_{2u}-globulin measurements in urine to confirm biochemically, a hyaline droplet nephropathy.

Monitoring for subchronic studies should include the following as necessary to ensure the best conditions to detect non-oncogenic toxicity:

(1) *Clinical observations*. Animals should be examined twice daily for overt signs of toxicity and for mortality. Animals should be examined in detail on a weekly basis with particular respect to skin and fur condition, eyes, mucosae, respiratory, circulatory and nervous system functions and general behaviour. These are standard to most profiles. Many subchronic studies do not have provision for the detailed examination of the eye, and some ophthalmic toxicology may be missed. It is useful to have, as a minimum, expert examination of the eyes by an ophthalmic veterinarian using biomicroscopy at the start and end of dosing. There is also increasing use of a functional observational battery (FOB) as a screen for the potential of a chemical to produce neurotoxicity (Chapter 34).

(2) *Body weight*. Body weights should be measured before dosing and at least weekly during the dosing and recovery periods. Body weight changes for the interweighing periods should be calculated. Body weight and body weight changes are sensitive indicators of the condition of the animals. Changes (usually loss) can be a consequence of alterations in food or water consumption, specific toxic effects or disease processes.

(3) *Food consumption*. This is a useful monitor if measured over 3 day or weekly intervals. Appropriate containers are needed to limit errors due to spillage. Food consumption data may be useful in the interpretation of body weight changes, and is of course essential if dosing is by incorporation in the diet in order to calculate consumed dosages.

(4) *Water consumption*. This measurement, over 3 or 7 day intervals, requires the use of individual water bottles for its determination. The information can be of considerable use in assessing body weight or urine volume changes.

(5) *Haematology*. Details of the use and application of peripheral blood haematology tests are given in Chapter 18. The following are typical measurements made:

- haemoglobin concentration;
- erythrocyte count;
- packed red blood cell volume (PCV);
- calculated values; mean corpuscular volume (MCV), mean corpuscular haemoglobin (MCH), mean corpuscular haemoglobin concentration (MCHC);
- leukocyte count—total and differential;
- platelet count;
- reticulocyte count;
- activated partial thromboplastin time.

(6) *Biochemical disturbances*. For detecting general biochemical disturbances (e.g. electrolytes) or to indicate specific organ/tissue damage, a multiplicity of tests are available (Chapter 17). The following measurements are typical for subchronic studies:

- glucose;
- urea nitrogen;
- creatinine;
- total protein, albumin and globulin (often with protein electrophoresis);
- bilirubin (total, conjugated and unconjugated);
- phosphorus;
- Ca^{2+}, Na^+, K^+, Cl^-, HCO_3^-;
- aspartate aminotransferase
- alanine aminotransferase
- creatine kinase
- sorbitol dehydrogenase
- γ-glutamyl transferase
- alkaline phosphatase
- glutamate dehydrogenase
- ornithine carbamyltransferase
- special studies (e.g. with organophosphates, measurement of acetylcholinesterase and butyrylcholinesterase).

(7) *Urinalysis*. Analysis of urine can yield valuable information not only on renal and urinary tract integrity, but also on acid–base balance and certain organ dysfunctions. Specimens should be collected separately, ideally using metabolic cages, over a specifically timed period (usually 16h). Typical measurements and observations include the following:

- volume;
- appearance;
- microscopy;
- pH;
- osmolality;
- protein;

- occult blood;
- glucose;
- ketones;
- bilirubin and urobilinogen;
- creatinine;
- α_{2u}-globulin;
- N-acetyl-β-D-glucosaminidase.

(8) *Necropsy and organ weights.* Necropsy examination with detailed inspection for gross pathology is required on all animals; those that die on study and sacrificed survivors at the interim, immediate post-treatment and recovery periods. Organs removed for weighing usually include brain, liver, kidneys, lungs, heart, spleen, thymus, adrenal glands and gonads. Whilst organ weights relative to body weight should be calculated, if changes in body weights have occurred these relative organ weight values may be misleading. For this reason it is also advisable to calculate organ weights relative to brain weight, since this is less variable and test materials that lead to a change in body weight do not generally affect brain weight.

(9) *Histology.* Light microscopic examination of all tissues and organs showing gross pathology should be undertaken. Many studies examine only other (no gross pathology) tissues from the high dose and control groups. Should histopathology be seen in the high-dose group, then tissues from the other treatment groups should be examined. Decisions on the need to examine tissues from recovery group animals will depend on the findings from the immediate post-dosing sacrifice group.

It is wise to remove as many tissues and organs as possible and keep them in fixative. Those to be examined are given in standard texts and regulatory guidelines, but investigators should carefully consider the needs for histology based on these and the nature of the study. Tissues not prepared for histology should be kept in fixative in case a subsequent need for their examination arises. Special staining techniques may be required based on the findings of the study overall, e.g. myelin stain with suspect neurotoxicity and Mallory Heidenhaim stain for hyaline droplet nephropathy.

CHRONIC TOXICITY STUDIES

A chronic study is conducted with the objective of exposure to the test material for the lifespan of the test species, or a significant proportion of it. Therefore, with the small laboratories animals conventionally used, the dosing extends over a period of about 2 years. The majority of these studies are conducted with the objective of determining the carcinogenic potential of the test material, and only in a relatively few cases is it necessary to extend a subchronic study into a chronic study based on the non-oncogenic toxicity potential of the test material. Nevertheless, most chronic studies are carried as a combined chronic toxicity and carcinogenicity study, since this allows a more definitive assessment of threshold and no-effects levels for known non-oncogenic effects. In this respect they give a more reliable estimate of safety margins in risk assessment procedures and the assignment of permissible exposure levels where there is long-term human, but controllable, exposure; e.g. pesticides, food additives and food contaminants. With respect to determining the carcinogenic potential of a material, this may be seen in one of several ways, or a combination of them. These are, in comparison with the controls, a decrease in latency to occurrence of tumours found in the controls, an increased incidence of tumours of the types seen in the controls, the development of tumours not seen in controls, and an increase in the multiplicity of tumours in individual animals. Dose–response relationships and statistical significance compared with the untreated controls are important interpretive considerations.

A decision to conduct a chronic study clearly requires a detailed analysis of the need for and advantages of the study. This will include considerations on the use and exposure pattern of the test material, findings from other toxicology studies, known dose–response relationships and their relevance to in-use situations, and the demands of regulatory agencies. For example, a material of well established non-oncogenic toxicity potential with positive findings in genetic toxicology studies will have a higher priority for chronic testing than a material of known non-oncogenic toxicity potential but shown not to be mutagenic or clastogenic in a number of genetic toxicology studies.

In view of the duration, labour-intensive nature and high cost of chronic toxicology studies, it is of the greatest importance that they be planned in fine detail to ensure that the objectives for conducting the study are met, including monitoring procedures, and that there is the maximum likelihood for survival over the test period of those animals not affected by known toxicity (e.g. detailed considerations on animal welfare standards and the exclusion of factors that would cause morbidity and mortality for reason unconnected with the test material). The widest representation of views should be obtained in the planning phase, including those of pathologists and statisticians, and with possible discussions involving the relevant regulatory agencies (national and international). As stated by Stevens and Mylecraine (1994), 'Doing the study right therefore requires that we concern ourselves with the demands of science *and* society—they need not be mutually exclusive'.

Detailed considerations for the conduct of chronic toxicology studies have been given (WHO, 1978; Stevens and Mylecraine, 1994). There should be at least three treatment groups and a control group. The control group should be at least equal to that of one of the treatment groups. Some investigators have used two (separate) control groups against which statistical comparisons can be made. In many cases the use of two control groups, with separate statistical evaluation, has led to interpretive complications due to, at least in part, to random differences in tumour incidence between the two control groups. It may be better, for comparative statistical purposes, to have a large-size single control group, possibly equal in numbers to the combined treatment groups. Essential to a study of latency is the use of several interim sacrifice groups; as a minimum these should be at 6, 12 and 18 months. However, others suggest a larger number of interim sacrifices, starting at 3 months. In this manner a comparison can be made between the first interim sacrifice and the findings from a previously conducted subchronic study, with respect to the quantitative aspects of the toxicity potential of the test material. Group size should be adequate for both survival considerations and subsequent detailed statistical analyses. At least 20 per sex per group should be used for the final sacrifice (2 year) group. Dose selection is usually based on an MTD defined by the subchronic study, which requires careful interpretation against the objectives and conditions for the chronic study. Monitoring for non-oncogenic end-points is normally the same as for the subchronic study, with additional procedures based on the findings from the subchronic study, and other known toxicology.

The results from repeated exposure studies clearly require to be interpreted in terms of metabolic and pharmacokinetic considerations, such as incremental increases in body or organ/tissue load required to initiate a toxic process, storage of parent material and/or metabolites and their rate of release from storage sites, development of repair processes, and the balance of induced metabolic activation and detoxification mechanisms. The mode of dosing may influence the toxic response, including route of exposure which will determine the overall rate of absorption and the potential for relative and absolute metabolic activation and detoxification. Also, the pharmacokinetic characteristics and potential for toxicity may depend on whether dosing is by repeated boluses (eg. gavage) or continuous administration (eg. drinking water or food). With the former, intermittent fluctuating high body loading is likely to be attained, and retention of parent material and metabolites will depend on their route(s) and rate of excretion. With sustained dosing, the attainment of a body and tissue/organ load to initiate and sustain a toxic process will be determined by the dynamic equilibrium between absorption, biodistribution, storage, and excretion. The same daily dose delivered by bolus or else by sustained dosing may result in differences in the quantitative expression of toxicity, and in some cases the nature of the toxic response. Additionally, and in contrast with acute studies, with the longer term repeated exposure studies there may be changing tissue sensitivity with increasing age, altered physiological and metabolic capacities, and the development of spontaneous disease processes. Thus, the interpretation of the findings from long-term repeated exposure studies should be against not only the apparent toxicity produced, but also against the possible influence of various changing biological parameters.

REFERENCES

Allaben, W. T. and Hart, R. W. (1998). Nutrition and toxicity modulation: the impact of animal body weight on study outcome. *Int. J. Toxicol.*, **17**, Suppl. 2, 1–3.

Anderson, D. (1998). Butadiene: species comparison for metabolism and genetic toxicology. *Mutat. Res.*, **405**, 247–258.

Ballantyne, B. (1978). The comparative short-term mammalian toxicology of phenarsazine oxide and phenoxarsine oxide. *Toxicology*, **10**, 341–361.

Ballantyne, B. (1989). Toxicology. In *Encyclopedia of Polymer Science and Engineering*, 2nd edn., Vol. 16. Wiley, New York, pp. 879–930.

Ballantyne, B. and Callaway, S. (1972). Inhalation toxicology and pathology of animals exposed to *o*-chlorobenzylidene malononitrile. *Med. Sci. Law*, **12**, 43–65.

Ballantyne, B., Norris, J. C., Dodd, D. E., Klonne, D. R., Losco, P. E., Neptun, D. A., Price, S. C. and Grasso, P. (1997). Short-term and subchronic repeated exposure studies with 5-ethylidene-2-norbornene vapor in the rat. *J. Appl. Toxicol.*, **17**, 197–210.

Benson, J., Lev, M. and Grand, C. G. (1956). Enhancement of mammary fibroadenomas in the female rat by a high fat diet. *Cancer Res.*, **16**, 135–137.

Bogers, M., Appelman, L. M., Feron, V. M., Beems, R. B. and Notten, W. R. F. (1987). Effects of the exposure profile on the inhalation toxicity of carbon tetrachloride in male mice. *J. Appl. Toxicol.*, **1**, 185–191.

Bond, J. A., Recio, L. and Andjelkovich, D. (1995). Epidemiological and mechanistic data suggest that 1,3-butadiene will not be carcinogenic in humans at exposures likely to be encountered in the environment or workplace. *Carcinogenesis*, **16**, 165–171.

Carroll, K. K. and Khor, H. T. (1975). Dietary fat in relation to tumorigenesis. *Prog. Biochem. Pharmacol.*, **10**, 303–353.

Chan, P. C. and Dao, T. L. (1981). Enhancement of mammary carcinogenesis by a high fat diet in Fischer, Long–Evans and Sprague–Dawley rats. *Cancer Res.*, **41**, 164–167.

Conybeare, G. (1980). Effect of quality and quantity of diet on survival and tumor incidence in outbred Swiss mice. *Food Cosmet. Toxicol.*, **18**, 65.

DePass, L. R., Weil, C. S., Ballantyne, B., Lewis, S. C., Losco, P. E., Reid, J. B. and Simon, G. S. (1986). Influence of housing conditions for mice on the results of a dermal oncogenicity bioassay. *Fundam. Appl. Toxicol.*, **7**, 601–608.

Dey, M. S., Breeze, R. A., Dey, R. A., Kreiger, R. I., Naser, L. J. and Renzl, B. E. (1982). Disposition and toxicity of paraquat delivered subcutaneously by injection and osmotic pump in the rat. *Toxicologist*, **2**, 96.

Ecobichon, D. J. (1992). *The Basis of Toxicity Testing*. CRC Press, Boca Raton, FL, pp. 61–82.

Grasso, P. (1988). Carcinogenicity tests in animals: some pitfalls that can be avoided. In Ballantyne, B. (Ed.), *Perspectives in Basic and Applied Toxicology*. Wright, Bristol, pp. 268–284.

Haseman, J. K. (1985). Issues in carcinogenicity testing: dose selection. *Fundam. Appl. Toxicol.*, **5**, 66–78.

Haseman, J. K. (1998). National Toxicology Program experience with dietary restriction: does the manner in which reduced body weight is achieved affect tumor incidence? *Int. J. Toxicol.*, **17**, Suppl. 2, 119–134.

Hatch, A., Balazo, T., Wiberg, G. S. and Grice, H. C. (1965). The importance of avoiding mental suffering in laboratory animals. *Anim. Welfare Inst. Rep.*, **14**, No. 3.

Hermansky, S. J., Yang, R. S. H., Garman R. H. and Leung, H-W (1999). Chronic toxicity and carcinogenicity studies of ethylenediamine. *Food Chem. Toxicol.*, in press.

Himmelstein, M. W., Acquavella, J. F., Recio, L., Medinski, M. A. and Bond, J. A. (1997). Carcinogenicity and epidemiology of 1,3-butadiene. *Crit. Rev. Toxicol.*, **27**, 1–128.

Johnson, M. K. (1992). Molecular events in delayed neuropathy: Experimental aspects of neuropathy target esterase. In, Ballantyne, B. and Marrs, T. C. (Eds), *Clinical and Experimental Toxicology of Organophosphates and Carbamates*. Butterworth-Heinemann, Oxford, pp. 90–113.

Kinkead, E. R., Pozzane, V. C., Geary, D. L. and Carpenter, C. P. (1971). The mammalian toxicology of ethylidene norbornene [5-ethylidenbicyclo(2,2,1)hept-2-ene]. *Toxicol. Appl. Pharmacol.*, **20**, 250–259.

Leakey, J. E. A., Seng, J. E., Barnas, C. R., Baker, V. M. and Hart, R. W. (1998). A mechanistic basis for the beneficial effects of caloric restriction on longevity and disease: consequences for the interpretation of rodent toxicity studies. *Int. J. Toxicol.*, **17**, Suppl. 2, 5–56.

Madhavan, T. V. and Gopalan, C. (1968). The effect of dietary protein on carcinogenesis by aflotoxin. *Arch. Pathol.*, **85**, 133–137.

Melnick, R. J., Jameson, C. W., Goehl, T. J., Maronpot, R. R., Collins, B. J., Greenwall, A., Harrington, F. W., Wilson, R. E., Tomaszewstei, R. E. and Argwal, D. R. (1987). Appliction of microencapsulation for toxicology studies: II. Toxicity of microencapsulation trichlormethylene in Fischer 344 rats. *Fundam. Appl. Toxicol.*, **8**, 432–442.

Melnick, R. L., Huff, J., Chou, B. J. and Miller, R. A. (1990). Carcinogenicity of 1,3-butadiene in (C57B1/6 × 3CH) F1 mice at low exposure concentrations. *Cancer Res.*, **50**, 6593–6599.

Miller, J. A. and Miller, E. C. (1953). The carcinogenic aminoazo dyes. *Adv. Cancer Res.*, **1**, 339–396.

NTP (1993). NTP Technical Report on Toxicity Studies of Glutaraldehyde Administered by Inhalation to F344/N and B6C3F₁ Mice. *NIH Publication 93-3348*. US Department of Health and Human Services, Public Health Service, National Institutes of Health, Washington, DC.

Ray, N. and Theeuwes, F. (1987). Implantable osmotically powered drug delivery system. In Johnson, A. and Lloyd-Jones, J. (Eds), *Drug Delivery Systems*. Ellis Horwood, Chichester. pp. 120–138.

Reddy, B. S., Narisawa, T., Vukusich, D., *et al.* (1976). Effects of quality and quantity of dietary fat and dimethyl hydrazine in colon carcinogenesis in rats. *Proc. Sci. Exp. Biol. Med.*, **151**, 237–239.

Roebuck, B. D., Yager, J. D. and Longnecker, D. S. (1981). Modulation of azaserine induced pancreatic carcinogenesis in the rat. *Cancer Res.*, **41**, 888–893.

Sontag, J. M., Page, N. P. and Safiotti, U. (1976). Guidelines for Carcinogen Bioassays in Small Rodents. *Department of Health and Human Services Publication NIH/76–801*. National Cancer Institute, Bethesda, MD.

Stevens, K. R. and Mylecraine (1994). Issues in chronic toxicology. In Hayes, A. W. (Ed), *Principles and Methods of Toxicology*. Raven Press, New York, pp. 673–695.

Toft, K., Olofsson T., Tunek, A. and Berlin, M. (1982). Toxic effects on mouse bone marrow caused by inhalation of benzene. *Arch. Toxicol.*, **51**, 295–302.

Tucker, M. J. (1979). The effect of long-term food restriction on tumors in rodents. *Int. J. Cancer*, **23**, 803–807.

Turturro, A., Hass, B., Hart, R. and Allaben, W. T. (1998). Body weight impact on spontaneous diseases in chronic bioassays. *Int. J. Toxicol.*, **17**, Suppl. 2, 79–99.

Tyler, T. and Ballantyne, B. (1988). Practical assessment and communication of chemical hazards in the workplace. In Ballantyne, B. (Ed.), *Perspectives on Basic and Applied Toxicology*. Wright, Bristol, pp. 330–378.

Walter, G. L. (1999). Effects of carbon dioxide inhalation on hematology, coagulation, and serum clinical chemistry values in rats. *Toxicologic Path.*, **27**, 217–225.

WHO (1978). Principles and methods for evaluating the toxicity of chemicals. Part 1. *Environmental Health Criteria No. 6*. World Health Organization, Geneva.

Wilmer, J. W. G. M., Wouterson, R. A., Appelman, L. M., Leeman, W. R. and Feron, V. J. (1987). Subacute (4-week) inhalation toxicity study of formaldehyde in male rats: 8-hour intermittent versus 8-hour continuous exposure. *J. Appl. Toxicol.*, **7**, 15–16.

Wilson, N. H. and Hayes, J. P. (1994). Short-term repeated dosing and subchronic toxicity studies. In Hayes A. W. (Ed.), *Principles and Methods of Toxicology*. Raven Press, New York, pp. 649–695.

Yang, R. S. H. and Tallant, M. J. (1982). Metabolism and pharmacokinetics of ethylenediamine in the rat following oral, endotracheal or intravenous administration. *Fundam. Appl. Toxicol.*, **2**, 252–260.

Yuan, J., Jameson, C. W., Goehl, T. J. and Collins, B. J. (1991). Molecular encapsulator: a novel vehicle for toxicology studies. *Toxicol. Methods*, **1**, 231–241.

Chapter 4
Toxicokinetics

A. G. Renwick

CONTENTS

INTRODUCTION

The generation of *in vivo* toxic effects, distal to the site of administration, requires two distinct aspects: absorption from the site of administration and delivery to the target, and cellular events mediated by the chemical at the target organ, or cell(s). Important aspects of delivery to the target include the duration of exposure, the magnitude of exposure and the potential for accumulation. Thus, the production of toxicity can be subdivided into *toxicokinetics* (the movement of the toxic chemical around the body) and *toxicodynamics* (the actions of the chemical within the target organ) **(Figure 1)**.

In recent years there has been increasing emphasis on the development of *in vitro* tests for specific organ toxicity, in order to reduce the numbers of animals given toxic doses of chemicals. However, the logical interpretation of the results of such *in vitro* tests places a greater requirement for the definition of the *in vivo* concentrations of the chemical that could be present in the target organ, the time course of exposure and the potential for accumulation during repeated dosing. Such information can only be obtained from the results of appropriate *in vivo* studies on the fate of the chemical within the body, that is, the toxicokinetics.

Toxicokinetics are also of importance in extrapolating both *in vitro* and *in vivo* animal data to man (see Chapter 13). The techniques used in toxicokinetics, such as the collection of timed blood and urine samples, can also be investigated in human volunteers provided, of course, that it is ethical to administer the chemical to humans. The basic processes involved in absorption, distribution and elimination, and their mathematical description/ quantitation given in this chapter, are common to all chemicals which are foreign to the body, irrespective of the biological activity, *e.g.* toxins, human and veterinary drugs, pesticides and food additives. The mathematical descriptions were developed to describe the fate of drugs in humans, and are termed *pharmacokinetics*. The use of a separate term toxicokinetics is of some value, because of the implications of data related to high-dose animal studies, but it should be appreciated that many of the best sources of information on 'toxicokinetics' are to be found in the 'pharmacokinetic' literature.

ADME STUDIES

The delivery of the chemical to the site of toxicity **(Figure 2)** depends on the processes of *absorption* from the site of administration into the general circulation and *distribution via* the blood to the site of action and all body tissues. The concentrations present at the site of action, and the duration of exposure, depend on the rate of *elimination* from the body, which may be by either *metabolism* or

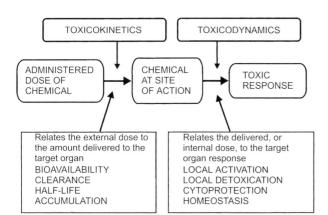

Figure 1 Relationship between toxicokinetics and toxic effects.

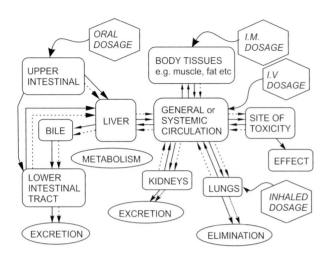

Figure 2 Delivery of chemicals to their site of action. This scheme assumes that the site of toxicity is not locally at the site of administration. Compounds absorbed from the gastrointestinal tract are transported *via* the hepatic portal vein to the liver before they enter the general circulation. Solid arrows refer to the parent compound, dotted arrows refer to metabolites.

excretion. Studies on absorption, distribution, metabolism and excretion, which are often referred to simply as ADME studies, form an essential first step in the evaluation of the fate of the chemical in the body (Glocklin, 1982). Usually ADME studies involve following the fate of a radiolabelled dose of the chemical by measuring the total radioactivity and the separation of radiolabelled metabolites in the excreta, and also the tissue distribution of total radioactivity by autoradiography at various times after dosing. Such studies clearly provide important information on the fate of the chemical in the body, but they provide only a part of the total study of the toxicokinetics of the compound. A radiolabelled compound is used to provide information on the total balance of all compound-related products whether or not they have been identified and characterized. Thus the strength of radiolabelled ADME studies is the use of *non-specific detection methods* which allow the detection of all compound-related products. However, this strength is also a weakness because it provides limited data on exposure of the body to the parent chemical itself or to specific identified metabolites. ADME studies also provide essential data on the extent of absorption, the pathways of metabolism and the routes of elimination. Identification of metabolites in excreta (and the circulation) and the definition of pathways of metabolism are essential for interspecies comparisons, for the establishment of specific analytical procedures and for indications of possible metabolic bioactivation.

Investigation of the kinetics of the parent molecule itself requires the use of a *specific detection method*, which not only separates the chemical from the normal (endogenous) constituents of the sample being analysed,

but also from any metabolites of the chemical that are formed *in vivo*. In cases where the toxicity of a chemical is due to a specific metabolite, toxicokinetic studies will need to define the extent of absorption of the parent chemical, its delivery to the site(s) of metabolism, the extent of formation of the metabolite and its delivery to the target organ **(Figure 2)**. Additional information essential to the interpretation of toxicity studies includes the influence of dose on the fate of the chemical and the extent of accumulation of the parent compound and/or active metabolites on repeated administration of the compound.

Toxicokinetics represent an important part of the safety evaluation of chemicals, but because the subject is perceived as being mathematically based it tends to be regarded as a difficult and rather unapproachable subject by biologists. This chapter will relate the basic pharmacokinetic parameters and constants to the underlying physiological and biochemical processes. This will be followed by a consideration of the types of experimental data that are needed in order to determine the various parameters. The chapter will conclude with a consideration of specific aspects related to the interpretation of high-dose, chronic animal studies.

PHARMACOKINETIC PARAMETERS AND CONSTANTS

Each of the basic processes involved in pharmacokinetics, *i.e.* absorption, distribution and elimination, may be described by parameters which define the *extent* to which the process occurs and the *rate* at which it occurs. These parameters are usually calculated from the concentrations of the chemical and/or its metabolites in biological fluids, such as whole blood, plasma or urine, measured at known times after the administration of known doses.

Absorption

Absorption is the process of transfer of the chemical from the site of administration into the general circulation. Absorption from the gastrointestinal tract is studied most frequently because this is the route of exposure of experimental animals *via* gavage dosing or by incorporation of the chemical into the diet. Oral administration is also the most common route by which humans are exposed to chemicals either as drugs or as intentional, incidental or accidental components of the diet. The process of absorption occurs whenever the compound is given by a route other than direct intravascular injection, for example, across the skin, from the airways, from subcutaneous sites and also from the peritoneal cavity.

Rate of absorption

The rate of absorption depends on both the nature of the chemical and the site of administration.

Lipid-soluble chemicals can readily dissolve in membranes and therefore diffuse across cell walls. In contrast, ionized molecules do not readily enter the lipid membrane matrix in the ionized form, and therefore only the non-ionized form freely diffuses across membranes **(Figure 3)**. For strong acids and bases at physiological pH (7.4), the non-ionized form on each side of the membrane is in equilibrium with the ionized form; the concentrations of the ionized form may be orders of magnitude higher than the concentration of the non-ionized, lipid-soluble form. Thus the transfer of highly ionized chemicals across cell membranes is very slow. For very strong acids and bases, and also quaternary amines (which have a fixed positive charge), the absorption rate across the intestinal wall may be slower than the rate of transfer along the bowel by peristalsis; under such circumstances a fraction of the dose may be lost in the faeces without ever being absorbed or available to produce systemic toxicity.

The rate of absorption also depends on the site of administration; for example absorption across the skin is usually extremely slow, because it involves transfer across the stratum corneum—the main permeability barrier of the body. In contrast, absorption from the airways tends to be rapid, because it involves transfer across a thin membrane which has a large surface area and a good blood supply.

Absorption from the gut is often complex because chemicals are absorbed less effectively from the stomach, with its smaller surface area and lower pH, than from the duodenum and jejunum. In consequence, there can be a delay before any appreciable absorption occurs, while

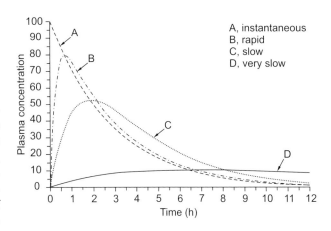

Figure 4 Plasma concentration–time curves of compounds showing different rates of absorption from the site of administration.

the compound is in the stomach lumen. However, once the dose has left the stomach, it reaches the large surface area of well perfused intestine, which can allow very rapid absorption.

The kinetic parameters which describe the absorption rate are the absorption rate constant (k_a) and its associated absorption half-life. These parameters assume that the rate of transfer of chemical into the plasma is proportional to the amount of chemical available to be absorbed, i.e. absorption is a first-order process (see later). This assumption is often a vast oversimplification, and absorption may be zero order or first order and often involves a lag phase prior to significant absorption **(Figure 4)**. In some cases absorption is complete and so rapid that the absorption rate constant cannot be calculated, and the plasma concentration–time curve resembles an intravenous dose **(Figure 4)**. A low, almost flat, profile is obtained when absorption is very slow **(Figure 4)**.

Extent of absorption

There are a number of reasons why all of the dose of a chemical introduced into the gut lumen may not be able to pass into the general circulation as the parent compound **(Table 1)**. The parameter which describes the extent of absorption is the *bioavailability* (*F*), which is defined as *the fraction of the dose which is transferred from the site of administration into the general circulation as the parent compound.*

Each of the processes in **Table 1** can cause a decrease in the amount of parent chemical able to reach the general circulation. Incomplete absorption (*F* <1.0) may be due to an inability of the chemical to cross the lipid barrier of the epithelial membrane so that the parent compound is unabsorbed and eliminated in the faeces (indicated by ADME data), or it may be due to metabolism prior to reaching the general circulation. The latter is referred to as *first-pass metabolism* since it usually occurs on the first

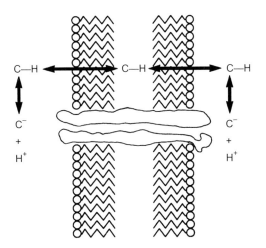

Figure 3 The transfer of an ionizable organic acid across a cell membrane. At equilibrium the concentration of the diffusible form (C-H) will be the same on each side of the membrane. The concentration of the ionized form (C⁻) will depend on the pK_a of the chemical and the pH of the solution.

Table 1 Reasons for incomplete absorption from the site of administration

Reason	Example
Incomplete dissolution	The formulation, *e.g.* tablet or suspension, is not completely dissolved during transit through the intestinal tract
Incomplete passage across absorptive epithelium	The compound is too polar to be absorbed completely before it is voided in the faeces (oral) or the unabsorbed dose is removed (transdermal). The rate of loss in exhaled air exceeds the rates of dissolution and absorption (inhaled gases)
Metabolism at the site of administration	The compound is metabolized or decomposes owing to the pH or enzymes present in the gut lumen (oral or rectal). Inactivation by lung enzymes (inhalation)
Metabolism between site of administration and the general circulation	The compound is metabolized by the gut wall or liver prior to entering the general circulation (oral dosage)

passage through the liver during the absorption process. This term is also used to describe metabolism at any of the presystemic sites listed in **Table 1**. First-pass metabolism can result in an apparent discrepancy between radiolabelled studies and toxicokinetic data. The former may demonstrate that all of a radiolabelled dose is absorbed and eliminated in urine, but the bioavailability of the parent compound may be considerably less than 1.0. The discrepancy arises from the non-specific nature of radiochemical measurements which measure parent compound plus metabolites.

Distribution

Distribution is the process of reversible transfer of the chemical from the general circulation into the body tissues. The process may be characterized as both rate and extent; the corresponding parameters are the distribution rate constant(s) (α, k_{12} and k_{21}) and the apparent volume of distribution (V). Measurement of these parameters requires knowledge of the amount of compound which enters the general circulation, and therefore distribution parameters can be defined only when the chemical has been given by direct intravascular injection. Thus intravenous dosage is essential for a full description of toxicokinetics, even for compounds such as food additives, for which there could never be parenteral dosage and for which parenteral *toxicity* studies are not necessary or useful.

Rate of distribution

Because distribution is usually rapid, the distribution rate constant is measured following the administration of a single rapid (bolus) intravenous dose **(Figure 5)**. The rate of distribution into tissues may be slow for two possible reasons. First, distribution will be slow if the chemical has a high affinity for and accumulates in a tissue or organ which is only slowly perfused, *e.g.* fat or muscle. For such a compound the rate at which the tissues and blood can reach equilibrium will be limited by the blood flow to the tissues. Second, the chemical

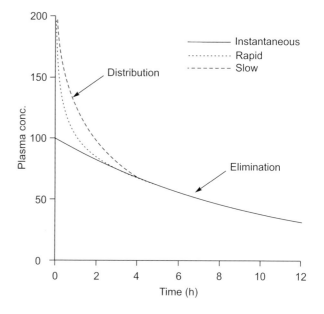

Figure 5 Plasma concentration–time curves following intravenous bolus doses of chemicals showing different rates of distribution from the blood into peripheral tissues.

may be polar so that its rate of entry into the intracellular fluid of all tissues will be limited by its solubility in the lipid of the membrane.

Extent of distribution

The tissues into which a chemical distributes can be identified by autoradiography but this technique cannot determine the overall extent to which a chemical has left the blood or plasma and entered the body tissues. In addition, autoradiography cannot differentiate between parent compound and metabolites, and cannot be used to provide data in humans. The apparent volume of distribution (V) is the parameter which relates the total amount of chemical in the body to the plasma concentration. It can be regarded as a dilution factor and represents the volume of plasma into which the chemical appears to have dissolved (see later).

The extent of distribution of a chemical from the blood into tissues depends on a number of variables:

- *Water solubility*   Water-soluble compounds, for example ethanol and caffeine, show limited uptake into adipose tissue or the central nervous system and are distributed to total body water.

- *Plasma protein binding*   Chemicals which reversibly bind to plasma proteins with a high affinity show reduced tissue distribution and are retained to a greater extent in the circulation. An equilibrium is established between the concentration unbound in plasma and that (unbound) in tissues **(Figure 6)**.

- *Tissue protein binding*   Chemicals with a high affinity for reversible binding to tissue proteins will show more extensive distribution. The blood:tissue equilibrium relates to the unbound chemical in each compartment **(Figure 6)**, and therefore the overall extent of distribution depends on the relative binding in tissues and blood.

- *Lipid solubility*   Lipid-soluble compounds are concentrated in adipose tissue, organs, such as the central nervous system, which have a high lipid content and the cytoplasmic membranes and endoplasmic reticulum of all cells in the body.

Information on the concentration of a compound in a specific tissue can be determined only by analysis of that tissue. The data in **Figure 7** show that cyclohexylamine rapidly enters the testes, which are the target for toxicity (Bopp *et al.*, 1986), and the concentrations in the testes are about four times higher than those in plasma. In contrast, the hydroxylated metabolites (3- and 4-amino-cyclohexanols) enter the testes less readily and there is not a high testes:plasma ratio even after chronic

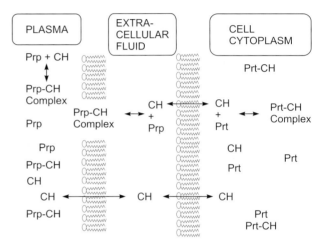

Figure 6 Plasma and tissue protein binding of chemicals. The chemical (CH) may bind as the ionized or non-ionized form to the plasma proteins (Prp) and tissue proteins (Prt). The total tissue: plasma ratio depends on the relative affinity of tissue and plasma protein binding.

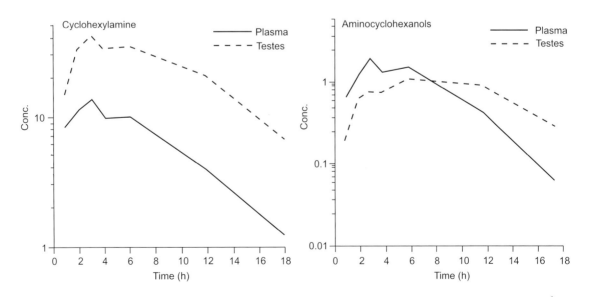

Figure 7 The concentrations of cyclohexylamine and its hydroxymetabolites (aminocyclohexanols) in the plasma μg ml^{-1} and testes μg g^{-1} of rats following a single oral dose (from Roberts and Renwick, 1989).

administration (Roberts *et al.*, 1989). These data illustrate that minor changes in molecular structure, such as the increase in polarity resulting from the hydroxylation of cyclohexylamine, can alter considerably the uptake into tissues, especially organs such as the brain and testes which have an efficient permeability barrier (blood–organ barrier).

Elimination

There are two principal mechanisms of elimination of foreign compounds from the body.

Metabolism eliminates the chemical from the body by converting it into a metabolite, which is a different chemical species. The resulting metabolite may itself undergo further metabolism or it may be removed from the body by an excretory process. However, from a toxicokinetic perspective, the parent compound has been eliminated as soon as it has been changed into the initial metabolite. Thus, in the analysis of the kinetics of the parent compound it is essential that the assay method separates the compound from all of its metabolites. The metabolism of foreign compounds has been the subject of numerous reviews and is discussed in detail in Chapter 6. The cytochrome P450 isoenzymes are in the endoplasmic reticulum and are important in the metabolism and elimination of lipid-soluble foreign compounds. Sometimes the initial metabolic step results in the generation of a toxic metabolite which is released into the circulation (Chapter 8), in which case measurements of the concentrations of parent compound provide information on the amount of substrate available for activation, but may not be the best estimate of body exposure to the toxic moiety. Under such circumstances toxicokinetics should concentrate on measurement of the toxic moiety itself in plasma and tissues, especially the target organ. When toxicity arises from the formation of an unstable reactive metabolite, exposure to the toxicant may be assessed by measuring the products formed from the unstable metabolite either in plasma, tissues or urine (a biomarker). For example, the extent of formation of the toxic quinoneimine metabolite of paracetamol can be assessed by measurement of the urinary excretion of the thio conjugates, *i.e.* the cysteine and mercapturic acid metabolites. Any bioactivation process within the target organ is part of the toxicodynamics, because it is not part of the movement of the chemical around the body (kinetics), and, of equal importance in relation to risk assessment, it cannot usually be estimated readily (or reliably?) in humans.

Excretion can occur *via* body fluids and waste products, *e.g.* faeces and expired air; the route of importance is determined largely by the physicochemical properties of the compound **(Table 2)**. When considering the toxicokinetics of a chemical, only the excretion of the chemical which is being measured is of importance. Confusion can arise when trying to relate studies with radiolabelled compounds to toxicokinetic data. For example, although all of the radioactivity may be eliminated in the urine, it is possible that this is all as metabolites and not as parent compound. Under such circumstances the renal clearance (see later) of the chemical itself will be negligible, and the kidneys will not be of importance in the elimination of the chemical *per se*.

The elimination of a chemical can be divided into the rate and extent of elimination.

Rate of elimination

The rate of elimination is limited by two biological processes:

- the ability of the organs of elimination to extract the chemical from the circulation and to remove it from the body by metabolism or excretion;
- the extent to which the chemical remains in the circulation and is available for elimination rather than

Table 2 Routes of elimination of foreign compounds

Route	Type of chemical
Expired air	Volatile compounds, *e.g.* gaseous anaesthetics, solvents, aerosol propellants
Saliva	Many low molecular weight compounds, but reabsorption occurs on passage down the gut
Bile	High molecular weight compounds, usually conjugated metabolites rather than the parent compound. Wide species differences exist in the molecular weight threshold for significant biliary excretion. Reabsorption and/or bacterial metabolism may occur in the lower bowel
Faeces	An important route for the elimination of compounds not absorbed from the gut and for compounds excreted in the bile. Some chemicals can pass from the circulation into the gut lumen by diffusion or active transport and thereby undergo elimination in the faeces
Urine	The major route of elimination for low molecular weight, polar compounds. Lipid-soluble compounds are filtered at the glomerulus, but reabsorbed on passage down the renal tubule, and such compounds are eliminated by metabolism and their metabolites removed in the urine and/or bile
Milk	Both water- and lipid-soluble compounds are present in milk. This route is usually of limited significance with respect to elimination from the mother but may be of critical importance with respect to exposure of the neonate
Hair	Quantitatively unimportant but the slow and directional growth of hair can allow an 'exposure history' to be determined based on the position of the chemical along the hair

entering tissues. If the compound has entered the body tissues to a major extent, so that at any time only a very small fraction of the total body load remains in the blood and is available for elimination, then the rate at which it is transferred back from the tissues into the circulation may become the main variable determining the elimination rate.

Extent of elimination

The extent of elimination is of less importance than the rate. Following a single dose, the extent of elimination will eventually be 100% of the dose. This is even true for chemicals which bind covalently to tissue macromolecules, because the parent compound is eliminated by the formation of the adduct. During chronic intake the body load increases until the extent of elimination per day equals the daily intake of the chemical.

DERIVATION OF PHARMACOKINETIC CONSTANTS

Most pharmacokinetic parameters are based on the measurement of the chemical in plasma samples collected at various times after dosing. In some cases the concentrations in whole blood or urine are used.

Basic Concepts

Before it is possible to describe the measurement of specific pharmacokinetic parameters it is necessary to define certain basic concepts.

Order of reaction

At low doses, most processes involved in toxicokinetics can be described as *first-order reactions* with respect to substrate. That is, the rate of reaction is proportional to the amount of substrate present. Examples include passive diffusion, metabolism, protein binding and excretion, in which an increase in concentration will increase the amounts of chemical which cross a membrane, undergo metabolism, *etc.* The equation for such reactions is:

$$\frac{dC}{dt} = kC .$$

where dC/dt is the rate of change in concentration, k is the rate constant and C is the concentration. The term k is the rate constant for the process being described by the change dC/dt and may be absorption, distribution or elimination; the greater the value of k, the greater is the rate of the process. The units of k are time^{-1} and k can be regarded as the natural logarithm of the proportion of

the chemical that is changed within one unit of time. For example, if $k = 0.693$ h^{-1} then the concentration will change by a factor of 2 (the anti-natural logarithm of 0.693) each hour.

Processes which involve an interaction of the chemical with a cellular protein, such as enzyme-catalysed metabolism, or active transport, may be saturated at very high concentrations of the chemical. Under these conditions the rate of change in concentration is not proportional to the concentration of substrate available. This is known as a *zero-order reaction*, which can be described by the equation:

$$\frac{dC}{dt} = k$$

The rate constant (k) of a zero-order reaction can be described in terms of mass (or concentration) per unit time (*e.g.* μg min^{-1}) and this value is a constant at all concentrations. A straight line is obtained when the data for a zero-order reaction are plotted on a linear axis (**Figure 8**, left). In contrast, for a first-order reaction the rate of change is proportional to the concentration; the rate of change is high at high concentrations (*i.e.* a steep slope) and the slope decreases with decrease in concentration. Thus first-order reactions result in exponential decreases, and can be described by exponential equations:

$$C_t = C_0 e^{-kt}$$

where C_t is the concentration at time t, C_0 is the initial concentration and t is the time after dosage; or taking natural logarithms,

$$\ln C_t = \ln C_0 - kt$$

Plotting the natural logarithm of the concentration (ln C_t) against time (t) will give a straight line with an intercept of $\ln C_0$ and a slope of $-k$ (**Figure 8**, right). If $\log_{10}$ is used, then the intercept is $\log_{10} C_0$ and the slope of $-k/2.303$. A zero-order decrease becomes non-linear when plotted on a logarithmic axis.

Half-lives

For first-order reactions the rate constant has units of time^{-1} (*e.g.* min^{-1}), which are difficult to visualize. Therefore, the rate of a first-order reaction is normally described by a parameter which is a reciprocal of k, and which therefore has units of time. A property of exponential decreases is that the time taken for any concentration on the curve to decrease by a factor of 2 (*i.e.* to halve) is a constant, and independent of concentration. This parameter is the half-life of the decrease and is related to k by the equation

$$t_{1/2} = \frac{0.693}{k}$$

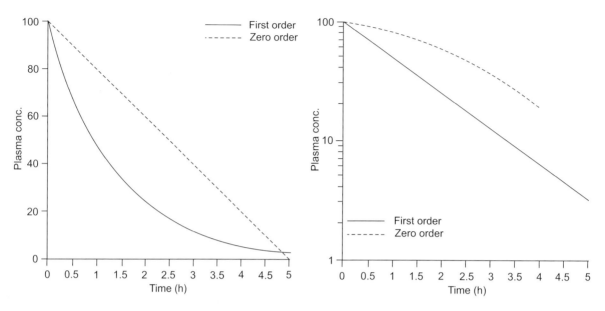

Figure 8 Graphical representations of first-order and zero-order decreases in concentrations plotted on linear and logarithmic axes.

This can be seen graphically for the first-order reaction in **Figure 8** where the concentrations decrease by a factor of 2 between successive hourly intervals, *i.e.* 100, 50, 25, 12.5, 6.25, 3.125, so that the half-life in this case is 1 h. The half-life is usually calculated from the slope of the decrease, *e.g.* the initial concentration in **Figure 8** is 100 and at 5 h the concentration is 3.125, *i.e.*

$$\ln 3.125 = \ln 100 - k \times 5$$

$$-k = \frac{\ln 3.125 - \ln 100}{5} = -0.693$$

$$k = 0.693 \text{ h}^{-1}$$

$$t_{1/2} = \frac{0.693}{0.693 \text{ h}^{-1}} = 1 \text{ h}$$

Real data are never calculated by taking two individual time points, but are fitted by a least-squares regression programme to the ln(concentration)–time curve and the slope is used to calculate the half-life.

Clearance

A clearance process is one in which the chemical is removed permanently from the circulation, *i.e.* by metabolism or excretion. Clearance is defined as *the volume of blood (or plasma) cleared of chemical per unit time*. Thus, on passage through an organ of elimination the blood can be cleared, either totally or partially, of the compound. The extent of uptake and removal is indicated by the decrease in concentration in the blood leaving the organ *via* the vein (C_v) compared with that entering *via* the artery (C_a). (The decrease must be due to removal, not simply distribution, which is reversible, and therefore such measurements are usually made at steady state; see later.) The removal by the organ is usually expressed as the *extraction ratio* (*ER*):

$$ER = \frac{(C_a - C_v)}{C_a}$$

If all of the chemical is removed then $C_v = 0$ and $ER = 1.0$, whereas if only 10% of the arterial concentration is removed $C_v = 0.9$ and $ER = 0.1$. If ER approaches 1.0 then all of the blood which flows through the organ of elimination will be cleared of the chemical. Thus the clearance (*CL*) will equal the blood (or plasma) flow through the organ (Q). If the extraction ratio is 0.1 then only one tenth of the organ blood flow will be cleared of the chemical, *i.e.*

$$CL = Q \bullet ER$$

The physiological significance of this is that the most important toxicokinetic parameter (*CL*) can be related to the blood flow to the organ of elimination (Q) and the capacity of the organs to extract the chemical (*ER*) and to remove it from the body (*e.g.* by metabolism). These processes are the basis for developing physiologically based pharmacokinetic (PBPK) models (see Chapter 7).

If the extraction ratio is low then uptake or extraction by the organ is dependent on the time available for uptake, *i.e.* the slower the organ blood flow (Q) the greater will be the extraction ratio (*ER*). Thus, a change in Q results in an opposite change in ER so that CL remains relatively constant and independent of organ blood flow. If a compound has a very high extraction ratio, then changes in organ blood flow will not significantly affect the extraction efficiency of the organ, and consequently clearance will be dependent on and be directly proportional to the organ blood flow.

There are mathematical models which characterize the relationship between CL, Q and ER (see Wilkinson,

1976). In the context of the present chapter, the importance of this relationship is that if the doses of the chemical given to animals are sufficient to alter organ perfusion, then this could influence the clearance of the chemical if it has a high extraction ratio.

Absorption

Rate of Absorption

Measurement of the rate of absorption requires information on the plasma (or blood) concentrations of the compound at frequent time intervals following a single dose administered to the site of absorption. The resulting data can be analysed in a number of ways. In the simple example shown in **Figure 9** the absorption occurs rapidly as a first-order process and the total concentration–time curve is dependent on two exponential terms, one for absorption (k_a) and one for elimination (k), *i.e.*

$$C_t = \frac{F \times \text{dose} \times k_a(e^{-kt} - e^{-kat})}{V \times (k_a - k)}$$

where F = bioavailability (see later) and V = apparent volume of distribution (see later). Because k_a exceeds k, the term e^{-kat} approaches zero at late time points, and the concentration–time curve is determined by a single exponential e^{-kt}. This is shown in **Figure 9** by the extrapolation line of the terminal data. If all of the dose had entered the circulation as a single bolus dose, then the concentration–time curve would have resembled this extrapolation line. The *difference* between the actual data obtained and the extrapolation line is due to the

absorption of the chemical into the circulation. The differences (or *residuals*) between the actual data and the extrapolation line are then plotted **(Figure 9)** in order to derive the absorption rate constant.

The absorption and elimination of chemicals rarely show this simple pattern and more complex equations may be necessary. For example, if there is a lag time (t_{lag}) between dosing and measurable concentrations then the time t in the equation given above has to be replaced by $t - t_{lag}$. In addition, if there is a clear distribution phase (see later), then a more complex equation involving three exponential terms may be required; in some cases the absorption rate can only be determined by comparison of oral and intravenous data. Readers are referred to Chapter 4 of Gibaldi and Perrier (1982) for further information. Characterization of the rate of absorption requires the collection of a number of blood samples (at least three or four) during the absorption phase.

In some cases the rate of absorption does not resemble either a first- or a zero-order input and the data cannot be fitted by any model. Under such circumstances the best estimate of the rate of absorption is the mean absorption time (MAT). This is calculated from plasma concentration–time curve data after *both* oral and intravenous dosing using statistical moments analysis (see Gibaldi and Perrier 1982; Chapter 11):

$$MAT = MRT_{oral} - MRT_{iv}$$

where MRT = mean residence time (see later under dose-dependent kinetics).

In the brief description above it is assumed that the compound is absorbed rapidly but eliminated slowly, for example a lipid-soluble compound requiring metabolism. For highly polar molecules, absorption from the gut may be slow whereas elimination from the blood, *via* the kidneys, may be rapid. However, the concentration–time curve still resembles that shown in **Figure 9**. The reason for this is that the exponential function which defines the later time points is always that with the lower rate constant whether it is k or k_a. Therefore, in the rate equation given above the value of $k_a - k$ will be negative when $k > k_a$, and at late time points e^{-kt} will approach zero and the concentration will be determined by $-e^{-kat}$. Thus, for slowly absorbed/rapidly eliminated compounds, the terminal slope is determined by k_a and the more rapid increase by k, a situation described as flip-flop kinetics. This type of profile is usually shown by transdermal absorption.

Both the rate and extent of absorption from the gastrointestinal tract can be influenced by a number of variables such as the nature and volume of the vehicle, the dose of compound (especially in relation to its solubility) and the presence of food in the gut lumen. Toxicokinetic studies should be performed under conditions which reflect the dosing regimen used in animal toxicity studies, *e.g.* gavage in corn oil or administration with diet.

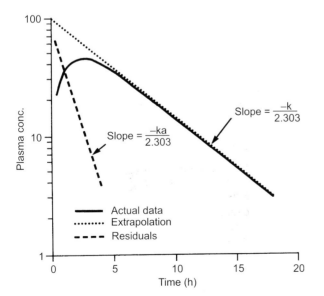

Figure 9 Plasma concentration–time curve following oral administration of a compound showing simple first-order absorption.

Extent of absorption

The fraction of the dose absorbed as the parent compound (or bioavailability, F) can be determined only by reference to conditions in which it is known that all of the dose enters the general circulation *as the parent compound*, *i.e.* by reference to an intravenous dose given as a bolus or as a slow infusion. Because of the different shapes of the concentration–time curves following oral and intravenous doses **(Figure 10)**, comparisons of the concentrations at single time points are meaningless.

The bioavailability can be calculated from the area under the plasma concentration–time curve (AUC) between administration and infinity following both routes of administration, *i.e.* if the doses are identical

$$F = \frac{\text{AUC}_{\text{oral}}}{\text{AUC}_{\text{iv}}}$$

This is illustrated in **Figure 10**. In many cases acute toxicity may prevent the administration of a high intravenous dose, while a high oral dose may be essential to obtain measurable plasma concentrations. Under such circumstances, different doses may be given by oral and intravenous routes and F is calculated as

$$F = \frac{\text{AUC}_{\text{oral}} \times \text{dose}_{\text{iv}}}{\text{AUC}_{\text{iv}} \times \text{dose}_{\text{oral}}}$$

The basis for this calculation is that plasma clearance (CL; see later) is the same after each of the two separate doses (oral and intravenous). In clinical studies this is ensured by studying the same subjects on two separate occasions. For animal toxicity studies it may be necessary to study different animals for each route, in which case the age and sex of the animals should be comparable. The AUC values must be calculated to infinity (see later), so that it is important that the concentration–time curves are followed for sufficient time to allow accurate measurement of the terminal half-life.

The use of AUC data assumes that there is no saturation of elimination, and that the intravenous dose with its possibly higher plasma concentrations does not produce cardiovascular, renal or metabolic effects which could alter the plasma clearance of the compound.

The bioavailability can also be calculated from urinary data. The percentage of the dose which is excreted in the urine *as the parent compound* is dependent on the amount of parent compound presented to the kidneys *via* the circulation, *i.e.* the percentage of the dose excreted in the urine to time t is proportional to the plasma AUC to time t. Thus bioavailability (F) can be calculated as

$$F = \frac{\% \text{ oral dose in urine as the parent compound}}{\% \text{ intravenous dose in urine as the parent compound}}$$

where the percentage dose is measured until no more parent drug is excreted (*i.e.* $t = $ infinity).

Distribution

Rate of distribution

The rate at which a compound distributes out of the blood into body tissues is usually rapid and can only be measured when the dose enters the circulation at a rate considerably greater than the rate of distribution. In effect, this means that usually the rate of distribution is measured following an intravenous bolus dose. The plasma concentration–time curve, following a bolus dose, depends on the rate and extent of distribution as well as the rate of elimination.

In the simplest case **(Figure 5**, bottom line), complete distribution occurs between dosing and the collection of the first blood sample, so that distribution is essentially instantaneous. Thus the concentration–time curve can be described by a single exponential term (k) dependent on elimination and the compound achieves instantaneous distribution within a single compartment **(Figure 11)**.

However, normally a distinct distribution phase can be detected **(Figure 5**, top two lines), during which the

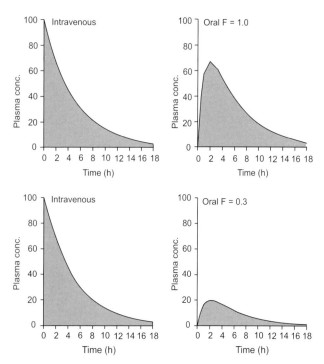

Figure 10 Comparison of areas under the plasma concentration–time curves for a compound showing complete absorption (F = 1.0; top panels) and a compound showing incomplete absorption (F = 0.3; bottom panels). The reason for the incomplete bioavailability, *e.g.* first-pass metabolism or poor absorption from the gut lumen, cannot be determined without additional information.

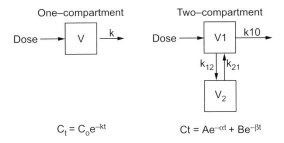

$$C_t = C_o e^{-kt} \qquad Ct = Ae^{-\alpha t} + Be^{-\beta t}$$

Figure 11 Simple one- and two-compartment models of distribution and elimination. More complex models involving three or more compartments with elimination from both central and peripheral compartments are sometimes necessary to provide a mathematical description of the plasma concentration–time curves. The relationships between α, β, k_{10}, k_{12} and k_{21} are given in the text.

chemical is undergoing *both* distribution and elimination. The tissues and blood eventually reach equilibrium and the concentration–time curve becomes a simple mono-exponential decrease determined by the elimination rate constant (k). For such compounds the body has to be regarded as comprising two compartments with the chemical achieving instantaneous equilibrium in compartment 1 (the central compartment) but taking a finite time for equilibration between compartment 1 and compartment 2 (the peripheral compartment) **(Figure 11)**. Thus two exponential terms are necessary: a rapid distribution rate (α) and the slower elimination rate (β). A more correct nomenclature for such multiple exponential rate constants is λ_1, λ_2, *etc.*, and λ_z, where these represent the rate constants for the fastest, next fastest and slowest rate, respectively. This nomenclature is receiving increasingly wide usage. The overall elimination rate (β or λ_z) or terminal half-life ($0.693/\beta$) is *not* equivalent to k_{10}; it is a composite term involving k_{10}, k_{21} and k_{12}.

The concentration in the peripheral compartment is zero initially, and then rises during the distribution phase until equilibrium is reached, following which the concentrations decrease is parallel with those in the general circulation **(Figure 12)**. The absolute concentration in the tissue will depend on the relative affinity of the blood and tissue for the compound **(Figure 6)**. Tissues with different relative affinities may be part of the same peripheral compartment because this is a mathematical concept, and the only parameter that is shared is the rate of equilibrium between blood and tissue **(Figure 12)**. Thus calculation of a mean concentration for the peripheral compartment is rarely of value. However, concentrations in the peripheral compartment can be predicted from a single post-equilibrium measurement and a knowledge of the terminal rate constant (β) in plasma.

The rate constants α and β and intercepts A and B can be calculated by the method of residuals **(Figure 13)**. The 'micro'-rate constants k_{10}, k_{12} and k_{21} can be calculated as

$$k_{21} = \frac{A\beta + B\alpha}{A + B}$$

$$k_{10} = \frac{\alpha\beta}{k_{21}}$$

$$k_{12} = \alpha + \beta - k_{21} - k_{10}$$

It should be appreciated that such manipulations of derived data exaggerate any errors in the measurements.

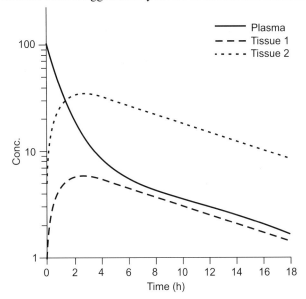

Figure 12 Concentration–time curve for a chemical in plasma (and tissues in the instantaneously equilibrating central compartment) and in two tissues which are part of the slowly equilibrating peripheral compartment.

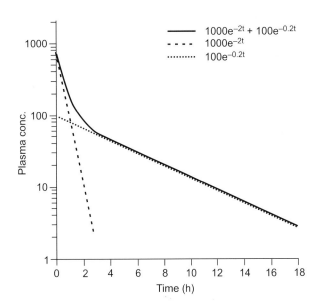

Figure 13 The use of the method of residuals to calculate distribution parameters. The terminal phase is given by $Be^{-\beta t}$ (in this case $100e^{-0.2t}$) and the differences between the plasma concentrations and this line give the distribution phase $Ae^{-\alpha t}$ (in this case $1000e^{-2t}$)

Accurate parameter estimates require that at least 3–4 blood samples are collected during each separate phase (e.g. α and β) and that the terminal phase is followed for as long as possible and for at least two half-lives. Some compounds may require three or more exponential terms (and compartments) to provide an adequate model.

Extent of distribution

The shape of the concentration–time curve following a single bolus intravenous dose is dependent on both the rate of distribution and the extent to which the dose is retained in the central compartment or distributed to the tissues. This is illustrated in **Figure 14**. For the top line ($C_t = 100e^{-2t} + 1000e^{-0.2t}$) only one tenth of the material is associated with the rapid phase of distribution to the tissues and the concentration–time curve almost resembles a mono-exponential decrease; the distribution phase could have been missed if the first sample had been taken at 1 h. For the lower line ($C_t = 1000e^{-2t} + 100e^{-0.2t}$) most of the dose undergoes the distribution phase, two phases are apparent and distribution clearly continues until about 3 h after the dose.

The extent of distribution is characterised by the *apparent volume of distribution* (V), which can be calculated using a number of different methods. V is the parameter which relates the concentration in plasma (C) to the total body load (A_b) with which it is in equilibrium, *i.e.*

$$V = \frac{A_b}{C}$$

Thus, for a one-compartment system which shows instantaneous equilibrium,

$$V = \frac{dose}{C_0}$$

where C_0 is the concentration at $t = 0$.

For a two-compartment system the situation is more complex. Dose/$(A + B)$ gives the volume of the central compartment only, because the constant A is derived prior to distribution and the attainment of equilibrium. The volume of distribution can be calculated as dose/B but this estimate does not take into account the volume of, or the amount of chemical in, the central compartment. The apparent volume of distribution usually calculated for two-compartment systems is V_β:

$$V_\beta = \frac{dose}{AUC \times \beta}$$

where AUC is the area under the plasma concentration–time curve between time = zero and infinity.

It must be emphasized that the volume of distribution is not a real volume, but is the volume of plasma

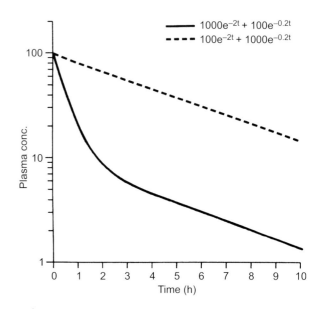

Figure 14 Plasma concentration–time curves for two compounds with the same rate constants (α and β) but with different proportions of the dose undergoing distribution.

(or blood if the concentration is measured in whole blood) in which the compound *appears* to have dissolved. If the concentration in plasma after equilibration with all the tissues is extremely low then the apparent volume of distribution (A_b/C or dose/C_0) will be extremely high. For example, highly lipid-soluble compounds may have an apparent volume of distribution of 50 l per kg body weight—a physiological impossibility. Thus all that the apparent volume of distribution really represents is the dilution factor between plasma concentration and body load. It provides an indication of the extent to which the compound has left plasma and entered the tissues, but it cannot provide information on uptake into specific tissues.

If a chemical enters a tissue but is eliminated without re-entering the general circulation, this is an elimination or clearance process and *does not contribute to the distribution parameters*.

Elimination

The overall rate of elimination (k or β) depends on two independent variables, the apparent volume of distribution (V) and the clearance (CL). This is illustrated in **Figure 15** by analogy with the emptying of a container of water. In the case of a single compartment the rate at which the level falls in the container will be proportional to the removal (flow) through the tap (analogous to the clearance) but inversely proportional to the volume of the container (analogous to the apparent volume of distribution), *i.e.*

$$\text{rate} \, \alpha \, \frac{CL}{V}$$

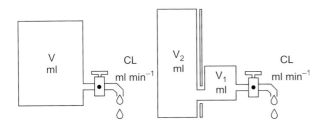

Figure 15 The relationship between volume, clearance and overall elimination. Rate of elimination is proportional to CL/V.

In the case of the two-compartment system (**Figure 15**, right) the rate at which the level falls in V_1 is dependent on CL and the size of $V_1 + V_2$.

Clearance

The clearance (CL) of a chemical is perhaps the single most important pharmacokinetic parameter. It is defined as

$$CL = \frac{\text{rate of elimination of the chemical}}{\text{plasma concentration}} \quad e.g. \frac{\mu g \; min^{-1}}{\mu g \; ml^{-1}}$$

For first-order reactions an increase in plasma concentration results in an increase in the rate of elimination, so that CL is constant. The units of CL are volume (time)$^{-1}$ (e.g. ml min^{-1}) and clearance represents the volume of plasma (or blood if concentrations are measured in whole blood) cleared of compound per unit time. The plasma clearance (CL) represents the sum of all individual clearance processes such as metabolism (CL_M), renal excretion (CL_R) and biliary excretion (CL_B):

$$CL = CL_M + CL_R + CL_B + \cdots$$

Plasma clearance is usually calculated from the area under the plasma concentration–time curve (AUC). The rate of elimination of the chemical from the body is the rate of change of body load (dA_b/dt), i.e.

$$CL = \frac{dA_b}{dt} \times \frac{1}{C}$$

or

$$CL \times C dt = dA_b$$

If this equation is integrated between time zero and infinity, the term dA_b (the change in body load) becomes the dose administered, while $C dt$ (which is the area under the concentration–time curve for the time interval dt) becomes the AUC:

$$CL \times AUC = dose$$

or

$$CL = \frac{dose}{AUC}$$

For this equation to be valid both the dose and AUC need to be defined properly.

Dose

The dose has to be fully available to the organs of elimination. Thus CL is calculated from the data following an *intravenous dose*, which can be given either as a bolus or as a slow infusion. If the dose is given orally then the true dose available to the organs of elimination is ($F \times$ dose administered) where F is the bioavailability, *i.e.*

$$CL = \frac{dose_{iv}}{AUC_{iv}} = \frac{dose_{oral} \times F}{AUC_{oral}}$$

Rearrangement of the above equation shows how the bioavailability can be calculated from AUC data and also explains why this calculation assumes that CL is a constant for the two different routes:

$$F = \frac{AUC_{oral} \times dose_{iv}}{dose_{oral} \times AUC_{iv}}$$

It is common to see papers give a parameter termed 'oral clearance', which is the dose/AUC for oral data; in reality this parameter is CL/F, and is of limited value because it depends on two variables, either of which could be influenced by physiological changes.

AUC

The AUC can be calculated by the trapezoidal rule between time zero and the last measured concentration, but needs to be extrapolated to infinity if the calculation of CL is to be valid. This is normally done by dividing the last measured concentration (C_{last}) by the terminal slope (β) which is derived from the terminal log-linear portion of the concentration–time curve. Consequently, it is essential for the samples to be collected until a log-linear decrease is defined clearly. The AUC can also be derived by fitting a suitable model to the data and calculating the AUC from the derived parameters, e.g. AUC $= C_0/k$ or AUC $= A/\alpha + B/\beta$.

Relationship of clearance to half-life

The relationship between clearance, the terminal slope and the apparent volume of distribution can be derived from the simple definition of clearance, *i.e.*

$$CL = \frac{dA_b}{dt} \times \frac{1}{C}$$

For a first-order reaction $dA_b/dt = kAb$,

$$CL = \frac{kA_b}{C}$$

From the definition of apparent volume of distribution $A_b = VC$,

$$CL = \frac{kVC}{C} = kV$$

or

$$k = \frac{CL}{V} \quad \text{and} \quad t_{1/2} = \frac{0.693V}{CL}$$

This derivation has been included to emphasize (a) that the terminal elimination rate constant is a composite parameter which is dependent on two independent, physiological variables, *i.e.* CL, which reflects the rate of extraction and removal from blood, and $1/V$, which reflects the amount of chemical remaining in the blood and available for clearance, and (b) that the interrelationship between CL, V and $t_{1/2}$ assumes that first-order kinetics apply, *i.e.* that the chemical does not show dose-dependent kinetics.

Renal clearance (CL_R) is the only specific clearance term that can be measured easily. CL_R may be defined as

$$CL_R = \frac{\begin{array}{c}\text{rate of elimination in urine}\\\text{(as the parent compound)}\end{array}}{\text{concentration in plasma}}$$

The rate of elimination in urine can be calculated by measuring the concentration of the chemical (C_u) in the volume of urine (V_u) produced in a known time interval (Δt). If the concentration in plasma at the mid-point of the urine collection (C_{mid}) is known, then CL_R can be calculated as

$$CL_R = \frac{C_u \times V_u}{\Delta t} \times \frac{1}{C_{mid}}$$

where $C_u \times V_u$ is the total amount excreted (A_{ex}) over the time interval Δt.

The product $\Delta t \times C_{mid}$ is the AUC of the plasma concentration–time curve for the time interval Δt. Therefore CL_R may be calculated also from plasma AUC data and the amount excreted unchanged (A_{ex}) over the same time interval, *i.e.*

$$CL_R = \frac{A_{ex0-t}}{AUC_{0-t}}$$

The terminal half-life can be calculated from serial timed urine collections without taking blood samples:

$$CL_R = \frac{\text{rate of urinary excretion}}{C_{mid}}$$

rate of urinary excretion $= C_{mid} \times CL_R$

CL_R is a constant for first-order reactions and therefore the rate of excretion at any time will be proportional to the plasma concentration. Therefore, the decrease in excretion rate with time will mirror the decrease in plasma concentration. Thus a graph of the natural logarithm of the excretion rate *vs* time will have a rate

constant and half-life the same as those in plasma. Alternatively, the half-life can be calculated from the amount remaining to be excreted using the sigma-minus method (see under trans-species comparisons). [It is not possible to derive total plasma clearance (CL), renal clearance (CL_R) or the apparent volume of distribution (V) without taking blood samples.]

Metabolic clearance (CL_M) cannot be measured readily but metabolism and renal excretion are the two principal routes of total clearance (CL) in many cases, and it can be *assumed* that

$$CL = CL_M + CL_R$$
$$CL_M = CL - CL_R$$
$$CL_M = \frac{\text{dose}}{AUC} - \frac{\text{amount excretion unchanged}}{AUC}$$
$$CL_M = \frac{(\text{dose} - \text{amount excreted unchanged})}{AUC}$$

INTERPRETATION OF CHRONIC HIGH-DOSE ANIMAL STUDIES

In many cases, regulatory decisions are based on the use of chronic high-dose animal studies to predict possible risk for man. However, such a protocol can lead to changes in clearance and accumulation that would not be anticipated from single dose studies.

Chronic Intake

During chronic intake the concentration of the chemical accumulates in the plasma and tissues, as illustrated in **Figure 16**. Both of the hypothetical compounds shown in **Figure 16** exhibit essentially instantaneous absorption and one-compartment kinetics with similar apparent volumes of distribution; therefore, the 10-fold difference in the elimination rate constant arises from a 10-fold difference in clearance. The compound in **Figure 16** for which $k = 0.2 \text{ h}^{-1}$ shows negligible concentrations remaining at 24 h when the next dose is given. In contrast, at 24 h the concentration of the compound for which $k = 0.02 \text{ h}^{-1}$ is 62% of the value at $t = 0$, so that there is marked accumulation with successive doses. Eventually a steady state will be reached in which the rate of elimination per 24 h equals the rate of administration, *i.e.*

rate of input = rate of elimination

$$\frac{D \times F}{T} = CL \times C_{ss} \quad \text{or} \quad C_{ss} = \frac{D \times F}{T \times CL}$$

where D = dose administered, F = bioavailability, T = dose interval, CL = clearance and C_{ss} = average plasma concentrations at the steady state.

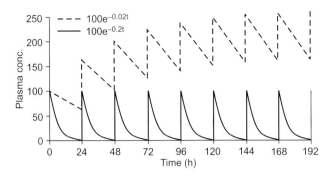

Figure 16 Accumulation of chemicals during chronic intake. In the two examples shown the compounds are given as single intravenous bolus doses every 24 h. Both compounds exhibit monoexponential decreases (i.e. $C_t = C_0 e^{-kt}$).

These determinants of C_{ss} can be deduced intuitively since C_{ss} is directly proportional to dose given and the fraction absorbed and inversely proportion to the interval between successive doses and the ability of the organism to eliminate the chemical.

This equation is based on the definition of clearance (i.e. CL = rate of elimination/C) applied to the steady-state condition when the rate of elimination exactly equals the rate of administration. Thus steady-state data can be used to calculate the value of CL, i.e.

$$CL = \frac{D \times F}{T \times C_{ss}}$$

$T \times C_{ss}$ is the AUC for a dose interval at the steady state, so that this equation can also be written as

$$CL = \frac{D \times F}{AUC_{0-T}}$$

This can be compared with the measurement of CL after a single dose, where

$$CL = \frac{D \times F}{AUC_{0-\infty}}$$

Thus the AUC_{0-T} at the steady-state and the average steady-state concentration (C_{ss}) can be calculated from the $AUC_{0-\infty}$ for a single dose:

$$AUC_{0-T}(\text{steady-state}) = AUC_{0-\infty} \text{ (single dose)}$$
$$C_{ss} = \frac{AUC_{0-\infty} \text{ (single dose)}}{T}$$

This is illustrated in **Figure 17**. *The AUC for a dose interval at the steady-state is the best estimate of exposure to the chemical* and can be determined without fitting any specific model to the data.

The increase to the steady state for a compound which shows a simple monoexponential decline after an

intravenous bolus dose is an inversion of the elimination phase, *i.e.* the percentage of the steady state achieved after administration for one, two, three, four and five half-lives is 50, 75, 87.5, 93.75, 96.875%, respectively, of the steady-state concentration (C_{ss}) or body load ($C_{ss} \times V$). Thus it takes approximately 4–5 times the elimination (terminal) half-life to approach the steady state. For a compound which shows a more complex plasma concentration–time curve **(Table 3)**, for example oral administration of a slowly absorbed compound such as saccharin, the percentage of the steady state at any time ($= t$) can be calculated from single dose data as $(AUC_{0-t}/AUC_{0-\infty}) \times 100$. Hence the time to steady-state can be assessed without the fitting of any model **(Figure 18)**.

The 'steady state' will be reached within the first 24 h of regular dosing for compounds which have a half-life of 6 h or less. However, there will be massive diurnal

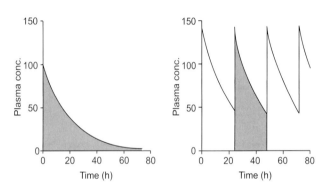

Figure 17 Relationship between $AUC_{0-\infty}$ for a single dose and AUC_{0-T} for a dose interval at the steady state.

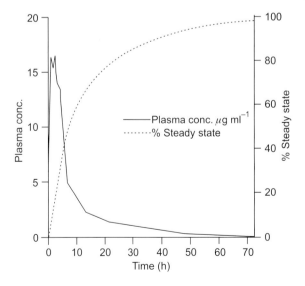

Figure 18 Relationship between single-dose kinetics and the development of the steady state during chronic administration. The percentage of the steady state at any time is the AUC to that time divided by the AUC to infinity times 100 (data from Table 3).

Table 3 Use of single dose data to predict the development of the steady state

Time (t) (h)	C (μg ml^{-1})	AUC$_{0-t}$ (μg ml^{-1}h)	%SS
0	0		
0.5	11.03	2.76	1.91
1	16.32	9.60	6.66
1.5	15.41	17.52	12.15
2	16.69	25.55	17.71
3	13.89	40.80	28.28
4	13.45	54.47	37.76
5	8.82	65.44	45.37
6	5.82	72.66	50.37
7	4.85	77.98	54.06
8	4.63	82.71	57.34
12	2.41	96.52	66.91
14	2.26	101.26	70.20
24	1.23	118.19	81.93
28	0.93	122.48	84.91
32	0.92	126.18	87.47
48	0.39	136.07	94.33
56	0.35	139.02	96.37
72	0.12	142.46	98.76
∞	–	144.25	100.00

The plasma concentration–time curve data are for a single dose of saccharin given orally to a human volunteer (data from Sweatman *et al.*, 1981). C = concentration in plasma; AUC$_{0-t}$ = area under concentration–time curve to the time of the plasma sample; %SS = percentage of steady state = (AUC$_{0-t}$/AUC$_{0-\infty}$) × 100.

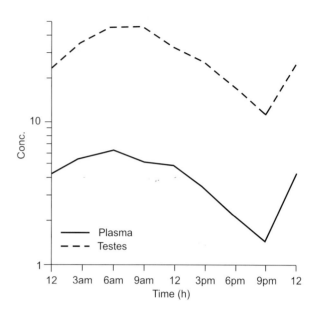

Figure 19 Concentration–time curves for cyclohexylamine in the plasma μg ml^{-1} and testes μg g^{-1} of rats given cyclohexylamine in the diet *ad libitum*. The animal room was dark between 9 pm and 6 am, during which time the animals consumed the diet. From Roberts and Renwick (1989).

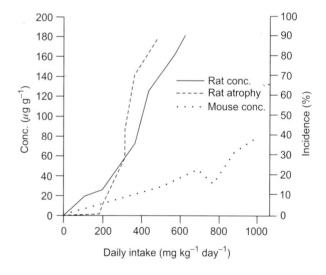

Figure 20 Concentrations of cyclohexylamine in the testes of rats and mice measured at 6 am (from Roberts and Renwick, 1989) in relation to the daily intake, and the corresponding dose–response for testicular atrophy in the rat (from Bopp *et al.*, 1986).

variations in concentration, as illustrated in **Figure 16**, where the half-life of one of the compounds is only $3.5 \text{h}(0.693/0.2 \text{ h}^{-1})$. Compounds which have long half-lives will accumulate during chronic intake but show less inter-dose fluctuation. These various aspects of chronic administration can be illustrated by toxicokinetic data for cyclohexylamine (which has a very short half-life) and the slowly eliminated organochlorine compounds (which are discussed later under trans-species comparisons).

Cyclohexylamine is a metabolite of the intense sweetener cyclamate (see Renwick, 1986) which produces testicular atrophy when administered to rats but not mice at doses of 200 mg kg^{-1} day^{-1} or more in a 90 day study (see Bopp *et al.*, 1986). The terminal half-life in rats was 4.6 h following a single oral dose of 200 mg kg^{-1} (Roberts and Renwick, 1989), so that negligible accumulation would be expected during chronic administration. Wide diurnal variations in plasma concentration would be expected. The concentration–time profile over 24 h during chronic dietary administration **(Figure 19)** was determined largely by the nocturnal feeding habits of the rat. The concentrations of cyclohexylamine in the testes increased rapidly following a single oral dose **(Figure 7)**, and therefore the testes represent part of the rapidly equilibrating central compartment. Therefore, the diurnal fluctuations detected in plasma would occur also in the target organ for toxicity **(Figure 19)**.

The area under the concentration–time curve is the best estimate of exposure of the whole body (if based on plasma concentrations) or the target organ (if based on tissue concentrations). For cyclohexylamine, the AUC values for both plasma and testes were about 2–3 times higher in rats than in mice. Therefore, the species difference in toxicokinetics contributes to the marked difference in sensitivity between rats and mice fed the same dietary concentration of cyclohexylamine

(Roberts *et al.*, 1989). This species difference was supported by data on the relationship between the concentration in the testes at steady state and the daily intake in the test animals **(Figure 20)**. For example, the concentration in the rat testes at the minimally effective intake of 200 mg kg^{-1} day^{-1} was approximately 30 μg g^{-1}, whereas at the clearly toxic daily intake of 400 mg kg^{-1} day^{-1} (Roberts *et al.*, 1989), the concentration in the testes was approximately 100 μg g^{-1}. In contrast, an intake of 400 mg kg^{-1} day^{-1}, which is non-toxic in mice (Roberts *et al.*, 1989), produced concentrations of only about 25 μg g^{-1} in the mouse testes. The concentration–intake data in the rat showed clear evidence of non-linearity at intakes greater than about 200 mg kg^{-1} day^{-1}. This non-linearity was also detected in plasma and probably contributed to the steep dose–response relationship for testicular atrophy in the rat **(Figure 20)**.

Dose-Dependent Kinetics

A non-linear relationship between dose and area under the plasma concentration–time curve is indicative of *dose-dependent* or *non-linear kinetics*, that is, the compound does not obey first-order kinetics at high doses. Non-linear kinetics can arise whenever an interaction between the chemical and a body constituent is saturated by the presence of excess chemical **(Table 4)**.

Non-linear kinetics can be detected by studying a range of single doses, but frequently non-linearity is detected during chronic administration when the accumulation of the compound causes saturation. If saturation of elimination occurs during chronic administration, then the clearance will be reduced and the area under the curve (AUC) for a dose interval will be increased (see above). Evidence of saturation of elimination is that the AUC for a dose interval at the steady state

exceeds the AUC to infinity of a single dose. In the example in **Figure 20**, the AUC for a dose interval at the steady state was not measured and non-linearity was based on a single measurement taken at 6 a.m. Therefore, the non-linearity in **Figure 20** could have been obtained for reasons other than a decrease in clearance, for example if high doses altered the pattern of food consumption or the rate of absorption of cyclohexylamine. In the case of cyclohexylamine, saturation of elimination had been demonstrated by single dose studies, but it should be appreciated that the data in **Figure 20** alone are indicative but not proof of saturation of elimination.

Sometimes chronic administration results in the induction of the enzymes which are responsible for foreign compound elimination. When this happens, the clearance will be increased during chronic administration, and therefore the AUC for a dose interval will be reduced compared with the AUC to infinity of a single dose.

It should be appreciated that age-related changes in physiological processes, such as renal blood flow, will occur during lifetime feeding studies. Therefore, it is possible that steady-state concentrations during a chronic bioassay may be age-dependent. The basic equation for average steady-state concentration (C_{ss}) still applies, *i.e.*

$$C_{ss} = \frac{\text{dose} \times F}{CL \times T}$$

Metabolic and physiological processes, such as renal blood flow, are immature in neonates (Blumer, 1990) and clearances may be lower than in mature individuals. The neonatal phase of a two-generation protocol may result in excessively high plasma concentrations of compounds fed in the diet due to the lower clearance, and also because of enhanced intake due to the higher food intake

Table 4 Possible sources of dose-dependent or non-linear kinetics

Site	Mechanism	Consequences at high dose
Absorption	Dissolution	Elimination of undissolved chemical in faeces; decrease in F
	Active uptake	Saturation of transport; delayed uptake; decrease in F
	First-pass metabolism	Increase in F
Distribution	Plasma protein binding	Increased availability to tissues: increase in V; increase in $t_{1/2}$
	Tissue protein binding	Increased retention in plasma; decrease in V; decrease in $t_{1/2}$
Metabolism	Saturation by substrate or cofactor depletion or product inhibition	Increase in AUC; decrease in clearance; increase in terminal half-life possible (*e.g.* cofactor depletion); increased renal excretion of parent compound; increased metabolism by alternative unsaturated pathways
Excretion	Saturation of renal tubular secretion	Increase in AUC; decrease in renal clearance; terminal half-life not affected (see text); increased metabolism
Cardiac output	Decreased organ perfusion due to cardio-vascular toxicity	Slower distribution; increase in AUC and decrease in clearance for compounds showing high renal or hepatic (metabolic) clearance, *i.e.* high extraction ratio

in neonates (per kg body weight). In ageing animals C_{ss} may increase owing to an age-related decrease in clearance. In the case of N-acetylprocainamide the systemic clearance ($\text{dose}_{iv}/\text{AUC}_{iv}$) in 12-month-old rats was only 40% of that in 3-month-old rats. However, the AUC oral showed a much less marked age-related change than the AUC_{iv} because bioavailability was also decreased in 12-month-old rats (Yacobi *et al.*, 1982). This illustrates that the AUC_{oral} is dependent on both the systemic clearance and the bioavailability and that these can vary independently.

If saturation of elimination is detected on giving increasing single doses, this is usually seen as delayed elimination at high plasma concentrations, but with the normal rate of elimination once the concentration decreases and first-order kinetics apply **(Figure 21)**. Under such circumstances the compound is said to obey Michaelis–Menten kinetics, that is,

$$\frac{dC}{dt} = \frac{V_{max} \times C}{K_m + C}$$

where dC/dt = the rate of change of concentration, V_{max} = maximum rate of the enzyme (or transport), K_m = Michaelis constant of the enzyme (affinity constant) and C = concentration available to the enzyme.

At low concentrations $K_m \gg C$ and therefore $K_m + C$ approximates to K_m:

$$\frac{-dC}{dt} = \frac{V_{max} C}{K_m} = \text{constant} \times C = \text{first-order reaction}$$

At high concentrations $C \gg K_m$ and therefore $K_m + C$ approximates to C:

$$\frac{dC}{dt} = \frac{V_{max} C}{C} = V_{max} = \text{zero-order reaction}$$

The true terminal half-life is measured when concentrations are very low and is not dose-dependent (see **Figure 21**). However, the measured half-life may indicate the possibility of saturation of elimination if the concentration–time curve is not followed for long enough, for example if measurements had been made for only 50 min after each dose in **Figure 21**.

The best indication of dose-dependent elimination is the calculation of the clearance as dose/AUC to infinity. This is illustrated in **Figure 21**, which gives data for a compound showing a single exponential decrease at low concentrations and where $K_m = 20$ units and $V_{max} = 1$ unit min^{-1}. The initial plasma concentration (C_0) is dependent only on the dose and the apparent volume of distribution (V) ($C_0 = \text{dose}/V$) and the three doses were in the ratio 1:5:10. However, the AUC values increased in the order 250:2242:6988, *i.e.* 1:9:28. Thus the clearance (dose/AUC) decreased in the ratio 1:0.56:0.36, but the terminal half-life was 15 min for each dose.

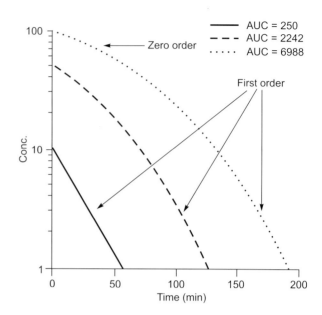

Figure 21 Plasma concentration–time curve for a compound showing saturation kinetics given at doses sufficient to give initial plasma concentrations of 10, 50 and 100 units. The compound is eliminated by a single saturable pathway.

A compound which shows non-linear toxicokinetics similar to those depicted in **Figure 21** is the solvent 1,4-dioxane (Dietz *et al.*, 1982), for which an increase in intravenous dose in rats from 3 to 1000 mg kg^{-1} (333-fold) caused a 4439-fold increase in AUC. The disproportionate increase in AUC of dioxane at high doses was associated with a decrease in the urinary excretion of the metabolite β-hydroxyethoxyacetic acid and an increase in the elimination of the solvent *per se* in the expired air. However, during chronic daily administration of $[^{14}\text{C}]$-dioxane, the body burden at steady state was only slightly higher after 1000 mg kg^{-1} day^{-1} compared with 10 mg kg^{-1} day^{-1} after allowing for differences in dose. These data suggest that the non-linear AUC difference between 1000 and 10 mg kg^{-1} as single doses overestimated the difference at steady state. Studies on enzyme activities suggested that dioxane at high doses induces its own metabolism (Dietz *et al.*, 1982), so that an increase in V_{max} compensated for saturation of the enzyme.

Non-linear kinetics can be demonstrated by the use of a time-based parameter derived from the AUC, *i.e.* the mean residence time (MRT). The mean residence time is the ratio of the area under the first moment of the concentration–time curve (AUMC) divided by the area under the concentration–time curve (AUC).

$$\text{MRT} = \frac{\text{AUMC}}{\text{AUC}}$$

The AUMC is derived by the trapezoidal rule applied to a graph of concentration times time ($C \times t$), for each sample, plotted against time (t) for that sample and therefore does not require fitting of any specific models to the data. Both the AUC and the AUMC data must be extrapolated to infinity for the above equation to be valid. Extrapolation of the AUMC from the last concentration–time point to infinity is achieved by the addition of

$$\frac{t_{last} \times C_{last}}{\beta} + \frac{C_{last}}{\beta^2}$$

where β is the terminal slope.

For the data in **Figure 21** the AUMC values for the increasing doses were 5606, 77 427 and 354 639 [which have units of concentration $\times (time)^2$] whereas the corresponding AUC values were 250, 2242 and 6988 (which have units of concentration $\times$ time). Thus the MRT values, which are AUMC/AUC, have units of time and for the data in **Figure 21** were 22.4, 35.3 and 50.7 min, thereby clearly demonstrating dose dependence. The MRT can be regarded as *the mean time for which any one molecule of the chemical will be present in the body*, and is analogous to but not identical with the half-life. The half-life ($t_{1/2}$) can be calculated as

$$t_{1/2} = MRT \times 0.693$$

In the case of the lowest dose in **Figure 21**, $t_{1/2}$ can be calculated as $22.4 \times 0.693 = 15$ min, which agrees with that derived from the terminal slope. Using the MRT to calculate the 'half-life' for the two higher doses is not logical since the half-lives obtained will be composite values based on the whole concentration–time curve which includes the zero-order component (for which a half-life is not appropriate). However, such a calculation would demonstrate dose-dependent, non-linear kinetics.

The statistical moment analysis can also be applied to an intravenous infusion (although a different correction is necessary—see Gibaldi and Perrier, 1982; Chapter 11) and to oral administration to calculate the MAT (see earlier). In addition, it is possible to use single dose data to calculate the volume of distribution at the steady state (V_{ss}), which is analogous to $V_\beta(CL/\beta)$, by the equation

$$V_{ss} = CL \times MRT = \frac{dose}{AUC} \times \frac{AUMC}{AUC}$$

Dose-dependent kinetics can arise from the saturation of a number of protein–chemical interactions **(Table 4)**. Therefore, non-linear relationships can produce a range of different changes to the plasma concentration–time profile. A number of different approaches can be taken to demonstrate dose-dependent kinetics, *e.g.*

(i) Divide the plasma concentration for each time point by the dose, and plot the resulting dose-adjusted data. For purely linear and first-order processes the adjusted data will be superimposable. A consistent

dose-dependent deviation indicates that non-linearity is present but does not indicate the reason.

(ii) Fit all doses to a common model and evaluate systematic changes in parameter estimates.

(iii) Measure metabolite formation either in plasma or urine. A dose-dependent change in the ratio of the AUC for the parent compound to the AUC of the metabolite (or percentage dose in urine) would indicate saturation of metabolism.

(iv) Measure tissue to plasma ratios for a range of doses to detect saturation of protein binding in either plasma or tissue.

Trans-Species Comparisons

The use of animal data to predict potential risks to humans, or to establish safe exposure levels, is based on the assumption that both the toxicodynamics and the toxicokinetics in animals are relevant to humans. There are wide differences between different animal species and between animals and humans in physiological processes, such as organ perfusion rates and in biochemical processes such as foreign compound metabolism. In consequence, all extrapolations from animals to humans must take into account differences in toxicokinetics. These differences are illustrated by data on chlorinated dibenzo-*p*-dioxins.

Chlorinated dibenzo-*p*-dioxins, such as 2, 3, 7, 8-tetra-chlorodibenzo-*p*-dioxin, (TCDD), are among the most toxic chemicals known and produce acnegenic, carcinogenic, foetotoxic, immunosuppressive and teratogenic effects (HMSO, 1989). There are wide inter-species differences in acute toxicity of TCDD, with the guinea pig being about 10–20 times more sensitive than the rat (Kociba *et al.*, 1976) or mouse (Beatty *et al.*, 1978; McConnell *et al.*, 1978), while the hamster appears to be the least sensitive species (Olson *et al.*, 1980a). The elimination half-life in guinea pigs (30 ± 6 days; Gasiewicz and Neal, 1979) is similar to that in rats (Rose *et al.*, 1976), and only about twice that in hamsters (15 ± 3 days; Olson *et al.*, 1980b). Differences in sensitivity to TCDD in different strains of rats cannot be related to differences in toxicokinetics (Pohjanvirta *et al.*, 1990). Thus the species and strain differences in acute toxicity are not related to the ability to eliminate the compound.

Because of the slow elimination of [^{14}C]TCDD, the elimination rate constant was calculated from the total amount of radioactivity recovered in urine and faeces each day using an adaptation of the *sigma minus method* (Gibaldi and Perrier, 1982). This method is based on measurements of the excretion of the parent compound until no more can be detected in the urine (and/or faeces). For each collection time interval the amount remaining to be excreted is calculated as (amount excreted as parent compound to infinity − amount excreted up to that time); a plot of the natural logarithm of the amount remaining to be excreted against the time at the end of the collection interval will have a slope of $-\beta$ (or $-\lambda_z$) with an intercept of the natural logarithm of the total amount excreted unchanged. This method is applicable even in cases where excretion of the parent compound is not the major route of elimination, because the amount of parent compound excreted at any time is proportional to the plasma concentration (C) and therefore the body load $(V$ times $C)$ of parent compound at that time. In the case of TCDD, the 'body burden' of TCDD remaining after each day was calculated as (dose administered $-$ total ^{14}C recovered in excreta to that time). A plot of the natural logarithm of the body burden against time was used to calculate the elimination half-life. This approach is particularly useful for calculating the elimination kinetics of compounds that are eliminated very slowly, and also has the advantage of being non-invasive; the method is illustrated in **Table 5** and **Figure 22**. It should be appreciated that in studies on slowly eliminated lipid-soluble compounds, such as TCDD, the radioactivity detected in the excreta may be present partly as metabolites (Neal *et al.*, 1982). Under such circumstances, the sigma minus method using excretion of total ^{14}C is only valid if the body burden is as parent compound and the metabolites, once formed, are eliminated rapidly, *i.e.* the rate-limiting step is the initial metabolism of the parent compound.

The octachloro analogue of TCDD (OCDD) is 100–1000 times less potent than TCDD (Couture *et al.*, 1988), but it shows even slower elimination in rats with a half-life of 3–5 months, so that even greater accumulation is

possible (Birnbaum and Couture, 1988). For compounds with such long half-lives, the steady state will not have been reached at the end of a 7 or 13 week study **(Figure 23)**. In addition, if there is a minimum body burden or plasma concentration necessary for toxicity, this may have been reached only a short time before killing the animal. Clearly, the interpretation of data from 'short-term' studies should take into account the half-life of

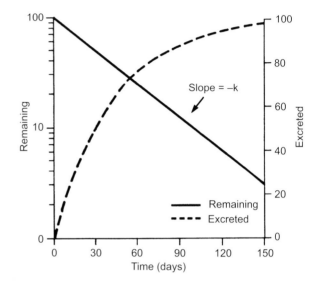

Figure 22 Calculation of the elimination rate constant from the cumulative elimination of the compound (see Table 5 for data). This analysis assumes that either the parent compound is excreted unchanged or that the formation of excretable metabolites is the rate-limiting step.

Table 5 Calculation of elimination rate constant by the sigma minus method

| Time[a] (days) | % Dose excreted (as parent compound plus metabolites) | | | | |
	Urine	Faeces	Total	Cumulative total	Amount remaining
0	0.0	0.0	0.0	0.0	100.0
2	1.8	2.7	4.5	4.5	95.5
4	1.7	2.6	4.3	8.8	91.2
6	1.6	2.5	4.1	12.9	87.1
8	1.6	2.4	4.0	16.9	83.1
10	1.5	2.2	3.7	20.6	79.4
15	3.5	5.2	8.7	29.3	70.7
20	3.1	4.6	7.7	37.0	63.0
25	2.8	4.1	6.9	43.9	56.1
30	2.4	3.7	6.1	50.0	50.0
40	4.1	6.2	10.3	60.3	39.7
50	3.3	4.9	8.2	68.5	31.5
60	2.6	3.9	6.5	75.0	25.0
70	2.0	3.1	5.1	80.1	19.8
80	1.6	2.5	4.1	84.2	15.8
100	2.4	3.5	5.9	90.1	9.9
120	1.4	2.2	3.6	93.7	6.3
150	1.3	1.9	3.2	96.9	3.1

The data are for the excretion of a compound which is eliminated slowly in both urine and faeces with approximately 60% of the dose excreted in faeces and 40% in urine. The method assumes that the elimination of metabolites is formation rate limited and that there is no accumulation of metabolites.
[a] Time at the end of the sequential collection intervals (e.g. 2 = 0–2, 30 = 25–30 and 150 = 120–150).

the compound, since a 90 day study may be a steady-state study for some compounds but not for others (see **Figure 23**). [Toxicologists not conversant with toxicokinetics might consider that, for compounds with such extremely long half-lives, animals given lower doses would eventually reach the same plasma concentrations and body loads as animals given higher doses but take longer to get there. This is *not* true, as illustrated by the data for TCDD (Rose *et al.*, 1976) and the theoretical consideration given in **Figure 23**.]

There are problems with extrapolation of the data for TCDD in rodents to possible human intakes. The half-life of TCDD in humans based on the elimination by occupationally exposed individuals is about 7 years (Wolfe *et al.*, 1988). Another report (Poiger, 1988) of the elimination of TCDD following self-administration of [³H]TCDD indicated that the half-life may be as long as 9 years. Using the value of 7 years it would take about 30–35 years of exposure for humans to reach steady state during constant intake. If the differences in half-life between animal species and humans are assumed to be due to differences in clearance, *i.e.* there are no significant differences in the apparent volume of distribution, then it is possible to compare theoretical steady-state body burdens under differing rates of administration. These are summarized in **Table 6** and indicate that the steady-state body burden of TCDD in man from environmental exposure would be approximately two orders of magnitude below those that would be present in monkeys during chronic toxicity studies. Clearly, this analysis indicates a reassuring safety factor of just over 100 between the minimal toxicity seen in the most sensitive species (the monkey) and potential human exposure.

The apparent safety margin based on body burden is probably a slight overestimate since the monkeys were treated for 4 years prior to mating, *i.e.* a period of 'only' 1.46 half-lives (2.74 years), so that the animals would have reached only 64% of the steady state at the time of

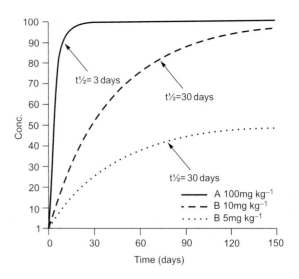

Figure 23 Accumulation of compounds during chronic administration. The compounds have similar apparent volumes of distribution but the clearance of A is 10 times greater than that of B, so that its half-life is 10 times less. Thus, daily intakes of 100 mg kg⁻¹ of A and 10 mg kg⁻¹ of B will give similar average steady-state concentrations while a dose of 5 mg kg⁻¹ of B will give an average steady-state concentration half of that at a dose of 10 mg kg⁻¹ day⁻¹.

reproduction. A similar percentage of the steady state would be reached by a human at approximately 10 years of age, whereas a woman giving birth at 25 years of age would have reached approximately 92% of the steady state. Thus, the apparent safety margin may have been overestimated by a factor of about 1.4. In contrast, if the limiting toxicity had been carcinogenicity in the rat then the steady state would have been approached in the animals after 4–5 months, *i.e.* after approximately 16% of the animal's life. In contrast, the steady state for humans given in **Table 6** would not have been approached until after 28–35 years, *i.e.* approximately 50% of the lifespan. Thus the test animals would have

Table 6 Inter-species comparisons of theoretical steady-state body burdens of TCDD at different rates of administration

Species	Half-life	Rate of administration	Steady-state body burden
Rat	30 days	$1.0\ \mu g\ kg^{-1}\ day^{-1\,a}$	$20\ \mu g\ kg^{-1\,a}$
		$0.1\ \mu g\ kg^{-1}\ day^{-1\,a}$	$2\ \mu g\ kg^{-1\,a}$
		$0.01\ \mu g\ kg^{-1}\ day^{-1\,b}$	$0.2\ \mu g\ kg^{-1}$
Guinea pig	30 days	$6\ ng\ kg^{-1}\ day^{-1\,c}$	$0.12\ \mu g\ kg^{-1}$
Monkey	1000 days[d]	$0.12\ ng\ kg^{-1}\ day^{-1\,e}$	$0.08\ \mu g\ kg^{-1}$
Man	7 years[f]	$0.0004\ ng\ kg^{-1}\ day^{-1\,g}$	$0.0007\ \mu g\ kg^{-1}$

[a] Data from Gehring and Young (1978) at toxic doses during a 90 day study. Used as the basis for calculation the steady-state body burdens in other species by correcting for half-life (assuming no species differences in the apparent volume of distribution).

$$\text{Body burden at steady state} = 20 \times \frac{\text{rate of administration (ng kg}^{-1}\text{day}^{-1})}{1000} \times \frac{\text{half}-\text{life (days)}}{30}$$

[b] Minimal effect level for carcinogenic effects (HMSO, 1989).
[c] Minimal effect level for immunotoxic effects (HMSO, 1989).
[d] Taken from HMSO (1989, p. 96).
[e] Minimal effect level for reproductive toxicity (HMSO, 1989).
[f] Taken from Wolfe *et al.* (1988).
[g] Daily intake from foods in West Germany (HMSO, 1989).

been exposed to the steady-state body burden for a considerably longer proportion of their lifespan than would be possible in humans.

The interpretation of the human epidemiological data on occupational exposures to TCDD is complex, both for comparisons between species and between occupational and environmental exposure. The body burdens arising from occupational exposures have usually been derived by back-extrapolation through time, based on a concentration measured some years after the period of high exposure (Hays *et al.*, 1997). Occupational exposure usually occurred at some time during the working life, which established a body burden; this body burden would then increase, be maintained or decrease, depending on whether it was below, equal to, or greater than the steady-state body burden associated with the subsequent environmental exposure. Quantitative comparisons between the profile of occupational exposure and either chronic animal studies or human environmental exposures are complicated by the selection of the correct body burden for comparison and the different shape of the exposure–time curve throughout life. Hays *et al.* (1997) compared total AUC values (over the lifetime), peak concentrations and average concentrations of TCDD in rats and humans with the corresponding tumour incidence (in liver and lung, respectively). The first of these measures (total AUC) is inappropriate, because of the difference in lifetime, while the second (peak concentration) is probably inappropriate for a 'promoter'. Comparisons of the average concentration during the lifetime is the most appropriate approach, but the period of exposure which would be above the average would represent an early high, short term and falling excess in the occupational cohort compared with a later, low, long-term and rising excess in the animal study.

An interesting safety issue that is partially resolvable by toxicokinetic considerations concerns the intake of TCDD and related compounds by human infants *via* maternal milk. The concentrations of TCDD in human milk exceed those in meat, eggs and cow's milk (HMSO, 1989), and therefore higher plasma concentrations and body burdens might be anticipated in infants. However, correspondingly higher body loads would only occur if the intake of human milk extended for 4–5 times the half-life of the compound, which in the case of TCDD would mean 30–35 years! Exposure *via* human milk is of such limited duration, with respect to the half-life of TCDD, that if the daily intake in infants *via* maternal milk (per kg body weight) was as much as 20 times that in adults, then the infant would only just have reached the adult steady-state plasma concentration and body burden after 6 months suckling (assuming a negligible body burden at birth). Therefore, in reality, exposure *via* maternal milk would not pose an extra risk to the neonate, but would simply act as a 'loading dose' so that the adult steady state would be achieved more rapidly, and then sub-

sequently maintained by the adult daily intake (Renwick and Walker, 1993).

This detailed analysis of the case of TCDD illustrates the critical role that toxicokinetics can play in the design and interpretation of toxicity studies, especially when the compound has a very long half-life. In addition, it should be appreciated that if as a result of the animal toxicity data it was decided that the exposure of humans should be reduced immediately to negligible levels, it would take about 7 years before the existing body burdens decrease by 50%, and about 30–40 years before they would become negligible. In reality, the persistence of TCDD in mammalian organisms compared with the environment (DiDomenico and Zapponi, 1986) indicates that the latter would be rate limiting in any attempted reduction of human body burdens.

The body burden of TCDD in humans in **Table 6** was calculated using a very simplistic analysis based on the body burdens of animals corrected for differences in clearance (assuming that differences in half-lives are due to differences in clearance) and intakes, but it is probably realistic. Most TCDD accumulates in fat and to some extent the liver, and so it can be assumed that the total body burden of a 70 kg human (0.0007 $\mu g\ kg^{-1} \times 70 = 0.049\ \mu g$) would be concentrated in about 10 kg of fat, *i.e.* approximately $0.005\ \mu g\ kg^{-1}$ of fat. This value is almost identical with that found in human body fat (approximately 6 ng kg^{-1}; HMSO, 1989, p. 44).

The use of animal data to predict the body load of TCDD in humans in **Table 6** is the simplest form of interspecies extrapolation. There are two principal methods by which more sophisticated extrapolations may be made, *i.e. allometry* and *physiologically based pharmacokinetic models*. The basis of both methods is that there are underlying similarities between mammalian species in the various processes involved in toxicokinetics. For example, (a) the intestine contains similar digestive enzymes and provides a large surface area for *absorption via* microvilli; (b) the compositions of blood and body tissues are similar across species with respect to fat and protein content so that tissue *distribution* should be similar; (c) the perfusion of the organs of *elimination* and the basic metabolic and excretory processes within these organs are similar. Hence reasonable estimates of human pharmacokinetic parameters should be derived from animal data after allowing for differences in body weight, cardiac output, *etc*. It should be emphasized that there are bound to be examples where clear species differences exist, especially with respect to specific pathways of metabolism, which render such extrapolations inappropriate (see risk assessment below).

Allometry is a mathematical extrapolation based on the body weight of animal (Calder, 1981). Thus the value of any parameter (P) is related to the mean body weight (W) of the species by an equation with two unknown variables:

$$P = aW^x$$

If the parameter estimate P is known in two or more species, then its value in a third species can be deduced from a simple regression equation of log P against log W. For example, the clearance values of the drug ceftizoxime in mice ($W = 23$ g), rats ($W = 180$ g), monkeys ($W = 7500$ g) and dogs ($W = 12\,000$ g) are 84.4, 208.8, 2670 and 2340 ml h^{-1}, respectively (Mordenti, 1985). A regression of log (clearance) against log (body weight) had a slope (x) of 0.573 and an intercept (log a) of 1.103, so that

$$P = 12.69\,W^{0.573}$$

Using this equation, the clearance values calculated for mice, rats, monkeys, dog and humans ($W = 70\,000$g) are 77, 249, 2108, 2760 and 7581 ml h^{-1}, respectively.

Inter-species comparisons of caffeine pharmacokinetics (Bonati *et al.*, 1985) showed that the apparent volume of distribution was linearly related to body weight (W) (*i.e.* $V = 0.79\,W^{1.00}$), whereas the plasma clearance (CL) showed a log-linear relationship (*i.e.* $CL = 6.26\,W^{0.739}$); the power term for clearance was similar to that for liver weight (L) (*i.e.* $L = 0.037\,W^{0.845}$).

Boxenbaum (1984) provided useful background information on the origins of allometry in pharmacokinetic scaling and extended this by the use of Dedrick plots in which plasma concentration–time curves in different species can be made superimposable if the concentration is corrected for dose (*e.g.* μg ml^{-1} per mg kg^{-1}) and the time is corrected for body weight (*e.g.* min kg$^{-0.25}$). The basis for this latter correction is conversion to 'physiological time', which in effect relates body weight to the lifespan of the animal. Thus, 100 min in the life of a 22 g mouse is physiologically equivalent to 751 min in the life of a 70 kg human. Although the approach of correcting pharmacokinetic data for the maximum potential lifespan helped to linearize the relationship between intrinsic clearance of caffeine and body weight (Bonati *et al.*, 1985), the authors concluded that 'no practical use can yet be suggested for the resulting good fit'. Bachmann (1989) applied allometry to the pharmacokinetics for a number of drugs in laboratory animals and humans. For each drug there was a linear relationship between the logarithm of the apparent volumes of distribution and the logarithm of body weights with correlation coefficients >0.95. The logarithm of the clearance was not as closely related to the logarithm of the body weight unless multiplied by the maximum lifespan potential (MLP) for each species. This is shown in **Figure 24**, which also illustrates the principle of allometric analysis. Bachmann proposed that the clearance in a species could be calculated from the $CL\times$ MLP regression since the term $CL \times$ MLP divided by body weight (BW) was relatively constant across species. It was suggested that if the mean $CL \times$ MLP/BW was calculated for three animal species

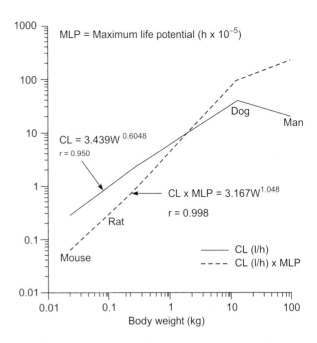

Figure 24 Inter-species scaling applied to the plasma clearance of phencyclidine (data taken from Bachmann, 1989).

this value could then be used to derive the clearance in a 70 kg human with an assumed MLP of 9.9×10^5 h (113 years).

An alternative approach is that of *physiologically based pharmacokinetic (PB-PK) modelling* (Gerlowski and Jain, 1983). The basis of the method is that each major organ system, plus any specialized sites such as targets for toxicity, are taken as representing a physiological compartment. Each separate compartment has its own blood flow, tissue volume, uptake process, affinity for the compound (*i.e.* partition coefficient) and elimination process as appropriate **(Figure 25)**. The kinetics of the compound are described by a series of flow-related equations, which can be solved following the incorporation of known physiological values and experimental estimates (*e.g.* partition coefficients). The main application of the technique is that species differences can be predicted based on known differences in perfusion rates, *etc.*; in cases where an important physiological value is not known for a species, this can be derived by allometry from species in which the values are known. Additional advantages of this technique are that it allows an assessment of the impact of altered physiology, *e.g.* ageing and renal function, on the toxicokinetics and target organ exposure, and that data from human studies, such as enzyme activities, can be incorporated directly into the model.

Simpler physiologically based models may be derived which are a compromise between tissue-based physiological compartments and traditional rapidly and slowly equilibrating compartments. For example, Andersen *et al.* (1987) utilized a mixture of specific physiological compartments, liver, fat, lung and gut, with two general

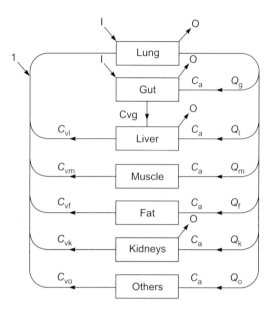

Figure 25 A physiologically based pharmacokinetic model. The rate of delivery to an organ such as muscle is given by the blood flow (Q_m) times the arterial concentration (C_a). The rate of removal from the organ is blood flow (Q_m) times the venous concentration (C_{vm}). Input functions (I) and output functions (O) can be first-order or Michaelis–Menten reactions. More complex models have been used, incorporating specific targets, such as bone marrow, or additional routes such as transdermal, in which case the skin becomes a discrete compartment.

compartments, 'richly perfused' and 'slowly perfused', in the analysis of the inhalation kinetics of dichloromethane.

The precision of a model similar to that used by Andersen *et al.* (1987) was investigated by Bois *et al.* (1990) for the saturable formation of the carcinogenic epoxide metabolite of tetrachloroethylene. The physiological model was coupled to a multistage model of carcinogenesis to predict cancer risk in humans exposed to 1 ng l^{-1} of tetrachloroethylene vapour. The median predicted incidence was 1.6 cancer per 10^6 and varying the parameter estimates within physiologically realistic bounds produced 5th and 95th percentile estimates of 0 and 6.8 per 10^6. The authors concluded that biases introduced by the choice of an inappropriate model greatly exceeded the errors due to variability in the parameters included in the model.

The pharmacokinetics of TCDD in the rat have been fitted using a simple physiologically based model, which allowed for enzyme induction (Leung *et al.*, 1990a). A similar model accurately predicted the influence of an inducing dose of TCDD on the concentration–time curve of the analogue 2-iodo-3, 7, 8-trichlorodibenzo-*p*-dioxin. Therefore, auto-induction during high-dose animal toxicity studies on TCDD can be taken into account by these models in predicting the behaviour of TCDD at the lower environment doses received by humans (Leung *et al.*, 1990b). A more complex physiological model has

been developed for the fate of TCDD in man (Kissel and Robarge, 1988). A number of assumptions were made in the model, but trial simulations showed that the most important variables were adipose:blood partition coefficients and adipose perfusion. The model also estimated intake and body exposure based on likely dietary sources, and accurately predicted the half-life and body burden in humans. The model also showed that the half-life was dependent on the relative amount of faecal output compared with adipose tissue storage. The potential value of this approach was demonstrated by simulations which showed that faecal output of TCDD was significantly enhanced by the ingestion of 10 g per day of a non-absorbable oil, and that this reduced both the half-life and steady-state concentration in adipose tissue.

A distinct advantage of PB-PK modelling is its ability to incorporate both *in vitro* enzyme activity data and *in vivo* organ blood flows to produce a composite model, which can avoid misleading conclusions. For example, the rate of *in vitro* bioactivation of furan was similar and very high in both mice and humans, but these high rates of metabolism would not be apparent *in vivo*, because they greatly exceeded the rate of liver perfusion (Kedderis and Held, 1996). In consequence, the species difference in bioactivation in the PB-PK model was determined largely by liver blood flow and not the difference in enzyme activity.

USE OF TOXICOKINETICS IN RISK ASSESSMENT

Assessments of the risks of exposure of human to chemicals are usually based on hazards identified in animal experiments and the associated dose–response curves for the effect. There are various approaches adopted by regulatory bodies for establishing 'acceptable' or 'safe' exposure for humans.

Low-dose risk extrapolation

This approach extrapolates from the incidence in the experimental dose–response range in animals down to a predefined negligible risk (10^{-5} or 10^{-6}). This process essentially defines a negligible risk in animals, unless inter-species differences are taken into account. A major advance with this approach has been the incorporation of toxicokinetic data, usually in the form of PB-PK modelling, to correct the experimental external dose to a target organ dose, and then to estimate the target organ dose in humans in relation to that in animals. However, such toxicokinetic refinements have not altered the vast uncertainties inherent in extrapolation at least four orders of magnitude away from the dose–response data. The outcome of such extrapolations is determined largely by the model selected rather than the biological data or its toxicokinetic refinement.

Margin of safety

This approach, which compares the doses in animals associated with toxicity and those in humans, is usually applied to occupational and environmental exposures. The adequacy of the 'safety margin' is then assessed based on the nature of the exposed human groups, the duration of exposure and the nature of the hazard. Again, PB-PK modelling has been used to refine the comparison (see analysis of **Table 6** above). The margin of safety is also compared with the safety factor of 100 which is used traditionally for non-cancer endpoints (see below). A refinement of the margin of safety approach is the exposure potency index, which is particularly useful for comparisons of the risks of different chemicals. The toxicity dose–response curve is used to calculate a fixed response (usually a 5% incidence) in experimental animals and the ratio is determined based on the body burden (or target organ dose from a PB-PK model) for the experimental animal and for humans.

Both physiologically based models and allometry can be of value to regulatory safety assessments (Scheuplein *et al.*, 1990). For example, physiologically based pharmacokinetic models have been applied to the regulatory risk assessment of trichloroethylene (Bogen, 1988) and 1,1,1-trichloroethane (Bogen and Hall, 1989), while both allometry (Beliles and Totman, 1989) and physiological models (Travis *et al.*, 1990) have been used to extrapolate data on benzene from rodents to humans. Physiologically based models are far more flexible than allometry, and more complex situations, such as exposure during lactation (Fisher *et al.*, 1990), can be taken into account.

Safety assurance procedures

This approach tends to be adopted for compounds which are required to undergo toxicity testing/risk assessment before approval and prior to human exposure. For some chemicals, such as medicines, the approval can be based on a risk:benefit analysis because of the clear benefit to the 'consumer'. However, for other chemicals such as food additives and pesticides, there are no direct health benefits to the consumer to offset against any possible health risk. Therefore, the establishment of a 'safe dose' in animals, and inter-species extrapolation to give a 'safe dose' in humans are of critical importance. The 'safe dose' in animals is the no observed adverse effect level (NOAEL), which is expressed as mg kg^{-1} body weight per day, and this is converted to the 'safe dose' for humans by dividing by a large safety factor. The 'safe dose' for humans is described as the acceptable daily intake (ADI), tolerable daily intake (TDI) or provisional tolerable weekly intake (PTWI). This is the approach adopted by bodies such as the WHO–FAO Joint Expert Committee on Food Additives (see WHO, 1987) and the Scientific Committee for Food of the European Union. Normally a 100-fold factor is used when the NOAEL is based on animal data and a 10-fold factor is used when the NOAEL is derived from a study in humans. In reality, the safety factor is an uncertainty factor which has to allow for possible differences between test species and humans and for possible human variability. Each 10-fold factor (inter-species and inter-individual) has to allow for toxicokinetic and toxicodynamic differences (Renwick, 1991) **(Figure 26)**. It has been proposed that the 10 × 10-fold factor should be considered as a four-way box **(Figure 27)** and values have been proposed for both toxicokinetic ad toxicodynamic aspects (Renwick, 1993) which when multiplied together give the original factors of 10 × 10. The rationale for this proposal was to allow relevant data on a chemical to replace part of the 'uncertainty', and thereby provide a more scientific basis for the determination of the 'safe' human dose. The values proposed were evaluated by a WHO Task Group, which considered the approach valuable but revised slightly the proposed default values (WHO, 1994) (see **Figure 27**). A recent extensive review has supported the revised WHO subdivision of the 10-fold factor for human variability and also analysed the extent to which this value provides adequate safety assurance (Renwick and Lazarus, 1998).

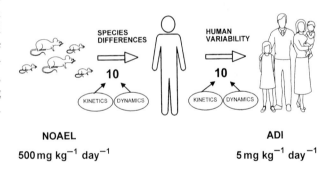

Figure 26 The use of a 100-fold safety or uncertainty factor to convert the no-observed adverse effect level (NOAEL) in animals into an acceptable steady intake (ADI) for humans (from Renwick, 1998).

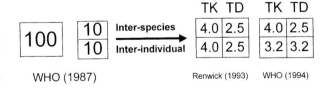

			TK	TD	TK	TD
100	**10**	Inter-species	4.0	2.5	4.0	2.5
	10	Inter-individual	4.0	2.5	3.2	3.2
WHO (1987)			Renwick (1993)		WHO (1994)	

TK - toxicokinetics
TD - toxicodynamics

Figure 27 The evolution of the 100-fold uncertainty factor (from Renwick, 1998).

There are a number of aspects which are critical to the replacement of a default by a chemical-specific value. These include:

(i) Separation of toxicokinetic and toxicodynamic aspects. The generation of appropriate data in humans is essential to replace either of the toxicokinetic defaults **(Figure 27)**. Human studies are usually limited to the determination of circulating concentrations, and therefore toxicokinetics stops at the delivery of chemical to the target sites; any process occurring within the target organ is therefore part of the toxicodynamics (including local metabolic bioactivation).

(ii) Identification of toxic compound. It is essential that the activity of the parent compound and metabolites is determined. The toxicokinetic comparison should be the delivery of the toxic moiety (which may be a metabolite) to the target organ in relation to the external dose of the parent compound.

(iii) Selection of the appropriate toxicokinetic parameters. In most cases this would be the AUC of the toxic moiety, but peak concentration may be more appropriate, especially for acute effects.

(iv) Selection of appropriate doses. Although toxicokinetic processes are essentially first order at low doses, it is possible that saturation may occur at the high doses used in animal studies. The correct comparison is between the toxicokinetics of the chemical in the test species at the NOAEL and in humans at the ADI/TDI that would be calculated in the absence of the toxicokinetic data.

(v) Dose metric. The 100-fold factor, and therefore the defaults shown in **Figure 27**, are applied to the external dose expressed in mg kg^{-1} body weight. If the dose is calculated on the basis of the body surface area, then this will be a form of allometry (see earlier). In humans, body weight and surface area are related by the equation

$$SA = W^{0.425} \times H^{0.725} \times 71.84$$

where SA = surface area, W = weight and H = height.

Inter-species comparisons often use simple equations in which the surface area is related to (bodyweight)$^{0.66}$ or (body weight)$^{0.75}$.

The use of surface area rather than body weight therefore appears to allow for species differences. The difference between body weight and surface area is equivalent to a factor of about eight for mice, four for rats and two for dogs; *i.e.* for a NOAEL in rats, the 'safe dose' for humans based on surface area would be four times lower than that expressed on the basis of body weight. Application of a 100-fold factor to a dose expressed on surface area would increase the normal inter-species safety margin (by a factor of four for rats) but would

reduce the inter-individual factor (by about 1.8-fold) in relation to the difference between adults and 1-year-old infants (Renwick, 1998). The rationale for the expression of dose on the basis of surface area is that this allows for physiological differences such as calorie intake, rates of intermediary metabolism and cardiac output. Although this is logical for dose selection for compounds subject to intermediary metabolism, such as certain cytotoxins used in cancer chemotherapy, it may not be appropriate for xenobiotic chemicals metabolized by pathways showing significant interspecies and inter-individual differences. Therefore, expression of dose in relation to surface area is *not* equivalent to allowing for species differences in toxicokinetics, and the replacement of defaults by specific chemical-related values is more appropriate. The fact that the inter-species default for toxicokinetics is similar to the simplistic correction by surface area emphasizes the need to develop a more refined approach to the use of uncertainty or safety factors (Renwick and Lazarus, 1998). The replacement of the defaults by relevant chemical-related data, or better still a specific PB-PK model, will give greater scientific credibility to a safety assurance process which at present appears arbitrary.

ADDITIONAL SOURCES OF INFORMATION

It has not been possible to cover the vast subject of toxicokinetics adequately within the confines of a single chapter. There are a number of text books and review articles to which readers are referred for further information, for the interpretation of more complex situations, and for sampling techniques. The following comments may help the reader choose an appropriate general text or review article; full references are gives in the reference list.

General Texts

Benet (1976)	Rather specialized but good background reading with respect to possible problems in geriatric animals.
Smyth and Hottendorf (1980)	Contains some useful examples, especially of problems of absorption.
Gibaldi and Perrier (1982)	The definitive text.
Curry and Whelpton (1983)	An experimental introduction to the subject.
Benet *et al.* (1984)	Based on a symposium, and therefore lacks the structure of Gibaldi and Perrier's or Rowland and

Greenblatt and Shader (1985)   Tucker's publications but contains some useful information.

Introductory text (do not be put off by the title!).

Clarke and Smith (1986)   Introductory text.

Rowland and Tucker (1986)   A more advanced text with useful chapters on inter-species scaling, dose-and time-dependent kinetics and response modelling.

Gabrielsson and Weiner (1997)   An altogether excellent textbook, clearly explained with large numbers of helpful diagrams.

Review Articles

Gehring and Young (1978)   Contains interesting examples from the work of the pioneers in the application of pharmacokinetics to problems of animal toxicology.

Wilkinson (1984)   A clearly written article which deals with first-pass metabolism and dose-dependent kinetics and introduces physiological approaches.

O'Flaherty (1985)   A consideration of dose-dependent metabolism.

Wilkinson (1987)   A comprehensive review of the application of clearance concepts to the elimination of foreign components; not toxicology orientated, but an excellent source of references (525).

Renwick (1989)   Similar to the present chapter but with an expanded section on dose-dependent kinetics, metabolite kinetics and worked examples.

Scheuplein et al. (1990)   An interesting article on the value of toxicokinetic data to regulatory agencies such as the FDA.

Pharmacokinetic data fitting

Drug Metabolism Reviews, Volume 15 (1984), contains a series of valuable but mathematically complex articles by leading workers in the field of pharmacokinetics. Topics covered include compartmental models (Segre; pp. 7–53), physiological models (Rowland; pp. 55–74), models in health and disease (Balant; pp. 75–102), non-compartmental statistical moments (Nuesch; pp. 103–131), the weighting of data for regression analysis (Peck, Sheiner and Nichols; pp. 133–148), population pharmacokinetics (Sheiner; pp. 153–171) and population pharmacokinetics applied to destructively obtained experimental data (Lindstrom and Birkes; pp. 195–264). This last paper proposes the derivation of pharmacokinetic parameters from observations of the concentrations in the plasma and tissues of killed animals; but the choice of an appropriately timed sampling protocol would be essential.

The book by Gabrielsson and Weiner (1997) contains useful sections on weighting of data, assessing goodness of fit and discriminating between different models.

Sampling Techniques

Waynforth (1980)   A textbook on surgical techniques in the rat.

Bakar and Niazi (1983)   A simple and reliable method for chronic venous cannulation in the rat.

Cocchetto and Bjornsson (1983)   Various methods of collecting rat body fluids; a useful review with 501 references.

REFERENCES

Andersen, M. E., Clewell, H. J., Gargas, M. L., Smith, F. A. and Reitz, R. H. (1987). Physiologically based pharmacokinetics and the risk assessment process for methylene chloride. *Toxicol. Appl. Pharmacol.*, **87**, 185–205.

Bachmann, K. (1989). Predicting toxicokinetic parameters in humans from toxicokinetic data acquired from three small mammalian species. *J. Appl. Toxicol.*, **9**, 331–338.

Bakar, S. L. and Niazi, S. (1983). Simple reliable method for chronic cannulation of the jugular vein for pharmacokinetic studies in rats. *J. Pharm. Sci.*, **72**, 1027–1029.

Beatty, P. W., Vaughn, W. K. and Neal, R. A. (1978). Effect of alteration of rat hepatic mixed-function oxidase (MFO) activity on the toxicity of 2,3,7,8-tetrachlorodibenzo-*p*-dioxin (TCDD). *Toxicol. Appl. Pharmacol.*, **45**, 513–519.

Beliles, R. P. and Totman, L. C. (1989). Pharmacokinetically based risk assessment of workplace exposure to benzene. *Regul. Toxicol. Pharmacol.*, **9**, 186–195.

Benet, L. Z. (1976). *The Effect of Disease States on Drug Pharmacokinetics*. American Pharmaceutical Association, Washington, DC.

Benet, L. Z., Levy, G. and Ferraiolo, B. L. (1984). *Pharmacokinetics: a Modern View*. Plenum Press, London.

Birnbaum, L. S. and Couture, L. A. (1988). Disposition of octachlorodibenzo-*p*-dioxin (OCDD) in male rats. *Toxicol. Appl. Pharmacol.*, **93**, 22–30.

Blumer, J. L. (1990). The effect of physiological competence on toxicity: the response of neonates. In Volans, G. N., Sims, J., Sullivan, F. M. and Turner, P. (Eds), *Basic Science in Toxicology*. Taylor and Francis, London, pp. 375–389.

Bogen, K. T. (1988). Pharmacokinetics for regulatory risk analysis: the case of trichloroethylene. *Regul. Toxicol. Pharmacol.*, **8**, 447–466.

Bogen, K. T. and Hall, L. C. (1989). Pharmacokinetics for regulatory risk analysis: the case of 1,1,1-trichloroethane (methylchloroform). *Regul. Toxicol. Pharmacol.*, **10**, 26–50.

Bois, F. Y., Zeise, L. and Tozer, T. N. (1990). Precision and sensitivity of pharmacokinetic models for cancer risk assessment: tetrachloroethylene in mice, rats and human. *Toxicol. Appl. Pharmacol.*, **102**, 300–315.

Bonati, M., Latini, R., Tognoni, G., Young, J. F. and Garattini, S. (1985). Inter-species comparison of *in vivo* caffeine pharmacokinetics in man, monkey, rabbit, rat and mouse. *Drug Metab. Rev.*, **15**, 1355–1383.

Bopp, B. A., Sonders, R. C. and Kesterson, J. W. (1986). Toxicological aspects of cyclamate and cyclohexylamine. *CRC Crit. Rev. Toxicol.*, **16**, 213–306.

Boxenbaum, H. (1984). Inter-species pharmacokinetic scaling and the evolutionary-comparative paradigm. *Drug Metab. Rev.*, **15**, 1071–1121.

Calder, W. M. (1981). Scaling of physiological process in homeothermic animals. *Annu. Rev. Physiol.*, **43**, 301–322.

Clarke, B. and Smith, D. A. (1986). *An Introduction to Pharmacokinetics*. Blackwell, Oxford.

Cocchetto, D. M. and Bjornsson, T. D. (1983). Methods for vascular access and collection of body fluids from the laboratory rat. *J. Pharm. Sci.*, **72**, 465–492.

Couture, L. A., Elwell, M. R. and Birnbaum, L. S. (1988). Dioxin like effects in male rats following exposure to octachlorodibenzo-*p*-dioxin (OCDD) during a 13-week study. *Toxicol. Appl. Pharmacol.*, **93**, 31–46.

Curry, S. H. and Whelpton, R. (1983). *Manual of Laboratory Pharmacokinetics*. Wiley, Chichester.

Dietz, F. K., Stott, W. T. and Ramsey, J. C. (1982). Nonlinear pharmacokinetics and their impact on toxicology: illustrated with dioxane. *Drug Metab. Rev.*, **13**, 963–981.

DiDomenico, A. and Zapponi, G. A. (1986). 2,3,7,8-Tetrachlorodibenzo-*p*-dioxin (TCDD) in the environment: human health risk estimation and its application to the Serveso case as an example. *Regul. Toxicol. Pharmacol.*, **6**, 248–260.

Fisher, J. W., Whittaker, T. A., Taylor, D. H., Clewell, H. J. and Andersen, M. E. (1990). Physiologically based pharmacokinetic modeling of the lactating rat and nursing pup: a multiroute exposure model for trichloroethylene and its metabolite, trichloroacetic acid. *Toxicol. Appl. Pharmacol.*, **102**, 497–513.

Gabrielsson, J. and Weiner, D. (1997). *Pharmacokinetic and Pharmacodynamic Data Analysis. Concepts and Application*. Swedish Pharmaceutical Press, Stockholm.

Gasiewicz, T. A. and Neal, R. A. (1979). 2,3,7,8-Tetrachlorodibenzo-*p*-dioxin tissue distribution, excretion, and effects on clinical chemistry parameters in guinea pigs. *Toxicol. Appl. Pharmacol.*, **51**, 329–339.

Gehring, P. J. and Young, J. D. (1978). Application of pharmacokinetic principles in practice. In Plaa, G. L. and Duncan, W. A. M. (Eds), *Proceedings of the First International Congress on Toxicology*. Academic Press, London, pp. 119–141.

Gerlowski, L. E. and Jain, R. K. (1983). Physiologically based pharmacokinetic modeling: principles and applications. *J. Pharm. Sci.*, **72**, 1103–1127.

Gibaldi, M. and Perrier, D. (1982). *Pharmacokinetics*, 2nd edn. Marcel Dekker, New York.

Glocklin, V. C. (1982). General considerations for studies of the metabolism of drugs and other chemicals. *Drug Metab. Rev.*, **13**, 929–939.

Greenblatt, D. J. and Shader, R. I. (1985). *Pharmacokinetics in Clinical Practice*. W. B. Saunders, London.

Hays, S. M., Aylward, L. L., Karch, N. J. and Paustenbach, D. J. (1997). The relative susceptibility of animals and humans to the carcinogenic hazard posed by exposure to 2,3,7,8-TCDD: an analysis using standard and internal measures of dose. *Chemosphere*, **34**, 1507–1522.

HMSO (1989). *Dioxins in the Environment*. Department of the Environment, Central Directorate of Environment Protection, Pollution Paper No. 27. Her Majesty's Stationery Office, London.

Kedderis, G. L. and Held, S. D. (1996). Prediction of furan pharmacokinetics from hepatocyte studies: comparison of bioactivation and hepatic dosimetry in mice, rats and humans. *Toxicol. Appl. Pharmacol.*, **140**, 124–130.

Kissel, J. C. and Robarge, G. M. (1988). Assessing the elimination of 2,3,7,8-TCDD from humans with a physiologically based pharmacokinetic model. *Chemosphere*, **17**, 2017–2027.

Kociba, R. J., Keeler, P. A., Park, C. N. and Gehring, P. J. (1976). 2,3,7,8-Tetrachlorodibenzo-*p*-dioxin (TCDD): results of a 13-week oral toxicity study in rats. *Toxicol. Appl. Pharmacol.*, **35**, 553–574.

Leung, H.-W., Paustenbach, D. J., Murray, F. J. and Andersen, M. E. (1990a). A physiological pharmacokinetic description of the tissue distribution and enzyme-inducing properties of 2,3,7,8-tetrachlorodibenzo-*p*-dioxin in the rat. *Toxicol. Appl. Pharmacol.*, **103**, 399–410.

Leung, H.-W., Poland, A., Paustenbach, D. J., Murray, F. J. and Andersen, M. E. (1990b). Pharmacokinetics of [^{125}I]-2-iodo-, 3,7,8-trichlorodibenzo-*p*-dioxin in mice: analysis with a physiological modeling approach. *Toxicol. Appl. Pharmacol.*, **103**, 411–419.

McConnell, E. E., Moore, J. A., Haseman, J. K. and Harris, M. W. (1978). The comparative toxicity of chlorinated dibenzo-*p*-dioxins in mice and guinea pigs. *Toxicol. Appl. Pharmacol.*, **44**, 335–356.

Mordenti, J. (1985). Pharmacokinetic scale up: accurate prediction of human pharmacokinetic profiles from animal data. *J. Pharm. Sci.*, **74**, 1097–1099.

Neal, R. A., Olson, J. R., Gasiewicz, T. A. and Geiger, L. E. (1982). The toxicokinetics of 2,3,7,8-tetrachlorodibenzo-*p*-dioxin in mammalian systems. *Drug Metab. Rev.*, **13**, 355–385.

O'Flaherty, E. J. (1985). Differences in metabolism at different dose levels. In Clayson, D. B., Krewski, D. and Munro, I. (Eds), *Toxicological Risk Assessment*, Vol. 1. CRC Press, Boca Raton, FL, pp. 53–90.

Olson, J. R., Holscher, M. A. and Neal, R. A. (1980a). Toxicity of 2,3,7,8-tetrachlorodibenzo-*p*-dioxin in the golden Syrian hamster. *Toxicol. Appl. Pharmacol.*, **55**, 67–78.

Olson, J. R., Gasiewicz, T. A. and Neal, R. A. (1980b). Tissue distribution, excretion and metabolism of 2,3,7,8-tetrachlorodibenzo-*p*-dioxin (TCDD) in the golden Syrian hamster. *Toxicol. Appl. Pharmacol.*, **56**, 78–85.

Pohjanvirta, R., Vartiainen, T., Uusi-Rauva, A., Monkkonen, J. and Tuomisto, J. (1990). Tissue distribution, metabolism, and excretion of ^{14}C – TCDD in a TCDD-susceptible and a TCDD-resistant rat strain. *Pharmacol. Toxicol.*, **66**, 93–100.

Poiger, H. (1988). Toxicokinetics of 2,3,7,8-TCDD in man: an update. Paper presented at Dioxin '88, Umeå, Sweden, 1988.

Renwick, A. G. (1986). The metabolism of intense sweeteners. *Xenobiotica*, **16**, 1057–1071.

Renwick, A. G. (1989). Pharmacokinetics in Toxicology. In Hayes, A. W. (Ed.), *Principles and Methods of Toxicology*, 2nd edn. Raven Press, New York, pp. 835–878.

Renwick, A. G. (1991). Safety factors and the establishment of acceptable daily intakes. *Food Addit. Contam.*, **8**, 135–150.

Renwick, A. G. (1993) Data-derived safety factors for the evaluation of food additives and environmental contaminants. *Food Addit. Contam.*, **10**, 275–305.

Renwick, A. G. (1998). Toxicokinetics in infants and children in relation to the ADI and TDI. *Food Addit. Contam.*, **15**, Suppl., 17–35.

Renwick, A. G. and Lazarus, N. R. (1998). Human variability and noncancer risk assessment—an analysis of the default uncertainty factor. *Regul. Toxicol. Pharmacol.*, **27**, 3–20.

Renwick, A. G. and Walker, R. (1993). An analysis of the risk of exceeding the acceptable or tolerable daily intake. *Regul. Toxicol. Pharmacol.*, **18**, 463–480.

Roberts, A. and Renwick, A. G. (1989). The pharmacokinetics and tissue concentrations of cyclohexylamine in rats and mice. *Toxicol. Appl. Pharmacol.*, **98**, 230–242.

Roberts, A., Renwick, A. G., Ford, G., Creasy, D. M. and Gaunt, I. F. (1989). The metabolism and testicular toxicity of cyclohexylamine in rats and mice during chronic dietary administration. *Toxicol. Appl. Pharmacol.*, **98**, 216–229.

Rose, J. Q., Ramsey, J. C., Wentzler, T. H., Hummel, R. A. and Gehring, P. J. (1976). The fate of 2,3,7,8-tetrachlorodibenzo-*p*-dioxin following single and repeated oral doses to the rat. *Toxicol. Appl. Pharmacol.*, **36**, 209–226.

Rowland, M. and Tucker, G. T. (1986). *Pharmacokinetics: Theory and Methodology*. Pergamon Press, Oxford.

Scheuplein, R. J., Shoaf, S. E. and Brown, R. N. (1990). Role of pharmacokinetics in safety evaluation and regulatory considerations. *Annu. Rev. Pharmacol. Toxicol.*, **30**, 197–218.

Smyth, R. D. and Hottendorf, G. H. (1980). Application of pharmacokinetics and biopharmaceutics in the design of toxicological studies. *Toxicol. Appl. Pharmacol.*, **53**, 179–195.

Sweatman, T. W., Renwick, A. G. and Burgess, C. D. (1981). The pharmacokinetics of saccharin in man. *Xenobiotica*, **11**, 531–540.

Travis, C. C., Quillen, J. L. and Arms, A. D. (1990). Pharmacokinetics of benzene. *Toxicol. Appl. Pharmacol.*, **102**, 400–420.

Waynforth, H. B. (1980). *Experimental and Surgical Technique in the Rat*. Academic Press, London.

WHO (1987). *Principles for the Safety Assessment of Food Additives and Contaminants in Food*. Environmental Health Criteria, **70**. World Health Organization, Geneva.

WHO (1994). *Assessing Human Health Risks of Chemicals: Derivation of Guidance Values for Health-based Exposure Limits*. Environmental Health Criteria, **170**. World Health Organization, Geneva.

Wilkinson, G. R. (1976). Pharmacokinetics in disease states modifying body perfusion. In Benet L. Z. (Ed.), *The Effect of Disease States on Drug Pharmacokinetics*. American Pharmaceutical Association, Academy of Pharmaceutical Sciences, Washington, DC, pp. 13–32.

Wilkinson, G. R. (1984). Pharmacokinetic considerations in toxicology. In Mitchell, J. R. and Horning, M. G. (Eds), *Drug Metabolism and Drug Toxicity*. Raven Press, New York, pp. 213–235.

Wilkinson, G. R. (1987). Clearance approaches in pharmacology. *Pharmacol. Rev.*, **39**, 1–47.

Wolfe, W., Miner, J. and Petersen, M. (1988). Serum 2,3,7,8-tetrachlorodibenzo-*p*-dioxin levels in air force health study participants—preliminary report. *J. Am. Med. Assoc.*, **259**, 3533–3535.

Yacobi, A., Kamath, B. L. and Lai, C.-M. (1982). Pharmacokinetics in chronic animal toxicity studies. *Drug Metab. Rev.*, **13**, 1021–1051.

Chapter 5
Biotransformation of Xenobiotics

John A. Timbrell

CONTENTS

INTRODUCTION

Xenobiotics which are absorbed into biological systems by passive diffusion are usually lipid soluble and consequently not ideally suited for excretion. For example, very lipophilic substances such as the polychlorinated biphenyls are very poorly excreted and, hence, may remain in a mammalian body for many years.

After a xenobiotic has been absorbed into a biological system, it may undergo biotransformation to products which are rapidly excreted and therefore elimination of the compound from the animal is facilitated. However, biotransformation may also change the biological activity of the substance. Hence the metabolic fate of the compound can have an important bearing on its toxic potential, its disposition in the body and its excretion.

The products of metabolism are usually more water soluble than the original compound. Indeed, in animals, biotransformation seems directed at increasing water solubility and, hence, excretion. For example, the analgesic drug paracetamol (acetaminophen) has a renal clearance value of 12 ml min^{-1}, whereas one of its major metabolites, the sulphate conjugate, is cleared at the rate of 170 ml min^{-1}.

Facilitating the excretion of a compound means that its biological half-life is reduced and, hence, its potential toxicity is kept to a minimum. Metabolism may also directly affect the biological activity of a foreign compound. For example, the drug succinylcholine causes muscle relaxation, but its action lasts only a few minutes because metabolism cleaves the molecule to yield inactive products **(Figure 1)**. However, in some cases metabolism increases the toxicity of a compound. There are now many examples of this (see below) which have been documented, but a relatively simple case is ethylene glycol. This is metabolized to oxalic acid, which is partly responsible for several of the toxic effects **(Figure 2)**.

Biotransformation is therefore an extremely important phase of disposition, as it may have a major effect on the biological activity of the compound, and by increasing polarity and so water solubility, thereby increase excretion.

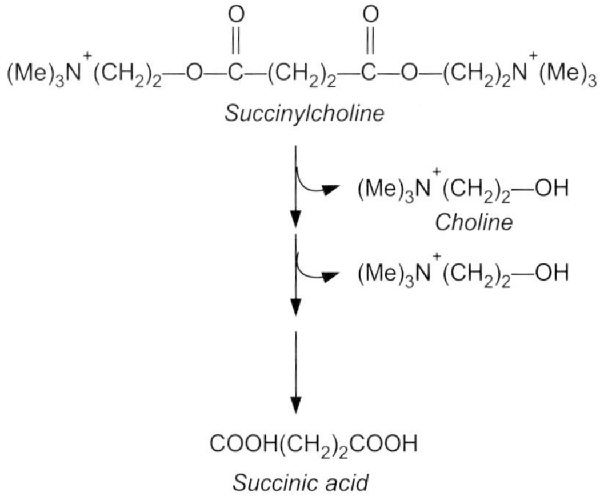

Figure 1 Metabolic hydrolysis of succinylcholine.

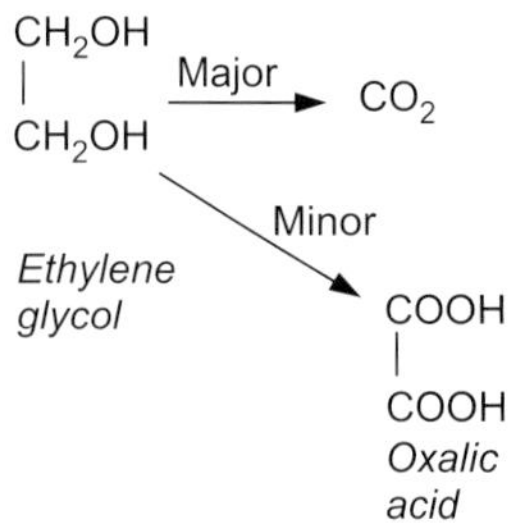

Figure 2 Metabolism of ethylene glycol.

Rarely, metabolism may decrease water solubility and so reduce excretion. For example, acetylation decreases the solubility of some sulphonamides in urine and so may lead to crystallization of the metabolite in the kidney tubules, causing tissue necrosis.

Biotransformation can generally be simply divided into phases 1 and 2, although further metabolism of conjugates has been termed phase 3. Phase 1 is the alteration of the original foreign molecule so as to add on a functional group which can then be conjugated in phase 2. This can best be understood by examining the example in **Figure 3**. The xenobiotic is benzene, a highly lipophilic molecule which is not readily excreted from the animal except, as it is volatile, in the expired air. Phase 1 metabolism converts benzene into a variety of metabolites, but the major one is phenol. The insertion of a hydroxyl group allows a phase 2 conjugation reaction to take place with the polar sulphate group being added. Phenyl sulphate, the final metabolite, is very water soluble and is readily excreted in the urine.

Some foreign molecules, such as phenol, already possess functional groups suitable for phase 2 reactions and therefore simply undergo a phase 2 reaction. The products of phase 2 biotransformations, such as glutathione conjugates, may be further metabolized in what are sometimes termed phase 3 reactions.

Biotransformation is almost always catalysed by enzymes and these are usually, but not always, found most abundantly in the liver in animals. The reason for this location is that most foreign compounds enter the body via the gastrointestinal tract and the portal blood supply from this organ goes directly to the liver (**Figure 4**). However, it is important to remember that (1) the enzymes involved with the metabolism of foreign compounds may be found in many other tissues as well as the liver (Krishna and Klotz, 1994); (2) the enzymes may be localized in one particular cell type in an organ; (3) unlike the enzymes involved in intermediary metabolism, those involved in the biotransformation of xenobiotics are generally non-specific and consequently are not always very efficient; (4) enzymes normally involved in intermediary metabolism may catalyse the biotransformation of a xenobiotic if the chemical structure happens to be suitable; and (5) a xenobiotic may undergo many different biotransformations and the relative importance of each of these may be affected by many factors.

The enzymes involved in biotransformation also have a particular subcellular localization: many are found in

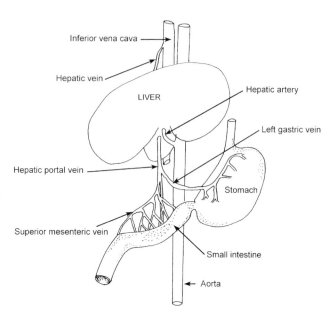

Figure 4 Blood supply to the liver (drawn by C. J. Waterfield).

the endoplasmic reticulum, some are located in the cytosol and a few are found in other organelles such as the mitochondrion.

The various types of metabolic reactions are shown in **Table 1**.

Table 1 The major biotransformation reactions

Phase 1		Phase 2
Oxidation	Aromatic	Sulphation
	Aliphatic	
	Heterocyclic	Glucuronidation
	Alicyclic	
	Of nitrogen	Glutathione
	Of sulphur	conjugation
	N-Hydroxylation	Acetylation
	Dealkylation	Amino acid
		conjugation
Reduction	Azo	Methylation
	Nitro	
Hydrolysis	Ester	
	Amide	
	Hydrazide	
	Carbamate	
Hydration		
Dehalogenation		

PHASE 1 REACTIONS

Oxidation Reactions

The majority of oxidation reactions which xenobiotics undergo are catalysed by one enzyme system, the cytochrome P450 monooxygenase system (Guengerich, 1991, 1994). However, there are a number of other

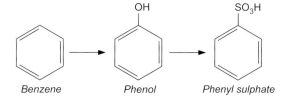

Figure 3 Benzene metabolism.

oxidative enzyme systems whose importance in the bio-transformation of xenobiotics is increasingly being recognized, and these will be discussed later in this chapter.

Cytochrome P450

Cytochrome P450 is a membrane-bound enzyme system located primarily in the smooth endoplasmic reticulum of the cell, although some forms of cytochrome P450 may be located in other organelles such as the mitochondria. After homogenization and fractionation of the cell, the enzyme system is isolated in the so-called microsomal fraction. The liver has the highest concentration of this enzyme, although it can be found in most tissues. The reactions catalysed by cytochrome P450 also require NADPH and molecular oxygen and the overall reaction is

$$SH + O_2 + NADPH + H^+ \rightarrow SOH + H_2O + NADP^+$$

where S is the substrate.

The sequence of metabolic reactions is shown in **Figure 5** and involves six distinct steps: (1) addition of substrate to the enzyme; (2) donation of an electron; (3) addition of oxygen and rearrangement; (4) donation of a second electron; and (5) loss of water. These steps are followed by (6) loss of the oxidized substrate.

The cytochrome P450 system is actually a collection of enzymes, all of which possess an iron atom in a porphyrin complex. These catalyse different types of oxidation reactions and under certain circumstances may catalyse other types of reaction such as reduction. There are three main gene families important in xenobiotic metabolism: *CYP1*, *CYP2* and *CYP3*. *CYP4* is involved in fatty acid metabolism. Within these there are subfamilies, which with the exception of *CYP2* contain one subfamily, i.e. *CYP1A*, *CYP3A* and *CYP4A*. *CYP2* has five subfamilies, *A*, *B*, *C*, *D* and *E*. These may be further divided into genes coding for single distinct enzyme proteins such as *CYP 1A1* and *CYP 1A2* (Nelson *et al.*, 1993). There may also be allelic variants giving rise to different proteins. The enzyme proteins CYP1A1, CYP1A2 and CYP2E1 seem to be highly conserved and similar in all species. Humans have about 15 different cytochrome P450 enzymes (Gonzalez, 1989; Wrighton and Stevens, 1992).

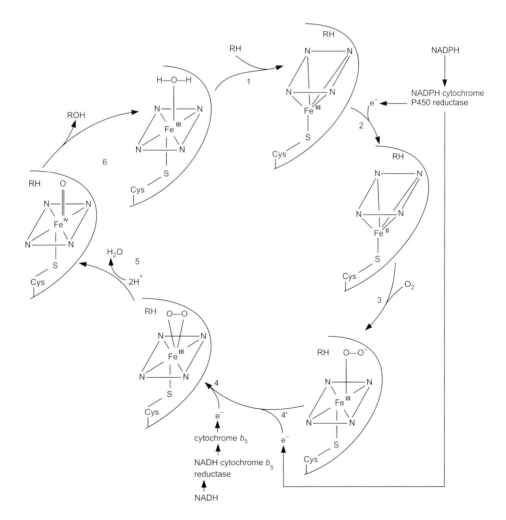

Figure 5 The cytochrome P450 system (Reproduced from Timbrell, 1991).

One important feature of the cytochrome P450 enzyme system is its broad and overlapping substrate specificities which reflect the enormous variety of chemicals which may be potential substrates. Furthermore, one substrate may be metabolized to more than one product by different forms of cytochrome P450. For example, the drug propranolol can be metabolized by CYP2D6 and CYP2C19 to 4-hydroxypropranolol and naphthoxylacetic acid, respectively. Sometimes the same form of cytochrome P450 may metabolize one drug to more than one product. For example, the drug methoxyphenamine can be metabolized by CYP2D6 either by *O*-demethylation or hydroxylation at the 5-position.

Another important feature of the enzyme is its inducibility (Okey *et al.*, 1986; Whitlock, 1989; Okey, 1990; Batt *et al.*, 1992). Thus, treatment of an animal with certain substances may lead to an increase in the synthesis of one or more isoenzymes of cytochrome P450, leading to an apparent increase in overall activity with respect to a particular substrate. There is now a large number of known inducers of different isoenzymes of cytochrome P450. Exposure of an animal to these substances clearly may have an effect on the metabolism of a compound and can influence its toxicity (this is discussed in more detail later in the chapter).

The major types of oxidation reaction catalysed by the cytochrome P450 system may be subdivided into aromatic hydroxylation of carbon, aliphatic hydroxylation of carbon, alicyclic hydroxylation of carbon, heterocyclic hydroxylation, epoxidation, *N*-, *S*- and *O*-dealkylation, *N*-oxidation, *N*-hydroxylation, *S*-oxidation, desulphuration, dehydrogenation, cleavage of esters and deamination.

Aromatic hydroxylations

Aromatic hydroxylation, such as occurs with benzene **(Figure 6)**, is a very common reaction for compounds containing an unsaturated ring. The initial products are phenols, but catechols, quinols and further hydroxylated products may be formed. One of the toxic effects of benzene is aplastic anaemia. This is believed to be due to an intermediate metabolite, possibly the hydroquinone, which may be formed in the bone marrow, the target site. Aromatic hydroxylation usually proceeds via an epoxide intermediate, also called an oxirane ring or arene oxide **(Figure 7)**, which involves the addition of oxygen across the unsaturated double bond. The formation of this intermediate may have important toxicological implications, for example the hepatotoxicity of bromobenzene (discussed in detail later in the chapter). Epoxides are often chemically reactive and fairly unstable. They may give rise to positively charged intermediates (electrophiles). The products formed *in vivo* will depend on the reactivity of the particular epoxide and they therefore may form a number of other metabolites, either phenols by chemical rearrangement or, following

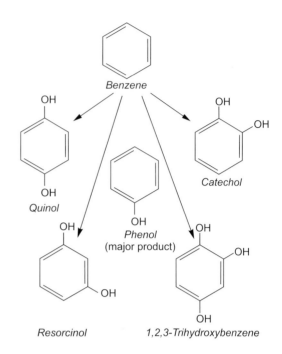

Figure 6 Routes of hydroxylation of benzene.

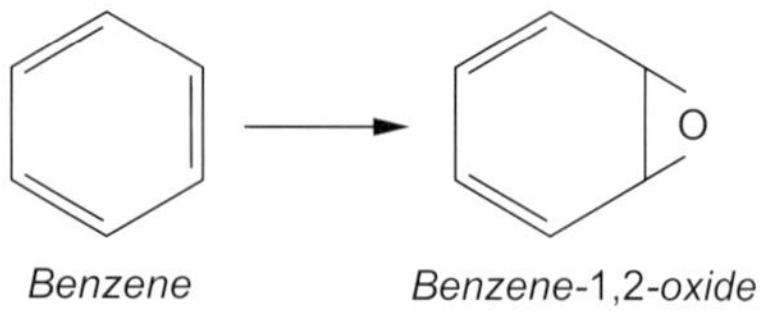

Figure 7 Oxidation of benzene to an epoxide.

further metabolism, dihydrodiols, glutathione conjugates and catechols. Destabilized epoxides, for example, will tend to form phenols by chemical rearrangement.

The reactivity of metabolic intermediates may well determine the toxicity of the compound in question. However, extremely reactive intermediates are likely to react with many cellular constituents in the close proximity of their formation. Less reactive intermediates may travel to distant sites within or even outside the cell and react with more critical cellular targets (Monks and Lau, 1988; Nelson and Pearson, 1990) (see below). Also, aromatic hydroxylation is influenced by the substituents on the ring. Thus, a nitro or other electron-withdrawing group will tend to direct hydroxylation to the *meta* and *para* positions, whereas an electron-donating group such as an amino group will be *ortho*- and *para*-directing.

Aliphatic Hydroxylations

Hydroxylation of unsaturated aliphatic compounds may also proceed with the formation of an epoxide across the unsaturated bond. For example, the toxic industrial intermediate vinyl chloride **(Figure 8)** undergoes such a biotransformation to yield chloroacetaldehyde. When

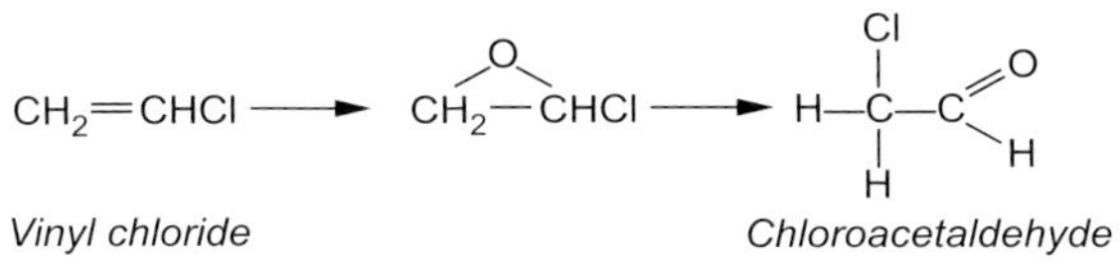

Vinyl chloride   Chloroacetaldehyde

Figure 8 Oxidation of vinyl chloride to an epoxide.

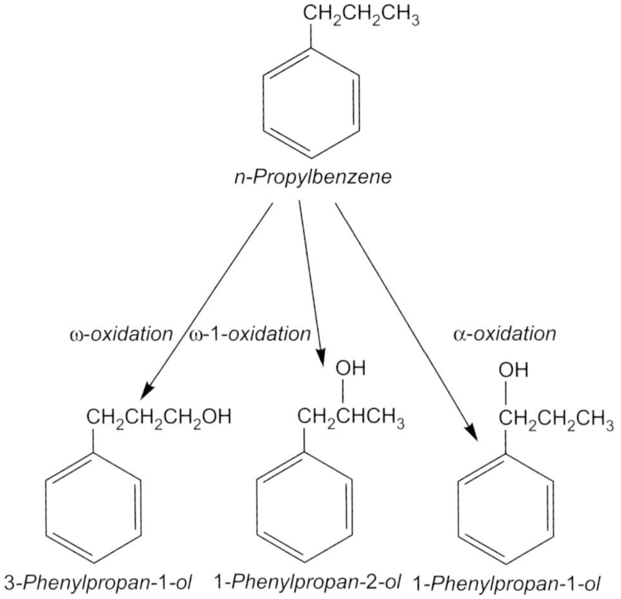

n-Propylbenzene

ω-oxidation   ω-1-oxidation   α-oxidation

3-Phenylpropan-1-ol   1-Phenylpropan-2-ol   1-Phenylpropan-1-ol

Figure 9 Hydroxylation of propylbenzene.

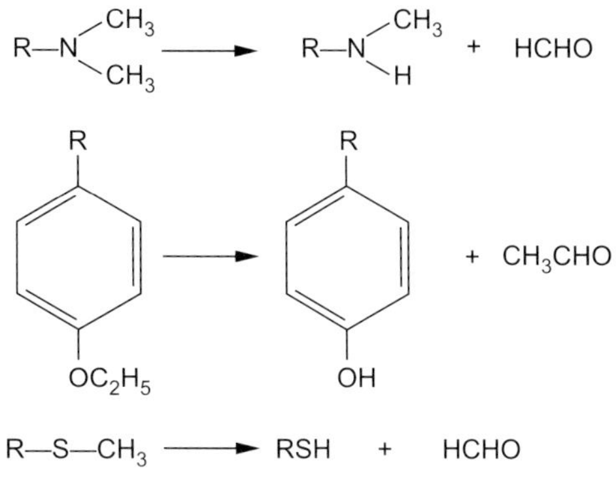

Figure 10 Dealkylation reactions.

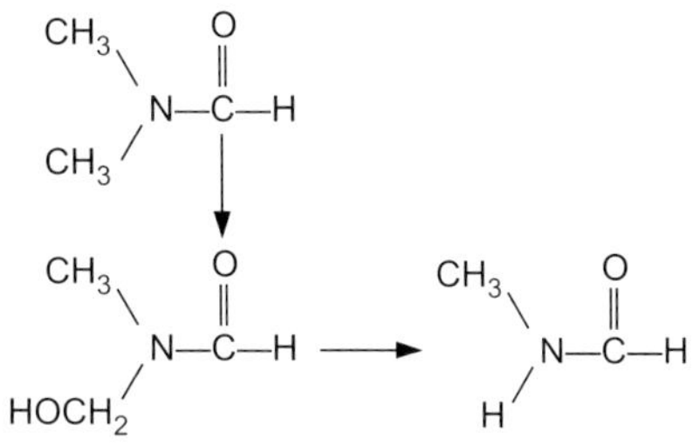

Figure 11 Dealkylation of dimethylformamide via a stable hydroxymethyl intermediate.

the epoxide opens, there may be a shift in the chlorine atom to the adjacent carbon (Hathway, 1984).

Hydroxylation of a saturated aliphatic moiety such as that in propylbenzene may occur at one of three positions **(Figure 9)**. Further metabolism will yield the aldehyde and then the acid from the 3-phenylpropan-1-ol. These further biotransformations may be catalysed by enzymes other than cytochrome P450. Fatty acids such as lauric acid are hydroxylated on the terminal (omega) and penultimate (omega−1) carbon.

Alicyclic Hydroxylations

Alicyclic rings may also undergo hydroxylation catalysed by cytochrome P450. For example, cyclohexane may be oxidized to cyclohexanol and then further to the *trans*-1,2-diol. Similarly, heterocyclic rings such as that in the drug hydralazine may be hydroxylated (see **Figure 19**). However, other enzymes may also be involved in this type of oxidation, such as the xanthine oxidases (see below).

N-, S- and O-Dealkylations

Alkyl groups attached to N, O or S atoms are removed by dealkylation reactions which involve oxidation of the alkyl group. The intermediate hydroxyalkyl compound

may be unstable and rearrange with loss of the respective aldehyde **(Figure 10)**. Sometimes stable hydroxyalkyl products are produced, for example, when dimethylformamide undergoes metabolism **(Figure 11)**. S-Dealkylation may also involve a factor from the cytosol and so may not be a straightforward microsomal reaction. The chain length will have a bearing on whether dealkylation or oxidation of the alkyl group occurs. The longer the chain length the more likely is oxidation of the terminal carbon atom to occur.

N-Hydroxylation, S-Oxidation, deamination, etc.

Nitrogen atoms in primary arylamines, arylamides and hydrazines may undergo hydroxylation which is catalysed by cytochrome P450 **(Figure 12)**. This reaction may result in a metabolic activation and so be responsible for toxicity (see below). Nitrogen atoms in xenobiotics may also be oxidized by other oxidases (see below).

Sulphur atoms can also be oxidized by microsomal monooxygenases to yield S-oxides and sulphones, such as in the pesticide aldicarb **(Figure 13)**. Sulphur atoms may also be removed oxidatively and replaced by oxygen such as in the metabolism of the insecticide parathion **(Figure 14)**. Similarly, halogen atoms may be removed via oxidative reactions, as shown for the metabolism of the anaesthetic halothane to trifluoroacetic acid **(Figure 15)**.

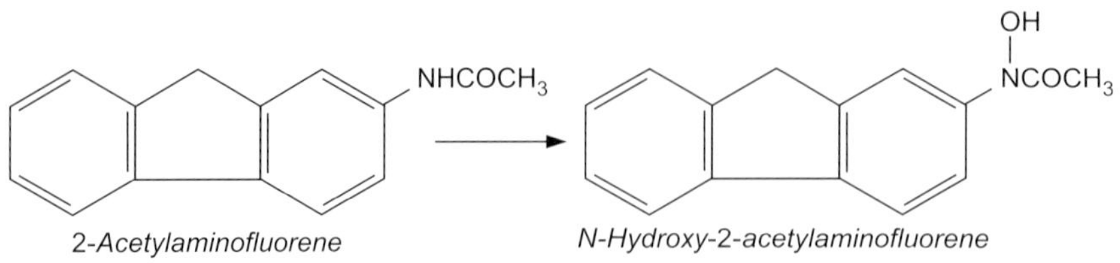

Figure 12 *N*-Hydroxylation of acetylaminofluorene.

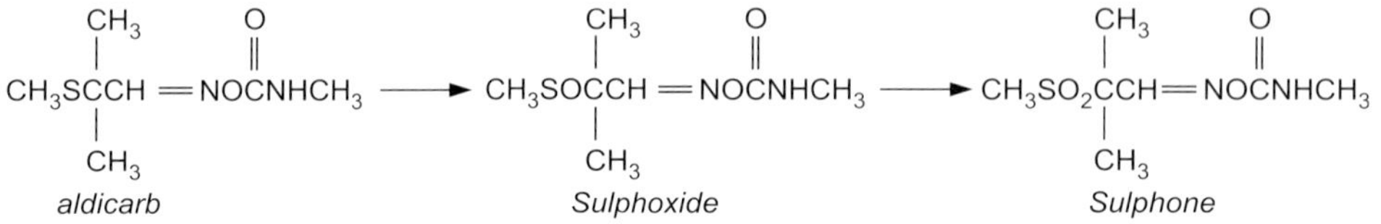

Figure 13 Oxidation of the pesticide aldicarb (Temik) to sulphoxide and sulphone metabolites.

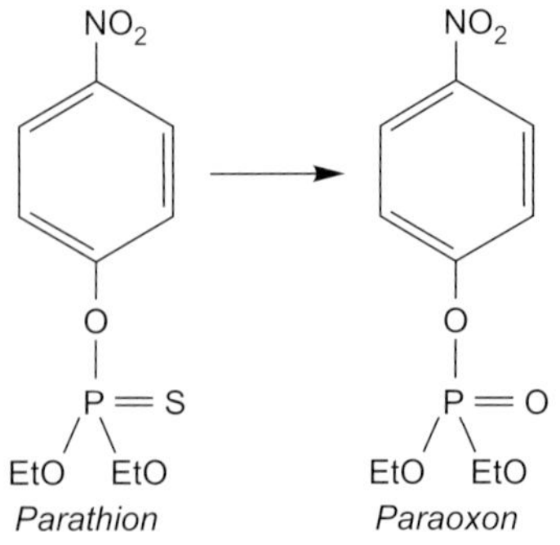

Figure 14 Oxidative desulphuration of parathion.

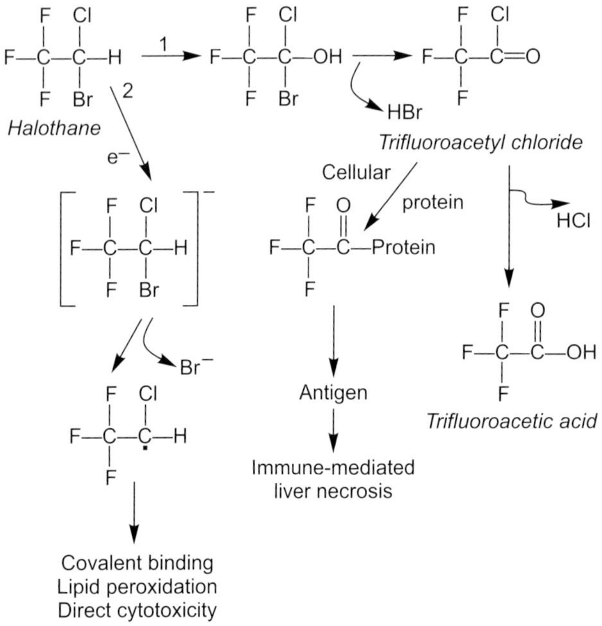

Figure 15 Metabolism of the anaesthetic halothane showing both oxidative (1) and reductive (2) pathways and their role in toxicity.

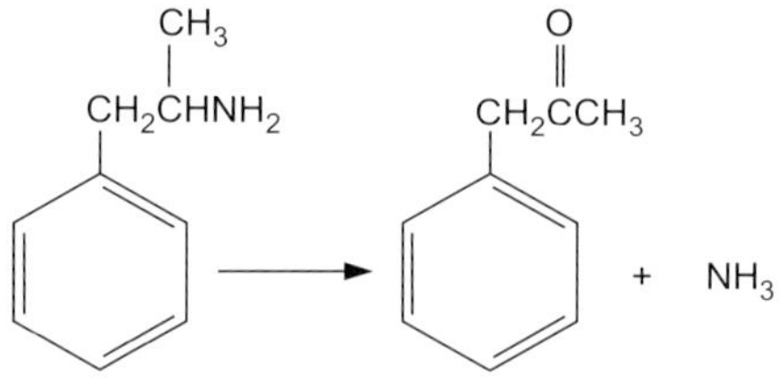

Figure 16 Deamination of amphetamine.

Amine groups can also be removed oxidatively via a deamination reaction which may be catalysed by cytochrome P450. For example, in the rabbit amphetamine is metabolized in this way to phenylacetone **(Figure 16)**. However, the initial attack is probably on the carbon atom to yield a carbinolamine, which can rearrange to the ketone with loss of ammonia as shown. Alternatively, the reaction may proceed via phenylacetone oxime, which has been isolated as a metabolite and for which there are several possible routes of formation. The phenylacetone oxime is hydrolysed to phenylacetone. *N*-Hydroxylation of amphetamine is also believed to take place and may also give rise to the observed metabolite, phenylacetone. The mechanism underlying the oxidative deamination of amphetamine has been a source of speculation and controvery but it illustrates that there may be several routes of biotransformation to yield a particular metabolite (Gorrod and Raman, 1989).

Non-Cytochrome P450-dependent Oxidations

Certain oxidation reactions are catalysed by enzymes other than the cytochrome P450 monooxygenase system, such as the microsomal flavin (FAD)-containing monooxygenases (Damani, 1988; Ziegler, 1993; Benedetti and Dostert, 1994; Cashman, 1995). This is responsible for the *N*-oxidation of tertiary amines such as dimethylaniline and trimethylamine **(Figure 17)**. The enzyme requires NADPH and molecular oxygen and proceeds

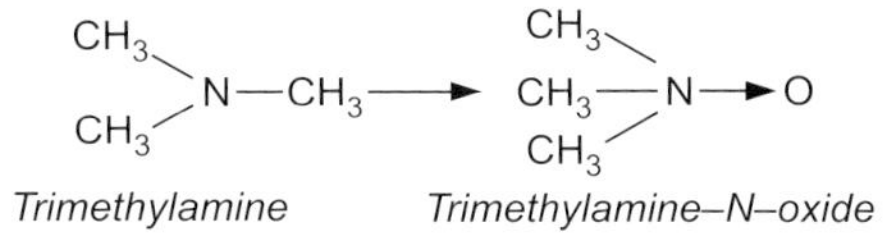

Figure 17 Oxidation of trimethylamine.

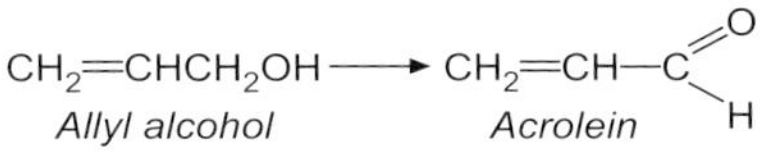

Figure 18 Oxidation of allyl alcohol.

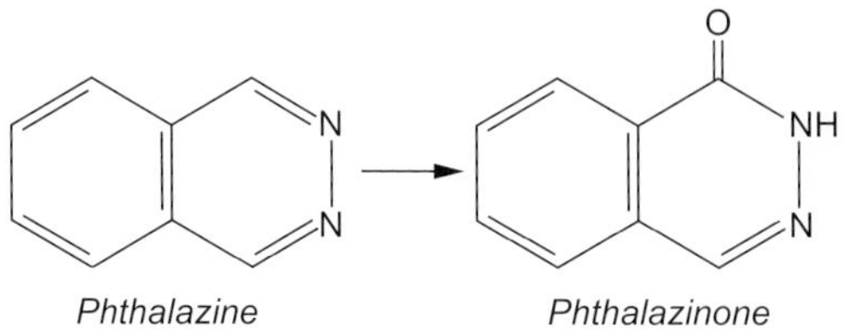

Figure 19 Oxidation of the hydralazine metabolite phthalazine.

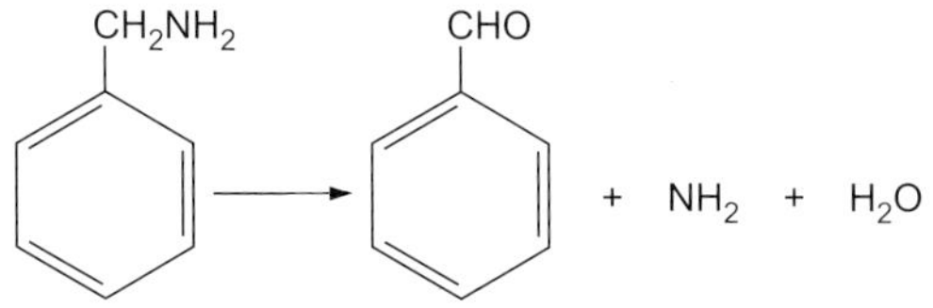

Figure 20 Oxidation of benzylamine by monoamine oxidase.

Figure 21 Oxidation of putrescine by diamine oxidase.

in six steps. The substrate specificity also includes secondary amines and sulphides, thioethers, thiols and thiocarbamates and even organophosphates.

Alcohols, both aliphatic and aromatic, may be oxidized by alcohol dehydrogenase **(Figure 18)**. This enzyme requires NADH and is cytosolic. The products from primary alcohols are aldehydes, whereas ketones are formed, more slowly, from secondary alcohols. The oxidation of an alcohol may result in a toxic metabolite being formed, such as that from allyl alcohol **(Figure 18)**. A microsomal ethanol-metabolizing system has also been demonstrated. This is known to be involved in the metabolism of ethanol and methanol.

Aldehydes may be further oxidized to acids by aldehyde dehydrogenase, another cytosolic enzyme which also requires NAD.

Other enzymes may also be involved in the oxidation of aldehydes, such as aldehyde oxidase and xanthine oxidase. These are also cytosolic enzymes which contain molybdenum and require flavoprotein cofactors (Beedham, 1988).

Xanthine oxidase also catalyses the oxidation of nitrogen heterocycles such as the purine hypoxanthine and also phthalazine to phthalazinone **(Figure 19)**. Aldehyde oxidase will also catalyse the latter reaction. Some amines such as tyramine, found in certain foodstuffs such as cheese, are substrates for the monoamine oxidases. These are mitochondrial enzymes found in a variety of tissues, including the liver. The oxidative deamination of amines via the monoamine oxidases yields an aldehyde product **(Figure 20)**. The action of monoamine oxidases may give rise to toxic products, however, such as the oxidation of allylamine to allylaldehyde in heart tissue and the oxidation of the contaminant of certain 'home-made' drugs, 1-methyl-4-phenyl-1,2,3,6-tetrahydropyridine (MPTP), to a toxic metabolite responsible for degeneration of the substantia nigra in the brain.

Diamines such as putrescine are metabolized by the soluble enzyme diamine oxidase to dialdehyde products **(Figure 21)**. Secondary and tertiary amines are less readily oxidized by these enzymes, dealkylation to the primary amine being preferred if it is possible.

Another group of enzymes which are involved in the oxidation of xenobiotics are the peroxidases (Eling *et al.*, 1983; Larsson *et al.*, 1988). There are a number of these enzymes in mammalian tissues: prostaglandin synthase, found in kidney, lung, intestine and spleen; lactoperoxidase, found in mammary glands; myeloperoxidase, found in liver Kupffer cells and neutrophils, where it is thought to be responsible for the oxidation of drugs such as hydralazine and procainamide (Uetrecht, 1992). It is also found in bone marrow cells, where it may be involved in the metabolic activation and therefore toxicity of benzene.

Uterine peroxidase has been suggested as being involved in the metabolic activation and toxicity of diethylstilboestrol.

The overall peroxidase catalysed reaction may be summarized as follows:

$$\text{peroxidase} + H_2O_2 \rightarrow \text{compound I}$$
$$\text{compound I} + RH_2 \rightarrow \text{compound II} +^{\bullet} R\dot{H}_2^{+}$$
$$\text{compound II} + RH_2 \rightarrow \text{peroxidase} +^{\bullet} RH_2^{+}$$

Probably the most important is prostaglandin synthase. This is known to catalyse the oxidation of *p*-phenetidine, a metabolite of the drug phenacetin, a process which may be involved in the nephrotoxicity of the drug. The prostaglandin synthase-catalysed oxidation of this compound gives rise to free radicals which may be responsible for binding to DNA. Horseradish peroxidase will also catalyse the oxidation of this compound.

Reduction

Reduction may be catalysed by either mammalian microsomal or cytosolic reductases and by the gut bacteria, which also possess reductases. The latter are clearly important for substances taken orally, where contact with gut microflora is likely. Apart from the gut flora, azo and nitro reduction are catalysed by enzymes in the liver, cytochrome P450 or NAD(P)H quinone oxidoreductase (DT diaphorase). Reduction takes place under anaerobic conditions and utilizes NADH or NADPH. FAD may also be involved, possibly as a non-enzymic electron donor. The most commonly encountered types of reductive reaction are the reduction of nitro and azo groups. However, aldehydes, ketones, disulphides, sulphoxides, quinones, N-oxides, alkenes, halogenated hydrocarbons and certain metals may also be reduced *in vivo*. The reduction of azo groups such as those present in the drug Prontosil **(Figure 22)** is a two-step reaction involving first reduction to a substituted hydrazine, followed by a second reduction and cleavage to yield the amine.

Reduction of nitro groups is also an important route of biotransformation, such as for the compound nitrobenzene **(Figure 23)**. Again this involves several steps, producing first a nitroso derivative, then a hydroxylamine and finally an amine. Reduction of nitro groups may be associated with toxicity. Nitrobenzene is haematotoxic in rats when given orally, causing methaemoglobinaemia and haemolysis, whereas given intraperitoneally or to rats without gut flora it is devoid of this toxicity. This is due to reduction of the compound in the gut to yield the nitroso and hydroxylamine metabolites which are responsible for toxicity to haemoglobin. Another example is nitroquinoline N-oxide, which is reduced to a hydroxylamine **(Figure 24)**, which is believed to be carcinogenic.

The less common reduction reactions include reduction of aldehyde and keto groups, epoxides and double bonds and may involve other enzymes such as alcohol dehydrogenase and carbonyl reductase, both of

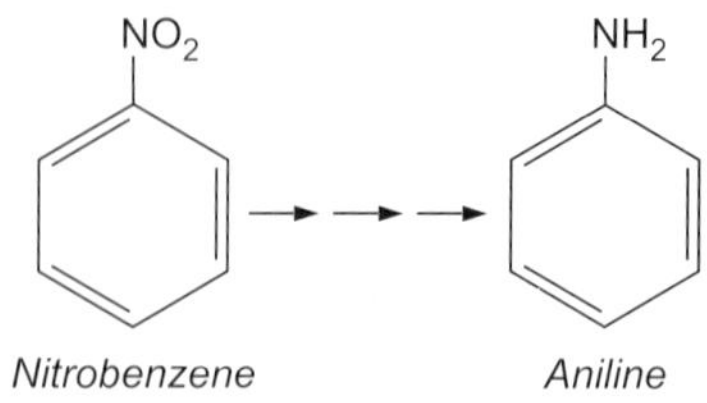

Figure 23 Reduction of nitrobenzene.

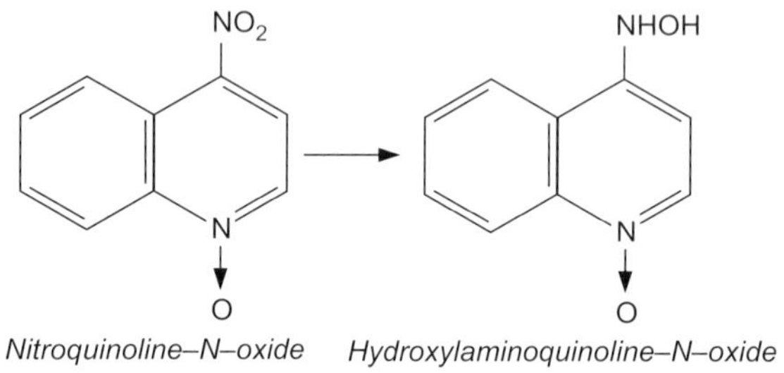

Figure 24 Reduction of the carcinogen nitroquinoline-*N*-oxide.

which are found in the liver cytosol as well as other tissues. Reduction of quinones involves DT diaphorase and disulphides, glutathione reductase and glutathione.

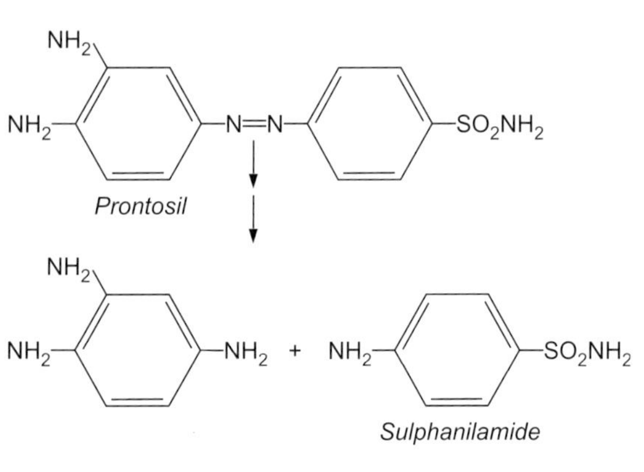

Reductive dehalogenation, catalysed by the microsomal enzymes, may also occur in the metabolism of halogenated compounds such as carbon tetrachloride and the anaesthetic halothane (see **Figure 40**, below, and **Figure 15**). The reductive route is believed to be responsible for the acute toxicity of halothane in rats when the oxygen tension is low. The reactive radical metabolites produced by the reductive pathway will bind covalently to liver protein and this may lead to toxicity. However, the oxidative pathway is probably more important in man under normal conditions of anaesthesia. This also gives rise to a reactive metabolite, trifluoroacetyl chloride. Both the oxidative and reductive pathways involve cytochrome P450. In the reductive mode the enzyme donates an electron to the substrate, which then loses bromide ion, and a second electron is donated, which produces a radical species which may either react with protein or rearrange to other metabolic products.

Similarly, reductive dechlorination is also involved in the toxicity of carbon tetrachloride. Here, again, cytochrome P450 donates an electron under reductive conditions and the products are chloride ion and the trichloromethyl radical (see **Figure 40**, below). This may then react further with oxygen to form the trichloromethylperoxy radical species, which is believed to cause damage to lipids in cell membranes. Alternatively, the trichloromethyl radical may abstract a hydrogen atom from any of a variety of sources (such as glutathione) resulting in the production of chloroform and another radical (such as the glutathionyl radical).

Figure 22 Reduction of the azo bond in Prontosil.

Hydrolysis

Esters (carboxylic acid and thioesters) and amides are hydrolysed by carboxylesterases and amidases, respectively, and there are a number of these enzymes occurring in a variety of tissues. They are usually found in the cytosol of cells, but microsomal esterases and amidases have also been described; some are also found in the plasma and carboxylesterases are also present in red blood cells. A typical amidase reaction is shown in **Figure 25**. Esterases have been classified as type A, B or C on the basis of activity towards phosphate triesters. Thus, B-type esterases are all inhibited by paraoxon and have a serine residue at the active site which may be phosphorylated. However, there are a number of different enzymes within this group with different specificities. Esterases also have amidase activity and vice versa, and so these two activities may be part of the same overall activity. Hydrazides and carbamates may also be hydrolysed by amidases. Amidases have an important role in the toxicity of the drugs isoniazid and phenacetin, where hydrolysis is an important step in the metabolic activation (see **Figure 44**).

Amides are generally hydrolysed more slowly than esters. However, electron-withdrawing substituents will weaken the amide bond, making it more susceptible to hydrolysis.

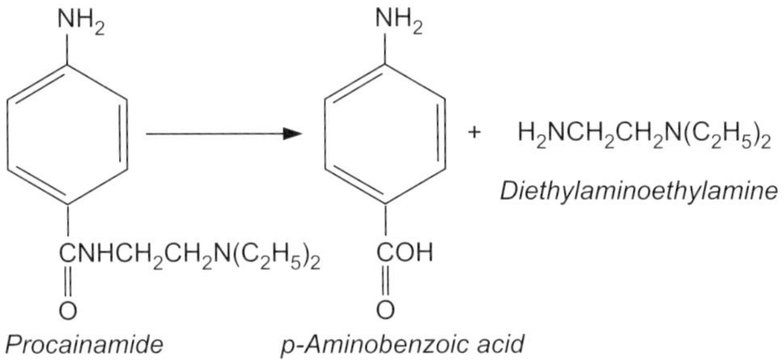

Figure 25 Hydrolysis of an amide, procainamide.

Hydration

Alkene epoxides and arene oxides, which are three-membered rings containing an oxygen atom, may be reactive metabolic intermediates although this is not always the case as there are stable epoxides. They may undergo hydration catalysed by the enzyme epoxide hydrolase There are three forms of this enzyme, two of which are located in the smooth endoplasmic reticulum, conveniently near to the cytochrome P450 system which produces the epoxide, and one cytosolic enzyme. Indeed, most tissues contain enzyme activity and in the liver and lung, for example, this may parallel the distribution of cytochrome P450 activity. Like the latter enzyme, epoxide hydrolase is also inducible. The reaction can

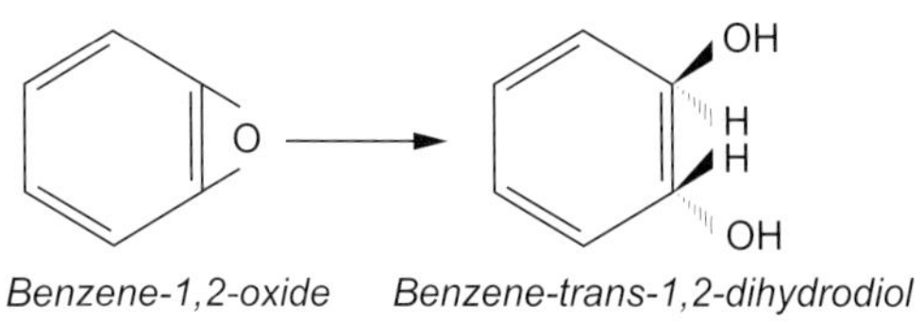

Figure 26 Hydration of an epoxide.

normally be regarded as a detoxication reaction, as the dihydrodiol products are usually much less chemically reactive than the epoxide **(Figure 26)**. The products are *trans*-diols. However, there are examples where the diol is further metabolized to a more toxic metabolite such as benzpyrene 7, 8-dihydrodiol. Both aromatic and aliphatic epoxides may be substrates for the enzyme.

PHASE 2 REACTIONS

Phase 2 reactions, also known as conjugation reactions, involve the addition of a readily available, polar endogenous substance to the foreign molecule. This polar moiety is conjugated either to an existing group or to one added in a phase 1 reaction. The polar moiety renders the foreign molecule more water soluble and so more readily cleared from the body and less likely to exert a toxic effect. The endogenous metabolites donated in phase 2 reactions include carbohydrate derivatives, amino acids, glutathione and sulphate. The mechanism involves formation of a high-energy intermediate: either the endogenous metabolite is activated as a high-energy derivative (type 1) or the substrate is activated (type 2).

Conjugation reactions

Sulphation

The addition of the sulphate moiety to a hydroxyl group is a major route of conjugation for foreign compounds, and also endogenous compounds, such as steroids, may also undergo sulphation. The reaction is catalysed by cytosolic sulphotransferase enzymes found particularly in the liver, gastrointestinal mucosa and kidney. The reaction also requires the coenzyme 3'-phosphoadenosine-5'-phosphosulphate (PAPS). This coenzyme is produced from inorganic sulphate ions and ATP in a two-stage reaction **(Figure 27)**. Other anions may replace sulphate in the first reaction but the products are unstable. This may lead to toxicity by the depletion of ATP. The available inorganic sulphate in the body may also be depleted by large doses of compounds such as paracetamol which are conjugated with sulphate (see below).

There are a number of different sulphotransferases, classified by the particular type of substrate, and some

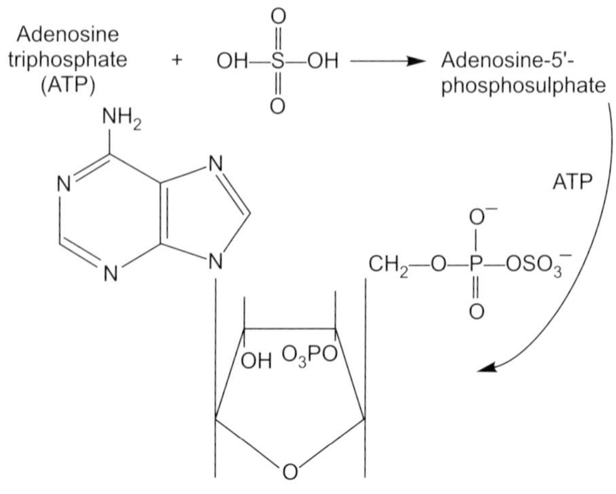

3'-Phosphoadenosine-5'-phosphosulphate (PAPS)

Figure 27 Formation of the sulphate donor PAPS.

of these exist in several forms. The product of sulphate conjugation is an ester which is very polar and water soluble. Both aromatic and aliphatic hydroxyl groups may be conjugated with sulphate, as may N-hydroxy

groups and amino groups **(Figure 28)**. Sulphate conjugation may be involved in the metabolic activation of compounds such as the carcinogen acetylaminofluorene (Mulder *et al.*, 1988) (see below).

Glucuronidation

The addition of glucuronic acid, a polar and water-soluble carbohydrate molecule, to hydroxyl groups, carboxylic acid groups, amino groups and thiols is a major route of phase 2 metabolism. Uridine diphosphate glucuronic acid (UDP Glucuronic acid) is the cofactor which donates glucuronic acid and, as with sulphation, the moiety added, glucuronic acid, is in a high-energy form as UDP Glucuronic acid. UDP Glucuronic acid is synthesized from glucose-1-phosphate in the cytosol in a two-step reaction **(Figure 29)**.

The addition of the glucuronic acid to the xenobiotic molecule is catalysed by one of four glucuronosyl transferases which are microsomal enzymes. The enzymes are inducible in animals treated with compounds such as phenobarbitone (Burchill and Coughtrie, 1992).

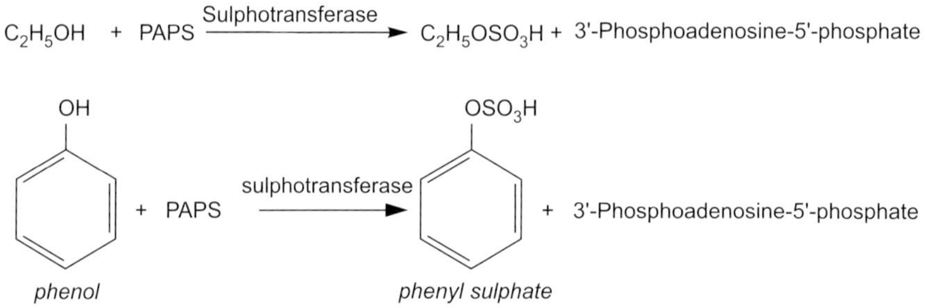

Figure 28 Conjugation of aromatic and aliphatic hydroxyl groups with sulphate.

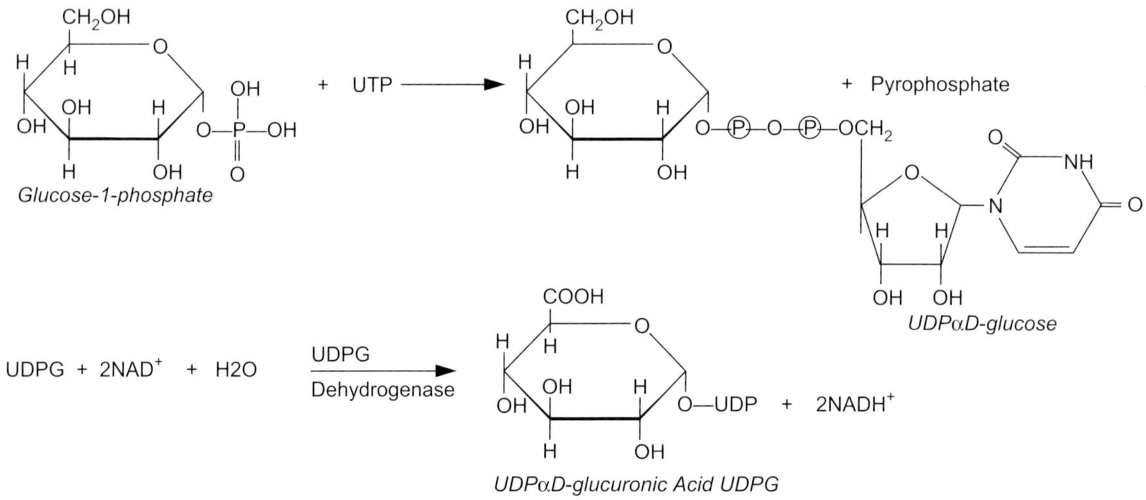

Figure 29 Formation of the glucuronic acid donor UDPG.

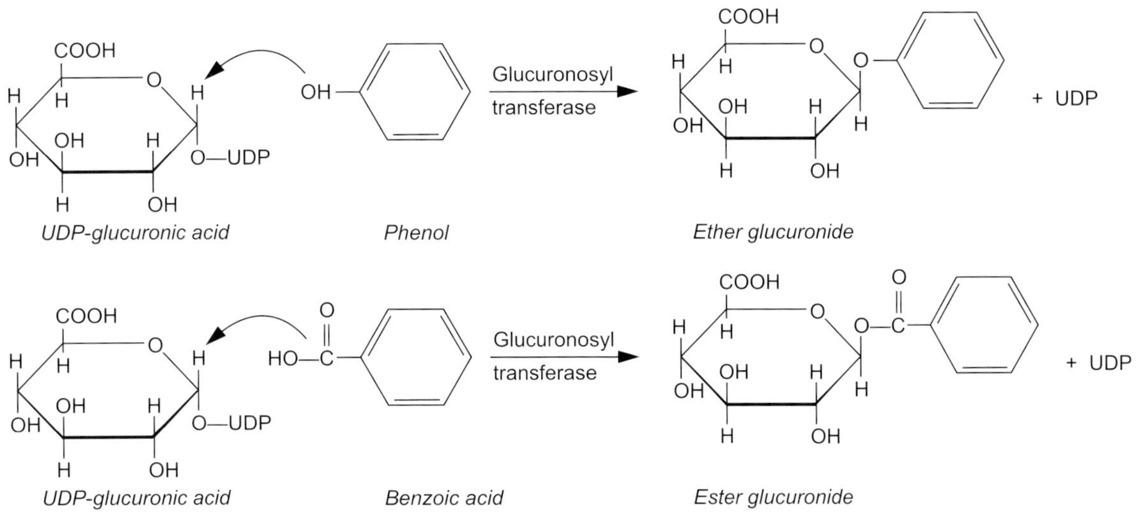

Figure 30 Formation of ether and ester glucuronide conjugates.

The reaction involves nucleophilic attack by the recipient atom (oxygen, sulphur or nitrogen) at the C-1 carbon atom of the glucuronic acid. This displacement reaction involves an inversion of configuration resulting in the product being in the β-configuration **(Figure 30)**.

As with sulphation, glucuronidation, although generally a detoxication reaction, may occasionally be involved in increasing toxicity, as with the conjugation of a metabolite of acetylaminofluorene (see below).

Glucose Conjugation

Other carbohydrates may also be involved in conjugation such as glucose, which is utilized by insects to form glucosides. Ribose and xylose may also be used in conjugation reactions.

Glutathione Conjugation

This group of reactions involves the addition of glutathione to a molecule, usually with the subsequent removal of two amino acids to leave a cysteine conjugate. This is then acetylated to yield a mercapturic acid or N-acetylcysteine conjugate **(Figure 31)**. Glutathione is a tripeptide (glutamylcysteinylglycine) found in most mammalian tissues, but especially the liver. It has a major protective role in the body, as it is a scavenger for reactive compounds of various types (Reed and Beatty, 1980). The sulphydryl (SH) group reacts with the reactive part of the foreign compound. Glutathione conjugation is a particularly important route of phase 2 metabolism from the toxicological point of view, as it is often involved in the removal of reactive intermediates. However, more recently this route has also been shown to be the cause of some toxic reactions (Van Bladeren et al.,

1988; Monks et al., 1990; Dekant and Vamvakas, 1993) (see below).

Normally the sulphydryl group of glutathione acts as a nucleophile and either displaces another atom (e.g. Cl) or group (e.g. nitro) or attacks an electrophilic site **(Figure 31)**. Consequently, glutathione may react either chemically or in enzyme-catalysed reactions with a variety of compounds which are reactive/electrophilic metabolites produced in phase 1 reactions (Ketterer, 1982). The reactions may be catalysed by one of a group of glutathione transferases (Armstrong, 1997). These are widely distributed enzymes which are located primarily in the soluble fraction of the cell but have also been detected in the microsomal fraction. The substrates include aromatic, heterocyclic, alicyclic and aliphatic epoxides, aromatic halogen and nitro compounds, alkyl halides and unsaturated aliphatic compounds. Although the specificity is not high for the xenobiotic, there is high specificity for glutathione.

The glutathione conjugate which is produced usually undergoes further metabolism which involves first a removal of the glutamyl residue, catalysed by γ-glutamyl transferase, then loss of glycine, catalysed by cysteinyl glycinase, and finally the cysteine moiety is acetylated to give the N-acetylcysteine conjugate or mercapturic acid **(Figure 31)**. The N-acetyltransferase which carries out this reaction is a microsomal enzyme found in liver and kidney but is not the same as the N-acetyltransferase which catalyses the acetylation of xenobiotic amine groups (see below). This further metabolism of conjugates such as illustrated for glutathione conjugates and cysteine conjugates (see below) has been termed phase 3 metabolism.

Glutathione conjugates, or the cysteinylglycine conjugate which results from them, may be excreted directly into the bile and further metabolism may take place in the gastrointestinal tract.

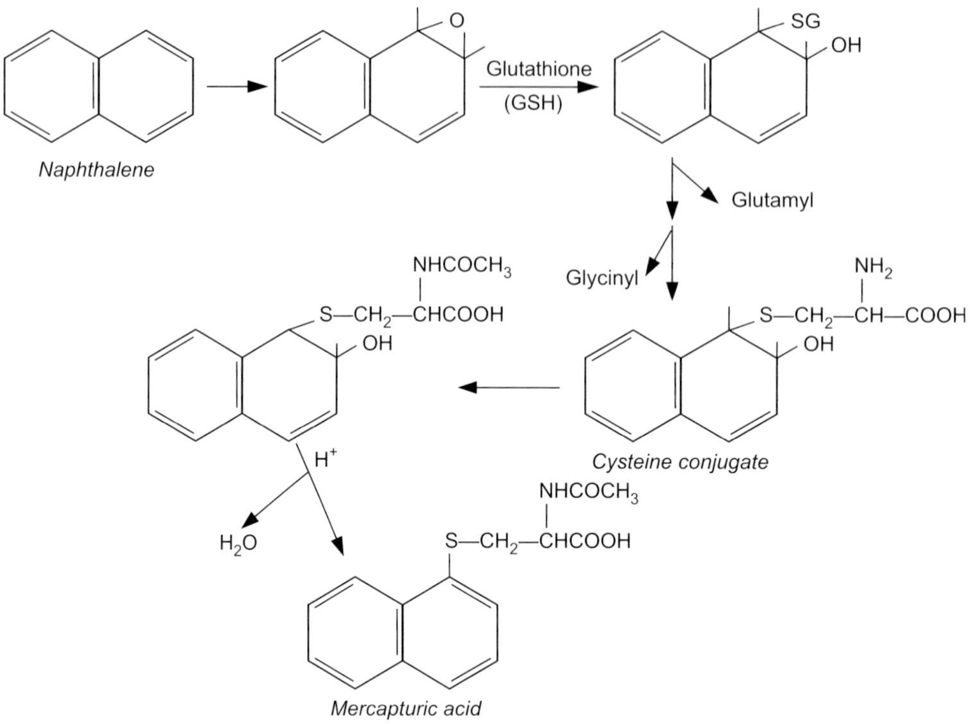

Figure 31 Metabolism of naphthalene to an *N*-acetylcysteine conjugate.

Cysteine Conjugate β-Lyase

This enzyme is responsible for the further metabolism of cysteine conjugates before they are acetylated. Only non-acetylated cysteine conjugates are substrates. The result is a thiol conjugate of the xenobiotic, pyruvic acid and ammonia. The thiol conjugate which results may in some cases prove to be toxic (see below).

Acetylation

This metabolic reaction is one of two types of acylation reaction and involves an activated conjugating agent, acetyl coenzyme A (acetyl CoA). It is also notable in that the product may be less water soluble than the parent compound. Acetylation is an important route of metabolism for aromatic amino compounds, sulphona-mides, hydrazines and hydrazides **(Figure 32)**. The enzymes involved are acetyltransferases and are found in the cytosol of cells in the liver, gastric mucosa and white blood cells. The enzymes utilize acetyl CoA as cofactor. The mechanism of the acetylation reaction involves first an acetylation of the enzyme, followed by addition of the substrate and then transfer of the acetyl group to the substrate. There are two enzymes (NAT 1 and NAT 2) in humans, rabbits and hamsters which differ markedly in activity and substrate specificity. NAT 1 is located in liver and gut whereas NAT 2 is found in most tissues. In humans the possession of a particular mutant isoenzyme is genetically determined

and gives rise to two distinct phenotypes known as 'rapid' and 'slow' acetylators. The acetylator phenotype has an important role in the toxicity of a number of drugs such as hydralazine, isoniazid and procainamide. These examples illustrate the importance of genetic factors in toxicology (Evans, 1992, 1993; Grant *et al.*, 1992; Kalow, 1992).

In addition to *N*-acetylation, a related reaction is *N, O*-transacetylation. This reaction applies to arylamines

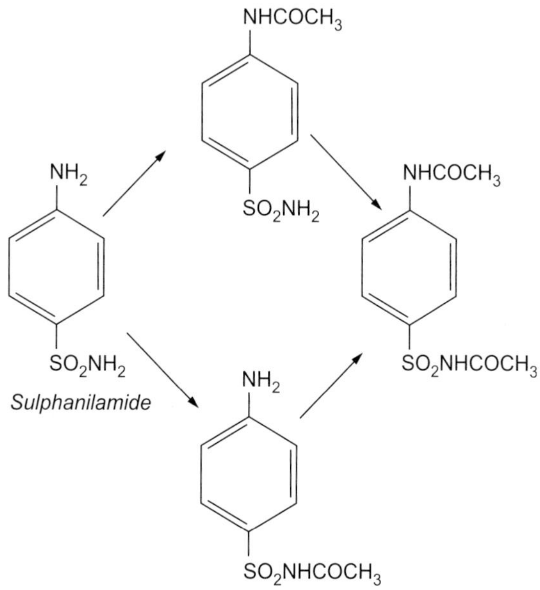

Figure 32 Acetylation of amino and sulphonamido groups.

which first undergo *N*-hydroxylation and then the hydro-xylamine group is acetylated to yield an arylhydroxamic acid (see **Figure 45** below). This may then transfer the acetyl group to another amine molecule or to the hydroxy group, to yield a highly reactive acyloxyarylamine which is capable of reacting, after a rearrangement, with pro-teins and nucleic acids (see below). The enzyme involved, an *N, O*-acyltransferase, is a cytosolic enzyme.

Amino Acid Conjugation

This is the second type of acylation reaction but in this type the xenobiotic itself is activated. Organic acids are the usual substrates for this reaction, with conjugation to an endogenous amino acid. The particular amino acid utilized depends on the species concerned and indeed species within a similar evolutionary group tend to utilize the same amino acid. Glycine is the most common amino acid used, but taurine, glutamine and ornithine are also utilized. The foreign carboxylic acid group is first activated by reaction with coenzyme A in a reaction which requires ATP and is catalysed by a mitochondrial ligase enzyme. The S-CoA derivative then reacts with the particular amino acid **(Figure 33)**. This second reaction is catalysed by an acyltransferase enzyme which is found in the mitochondria. Two enzymes have been purified, each utilizing a different group of CoA derivatives.

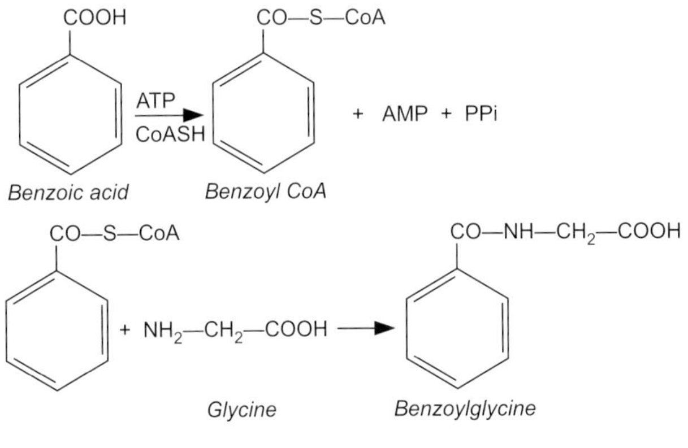

Figure 33 Conjugation of an aromatic acid with glycine.

Methylation

Hydroxyl, amino and thiol groups in both exogenous and endogenous compounds may be methylated by one of a series of methyltransferases **(Figure 34)**. These enzymes are normally found in the cytosol, although a microsomal *O*-methyltransferase and an *S*-methyl-transferase have been described. The cofactor required is *S*-adenosylmethionine, which is the methyl donor. As with acetylation, the methylation reaction tends to decrease rather than increase the water solubility of the

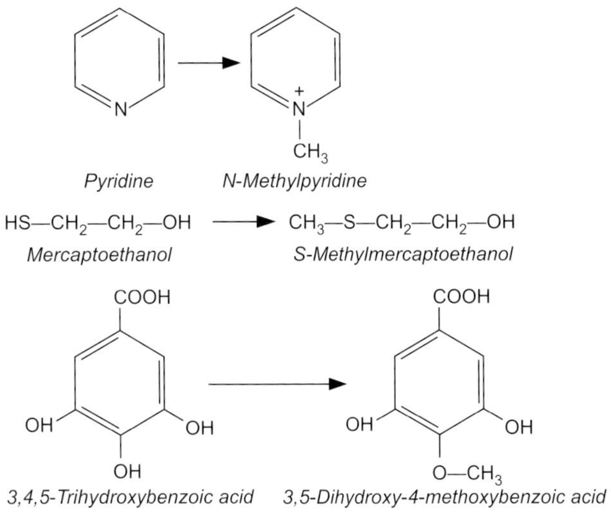

Figure 34 Methylation reactions.

molecule. A number of metals such as mercury may also be methylated by microorganisms, a reaction which changes both the toxicity of mercury and its physico-chemical characteristics and, hence, its environmental behaviour.

There are other minor reactions which a foreign mole-cule may undergo, but for information about these the interested reader should consult one of the texts or reviews given in the References. An important point, however, is that although a molecule is foreign to a living organism, it may still be a substrate for an enzyme involved in normal metabolic pathways, provided that its chemical structure is appropriate. For example, a foreign compound which is a halogenated fatty acid derivative may be metabolized by the *β*-oxidation path-way but might potentially interfere with that pathway. The possible involvement of enzymes of intermediary metabolism therefore widens the scope of potential meta-bolic reactions. Foreign compounds can be metabolized by a number of different enzymes simultaneously in the same animal and so there may be many different meta-bolic routes and metabolites. The balance between these routes can often determine the toxicity of the compound.

For more information on the metabolism of foreign compounds, the reader should consult the more detailed texts given in the References.

FACTORS AFFECTING METABOLISM

Factors which affect metabolism may often affect the toxicity of a compound, either by changing the rate of removal of the parent compound or by altering the pat-tern of metabolism. Different species will often metabol-ize compounds differently, and so show differences in toxicity. Environmental factors such as dietary constitu-ents and drugs taken by humans may influence the metabolism, and so alter the toxicity of a particular substance (Shimada *et al.*, 1994). In man genetic factors may play an important role in drug effects (Meyer 1998) and in determining which metabolic pathway is utilized and therefore whether a compound is toxic or not (Weber, 1987; Sitar, 1989; Alvan, 1992; Evans, 1992; Kalow, 1992; Meyer, 1994).

The multiple forms of cytochrome P450 may underly the species differences in metabolism (Berthou *et al.*, 1992) and may be relevant to the effects of age, sex, nutrition, strain and genetic differences. Different tissues may contain different isoenzymes and, hence, be differently susceptible to certain toxic compounds.

Table 2 Species differences in the hydroxylation of aniline

Species	% of dose excreted	
	o-Aminophenol	*p*-Aminophenol
Gerbil	3	48
Guinea pig	4	46
Golden hamster	6	53
Chicken	11	44
Rat	19	48
Ferret	26	28
Dog	18	9
Cat	32	14

Data from Parke (1968).

Species

Different species are utilized in the safety evaluation of chemicals, and in the environment widely different species may all be exposed to a chemical. These species may react very differently to xenobiotics. Indeed, this difference in sensitivity is exploited in pesticides. Insecticides such as organophosphorus compounds and DDT are much more toxic to insects than to humans and other mammals. In the case of malathion this is due to a metabolic difference **(Figure 35)**.

There are many species differences in metabolism which have been documented (Caldwell, 1980), but this section will mainly concentrate on those which are significant as far as toxicity is concerned.

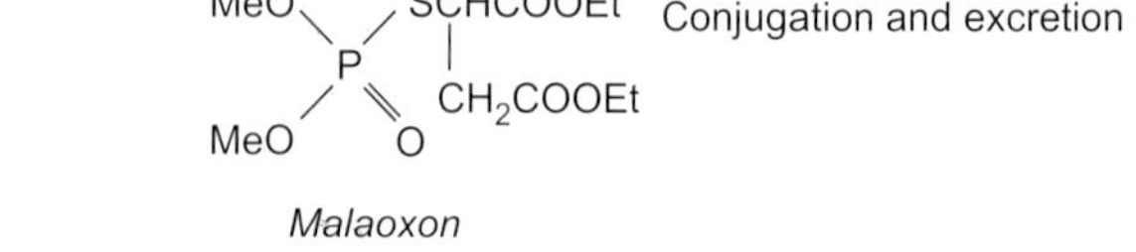

Figure 35 Metabolism of malathion.

Phase 1 Reactions

There are often quantitative differences between species in oxidation reactions but qualitative differences are perhaps less common. It is difficult to find a species pattern in these differences. These differences may often be the result of different combinations of cytochrome P450 enzymes.

The aromatic hydroxylation of aniline has been shown to vary between various species **(Table 2)**, and those

species such as the cat which produce more *o*- as opposed to *p*-aminophenol are more susceptible to the toxicity. The trend in this case is for carnivores to favour *ortho*- rather than *para*-hydroxylation. Another example of quantitative differences in metabolism between species is in the metabolism of ethylene glycol to oxalate **(Figure 2)**. The toxicity is partly due to the oxalic acid produced by the oxidative pathway and the toxicity correlates with the production of oxalate. Here again the cat is the species most susceptible to the toxicity, producing the most oxalate, followed by the rat, with the rabbit producing the least.

The *N*-oxidation of paracetamol (see below) also shows quantitative differences in metabolism between species, which accounts for species differences in hepatotoxicity. Thus, the rat is relatively resistant to the toxicity and metabolizes less via the toxic pathway, whereas the hamster is very susceptible. In contrast, the rat is well able to carry out *N*-hydroxylation of acetylaminofluorene **(Figure 12)**, a step which is necessary for the carcinogenicity of the compound (see also **Figure 45** below).

In the metabolism of the drug hexobarbitone (hexobarbital) there are striking differences between species, which correlate with the pharmacological effect **(Table 3)**. The overall metabolic rate tends to decrease as the size of the species increases, and this would be expected to have some bearing on drug metabolism. In this example this is approximately true, apart from the rat and rabbit being transposed.

Another Phase 1 reaction which shows a striking species difference that is a cause of selective toxicity is hydrolysis. Thus, the insecticide malathion is readily hydrolysed in mammals but in the insect the carboxylesterase enzyme is absent and oxidative metabolism is the major route **(Figure 35)**. This route leads to the production of malaoxon, which is toxic because it binds to the active site of cholinesterases.

Phase 2 Reactions

A number of Phase 2 reactions also show well characterized species differences. For example, the metabolism of

Table 3 Species differences in the metabolism and duration of action of hexobarbitone (hexobarbital)

Species	Duration of action (min)	Plasma half-life (min)	Relative enzyme activity (μg g^{-1} h^{-1})	Plasma level on awakening (μg ml^{-1})
Mouse	12	19	598	89
Rabbit	49	60	196	57
Rat	90	140	135	64
Dog[a]	315	260	36	19

Data from Quinn *et al.* (1958).
[a] Dose in dogs, 50 mg kg^{-1}; other species, 100 mg kg^{-1}.

phenols in most mammals, and also birds, amphibians and reptiles but not fish, usually involves conjugation with either glucuronic acid or sulphate, depending on the species, but most species utilize a mixture of these two routes. The cat, however, cannot utilize glucuronic acid and the pig cannot usually conjugate with sulphate. There are also clear differences in the conjugation of organic acids. Carnivores favour glucuronic acid conjugation, herbivores favour amino acid conjugation, whereas omnivores utilize both. Which amino acid is utilized also varies, and although glycine is the most common, glutamine and taurine may be used and reptiles utilize ornithine, whereas insects utilize arginine.

Strain of Animal

Different inbred strains of the same animal may show variations in metabolism, just as different species may vary in their response to toxic compounds and in the way they metabolize them. For example, different strains of mice vary widely in their ability to metabolize barbiturates and consequently the magnitude of the pharmacological effect varies between these strains **(Table 4)**. Similarly, variations between human individuals may also occur but will be considered separately in this chapter (see below).

Table 4 Strain differences in the duration of action of hexobarbitone (hexobarbital) in mice

Strain	Numbers of animals	Mean sleeping time $\pm$ SD (min)
A/NL	25	48 $\pm$ 4
BALB/cAnN	63	41 $\pm$ 2
C57L/HeN	29	33 $\pm$ 3
C3HfB/HeN	30	22 $\pm$ 3
SWR/HeN	38	18 $\pm$ 4
Swiss (non-inbred)	47	43 $\pm$ 15

Data from Jay (1955).

Sex

There can also be variation in the responses between males and females due to metabolic and hormonal dif-ferences. Males in some species metabolize compounds more rapidly than females, although this difference is not found in all species. The difference in susceptibility to chloroform-induced liver damage between male and female rats is an example of a sex difference which has a metabolic and hormonal basis, thought to be due to the effects of testosterone on liver microsomal enzyme activity. Thus, treatment of females with testosterone decreases the LD_{50} and treatment of males with oestradiol increases the LD_{50} of chloroform. Similarly, there is a sex difference in the nephrotoxicity of chloroform in mice, with male mice being more susceptible. This difference can be removed by castration and restored by administration of androgens to the males. It may be that testosterone is increasing the microsomal enzyme-mediated metabolism of chloroform to toxic metabolites (Pohl, 1979).

Other examples are the metabolism of ethylmorphine and hexobarbitone (hexobarbital), which are clearly under hormonal control in the male rat. Castration of the animals significantly reduces the metabolism of both compounds. However, the normal rate of metabolism can be restored by the administration of androgens to the castrated animals.

Genetic Factors

Genetic variation in metabolism within the human population probably underlies much of the variability in response of that population to the toxic effects of foreign compounds (Meyer, 1994, 1998; Tucker, 1994). There are now many examples of toxic drug reactions which occur particularly in individuals who have a genetic defect or genetic difference in metabolism. Perhaps the best known example of genetic variability in man is the acetylator phenotype (Weber, 1987; Evans, 1992; Grant *et al.*, 1992). In this example the acetylation reaction (see above) shows genetic variations which are due to the presence of mutations in the gene coding for the *N*-acetyltransferase, NAT 2. These mutations give rise to enzymes with differing activities and result in two distinct populations, the rapid and slow acetylator phenotypes. NAT 2 has therefore been termed a polymorphic enzyme. However, recent evidence suggests that NAT 1 may also show bimodal variation. The slow acetylator phenotype, which occurs to a variable extent in the population, depending on the racial origin **(Table 5)**, is an important factor in a number of adverse drug reactions **(Table 6)**. For example, the lupus syndrome induced by the drug hydralazine only occurs in slow acetylators. The metabolism of the drug is influenced by the acetylator phenotype, with more being metabolized by an oxidative pathway in the slow acetylators (Timbrell *et al.*, 1984). However, it is not yet known whether this is responsible for the toxic effect but oxidation by myeloperoxidase in neutrophils has been implicated (Uetrecht, 1992).

The acetylator phenotype is also believed to be a factor in isoniazid toxicity (see below) and bladder cancer, which occurs in workers exposed to aromatic amines. Thus, there is an increased incidence of the cancer in slow acetylators. This is postulated to be due to the decreased ability of slow acetylators to detoxify the aromatic amines by acetylation (Cartwright *et al.*, 1982; Mommsen *et al.*, 1985; Kadlubar, 1994). However, one recent study did not find any evidence that the slow acetylator phenotype was more susceptible to benzidine-induced bladder cancer (Hayes *et al.*, 1993).

Another genetic factor in metabolism is polymorphism in the hydroxylation of debrisoquine **(Figure 36)** (Gonzalez *et al.*, 1988; Eichelbaum and Gross, 1990). This variation in oxidation has now been shown for a number of other drugs, such as phenytoin, sparteine and phenformin. Again there are two phenotypes, designated poor metabolizers and extensive metabolizers. Unlike the acetylator phenotype, however, the poor metabolizer phenotype is relatively uncommon, only occurring in about 5–10% of a Caucasian population. In some cases toxic reactions are associated with the poor metabolizer status. The difference between the poor metabolizers and extensive metabolizers is believed to be due to differences in the isozymes of cytochrome P450 present in the particular subject. It has been shown (Gonzalez and Meyer, 1991) that poor metabolizer individuals have a deficiency in liver cytochrome P450 2D6 resulting from various mutations in the *CYP 2D6* gene. It seems that there are two cytochrome P450 isozymes catalysing the oxidation of debrisoquine and similar substrates, with different affinities and capacities for a particular substrate. The extensive metabolizers may have both the isozymes, whereas the poor metabolizers may be deficient in the high-affinity isozyme. It also seems likely that only one of these isozymes is controlled by the polymorphism.

Environmental Factors

Exposure of animals to chemical substances via the environment, such as in the diet, air or water, may influence the metabolism and therefore the toxic response to the chemical of interest. Humans may be receiving medication with several drugs when exposure to an industrial

Table 5 Acetylator phenotype distribution in various ethnic groups

Ethnic group	Rapid acetylators (%)	Drug
Eskimos	95–100	INH
Japanese	88	INH
Latin Americans	70	INH
Black Americans	52	INH
White Americans	48	INH
Africans	43	SMZ
South Indians	39	INH
Britons	38	SMZ
Egyptians	18	INH

Data from Lunde *et al.* (1977).

Table 6 Toxicities related to the acetylator phenotype

Xenobiotic	Adverse effect	Incidence
Isoniazid	Peripheral neuropathy	Higher in slow acetylators
Isoniazid	Hepatic damage	Higher in slow acetylators
Procainamide Hydralazine	Lupus erythematosus	Higher in slow acetylators
Phenelzine	Drowsiness/ nausea	Higher in slow acetylators
Aromatic amines	Bladder cancer	Higher in slow acetylators

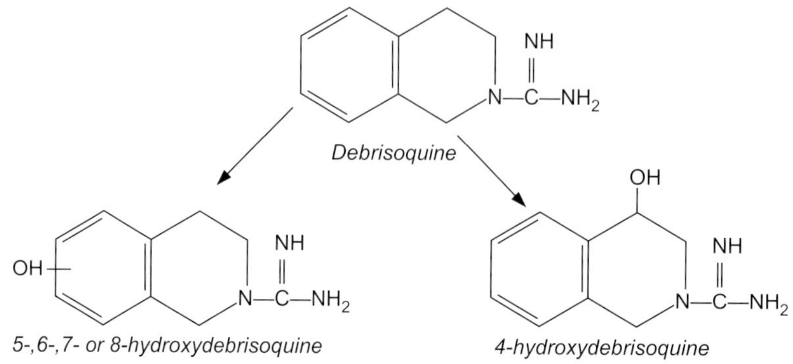

Figure 36 Metabolism of debrisoquine.

chemical occurs, for instance. The intake of one drug may affect the metabolism of another. For example, overdoses of paracetamol are more likely to cause serious liver damage if the victim is also exposed to large amounts of alcohol or barbiturates. Both of these drugs influence drug-metabolizing enzymes and thereby increase the metabolism and, in turn, the toxicity of paracetamol (see below).

The diet contains many substances, such as the naphthoflavones found in certain vegetables, which may influence the enzymes involved in drug metabolism. Cigarette smoking is also known to affect drug metabolism. One way in which a particular substance may influence the metabolism of another is by increasing the apparent activity of the drug-metabolizing enzymes. This is known as induction. The induction of the microsomal monooxygenases, as well as a number of other enzymes, is now a well known phenomenon and is caused by a large variety of compounds (Batt *et al.*, 1992). It occurs in many species. However, these different inducers induce different cytochrome P450 enzymes and are therefore of importance for different types of substrates.

The first type of microsomal enzyme inducer to be described was the barbiturate phenobarbitone. When animals are exposed to repeated doses of this compound, there are a number of changes which can be observed. The liver of the animal exposed increases in weight, there is an increase in liver blood flow and the smooth endoplasmic reticulum proliferates. These changes are accompanied by an increase in the total amount of cytochrome P450 in the liver. The activity of other enzymes found in the endoplasmic reticulum also increases.

The effect of enzyme induction is that the metabolism of certain foreign compounds is increased. At the molecular level there is an increase in protein synthesis and underlying this an increase in mRNA synthesis. Since the initial discovery that phenobarbitone induced the enzymes responsible for its own metabolism, many other inducers have been discovered and studied, and some of these have been found to be different types of inducer. These different inducers induce different isoenzymes of cytochrome P450 and do not necessarily cause all the changes observed with phenobarbitone induction,

such as the increase in liver weight and blood flow. The inducers currently known can be divided into five types: (i) the barbiturate type; (ii) the polycyclic aromatic hydrocarbon type; (iii) the isoniazid type; (iv) the steroid type typified by pregnenolone carbonitrile; and (v) the clofibrate type. Each of these induces a different form or forms of the enzyme. These can in some cases be distinguished and detected on the basis of catalytic activity *in vivo* or *in vitro* as well as increased amounts of protein. There are also inducers which have a broader inducing ability, such as the compound Arochlor 1254, which may be both a barbiturate type and a polycyclic hydrocarbon type of inducer. Some of the enzymes induced may be constitutive whereas others induced by some of these compounds may represent only a small proportion of the total cytochrome P450 present in the uninduced animal. In this case the induction may cause a large shift in the metabolic profile rather than a simple increase in the overall rate of metabolism. Thus, for the polycyclic hydrocarbon type of inducers the form of cytochrome P450 induced normally only represents about 5% of the total enzyme, whereas after induction the amount may be increased by a factor of 16. Furthermore, induction is not confined to the hepatic enzymes, those in other tissues may also be induced. The effect of different inducers on the metabolism of different compounds can be seen from the data in **Table 7**. Clearly, although all these compounds are inducers of cytochrome P450, the effects on different substrates for the enzyme are different. These differential effects even extend to different isomers **(Table 8)**. This can be rationalized by the fact that there are many different isoenzymes and that these are induced by different compounds.

In addition to influencing the metabolism of foreign compounds, enzyme induction may have effects on the metabolism of endogenous compounds and so disrupt normal physiological processes.

The mechanisms underlying induction are not all entirely clear but it is known to be a cellular response, which can be studied in isolated hepatocytes, for example. Indeed, the mechanisms seem to vary between the different types and may involve transcriptional activation (e.g. CYP1A1) or enzyme stabilization (CYP2E1).

Table 7 Effects of different inducers on the metabolism of various substrates (units: nmol product per min per nmol cytochrome P450)

Substrate	Inducer[a]				
	Control	Pb	PCN	3MC	ARO
Ethylmorphine	13.7 ± 0.8	16.8 ± 4.3	24.9 ± 3.5	6.4 ± 0.5	9.5 ± 1.2
Aminopyrine	9.9 ± 0.8	13.9 ± 1.7	9.7 ± 1.3	7.6 ± 1.8	13.7 ± 1.2
Benzphetamine	12.5 ± 1.2	45.7 ± 14.0	6.6 ± 0.7	5.7 ± 1.1	15.8 ± 2.7
Caffeine	0.5 ± 0.1	0.7 ± 0.1		0.5 ± 0.1	0.6 ± 0.1
Benzo[a]pyrene	0.1	01.	0.1	0.3	

Data from Powis *et al.* (1977).
[a] Pb, phenobarbitone; PCN, pregnenolone-16α-carbonitrile; 3MC, 3-methylcholanthrene; ARO, Arochlor 1254.

Table 8 Differential effect of cytochrome P450 inducers on the hydroxylation of warfarin isomers (units: nmol metabolite formed per nmol cytochrome P450)

	Hydroxylated warfarin metabolites			
	R-Isomer		S-Isomer	
	7-OH	8-OH	7-OH	8-OH
Control	0.22	0.04	0.04	0.01
Phenobarbitone	0.36	0.07	0.09	0.02
3-Methylcholanthrene	0.08	0.50	0.04	0.04

Data from Table 3.6 in Gibson and Skett (1986).

The synthesis of new protein is involved, as the induction process can be prevented by inhibitors of protein synthesis. Synthesis of RNA is required but not of DNA, and so it seems that the effect is at the level of transcription. For the polycyclic hydrocarbon type of inducer, studied using tetrachlorodibenzodioxin (dioxin), which is an exquisitely potent inducer, it seems that there is a cytosolic receptor which binds the inducer. The inducer–receptor complex is then transported to the nucleus and there enhances transcription of the *CYP1A1* gene and other genes such as *CYP1A2*, glutathione transferase and glucuronosyl transferase. This causes mRNA coding for cytochrome P450 1A1 and other enzymes to be synthesized. This then allows increased synthesis of the particular cytochrome P450 enzymes for which the mRNA is coded. This involves inducer-dependent derepression and activation of gene expression (Okey, 1990; Waxman and Azaroff, 1992; Whitlock, 1993). However, to date no receptor for the barbiturate type of inducer has been found although evidence suggests that the induction may involve inducer-dependent derepression and activation of gene expression as for the polycyclic hydrocarbon type. The peroxisome-proliferator (clofibrate) type of induction (CYP4A) also involves a receptor (Muerhoff *et al.*, 1992).

Consequences of Induction

Induction of drug-metabolizing enzymes may lead to an alteration in the metabolism of a compound, which may then result in the toxicity being either increased or decreased. Prediction of which will occur is possible only with a knowledge of the metabolism and mechanism of toxicity of the compound in question. In some of the examples at the end of this chapter the effect of inducers will also be discussed.

Inhibition of Metabolism

Just as some of the enzymes involved in biotransformation may be induced, so these enzymes may also be inhibited, and this can have major consequences for toxicity (Netter, 1987; Halpert *et al.*, 1994). Such inhibi-

tions are sometimes of major importance clinically with the interaction between drugs and are probably more important than induction effects. Inhibition generally requires only a single dose of a compound rather than the repeated doses which are required for induction. The environmental impact of inhibition is, however, probably less than that of induction. Inhibition also may be relevant to the toxic effects of substances encountered in the workplace. For example, workers exposed to the solvent dimethylformamide seem more likely to suffer alcohol-induced flushes than those not exposed, possibly owing to the inhibition of alcohol metabolism.

There are many different types of inhibitor of the microsomal monooxygenase system. Thus, there are inhibitors which appear to bind as substrates and are competitive inhibitors, such as dichlorobiphenyl, which inhibits the O-demethylation of p-nitroanisole. There are those inhibitors which are metabolized to compounds which bind strongly to the active site of the enzyme, such as piperonyl butoxide, which probably acts by forming an inactive complex with cytochrome P450, which becomes irreversibly inhibited. There are indeed many compounds which form such inhibitory complexes with cytochrome P450, including some commonly used drugs, such as triacetyloleandomycin. Some inhibitors destroy cytochrome P450, such as carbon tetrachloride, cyclophosphamide, carbon disulphide and allylisopropylacetamide. Finally, there are those which interfere with the synthesis of the enzyme, such as cobalt chloride, which inhibits cytochrome P450 *in vivo* by interfering with the synthesis of the haem portion of the enzyme.

Other toxicologically relevant enzymes involved in biotransformation which also may be inhibited are the esterases, which are inhibited by organophosphorus compounds. Inhibition of monoamine oxidases by drugs such as iproniazid is important clinically, because it results in a decreased metabolism of naturally occuring amines such as tyramine which may be ingested in the diet. These amines may thereby accumulate and can have profound physiological effects such as causing an increase in blood pressure, which in some cases may be fatal.

Pathological State

The influence of disease states on metabolism and toxicity has not been well explored. Diseases of the liver might be expected to affect metabolism, but in practice different liver diseases can influence metabolism differently (Hoyumpa and Schenker, 1982; Howden *et al.*, 1989; Kraul *et al.*, 1991). Indeed, some metabolic pathways are unaffected by liver damage. For example, the glucuronidation of paracetamol, morphine and oxazepam was not found to be affected by liver cirrhosis in human subjects. Conversely, the oxidation of a number of drugs such as barbiturates, antipyrine and methadone and the conjugation of salicylates with glycine were all depressed by cirrhosis. Disease states such as influenza are also known to affect drug metabolising enzymes, possibly via the production of interferon in response to the infection (Azri and Renton, 1991).

Age

In general, animals at the extremes of age—neonates and geriatrics—are less able to metabolize foreign compounds than are adult animals between these extremes (Besunder et al., 1988; Kinirons and Crome, 1997). However, the development of drug-metabolizing ability is complex and depends on the particular substrate, and is influenced also by sex and species (Horbach et al., 1992). For example, in the rat phase 1 metabolic activity may develop only after weaning for some demethylation reactions but the p-hydroxylation of aniline develops from birth. With phase 2 reactions, again, some are low at birth, such as glucuronidation, whereas acetylation and sulphation are at adult levels, even in the foetus in the guinea pig.

In rats monooxygenase activity begins to decline when the animals reach 1 year of age.

These effects on drug metabolism may be translated into differences in toxicity, but it is not always the young animal which is more susceptible. For example, paracetamol is less hepatotoxic in young mice than in adults. This may be due to the fact that the development of the cytochrome P450 system required to activate paracetamol (see below) reaches maximum, adult levels more slowly than hepatic glutathione levels (Hart and Timbrell, 1979).

Diet

Although there is a paucity of information in this area, it is clear that dietary deficiencies can affect the metabolism of foreign compounds by altering the enzymes involved (Gibson and Skett, 1994). Thus, a low-protein diet will generally decrease the activity of the monoxygenases and decrease the content of cytochrome P450. For example, rats fed a low-protein (5%) diet show 50% of the in vitro microsomal enzyme activity of rats fed a normal diet (20% protein). The effect occurs within 24 h and the enzyme activity is minimal after 4 days. In vivo findings are in agreement with these observations. The decrease in microsomal enzyme activity due to a low-protein diet may result in reduced toxicity. For example, carbon tetrachloride hepatotoxicity is less in protein-deficient rats than normal animals. However, other changes may occur which have the opposite effect, and so paracetamol is more hepatotoxic in protein-deficient animals, possibly owing to decreased hepatic glutathione levels. As with protein deficiency, a dietary deficiency in lipid

such as linoleic acid also tends to decrease levels of cytochrome P450.

Changes in carbohydrate seem to have few effects on drug metabolism, although an increase in glucose intake seems to decrease hepatic cytochrome P450 and inhibit barbiturate metabolism.

The effects of starvation seem to be variable, with some microsomal enzyme activities being increased and others decreased. Deficiencies in vitamins in general also reduce the activity of the monooxygenases, although there are exceptions to this.

Chiral Factors in Metabolism

The importance of chiral factors in metabolism and toxicity has been recognized only relatively recently. The presence of a chiral centre in a molecule, giving rise to isomers, may influence the routes of metabolism and toxicity of that compound. Alternatively, metabolism may yield a specific isomer as a product from a molecule without a chiral centre. For example, it has now been found that only the glutaminic acid derived from the S-(−)-enantiomer of thalidomide is embryotoxic, and not that formed from the R-(+)-enantiomer.

Benzo[a]pyrene is metabolized stereoselectively by a particular cytochrome P450 isozyme, P450/A/, to the (+)-(7R, 8S)-oxide, which, in turn, is metabolized by epoxide hydrolase to the (−)-(7R, 8R)-dihydrodiol. This metabolite is further metabolized to (+)-benzo[a]pyrene-(7R, 8S)-dihydrodiol-(9S, 10R)-epoxide, in which the hydroxyl group and epoxide are trans and which is more mutagenic than are other enantiomers. This diol-epoxide metabolite is not a substrate for epoxide hydrolase and consequently is not detoxified by this route and is highly mutagenic. The (−)-(7R, 8R)-dihydrodiol of benzo[a]pyrene is ten times more tumorigenic than is the (+)-(7S, 8S)-dihydrodiol.

It was felt that in this case the configuration was more important for tumorigenicity than the chemical reactivity.

The hydroxylation of the drug bufuralol (Figure 37) in the 1-position only occurs with the (+)-isomer, whereas for hydroxylation in the 4- and 6-positions the (−)-isomer is the substrate. Glucuronidation of the side-chain hydroxyl group is specific for the (+)-isomer. A further complication in human subjects is that the 1-hydroxylation is under genetic control, being dependent on the debrisoquine hydroxylator status. The selectivity for the isomers for the hydroxylations is virtually abolished in poor metabolizers. In addition to cytochrome P450, other enzymes are specific for or form specific isomers. Thus, epoxide hydrolase forms trans-dihydrodiols from cyclic epoxides and glutathione transferases are also stereospecific enzymes.

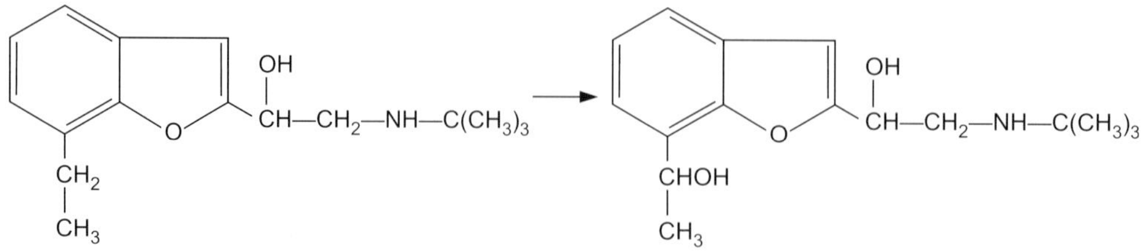

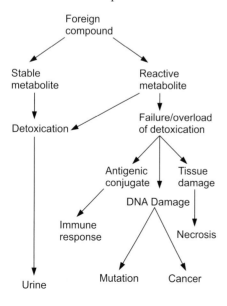

Figure 37 Stereo-selective hydroxylation of bufuralol.

TOXICATION VERSUS DETOXICATION

The biotransformation of foreign compounds is often regarded as detoxication because it usually converts compounds into more water-soluble, readily excreted substances. This tends to decrease the exposure of the animal to the compound and so tends to decrease the toxicity. However, in some cases the reverse occurs and a metabolite is produced which is more toxic than the parent compound. There are many factors which affect this, such as the dose, availability of cofactors and the relative activity of the various drug-metabolizing enzymes. There may also be several, competing pathways of metabolism—some leading to detoxication, others to toxicity. Factors which alter the balance between these competing pathways will alter the eventual toxicity. This balance between toxication and detoxication pathways **(Figure 38)** is very important in toxicology and underlies some of the factors which affect toxicity (Nelson and Harvison, 1987; Monks and Lau, 1988; Nelson, 1995). Although in many cases the toxic metabolites are generated by the enzymes involved in phase 1 pathways, there are now a number of examples where phase 2 conjugation reactions are involved in toxication as opposed to detoxication processes.

Paracetamol

A prime example of the role of competing metabolic pathways in toxicity and the importance of endogenous cofactors is afforded by the drug paracetamol (acetaminophen) (Monks and Lau, 1988). This widely used drug is unfortunately sometimes taken in overdose. Such overdoses cause centrilobular hepatic necrosis in man and experimental animals, and a wealth of research has revealed that this toxicity is due in part to metabolism of the drug.

There are three pathways of metabolism for paracetamol **(Figure 39)**, of which the two most important quantitatively are sulphate and glucuronic acid conjugation. The third, resulting in conjugation with glutathione, only represents a few per cent of the dose in humans. This latter pathway involves an initial reaction catalysed by cytochrome P450, producing a reactive metabolite which is normally detoxified by conjugation with glutathione. The resulting glutathione conjugate is then further

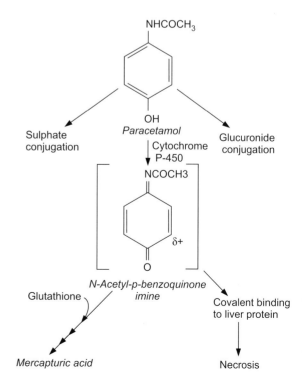

Figure 38 Some of the various consequences of biotransformation

Figure 39 Metabolism of paracetamol.

metabolized to a cysteine conjugate which is acetylated and excreted as a N-acetylcysteine conjugate or mercapturic acid.

Hepatotoxicity ensues when a sufficiently large dose of paracetamol is taken to deplete the liver of the majority of the glutathione (to 20% or less in experimental animals). This means that the reactive metabolite is able to react with cellular macromolecules such as protein, covalently bind to these macromolecules and cause hepatic necrosis. The nature of the reactive metabolite has received much attention but seems to be a quinoneimine (N-acetyl-p-benzoquinoneimine; NAPQI), although the exact mechanism of formation is not certain (Nelson, 1995).

In liver microsomal incubations both *in vitro* and *in vivo*, radiolabelled paracetamol binds covalently to protein, and the major adduct isolated from these protein conjugates is 3-cystein-S-yl-4-hydroxyaniline. A number of protein targets have been isolated, in particular a 55–58 kDa cytosolic protein and a 100 kDa protein which is N-10-formyltetrahydrofolate dehydrogenase. Arylation of this protein correlates with loss of enzyme activity. (Pumford *et al.*, 1997). Mitochondrial protein targets such as glutamate dehydrogenase have also been identified. Again, arylation is associated with loss of enzyme activity (Pumford *et al.*, 1997). The loss of enzyme activity may contribute to the development of toxicity such as the detoxication of ammonia. However, as yet unidentified targets such as a 58 kDa protein may also play a role in the development of the toxicity and it is likely a number of separate events are involved (Cohen and Khairallah, 1997).

It seems, however, that an electrophilic metabolite is involved in some way in the hepatotoxicity. It is clear that the NAPQI is a cytotoxic, reactive metabolite of paracetamol, produced via an oxidation reaction catalysed by one of several cytochrome P450 enzymes, including CYP1A1, CYP1A2, CYP2E1, CYP3A1 and CYP3A2. Recent evidence suggests that Kupffer cells and nitric oxide are also involved in the metabolic activation (Pike *et al.*, 1998). The reactive metabolite produced will react with glutathione. It reacts with glutathione in two ways: (1) by forming a conjugate and (2) by oxidizing glutathione and being itself reduced back to paracetamol. NADPH can also reduce NAPQI back to paracetamol in a reaction which may involve glutathione reductase. The reactive metabolite can also react with cysteine residues in proteins via either arylation or oxidation of the cysteine SH.

Deacetylation of paracetamol can also occur, giving rise to *p*-aminophenol and subsequent metabolites. *p*-Aminophenol is a known nephrotoxin, and this might account for the nephrotoxicity seen after overdoses of paracetamol and occasionally reported with chronic dosage.

There are two main detoxication pathways for paracetamol: conjugation with (1) glucuronic acid and (2) sulphate. The oxidative pathway(s) leading to the mer-

capturic acid accounts for about 5% in man. The deacetylation pathway is also presumably minor. However, this balance may be altered in a number of ways. Large doses of paracetamol may deplete animals of sulphate as well as glutathione. Metabolism may thereby be diverted through the oxidative pathway catalysed by the cytochrome P450 enzymes and more will be conjugated with glucuronic acid (**Figure 39**). Factors which affect the activity of the microsomal enzymes such as inducing agents will also alter this balance. For example, pretreatment of animals with phenobarbitone will increase the hepatotoxicity in some species (rats) by increasing the amount metabolized via the cytochrome P450 pathway. However, this pretreatment will also increase the activity of glucuronosyl transferase and in some species (hamsters) this effect will decrease the hepatotoxicity. In the hamster the oxidative pathway is quantitatively of greater importance than in the rat, a factor which underlies the large difference in susceptibility to the hepatotoxicity between these two species.

Carbon Tetrachloride

Carbon tetrachloride is a potent hepatotoxin which has been extensively studied. The major toxic effect it causes is centrilobular hepatic necrosis which is dependent upon metabolism via the cytochrome P450 system. However, the enzyme system is acting as a reductase in this instance. Cytochrome P450 donates an electron to the carbon tetrachloride molecule and thereby allows the homolytic cleavage of a carbon–chlorine bond (**Figure 40**). This yields the trichloromethyl radical and a chloride ion. The trichloromethyl radical may then react with oxygen to give the trichloromethylperoxy radical. Alternatively, the trichloromethyl radical can abstract a hydrogen atom from polyunsaturated lipids and thereby form a lipid radical and a stable product, chloroform. The lipid radical can then proceed to react with other cellular constituents and cause a cascade of disturbances within the cell, including peroxidation of lipids. Alternatively, the trichloromethyl radical can react covalently with lipids and proteins. The trichloromethylperoxy

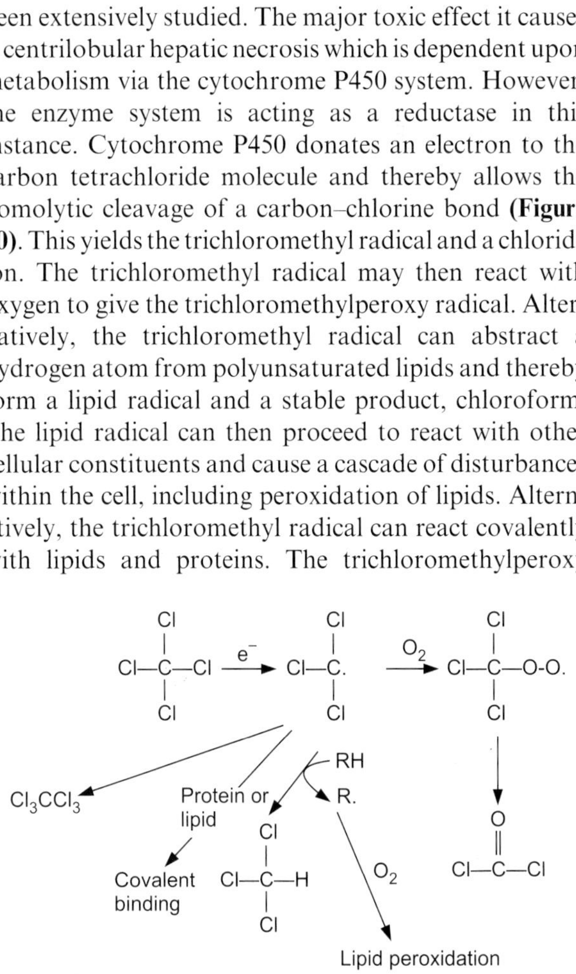

Figure 40 Metabolism of carbon tetrachloride.

radical is believed to be the reactive metabolite responsible for lipid peroxidation.

The oxygen concentration is important for the formation of the trichloromethylperoxy radical and the lipid peroxidation. As carbon tetrachloride is metabolically activated by cytochrome P450 in the smooth endoplasmic reticulum, the reactive radicals formed are able to react with the enzyme itself and the lipids of the endoplasmic reticulum. The result is that cytochrome P450 is destroyed by carbon tetrachloride. Consequently, if animals are given a small dose of carbon tetrachloride (0.05 ml kg^{-1}), a subsequent larger dose is less toxic than the same dose administered to a control animal (Glende, 1972). This is because the form of cytochrome P450 which activates carbon tetrachloride is destroyed. Carbon tetrachloride is thus hepatotoxic only when it can be metabolically activated (Sesardic *et al.*, 1989).

Bromobenzene

Bromobenzene is another hepatotoxic compound but one which may also damage the kidneys, and the involvement of metabolism in these two toxic effects is different. Bromobenzene metabolism affords an interesting example of the importance of competing pathways of detoxication versus toxication and of the way in which metabolic pathways may be switched by inducers.

Bromobenzene is metabolically activated by oxidation, catalysed by cytochrome(s) P450, to yield an intermediate 3,4-epoxide **(Figure 41)**. This epoxide is chemically reactive but may be detoxified in two ways. The first involves conjugation with glutathione **(Figure 41)**, eventually giving rise to a mercapturic acid conjugate which is excreted in the urine. The cytosolic glutathione transferases seem to be involved in the conjugation of the epoxide with glutathione rather than the microsomal glutathione transferases or a direct chemical reaction with glutathione. The second route of detoxication is metabolism to the dihydrodiol mediated by epoxide hydrolase. Just as with paracetamol, a sufficiently large dose of bromobenzene will deplete the liver of glutathione and, hence, the reactive epoxide will bind to tissue macromolecules, a process which seems to underly the liver necrosis.

There is another oxidation pathway, however, also catalysed by cytochrome(s) P450, which gives rise to another epoxide, the 2,3-epoxide, which is believed to be non-toxic. The evidence for this comes from the effect of inducers on the toxicity and metabolism, and illustrates switching of metabolic pathways. Pretreatment of animals with phenobarbitone increases metabolism via the 3,4-epoxide pathway and increases the toxicity. Conversely, pretreatment with 3-methylcholanthrene increases metabolism via the 2,3-epoxide pathway, as indicated by an increased excretion of *o*-bromophenol, and decreases the toxicity **(Table 9)**. Also, mice which

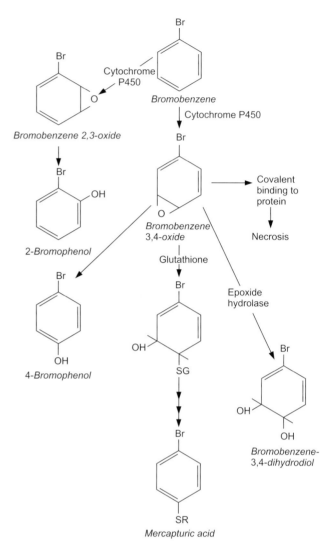

Figure 41 Some of the metabolic pathways for bromobenzene.

Table 9 Effect of induction with 3-methylchlolanthrene on the metabolism of bromobenzene in rats

Metabolite	% Total urinary metabolites	
	Control	3-MC treated
4-Bromophenylmercapturic acid	72	31
4-Bromophenol	14	20
4-Bromocatechol	6	10
4-Bromophenyldihydrodiol	3	17
2-Bromophenol	4	21

Data from Zampaglione *et al.* (1973).
Dose of bromobenzene 10 mmol kg^{-1}

have the cytochrome P450 isoenzyme which catalyses the formation of the 3,4-epoxide show greater hepatic damage after doses of bromobenzene than do those which who do not. *In vitro* the 3,4-epoxide binds to microsomal protein and seems to prefer to bind to

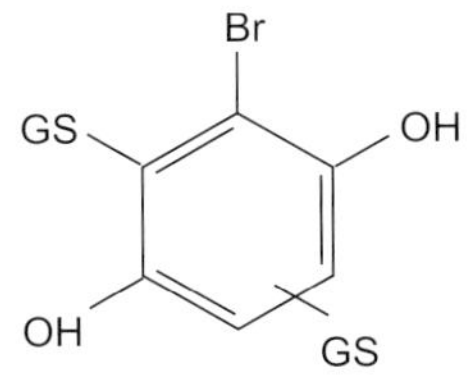

Figure 42 Diglutathione conjugate of bromobenzene.

histidine residues, whereas the 2,3-epoxide binds to hae-moglobin and prefers to bind to the cysteine residues. It is suggested that the 2,3-epoxide is more stable than the 3,4-epoxide and therefore reacts with a different target protein. However, the 3,4-epoxide was detected in both blood *in vivo* and hepatocyte incubation medium *in vitro* when animals or hepatocytes were exposed to bromo-benzene. Clearly the reactive intermediate has sufficient stability to move within the hepatocyte and even leave the cell. There would seem to be an optimum reactivity for the epoxide in order for it to be toxic and react with critical sites on macromolecules. Reactive metabolites which are chemically too reactive will tend to interact with biological molecules indiscriminately and may never reach critical target molecules. Further meta-bolism of the bromophenols may also occur, to give bromoquinols and bromocatechols. 2-Bromohydroqui-none will deplete glutathione in both liver and kidney but only causes pathological damage in the kidney. It is believed that the diglutathione conjugate of bromohy-droquinone **(Figure 42)** is the nephrotoxic agent.

Methanol

Methanol is a widely used and readily available solvent which is often found in combination with ethanol. Con-sequently, it sometimes features in poisoning cases. The toxicity of methanol illustrates the role of metabolism in toxicity where a chemically reactive metabolite does not seem to be involved. Also, a species difference in detox-ication is revealed. It also illustrates the importance of understanding the mechanism of toxicity in order to treat the poisoned patient in a rational way. Methanol is toxic mainly as a result of its metabolism to formic acid **(Figure 43)**. This is a two-step reaction, with metabolism to for-maldehyde being catalysed by either alcohol dehydro-genase or catalase. The second metabolic step to give formic acid is catalysed by either aldehyde dehydrogen-ase or formaldehyde dehydrogenase, an enzyme which requires glutathione.

The formic acid damages the optic nerve, seemingly by inhibiting the mitochondrial enzyme cytochrome

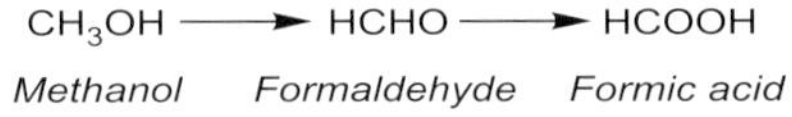

$$CH_3OH \longrightarrow HCHO \longrightarrow HCOOH$$
Methanol   Formaldehyde   Formic acid

Figure 43 Metabolism of methanol.

oxidase and, hence, reducing the level of ATP available to the nerves. Humans and certain other primates are much more susceptible than are rodents to the toxicity of methanol. It seems that this is due at least in part to the accumulation of formic acid in the susceptible species compared with the non-susceptible species. Formic acid may be detoxified by the action of tetrahydrofolate, giv-ing 10-formyltetrahydrofolate. This detoxication seems to be more efficient in rodents than in susceptible prim-ates. Because the metabolism is clearly important in the toxicity, treatment of the poisoning involves blocking the first step in the metabolic pathway by using ethanol as a competitive inhibitor of alcohol dehydrogenase. Another alcohol which is metabolized via alcohol dehy-drogenase leading to toxicity is allyl alcohol. This com-pound causes periportal liver necrosis when administered to animals. This is believed to be due to oxidation to allyl aldehyde catalysed by alcohol dehy-drogenase **(Figure 18)**.

Allylaldehyde is reactive and may cause toxicity by reacting with critical macromolecules in the cell. Glu-tathione conjugation is likely, as an *N*-acetylcysteine conjugate is excreted in the urine. Elegant work using deuterium-labelled allyl alcohol showed that oxidation was necessary for the toxicity (Patel *et al.*, 1983).

Isoniazid

Isoniazid is a widely used antitubercular drug which may cause hepatic damage in some patients receiving it. There are several routes of metabolism but the most important route is the acetylation reaction **(Figure 44)**. The acetyl-isoniazid that results from this is further metabolized by hydrolysis to yield acetylhydrazine and isonicotinic acid. Acetylhydrazine has been shown to be hepatotoxic in experimental animals and this is due to further meta-bolism via a cytochrome P450-mediated pathway **(Figure 44)**. The product is suggested to be a *N*-hydroxylated metabolite which on loss of water would yield a diazene, which can fragment to a reactive intermediate. This may be either a radical or a carbonium ion which may react with proteins and cause hepatic necrosis. This pathway is induced by phenobarbitone, which also increases the covalent binding of the acetyl group to protein and the hepatotoxicity of acetylhydrazine. However, acetyl-hydrazine may also be further metabolized by a different route, a second acetylation step, which is a detoxication reaction. Both the primary acetylation step, giving acet-ylisoniazid, and this second step are influenced by the acetylator phenotype (see above). Therefore, although rapid acetylators produce more acetylisoniazid and therefore more acetylhydrazine, this is then more extens-ively removed by acetylation to diacetylhydrazine in the rapid acetylator. When the plasma level of acetylhydra-zine in human subjects after a dose of isoniazid was determined, it was found that the slow acetylator has a

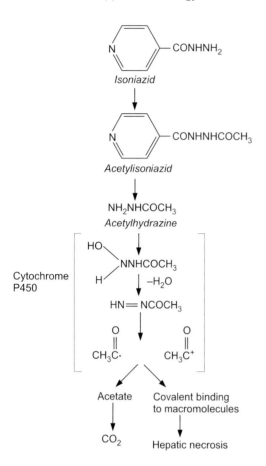

Figure 44 Part of the biotransformation of isoniazid.

greater exposure to acetylhydrazine. This example illustrates both the importance of competing detoxication and toxication routes of metabolism and also the influence which genetic factors may have on toxicity (Timbrell, 1988).

Aromatic amines

Another example in which acetylation features is the carcinogenicity of aromatic amines. For some aromatic amines acetylation is a detoxication reaction. For example, 2-naphthylamine and benzidine both cause bladder cancer in man and it seems likely that the acetylation reaction reduces the carcinogenicity. Acetylated derivatives of benzidine are less reactive towards DNA and cause less damage to this macromolecule than does the parent compound. Several studies have shown that the slow acetylator is more at risk than is the fast acetylator from developing bladder cancer, especially those whose work may expose them to aromatic amines, although data from a more recent study found no such increased risk (Hayes *et al.*, 1993). However, acetylation may be an activation step, involved in the toxic pathway for some compounds, such as aminofluorene. There are several metabolic pathways involving acetylation and *N*-hydro-

xylation yielding *N*-acetoxyaminofluorene **(Figure 45)**. The acetylation steps seem to involve similar but possibly distinct enzymes, either *N*-acetyltransferase (NAT), arylhydroxamic acid acetyl transferase (AHAT) or *N*-hydroxy-*O*-acetyl transferase (NHOAT). The *N*-acetoxyaminofluorene may rearrange to yield a reactive nitrenium ion which can react with DNA to give covalent adducts such as *N*-(deoxyguanosin-8-yl)-2-aminofluorene **(Figure 45)**. This has been shown both *in vitro* and *in vivo*. Alternatively, *N*-hydroxyacetylaminofluorene may be sulphated on the hydroxyl group and this has also been shown to be an activation step and may be involved in hepatocarcinogenesis, at least in mice. However, using hepatocytes from rabbits which were phenotyped as either rapid or slow acetylators, it was found that the rapid acetylators were more susceptible to DNA damage from aminofluorene, which suggests a role for acetylation. It seems likely that there are several routes for the metabolic activation of acetylaminofluorene in which acetylation, sulphation and glucuronidation may play a part, with variation in the predominant pathways between organs and species. This example, however, illustrates the role that phase 2 metabolic pathways may have in metabolic activation.

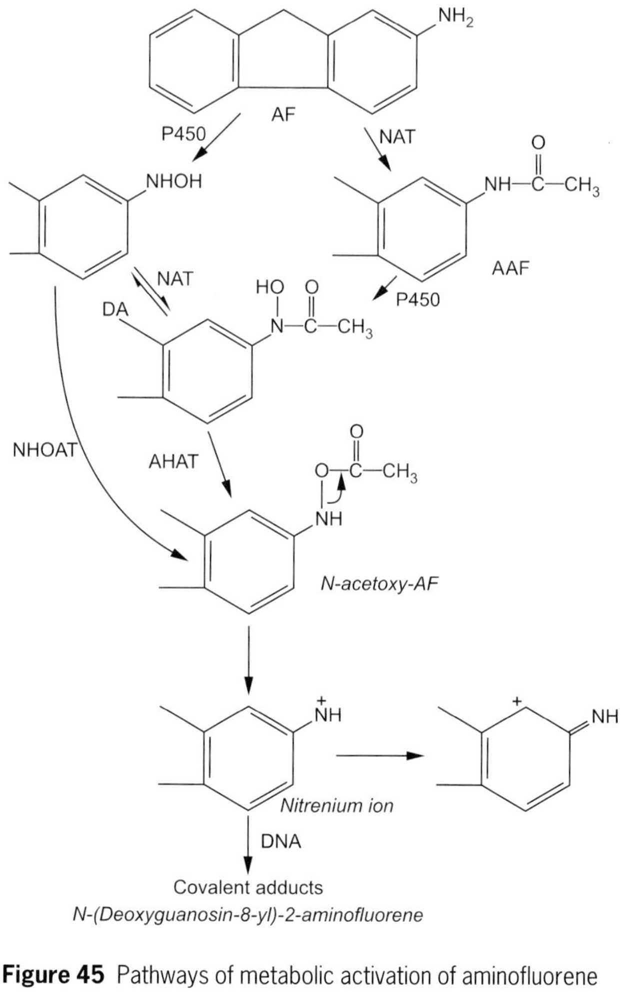

Figure 45 Pathways of metabolic activation of aminofluorene

Haloalkanes

The toxicity of haloalkanes illustrates the role of glutathione conjugation in metabolic activation as opposed to detoxication. Several different haloalkanes are known to be metabolically activated by conjugation with glutathione. For example, the compounds 1,2-dichloroethane and 1,2-dibromoethane are both conjugated with glutathione in a reaction catalysed by glutathione transferase **(Figure 46)**. The resultant haloethylglutathione conjugate can undergo loss of the halogen and rearrangement to yield a charged episulphonium ion which can react with DNA. Incubation of 1,2-dibromothane with DNA and glutathione transferase gives the adduct S-[2-(N-guanyl)ethyl]glutathione. This interaction is believed to be responsible for the mutagenicity of these compounds.

Some haloalkanes are nephrotoxic and glutathione conjugation has been shown to mediate this toxic effect also. For example, hexachlorobutadiene is conjugated with glutathione, which is then further metabolized to a cysteine conjugate **(Figure 47)**. This cysteine conjugate may then undergo further metabolism, either acetylation, deamination or cleavage by the action of the enzyme cysteine conjugate β-lyase. This gives rise to a thiol conjugate which has been shown to be nephrotoxic and is able to bind covalently to protein (Dekant and Vamvakas, 1996).

In addition to enzymes commonly associated with drug metabolism, sometimes enzymes normally involved in intermediary metabolism may be responsible for metabolic activation. Thus, a metabolite of valproic acid (2-*n*-propyl pent-4-enoic acid) is believed to be involved in the hepatotoxicity sometimes caused by this drug. This metabolite, Δ^4-VPA, irreversibly inhibits enzymes of the β-oxidation system and destroys cytochrome P450. This reactive metabolite may be involved in the hepatotoxicity of the drug. Further metabolism, gives 3-oxo-Δ^4-VPA

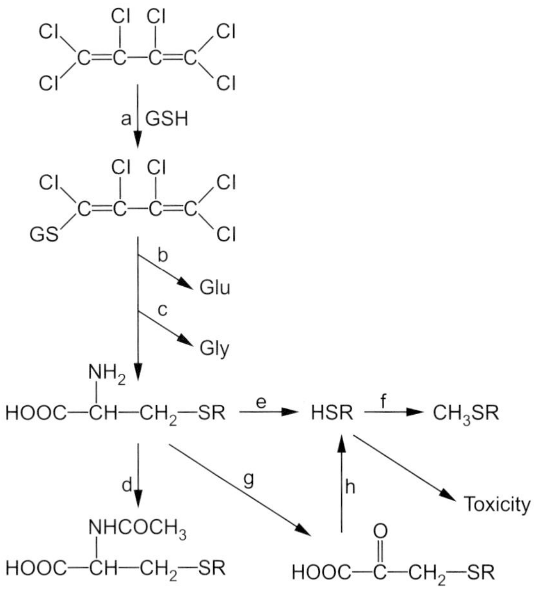

Figure 47 Metabolic activation of hexachlorobutadiene involving the action of β-lyase. The toxicity indicated is nephrotoxicity. R represents the 1, 2, 3, 4, 4-pentachlorobutadienyl moiety. GSH, glutathione; Glu, glutamate; Gly, glycine. The letters a–h represent the enzymes involved in the particular reactions: a, glutathione transferase; b, glutamyl transferase; c, dipeptidase; d, *N*-acetyltransferase; e, β-lyase; f, thiol *S*-methyltransferase; g, deaminase; h, thiopyruvate lyase.

which inhibits the enzyme 3-ketoacyl-CoA thiolase, the terminal enzyme of the fatty acid oxidation system (Baillie and Sheffels, 1995). However, recent *in vitro* evidence suggests that reactive oxygen species may also be involved in the toxicity (Tabatei *et al.*, 1998).

Thus, in conclusion, it can be seen that biotransformation is often a crucial aspect of the toxicity of a compound and may in a variety of circumstances be the cause of toxicity rather than a process of detoxication.

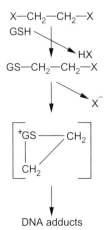

Figure 46 Formation of a reactive metabolite of a haloalkane from a glutathione conjugate.

REFERENCES

Alvan, G. (1991). Clinical consequences of polymorphic drug oxidation. *Fund. Clin. Pharmacol.*, **5**, 209–228.

Armstrong, N. R. (1997). Structure, catalytic mechanism and evolution of the glutathione transferases. *Chem. Res. Toxicol.*, **10**, 2–18.

Azri, S. and Renton, K. W. (1991). Factors involved in the depression of hepatic mixed function oxidase during infection with Listeria monocytogenes. *Int. J. Immunopharmacol.*, **13**, 197–204.

Baillie, T. A. and Sheffels, P. R. (1995). Valproic acid. Chemistry and biotransformation. In Levy, R. H., Mattson, R. H. and Meldrum, B. S. (Eds), *Antiepileptic Drugs*, 2nd edn. Raven Press, New York.

Batt, A. M., Siest, G., Magdalou, J. and Galteau, M.-M. (1992). Enzyme induction by drugs and toxins. *Clen. Chem. Acta.*, **209**, 109–121.

Beedham, C. (1988). Molybdenum hydroxylases. In Gorrod, J. W., Oelschlager, H. and Caldwell, J. (Eds), *Metabolism of Xenobiotics*. Taylor and Francis, London, pp. 51–58.

Benedetti, M. S. and Dostert, P. (1994). Contribution of amine oxidases to the metabolism of xenobiotics. *Drug Metab. Rev.*, **26**, 507–535.

Berthou, F., Guillois, B., Riche, C., Dreano, Y., Jacqz-Aigrain, E. and Beaune, P. H. (1992). Interspecies variation in caffeine metabolism related to cytochrome P4501a enzymes. *Xenobiotica*, **22**, 671–680.

Besunder, J. B., Reed, M. D. and Blumer, J. (1988). Principles of drug biodisposition in the neonate. *Clin. Pharmacokinet.*, **14**, 189–216.

Burchill, B. and Coughtrie, M. W. H. (1992). UDP-glucuronosyltransferases. In Kalow, W. (Ed.), *Pharmacogenetics of Drug Metabolism*. Pergamon Press, New York, pp. 195–225.

Caldwell, J. (1980). Comparative aspects of detoxication in mammals. In Jakoby, W. B. (Ed.), *Enzymatic Basis of Detoxication*, Vol. **1**. Academic Press, New York, pp. 85–111.

Cartwright, R. A., Glashan, R. W., Rogers, H. J., Ahmad, R. A., Barham-Hall, D., Higgins, E. and Kahn, M. A. (1982). Role of *N*-acetyltransferase phenotypes in bladder carcinogenesis: a pharmacogenetic approach to bladder cancer. *Lancet*, **ii**, 842–846.

Cashman, J. R. (1995). Structural and catalytic properties of the mammalian flavin-containing monoxygenase. *Chem. Res. Toxicol.*, **8**, 165–181.

Cohen, S. D. and Khairallah, E. A. (1997). Selective protein amylation and acetaminophen-induced hepatotoxicity. *Drug. Metab. Rev.*, **29**, 59–71.

Damani, L. A. (1988). The flavin-containing monooxygenase as an amine oxidase. In Gorrod, J. W., Oelschlager, H. and Caldwell, J. (Eds), *Metabolism of Xenobiotics*. Taylor and Francis, London, pp. 59–70.

Dekant, W. and Vamvakas, S. (1993). Glutathione-dependent bioactivation of xenobiotics. *Xenobiotica*, **23**, 873–887.

Dekant, W. and Vamvakas, S. (1996). Biotransformation and membrane transport in nephrotoxicity. *Crit. Rev. Toxicol.*, **26**, 309–334.

Eichelbaum, M. and Gross, A. S. (1990). The genetic polymorphism of debrisoquine/sparteine metabolism—clinical aspects. *Pharmacol. Ther.*, **46**, 377–394.

Eling, T., Boyd, J., Reed, G., Mason, R. and Sivarajoh, K. (1983). Xenobiotic metabolism by prostaglandin endoperoxide synthetase. *Drug Metab. Rev.*, **14**, 1023–1053.

Evans, D. A. P. (1992). *N*-Acetyltransferase. In Kalow, W. (Ed.), *Pharmacogenetics of Drug Metabolism*. Pergamon Press, New York, pp. 95–178.

Gibson, G. G. and Skett, P. (1986). *Introduction to Drug Metabolism*. Chapman and Hall, London.

Glende, E. A. (1972). Carbon tetrachloride-induced protection against carbon tetrachloride toxicity. The role of the liver microsomal drug-metabolising system. *Biochem. Pharmacol.*, **21**, 1679–1702.

Gonzalez, F. J. (1989). The molecular biology of cytochrome P450s. *Pharmacol. Rev.*, **40**, 243–288.

Gonzalez, F. J., Skoda, R. C., Kimura, S., Umeno, M., Zanger, U. M., Nebert, D. W., Gelboin, H. V., Hardwick, J. P. and Meyer, U. A. (1988). Characterisation of the common genetic defect in humans deficient in debrisoquine metabolism. *Nature*, **331**, 442–446.

Gonzalez, F. J. and Meyer, U. A. (1991). Molecular genetics of the debrisoquine/sparteine polymorphism. *Clin. Pharmacol. Ther.*, **50**, 233–238.

Gorrod, J. W. and Raman, A. (1989). Imines as intermediates in oxidative aralkylamine metabolism. *Drug Metab. Rev.*, **20**, 307–339.

Grant, D. M., Blum, M. and Meyer, U. A. (1992). Polymorphisms of *N*-acetyltransferase genes. *Xenobiotica*, **22**, 1073–1081.

Guengerich, F. P. (1991). Reactions and significance of cytochrome P450 enzymes. *J. Biol. Chem.*, **266**, 10019–10022.

Guengerich, F. P. (1994). Catalytic selectivity of human cytochrome P450 enzymes: relevance to drug metabolism and toxicity. *Toxicol. Lett.*, **70**, 133–138.

Halpert, J. R., Guengerich, F. P., Bend, J. R. and Correia, M. A. (1994). Contemporary issues in toxicology: selective inhibitors of cytochromes P450. *Toxicol. Appl. Pharmacol.*, **125**, 163–175.

Hart, J. G. and Timbrell, J. A. (1979). The effect of age on paracetamol hepatotoxicity in mice. *Biochem. Pharmacol.*, **28**, 3015–3017.

Hayes, R. B., Bi, W., Rothman, N., Broly, F., Caporaso, N., Feng, P., You, X., Yin, S., Woosley, R. L. and Meyer, U. A. (1993). *N*-Acetylation phenotype and genotype and risk of bladder cancer in benzidine-exposed workers. *Carcinogenesis*, **14**, 675–678.

Horbach, G. J. M. J., van Asten, J. G., Rietjens, I. M. C. M., Kremers, P. and van Bezooija, C. F. M. (1992). The effect of age on inducbility of various types of rat liver cytochrome P450. *Xenobiotica*, **22**, 515–522.

Hoyumpa, A. M. and Schenker, S. (1982). Major drug interactions: effect of liver disease alcohol and malnutrition. *Annu. Rev. Med.*, **33**, 113–150.

Howden, C. W., Birnie, G. G. and Brodie, M. J. (1989). Drug metabolism in liver disease. *Pharmacol. Ther.*, **40**, 439–474.

Jay, G. E. (1955). Variation in response of various mouse strains to hexobarbital (EVIPAL). *Proc. Soc. Exp. Biol. Med.*, **90**, 378–380.

Kadlubar, F. F. (1994). Biochemical individuality and its implications for drug and carcinogen metabolism: recent insights from acetyltransferase and cytochrome PA4501A2 phenotyping and genotyping in humans. *Drug Metab. Rev.*, **26**, 37–46.

Ketterer, B. (1982). The role of non-enzymatic reactions of glutathione in xenobiotic metabolism. *Drug Metab. Rev.*, **13**, 161–187.

Kihara, T., Toda, A., Imesue, I., Ono, N., Shigematsu, H., Soeda, S. and Shimeno, H. (1998). Effect of interleukin 1β-induced fever on hepatic drug metabolism in rats. *Xenobiotica*, **28**, 559–569.

Kinirons, M. T. and Crome, P. (1997). Clinical pharmacokinetic considerations in the elderly. *Clin. Pharmacokinet.*, **33**, 302–312.

Kraul, H., Truckenbrodt, J., Huster, A., Topfer, R. and Hoffmann, A. (1991). Comparison of *in vitro* and *in vivo* biotransformation in patients with liver disease of differing severity. *Eur. J. Clin. Pharmacol.*, **41**, 475–480.

Krishna, D. R. and Klotz, U. (1994). Extrahepatic metabolism of drugs in humans. *Clin. Pharmacokinet.*, **26**, 144–160.

Larsson, R., Boutin, J. and Moldeus, P. (1988). Peroxidase-catalysed metabolic activation of xenobiotics. In Gorrod, J. W., Oelschlager, H. and Caldwell, J. (Eds), *Metabolism of Xenobiotics*. Taylor and Francis, London, pp. 43–50.

Lunde, P. K. M., Frislide, K. and Hansteen, V. (1977). Disease and acetylation polymorphism. *Clin. Pharmacokinet.*, **2**, 182–197.

Meyer, U. A. (1994). The molecular basis of genetic polymorphisms of drug metabolism. *J. Pharm. Pharmacol.*, **46**, Suppl. 1, 409–415.

Meyer U. A. (1998). Medically relevant genetic variation of drug effects. In S. Stearns (Ed.), Evolution in Health and Disease. Oxford University Press.

Mommsen, S., Barfod, N. M. and Aagaard, J. (1985). *N*-Acetyltransferase phenotypes in the urinary bladder carcinogenesis of a low risk population. *Carcinogenesis*, **6**, 199–201.

Monks, T. I. and Lau, S. S. (1988). Reactive intermediates and their toxicological significance. *Toxicology*, **52**, 1–53.

Monks, T. J., Anders, M. W., Delcant, W., Stevens, J. L., Lau, S. S. and Van Bladeren, P. J. (1990). Contemporary issues in toxicology: glutathione conjugate mediated toxicities. *Toxicol. Appl. Pharmacol.*, **106**, 1–19.

Muerhoff, A. S., Griffin, K. J. and Johnson, E. F. (1992). The peroxisome proliferator-activated receptor mediates the induction of CYP4A6, a cytochrome P450 fatty acid χ-hydroxylase, by clofibric acid. *J. Biol. Chem.*, **267**, 10951–10953.

Mulder, G. I., Kroese, E. D. and Meerman, J. H. N. (1988). The generation of reactive intermediates from xenobiotics by sulphate conjugation and their role in drug toxicity. In Gorrod, J. W., Oelschlager, H. and Caldwell, J. (Eds), *Metabolism of Xenobiotics*. Taylor and Francis, London, pp. 24–250.

Nelson, D. R., Kamataki, T., Waxman, D. J., Guengerich, F. P., Eastabrook, R. W., Feyereisen, R., Gonzalez, F. J., Coon, M. J., Gunsalus, I. C. and Goto, H. O. (1993). The P450 superfamily: update on new sequences gene mapping accession numbers, early trivial names, and nomenclature. *DNA Cell Biol.*, **12**, 1–51.

Nelson, S. D. (1995). Mechanisms of the formation and disposition of reactive metabolites that can cause acute liver injury. *Drug Metab. Rev.*, **27**, 147–177.

Nelson, S. D. and Harvison, P. J. (1987). Roles of cytochrome P-450 in chemically induced cytotoxicity. In Guengerich, F. P. (Ed.), *Mammalian Cytochromes P450*. CRC Press, Boca Raton, FL, pp. 19–80.

Nelson, S. D. and Pearson, P. G. (1990). Covalent and noncovalent interactions in acute lethal cell injury caused by chemicals. *Annu. Rev. Pharmacol. Toxicol.*, **30**, 169–195.

Netter, K. J. (1987). Mechanisms of oxidative drug metabolism and inhibition. *Pharmacol. Ther.*, **33**, 1–9.

Okey, A. B. (1990). Enzme induction in the cytochrome P450 system. *Pharmacol. Ther.*, **45**, 241–298.

Okey, A. B., Roberts, E. A., Harper, P. A. and Denison, M. S. (1986). Induction of drug metabolising enzymes; mechanisms and consequences. *Clin. Biochem.*, **19**, 132–141.

Parke, D. V. (1968). *The Biochemistry of Foreign Compounds*. Pergamon. Press, Oxford.

Patel, J. M., Gordon, W. P., Nelson, S. D. and Leibman, K. C. (1983) Comparison of hepatic biotransformation and toxicity of allyl alcohol and [1,1, $-^2H_2$]allyl alcohol. *Drug Metab. Dispos.*, **11**, 164–166.

Pike, S. L., Pumford, N. R., Mayeux, P. R., Niesman, M. and Hinson, J. A. (1998). The Kuppffer cell inactivator gadolinium chloride eliminates acetaminophen-induced hepatotoxicity and hepatic nitrotyrosine-protein adducts in mice. *ISSX Proceedings*, volume 13, **304**.

Pohl, L. R. (1979). Biochemical toxicology of chloroform. *Rev. Biochem. Toxicol.*, **1**, 79–107.

Powis, G., Talcott, R. E. and Schenkman, J. B. (1977). Kinetic and spectral evidence for multiple species of cytochrome P-450 in liver mierosomes. In Ullrich, V., Roots, A., Hildentrandt, A., Estabrook, R. W. and Conney, A. H. (Eds), *Microsomes and Drug Oxidations*, Pergamon. Press, New York, pp. 127–135.

Pumford, N. R., Halmes, N. C. and Hinson, J. A. (1997). Covalent binding of xenobiotics to specific proteins in liver. *Drug. Metals. Rev.*, **29**, 39–57.

Quinn, G. P., Axelrod, J. and Brodie, B. B. (1958). Species, strain and sex differences in metabolism of hexobarbitone, amidopyrine, antipyrine and aniline. *Biochem. Pharmacol.*, **1**, 152–159.

Reed, D. J. and Beatty, P. W. (1980). Biosynthesis and regulation of glutathione: toxicological implications. *Rev. Biochem. Toxicol.*, **2**, 213–241.

Sesardic, D., Rich, K. L., Edwards, R. J., Davies, D. S. and Boobis, A. R. (1989). Selective destruction of cytochrome P-450d and associated monooxygenase activity by carbon tetrachloride in the rat. *Xenobiotica*, **19**, 795–811.

Shimada, T., Yamazaki, H., Mimura, M., Inui, Y. and Guergerich, F. P. (1994). Interindividual variations in human liver cytochrome P450 enzymes involved in the oxidation of drugs carcinogens and toxic chemicals: studies with liver microsomes of 30 Japanese and 30 Caucasians. *J. Pharmacol. Exp Ther.*, **270**, 414–423.

Sitar, D. S. (1989). Human drug metabolism *in vivo*. *Pharmacol. Ther.*, **43**, 363–375.

Tabatabaei, A. R., Farrell, K. and Abbott, F. S. (1998). Role of reactive oxygen species in the mechanism of valproic acid-induced toxicity on lymphocytes of a patient with a history of severe valproic acid hepatotoxicity. *ISSX Proceedings*, volume 13, **314**.

Testa, B. (1989). Mechanisms of chiral recognition in xenobiotic metabolism and drug–receptor interactions. *Chirality*, **1**, 7–9.

Timbrell, J. A. (1988). Acetylation and its toxicological significance. In Gorrod, J. W., Oelschlager, H. and Caldwell, J. (Eds), *Metabolism of Xenobiotics*. Taylor and Francis, London, pp. 259–266.

Timbrell, J. A., Facchini, V., Harland, S. J. and Mansilla-Tinoco, R. (1984). Hydralazine-induced lupus: is there a toxic pathway? *Eur. J. Clin. Pharmacol.*, **27**, 555–559.

Tucker, G. T. (1994). Clinical implications of genetic polymorphism in drug metabolism. *J. Pharm. Pharmacol.*, **46**, Suppl. 1, 417–424.

Uetrecht, J. P. (1992). The role of leukocyte generated metabolites in the pathogenesis of idiosyncratic drug reactions. *Drug Metab. Rev.*, **24**, 299–366.

Van Bladderen, P. J., den Besten, C., Bruggeman, I. M., Mertens, J. J. W. M., van Ommen, B., Spenkelink, B., Rutten, A. L. M., Temmink, J. H. M. and Vos, R. M. E. (1998). Glutathione conjugation as a toxication reaction. In Gorrod, J. W., Oelschlager, H. and Caldwell, J. (Eds), *Metabolism of Xenobiotics*. Taylor and Francis, London, pp. 267–274.

Waxman, D. J. and Azaroff, L. (1992). Phenobarbital induction of cytochrome P450 gene expression. *Biochem. J.*, **281**, 577–592.

Whitlock, J. P. (1989). The control of cytochrome P450 gene expression by dioxin. *Trends Pharmacol. Sci.*, **10**, 285–288.

Whitlock, J. P. (1993). Mechanistic aspects of dioxin action. *Chem. Res. Toxicol.*, **6**, 754–763.

Wrighton, S. A. and Stevens, J. C. (1992). The human hepatic cytochromes P450 involved in drug metabolism. *Crit. Rev. Toxicol.*, **22**, 1–21.

Zampaglione, N., Jollow, D. J., Mitchell, J. R., Stripp, B., Hamrick, M. and Gillette, J. R. (1973). Role of detoxifying enzymes in bromobenezene-induced liver necrosis. *J. Pharmacol. Exp. Ther.*, **187**, 218–227.

Ziegler, D. M. (1993). Recent studies on the structure and function of multisubstrate flavin-containing monoxygenases. *Annu. Rev. Pharmacol. Toxicol.*, **33**, 179–199.

FURTHER READING

Evans, D. A. P. (1993). *Genetic Factors in Drug Therapy: Clinical and Molecular Pharmacogenetics*. Cambridge, Cambridge University Press.

Gibson, G. G. and Skett, P. (1994). *Introduction to Drug Metabolism*, 2nd edn. Chapman and Hall, London.

Gorrod, J. W., Oelschlager, H. and Caldwell, J. (Eds) (1988). *Metabolism of Xenobiotics*. Taylor and Francis, London.

Guengerich, F. P. (Ed.) (1987). *Mammalian Cytochromes P450*. CRC Press, Boca Raton, FL, pp. 19–80.

Hathway, D. E. (1984). *Molecular Aspects of Toxicology*. Royal Society of Chemistry, London.

Hathway, D. E., Brown, S. S., Chasseaud, L. F. and Hutson, D. H. (Eds) (1970). *Foreign Compound Metabolism in Mammals*, Vols 1–6. Chemical Society, London.

Hawkins, D. R. (Ed.) (1988). *Biotransformations*, Vols 1–7. Royal Society of Chemistry, London.

Houston, J. B. (1994). Utility of *in vitro* drug metabolism data in predicting *in vivo* metabolic clearance. *Biochem. Pharmacol.*, **47**, 1469–1479.

Jakoby, W. B. (Ed.) (1980). *Enzymatic Basis of Detoxication*, Vol. 1. Academic Press, New York.

Jakoby, W. B. and Ziegler, D. M. (1990) The enzymes of detoxication. *J. Biol. Chem.*, **265**, 20715–20719.

Kalow, W (Ed.) (1992). *Pharmacogenetics of Drug Metabolism*. Pergamon Press, New York.

Mulder, G. J. (Ed.) (1990). *Conjugation Reactions in Drug Metabolism*. Taylor and Francis, London.

Nebert, D. W. (1989). The Ah locus: genetic differences in toxicity, cancer, mutations and birth defects. *CRC Crit. Rev. Toxicol.*, **20**, 153–174.

Timbrell, J. A. (1991). *Principles of Biochemical Toxicology*, 2nd edn. Taylor and Francis, London.

Weber, W. W. (1987). *The Acetylator Genes and Drug Response*. Oxford University Press, New York.

Williams, R. T. (1959). *Detoxication Mechanisms*. Chapman and Hall, London.

Ziegler, D. M. (1991). Unique properties of the enzymes of detoxification. *Drug Metab. Dispos.*, **19**, 847–852.

Chapter 6
The Biochemical Basis of Toxicity

John Caldwell and Jeremy J. Mills

CONTENTS

INTRODUCTION

One of the major aims of toxicology is to understand the ways in which chemicals exert harmful effects on the body and to use this information to ameliorate such effects. In recent years, toxicology has developed from an activity relying principally on the tools of classical pathology to observe and classify harmful effects, to become a discipline increasingly able to explain the effects of toxic compounds in molecular and mechanistic terms. There are now applied to problems in toxicology the techniques and concepts from a wide range of basic sciences, as a response to general concerns about the impact of the chemical environment upon human health. The development of modern toxicology can be traced initially to the tragedy of thalidomide and the realization that chemicals have a major influence on our well- being. Further key molecules in the development of our understanding of the toxicity of chemicals (as opposed to a mechanistic understanding of chemical carcinogenicity) are paracetamol (acetaminophen), bromobenzene, paraquat and the phthalate plasticizers. Mechanistic explanations of toxic phenomena are critically important as they: (1) account for the origin of toxicity; (2) aid treatment and prevention of toxicity by chemical or biological means; (3) provide a rational basis for the validity of animal data to anticipate the consequences of human exposure to a particular chemical; and (4) indicate the likely variability between members of the population in toxic responses.

This chapter will describe important mechanisms of toxicity, with particular emphasis on those of widespread occurrence, since specialized areas such as reproductive and immunological toxicity are dealt with elsewhere in this volume, exemplify the use of such approaches to chemical safety evaluation, and outline the basis for inter-individual differences in chemical susceptibility.

MECHANISMS OF TOXICITY

Most toxic compounds which are chemically stable give rise to characteristic effects by interfering with various biochemical or physiological homeostatic mechanisms. It is thus essential to appreciate that the toxicologist must have as full an understanding of the pharmacology of toxic compounds as possible. Up to 90% of all adverse reactions to therapeutic drugs arise from pharmacological responses (Rawlins, 1981) so that it is critical to examine their so-called secondary pharmacology (or safety pharmacology). In many cases, the primary action of the drug, that which is of therapeutic benefit, is studied in great detail, but too little attention is paid to the other sites at which the drug may act. As a result, inappropriate exposure to the drug in patients, resulting from overdose or in those with aberrant pharmacokinetics, serves to reveal further effects of the drug. In a number of cases this has had tragic consequences, e.g. the cardiac arrhythmias induced by terfenadine when the unchanged drug enters the circulation as a result of drug–drug or drug–food interactions (Ishizaki, 1996; Woosley, 1996) and the lactic acidosis induced by phenformin in those genetically unable to metabolize the drug (Oates *et al.*, 1981; McGuinness and Talbert, 1993). Even for chemicals with no defined therapeutic application, it is still critical to have a proper knowledge of the biochemical and molecular targets with which the compound can interact. Many adverse events are the consequence of disturbance of normal physiology and do not result in a permanent alteration to cell function or in cell death.

The cellular consequences of chemical exposure can be considered under two broad headings, modification of the regulation of cell division with harmful consequences, or causing the death of cells. It has been understood for many years that unrepaired, non-lethal genetic alteration to somatic cells results in mutation (Williams and Weisburger, 1991), ultimately expressed as carcinogenesis. More recently, it has become clear that compounds not interacting directly with the genome can also produce cancer by so-called epigenetic mechanisms (Williams and Weisburger, 1991; see also Chapter 51). These may involve a proliferative response of epithelial cells to cytotoxicity, as is suggested to occur with high-dose carcinogens such as allyl isothiocyanate (see below) and chloroform, or a more direct action to enhance the rate of cell division seen with promoters such as phorbol esters and the peroxisome proliferators (Butterworth *et al.*, 1991). Increased cell replication, however caused, brings with it an increased chance of an unrepaired DNA lesion becoming fixed as a mutation. It has long been suspected that hyperplasia precedes neoplasia but the inevitability or otherwise of such a progression has never been established on pathological grounds alone.

There occurs a considerable extent of 'normal' damage to DNA by reactive oxygen species in the cell and it has been suggested that the non-genotoxic carcinogens act by enhancing the likelihood of this normal damage being fixed as a mutation, leading to cancer (Ames *et al.*, 1993). This can be seen in rodent models with phenobarbitone (phenobarbital), where drug treatment alters the expression of critical regulatory genes in the mitoinhibitory pathways of the liver, creating a selective pressure for cells with mutations in the mitoinhibitory signalling system to thrive and progress to full neoplasia (Mills *et al.*, 1995).

Cytotoxicity, the cause of cell death, has two distinct origins, *necrosis* and *apoptosis*, either of which may be the consequence of exposure to a harmful chemical. Whichever mechanism operates, it must be appreciated that the number of cells which must be killed before the function of a tissue or organism is noticeably impaired is highly variable. Some cell types, notably the epithelia including the liver, have the ability to regenerate in response to insult while others, most notably neurons, cannot. Some organs, such as the liver, lung and kidney, have a substantial reserve capacity in excess of normal requirements and normal body function can be maintained in the presence of marked impairment.

Necrosis is generally caused by marked alteration to a cell's energy-yielding biochemistry, either through enzyme inhibition or damage to proteins. The induction of apoptosis, or programmed cell death, like carcinogenicity, may be either genotoxic (the result of mutation) or epigenetic, the result of the activation of specific genes via cellular receptors or mutation, and gives rise to an acceleration of the normal turnover of cells. One characteristic of apoptotis is the general absence of an inflammatory reaction in response to cell death as the liberated cell contents and genetic material are being phagocytosed by surrounding cells. Inflammation, which is frequently seen as a response to necrotic cell death, can involve infiltration by components of the cell-mediated immune response, particularly scavenging macrophages.

Having established the fundamental differences between toxic chemicals which act (1) through physiological mechanisms, (2) through cytotoxicity or (3) by causing proliferative lesions, we may now consider some basic mechanisms through which toxic chemicals may act.

RECEPTOR-MEDIATED EVENTS

Anything other than the most cursory description of receptor-mediated events is outside present consideration. However, it is important to appreciate that actions at the receptors for neurotransmitters and hormones, either as agonists or as antagonists of the physiological ligand, underlie numerous toxic responses. This is most clearly the case with neurotoxins, acting within and outside the central nervous system (CNS). In addition, it is now understood that a variety of toxic effects completely unrelated to any conceivable therapeutic or otherwise beneficial activity are mediated through receptor interactions. Interest has concentrated on the cytosolic receptors of the steroid hormone type and it is now clear that dioxin (TCDD) exerts most of, if not all, of its toxic effects by binding to a specific receptor of the steroid hormone type (Lilienfield and Gallo, 1989). More recently, a family of three cytosolic binding proteins have been identified as peroxisomal proliferator receptors which have DNA-binding domains and which appear to activate gene transcription in the nucleus in a way analogous to the steroid hormones (Green, 1992).

DISTURBANCE OF EXCITABLE MEMBRANE FUNCTION

Excitable membranes are critical to the function of nerve and muscle, most notably in their ability to generate and propagate action potentials. This depends on the normal activity of ion channels and membrane ion pumps, which can be influenced by a variety of toxic compounds. The neurotoxicity of DDT is the result of interference with closing of sodium channels (Joy, 1982). Most organic solvents are ethanol-like CNS depressants whose actions appear to be non-specific membrane effects (Rall, 1991).

DISTURBANCE OF NORMAL BIOCHEMICAL PROCESSES

The cells of the body maintain their function by a variety of closely coordinated synthetic and catabolic processes. The energy requirements of the body are met by the oxidation of carbohydrates and lipids, coupled to the synthesis of ATP by oxidative phosphorylation. The availability of oxygen to the tissues is obviously influenced by compounds affecting the transport of oxygen in the blood, e.g. those causing methaemoglobinaemia (Kiese, 1977), while the synthesis of ATP may be inhibited by uncoupling oxidative phosphorylation by compounds such as salicylate (Brenner and Simon, 1982). Under these circumstances, not only is there a loss of function owing to lack of ATP but also a marked rise in body temperature arising from excess heat production; this pyrexia can be fatal.

A number of compounds, notably quinones, are able to initiate redox cycling **(Figure 1)** with harmful consequences for the cell (Sies and Cadenas, 1983). These compounds are reduced by taking up an electron from NADPH to give a radical, which is then oxidized by molecular oxygen, returning the molecule to its original oxidized state and producing a series of reactive oxygen species from the primary product, superoxide anion radical O_2^-. These species include hydrogen peroxide, hydroxyl radical $OH^\bullet$, singlet oxygen $^1O_2$ and lipid peroxides. These are powerful oxidizing agents and can initiate a wide range of toxic responses including mutagenesis and carcinogenesis as a result of interactions with DNA, membrane damage by lipid peroxidation and biochemical disorders by enzyme inactivation. This underlies both the therapeutic and toxic actions of quinone drugs such as the anthracyclines, adriamycin and bleomycin, and the toxicity of agents such as paraquat and cephalosporin antibiotics (see below). The magnitude of any toxic response to such compounds is moderated by a variety of cellular defences such as glutathione peroxidase, catalase and superoxide dismutase, and endogenous antioxidants, notably vitamins A, C and E.

ALTERED CALCIUM HOMEOSTASIS

Calcium ions have critical roles in cellular function and the intracellular levels and locations of calcium ions are tightly controlled by a variety of compartmentation processes and transport mechanisms. Various toxic chemicals can disrupt these with marked deleterious effects on

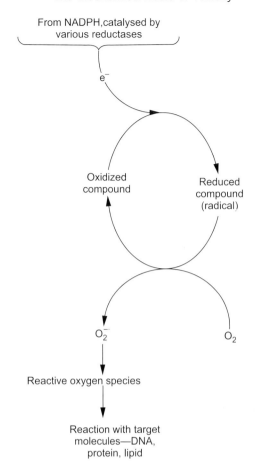

Figure 1 Formation of reactive oxygen species by redox cycling.

the cell (Orrenius *et al.*, 1989). Increases in free intracellular calcium concentrations lead to changes to the cytoskeleton, blebbing and ultimately leakage of the plasma membrane, impaired mitochondrial function and activation of calcium-dependent degradative enzymes (proteases, phospholipases, endonucleases). Chemicals can raise the intracellular calcium concentration in two ways, either by enhancing its influx (mainly caused by hormones and other chemicals acting via cytosolic receptors to enhance protein synthesis) or by impairing calcium transport. This latter mechanism is involved with the main chemicals inducing oxidative damage to the cell, e.g. free radicals, quinones and peroxides.

COVALENT BINDING TO CELLULAR MACROMOLECULES

It is now well understood that a great many toxic chemicals exert their effects by the covalent linkage of reactive metabolites to essential macromolecules of the cell (Brodie *et al.*, 1971). These include proteins, notably enzymes and membrane structural elements, lipids and nucleic acids (see below). This generally involves electrophilic metabolites binding to nucleophilic sites such as thiol, amino and hydroxy groups in the side-chains of proteins and is essentially irreversible, depending solely on the turnover of the macromolecule in question for the repair of the lesion. In addition, other toxins may bind to protein so as to impair normal function without being converted first to reactive intermediates This is best exemplified by the binding of metal ions to protein thiols, e.g. mercury ions in the kidney (Klaassen, 1991). Damage to lipids may take two forms, either covalent binding of reactive intermediates to free hydroxyl groups of lipids or the initiation of lipid peroxidation by free radicals derived from the compound *per se* or active oxygen species (superoxide, hydroxyl radical, etc.) produced by reactions such as redox cycling (see above).

GENOTOXICITY

Electrophilic compounds, generally formed by the oxidative metabolism of xenobiotics, are able to interact with various nucleophilic sites in DNA, principally O-6, N-7, N-2 and C-2 of guanine (Miller and Miller, 1985). Other compounds may interact with DNA by intercalation between the strands. In both cases, unless this DNA damage is repaired successfully, these interactions may alter gene expression: this is termed 'genotoxicity'. The unrepaired/incorrectly repaired DNA damage may cause the death of the cell, but more frequently the result is a somatic mutation which can be the initiating event for a process ultimately leading to the development of cancer. Most compounds which are genotoxic in mammals are also mutagenic in bacteria, subject to the availability of an appropriate metabolic system for activation (Ashby and Tennant, 1988). It is important to appreciate that not all carcinogens are genotoxic and that proliferative lesions may also arise through mechanisms influencing cell division not operating at the genomic level. Such compounds are termed 'non-genotoxic' or 'epigenetic' carcinogens (see Chapter 51).

TISSUE SPECIFICITY OF TOXICITY

All the tissues and organs of the body are to a greater or lesser extent susceptible to toxicity, but the effects of most toxic chemicals focus on one or more tissues or organs, the so-called target organs of toxicity. The examination of the reasons responsible for this specificity of action has proved extremely informative in developing a mechanistic understanding of the origin of the toxic response. In broad terms, the susceptibility of particular tissues and organs is a consequence of one or more of three factors:

- Tissue distribution of the chemical;
- Metabolic activation to toxic products within specific tissues;
- Biochemical differences between tissues exposed to the toxin.

Each of these may be illustrated by a considerable number of examples.

Role of Tissue Distribution

It is obviously the case that for a compound to exert a toxic effect it must be present at the site of action. The magnitude of any toxic effect will be dependent on the concentration of toxin to which the relevant target is exposed. This is the case for both reversible effects mediated by classical receptors and described by sigmoid dose–response curves (Ross, 1991), and for effects mediated through the formation of macromolecular adducts, where the concentration of adducts becomes the relevant index of exposure (Monro, 1992). There are a substantial number of cases in which the occurrence of toxicity is directly related to the ability of a particular site to concentrate a toxic chemical, some examples are listed in **Table 1**. These may variously involve specific active uptake mechanisms, tissue-specific binding processes or physicochemical concentration due to pH and ionization.

The pulmonary epithelium has the ability to concentrate from the peripheral circulation and metabolize during the first pass a variety of endogenous compounds present in the circulation, including biogenic amines and prostanoids (Youdim *et al.*, 1980), activities which probably arise from the need to protect the heart from the stimulant actions of the substrates. In addition, a variety of xenobiotics are also taken up and this has been most intensively studied with the herbicide paraquat. This very toxic chemical is taken up by a specific polyamine transport mechanism, whose endogenous substrate appears to be putrescine, seemingly in the alveolar type I and II cells and the Clara cells (Smith *et al.*, 1989). The result is that these cells in the lung are exposed to much higher concentrations of paraquat than other tissues and it is these cell types which are selectively damaged by paraquat as a consequence of reactive oxygen species produced by redox cycling (see above).

Table 1 Examples of chemicals whose toxicity is related to the ability of target organs to concentrate them

Compound	Tissue
Paraquat	Lung
Gentamicin, cephalosporins, sulphonamides	Kidney
Chloroquine	Eye
Kanamycin	Ear
Streptozotocin	Pancreas

The process of renal excretion involves the filtration, at the glomerulus, of all small molecules present in plasma followed by the progressive modification of the composition of the filtrate into urine by tubular reabsorption and secretion mechanisms. The aminoglycoside antibiotics, typified by gentamicin, are reabsorbed by the same mechanism as low molecular weight proteins and concentrated in the proximal tubular cell, bound to a number of organelles from which they are only slowly mobilized (Weinberg, 1988). The half-life for the loss of aminoglycosides from the renal cortex may be 100 times longer than the plasma elimination half-life. Some 10% of all cases of acute renal failure have been attributed to the aminoglycosides (Bennett, 1983) and their nephrotoxicity is the result of a variety of biochemical abnormalities, most notably inhibition of phospholipases (Humes and O'Connor, 1988).

The cephalosporins are also concentrated within the renal cortex, being taken up by the same active transport process as p-aminohippurate (Wold, 1981). However, they are not transported out of the cell across the luminal membrane and so accumulate within the proximal tubular cell. The incidence and severity of the nephrotoxicity of cephalosporins correlate directly with their concentration within the renal cortex. A variety of mechanisms have been associated with nephrotoxicity and the most attractive of these involves redox cycling and the generation of reactive oxygen species (Kuo et al., 1983).

In contrast, the nephrotoxicity of the sulphonamides is readily explicable on the basis of the physicochemical properties of their metabolites. Many of these are metabolized by N-acetylation, and the conjugates are readily excreted into the urine. However, they are poorly water-soluble and can crystallize out in the lumen of the nephron, leading to nephrotoxicity by mechanical blockage of the tubules (Caldwell, 1982).

In recent years, there has been great interest in the ability of a number of chemically inert and otherwise unremarkable molecules to give rise to a characteristic nephropathy and renal carcinoma in the male rat (US EPA, 1991). This is associated with the accumulation of droplets of a specific protein, $\alpha_2\mu$-globulin, in the kidneys. A list of compounds causing this notable renal toxicity, now generally referred to as '$\alpha_2\mu$-globulin nephropathy', is given in **Table 2**. None of these is genotoxic in a variety of short-term tests but it seems likely that they cause renal neoplasia after long-term, high-dose exposure as a result of the accumulation of hyaline protein droplets in the P2 segment of the renal tubule. The renal tumours are seen only in male rats, and not in female rats or in mice of either sex.

$\alpha_2\mu$-Globulin is a low molecular weight protein, approximately 18 000 Da, whose synthesis under androgenic control is specific to the liver of male rats. Under normal conditions, it is filtered in the kidney, reabsorbed to the extent of about 50–60% in the proximal tubule, and degraded by lysosomal enzymes there. However, a range

Table 2 Compounds giving rise to $\alpha_2\mu$-globulin nephropathy in male rats but not female rats or other species

1,4-Dichlorobenzene
Unleaded petrol
d-Limonene
Isophorone
Dimethyl methylphosphonate
Pentachloroethane
JP-4 jet fuel
JP-5 shale-derived jet fuel
Decalin (decahydronaphthalene)

Source: EPA (1991), and references therein.

of simple hydrocarbons are able to bind to $\alpha_2\mu$-globulin with remarkable consequences. The protein–hydrocarbon complex is filtered and reabsorbed by the kidney in the same way, but it is resistant to lysosomal breakdown and thus accumulates in the proximal tubular segment of the nephron. As more and more accumulates, the protein assumes the form of hyaline droplets, which are crystalline inclusion bodies. These lead to compensatory cell proliferation which in the long term acts as a tumour promoter. This mechanism is now accepted to be a male rat-specific event with no significance for the safe human use of causative compounds (Flamm and Lehmann-McKeeman, 1991).

The pigment melanin is found in the skin and a variety of other tissues, notably the retina of the eye and the inner ear. Studies in animals of the tissue distribution of radiolabelled compounds, most notably by whole-body autoradiography, have revealed that a significant number of compounds are concentrated in tissues rich in melanin (Ings, 1984). The role of melanin in this selective uptake may be most conveniently investigated by the comparison of tissue distribution in pigmented animals and albinos, which lack melanin. There appear to be two distinct modes of binding to melanin, differentiated on the basis of the half-life of the bound residue (Ings, 1984). When the half-life for depletion is up to 28 days, there occurs tight binding, but the drug–melanin complex is reversible and seems not to have toxicological sequelae. There is a much smaller number of cases in which occurs a much tighter, possibly covalent, linkage between the drug and melanin, and here the turnover of the complex is essentially that of melanin itself. This pattern of melanin binding is generally associated with toxicity.

A number of compounds, most notably chloroquine and certain phenothiazines, produce a retinopathy which involves visual disturbance progressing to colour and night blindness. The effects of chloroquine are essentially irreversible because of the extremely long residence of the drug, bound to melanin, in the eye, and the intensity of effects are directly related to the duration and size of dosage (Bernstein et al., 1963; Burns, 1966). Although chlorpromazine only rarely causes retinopathy, certain other phenothiazines, notably thioridazine, have proved much more retinotoxic, and one experimental member of this class caused blindness in volunteers (Boet, 1970). It is clear from tissue distribution and *in vitro* studies that this retinopathy is directly related to the very tight binding of the phenothiazine to melanin (Potts, 1962).

Kanamycin, neomycin and other aminoglycosides cause hearing disturbance, including tinnitus, loss of hearing acuity and frank deafness. This is 'nerve deafness' not involving mechanical damage to the ear and has been associated with binding to melanin in the stria vascularis of the inner ear, the site of toxicity (Denckner *et al.*, 1973).

METABOLIC ACTIVATION

Most toxic chemicals are unreactive and require metabolic activation to unveil their toxicity, in one of the following ways:

■ Formation of chemically stable metabolites, which may have increased or changed activity relative to the parent compound.

■ Formation of chemically reactive metabolites, most commonly electrophiles, able to interact with cellular constituents, leading to toxicity.

■ Formation, as by-products, of excess quantities of harmful endogenous compounds, notably active oxygen species.

The consequences for the cell of the formation of a reactive intermediate are governed by its inherent reactivity, and by the balance of the activities of enzymes responsible for its formation and inactivation.

The reactivity of metabolites obviously covers a wide spectrum, from those which are essentially inert end-products whose fate will depend on their physicochemical properties, to those which are so reactive that they exist only in the active site of the enzymes catalyzing their formation. Such extremely reactive intermediates may act as suicide substrate inactivators of enzymes (Ortiz de Montellano *et al.*, 1981). We must next consider intermediates with lifetimes long enough to allow them to leave the immediate vicinity of the relevant enzyme and to which essential cellular organelles are exposed. Most of these are electrophiles which have been classified into 'hard' and 'soft' reactants (Ketterer, 1988). 'Hard' electrophiles react very well with nucleophilic sites such as the S atom of methionine in proteins and with nucleophilic N, O and C atoms in nucleic acid bases, but have poor reactivity with glutathione (GSH) and protein thiols. 'Soft' electrophiles, on the other hand, react with thiols in glutathione and protein but not with other nucleophilic sites in biological macromolecules. Hard electrophiles are typically genotoxic intermediates such as the ultimate carcinogens *N*-sulphonyloxymethyl-4-aminoazobenzene and benzo[*a*]pyrene-7,8-diol-9,

10-oxide (Djuric *et al.*, 1987; Coles *et al.*, 1988), while soft electrophiles are typified by *N*-acetyl-*p*-benzoquino-neimine (NAPQI), the cytotoxic (but not genotoxic) metabolite responsible for the hepatotoxicity of paracetamol (acetaminophen). A numerical classification of 'hardness' and 'softness' is given by the second-order rate constant for the reactivity of the electrophile with GSH. For NAPQI, the rate constant is 3×10^{-4} M s^{-1}, for the mutagenic but not carcinogenic epoxide of 1-nitropyrene it is 1.5 M s^{-1}, while those for *N*-sulpho-nyloxymethyl-4-aminoazobenzene and benzo[*a*]pyrene-7, 8-diol-9, 10-oxide cannot be determined.

The cell possesses a number of enzymes which act to inactivate and detoxify reactive intermediates. Probably the most important of these in quantitative terms is GSH conjugation, in which the nucleophilic thiol of GSH (the tripeptide γ-glutamylcysteinylglycine) reacts with an electrophile, frequently under the catalysis of one or more of the glutathione *S*-transferases (GSTs). The reaction types involve attack on electrophilic centres (Caldwell, 1982), such as carbon atoms in strained oxirane rings, addition to α, β-unsaturated compounds and with carbonium ions. Electrophilic nitrogen atoms, including nitroso compounds and nitrate esters, and the electrophilic oxygen atoms in organic hydroperoxides are also attacked. The extent to which a particular reaction is catalysed by the GSTs varies very widely and represents one discernible influence on the biological properties of their substrates. Thus, benzo[*a*]pyrene-7, 8-diol-9, 10-oxide is a good substrate for a number of hepatic GSTs and this, together with the high concentration of GSH in the liver, accounts for its lack of hepato-carcinogenicity in the rat (Ketterer, 1988). Aflatoxin B$_1$-2, 3-oxide is a very poor substrate, which is consistent with its hepatocarcinogenicity under normal circumstances (Ketterer, 1988); interestingly, induction with ethoxyquin of the GSTs, catalysing its GSH conjugation, has a marked protective effect.

The cytochrome P450-catalysed oxidation of double bonds in alkenes and aromatic rings almost invariably produces an oxirane (arene oxide for aromatic rings, epoxide for alkenes) as the obligatory intermediate (Jerina *et al.*, 1970; Ortiz de Montellano, 1985). Arene oxides generally rearrange via the 'NIH shift' to phenols, but these and alkene oxides can exist free within the cell. Oxiranes are highly strained three-membered rings in which one or other of the carbon atoms can have marked electrophilic character depending on the substitution around the ring. Like other types of electrophiles, the reactivity of oxiranes covers a wide spectrum, from very stable cases such as carbamazepine 10, 11-oxide, which is a major urinary metabolite of this anticonvulsant (Faigle and Feldmann, 1982), to the very reactive, such as aflatoxin B$_1$-2,3-oxide as quoted above. In addition to undergoing GSH conjugation, the oxirane ring is readily opened by water, generally catalysed by an epoxide hydrolase (Ota and Hammock, 1980). Two distinct forms of this enzyme exist, one in the cytosol and the other in the endoplasmic reticulum, the form involved in the metabolism of a particular substrate being determined by its structure. The activities of these enzymes represent a second major cellular defence mechanism against the toxic consequences of a reactive oxirane intermediate, and in *in vitro* cytotoxicity and mutagenicity tests inhibition of epoxide hydrolases has been used to show the harmful consequences of an epoxide intermediate (Guest and Dent, 1980; Marshall and Caldwell, 1992).

Reactive metabolic intermediates are generally 'short-range toxins' and their extreme reactivity (half-lives between 10 s and 1 min) strongly suggests that their toxicity involves reactions specific to particular tissues. However, although the liver is the major site of metabolism of xenobiotics in the body, it is relatively rarely a target organ for toxicity. It seems likely that in a number of cases reactive metabolites formed in the liver are in fact sufficiently stable to be transported to other organs where toxicity is expressed. In a small number of cases, it is apparent that metabolic activation is multiphasic, with a first step in the liver followed by further reactions in the target organ itself.

It must be remembered that not all toxic metabolites are reactive intermediates. On occasion, chemically stable products can be involved in toxicity, through their action at receptors, by physicochemical means, such as the renal toxicity of the sulphonamides (see above), or by retention in the body.

An example of activation by oxidation not involving an electrophile or a free radical is seen in the case of the solvent *n*-hexane (Bus, 1985). This is well known to produce a characteristic neuropathy, described as a 'dying back' of the axons of peripheral nerves, as well as testicular atrophy. These two toxic manifestations follow different time courses. The first clues that there might be a metabolic basis to this neuropathy was given by the fact that methyl *n*-butyl ketone (2-hexanone) gave pathologically similar effects, and it was then demonstrated that *n*-hexane and 2-hexanone had a number of common metabolites. It is now clear that *n*-hexane is metabolized by sequential ($\omega - 1$)-hydroxylation at both ends of the chain (C-2 and C-5), so that hexane-2,5-dione is a common metabolite of both *n*-hexane and 2-hexanone. Various studies involving the feeding of a number of metabolites indicate that hexane-2,5-dione is the common neurotoxic metabolite of these solvents. Work with a range of related materials has shown that γ-diketones (1, 4-diketones) or compounds metabolized to γ-diketones all give rise to axonopathies by binding to critical lysine residues in axonal proteins by Schiff base formation, leading to stable pyrrole derivatives.

Although most metabolic processes favour excretion from the body as a result of increases in polarity and water solubility, a small number of metabolites show increased lipophilicity relative to the parent compound

4,4'-Bis(methylsulphonyl)-2,2',5,5'-tetrachlorobiphenyl

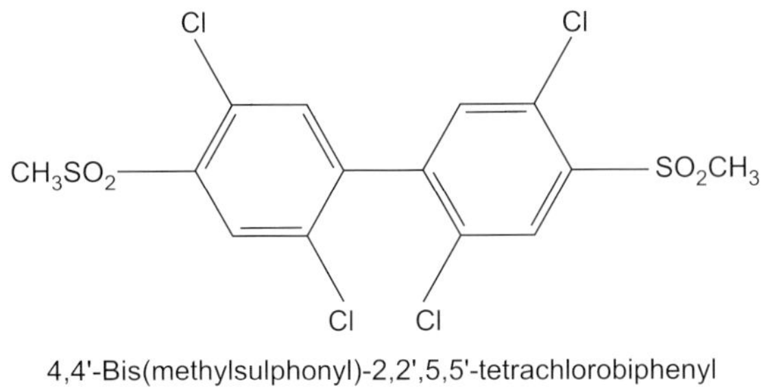

Figure 2 4, 4'-Bis(methylsulphonyl)-2,2',5,5'-tetrachlorobiphenyl, the lipophilic and pneumotoxic metabolite of 2,4,5, 2', 4', 5'-hexachlorobiphenyl.

and are retained in the body thereby. This is well established for a range of carboxylic acids and alcohols which are esterified with various lipids of the body (Caldwell and Marsh, 1983), and is also the case with certain end-products of the metabolism of glutathione conjugates. Glutathione conjugates undergo extensive metabolism by hydrolysis to the corresponding *S*-substituted cysteine, which may be *N*-acetylated to give a mercapturic acid, readily cleared in the urine of many species (Caldwell, 1982). However, the cysteine conjugates may also undergo other reactions of *S*-oxidation, transamination, and the so-called 'thiomethyl shunt' (Caldwell *et al.*, 1989). This involves the cleavage of the cysteine conjugate by β-lyase to yield a thiol which is then methylated (Jakoby and Stevens, 1983). The thiomethyl conjugates so formed often undergo *S*-oxidation to give very lipophilic sulphones (Jakoby and Stevens, 1983). An example of the toxicological significance of this pathway is given by the metabolism of the polychlorinated biphenyl (PCB) 2, 4, 5, 2', 4', 5'-hexachlorobiphenyl. This PCB is metabolized to a bisglutathionyl conjugate, which is progressively transformed as outlined to the very lipophilic 4, 4'-bis(methylsulphonyl)-2, 2', 5, 5'-tetrachlorobiphenyl (**Figure 2**) (Brandt *et al.*, 1985). This accumulates in lung and kidney of mice and rats and was associated, in lung at least, with binding to a cytosolic protein. It is well known that PCBs accumulate in the tissues of various species exposed environmentally, the tissue residues generally being in the form of methylsulphones. Many of these methylsulphones are concentrated in the lung, which is of interest as the lung is a target organ for PCB toxicity in humans, as was shown in the Yusho incident in Japan, an epidemic of human PCB intoxication.

Metabolic Activation at the Site of Toxicity

Most examples in which the toxicity of a compound is accounted for by metabolism within the site of toxicity are indeed seen in the liver. The liver necrosis caused by compounds such as paracetamol (acetaminophen) and carbon tetrachloride is the result of their metabolic activation in the liver. Paracetamol necrosis results from the cytochrome P450-mediated formation of NAPQI in quantities sufficient to exceed the capacity of the glutathione conjugation mechanism to protect the hepatocyte (Prescott and Critchley, 1983). This knowledge has permitted the rational treatment of paracetamol overdose, many cases of which are fatal unless treated in time by agents such as N-acetylcysteamine, which enhance the cell's protective pools of nucleophilic thiols (Prescott and Critchley, 1983).

The volatile general anaesthetic halothane is similarly activated by cytochrome P450 to a very reactive trifluoracylating species whose toxicity is a consequence of the organism's immune response to the trifluoracylated proteins produced by the hepatocyte (Kenna, 1991). A single exposure to halothane has no harmful consequences, but can sensitize individuals so that subsequent doses can result in a fulminant hepatitis which has proved fatal (Stock and Strunin, 1985).

The hepatotoxicity of carboxylic acid non-steroidal anti-inflammatory drugs (NSAIDs) has been known for many years, from the early examples of ibufenac, withdrawn in 1964 after a year on the market due to jaundice, and benoxaprofen, which caused the deaths of a number of elderly patients in the early 1980s (Taggart and Alderdice, 1982). Over the years, many drugs in this class have shown this form of toxicity in humans, resulting in termination of their clinical development or precipitate withdrawal from the market. One feature of all of these drugs was that their hepatotoxicity was not evident from standard animal toxicity tests.

A major pathway of metabolism of these carboxylic acid drugs is conjugation with glucuronic acid, giving acyl glucuronides, which, in animals at least, are preferentially cleared through the bile (Smith, 1973). Unlike other glucuronides, these are reactive intermediates (Spahn-Langguth and Benet, 1992) which can either function as acyl donors to suitable nucleophiles or glycate proteins by the formation of Schiff's bases between amino groups on proteins and the free aldehyde of the sugar ring, liberated by the acyl migration reaction which is a feature of their chemistry. A number of these agents give rise to NSAID–protein adducts, the formation of which is glucuronidation-dependent (Wade et al., 1997). In the cases of diclofenac and sulindac, the most hepatotoxic NSAIDs in general prescription use (Katz and Love, 1992), these adducts have been localized to the bile canalicular plasma membrane (Somchit et al., 1998a, b) and their molecular weights are similar to those of the major transporter proteins responsible for bile formation (Wade et al., 1997; Somchit et al., 1998, 1999). Both sulindac and diclofenac cause a dose-dependent cholestasis upon repeated administration, with reduction in bile acid excretion and hepatocellular necrosis (Somchit et al., 1997a, b). The protein adducts, DNA fragmentation and up-regulation of BAX protein

(both markers for apoptosis) were all co-localized in the centrilobular hepatocytes. It is known that cholestasis induces apoptosis in the liver (Patel and Gores, 1997). It thus seems likely that there is a link between the formation of these NSAID–protein adducts and apoptosis via accumulation of bile acid in hepatocytes. This work now provides for the first time an animal model of the hepatotoxicity of these drugs. In conventional toxicity studies of NSAIDs, the gastro-intestinal bleeding which occurs as a result of the inhibition of synthesis of cytoprotective prostaglandins is severely dose limiting. However, in all these newer studies, the NSAIDs were given by i.p. injection, which allowed the use of higher doses without the problem of gastro-intestinal toxicity.

Tissue- or cell-specific activation of toxins also occurs outside the liver and one notable set of examples is seen in the lung. The lung is a highly heterogeneous organ, with over 40 cell types, and a number of indoles and furans are markedly pneumotoxic. These are selective for the Clara cells of the pulmonary epithelium, which contain very large amounts of a number of cytochrome P450 isozymes able to form reactive and cytotoxic epoxides from compounds such as the furan 4-ipomeanol (Boyd, 1977).

1 - Methyl - 4 - phenyl - 1, 2, 3, 6 - tetrahydropyridine (MPTP) is a neurotoxin first identified in illicitly synthesized samples of the opiate pethidine (meperidine). It causes selective destruction of dopaminergic neurons in the substantia nigra and produces a syndrome essentially indistinguishable from idiopathic Parkinsonism (Jenner and Marsden, 1987). MPTP is highly lipophilic and readily crosses the blood–brain barrier. Within the brain, it is oxidized in two steps by the 'B' form of monoamine oxidase (MAO-B) (Singer et al., 1987) to the pyridinium species MPP$^+$ **(Figure 3)**, which inhibits mitochondrial respiration. This is a substrate for the dopamine uptake pump and is very toxic to nigral neurons in culture. MPP$^+$ destroys dopaminergic neurons when injected stereotactically into the substantia nigra, indicating it to be the ultimate neurotoxin of MPTP. The neurotoxicity of MPTP, which is irreversible, can be prevented by MAO-B inhibitors and dopamine uptake blockers, which prevent the formation of MPP$^+$ and its access to its site of action (Jenner, 1989). There is a very marked species difference in susceptibility to MPTP. Old World monkeys and humans are far more susceptible (Kramer et al., 1998) than mice, since there is a much more extensive first-pass excretion for MPTP in rodents following central nervous system exposure.

Streptozotocin, a methylnitrosourea antitumour drug, is a widely used experimental tool for the induction of diabetes. It is also a pancreatic carcinogen which causes the selective destruction of the pancreatic islet cells, thereby preventing insulin release. Although the nitrosoureas are non-selective in their action, the glucose moiety apparently targets streptozotocin to the pancreas

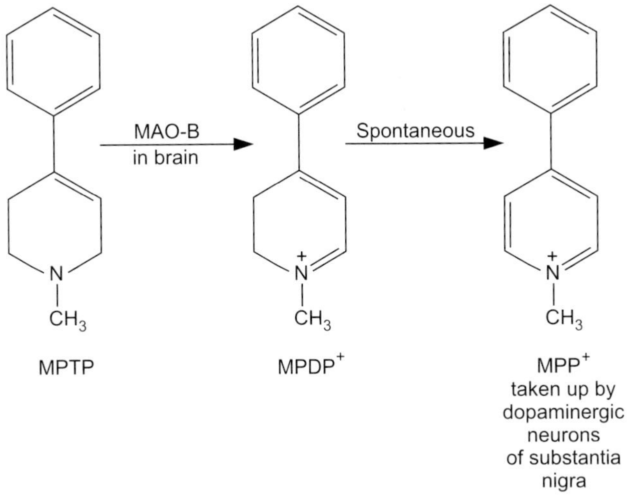

Despite its presumed high reactivity, the epoxide is able to escape from hepatocytes and is transported to the other tissues where part of its toxicity is expressed (Monks *et al.*, 1984). Bromobenzene 3,4-oxide can be detected in rat blood after administration of bromobenzene and although its half-life is very short (approximately 13.5 s), this is longer than the circulation time of the rat (5–10 s), which means that the hepatically generated epoxide is available to the lung and other tissues (Lau *et al.*, 1984).

Metabolic Activation as a Consequence of Multiple Reactions in Multiple Tissues

This is typified by the nephrotoxicity of the halogenated solvent hexachlorobutadiene (Anders *et al.*, 1988) which is mediated through its glutathione conjugate and involves successive transformation in different organs, finishing in the kidney **(Figure 4)**. The major site of

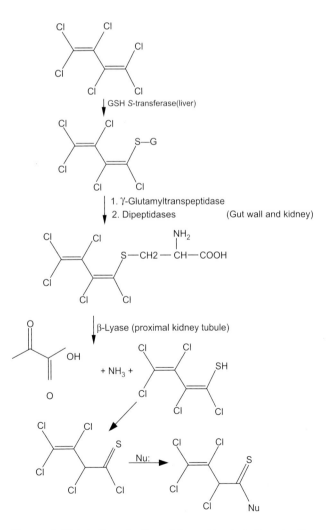

Figure 4 Metabolic activation of hexachlorobutadiene by the catabolism of its glutathione conjugate to a nephrotoxic electrophilic thiol.

and releases the toxic and carcinogenic nitrosourea there (Srivastava *et al.*, 1982).

TRANSPORT OF REACTIVE INTERMEDIATES AROUND THE BODY FROM THEIR SITE OF FORMATION TO THEIR SITE OF ACTION

Extrahepatic Toxins Whose Metabolic Activation Occurs in the Liver

Although, as has already been mentioned, reactive intermediates are generally thought of as 'short-range toxins', it is now clear that a number of these are sufficiently stable to leave their site of formation and be transported to remote sites where they exert their toxicity. An early example of this is seen with the pyrrolizidine alkaloids present in various plants from the *Senecio*, *Heliotropium* and *Crotalaria* species, which all too often contaminate human and animal foodstuffs (Culvenor, 1980). These alkaloids are typified by monocrotaline, which is highly toxic to liver and lung through its metabolite dehydromonocrotaline. *In vitro* studies show that only the liver has the ability to activate monocrotaline and its pneumotoxicity is due to the transport of the metabolite from the site of formation in the liver to the lung (Mattocks, 1972).

One of the earliest cases of the toxicity of a compound being directly related to its conversion to a reactive intermediate was bromobenzene, which is converted into bromobenzene 3,4-oxide. This binds covalently to hepatic macromolecules and this is presumed to underlie its hepatotoxicity (Brodie *et al.*, 1971). In addition to having effects on the liver, bromobenzene is covalently bound and has toxic effects in a range of extrahepatic tissues.

Figure 3 Metabolic activation of MPTP by MAO-B in the brain.

formation of the glutathione conjugate, which occurs by displacement of a chlorine atom by the sulphur atom of glutathione, is the liver. The conjugate is then hydrolysed by the liver, gut flora and kidney to the corresponding *S*-substituted cysteine which is the proximate nephrotoxin. The cysteine conjugate is a substrate for the cysteine conjugate β-lyase of kidney, which produces a reactive thiol which is the ultimate toxic metabolite. The tissue-specific expression of toxicity of hexachlorobutadiene thus involves metabolism first in the liver, giving a metabolite which is transported to the kidney, and then in the target organ, the kidney.

The urinary bladder is the target for the carcinogenicity of allyl isothiocyanate (AITC) and 2-naphthylamine. In both cases, the physicochemical conditions within the bladder result in the reversal of their metabolism, so that the urothelium is exposed to toxic compounds. AITC, the pungent flavour principle of mustard and horseradish, has been shown to be a bladder carcinogen in male, but not female, rats (NTP, 1982). No effects were seen in the bladders of mice. The interpretation of the significance of the animal carcinogenicity data for the human safety of AITC is problematic in the absence of a clear mechanism for tumorigenesis: the mutagenicity of AITC is far from clear (NTP, 1982), making a genotoxic mechanism unlikely. There is a strong possibility that a knowledge of the metabolism of AITC is relevant. AITC is detoxified by GSH conjugation in the liver and the glutathione conjugate is transformed to the corresponding mercapturic acid (*N*-acetylcysteine) (Ioannou *et al.*, 1984). This conjugation is reversible **(Figure 5)**, so that AITC can be released at another site in the body where GSH concentrations are lower and/or pH favours the release of the free isothiocyanate (van Bladeren *et al.*, 1987). It is reasonable to hypothesize that the tumours originate from chronic irritation of the bladder epithelium by AITC, a known strong irritant to skin and mucous membranes, which is liberated from its labile mercapturic acid conjugate under the conditions (temperature, basic pH, low or absent GSH levels, etc.) in the bladder. This prolonged irritation leads to hyperplasia and thence to neoplasia. It

has been suggested that the restriction of tumours to the male rat is related to the much lower urine flow in that sex (Ioannou *et al.*, 1984). Although knowledge of the metabolism of AITC is fragmentary, it is clear that major differences exist between its fate in rats and mice (Ioannou *et al.*, 1984).

AITC undergoes very extensive conjugation with glutathione in all species, but the subsequent fate of the glutathione conjugate is very variable. It is known that the further metabolism of the *S*-substituted cysteines produced by hydrolysis of glutathione conjugates shows very marked inter-species variability: while the major pathway in rats is almost invariably *N*-acetylation, yielding the mercapturic acid, in the mouse there occurs substantial transamination of the cysteine conjugate, giving thioglycollic and thioacetic acids (Caldwell *et al.*, 1989). In the case of isothiocyanate conjugates, these will cyclize to yield thiazolidin-2-thiones (Görler *et al.*, 1982). These may be expected to have very different reactivities from the mercapturic acid, which may account for the species specificity of tumour occurrence. The likely mechanism of tumorigenicity is thus a secondary mechanism, not involving genotoxicity, and which would be expected to show a dose threshold. The maximum human dose of AITC is limited by its very strong taste (Fenwick *et al.*, 1982). This dose is far smaller than those which gave rise to a small number of tumours in one relevant species, in one sex only. There is therefore a sufficient margin of safety for the use of this popular flavour.

2-Naphthylamine is a genotoxic carcinogen which is activated by *N*-hydroxylation. Sulphation and/or acetylation of *N*-hydroxy-2-naphthylamine lead to nitrenium ions which give rise to DNA adducts and, ultimately, tumours in a variety of organs. In a detoxication reaction, *N*-hydroxy-2-naphthylamine is *N*-glucuronidated

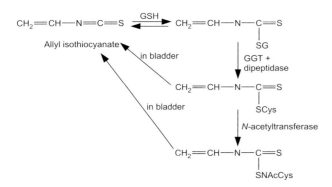

Figure 5 Reversible glutathione conjugation of allyl isothiocyanate, the basis for its toxicity to the urinary bladder.

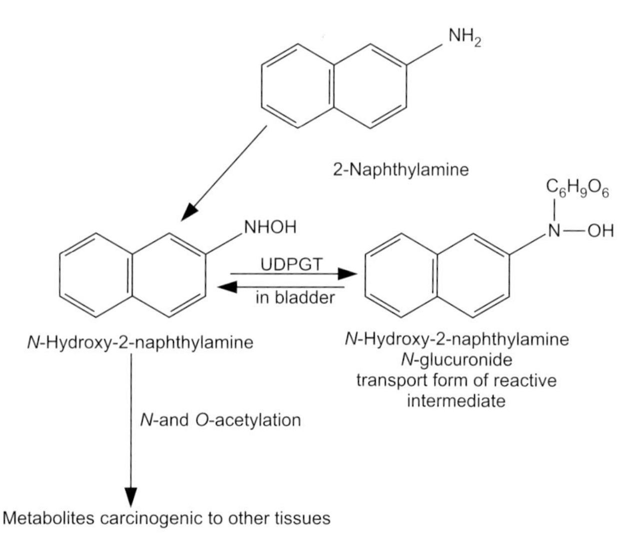

Figure 6 Metabolism of 2-naphthylamine, showing how the *N*-glucuronide of *N*-hydroxy-2-naphthylamine acts as a stable transport form for this reactive metabolite to the urinary bladder.

and the conjugate acts as a stable transport form which is excreted in the urine (Kadlubar *et al.*, 1977). The pH (~5) within the bladder of the average person eating a Western diet is low enough to break down the *N*-glucuronide, releasing the genotoxic *N*-hydroxy-2-naphthylamine in the lumen so as to allow it to attack the urothelium (Kadlubar *et al.*, 1977). This sequence of reactions is outlined in **Figure 6**.

INDIVIDUALIZATION OF CHEMICAL RESPONSES

The establishment of conditions under which a chemical may be safely and effectively used depends upon preclinical animal and *in vitro* studies and the judgmental extrapolation of these data to the human situation. We therefore need to 'humanize' safety evaluation to reduce the subjectivity inherent in this process and increase confidence in the data package as an indicator of the potential risk to human populations.

In terms of metabolism, it is now possible to work with human tissue preparations (microsomes, hepatocytes, liver slices, etc.) to establish the major pathways of metabolism of the chemical. Furthermore, the application of molecular biology techniques has permitted the elucidation of the roles of individual isozymes of the human cytochrome P450 system and other drug-metabolizing enzymes in ways not previously possible. The cDNAs for many human drug-metabolizing enzymes have now been cloned and expressed in a variety of bacterial, fungal and mammalian cell lines. These expressed enzymes, used in cell homogenates or the intact cell lines themselves, provide a range of powerful new tools for metabolic studies which have direct relevance to the human situation. The information derived from such studies can be used to anticipate the sources and likely magnitude of population variability in metabolic activation, toxicokinetics and response. The accumulation of this type of detailed mechanistic knowledge of the toxic action of chemicals, and the use of modern molecular biology tools, have created a spring-board allowing investigations of inter- and intra-species differences. The relative ease by which DNA sequence information can now be obtained has enabled functional polymorphisms in metabolizing enzyme systems to be determined and quantitated. The incorporation of molecular analysis with histopathological analysis has enabled linkages and causal relationships to be formed between particular genetic conformations and a biological outcome. Polymorphisms in the human P450 system, particularly CYP2C19 and 2D6, can have a significant impact on drug metabolism within human populations (Smith *et al.*, 1995). Recently, the presence of particular polymorphisms in the GST enzyme metabolism system has been shown to alter susceptibility to cancer formation, particularly lung cancer in smokers (Strange *et al.*, 1998). The identification of the particular isozymes responsible for the metabolism of a chemical allows intelligent anticipation of genetic, environmental, physiological and pathological factors which will influence the its metabolic fate. Since in so many cases variations in metabolism are associated with variation in toxic susceptibility, this approach will contribute to more reliable safety evaluation.

Safety evaluation is also substantially improved by the application of comparative animal versus human exposure data derived from toxicokinetic and human volunteer studies to establish exposure-based safety margins. These are inherently superior to the use of dose multiples. Similarly, the use of molecular and mechanistic information on specific toxicities also enhances the reliability of animal data as an indicator of human safety. In particular, these latter data have played an important role in recent times in the avoidance of both 'false-positive' and 'false-negative' conclusions from animal studies. Thus, it is now well established that rodents overestimate the risk to humans from hepatic enzyme inducers, which are well known to be hepatocarcinogens in rats and mice but not in humans. A similar picture emerges with the peroxisome proliferators. Another example is seen in the case of the hydrocarbons which bind to $\alpha_2\mu$-globulin and result in renal cell carcinoma in the male rat (see above). It is also to be appreciated that rodents underestimate the risk to humans from tamoxifen and, possibly, other antiestrogens. While these compounds can be liver carcinogens in rodents (Greaves *et al.*, 1993), this is not seen in humans. However, women taking tamoxifen show an excess incidence of endometrial carcinoma, a tumour type so far not seen rodents (Ugwumadu *et al.*, 1998).

With increasing understanding of the molecular basis of human toxicity, the techniques of transgenesis offer the opportunity to establish 'designer species' in which the toxic end points will be of more direct human relevance. At the moment, this approach has been used in the area of chemical carcinogenesis, but the models derived thus far do not use human transgenes. However, the technology permits this innovation, which we may expect to be utilized in the near future. Transgenic animals could be used in several ways to determine mechanisms of chemical toxicity. For example, a human drug-metabolizing enzyme gene could be directly introduced into a mouse and the effects on toxic response evaluated. Alternatively, specific genes could be deleted from the mouse genome and the consequences for toxic responses determined. As a variety of toxic chemical agents can modulate patterns of gene expression within target cells, these transgenic models could be used to screen for responses to different types of toxic insult (Wolf and Henderson, 1998).

Despite our best efforts, it is the case that animal models are not adequate for the evaluation of the toxicity of a number of drugs and there are still instances of compounds toxic in humans in ways which were not anticipated from animal studies. In some cases, this is due to the fact that the exposure and/or toxic end-point used in animals did not reflect properly the human situation. In these cases, it is possible to design a better animal test, something which has recently been achieved in the case of NSAID hepatotoxicity. However, there remain a number of human safety issues without animal models, which are mostly organ-specific toxicity. Examples include blood dyscrasices, immunotoxicity and cutaneous reactions.

humans are seen to be at least as sensitive as test animals to a given compound.

Finally, it must be realized that the use of mechanistic approaches is not limited to their *post hoc* use to explain unwanted effects in toxicity tests. These approaches allow for the first time the design of improved tests whose end-points are far more relevant to the human situation and which allow the more economic and ethical deployment of test animals and other resources to support the safer and more effective use of chemicals in the human population.

CONCLUDING COMMENTS

The coverage of this chapter has hinted at the state of knowledge concerning various mechanisms of toxicity. The efforts of a number of disparate scientific disciplines, both chemical and biological, have combined to allow an understanding of the origin of a number of toxic reactions. There has been rapid progress in recent years, and the applications of the techniques and concepts of molecular biology currently going on will enable this to continue.

It is important to appreciate that there remains a considerable problem in discerning cause and effect as far as toxicology is concerned, which may be illustrated by the phenomenon of lipid peroxidation. This represents an important primary mechanism of cytotoxicity for a number of compounds, but it is also a general feature of dying cells. To delineate whether it is indeed a mechanism of toxicity or is simply the consequence of cell death caused in some other way is problematic indeed, and it is all too easy to be misled.

Molecular biology affords the opportunity to look for the first time at toxic mechanisms at the most fundamental level. This includes cytotoxicity, particularly now that programmed cell death, or apoptosis, is accessible to experiment. New insights are also possible into proliferative lesions, most importantly cancer, as knowledge develops of cellular regulatory processes. Basic mechanisms of reproductive toxicity are approachable for the first time with increased understanding of developmental biology.

The practical significance of a mechanistic basis of toxicity is that, first and foremost, it allows properly informed safety assessments to be made. The recognition of qualitative and/or quantitative differences in the occurrence of a toxic mechanism or a particular metabolic pathway between species and/or exposure situations provides a scientifically acceptable and objective basis for the extrapolation of data, most notably from animals to humans. This may be favourable, in that it may show that animal data overestimate human risk, as is the case with the peroxisome proliferators and *d*-limonene (see above), but in other cases, such as paracetamol,

REFERENCES

Ames, B. N., Shigenaga, M. K. and Gold, L. S. (1993). DNA lesions, inducible DNA repair and cell division: three key factors in mutagenesis and carcinogenesis. *Environ. Health Perspect.*, **101**, Suppl. 5, 35–44.

Anders, M. W., Lash, L., Dekant, W., Elfarra, A. A. and Dohn, D. R. (1988). Biosynthesis and biotransformation of glutathione S-conjugates into toxic metabolites. *CRC Crit. Rev. Toxicol.*, **18**, 311–341.

Ashby, J. and Tennant, R. W. (1988). Chemical structure, *Salmonella* mutagenicity and extent of carcinogenicity as indicators of genotoxic carcinogenesis. *Mutat. Res.*, **204**, 17–115.

Bennett, W. M. (1983). Aminoglycoside nephrotoxicity. *Nephron*, **35**, 73–77.

Bernstein, H. N., Zvaifler, N., Rubin, M. and Mansour, A. M. (1963). The ocular deposition of chloroquine. *Invest. Ophthalmol.*, **2**, 381–392.

Boet, D. J. (1970). Toxic effects of phenothiazines on the eye. *Doc. Ophthamol.*, **28**, 1–69.

Boyd, M. R. (1977). Evidence for the Clara cell as a site of cytochrome P-450-dependent mixed function oxidase activity in lung. *Nature*, **269**, 713.

Brandt, I., Lund, J., Bergman, A., Klasson-Wheler, E., Poellinger, L. and Gustafsson, J.-Å. (1985). Target cells for the polychlorinated biphenyl metabolite 4,4′-bis(methylsulfonyl)-2,2′,5,5′-tetrachlorobiphenyl in lung and kidney. *Drug Metab. Dispos.*, **13**, 490–496.

Brenner, B. E. and Simon, R. R. (1982). Management of salicylate intoxication. *Drugs*, **2A**, 335–340.

Brodie, B. B., Reid, W. D., Cho, A. K., Sipes, I. G., Krishna, G. and Gillette, J. R. (1971). Possible mechanism of liver necrosis caused by aromatic organic compounds. *Proc. Natl. Acad. Sci. USA*, **68**, 160.

Burns, C. A. (1966). Ocular effects of indomethacin. Slit lamp and electroretinographic (ERG) study. *Invest. Ophthalmol.*, **5**, 325.

Bus, J. S. (1985). Alkanes. In Anders, M. W. (Ed.), *Bioactivation of Foreign Compounds*. Academic Press, New York, pp. 111–120.

Butterworth, B. E., Slaga, T., Farland, W. and McClain, M. (Eds) (1991). *Chemically-Induced Cell Proliferation: Implications for Risk Assessment*. Wiley-Liss, New York.

Caldwell, J. (1982). The conjugation reactions in foreign compound metabolism: definition, consequences and species differences. *Drug Metab. Rev.*, **13**, 745–778.

Caldwell, J. and Marsh, M. V. (1983). Interrelationships between xenobiotic metabolism and lipid biosynthesis. *Biochem. Pharmacol.*, **32**, 1667–1672.

Caldwell, J., Weil, A. and Tanaka, Y. (1989). Species differences in xenobiotic conjugation. In Kato, R., Estabrook, R. W. and Cayen, M. N. (Eds), *Xenobiotic Metabolism and Disposition*. Taylor and Francis, London, pp. 217–224.

Coles, B., Wilson, I., Workman, P., Hinson, J. A., Nelson, S. D. and Ketterer, B. (1988). The spontaneous and enzymatic reaction of *N*-acetyl-*p*-benzoquinoneimine with glutathione: a stopped-flow kinetic study. *Arch. Biochem. Biophys.*, **24**, 257–260.

Culvenor, C. C. J. (1980). Toxicology of pyrrolizidine alkaloids. In Smith, R. L. and Bababunmi, E. A. (Eds), *Toxicology in the Tropics*. Taylor and Francis, London, pp. 124–137.

Denckner, L., Lindqvist, N. G. and Ullberg, S. (1973). Mechanism of drug-induced chronic otic lesions. *Experientia*, **29**, 1362.

Djuric, Z., Coles, B., Fifer, E. K., Ketterer, B. and Beland, F. A. (1987). *In vivo* and *in vitro* formation of glutathione conjugates from the K-region epoxides of 1-nitropyrene. *Carcinogenesis*, **8**, 1781–1786.

EPA (1991). $\alpha_2\mu$-*Globulin: Association with Chemically Induced Renal Toxicity and Neoplasia in the Male Rat*. United States Environmental Protection Agency, Washington, DC.

Faigle, J. W. and Feldmann, K. F. (1982). Carbamazepine biotransformation. In Woodbury, D. M., Penry, J. K. and Pippenger, C. E. (Eds), *Antiepileptic Drugs*, 2nd edn. Raven Press, New York, pp. 483–495.

Fenwick, G. R., Heaney, R. K. and Mullin, W. J. (1982). Glucosinolates and their breakdown products in food and food plants. *CRC Crit. Rev. Food Sci. Nutr.*, **18**, 123–201.

Flamm, W. G. and Lehmann-McKeeman, L. D. (1991). The human relevance of the renal tumor-inducing potential of *d*-limonene in male rats: implications for risk assessment. *Regul. Toxicol. Pharmacol.*, **13**, 70–86.

Görler, K., Krumbiegel, G. and Mennicke, W. H. (1982). The metabolism of benzyl isothiocyanate and its cysteine conjugate in guinea-pigs and rabbits. *Xenobiotica*, **12**, 535–542.

Greaves, P., Goonetilleke, R., Nunn, G., Topham, J., and Orton, T. (1993). Two-year carcinogenicity study of tamoxifen in Alderley Park Wistar-derived rats. *Cancer Res.*, **53**, 3919–3924.

Green, S. (1992). Receptor-mediated mechanisms of peroxisome proliferation. *Biochem. Pharmacol.*, **43**, 393–401.

Guest, D. and Dent, J. G. (1980). Effects of epoxide hydratase inhibitors in forward and reverse bacterial mutagenesis assay systems. *Environ. Mutagen.*, **2**, 27–34.

Humes, H. D. and O'Connor, R. P. (1988). Aminoglycoside nephrotoxicity. In Schrier, R. W. and Gottschalk, C. (Eds), *Diseases of the Kidney*, 4th edn, Vol. 2. Little, Brown, Boston, pp. 1229–1273.

Ings, R. M. J. (1984). The melanin binding of drugs and its implications. *Drug Metab. Rev.*, **15**, 1183–1212.

Ioannou, Y. M., Burka, L. T. and Matthews, H. B. (1984). Allyl isothiocyanate: comparative disposition in rats and mice. *Toxicol. Appl. Pharmacol.*, **75**, 173–181.

Ishizaki, T. (1996). Strategic proposals to avoid drug interactions during drug development: a lesson from a terfenadine-related drug interaction. *J. Toxicol. Sci.*, **21**, 301–303.

Jakoby, W. B. and Stevens, J. (1983). Cysteine conjugate β-lyase and the thiomethyl shunt. *Biochem. Soc. Trans.*, **12**, 3–35.

Jenner, P. (1989). MPTP-induced Parkinsonism: chemical basis of an age-related disease. In Volans, G. N., Sims, J., Sullivan, F. M. and Turner, P. (Eds), *Basic Science in Toxicology: Proceedings of the Vth International Congress of Toxicology*. Taylor and Francis, London, pp. 615–625.

Jenner, P. and Marsden, C. D. (1987). MPTP-induced parkinsonism in primates and its use in the assessment of novel strategies for the treatment of Parkinson's disease. In Rose, F. C. (Ed.), *Parkinson's Disease. Clinical and Experimental Advances*, Vol. 87. John Libbey, London, pp. 149–162.

Jerina, D. M., Daly, J. W., Witkop, B., Zaltzman-Nirenberg, P. and Udenfriend, S. (1970). 1,2-Naphthalene oxide as an intermediate in the microsomal hydroxylation of naphthalene. *Biochemistry*, **9**, 147–156.

Joy, R. M. (1982). Chlorinated hydrocarbon insecticides. In Ecobichon, D. J. and Joy, R. M. (Eds), *Pesticides and Neurological Disorders*. CRC Press, Boca Raton, FL, pp. 91–150.

Kadlubar, F. F., Miller, J. A. and Miller, E. C. (1977). Hepatic microsomal *N*-hydroxyarylamines in relation to urinary bladder carcinogenesis. *Cancer Res.*, **37**, 805–814.

Katz, L. M., and Love, P. Y. (1992). NSAIDs and the liver. In Famaey, J. P. and Paulus, H. E. (Eds), *Therapeutic Applications of NSAIDs: Sub-populations and New Formulations*. Marcel Dekker, New York, pp. 247–263.

Kenna, J. G. (1991). The molecular basis of halothane induced hepatitis. *Biochem. Soc. Trans.*, **19**, 191–195.

Ketterer, B. (1988). Protective role of glutathione and glutathione transferases in mutagenesis and carcinogenesis. *Mutat. Res.*, **202**, 343–361.

Kiese, M. (1977). *Methemoglobinemia, a Comprehensive Treatise*. CRC Press, Boca Raton, FL.

Klaassen, C. D. (1991). Heavy metals and heavy metal antagonists. In Gilman, A. G., Rall, T. W., Nies, A. S. and Taylor, P. (Eds), *Goodman and Gilman's The Pharmacological Basis of Therapeutics*, 8th edn. Pergamon Press, New York, pp. 1592–1614.

Kramer, P. J., Caldwell, J., Hofmann, A., Tempel, P. and Weisse, G. (1998). Neurotoxicity risk assessment of MPTP (*N*-methyl-4-phenyl-1,2,3,6-tetrahydropyridine) as a synthetic impurity of drugs. *Hum. Exp. Toxicol.*, **17**, 283–293.

Kuo, C. H., Maita, K., Sleight, S. D. and Hook, J. B. (1983). Lipid peroxidation: a possible mechanism of cephaloridine-induced nephrotoxicity. *Toxicol. Appl. Pharmacol.*, **67**, 78–88.

Lau, S. S., Monks, T. J. and Gillette, J. R. (1984). Detection and half-life of bromobenzene-3,4-oxide in blood. *Xenobiotica*, **14**, 539–543.

Lilienfield, D. E. and Gallo, M. A. (1989). 2,4-D, 2,4,5-T and 2,3,7,8-TCDD: an overview. *Epidemiol Rev.*, **11**, 28–58.

Marshall, A. D. and Caldwell, J. (1992). Influence of modulators of epoxide metabolism on the cytotoxicity of *trans*-anethole in freshly isolated rat hepatocytes. *Food Chem. Toxicol.*, **30**, 376–473.

Mattocks, A. R. (1972). Toxicity and metabolism of *Senecio* alkaloids. In Harborne, J. (Ed.), *Phytochemical Ecology*. Academic Press, New York, pp. 179–200.

McGuiness, M. E. and Talbert, R. L. (1993). Phenformin-induced lactic acidosis: a forgotten adverse drug reaction. *Ann. Pharmacother.*, **27**, 1183–1187.

Miller, E. C. and Miller, J. A. (1985). Some historical perspectives on the metabolism of xenobiotic chemicals to reactive electrophiles. In Anders, M. W. (Ed.), *Bioactivation of Foreign Compounds*. Academic Press, New York, pp. 3–28.

Mills, J. J., Jirtle, R. L., and Boyer, I., (1995). Mechanisms of tumor promotion. In Jirtle, R. (Ed.), *Liver Regeneration and Carcinogenesis: Molecular and Cellular Mechanisms*. Academic Press, New York, pp. 199–225.

Monks, T. J., Lau, S. S. and Gillette, J. R. (1984). Diffusion of reactive intermediates out of hepatocytes: studies with bromobenzene. *J. Pharmacol. Exp. Ther.*, **228**, 393–399.

Monro, A. M. (1992). What is an appropriate measure of exposure when testing drugs for carcinogenicity in rodents? *Toxicol. Appl. Pharmacol.*, **112**, 171–181.

NTP (National Toxicology Program) (1982). *NTP Technical Report on the Carcinogenesis Bioassay of Allyl Isothiocyanate*. DHHS Publication (NIH) 83-1790. Department of Health and Human Services, Washington, DC.

Oates, N. S., Shah, R. R., Idle, J. R., and Smith, R. L. (1981). Phenformin-induced lacticacidosis associated with impaired debrisoquine hydroxylation. *Lancet*, **i**, 837–838.

Orrenius, S., McConkey, D. J. and Nicotera, P. (1989). The role of calcium in neurotoxicity. In Volans, G. N., Sims, J., Sullivan, F. M. and Turner, P. (Eds), *Basic Science in Toxicology: Proceedings of the Vth International Congress of Toxicology*. Taylor and Francis, London, pp. 629–635.

Ortiz de Montellano, P. R. (1985). Alkenes and alkynes. In Anders, M. W. (Ed.), *Bioactivation of Foreign Compounds*. Academic Press, New York, pp. 121–155.

Ortiz de Montellano, P. R., Mico, B. A., Mathews, J. M., Kunze, K. L., Miwa, G. T. and Lu, A. Y. H. (1981). Selective inactivation of cytochrome P-450 isozymes by suicide substrates. *Arch. Biochem. Biophys.*, **210**, 717–728.

Ota, K. and Hammock, B. D. (1980). Cytosolic and microsomal epoxide hydrolases: differential properties in mammalian liver. *Science*, **207**, 1479–1480.

Patel, P. and Gores, GJ. (1997). Inhibition of bile salt-induced hepatocyte apoptosis by the antioxidant lazareid U83836E. *Toxicol. Appl. Pharmacol.*, **142**, 116–122.

Potts, A. M. (1962). The concentration of phenothiazines in the eyes of experimental animals. *Invest. Ophthalmol.*, **1**, 522–530.

Prescott, L. F. and Critchley, J. A. J. H. (1983). The treatment of acetaminophen poisoning. *Annu. Rev. Pharmacol.*, **23**, 87–101.

Rall, T. W. (1991). Hypnotics and sedatives: ethanol. In Gilman, A. G., Rall, T. W., Nies, A. S. and Taylor, P. (Eds), *Goodman and Gilman's The Pharmacological Basis of Therapeutics*, 8th edn. Pergamon Press, New York, pp. 345–382.

Rawlins, M. D. (1981). Adverse reactions to drugs. *Br. Med. J.*, **282**, 974–976.

Ross, E. M. (1991). Pharmacodynamics: mechanisms of drug action and the relationship between drug concentration and effect. In Gilman, A. G., Rall, T. W., Nies, A. S. and Taylor, P. (Eds), *Goodman and Gilman's The Pharmacological Basis of Therapeutics*, 8th edn. Pergamon Press, New York, pp. 33–48.

Sies, H. and Cadenas, E. (1983). Biological basis of detoxication of oxygen free radicals. In Caldwell, J. and Jakoby, W. B. (Eds), *Biological Basis of Detoxication*. Academic Press, New York, pp. 181–211.

Singer, T. P., Castagnoli, N., Jr, Ramsay, R. R. and Trevor, A. J. (1987). Biochemical events in the development of Parkinsonism induced by 1-methyl-4-phenyl-1,2,3,6-tetrahydropyridine. *J. Neurochem.*, **49**, 1–8.

Smith, G., Stanley, L., Sim, E., Strange, R., and Wolf, C. (1995). Metabolic polymorphisms and cancer susceptibility. Genetics and cancer: a second look. *Cancer Surv.*, **25**, 27–65.

Smith, L. L., Lewis, C., Wyatt, I. and Cohen, G. M. (1989). The importance of epithelial uptake mechanisms in lung toxicity. In Volans, G. N., Sims, J., Sullivan, F. M. and Turner, P. (Eds), *Basic Science in Toxicology: Proceedings of the Vth International Congress of Toxicology*. Taylor and Francis, London, pp. 233–241.

Smith, R. L. (1973). *The Excretory Function of Bile*. Chapman and Hall, London.

Somchit, N., Wade, L. T., Goldin, R. D., Ramsey, L. A., Kenna, J. G. and Caldwell, J. (1997a). Hepatotoxicity in rats treated chronically with the nonsteroidal anti-inflammatory drug diclofenac but not ibuprofen. *ISSX Proc.* **11**, 105.

Somchit, N., Wade, L. T., Ramsey, L. A., Goldin, R. D., Kenna, J. G. and Caldwell, J. (1997b). Hepatotoxicity and hepatic protein adduct formation in rats dosed i.p. with diclofenac. *Hum. Exp. Toxicol.*, **16**, 401.

Somchit, N., Wade, L. T., Goldin, R. D., Kenna, J. G. and Caldwell, J. (1998). Sulindac-associated liver injury: an animal model. *Br. J. Clin. Pharmacol.*, **45**, 503P.

Somchit, N., Wade, L. T., Kenna, J. G. and Caldwell, J. (1999). Glucuronidation mediates protein adduct formation in livers of rats treated with the nonsteroidal anti-inflammatory drug diclofenac, but not in livers of rats given ibuprofen. Submitted.

Spahn-Langguth, H., and Benet, L. (1992). Acyl glucuronides revisited: is the glucuronidation process a toxification as well as a detoxification mechanism. *Drug Metab. Rev.*, **24**, 5–47.

Srivastava, L. M., Bora, P. S. and Bhatt, S. D. (1982). Diabetogenic action of streptozotocin. *Trends Pharmacol. Sci.*, **3**, 376.

Stock, J. G. L. and Strunin, L. (1985). Unexplained hepatitis following halothane. *Anesthesiology*, **63**, 424–439.

Strange, R., Lear J., and Fryer, A. (1998). Glutathione S-transferase polymorphisms: influence on susceptibility to cancer. *Chem.-Biol. Interact.*, **111**, 351–364.

Taggart, H. M., and Alderdice, J. M. (1982). Fatal cholestatic jaundice in elderly patients taking benoxaprofen. *Br. Med. J. (Clin. Res. Ed.)*, **284**, 1372.

Ugwumadu, A. H. N., Carmichael, P. L. and Neven, P. (1998). Tamoxifen and the female genital tract. *Int. J. Gynecol. Cancer*, **8**, 6–15.

Van Bladeren, P. J., Bruggeman, I. M., Jongen, W. M. F., Scheffer, A. G. and Temmink, J. H. M. (1987). The role of conjugating enzymes in toxic metabolite formation. In Benford, D. J., Bridges, J. W. and Gibson, G. G. (Eds), *Drug Metabolism—From Molecules to Man*. Taylor and Francis, London, pp. 151–170.

Wade, L. T., Kenna, J. G. and Caldwell, J. (1997). Immunochemical identification of mouse hepatic protein adducts derived from the non-steroidal anti-inflammatory drugs diclofenac, sulindac and ibuprofen. *Chem. Res. Toxicol.*, **10**, 546–555.

Weinberg, J. M. (1988). The cellular basis of nephrotoxicity. In Schrier, R. W. and Gottschalk, C. (Eds), *Diseases of the Kidney*, 4th edn, Vol. 2. Little, Brown, Boston, pp. 1137–1195.

Williams, G. M. and Weisburger, J. H. (1991). Chemical carcinogenesis. In Amdur, M. O., Doull, J. and Klaassen, C. D. (Eds), *Casarett and Doull's Toxicology*, 4th edn. Pergamon Press, New York, pp. 127–200.

Wold, J. S. (1981). Cephalosporin nephrotoxicity. In Hook, J. B. (Ed.), *Toxicology of the Kidney*. Raven Press, New York, pp. 251–266.

Wolf, C. and Henderson, C. J. (1988). Use of transgenic animals in understanding molecular mechanisms of toxicity. *J. Pharm. Pharmacol.*, **50**, 567–574.

Woosley, R. L. (1996). Cardiac actions of antihistamines. *Annu. Rev. Pharmacol. Toxicol.*, **36**, 233–252.

Youdim, M. B. H., Bakhle, Y. S. and Ben-Harari, R. R. (1980). Inactivation of monoamines by the lung. In *Metabolic Activities of the Lung*. Ciba Foundation Symposium 78 (new series). Excerpta Medica, Amsterdam, pp. 105–122.

Chapter 7
Physiologically Based Pharmacokinetic Modelling

Hon-Wing Leung

C O N T E N T S

INTRODUCTION

Pharmacokinetic (PK) models are used to make a rational prediction of the disposition of a chemical throughout the body. PK modelling has evolved over the past several decades. An early approach assumed that data on the internal environment of a chemical, e.g. tissue concentrations, cannot be obtained without employing invasive techniques. These PK models were developed to predict concentrations of chemicals in readily accessible media, such as blood and excreta. The plasma concentration, as an index of bioavailability, is assumed to mimic the biological effect in the entire system. Evidently this kind of approach cannot provide information on the concentration–time course of a chemical at the target site, which is not necessarily reflected by the blood concentration.

In recent years, biologically based models which apply first principles such as material balance and incorporate physiological parameters have been developed, initially to describe the kinetics of therapeutic drugs (Himmelstein and Lutz, 1979), then to environmental chemicals (Leung, 1991). These models include the exact physiology and anatomy of the animal species being described, in addition to parameters such as blood flow, ventilation rates, metabolic constants, tissue solubilities and binding to macromolecules. These models are commonly known as physiologically based pharmacokinetic (PBPK) models, and those for environmental toxicants are summarized in **Table 1**.

Classical Versus Physiological Pharmacokinetics

In early PK modelling, the whole body was treated as a single compartment. More sophisticated models are created by the addition of peripheral compartments. In a multicompartment model the concentration–time course in the central compartment is typically curvilinear with a terminal linear portion. By the method of residuals or feathering, this kinetic behaviour is mathematically resolved into decaying exponential terms to account for the curvature of the data. The number of exponential terms corresponds to the number of compartments in the model, each representing an exchange between a peripheral tissue or organ with the central compartment. Obviously, compartmentalization by such a rigid curve stripping process is a rather abstract mathematical construct and lacks physiological relevance.

In recent years, physiological modelling has emerged as a pre-eminent approach to PK modelling (Clewell and Andersen, 1985). However, it must be emphasized that classical and physiological PK are not fundamentally incompatible; in fact, they share a common connection. The difference between them lies in the kinds of parameters on which the models are developed, and consequently they differ in their applications. In classical PK modelling, no attempt is made to assign physiological correlates to model parameters. A compartment is simply considered as a kinetically homogeneous volume with transfer constants in and out of the compartment. In physiological PK modelling, a compartment is treated

Table 1 Physiologically based pharmacokinetic models for environmental toxicants

Chemical	Reference	Chemical	Reference
Acetone[a]	Morris *et al.* (1993)	2, 2', 4, 4', 5, 5'-Hexabromobiphenyl	Tuey and Matthews (1980)
Acrylonitrile[a]	Gargas *et al.* (1995)	Hexachlorobenzene[a]	Roth *et al.* (1993)
Arsenic[a]	Mann *et al.* (1996)	Hexane[a]	Perbellini *et al.* (1986)
Benzene[a]	Medinsky *et al.* (1989)	2-Iodo-3,7,8-trichlorodibenzo-*p*-dioxin	Leung *et al.* (1990)
Benzoic acid	Macpherson *et al.* (1996)	Isoamyl alcohol	Morris *et al.* (1993)
Benzo[*a*]pyrene	Roth and Vinegar (1990)	Isofenphos	Knaak *et al.* (1990)
Bromobenzene	Morris *et al.* (1993)	Kepone[a]	Bungay *et al.* (1981)
Bromodichloromethane	Lilly *et al.* (1997)	Lead[a]	Dalley *et al.* (1990)
Buta-1,3-diene[a]	Johanson and Filser (1993)	Lindane	DeJongh and Blaauboer (1997)
2-Butoxyethanol[a]	Johanson (1986)	Methanol[a]	Horton *et al.* (1992)
Carbon tetrachloride[a]	Paustenbach *et al.* (1988)	2-Methoxyethanol	Clarke *et al.* (1993)
Chlorfenvinphos	Ikeda *et al.* (1992)	Methoxyacetic acid[a]	Terry *et al.* (1995)
Chloroalkanes	Gargas and Clewell (1990)	Methylmercury[a]	Farris *et al.* (1993)
Chloroform[a]	Corley *et al.* (1990)	Methyl ethyl ketone	Liira *et al.* (1990)
Chloropentafluorobenzene[a]	Vinegar *et al.* (1990)	Methyl *tert*-butyl ether[a]	Borghoff *et al.* (1996)
Chromium	O'Flaherty (1996)	Nickel	Menzel (1988)
1,2-Dichlorobenzene	Hissink *et al.* (1997)	Nicotine[a]	Plowchalk *et al.* (1992)
1,2-Dichloroethane[a]	D'Souza *et al.* (1987)	Parathion	Sultatos (1990)
1,1-Dichloroethylene[a]	Andersen (1987)	Pentachloroethane	Nichols *et al.* (1994)
1,2-Dichloroethylene	Barton *et al.* (1995)	Physostigmine	Somani *et al.* (1991)
Dichloromethane[a]	Andersen *et al.* (1987a)	Polychlorinated biphenyls	Lutz *et al.* (1984)
2,4-Dichlorophenoxyacetic acid[a]	Kim *et al.* (1994)	Soman	Langenberg *et al.* (1997)
2,2-Dichloro-1,1,1-trifluoroethane[a]	Vinegar *et al.* (1994)	Styrene[a]	Ramsey and Andersen (1984)
Dieldrin	Lindstrom *et al.* (1974)	Toluene[a]	Tardif *et al.* (1993)
Diisopropylfluorophosphate	Gearhart *et al.* (1990)	2,3,7,8-Tetrabromodibenzo-*p*-dioxin[a]	Kedderis *et al.* (1993b)
5, 5'-Dimethyloxazolidine-2,4-dione[a]	O'Flaherty *et al.* (1992)	2,3,7,8-Tetrachlorodibenzofuran[a]	King *et al.* (1983)
1,4-Dioxane[a]	Leung and Paustenbach (1990)	2,3,7,8-Tetrachlorodibenzo-*p*-dioxin[a]	Leung *et al.* (1988)
Ethanol	Pastino *et al.* (1997)	Tetrachloroethylene[a]	Chen and Blancato (1987)
Ethyl acrylate	Frederick *et al.* (1992)	1,1,1-Trichloroethane[a]	Reitz *et al.* (1988)
Ethyl acetate	Morris *et al.* (1993)	Trichloroethylene[a]	Andersen (1987)
Ethylene oxide	Krishnan *et al.* (1992)	1,1,2-Trichloro-1,2,2-trifluoroethane	Auton and Woollen (1991)
Fluoride	Rao *et al.* (1995)	Vinyl chloride[a]	Barton *et al.* (1995)
Fluazifop-butyl[a]	Auton *et al.* (1993)	Vinylidene fluoride	Medinsky *et al.* (1990)
Furan[a]	Kedderis *et al.* (1993a)	Xylene[a]	Morris *et al.* (1993)

[a] These chemicals have more than one model. The reference identifies the model appearing the earliest in the published literature.

as individual organs or tissues arranged in a precise anatomical configuration connected by the cardiovascular system. The transfer of chemicals between compartments is governed by actual blood flow rates and tissue solubilities (partition coefficients).

Because of a lack of biological constraints with conventional PK modelling, empirical data can be fitted by freely varying the model parameters. These best estimates of parameter values can then be statistically compared across experimental conditions, treatments or chemicals to establish whether apparent differences are significant. In contrast, in physiological PK modelling any major discrepancies between the physiological model prediction and experimental data will necessitate the reformulation of the model to account for the observed behaviour. Since classical models are constructed without conforming to anatomical reality, they cannot account for physiological or biochemical alterations such as body and organ weight changes (tissue growth or atrophy) or enzyme induction and inhibition. While both classical and physiological models are capable of predicting tissue doses, albeit to different extents, classical models do not lend themselves to interspecies extrapolation of such dose–effect data (Monro, 1994).

THEORY AND PRINCIPLE OF PHYSIOLOGICAL MODELLING

The transfer of a chemical out of a single compartment follows Fick's law of simple diffusion, which states that the flux of a chemical is proportional to its concentration gradient. The differential rate equation describing this first-order process can be written as follows:

$$dC/dt = K \cdot \Delta C/V \qquad (1)$$

where C is the concentration of chemical in the compartment, K is the transfer constant, V is the volume of the compartment and ΔC is the concentration gradient.

If the transfer is perfusion-or flow-limited, then the transfer constant is the rate of blood flow (Q) to the compartment. It follows, therefore, that

$$dC/dt = Q(C_a - C_v)/V \qquad (2)$$

where C_a is the concentration of the chemical in the arterial blood entering the compartment and C_v is the concentration of the chemical in the venous blood leaving the compartment.

Since chemicals do not equilibrate freely in body fluids but, depending on their physicochemical properties, may be sequestered in tissue lipids, the concentration determined experimentally from a tissue sample is a composite of both the free and the sequestered form. Since transfer of a chemical in a tissue compartment is assumed to be flow-limited, the chemical concentration in the venous blood exiting from a tissue is equal to the concentration in the tissue fluid, i.e. the so-called free form. The partitioning of the chemical between the body fluid and tissue lipids is governed by tissue solubility or partition coefficient, P, as follows:

$$P = C/C_v$$

Substituting this into Equation 2, one obtains

$$dC/dt = Q(C_a - C/P)/V \qquad (3)$$

Equation 3 represents the fundamental relationship on which all PBPK models are constructed. The expression for all non-metabolizing, non-eliminating and non-binding tissue compartments will have this same mathematical form. The expressions for blood and other eliminating tissues such as liver, kidney and lung are more complex, but are based on the same principles of flow, mass conservation and partitioning.

DEVELOPMENT OF PHYSIOLOGICAL PHARMACOKINETIC MODELS

The development of a PBPK model is a highly integrative process. **Figure 1** depicts the flow processes in the development of a PBPK model. The first step involves

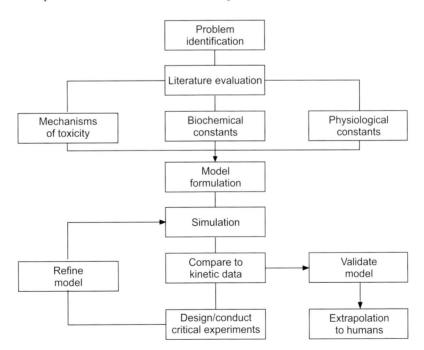

Figure 1 Flow chart of the development of a physiologically based pharmacokinetic model. Problem identification: the finding of a particular toxicity, in a particular organ, in a particular species. Literature evaluation: the integration of available information about the mechanism of toxicity, the pathways of chemical metabolism, the nature of the toxic chemical species, the tissue-binding characteristics and the physiological parameters of the target species. From these data a model is developed to estimate the appropriate measure of tissue exposure for a wide variety of exposure conditions. Reprinted with permission from National Academy Press, Washington, DC.

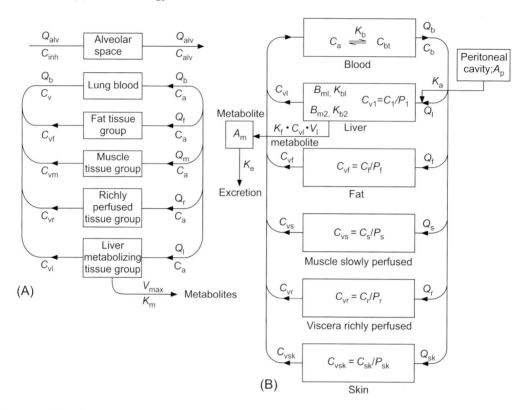

Figure 2 Two examples of physiologically based pharmacokinetic model depicting the schematic of their model structures. Q_{alv} = alveolar ventilation rate; C_{alv} = alveolar concentration. (A) A volatile chemical: 1,4-dioxane. (B) A non-volatile chemical: 2,3,7,8-tetrachlorodibenzo-p-dioxin. C_b = concentration of free dioxin in blood; C_{bt} = concentration of total dioxin (free and bound) in blood; K_b = binding constant in blood; B_{ml} = binding capacity to Ah receptor; B_{m2} = binding capacity to Ah receptor; K_{b1} = binding constant to Ah receptor; K_{b2} = binding constant to microsomal protein; K_a = absorption constant from gastro-intestinal tract to liver.

defining the nature of the problem and reviewing the literature to assess the impact of mechanism on the choice of tissue dosimetrics. The actual model formulation is divided into four interwoven steps, as follows.

Selection of Appropriate Tissue Compartments

The most natural approach to the choice of tissue compartments in PBPK modelling is to model a whole body by describing every organ and tissue. However, such detailed models, aside from the prohibitive labour and expense to develop them, are not required in most circumstances. The selection should be governed by the degree of detail necessary to provide a satisfactory depiction of the events. A knowledge of the chemical's mode and mechanism of action and its physicochemical properties will help make such a judgement. For instance, if a substance is known to accumulate in, bind to, be metabolized by, or be toxic to specific organs or tissues, these should form the integral compartments of the model that are described in detail. If a chemical is highly lipophilic, then the adipose tissues should be described as a separate compartment. Other 'non-target' organs and tissues may

be lumped together with respect to similar kinds or properties, e.g. richly perfused tissues representing kidneys and other visceral organs, slowly perfused tissues representing skin and muscle. The tissues or organs in the same body group are considered to have common kinetic behaviour and can be described by a single concentration profile. Naturally, if the grouping is carried out to the extreme, it degenerates to the classical one-compartment model, where the entire body is assumed to have uniform concentration. This phenomenon is most likely only if a chemical is relatively slow acting, is hydrophilic and has no complex biochemical mechanism such as active transport or macromolecular binding. **Figure 2** shows two examples of PBPK model structure for a volatile chemical, e.g. 1,4-dioxane (Leung and Paustenbach, 1990), and a non-volatile chemical, e.g. 2,3,7,8-tetrachlorodibenzo-p-dioxin (Leung et al., 1988).

Formulation of the Mathematical Relationship

After the model structure has been decided, differential rate equations are written to describe the transport, metabolism, binding and clearance for each compartment. The derivation of the basic form of the equation for non-metabolizing, non-eliminating tissues has been described previously (Equation 3).

For blood, the efferent blood from each tissue compartment is assumed to combine simultaneously to yield a mixed venous blood concentration (C_b) returning to the lungs at a flow-rate equal to the cardiac output (Q_b), as follows:

$$dC_b/dt = \sum (Q_i \cdot C_{vi})/Q_b$$

where i = name of tissue compartment.

For metabolizing tissues such as the liver, depending on the number and type of metabolic pathways, the basic differential equation is modified by the inclusion of terms describing a first-order metabolic process (K_f) or saturable Michaelis–Menten-type enzyme kinetics (K_m and V_{max}), or both:

$$V(dC/dt) = Q(C_a - C/P) - K_f(C/P) - (V_{max} \cdot C/P)/(K_m + C/P)$$

For tissues which exhibit specific binding, in addition to the amount partitioned by solubility, the total tissue concentration will also include the portion in bound form, as follows:

$$V/Q \cdot (dC/dt) = C_a - \{(C \cdot V)/[(V \cdot P) + B/(K_b + C_v)]\}$$

where B = binding capacity and K_b = equilibrium dissociation constant.

Hence, the formulation of the mathematical equations is fairly simple. The key consideration is to maintain a mass balance within each tissue compartment and also the entire model by carefully accounting for the inputs and outputs of the chemical.

Determining Model Parameter Values

The next step in the development of a PBPK model involves obtaining or determining the necessary model parameter values. Three classes of parameters are required: (1) anatomical and physiological variables such as organ and tissue volumes and blood flow-rates; (2) thermodynamic parameters such as tissue solubility (partition coefficients) and binding constants; and (3) biochemical parameters such as absorption, excretion and metabolic constants. Values for organ/tissue volumes, blood flows and ventilation rates can be readily obtained from the literature (Arms and Travis, 1988). Values not available may be scaled allometrically (Rowland, 1985). Analysis of organ weights and other physiological parameters have led to numerous equations of the type

$$X = \alpha W^\beta$$

where X = the parameter of interest, W = body weight and α and β are numerical constants. In general, organ size is directly proportional to body weight and $\beta \approx 1$. For body surface area, flow-rates and metabolic and clearance rates, they tend to vary to a fractional power of the body weight, and $\beta \approx \frac{2}{3} - \frac{3}{4}$. Like all procedures concocted to substitute for missing information, they only provide a best guess in the absence of data. When specific information becomes available, it should be used to adjust or to supplant the procedure (O'Flaherty, 1989).

Tissue–air partition coefficients for volatile chemicals can be determined by headspace analysis with the vial equilibration technique, using tissue preparations or homogenates (Fiserova-Bergerova and Diaz, 1986; Gargas et al., 1989; Mattie et al., 1994). As a rough approximation, a simple correlation approach based on other physiochemical properties such as water solubility and vapour pressure (Paterson and Mackay, 1989) or n-octanol–water partition coefficient (DeJongh et al., 1997) may be used. Tissue–blood partition coefficients are calculated from the tissue–air partition coefficients by dividing by the corresponding blood–air partition coefficient:

$$P_i = P_{Ai}/P_{Ab}$$

where P_{Ai} = tissue–air partition coefficient and P_{Ab} = blood–air partition coefficient. The metabolic constants V_{max} and K_m can also be estimated using a similar vial equilibration technique with tissue homogenates in vitro (Sato and Nakajima, 1979) or with an in vivo technique by measuring gas uptake (Gargas et al., 1986; Filser, 1992) or the exhalation rates of animals in an exposure chamber (Gargas and Andersen, 1989). **Figure 3** shows the apparatus used for these experiments. In the gas uptake study a closed recirculated exposure system is used to generate a series of uptake curves at a range of initial concentrations. The shapes of these curves are a function of P_i, V_{max} and K_m. Tissue partition coefficients are experimentally determined by the vial equilibration technique and incorporated into a PBPK model, which is then used to simulate the uptake process. An optimal fit of the family of uptake curves is then obtained by adjusting the biochemical constants for metabolism of the chemical. For materials of low vapour pressure which exhibit increasing blood and tissue solubilities, animals are first exposed by constant-concentration inhalation and then placed in exhaled breath chambers with a fresh air flow. The chemical concentration in the chamber is analysed serially. The metabolic constants are estimated with the PBPK model by optimizing the fit of the elimination curves. For non-volatile chemicals, tissue–blood partition coefficients may be estimated by using a vial equilibration (Murphy et al., 1995), an

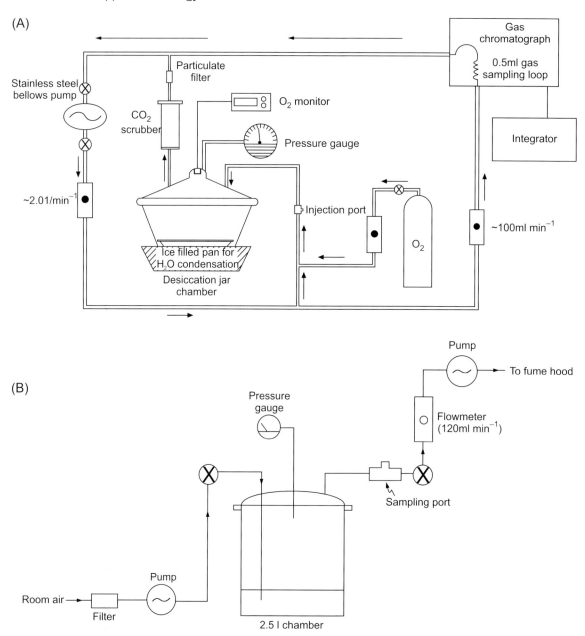

Figure 3 Schematic diagram of the apparatus used to determine metabolic constants *in vivo*. (A) Gas uptake for highly volatile chemicals; (B) exhaled breath chamber for less volatile chemicals. Reprinted with permission from Academic Press, Orlando, FL.

equilibrium dialysis (Lin *et al.*, 1982) or a filtration/extraction technique (Jepson *et al.*, 1994) *in vitro*, by single-pass perfusion of isolated organs *in situ* (Sultatos *et al.*, 1990), by bolus intravenous injection (Lam *et al.*, 1982) or by whole-body constant intravenous infusion *in vivo* (Chen and Gross, 1979). Metabolic constants for non-volatiles are determined with traditional enzyme assays by measuring the rate of disappearance of the substrate or the formation of product in tissue homogenates *in vitro* or in exposed animals.

In general, *in vivo* metabolic constants are difficult to determine empirically, and for ethical reasons it is nearly impossible to determine them for humans. In situations where only *in vivo* metabolic constants are available for the laboratory animal, V_{max} for humans may be scaled allometrically according to the fractional power rule. Alternatively, when *in vitro* data are available, the human *in vivo* V_{max} may be estimated, as has been demonstrated for methylene chloride (Reitz *et al.*, 1989). The Michaelis constant K_m generally is considered to be invariant among animal species.

Absorption rate constants are estimated from the rising portion of the blood concentration–time curve, and bioavailability is determined from the area under the blood curve following intravenous and other routes of administration.

Model Validation and Reformulation

Once the PBPK model has been configured and the requisite model parameters have been collected, the model is subjected to validation against kinetic, metabolic and toxicity information. This is accomplished by comparing the model predictions with experimental results. These exercises can suggest additional experiments to collect crucial data for verifying or improving model performance. When the model fails to simulate accurately known kinetic and toxicity behaviour despite modification of the model parameters consistent with physiological limits, it suggests that there may be additional mechanism(s) of action unaccounted for by the present model formulation. In such an instance, the model structure will need to be reformulated to justify the discrepancies. Obviously, there are multiple ways to restructure a PBPK model if the objective is simply to improve the goodness of fit to the experimental results. However, model reformulation should be guided by plausible biological mechanisms, which can be verified experimentally. A model is validated when it is successful in simulating the empirical results. The more extensive the database against which a PBPK model is validated, the more robust it is. A validated model can be used to make predictions of responses for a variety of exposure conditions, including ones which are difficult to perform experimentally. It also provides a means of predicting human kinetic behaviour when the biochemical constants and tissue-binding characteristics of the chemical have been determined in human tissues.

APPLICATIONS OF PBPK MODELLING IN TOXICOLOGY

Health Risk Assessment

The most common application of PBPK modelling in toxicology is dosimetric scaling in human health risk assessment (Leung and Paustenbach, 1995). For ethical reasons, most toxicological data are traditionally derived from experimentations with laboratory animals. High exposure levels are also frequently employed to maximize the likelihood of observing effects. In order to assess the human health risk from exposure to a chemical from the animal toxicity data, it will be necessary to make extrapolations of the toxic response from (1) the test species to human, (2) high to low exposure levels and (3) the test route to another route of exposure.

Historically, exposure is expressed as the dose administered in proportion to body weight. This dosimetric method assumes that the response of the biological system is directly proportional to the initial concentration of the test material, which in turn correlates with the body volume. Interspecies dose adjustment is scaled according to an animal's body mass. A variation based on a similar concept of initial whole-body concentration is to scale according to body surface area (Freireich et al., 1966). This latter scaling approach has lately become the method of choice for many risk assessment applications, e.g. the US Environmental Protection Agency's Carcinogen Assessment Group. Despite its popularity, this form of dosimetric scaling is only marginally accurate for intraspecies extrapolation and is rarely acceptable for interspecies extrapolation. The apparent unreliability of this approach is due to its failure to consider pharmacokinetic differences between species. The premise for this form of scaling assumes that the intensity of the toxic response correlates with the external exposure concentration or the amount of chemical administered. However, toxicity is not caused simply by the amount of chemical administered, but by the concentration of the chemical reaching the target tissues. Owing to the modifying effects of absorption, distribution, metabolism and excretion processes, target tissue dose is not always directly related to the amount of chemical administered. Another area where pharmacokinetics are important is in extrapolation of biological response from high to low dose. At low exposure levels typically associated with environmental conditions, pharmacokinetic processes generally proceed at rates directly proportional to the chemical concentration. However, at the high doses used in toxicity studies, many pharmacokinetic processes, especially metabolism, have a finite capacity and may become saturated. **Figure 4** compares the interspecies scaling of doses, using the body volume correction and the PBPK approach.

One other important application of PBPK modelling in toxicological risk assessment is extrapolation from one route of exposure to another. Inter-route extrapolation is necessary because the bulk of toxicity testing has been conducted with the oral route, whereas environmental

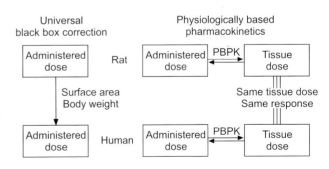

Figure 4 Comparison of approaches used in interspecies scaling. The universal black-box correction scales the externally administered dose from animal to human on the basis of body size (body weight or body surface area). In the PBPK approach, the equivalent human administered dose is estimated through a linkage of the internal tissue dose calculated by the respective animal and human PBPK models.

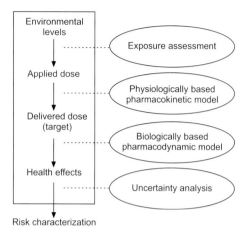

Figure 5 The roles of physiologically based pharmacokinetic and biologically based pharmacodynamic modelling in a refined health risk assessment paradigm.

and occupational exposures typically occur by inhalation or skin contact. The general aspects of route-to-route extrapolation using PBPK modelling have been described (Gillette, 1987). Specific examples include the dermal to inhalation extrapolation of organic chemical vapours (McDougal *et al.*, 1986), inhalation to oral extrapolation of trichloroethylene (Fisher, 1990) and methylene chloride (Angelo and Pritchard, 1987) and oral to dermal extrapolation of ethyl acrylate (Frederick *et al.*, 1992).

PBPK modelling provides a means of estimating the tissue doses of chemicals and their metabolites over a wide range of exposure conditions in different animal species. It can provide a biologically based means of extrapolating from the animal results to predict effects in human populations. These techniques have been applied to the human cancer risk assessment of methylene chloride (Andersen *et al.*, 1987a), ethylene dichloride (D'Souza *et al.*, 1987), perchloroethylene (Chen and Blancato, 1987), trichloroethylene (Bogen, 1988), 1,4-dioxane (Leung and Paustenbach, 1990), chloroform (Reitz *et al.*, 1990), ethyl acrylate (Frederick *et al.*, 1992) and vinyl chloride (Reitz *et al.*, 1996).

In a refined risk assessment paradigm **(Figure 5)**, a risk assessor conducts an evaluation of the environmental levels and the extent of exposure (frequency and duration) which provides an estimate of the administered dose. From the administered dose, a PBPK model is then used to estimate the delivered dose. In the next step, a biologically based pharmacodynamic model is used to provide the connection between the biological effective dose and the toxic response, ultimately yielding a risk estimate. Finally, an uncertainty analysis of the model parameters completes the health assessment by providing the confidence limits around the risk estimates.

Refining Experimental Design in Toxicity Testing

Metabolism plays a salient role in regulating the toxicity of a multitude of chemicals. Almost all metabolic and many excretory processes utilize specific enzymes or binding proteins which have limited capacity and may become saturated at high substrate concentrations. When these processes are saturated, internal dose parameters, such as area under the tissue curve or the amount of metabolite formed during inhalation exposure, are not linearly related to the externally administered dose or inspired concentration (Andersen, 1981). PBPK analysis of the dose-dependent processes provides an understanding of the relationship between external and internal dosimetrics under various exposure conditions. Recognition of these complex kinetic behaviours is essential to the proper design of toxicological experimentation. It is particularly relevant for dose selection in contemporary cancer bioassays, which emphasize the use of a maximum tolerated dose (MTD). The development of a comprehensive pharmacokinetic description to examine the influence of saturable processes on the delivery of a chemical to target tissues will aid in the correct selection of dosing regimen and test species. Although some *in vivo* animal experimentation will always be necessary to test the accuracy of the predicted behaviour by the PBPK model, this limited work requires fewer animals than conventional experimentation for assessing pharmacokinetic behaviour (Clewell and Andersen, 1985). Thus, a PBPK guided study design for chronic toxicity testing will enhance the information content of the experiment, while reducing the number of laboratory animals used.

Evaluating Metabolic Interactions in Chemical Mixtures

In addition to uses for improving toxicity study design, PBPK models have been used to examine chemical interactions. An early example of this is the work of Andersen (1987) with a dichloroethylene and trichloroethylene mixture. In this approach, a PBPK model is first constructed for the two chemicals individually, then linked via a mass-balanced differential rate equation for the liver compartment that has been generalized to account for the various mechanisms of metabolic interaction. The PBPK models are then tested by optimizing the fit to a series of uptake data in a closed-chamber inhalation exposure to the chemical mixture. These kinetic analyses, coupled with *in vitro* interaction data, can help to delineate the correct mechanistic possibility. The advantage of this PBPK approach is that analysis of the gas uptake data instead of the hepatic metabolism data greatly simplifies the evaluation of the kinetic interactions. Furthermore, a validated metabolic interaction model can be used to predict the outcomes of exposures to chemical mixtures of various proportions. This would have been almost impossible if it were to be tested experimentally, considering the large number of permutations. Other examples of analyses of metabolic interaction utilizing PBPK modelling include binary mixtures of hexane with methyl *n*-butyl ketone or hexane-2,5-dione (Mumtaz *et al.*, 1993), trichloroethylene–ethanol (Sato *et al.*, 1991b), benzene–toluene (Purcell *et al.*, 1990), toluene–*m*-xylene (Tardif *et al.*, 1993), carbon tetrachloride–chlordecone (kepone) (El-Masri *et al.*, 1996) and carbon tetrachloride–methanol (Evans and Simmons, 1996) and ternary mixtures of alkylbenzenes (Tardif *et al.*, 1997) and vinyl chloride–trichloroethylene–1,2-dichloroethylene (Barton *et al.*, 1995).

Establishing and Adjusting Occupational Exposure Limits

PBPK modelling has also been applied to evaluate the hazards of chemicals in the occupational setting.

Occupational exposures to industrial chemicals traditionally have been evaluated by monitoring the airborne concentration of the chemicals. However, air monitoring does not represent the absorbed dose, since it ignores modifying processes such as bioavailability and metabolism. In addition, routes of exposure other than inhalation may contribute to the total body burden. In order to determine accurately the actual received dose, biological monitoring techniques can be used. Reference standards known as biological exposure indices (BEIs), defining the acceptable levels of chemical substances in biological media, have been established. PBPK models are well suited for setting BEIs, because they can readily be used to estimate chemical concentrations in a variety of body fluids or tissues corresponding to the airborne exposure concentrations. This is achieved by exercising the PBPK models at an exposure scenario corresponding to an 8 h inhalation at the airborne exposure limit (Leung and Paustenbach, 1988; Leung, 1992). Most occupational exposure limits are set for the average or standard worker. PBPK models, however, can accommodate individual physiological variations such as body weight, body fat content and metabolic rate. Theoretically, with the aid of PBPK modelling, one can develop custom exposure limits specifically tailored to a particular worker.

Recently, the PBPK modelling approach has been advocated for setting occupational exposure limits (OELs) for work shifts of longer duration than the standard 8 h per day, 5 days per week work schedule (Andersen *et al.*, 1987b). The rationale for adjusting OELs for unusual work shifts is to ensure that workers are not placed at greater risk than those working a standard shift. Therefore, central to the development of a PBPK model for adjusting OELs for non-conventional

work shifts is the quantification of the degree of risk associated with the standard work shift such that the calculated OEL for the longer schedule poses no more than an equivalent risk. The selection of an appropriate risk index depends on a chemical's mechanism of toxicity. For most systemic toxicants, the risk index is the integrated tissue dose, i.e. the concentration and time ($C \times t$) cross-product. An important advantage of PBPK models is their ability to track the areas under the tissue or metabolism curves. Assuming that the area under the blood curve is the proper risk index associated with styrene exposure, Andersen *et al.* (1987b) determined that a 12 h exposure to 64 ppm was equivalent to an 8 h exposure to 100 ppm. In another example, blood carboxyhaemoglobin level was identified as the appropriate risk index for methylene chloride exposure. The OEL for non-standard work shifts is determined by maintaining the end-of-shift blood carboxyhaemoglobin concentration at a level no greater than those observed after exposure to the 8 h time-weighted average OEL.

Evaluating the Performance of Personal Protective Equipment

Traditionally, the performance of personal protective equipment such as a respirator is evaluated by measuring simultaneously the chemical concentration inside and outside the respirator. There are several problems with this approach: (1) it is cumbersome for the worker to carry around two air sampling trains; (2) air sampling over the work shift only gives a snapshot of the concentration, and does not provide a concentration–time profile; (3) since the exposure concentration rather than the absorbed dose is measured, it will underestimate the overall protection (e.g. skin absorption) offered by the protective equipment. PBPK modeling may provide a means to overcome some of these problems. The approach (Crank and Vinegar, 1992) involves measuring the post-expired breath at the end of the work shift, and using a PBPK model to estimate retrospectively the actual exposure concentration (i.e. the concentration leaking through the protective equipment). The PBPK model is exercised to identify combinations of exposure duration and concentration which will result in an accurate simulation of the expired breath data. Comparison of the model-predicted exposure concentration and the ambient exposure concentration will yield the protection factor of the protective equipment.

UNCERTAINTIES AND LIMITATIONS IN PBPK MODELLING

Since modelling is based on data which have inherent errors, any model will have a certain degree of uncertainty associated with it. There are two important areas of uncertainties in the development of PBPK models. The first concerns the selection of the proper model and the second deals with the model parameters estimated (Sato *et al.*, 1991a). When a PBPK model is used to make predictions, it should reflect these uncertainties in terms of confidence limits in the values predicted by the model, and the confidence regions around the estimated parameters. As shown in **Figure 1**, the first step in PBPK modelling is to define the problem to be solved. The next step is to postulate several plausible physiological mechanisms to describe the data set. The third step is to use the data to discriminate between candidate models. The selection of the best model and the estimation of model parameters can be guided by statistical analysis, often with the aid of computer programs (Blau and Neely, 1987). Since small changes in input data or in the goodness of fit to a set of experimental data may significantly affect the predicted output and, in turn, the risk estimate when the PBPK model is used to support quantitative risk assessment, the uncertainties associated with PBPK model parameters should be carefully analysed. The systematic testing of the effects of the model parameters on the model predictions in PBPK modelling is called sensitivity/variability analysis (Cohn, 1987). This procedure of uncertainty evaluation in input parameters has been shown with PBPK models for methylene chloride (Portier and Kaplan, 1989), soman (Maxwell *et al.*, 1988), tetrachloroethylene (Farrar *et al.*, 1989), benzene (Spear *et al.*, 1991) and carbon tetrachloride (Evans *et al.*, 1994). Finally, a PBPK model is developed to provide insight to specific questions, and should never be used for extrapolation beyond its intended purpose. Furthermore, its use for prediction should come only after a through validation process.

REFERENCES

Andersen, M. E. (1981). Saturable metabolism and its relationship to toxicity. *CRC Crit. Rev. Toxicol.*, **9**, 105–150.

Andersen, M. E., (1987). Quantitative evaluation of the metabolic interactions between trichloroethylene and 1,1-dichloroethylene *in vivo*. *Toxicol. Appl. Pharmacol.*, **89**, 149–157.

Andersen, M. E., Clewell, H. J., III, Gargas, M. L., Smith, F. A. and Reitz, R. H. (1987a). Physiologically based pharmacokinetics and the risk assessment process for methylene chloride. *Toxicol. Appl. Pharmacol.*, **87**, 185–205.

Andersen, M. E., MacNaughton, M. G., Clewell, H. J., III, and Paustenbach. D. J. (1987b). Adjusting exposure limits for long and short exposure periods, using a physiological pharmacokinetic model. *Am. Ind. Hyg. Assoc. J.*, **48**, 335–343.

Angelo, M. J. and Pritchard, A. B. (1987). Route-to-route extrapolation of dichloromethane exposure using a physiological pharmacokinetic model. In *Drinking Water and Health, Vol. 8, Pharmacokinetics in Risk Assessment*. National Academy Press, Washington, DC, pp. 254–264.

Arms, A. D. and Travis, C. C. (1988) *Reference Physiological Parameters in Pharmacokinetic Modelling*. US EPA 600/6-88/004. Final Report. (Available from NTIS, PB88–196019).

Auton, T. R. and Woollen, B. H. (1991). A physiologically based mathematical model for the human inhalation pharmacokinetics of 1,1,2-trichloro-1,2,2-trifluoroethane. *Int. Arch. Occup. Environ. Health*, **63**, 133–138.

Auton, T. R., Ramsey, J. D. and Woollen, B. H. (1993). Modelling dermal pharmacokinetics using *in vitro* data. Part I. Fluazifop-butyl in the rat. *Hum. Exp. Toxicol.*, **12**, 199–206.

Barton, H. A., Creech, J. R., Godin, C. S., Randall, G. M. and Seckel, C. (1995). Chloroethylene mixtures: pharmacokinetic modeling and *in vitro* metabolism of vinyl chloride, trichloroethylene, and *trans*-1,2-dichloroethylene in rat. *Toxicol. Appl. Pharmacol.*, **130**, 237–247.

Blau, G. E. and Neely, W. B. (1987). Dealing with uncertainty in pharmacokinetic models using Simusolv. In *Drinking Water and Health, Vol. 8, Pharmacokinetics in Risk Assessment*. National Academy Press, Washington, DC, pp. 185–207.

Bogen, K. T. (1988). Pharmacokinetics for regulatory risk analysis: the case of trichloroethylene. *Regul. Toxicol. Pharmacol.*, **8**, 447–466.

Borghoff, S. J., Murphy, J. E. and Medinsky, M. A. (1996). Development of a physiologically based pharmacokinetic model for methyl tertiary-butyl ether and tertiary-butanol in male Fischer-344 rats. *Fundam. Appl. Toxicol.*, **30**, 264–275.

Bungay, P. M., Dedrick, R. L. and Matthews, H. B. (1981). Enteric transport of chlordecone (Kepone) in the rat. *J. Pharmacokinet. Biopharm.*, **9**, 309–341.

Chen, C. W. and Blancato, J. N. (1987). Role of pharmacokinetic modelling in risk assessment: perchloroethylene as an example. In *Drinking Water and Health, Vol. 8, Pharmacokinetics in Risk Assessment*. National Academy Press, Washington, DC, pp. 369–390.

Chen, H. S. G. and Gross, J. F. (1979). Estimation of tissue-to-plasma partition coefficients used in physiological pharmacokinetic models. *J. Pharmacokinet. Biopharm.*, **7**, 117–125.

Clarke, D. O., Elswick, B. A., Welsch, F. and Conolly, R. B. (1993). Pharmacokinetics of 2-methoxyethanol and 2-methoxyacetic acid in the pregnant mouse: a physiologically based mathematical model. *Toxicol. Appl. Pharmacol.*, **121**, 239–252.

Clewell, H. J., III, and Andersen, M. E. (1985). Risk assessment extrapolations and physiological modelling. *Toxicol. Ind. Health*, **1**, 111–122.

Cohn, M. S. (1987). Sensitivity analysis in pharmacokinetic modeling. In *Drinking Water and Health, Vol. 8, Pharmacokinetics in Risk Assessment*, National Academy Press, Washington, DC, pp. 265–272.

Corley, R. A., Mendrala, A. L., Smith, F. A., Staats, D. A., Gargas, M. L., Conolly, R. B., Andersen, M. E. and Reitz, R. H. (1990). Development of a physiologically-based pharmacokinetic model for chloroform. *Toxicol. Appl. Pharmacol.*, **103**, 512–527.

Crank, W. D. and Vinegar, A. (1992). A physiologically based pharmacokinetic model for chloropentafluorobenzene in primates to be used in the evaluation of protective equipment against toxic gases. *Toxicol. Ind. Health*, **8**, 21–35.

Dallas, C. E., Ramanathan, R., Muralidhara, S., Gallo, G. M. and Bruckner, J. V. (1989). The uptake and elimination of

1,1,1-trichloroethane during and following inhalation exposures in rats. *Toxicol. Appl. Pharmacol.*, **98**, 385–397.

Dalley, J. W., Gupta, P. K. and Hung, C. T. (1990). A physiological pharmacokinetic model describing the disposition of lead in the absence and presence of L-ascorbic acid in rats. *Toxicol. Lett.*, **50**, 337–348.

DeJongh, J. and Blaauboer, B. J. (1997). Simulation of lindane kinetics in rats. *Toxicology*, **122**, 1–9.

DeJongh, J., Verhaar, H. J. M. and Hermans, J. L. M. (1997). A quantitative property–property relationship (QRPR) to estimate *in vitro* tissue-blood partition coefficients of organic chemicals in rats and humans. *Arch. Toxicol.*, **72**, 17–25.

D'Souza, R. W., Francis, W. R., Bruce, R. D. and Andersen, M. E. (1987). Physiologically based pharmacokinetic model for ethylene dichloride and its application in risk assessment. In *Drinking Water and Health, Vol. 8, Pharmacokinetics in Risk Assessment*. National Academy Press, Washington, DC, pp. 286–301.

El-Masri, H. A., Thomas, R. S., Sabados, G. R., Phillips, J. K., Constan, A. A., Benjamin, S. A., Andersen, M. E., Mehendale, H. M. and Yang, R. S. H. (1996). Physiologically based pharmacokinetic/pharmacodynamic modeling of the toxicologic interaction between carbon tetrachloride and kepone. *Arch. Toxicol.*, **70**, 704–713.

Evans, M. V. and Simmons, J. E. (1996). Physiologically based pharmacokinetic estimated metabolic constants and hepatotoxicity of carbon tetrachloride after methanol pretreatment in rats. *Toxicol. Appl. Pharmacol.*, **140**, 245–253.

Evans, M. V., Crank, W. D., Yang, H-M. and Simmons, J. E. (1994). Applications of sensitivity analysis to a physiologically based pharmacokinetic model for carbon tetrachloride in rats. *Toxicol. Appl. Pharmacol.*, **128**, 36–44.

Farrar, D., Allen, B., Crump, K. and Shipp, A. (1989). Evaluation of uncertainty in input parameters to pharmacokinetic models and the resulting uncertainty in output. *Toxicol. Lett.*, **49**, 371–385.

Farris, F. F., Dedrick, R. L., Allen, P. V. and Smith, J. C. (1993). Physiological model for pharmacokinetics of methyl mercury in the growing rat. *Toxicol. Appl. Pharmacol.*, **119**, 74–90.

Filser, J. G. (1992). The closed chamber technique—uptake, endogenous production, excretion, steady-state kinetics and rates of metabolism of gases and vapors. *Arch. Toxicol.*, **66**, 1–10.

Fiserova-Bergerova, V. and Diaz, M. L. (1986). Determination and prediction of tissue-gas partition coefficients. *Int. Arch. Occup. Environ. Health*, **58**, 75–87.

Fisher, J. W. (1990). Using inhalation kinetic data in route-to-route extrapolation: a physiological models for oral absorption of trichloroethylene. In Gerrity, T. R. and Henry, C. J. (Eds), *Principles of Route-to-Route Extrapolation for Risk Assessment*. Elsevier, New York, pp. 297–311.

Frederick, C. B., Potter, D. W., Chang-Mateu, M. I. and Andersen, M. E. (1992). A physiologically based pharmacokinetic and pharmacodynamic model to describe the oral dosing of rats with ethyl acrylate and its implications for risk assessment. *Toxicol. Appl. Pharmacol.*, **114**, 246–260.

Freireich, E. J., Gehan, E. A., Rall, D. P., Schmidt, L. H. and Skipper, H. E. (1966). Quantitative comparison of toxicity of anticancer agents in mouse, rat, hamster, dog, monkey and man. *Cancer Chemother. Rep.*, **50**, 219–244.

Gargas, M. L. and Andersen, M. E. (1989). Determining kinetic constants of chlorinated ethane metabolism in the rat from rates of exhalation. *Toxicol. Appl. Pharmacol.*, **99**, 344–353.

Gargas, M. L. and Clewell, H. J., III (1990). Gas uptake inhalation techniques and the rates of metabolism of chloromethanes, chloroethanes, and chloroethylenes in the rat. *Inhal. Toxicol.*, **2**, 295–319.

Gargas, M. L., Andersen, M. E. and Clewell, H. J., III (1986). A physiologically based simulation approach for determining metabolic constants from gas uptake data. *Toxicol. Appl. Pharmacol.*, **86**, 341–352.

Gargas, M. L., Burgess, R. J., Voisard, D. E., Cason, G. H. and Andersen, M. E. (1989). Partition coefficients of low-molecular weight volatile chemicals in various liquids and tissues. *Toxicol. Appl. Pharmacol.*, **98**, 87–99.

Gargas, M. L., Andersen, M. E., Teo, S. K. O., Batra, R., Fennell, T. R. and Kedderis, G. L. (1995). A physiologically based dosimetry description of acrylonitrile and cyanoethylene oxide in the rat. *Toxicol. Appl. Pharmacol.*, **134**, 185–194.

Gearhart, J. M., Jepson, G. W., Clewell, H. J., III, Andersen, M. E., and Conolly, R. B. (1990). Physiologically based pharmacokinetic and pharmacodynamic model for the inhibition of acetylcholinesterase by diisopropylfluorophosphate. *Toxicol. Appl. Pharmacol.*, **106**, 295–310.

Gillette, J. R. (1987). Dose, species, and route extrapolation: general aspects. In *Drinking Water and Health, Vol. 8, Pharmacokinetics in Risk Assessment*. National Academy Press, Washington, DC, pp. 96–158.

Himmelstein, K. J. and Lutz, R. J. (1979). A review of the applications of physiologically based pharmacokinetic modeling. *J. Pharmacokinet. Biopharm.*, **7**, 127–145.

Hissink, A. M., Van Ommen, B., Kruse, J. and Van Bladeren, P. J. (1997). A physiologically based pharmacokinetic (PB-PK) model for 1,2-dichlorobenzene linked to two possible parameters of toxicity. *Toxicol. Appl. Pharmacol.*, **145**, 301–310.

Horton, V. L., Higuchi, M. A. and Rickert, D. E. (1992). Physiologically based pharmacokinetic model for methanol in rats, monkeys, and humans. *Toxicol. Appl. Pharmacol.*, **117**, 26–36.

Ikeda, T., Tsuda, S. and Shirasu, Y. (1992). Pharmacokinetic analysis of protection by an organophosphorus insecticide, chlorfenvinphos, against the toxicity of its succeeding dosage in rats. *Fundam. Appl. Toxicol.*, **18**, 299–306.

Jepson, G. W., Hoover, D. K., Black, R. K., McCafferty, J. D., Mahle, D. A. and Gearhart, J. M. (1994). A partition coefficient determination method for nonvolatile chemicals in biological tissues. *Fundam. Appl. Pharmacol.*, **22**, 519–524.

Johanson, G. (1986). Physiologically-based pharmacokinetic modeling of inhaled 2-butoxyethanol in man. *Toxicol. Lett.*, **34**, 23–31.

Johanson, G. and Filser, J. G. (1993). A physiologically based pharmacokinetic model for butadiene and its metabolite butadiene monoxide in rat and mouse and its significance for risk extrapolation. *Arch. Toxicol.*, **67**, 151–163.

Kedderis, G. L., Carfagna, M. A., Held, S. D., Batra, R., Murphy, J. E. and Gargas, M. L. (1993a). Kinetic analysis of furan biotransformation by F-344 rats *in vivo* and *in vitro*. *Toxicol. Appl. Pharmacol.*, **123**, 274–282.

Kedderis, L. B., Mills, J. J., Andersen, M. E. and Birnbaum, L. S. (1993b). A physiologically based pharmacokinetic model for 2,3,7,8-tetrabromodibenzo-*p*-dioxin (TBDD) in the rat: tissue distribution and CYP1A induction. *Toxicol. Appl. Pharmacol.*, **121**, 87–98.

Kim, C. S., Gargas, M. L. and Andersen, M. E. (1994). Pharmacokinetic modeling of 2,4-dichlorophenoxyacetic acid (2,4-D) in rat and in rabbit brain following single dose administration. *Toxicol. Lett.*, **74**, 189–201.

King, F. G., Dedrick, R. L., Collins, J. M., Matthews, H. B. and Birnbaum, L. S. (1983). A physiological model for the pharmacokinetics of 2,3,7,8-tetrachlorodibenzofuran in several species. *Toxicol. Appl. Pharmacol.*, **67**, 390–400.

Knaak, J., al-Bayati, M., Raabe, O. and Blancato, J. (1990). *In vivo* percutaneous absorption studies in the rat: pharmacokinetics and modeling of isofenphos absorption. In Scott, R. C., Guy R. H. and Hardgraft, J. (Eds), *Prediction of Percutaneous Penetration: Methods, Measurements, Modeling*. IBC, London, pp. 1–18.

Krishnan, K., Gargas, M. L., Fennell, T. R. and Andersen, M. E. (1992). A physiologically based description of ethylene oxide dosimetry in the rat. *Toxicol. Ind. Health*, **8**, 121–140.

Lam, G., Chen. M. L. and Chiou, W. L. (1982). Determination of tissue to blood partition coefficients in physiologically-based pharmacokinetic studies. *J. Pharm. Sci.*, **71**, 454–456.

Langenberg, van Dijk, C., Sweeney, R. E., Maxwell, D. M., De Jong, L. P. A. and Benschop, H. P. (1997). Development of a physiologically based model for the toxicokinetics of C(±)P(±)-soman in the atropinized guinea pig. *Arch. Toxicol.*, **71**, 320–331.

Leung, H. W. (1991). Development and utilization of physiologically based pharmacokinetic models for toxicological applications. *J. Toxicol. Environ. Health*, **32**, 247–267.

Leung, H. W. (1992). Use of physiologically based pharmacokinetic models to establish biological exposure indexes. *Am. Ind. Hyg. Assoc. J.*, **53**, 369–374.

Leung, H. W. and Paustenbach, D. J. (1988). Application of pharmacokinetics to derive biological exposure indexes from threshold limit values. *Am. Ind. Hyg. Assoc. J.*, **49**, 445–450.

Leung, H. W. and Paustenbach, D. J. (1990). Cancer risk assessment of dioxane based upon a physiologically-based pharmacokinetic approach. *Toxicol. Lett.*, **51**, 147–102.

Leung, H. W. and Paustenbach, D. J. (1995). Physiologically based pharmacokinetic and pharmacodynamic modeling in health risk assessment and characterization of hazardous substances. *Toxicol. Lett.*, **79**, 55–65.

Leung, H. W., Ku, R. H., Paustenbach, D. J. and Andersen, M. E. (1988). A physiologically based pharmacokinetic model for 2,3,7,8-tetrachlorodibenzo-*p*-dioxin in C57BL/6J and DBA/2J mice. *Toxicol. Lett.*, **42**, 15–28.

Leung, H. W., Poland, A., Paustenbach, D. J., Murray, F. J. and Andersen. M. E. (1990). Pharmacokinetics of [125I]-2-iodo-3,7,8-trichlorodibenzo-*p*-dioxin in mice: analysis with a physiological modeling approach. *Toxicol. Appl. Pharmacol.*, **103**, 411–419.

Liira, J., Johanson, G. and Riihimaki, V. (1990). Dose-dependent kinetics of inhaled methylethylketone in man. *Toxicol. Lett.*, **50**, 195–201.

Lilly, P. D., Andersen, M. E., Ross, T. M. and Pegram, R. A. (1997). Physiologically based estimation of *in vivo* rates of bromodichloromethane metabolism. *Toxicology*, **124**, 141–152.

Lin, J. H., Sugiyama, Y., Awazu, S. and Hanano, M. (1982). *In vitro* and *in vivo* evaluation of the tissue-to-blood partition

coefficient for physiological pharmacokinetic models. *J. Pharmacokinet. Biopharm.*, **10**, 637–647.

Lindstrom, F. T., Gillet, J. W. and Rodecap, S. E. (1974). Distribution of HEOD (dieldrin) in mammals: 1, preliminary model. *Arch. Environ. Contam. Toxicol.*, **2**, 9–42.

Lutz, R. J., Dedrick, R. L., Tuey, D., Sipes, I. G., Anderson, M. W. and Matthews, H. B. (1984). Comparison of the pharmacokinetics of several polychlorinated biphenyls in the mouse, rat, dog, and monkey by means of a physiological pharmacokinetic model. *Drug Metab. Dispos.*, **12**, 527–535.

Macpherson, S. E., Barton, C. N. and Bronaugh, R. L. (1996). Use of *in vitro* skin penetration data and a physiologically based model to predict *in vivo* blood levels of benzoic acid. *Toxicol. Appl. Pharmacol.*, **140**, 436–443.

Mann, S., Droz, P. O. and Vahter, M. (1996). A physiologically based pharmacokinetic model for arsenic exposure. *Toxicol. Appl. Pharmacol.*, **137**, 8–22.

Mattie, D. R., Bates, G. D., Jr, Jepson, G. W., Fisher, J. W. and McDougal, J. N. (1994). Determination of skin: air partition coefficients for volatile chemicals: experimental method and applications. *Toxicol. Appl. Pharmacol.*, **22**, 51–57.

Maxwell, D. M., Vlahacos, C. P. and Lenz, D. E. (1988). A pharmacodynamic model for soman in the rat. *Toxicol. Lett.*, **43**, 175–188.

McDougal, J. N., Jepson, G. W., Clewell, H. J., III, MacNaughton, M. G. and Andersen, M. E. (1986). A physiological pharmacokinetic model for dermal absorption of vapors in the rat. *Toxicol. Appl. Pharmacol.*, **85**, 286–294.

Medinsky, M. A., Sabourin, P. J., Lucier, G., Birnbaum. L. S. and Henderson. R. F. (1989). A physiological model for simulation of benzene metabolism by rats and mice. *Toxicol. Appl. Pharmacol.*, **99**, 193–206.

Medinsky, M. A., Bechtold, W. E., Birnbaum, L. S. and Henderson. R. F. (1990). Measurement of steady-state blood concentrations in B6C3F1 mice exposed by inhalation to vinylidene fluoride. *Toxicology*, **64**, 255–263.

Menzel. D. B. (1988). Planning and using PBPK models: an integrated inhalation and distribution model for nickel. *Toxicol. Lett.*, **43**, 67–83.

Monro, A. (1994). Drug toxicokinetics: scope and limitations that arise from species differences in pharmacodynamic and carcinogenic responses. *J. Pharmacokinet. Biopharm.*, **22**, 41–57.

Morris, J. B., Hassett, D. N., and Blanchard, K. T. (1993). A physiologically based pharmacokinetic model for nasal uptake and metabolism of nonreactive vapors. *Toxicol. Appl. Pharmacol.*, **123**, 120–129.

Mumtaz, M. M., Sipes, I. G., Clewell, H. J. and Yang, R. S. H. (1993). Risk assessment of chemical mixtures: biologic and toxicologic issues. *Fundam. Appl. Toxicol.*, **21**, 258–269.

Murphy, J. E., Jenszen, D. B. and Gargas, M. L. (1995). An *in vitro* method for determination of tissue partition coefficients of non-volatile chemicals such as 2,3,7,8-tetrachlorodibenzo-*p*-dioxin and estradiol. *J. Appl. Toxicol.*, **15**, 147–152.

Nicholas, J., Rheingans, P., Lothenbach, D., McGeachie, R., Skow, L. and McKim, J. (1994). Three-dimensional visualization of physiologically based kinetic model outputs. *Environ. Health Perspect.*, **102**, 952–956.

O'Flaherty, E. J. (1989). Interspecies conversion of kinetically equivalent doses. *Risk Anal.*, **9**, 587–598.

O'Flaherty, E. J. (1996). A physiologically based model of chromium kinetics in the rat. *Toxicol. Appl. Pharmacol.*, **138**, 54–64.

O'Flaherty, E. J., Scott, W., Schreiner, C. and Beliles, R. P. (1992). A physiologically based kinetic model of rat and mouse gestation: disposition of a weak acid. *Toxicol. Appl. Pharmacol.*, **112**, 245–256.

Pastino, G. M., Asgharian, B., Roberts, K., Medinsky, M. A. and Bond, J. A. (1997). A comparison of physiologically based pharmacokinetic model predictions and experimental data for inhaled ethanol in male and female B6C3F₁ mice, F344 rats, and humans. *Toxicol. Appl. Pharmacol.*, **145**, 147–157.

Paterson, S. and Mackay, D. (1989). Correlation of tissue, blood and air partition coefficients of volatile organic chemicals. *Br. J. Ind. Med.*, **46**, 321–328.

Paustenbach, D. J., Clewell, H. J., III, Gargas, M. L. and Andersen, M. E. (1988). A physiologically based pharmacokinetic model for inhaled carbon tetrachloride. *Toxicol. Appl. Pharmacol.*, **96**, 191–211.

Perbellini, L., Mozzo, P., Brugnone, F. and Zedde, A. (1986). Physiologicomathematical model for studying human exposure to organic solvents: kinetics of blood/tissue *n*-hexane concentrations and of 2,5-hexanedione in urine. *Br. J. Ind. Med.*, **43**, 760–768.

Plowchalk, D. R., Andersen, M. E. and DeBethizy, J. D. (1992). A physiologically based pharmacokinetic model for nicotine disposition in the Sprague–Dawley rat. *Toxicol. Appl. Pharmacol.*, **116**, 177–188.

Portier, C. J. and Kaplan, N. L. (1989). Variability of safe estimates when using complicated models of the carcinogenic process. A case study: methylene chloride. *Fundam. Appl. Toxicol.*, **13**, 533–544.

Purcell, K. J., Cason, G. H., Gargas, M. L., Andersen, M. E. and Travis, C. C. (1990). *In vivo* metabolic interactions of benzene and toluene. *Toxicol. Lett.*, **52**, 141–152.

Ramsey, J. C. and Andersen, M. E. (1984). A physiologically-based description of the inhalation pharmacokinetics of styrene in rats and humans. *Toxicol. Appl. Pharmacol.*, **73**, 159–175.

Rao, H. V., Beliles, R. P., Whitford, G. M. and Turner, C. H. (1995). A physiologically based pharmacokinetic model for fluoride uptake by bone. *Regul. Toxicol. Pharmacol.*, **22**, 30–42.

Reitz, R. H., McDougall, J. N., Himmelstein, M. W., Nolan, R. J. and Schumann, A. M. (1988). Physiologically based pharmacokinetic model with methylchloroform: implications for interspecies, high dose/low dose and dose route extrapolations. *Toxicol. Appl. Pharmacol.*, **95**, 185–199.

Reitz, R. H., Mendrala, A. L. and Guengerich, F. P. (1989). *In vitro* metabolism of methylene chloride in human and animal tissues: use in physiologically based pharmacokinetic models. *Toxicol. Appl. Pharmacol.*, **97**, 230–246.

Reitz, R. H., Mendrala, A. L., Corley, R. A., Quast, J. F., Gargas, M. L., Andersen, M. E., Staats, D. and Connolly, R. B. (1990). Estimating the risk of liver cancer associated with human exposures to chloroform using physiologically based pharmacokinetic modeling. *Toxicol. Appl. Pharmacol.*, **105**, 443–459.

Reitz, R. H., Gargas, M. L., Andersen, M. E., Provan, W. M. and Green, T.L. (1996). Predicting cancer risk from vinyl chloride exposure with a physiologically based pharmacokinetic model. *Toxicol. Appl. Pharmacol.*, **137**, 253–267.

Roth, R. A. and Vinegar, A. (1990). Action by the lungs on circulating xenobiotic agents, with a case study of physiologically based pharmacokinetic modeling of benzo (*a*)pyrene disposition. *Pharmacol. Ther.*, **48**, 143–155.

Roth, W. L., Freeman, R. A. and Wilson, A. G. E. (1993). A physiologically based model for gastrointestinal absorption and excretion of chemicals carried by lipids. *Risk Anal.*, **13**, 531–543.

Rowland, M. (1985). Physiologic pharmacokinetic models and interanimal species scaling. *Pharmacol. Ther.*, **29**, 49–68.

Sato, A. and Nakajima, T. (1979). A vial-equilibration method to evaluate the drug metabolizing enzyme activity for volatile hydrocarbons. *Toxicol. Appl. Pharmacol.*, **47**, 41–46.

Sato, A., Endoh, K., Kaneko, T. and Johanson, G. (1991a). A simulation study of physiological factors affecting pharmacokinetic behaviour of organic solvent vapours. *Br. J. Ind. Med.*, **48**, 342–347.

Sato, A., Endoh, K., Kaneko, T. and Johanson, G. (1991b). Effects of consumption of ethanol on the biological monitoring of exposure to organic solvent vapours: a simulation study with trichloroethylene. *Br. J. Ind. Med.*, **48**, 548–556.

Somani, S. M., Gupta, S. K., Khalique, A. and Unni, L. K. (1991). Physiological pharmacokinetic and pharmacodynamic model of physostigmine in the rat. *Drug Metab. Dispos.*, **19**, 655–660.

Spear, R. C., Bois, F. Y., Woodruff, T., Auslander, D., Parker, J. and Selvin, S. (1991). Modeling benzene pharmacokinetics across three sets of animal data: parametric sensitivity and risk implications. *Risk Anal.*, **11**, 641–654.

Sultatos, L. G. (1990). A physiologically based pharmacokinetic model of parathion based on chemical-specific parameters determined *in vitro*. *J. Am. Coll. Toxicol.*, **9**, 611–619.

Sultatos, L. G., Kim, B. and Woods, L. (1990). Evaluation of estimations *in vitro* of tissue/blood distribution coefficients for organothiophosphate insecticides. *Toxicol. Appl. Pharmacol.*, **103**, 52–55.

Tardif, R., Lapare, S., Krishnan, K. and Brodeur, J. (1993). A physiologically based modelling of the toxicokinetic interaction between toluene and *m*-xylene in the rat. *Toxicol. Appl. Pharmacol.*, **120**, 266–273.

Tardif, R., Charest-Tardif, G., Brodeur, J. and Krishnan, K. (1997). Physiologically based pharmacokinetic modelling of a ternary mixture of alkyl benzenes in rats and humans. *Toxicol. Appl. Pharmacol.*, **144**, 120–134.

Terry, K. K., Elswick, B. A., Welsch, F. and Conolly, R. B. (1995). Development of a physiologically based pharmacokinetic model describing 2-methoxyacetic acid disposition in the pregnant mouse. *Toxicol. Appl. Pharmacol.*, **132**, 103–114.

Tuey, D. B. and Matthews, H. B. (1980). Distribution and excretion of 2, 2′, 4, 4′, 5, 5′-hexabromobiphenyl in rats and man: pharmacokinetic model predictions. *Toxicol. Appl. Pharmacol.*, **53**, 420–431.

Vinegar, A., Winsett, D. W., Andersen, M. E. and Conolly, R. B. (1990). Use of a physiologically based pharmacokinetic model and computer simulations for retropective assessment of exposure to volatile toxicants. *Inhal. Toxicol.*, **2**, 119–128.

Vinegar, A., Williams, R. J., Fisher, J. W. and McDougal, J. N. (1994). Dose-dependent metabolism of 2,2-dichloro-1,1,1-trifluoroethane: a physiologically based pharmacokinetic model in the male Fischer 344 rat. *Toxicol. Appl. Pharmacol.*, **129**, 103–113.

ADDITIONAL READING

Clewell, H. J., III, and Andersen, M. E. (1989). Biologically motivated models for chemical risk assessment. *Health Phys.*, **57**, 129–137.

D'Souza, R. W. and Boxenbaum, H. (1988). Physiological pharmacokinetic models: some aspects of theory, practice and potential. *Toxicol. Ind. Health*, **4**, 151–171.

Thomas, R. S., Lytle, W. E., Keefe, T. J., Constan, A. A. and Yang, R. S. H. (1996). Incorporating Monte Carlo simulation into physiologically based pharmacokinetic models using advanced continuous simulation language (ACSL): a computational method. *Fundam. Appl. Toxicol.*, **31**, 19–28.

Chapter 8

Current Molecular and Cellular Concepts in Toxicology

Ian A. Cotgreave, Ralf Morgenstern, Bengt Jernström and Sten Orrenius

C O N T E N T S

INTRODUCTION AND HISTORICAL PERSPECTIVES

Our rapid approach to a new millennium of scientific endeavour heralds a growing appreciation of the wondrous complexity and integrity of biological systems. An holistic view of biological phenomena is being spurned by a combination of rapid technical advancement in biochemistry and molecular biology and some timely conceptual leaps in cell biology. These exciting developments are also currently making inroads into the science of toxicology, particularly in molecular and cellular concepts of the mechanisms of toxicity of xenobiotics.

Much of our present appreciation of cytotoxicity has been derived from attempts to define specific mechanisms of toxicity, particularly with respect to the induction of acute, necrotic cytotoxicity. However, a somewhat reductionst approach has, in the past, fostered the rather categorical view that the toxicity observed in specific cells in an intact animal is derived from a 'chain reaction' of events initiated at a 'point of insult' and rolling in a predestined manner along to the observed cytotoxicity 'end-point', classically the loss of cell viability **(Figure 1)**.

Thousands of biochemical reactions occur simultaneously in a cell and the correct integration and regulation of these are essential both to the maintenance of 'life' in a particular cell and in the expression of phenotypically specialized functions, which is the hallmark of cellular cooperation in complex tissues. Thus, classically, and rather simplistically, a basic molecular definition of toxicity can be considered in terms of a 'lowest common denominator' concept. This may constitute an alteration to the level of one particular biochemical intermediate, or in a single alteration to the function of a particular macromolecule. As biochemical events are under strict regulation and are highly integrated in the intracellular milieu, the molecular consequences of such singular alterations can quickly multiply, placing entire biochemical processes at jeopardy. At the molecular level these amplifications can occur rapidly, at rates too fast for the experimentalist to resolve temporally-specific combinations of alterations. In the toxicological setting, these alterations are often initiated by insult from chemical

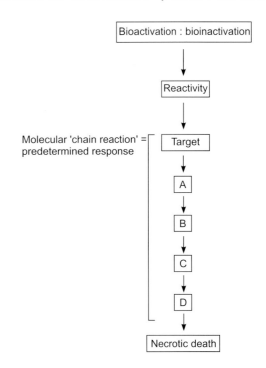

Figure 1 The simple 'straight-line' model of a molecular mechanism of toxicity. The mechanism relies on bioactivation of a foreign compound to a reactive intermediate which initiates a chain of molecular events by initial interaction with one or more cellular macromolecules.

agents, either as they are or as a result of bioactivation to reactive intermediates via the metabolic machinery of the cell (see Chapters 5 and 6).

As an illustrative example of the traditional view of molecular events in toxicity, and one illustrating the *modus operandi* of investigations during the 1980s, a great deal of effort was expended in defining molecular events occurring during the metabolism of many xenobiotics which either directly resulted in the formation of chemically reactive electrophiles or indirectly resulted in increased oxidant burden, or oxidative stress, in the cell by metabolically-driven 'redox cycling'. One typical class of agents studied were those bearing quinonoid structures.

Much early interest was drawn to the effect of quinones, such as menadione **(Figure 2)**, on cellular calcium homeostasis as a central component in the molecular mechanism of toxicity (Jewell *et al.*, 1982; Bellomo *et al.*, 1982). Incubation of hepatocytes with menadione caused sharp, concentration-dependent increases in intracellular Ca^{2+} concentrations, which were postulated to be central to the mechanisms of toxicity of the compound, particularly at concentrations of the quinone causing irreversible elevations. This event was identified to coincide with the induction of intracellular oxidative stress (Smith *et al.*, 1984) and the oxidation of cellular thiols (Di Monte *et al.*, 1984). 'Upstream' from these initial, rather central observations, efforts were then made to identify which macromolecular structure(s) were affected by the electrophiles and what was the rela-

tionship of this macromolecular damage to loss of Ca^{2+} homeostasis. Similarly, efforts were made to determine the 'downstream' metabolic consequences of elevated intracellular Ca^{2+} on the metabolic machinery of the cell. This resulted in a rather linearized vision of the mechanisms of quinone-induced necrosis in hepatocytes, originating in oxidation of critical thiol groups in calcium ion pump proteins, Ca^{2+} ATPases, in the plasma membrane (Bellomo *et al.*, 1983; Nicotera *et al.*, 1985), endoplasmic reticulum (Moore *et al.*, 1987a) and mitochondrion (Moore *et al.*, 1987b). A sustained, unregulated elevated calcium level in the cell was then shown to be associated with the activation of lipases and proteases (McConkey *et al.*, 1989; Orrenius *et al.*, 1989), resulting in cellular necrosis. Some attempts were also made to expand this view of the mechanism somewhat, by superimposing other effects of the quinone and of the oxidative stress derived from intracellular redox cycling on mitochondrial function, particularly the production of ATP and reduced nucleotides (Moore *et al.*, 1986) **(Figure 2)**. It will be noted, however, that it was not easy to determine the relative importance of each of these components of the overall process, nor was a clear temporal relationship between all of these molecular events amenable to the contemporary investigative tools.

In contrast to this rather simplistic view of molecular events in toxicity, we are now beginning to appreciate that a number of other 'players' are also involved in these processes, linking together in a 'network' of regulatory

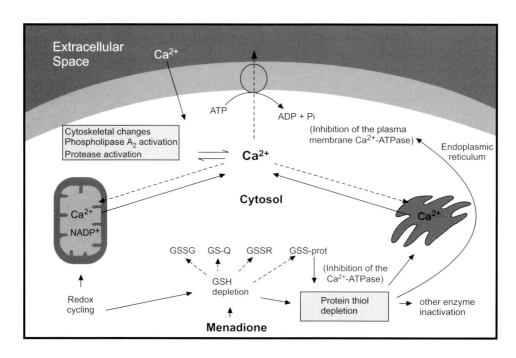

Figure 2 The molecular mechanism of menadiones cytotoxicity *anno* 1987. Menadione was shown to be acutely cytotoxic to isolated hepatocytes in association with elevated intracellular calcium concentrations. These arise from the development of oxidative stress in the cells by intracellular redox cycling, and the subsequent oxidation of cellular thiols, some in critical calcium pumps, and other redox alterations, particularly to mitochondrial pyridine nucleotide pools. The 'death effector' molecules are a variety of calcium-sensitive lipases and proteases.

devices which the cell may employ, or not, in order to conduct biochemical and biological 'decision making' as to the outcome of the insult. To this end, one major issue which has recently fuelled developments in this area of toxicology is the identification of apoptotic processes controlling 'self-deletion' of cells (McConkey *et al.*, 1996; McConkey and Orrenius, 1997) (see Chapter 9). Of equal importance has been the identification of the ability of biological systems to instigate adaptive biochemical and cytological responses to a variety of physically and chemically stressful stimuli, in both the intra- and extracellular environments (Ronai *et al.*, 1990; Dawson *et al.*, 1993; Pruett *et al.*, 1993; Leppa and Sistonen, 1997; Maines 1997). Thus, we are beginning to realise that cells are constantly subjected to changes in their physical and (bio)chemical environments, and that they are able to direct adaptive responses, many emanating from selective alterations to expression of genes, aimed at responding, in a 'pre-programmed' manner, either to increase the chances of survival and continued function of the affected cell or to initiate self-deletion in a controlled manner **(Figure 3)**.

Against these rapidly developing concepts, it is the purpose of this chapter to provide, using selective examples, those molecular and cellular concepts operating in a rather holistic vision of the complex patterns of events involved in directing the fate of the cells following toxic insult.

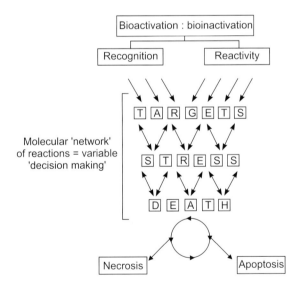

Figure 3 The 'network' theory of molecular mechanisms of toxicity. In this model, interaction of both bioactivated and inert molecules with specific combinations of cellular macromolecules initiates parallel series of reactions directed towards damage and disorder in the cells. Superimposed upon these processes are cellular homeostatic principles of repair and adaptation, so-called 'stress responses', which partake in the overall molecular decision making involved in either progression to cytotoxicity or survival of the affected cell. In the model, molecular decisions are also made in directing the mode of cell death, by either necrotic or apoptotic mechanisms.

FUNDAMENTAL MOLECULAR CONCEPTS IN TOXICITY.

Metabolism, reactivity and cytoprotection

In an evolutionary perspective, toxic insult is a natural facet in the co-evolution of plants and herbivores, which can be ultimately projected to chemical and physical interactions between 'parasite' and 'host' (Ames *et al.*, 1990) Clearly, complex multi-cellular organisms have evolved various overlapping functions in the defence of the individual against chemicals foreign to its biology, so-called xenobiotics. Thus, cells harbour different metabolic capacities (Pelkonen and Raunio, 1997) and mechanisms to sense and adapt (Van Bladeren, 1997) to changing environments on either side of their plasma membranes. In the case of the human being, this protective system has evolved so successfully that it allows the individual to ingest a multitude of potentially harmful allelochemicals of plant origin (Ames *et al.*, 1990) and man-made chemicals in gram amounts (e.g. paracetamol).

It is now well established that reactive intermediates, which are chemically capable of damaging cellular constituents (see below), are formed during the metabolism of foreign compounds (Pumford and Halmes, 1997). This 'bioactivation' should be generally regarded as normal, where reactive intermediates are being removed either directly, by detoxification enzymes (Wilkinson and Clapper, 1997), or after reaction with cellular constituents, by macromolecular repair processes (Yarosh and Kripke, 1996). In fact, many allelochemicals indeed 'signal' their presence via bioactivation and reaction with macromolecules and can themselves induce detoxication processes, thus protecting the organism, as is the case with anti-carcinogens (Kensler, 1997). From a cellular point of view, it is important to be able to 'sense' the normal situation, adjusting expression levels and/or activities of detoxification enzymes, and to react to a situation when the detoxification capacity is overwhelmed. These situations involve a number of physical and chemical concepts including the recognition of molecular shape and reactivity of xenobiotics and their metabolites, sensing modification to the levels (e.g. depletion of enzyme substrates) and/or activities of endogenous molecules, the induction of appropriate stress responses and, ultimately, either increased survival via induction of defence mechanisms or the loss of the cell by necrotic or apoptotic processes (see below).

Before briefly detailing those metabolic principles generally involved in bioactivation, it should be stated that many endogenous molecules are also metabolized by the same enzyme systems as are foreign chemicals, creating the possibility of mutual interaction in disease states

(Bolton and Shen, 1996; Iverson *et al.*, 1996). In fact, reactive intermediates also arise during the metabolism of endogenous compounds, e.g. reactive oxygen metabolites created during normal metabolism (Brumell *et al.*, 1996).

Reactive intermediates formed from xenobiotics that arise in the cell are central to the concept of cytotoxicity (Guengerich, 1993). However, reactive chemicals can also enter the body directly, e.g. ozone and nitrogen dioxide via the airways (Krishna *et al.*, 1996), or be transported between organs and cells (Koob and Dekant, 1991). These molecules can more or less specifically react with cellular constituents. As most reactive intermediates are electrophiles, cellular nucleophilic groups in protein, DNA and lipids are targets, matters which will be dealt with in more detail below.

One central component in the bioactivation scenario of relevance to the present discussion is the production of reactive, reduced metabolites of oxygen during both endogenous metabolism, i.e. the activity of cellular haemoproteins, and during the metabolism of reactive xenobiotics by processes such as 'redox cycling'. A situation of intracellular 'oxidative stress' results from an imbalance between oxidative events (unavoidably occurring in an aerobic milieu) and the corresponding antioxidant defence systems (Halliwell and Gutteridge, 1989). Superoxide dismutase, catalase and various glutathione peroxidases are central in the maintenance of low levels of the superoxide anion radical, hydrogen peroxide, nitric oxide and lipid hydroperoxides (Halliwell and Gutteridge, 1989). Dietary components (e.g. vitamin C and E, selenium and carotenoids) are also incorporated into the cellular antioxidant network, making it one of the most elaborate defence networks in biological systems (Halliwell and Gutteridge, 1989).

There is now a large body of literature which shows that, during the process of toxic insult, cellular homeostasis is compromised, commonly resulting in oxidative stress. Both redox cycling xenbiotics and reactive electrophiles can deplete cellular reducing equivalents, notably GSH, and, thus, compromise the ability of cells to reduce hydrogen peroxide and lipid hydroperoxides. An unchecked accumulation of these compounds leads to damage of cellular constituents, particularly the process of lipid peroxidation which gives rise to products that are strongly electrophilic and cytotoxic (e.g. hydroxyalkenals) (Esterbauer, 1993). This situation can now be defined as one of 'oxidant-mediated degradation'. On the other hand, it is now becoming appreciated that the term oxidative stress should be somewhat redefined to accommodate emerging evidence for a central role for endogenously these reactive oxygen and nitrogen intermediates in the correct regulation of normal processes in the cell, so-called 'oxidant-mediated regulation' (Cotgreave and Gerdes, 1998). Examples of this include the activity of redox-sensitive transcription factors (Nakamura *et al.*, 1997), the vasodilatory function of

nitric oxide (Joyner and Dietz, 1997) and use as regulators for lipoxygenases (Ursini *et al.*, 1997).

On a more integrated biological level, physiological processes, such as inflammation and pathophysiological conditions such as ischaemia–reperfusion, are also accompanied by oxidative stress (Halliwell and Gutteridge 1989). Hence these processes demand that cells can cope with, and respond correctly to, the degree of insult experienced locally. This is especially relevant as it is generally considered biologically harmful to surrounding healthy tissues if a group of cells undergo uncontrolled necrosis, releasing reactive substances resulting from oxidative stress, instead of controlled apoptosis (see below).

Having stated the importance of oxidative stress in toxicity and the decisive role of the antioxidant network in controlling events that occur in it, one must finally stress, however, that the exposure of biological systems to the vast and changing variety of xenobiotics is clearly different in its complexity to the situation of oxidative stress, where a limited number of key reactive oxygen species and secondary reactive compounds are formed. This has presented considerable pressure throughout evolution to develop detoxification systems able to cope with this adequately. Thus, xenobiotic detoxification enzymes are numerous and display broad specificity, e.g. phase I enzymes such as the cytochrome(s) P450 and the phase II conjugation glucuronyl-, sulpho- and glutathione-S-transferases, whereas the defence against oxidative stress involves relatively fewer enzymes. However, it should be remembered that some secondary products of oxidative stress, e.g. lipid and DNA hydroperoxides and reactive lipid breakdown products such as aldehydes, are substrates for both glutathione peroxidases and glutathione-S-transferases, thus linking again the two detoxification processes. Vital to this defence is glutathione.

Molecular 'targets' for reactive intermediates and their metabolic repair

One of the central buttresses in the study of molecular mechanisms of toxicity has been the concept that toxic agents, or their metabolites, interact with one or many macromolecular structures in cells, forming more or less stable complexes which, if unrepaired, can alter the defined function of the structure(s) affected (see Chapter 6). This, in turn, forces integrated biochemical processes out of step with each other, increasing the overall entropy of the cell. Such interactions may involve either direct covalent bond formation between the parent substance and/or metabolite and a protein, lipid and/or nucleic acid, often dependent on considerable parent chemical reactivity, or non-covalent interactions. In the latter case in particular, a high degree of molecular 'recognition' between the two interacting species is a prerequisite in the process. Of equal importance, it is now also apparent that each class of macromolecules is served by homeo-static repair mechanism(s), whose activities must be considered in the overall toxicity mechanism. In the next section we will briefly discuss the concept of 'molecular targets', using selected examples illustrating reactive intermediate interactions with cellular proteins and nucleic acids.

Proteins as molecular targets for reactive intermediates

Proteins contain a large number of nucleophilic sites which may undergo modification by reaction with electrophilic agents. Indeed, many amino acids undergo post-translation modification during natural processing of proteins to their functional states (Rando, 1996; Zhang and Casey, 1996). Of these chemical groups, the ionizable sulphydryl group of protein cysteinyl residues occupies a special position, based on its favourable redox chemistry under physiological conditions and the relatively high nucleophilicity of the thiolate anionic form of this functional group (Cotgreave et al., 1990). It should be stated at the outset, however, that the reaction between an electrophilic xenobiotic and nucleophilic protein thiols is controlled by a large number of chemical and physical factors, with respect both to the agent involved and to the protein undergoing modification. These factors include the correct partitioning of the agent in and around the intracellular milieu, correct access, proximity and orientation of the agent with respect to potential thiol reaction sites in proteins and the ionization status of the reacting thiol, which is mainly governed by the local electrostatic environment in the protein (Torchinski, 1981). It is imperative to understand that all protein thiols are not of equivalent nucleophilicity under physiological conditions and that most protein thiols will react with individual characteristics in proteins in intact cellular systems.

During the 1980s, many instances of xenobiotic adduct formation to cellular protein thiols were documented. As an example, work conducted in our institute with the analgesic drug paracetamol, or acetaminophen, clearly showed that the reactive intermediate, N-acetyl-p-benzoquinone imine (NABQI) (Dahlin et al., 1984), generated by a cytochrome P450-dependent reaction, forms adducts with hepatocellular proteins, via reaction with native thiol groups (Rundgren et al., 1988). In analogy with the case of manadione, this was clearly associated with the inhibition of a variety of key enzymes and ion pumps in the cells, including plasma membrane and endoplasmic reticulum Ca^{2+} ATPases and a number of enzymes controlling mitochondrial integrity and function (Nicotera et al., 1989). With the appropriate development of selective analytical techniques involving the derivatization of cellular protein thiols with the mem-

brane-permeable, thiol-reactive fluorigen monobromo-bimane, accompanied by the derivation of antibodies to proteins adducted with NAPQI, some selectivity of S-alkylation of hepatocellular protein was detected for NAPQI under conditions of acute necrotic toxicity (Bartolone et al., 1988). However, other studies showed that the bulk of the alkylation occurs rather indiscriminately (Weis et al., 1992).

In view of the methodological difficulties, however, to date few attempts have been made to correlate altered protein function finitely with the formation of a particular S-alkyl group in a specific protein. Similarly, it must be stated that no enzymatic repair mechanisms have been defined which are capable of regenerating reduced thiol groups from corresponding S-alkyl derivatives. However, the cell is able to respond to such damage via facilitated degradation of protein (Beynon and Bond, 1986). The efficiency of this reparative process in the overall scheme of toxicity is, however, constitutively dependent on the resynthesis of new, functional proteins.

Another, more subtle, manner in which toxic substances can affect protein thiol homeostasis is via their redox modification. Over the years, a number of lines of evidence have emerged supporting a fundamental role for redox modification of certain proteins in normal cellular biochemistry and physiology, as well as in pathophysiological processes. Of particular interest is the possibility that the most abundant low molecular weight thiol-containing endogen glutathione (GSH) is able to interact with protein cysteine in a reversible manner.

Several lines of evidence have emerged supporting this concept (Ziegler, 1985; Gilbert, 1990). Many purified proteins have been shown to be sensitive to thiol–disulphide interchange reactions. These include enzymes involved in intermediate metabolism, such as glucose-6-phosphate dehydrogenase and carbonic anhydrase, some involved in signal transduction, such as 5'-lipoxygenase and guanylate cyclase, and even enzymes of protein catabolism, such collagenase and trypsin (Cotgreave et al., 1990). These discoveries are continuing and notable recent additions to this list include the homodimeric HIV-1 protease, with suggestions that the action of this protease may be partially regulated by redox changes to its cysteines by S-glutathionylation (Davis et al., 1996).

The occurrence of GSH–protein mixed disulphides in cells and tissues has long been utilized as strong evidence that these processes have significance in intact biological systems (Ziegler, 1985; Cotgreave et al., 1989). However, most of the early observations of bulk quantities of GSH bound to cellular protein were made in association with the development of intracellular oxidative stress (Bellomo et al., 1987; Nakagawa et al., 1992). GSH–protein mixed disulphides have also been demonstrated in a variety of tissues, again mostly during oxidative stress. For instance, mixed disulphide formation has been recently shown to be associated with embryo toxicity elicited by oxidative stress during organogenesis in the rat conceptus (Hiranruengchok and Harris, 1995). Additionally, the accumulation of protein–GSH mixed disulphides in lens crystallins has long been proposed to be a molecular linker between oxidative stress and the development of cataracts, particularly in relation to diabetes (Luo *et al.*, 1995). Several lines of evidence are also emerging that mixed disulphide formation is of importance in the response of the mitochondrion to oxidative stress (Cohen *et al.*, 1997), particularly in mitochondrial membrane permeability changes induced by peroxides and peroxynitrite as an early event in the induction of apoptosis (Scarlett *et al.*, 1996).

Attempts have been made to determine the specificity of these *S*-glutathionylation reactions at the protein level. Patterns of *S*-glutathionylated proteins have been noted in many cell types formed during oxidative stress in intact cells (Grimm *et al.*, 1985). Such pattern recognition has, in most cases, been extended to identification of the major *S*-glutathionylated proteins. Thus, carbonic anhydrase III was identified as a substrate in hepatocytes during quinone-, peroxide-and neutrophil-promoted oxidative stress (Chai *et al.*, 1991). Other substrates include creatine kinase and glycogen phosphorylase b (Park and Thomas, 1989) in oxidant-treated myocytes and glyceraldehyde-3-phosphate dehydrogenase in peroxide-treated endothelial cells (Schuppe-Koistinen *et al.*, 1994) and in monocytes during the endogenous oxidative burst (Ravichandran *et al.*, 1994). Another common substrate identified in both endothelial cells (Schuppe-Koistinen *et al.*, 1995) and gastric mucosal cells (Rokutan *et al.*, 1994) is the structural protein actin. Here, reversible *S*-glutathionylation of the protein has been associated with alterations to the cytoskeletal organization of the cells in response to oxidative stress.

One important series of evidence which supports a central role for *S*-glutathionylation of cellular protein as a link between oxidative stress and alterations to cellular phenotype is the demonstration that the processes are generally reversible. The reversibility of *S*-glutathionylation of protein after oxidative stress has clearly been demonstrated in a number of cell types (Schuppe-Koistinen *et al.*, 1994a; Seres *et al.*, 1996). Several studies have shown that the reductive cleavage of mixed disulphides in intact cells involves both NADH- and NADPH-dependent processes involving 'dethiolase' enzymes with properties similar to those of mammalian thioredoxin (TRX)–thioredoxin reductase (TRXred) system and that of glutaredoxin (GRX) (Park and Thomas, 1989). More recent work has clearly implicated roles for both TRX and GRX in the reductive cleavage of GSH–protein mixed disulphides in intact cells (Fernando *et al.*, 1992, Jung and Thomas, 1996). The latter work clearly delineated GRX as the primary catalyst of mixed disulphide cleavage. This is not surprising in view of the affinity of TRX (Holmgren and Åslund, 1995) and PDI (Freedman *et al.*, 1995) for inter- and intra-peptide disulphides, and the established preference

of GRX for mixed disulphides between GSH and proteins (Gravina and Mieyal, 1993), selectivity dictated by the presence of the γ-L-glutamyl-L-cysteinyl moiety of GSH in the disulphide (Rabenstein and Millis, 1995).

Another more discrete line of evidence for a physiological function of reversible *S*-glutathionylation of proteins arises from the association of *S*-glutathionylation with the initiation and maintenance of complex, integrated physiological processes. Indeed, the efficient reversible regulation of mixed disulphide formation in intact cells has led to suggestions that the reactions may serve as a quantitatively relevant antioxidant function in cells (Thomas *et al.*, 1995), particularly endothelial cells (Schuppe-Koistinen *et al.*, 1994b). Indeed, it may be suggested that the efficiency of this freely reversible redox process may constitute a primitive, non-specific cellular glutathione peroxidase activity.

This basic property of cellular systems may have served as an evolutionary stimulus to the development of specific glutathione peroxidase proteins. Increased levels of mixed disulphide formation have also been shown to prime monocytes for the production of reactive oxygen species during the stimulated respiratory burst (Moriguchi *et al.*, 1996). However, perhaps the most important issue which may, in the future, find a place in this list of biological end-points containing links with reversible modification of cellular proteins extends to processes controlling cell proliferation, under both physiological and pathophysiological conditions. There is emerging evidence suggesting that reversible interactions of GSH with selected cellular proteins may be an important molecular link between the occurrence of oxidative stress in cells and the control of cell proliferation, at the levels of both mitogenesis and apoptosis (Cotgreave and Gerdes, 1998).

Nucleic acids as molecular targets

The genetic material is composed of deoxyribonucleic acid (DNA) and the structure and strict orderliness of these macromolecules are the basis for the existence of all organisms living today. A human diploid cell contains about 6×10^9 base pairs (bp), corresponding to about 2 m of nuclear DNA linearly arranged in a double helical structure. In order to be accommodated in the limited space of the nucleus, DNA, theoretically occupying a volume corresponding to about 6×10^{-12} cm^3, has to be packed in an increasing order of complexity. First, DNA is organized in nucleosomes in which 145–147 bp are wrapped around an octameric core of basic proteins, two each of histones H2A, H2B, H3 and H4, to form a disk-like nuclesome core particle (Luger *et al.*, 1997). This highly conserved complex occurs essentially every 200 ± 40 bp throughout the genome. Thus, the nuclesome core particles are separated by linkers of a variable number of bp to form a 'beads on a string' type of organization (McGhee and Felsenfeld, 1980). Histone

H1, which is localized where DNA enters and then leaves the nucleosome core particle, allows further condensation (about 30–40-fold) of DNA by close packing of nucleosomes on top of each other forming 30 nm thick fibers (Felsenfeld and McGhee, 1986).

These fibres form higher orders of structure which constitute the chromatin in the interphase cell. In addition to being complexed with histones, DNA in chromatin is associated with non-histone proteins, which are proteins with a wide range of functions. The DNA:histone:non-histone protein ratio is about 1:1:1, hence the chromatin is composed of one part of DNA and two parts of proteins, based on weight. Chromatin is divided into heterochromatin and euchromatin. The latter constitutes the major part of the chromatin and is more dispersed than heterochromatin. Gene activities such as replication, repair and transcription are associated with euchromatin and are believed to take place at the inner nuclear membrane to which loops of chromatin fibres containing about 30–100 kbp are attached (Berezney et al., 1996). Genetically active chromatin usually constitutes not more than a few per cent of total chromatin.

In addition to nuclear DNA, cytoplasmic DNAs are a crucial part of eukaryotic cells. It is an integral part of the mitochondria and is inherited in a non-Mendelian fashion from the female. The genome of the mitochondria is not associated with structural histone proteins as expected, considering its similarity with prokaryotes and suggested origin (Gray, 1989). Essential enzymes involved in respiration are among other proteins coded for by the mitochondrial genome (Attardi, 1985).

More than 15 potential nucleophilic sites are present in the nucleotide bases of DNA. Accordingly, in the total nuclear DNA of a human cell about 50×10^9 base targets for electrophilic attack are present. In addition, the phosphorus atoms of the phophodiester linkages are also potential targets for modification. The nucleophilic base sites are in principle accessible either via the minor groove (N-1 and N-3 of dA and O^2, and N-3 of dT, N-1, N-3 and N^2 of dG, and O^2 and N-3 of dC) or via the major groove (N^2 and N-7 of dA and O^4 of dT, and C-8 and N-7 and O^6 in dG and N^4 in dC). However, these potential targets are not freely available for interactions with electrophiles owing to the complex structural organization of DNA.

Rather than being randomly distributed throughout the genome, the nucleophilic sites available for reactions are strongly restricted by a number of factors. Such factors include the histone and non-histone proteins associated with nuclear DNA, the extent of chromatin condensation (i.e. euchromatin vs heterochromatin or chromosomes), whether DNA is involved in replication or transcription, or the distance of a potential target and the site of formation of the electrophile. Thus, since most reactive electrophiles are formed either in the ER or in the vicinity of the nuclear membrane and usually have short half-lives, a target close to the nuclear inner membrane is more likely to be modified than a corresponding target remote from the nuclear membrane. Furthermore, since gene activities are believed to take place at or close to the nuclear inner membrane (Berezney et al., 1996) and, consequently, the DNA is in a relatively 'loose' state, targets in this fraction of the genome are more prone to be modified than others. Another factor to consider with regard to adduct formation is the organization of DNA in nucleosomes. DNA associated with the histone octamer is in general less susceptible than DNA constituting the linkers. Moreover, the preference for the minor groove at d(A + T)-rich regions to interact with the histone octamer (Travers, 1987) renders such targets less accessible than dG and dC.

Two classes of electrophilic molecules can be distinguished which are able to interact with DNA. One class of molecules contains an atom with a partial or full positive charge and another class of molecules contains one or more unpaired electrons in their outer orbital. The former class of electrophiles are most often formed by metabolic activation involving cytochrome(s) P450, whereas the latter class, or free radicals, are formed either by homolytic fission of a covalent bond or by accepting or losing an electron. This may occur either spontaneously or by the assistance of reductases. Both classes of electrophiles interact with nucleophilic centres in DNA. A wide variety of electrophilic intermediates exist, ranging from small-sized hydroxyl radicals to large homo- or heterocyclic hydrocarbons. Furthermore, the electrophilic centre may involve oxygen, nitrogen, carbon, sulphur and various metals.

For instance, dimethylnitrosamine alkylates DNA (e.g. at position O^4 in dT and O^6 and N-7 in dG) following metabolic activation and formal production of a methylcarbocation (Archer and Labuc, 1985). Aromatic amines react with DNA (e.g. C-8, O^6 and N^2 in dG) following metabolism to hydroxylamines and formal production of nitrenium ions and carbocations (Kriek and Westra, 1978). Simple, unsaturated alkenes may form epoxides and give rise to subsequent formation of DNA adducts at the N-7 position of dG (Hemminki et al., 1980). More complex hydrocarbons, such as polycyclic aromatic hydrocarbons, are sequentially metabolized to so-called bay- and fjord region diol epoxides, which react preferentially with the exocyclic amino groups of dA or dG via cis or trans addition (Geacintov et al., 1997). Halogenated alkenes may form reactive S-episulphonium ions through a two-step reaction with glutathione and subsequent adduct formation at N-7 of dG (Koga et al., 1986). Radicals derived from oxygen, such as the hydroxyl radical, may react with dG at the C-8 position in dG forming 8-hydroxy-dG or with the pyrimidines to yield various hydroxylated products (Floyd, 1990).

Since all cellular activities and processes have their origin in the genome, uncontrolled DNA modification and adduct formation may have a number of unwanted and harmful effects. One specific adduct may initiate a cascade of events. The most obvious effect of adducts are the interference with proper replication and transcription. For instance, alkylation of O^6 in dG or O^4 in dT abolishes proper base pairing with dC and dA, respectively, during replication, but may base pair with dT and dA, respectively (Singer and Essigmann, 1991). These changes result in transition mutations and, if these occur in critical positions in oncogenes or suppresser genes, cell transformation and tumours may eventually be formed. Alkylation of the phophodiesters in DNA may affect the charge distribution and influence protein–DNA interactions. Bulky adducts, such as those derived from aromatic amines and polycyclic aromatic hydrocarbons, do not in general abolish the possibility of proper base pairing but interfere with the replication machinery in a hitherto unknown way. However, independently of whether such adducts are localized at the exocyclic amino groups of dA or dG, at C-8 or N-7 of dG, transversion mutations (i.e. GC → TA or AT → TA) are preferentially formed following replication (Loechler, 1996).

DNA adducts may be harmless to resting cells but acutely toxic to dividing cells by blocking DNA replication. Since bulky adducts may differ in their spatial orientation and may adopt different conformations (Geacintov et al., 1997), an intricate interplay between mutagenicity and acute toxicity exists. Bulky adducts localized in genes undergoing transcription inhibit elongation (Choi et al., 1994) and, thus, the production of complete RNA molecules and the further processing of functioning proteins. Adducts may interfere with transcription in an alternative way by interfering with the interaction of general or specific transcription factors with their binding sequences in DNA (Persson et al., 1996). In this case, altered gene expression and gene 'dosage' may be the consequence.

A great number of factors are known or expected to influence adduct formation. The most trivial factor is the cellular uptake of the compound giving rise to electrophiles and DNA adducts. This factor is fulfilled by the fact that most adduct precursors are highly lipophilic and, thus, are easily taken up by the cells by passive diffusion. Another crucial factor is the balance between the process of metabolic activation, i.e. the balance between the rate of electrophile formation and the process of electrophile elimination. If the rate of formation is higher than the rate of elimination of electrophiles, these may accumulate and find their way to DNA targets. Similarly, if the reverse is true, no DNA adduct formation is expected. Other factors are associated with the transport of electrophiles from their site of formation to their targets. Low molecular weight nucleophiles, in addition to those associated with various proteins, are expected to capture electrophiles en route to the nucleus. The same can be expected from a number of processes involving enzymes participating in conjugation reactions.

As mentioned above, the structural organization of DNA, in conjunction with a clear preference of certain electrophilic intermediates for specific targets in DNA, are important factors underlying the non-random adduct formation seen when analysing the adduct distribution. Another important factor is the size and stereochemical properties of the DNA-interacting molecule. The effect of size is well illustrated by the adduct distribution of dimethyl- and diethylnitrosamine. The former demonstrates a high preference for N-7 alkylation of dG, whereas the more bulky diethyl analogue reacts substantially less at this position of dG but rather forms phosphotriesters (Pegg, 1984). The importance of stereochemical factors can be illustrated by compounds such as the polycyclic aromatic hydrocarbons. Aflatoxin B_1, a potent toxin and carcinogen produced by the mould *Aspergillus flavus*, can in principle be activated to a pair of epoxide enantiomers (the *endo-* and *exo-* isomers). The *exo-*isomer binds almost exclusively to the N-7 position in dG and with the bound residue intercalated on the 5'-end of the adducted base (Raney et al., 1993). The chemically equally reactive *endo-*isomer shows no reactivity at all. This illustrates the importance of a well defined pre-reaction complex between the electrophile and the DNA target. Another example is the polycyclic aromatic hydrocarbon benzo[*a*]pyrene, a well studied environmental mutagen and carcinogen. This compound is activated to diol epoxide intermediates which can exist in a pair of diastereomers and each of these as a pair of enantiomers. Thus, in total, four stereoisomers are possible. These compounds react either via *cis* or *trans* addition with a high preference to the exocyclic amino group in dG (Jernström and Gräslund, 1994). Owing to the chirality of the molecules, the structures of the adducts differ greatly, and so do the biological responses. For instance, the *trans* adduct of the most mutagenic and carcinogenic isomer is localized in the minor groove of DNA and with the chromophore directed towards to 5'-side of the adducted strand. The corresponding enantiomer is also localized in the minor groove but directed towards the 3'-side (Jernström and Gräslund, 1994). This adduct is considerably less mutagenic and carcinogenic, but more toxic. This may be due to a more efficient inhibition of DNA replication considering the direction of DNA synthesis (3' → 5').

Since the physical interaction between a lipophilic compound and DNA precedes the formation of the pre-reaction complex and adduct formation, both DNA configuration, double-stranded vs single-stranded form, and the base sequence context adjacent to the reaction target are additional factors which influence the adduct distribution. In addition, in a normal, well functioning cell, the formation and accumulation of covalent adducts is restricted by surveillance systems such as different DNA repair processes.

Molecular target recognition and interactions not dependent on metabolic activation

In the above examples, one common factor is the formation of novel covalent interactions between often bioactivated foreign chemicals and nucleophilic sites on macromolecules. This is, however, not the only prerequisite to such effects and substances may directly 'fit' into binding sites on macromolecules. Indeed, this is the basis of most of the pharmacological activity of foreign chemicals. As one example of this currently receiving considerable attention, large families of rather metabolically inert polychlorinated aromatic compounds exist, which elicit some of their systemic toxicity by disturbing the normal biological regulation elicited by hormones and other signal substances. Thus, polychlorinated biphenyls (PCBs), their hydroxylated metabolites, and many other organochlorine insecticides elicit sex steroid-mimetic activity by binding to specific receptors belonging to the oestrogen receptor family (Safe and Sacharewsky, 1997). Indeed, the estrogenic activity of many of these agents is of considerable toxicological concern at the moment in terms of the risks for breast cancer in exposed human populations. Similarly, many dioxins, including 2,3,7,8-tetrachlorodibenzo-p-dioxin (TCDD) (Birnbaum, 1994), and dietary agents such as indolcarbazoles (Kleman et al., 1994), bind to the aryl hydrocarbon (ah) receptor (Poellinger, 1996), resulting in a cascade of signal transduction events involving heat shock proteins (HSPs), aryl hydrocarbon nuclear translocator protein (arnt) and other specific elements of the MAPP kinase pathway (Pratt, 1997). These ultimately result in altered expression of a wide variety of genes, including those of hormones and associated receptors and metabolic regulators. Thus, TCDD has been shown to affect the circulatory levels of, for example, thyroid hormones (T3 and T4) (Schuur et al., 1997), luteinizing hormone (LH) and follicle-stimulating hormone (FSH) (Li, X. et al., 1997) and melatonin (Pohjanvirta et al., 1996).

In addition to these xenobiotic–protein interactions, direct interactions can occur between foreign compounds and nucleic acids, particularly DNA. A great number of compounds have been shown to form physical complexes with DNA. Such compounds include intercalating substances such as aminoacridines and ethidium bromide, and other less complex dyes (Waring, 1986) or molecules containing an intercalating part and branched substituents composed of carbohydrate or peptide residues (Geierstanger and Wemmer, 1995). Examples of these are antibiotics such as actinomycin D and mitramycin. Other compounds form physical complexes with DNA by interacting with one of the grooves, in particular the minor one. Diaminopropidium iodide (DAPI) and netropsin are typical examples of non-intercalating agents that exhibit a great preference for interacting in the minor groove at AT-rich sequences. These compounds are positively charged and their preference is probably due to the negative electrostatic potential of AT tracts (Geierstanger and Wemmer, 1995). Various biochemical/biological effects of agents which interact physically with DNA are evident since these compounds include both antibiotics and chemotherapeutic agents.

CELLULAR CONCEPTS OF TOXICITY

Apoptosis and necrosis

At the cellular level, the lowest common denominator of toxicity which has been traditionally utilized is that of loss of cellular integrity, resulting in necrotic cytolysis. This is amply exemplified by the work discussed in the Introduction. However, more recently several other concepts have evolved in the area which further complicate our initial rather simplistic interpretations of cellular toxicity mechanisms. These include the activation of apoptotic and programmed cell death mechanisms, subjects which will be specifically dealt with in Chapter 9.

Apoptosis is a regulated form of cell death which counterbalances mitosis during normal physiological regulation of cell populations in tissues (McConkey et al., 1996). Apoptosis can also be inadvertently initiated during toxic insult by apogenic substances (Corcoran et al., 1994), and is operative during the development of a variety of disease states (Orrenius, 1995). Alternately, suppression of apoptosis through, for example, interference in cell signalling, can result in abberant accumulation of cells in the development of a number of pathologies, most notably in cancer (Rowan and Fisher, 1997).

The complex biochemical and cellular processes governing the process of apoptosis are now becoming clear. These include activation of nascent components in signal transduction pathways, and also the induction of altered gene expression. Several key biochemical components have been identified in the apoptotic process, including cytoskeletal rearrangements, such as the dismantling of nuclear scaffold structures (Zhivotovsky et al., 1997b), the fragmentation of nuclear DNA (Zhivotovsky et al., 1994), the rearrangement of plasma membrane phospholipid organization (Fadok et al., 1992), the activation of specific membrane-associated receptors and accompanying signal transduction devices, such as the TNF-α receptor family (Darnay and Aggarwal, 1997), and alterations to mitochondrial function, such as the depolarization of mitochondrial membranes and the release of cytochrome c (Wallace et al., 1997). A central role for oxidative stress and alterations to intracellular cacium homeostatis has also been proposed (McConkey and Orrenius, 1997). Thus, many central components in both the signal transduction mechanisms relaying

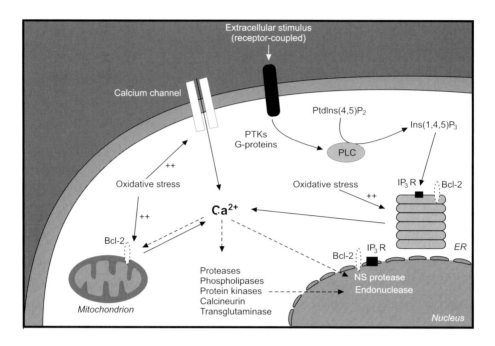

Figure 4 Changes in intracellular calcium concentration play a central role in some apoptotic processes, particularly during the generation of intracellular oxidative stress.

pro-apoptotic stimuli into cells and in the biochemical 'executioners' carrying out the apoptotic programme are reliant on fluxes in intracellular calcium concentrations **(Figure 4)**.

All of the above aspects of apoptotic processes are adequately detailed in Chapter 9. However, one area of research which is not only revealing key players in apoptotic processes, but also elegantly illustrates the power of patterning in biochemical regulation, is the case of the growing family of proteolytic proteins, the caspases.

Caspases are a class of cysteine protease with 'aspase' (aspartic acid-specific) activity, that play a critical role during apoptosis (Alnemri *et al.*, 1996). Although the term caspase refers to the human enzymes, many animal species possess homologues of this enzyme. At least 10 of these proteases have been identified in human cells (Zhivotovsky *et al.*, 1997a) **(Figure 5)**. The enzymes are normally present as proenzymes in the cytoplasm and, upon activation, the caspases cleave a variety of cellular proteins whose relationship to the death process is often unclear. However, a recent study into the substrate specificities of caspase family members has divided these proteases into three distinct groups. Two of these caspase families appear to be associated with different phases of the apoptotic process (Thornberry *et al.*, 1997). Several of the target proteins reside in the nucleus and are related to DNA repair mechanisms. Since the dormant caspases are present in the cytoplasm, it is generally assumed that, after activation, they must be imported into the nucleus in order to cleave nuclear proteins. This hypothesis is supported by findings with reconstituted systems, in which apoptotic degradation of nuclei isolated from untreated cells is achieved by incubation with the S-100 cytosolic fraction from apoptotic cells (Lazebnik *et al.*, 1993; Schlegel *et al.*, 1996). This suggests that nuclei are accessible to activated proteases and/or endonucleases present in the cytosol of apoptotic cells. Indeed, a caspase-activated endonuclease that can cleave chromatin at internucleosomal sites has been identified recently in the cytoplasm (Enary *et al.*, 1998).

Caspases are synthesized in a precursor form, and an apoptotic signal then converts the pro-caspase into the mature enzyme (Zhivotovsky *et al.*, 1997a). At least two pro-caspases, pro-caspase-8 and -1, are activated via oligomerization-induced autoproteolysis (Yang *et al.*, 1998). In contrast, pro-caspase-3, the best characterized executioner caspase, does not initiate activation in an autocatalytic manner. Activation of this enzyme requires an initiating first-step cleavage, probably by other pre-existing cellular caspases, followed by a second auto-proteolytic step.

In a search for biochemical components involved in caspase cascade activation, three apoptotic protease-activating factors (Apaf 1–3) were recently purified from a cell-free system based on cytosol from normal cells (Liu, X., *et al.*, 1996; Li, P. *et al.*, 1997; Zou *et al.*, 1997). One of these proteins (Apaf-2) was recognized as cytochrome *c*. Apaf-1 has a shared similarity with the pro-domain of CED-3 and CED-4 (the genes responsible for programme cell death in *C. elegans*) and Apaf-3 was identified as a member of the caspase family, pro-caspase-9. The binding of Apaf-3 to Apaf-1 is dependent on the presence of cytochrome *c* and dATP (ATP). This event leads to pro-caspase-9 activation. Activated

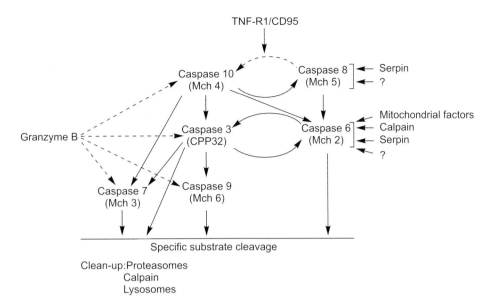

Figure 5 Molecular interactions between caspases in apoptosis. Delicate patterns of interaction exist between cellular caspases, which control the death effector stage of apoptosis. Auto-regulatory cleavage loops are apparent but it should be noted that the relative importance of each interaction in the cascade depends on the apogenic signal employed and, importantly, the cell type involved.

caspase-9 in turn cleaves and activates pro-caspase-3. Thus, cytochrome *c* plays a cofactor role in the activation of the proteolytic cascade. Although holocytochrome *c* is a mitochondrial protein, it has been demonstrated that following exposure of cells to apoptotic stimuli, cytochrome *c* is rapidly released from mitochondria into the cytosol (Kharbanda *et al.*, 1997; Kluck *et al.*, 1997a; Yang *et al.*, 1997). Additional experiments showed that cytochrome *c* release in apoptotic cells can precede changes in mitochondrial membrane potential (Kluck *et al.*, 1997a; Yang *et al.*, 1997). It was further reported that anti-apoptotic proteins of the Bcl-2 family prevent this translocation of cytochrome *c* from mitochondria to cytosol and thereby interfere with the subsequent activation of cytosolic caspases and apoptosis (Kluck *et al.*, 1997a; Yang *et al.*, 1997). It has recently been demonstrated that addition of exogenous cytochrome *c* to cytosolic extracts from normal cells induces caspase activation (Liu, X. *et al.*, 1996). Cytosolic caspase activation was only observed with intact holocytochrome *c* (Kluck *et al.*, 1997b, Hampton *et al.*, 1998). Neither heat-denatured cytochrome *c* nor enzyme-degraded cytochrome *c* (microperoxidase-11, the haem group of cytochrome *c* with amino acids 11–21) was able to substitute for holocytochrome *c* (Kluck *et al.*, 1997b; Hampton *et al.*, 1998). Cytochrome P450, cytochrome *b₅*, haemoglobin, biotinylated cytochrome *c* and apocytochrome *c* were also ineffective in this respect, showing the importance of the presence of unmodified cytochrome *c* in this reaction (Hampton *et al.*, 1998).

Although it appears that caspase family members play a most important role in promoting apoptotic cell death,

evidence has been advanced that other proteases are also involved in sequential or parallel steps of apoptosis. For example, the relative contribution of the proteolytic activity of calpain and also proteasomes to the apoptotic process may vary between different types and triggers of apoptosis (Zhivotovsky *et al.*, 1997a).

Irrespective of whether apoptotic or necrotic mechanisms are operating in cells suffering toxic insult, the net effect is that cells with defined phenotype are removed from the tissue or organ. In the former case, however, the cytolytic necrosis results in the activation of an inflammatory response which can amplify the damage in the affected tissue, events which may also spread to other organs if the inflammatory state perpetuates. Hence it must be considered advantageous, from a biological point of view, to possess areas of common interface between apoptosis and necrosis, which may allow some molecular control in directing intoxicated cells away from necrosis into apoptotic deletion. Indeed, increasing evidence is suggesting that the two forms of cell demise share similar characteristics, at least in the signalling and early progression phase.

We are only now beginning to understand those factors which govern molecular switching between necrosis and apoptosis. One of the initial observations in this field clearly identified the basic pharmacological/toxicological principles of dose and time of exposure as molecular 'weigh-masters'. Thus, incubation of RINm5F cells with the redox-cycling quinone 2,3-dimethoxy-1,4-naphthoquinone was shown either to stimulate cell proliferation, trigger apoptosis or cause necrosis, with increasing dose and/or duration of the exposure (Dypbukt *et al.*, 1994).

In later experiments with neuronal cells it was again clear that the mode of cell killing exerted during NMDA-induced excitotoxicity, thought to be involved in a number of neurodegenerative diseases including focal ischaemia, trauma, epilepsy, Huntington's disease and Alzheimer's disease, was dependent on the intensity and levels of NMDA exposure. Additionally, NMDA receptor-mediated neurotoxicity was shown to depend, in part, on the generation of nitric oxide ($NO^\bullet$) and superoxide anion ($O_2^{-\bullet}$), which react to form peroxynitrite ($OONO^-$) in the cells. Again, the mode of cell killing was greatly dependent on the level of oxidative stress imposed on the neuronal cell cultures by peroxynitrite (Leist *et al.*, 1997a). Collectively, in addition to providing some of the first data on a role of dose and time of exposure in switching between apoptosis and necrosis, these experiments give strong evidence for a central role of intracellular oxidative stress in apoptosis.

Knowledge of other more specific factors involved in the molecular interface between apoptosis and necrosis is beginning to evolve. Studies indicate that glutamate, released from neurones during ischaemia, can induce either early necrosis or delayed apoptosis in cultures of cerebellar granule cells. During and shortly after exposure to glutamate, a sub-population of the cells was shown to die by necrosis, characterised by acute collapse of the mitochondrial membrane potential. Cells surviving the early necrotic phase recovered mitochondrial potential and mitochondrial energy (ATP) levels. However, later, these cells underwent apoptosis, as shown by the formation of apoptotic nuclei and by chromatin degradation into high and low molecular weight DNA fragments. These results suggest that mitochondrial function is a critical factor that determines the mode of neuronal death in excitotoxicity (Ankarcrona *et al.*, 1995).

In narrowing the scope of critical switching alterations even further, a central role for the absolute level of ATP in the cell is emerging. Thus, apogenic treatment of human T cells, previously depleted of their ATP, resulted in necrotic cytotoxicity. However, selective and graded repletion of the extra-mitochondrial ATP pool with glucose prevented necrosis and restored the ability of the cells to undergo apoptosis. Pulsed ATP/depletion/repletion experiments also showed that ATP generation, either by glycolysis or by the mitochondria, was required for the active execution of the final phase of apoptosis, which involves nuclear condensation and DNA degradation (Leist *et al.*, 1997b). These results indicate a critical weigh-master role for ATP in directing the mode of cell death, with apoptosis being logically favoured by the presence of sufficient ATP to drive energy-requiring and coordinated processes in the apoptotic programme (Leist and Nicotera, 1997) **(Figure 6)**. These findings have now gained support in other systems (Eguchi *et al.*, 1997; Pang and Gedes, 1997). Many other studies have provided overwhelming evidence placing mitochondrial

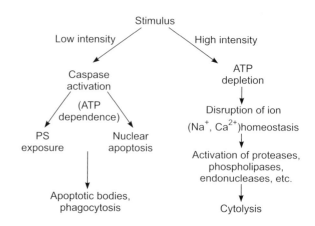

Figure 6 The 'weigh-master' role of cellular ATP in dictating the mode of cell death in intoxicated cells. The absolute levels of intracellular ATP maintained during toxic insult may determine the mode of cell death. Situations causing serious depletion of ATP may favour death by necrosis, i.e. random, chaotic degeneration, whereas moderate ATP depletion may favour the execution of energy-requiring processes associated with apoptosis, i.e. organized degeneration.

function at the heart of apoptotic processes, particularly the role of membrane potential and cytochrome *c* release. These are dealt with in more detail in Chapter 9.

CELLULAR STRESS RESPONSES

Functioning as a buffer in the molecular decision making governing the eventual outcome of a toxic insult **(Figure 2)**, is the ability of biological systems to mount an adaptive response to the stress. This may occur by re-routing existing resources in the cell, e.g. enzyme redundancy or the activation of parallel metabolic alternatives such as that seen in oxidative stress-dependent rerouting of glucose metabolism away from glycolysis and into pentose phosphate metabolism (Brigelius, 1985). However, most adaptive responses in biological systems result from selective alterations in the expression in the pattern of cellular gene expression. On the one hand this may involve the induction of genes whose products provide protective action in the cell, stimulate reparative processes and/or inhibit the intiation of apoptotic processes. On the other hand, specific gene supressions may also be envisaged as a component of the cellular adaptation. Adaptation may also involve selective alterations in the patterns of expressions controlling apoptotic processes resulting in the deletion of cells unable to conduct their normal physiological functions and/or beyond reparative rescue.

The concept of cellular stress response has been developed as a result of observations of biochemical and genetic reflexes in cells as a result of exposure to a variety of physical and chemical alterations to their environment.

Physical stress

Some of the initial evidence came from the adaptive alterations to cellular biochemistry exhibited by cells in response to heat shock (Leppa and Sistonen, 1997). It is now clear that the cell is able to alter the availability of a variety of cellular components, mostly proteins, in order to cope with the effects of aberrant temperature. The response to heat shock is a ubiquitous phenomenon amongst all eukaryotic cells and is a primitive sensor-response mechanism reacting to this fundamental 'danger' in biological systems. The archetypal components were termed 'heat shock proteins' or HSPs (Schedl et al., 1978) and are now known constitute a family of about 15 proteins exhibiting molecular chaperone activity (Morimoto et al., 1996). In addition, it is now becoming clear that these proteins are a part of everyday cellular life, performing important endogenous functions in the absence of heat shock. These chaperone proteins are rapidly induced by heat shock and the pattern of proteins induced is both cell-specific and dependent on the grade and duration of the shock. The proteins mostly function by stabilizing partially or 'quasi'-folded proteins (Freeman and Morimoto, 1996) and they are thought to contribute greatly to the molecular decision making as to whether cellular proteins should be degraded, repaired or allowed to aggregate, the last of which is a phenomenon often associated with terminal cytotoxicity. Indeed, the interaction between HSPs and quasi-folded proteins is a level of regulation of protein function which has generally not been considered previously. The HSPs are also actively involved in the re-folding of proteins into their native tertiary structures (Freeman and Morimoto, 1996).

In mounting the stress response, inducible heat shock factors (HSFs) have been identified (Morimoto et al., 1996; Kanei-Ishii et al., 1997), which function as molecular linkers between the physical stress and the transcription of chaperone proteins. Interestingly, anti-inflammatory drugs, such as corticosteroids and nonsteroidal agents, have been shown to increase HSF-1 expression, thus lowering the temperature at which cells react with a heat shock response (Lee et al., 1995).

Another physical factor to which most terrestrial organisms have always been exposed is UV radiation. Exposure to UVB has been shown to induce adaptive alterations to gene expression in the skin, particularly within keratinocytes. UVB-induced activation of the Rel/NF$_\kappa$b signalling pathway in keratinocytes has been shown to be involved in the molecular mechanism of signal transduction from the 'reception' of the stimulus to the level of the genome (Tobin et al., 1996). The cREL/Nf$_\kappa$b system seems to be stimulated by UVB through a tight cascade of events starting at the TNF-α receptor on the cell surface. Despite this, the identity of the initial 'energy transducer' is still unknown, but it is clear that the signal propagates by rapid association of TRAF-2 to the receptor (Tobin et al., 1998). This complex then activates I$_\kappa$b kinase, in turn releasing the active REL-A/cREL dimer for nuclear translocation.

Electrophilic stress

The treatment of cells with electrophilic agents has been shown to induce adaptive responses which help to direct the fate of the affected cells. As an illustrative example of this, the treatment of animals with the nephrotoxin dichlorovinylcysteine (DCVC) results in DNA binding of the molecule, which is mirrored by the simultaneous induction of a wide variety of stress-related genes, such as c-myc, c-fos, GADD153 and HSP70. The ornithine decarboxylase gene was also identified as a target in the DCVC-induced apoptotic pathway involving c-myc expression. However, histochemical evidence suggests that the proximal epithelial cells traverse from symptoms of classical apoptosis at early time points in the insult to clearly necrotic changes later. Interestingly, the closely related analogue tetrafluoroethylenecysteine (TFEC) does not cause DNA damage, is incapable of inducing c-myc and never gives rise to apoptosis in the proximal tubule of the kidney (Zhan et al., 1997). This elegantly illustrates that gene products such as c-myc, normally considered to be pro-proliferatory in its activity, may have multiple functions, depending on which combinations of other growth-regulatory gene products are present.

These halogenated chemicals cause a variety of changes to kidney epithelial cells, some of which are clearly indicative of the induction of intracellular oxidative stress. These include changes to cellular calcium compartmentation (Chen et al., 1994), the induction of lipid peroxidation and the oxidation of cellular thiols, particularly in proteins (Liu, H. et al., 1996). In model studies with the the thiol alkylator iodoacetamide, a variety of acute effects were induced in kidney epithelial cells, which are rather contradictory in their nature. In addition to causing acute necrotic or apoptotic injury in cells, adaptive inductions of stress proteins were also detected, which were associated with increased resistance of surviving cells to subsequent insult (Liu et al., 1997). One of the initially identified components of this adaptive response was HSP70. Iodoacetamide induces the expression of HSP70 via an activation of HSF-1. The alkylation of proteins was not, however, sufficient to induce the expression, but the counteracting effects of DTT suggested that the accumulation of oxidized (disulphide-linked) proteins in the cell served as the molecular trigger to the response (Liu, H. et al., 1996). However, subjecting the cells to heat shock alone fails to induce tolerance to the alkylator in renal epithelial cells. Further studies then identified that the chaperone molecules grp78 and grp94, endoplasmic equivalents of the soluble chaperones HSP70 and HSP90, respectively, and calreticullin, are all induced during iodoacetamide treatment of cells. The induction of these endoplasmic reticulum (ER) stress components were critical to the adaptive response of the cells to electrophilic insult, contributing to preventing disturbances in intracellular calcium (Liu *et al.*, 1997). Interestingly, the same group had previously shown that some of these proteins were actually targets for alkylation during the stress (Bruschi *et al.*, 1993). By monitoring the effects of ER stress on parameters associated with the induction of apoptosis and necrosis, these studies clearly position intracellular calcium in the molecular decision making resulting from stress modulation of apoptosis and necrosis. Hence, it is apparent that the actual loss of ER calcium during insult is associated with induction of apoptotic events, whilst a sustained rise in cytosolic calcium is associated with the induction of necrotic cell death. Thus, events able to buffer intracellular calcium will prevent necrotic toxicity, whereas agents able to prevent ER calcium loss are predicted to prevent apoptotic deletion in these cells.

Reductive stress

In a related series of experiments, a sharp interface between the adaptive alterations to ER stress proteins caused by alkylation agents and effects of agents affecting the cellular protein thiol redox balance were also provided by the demonstration that both oxidized and reduced thiols affect the expression of ER stress components at the genomic level. Thus, the induction of so-called reductive stress by incubation of cells with reduced thiols has been shown to activate the ER stress responses detailed above. The dithiol dithiothreitol (DTT) was particularly active in these inductive events (Halleck *et al.*, 1997a). Treatment of kidney epithelial cells with DTT also induced the expression of GADD 153, a protein normally associated with induction of 'genomic stress', for instance via the induction of multiple mutations. The induction was direct and not due to the production of oxidants in the cell by autoxidation of the thiol groups in the agent. Interestingly, other studies have shown that the oxidized form of DTT, *trans*-4,5-dihydroxy-1,2-dithiane, is also able to induce the ER response elements in renal epithelial cells, but not the classical heat shock element HSP70 (Halleck *et al.*, 1997b). In these experiments, oxidized DTT did not induce oxidative stress in the cells. However, it was shown to force the cells into consumption of reducing equivalents, indicating the involvement of cellular oxidoreductases in dictating the generation of reductive stress.

Oxidative stress

In terms of stress responses, one of the major phenomena identified in the area is that of oxidative stress. An imbalance in the pro-oxidant to antioxidant ratio in cells results in a build-up of oxidants in the cell and the generation of a state of oxidative stress. The concept of oxidative stress has been debated ostensibly in the context of the induction of necrotic cell lesions, as discussed earlier. Similarly, oxidative stress is being implicated in the execution of apoptotic programming (see earlier), as well as a factor involved in the stimulation of cellular proliferation (Payne *et al.*, 1995; Cotgreave and Gerdes, 1998). For the purposes of the discussion here, we will now detail some of the salient points implicating oxidative stress in adaptive processes involved in deciding the fate of cells undergoing toxic insult.

Some of the early observations in the 1980s clearly showed that cells exposed to pro-oxidants, such as hyperbaric oxygen, induced adaptive responses contributing to increased tolerance to the insult by the induction of antioxidant defence enzymes (Cotgreave *et al.*, 1988). However, it was not until the turn of this decade that clues as to the molecular sensors involved were revealed. These were in the form or redox-sensitive transcription factors, such as AP-1, $Nf_\kappa b$, p_{53} and SP-1, whose DNA-binding activity and stimulatory effects on gene expression are reliant on the redox status of cysteinyl thiols in their structures (Sun and Oberley, 1996). Many genes have now been identified whose expression can be directly or indirectly modulated by redox alterations to transcription factors. These include antioxidant enzymes, adhesion molecules, cytokines, stress proteins, proteins involved in transcription and proteins involved in the regulation of cell cycle (Curran, 1992).

An illustrative example of the role of oxidative stress in deciding the fate of cells comes from observations in experimental models of hippocampal responses to ischaemia. This model allows for studies in adaptive responses primarily because of differential responses exhibited by locally juxtaposed areas of the tissue in this area of the brain (Nellgard *et al.*, 1991). Thus, septal and thalamic cells of the C1 region undergo slow apoptotic deletion in response to hypoxia, whereas nearby granular cells in the C3 region are very resistant to the induction of such damage (Petito *et al.*, 1997). Fundamental differences in cell signalling and adaptive gene expression exist in these two areas of the brain in response to ischaemia, which determine progression to apoptosis in the C1 region and which promote survival in the C3 region. Genes such as *HSP70*, *c-fos*, *c-jun*, P_{53}, *BAX* and BCL_2 all seem to be involved in the molecular decision processes involved in directing these selective responses, but at present we are unable to define role(s) for each of these gene products in the overall patterns of expression detected. However, in terms of patterns of expression, it seems that the duration of expression of early response genes is coupled to the outcome of the stress response. Thus, rapid and transient over-expression of several of these genes is associated with the resistant phenotype of the C3 region, whereas sustained over-expression seems to be a prelude to apoptosis in the C1 region (Kamme and Wieloch, 1996a, b; Clark *et al.*, 1997; Parsadanian *et al.*, 1998).

Common Features in Stress Responses

As we begin to develop a more holistic view of molecular events in stress responses, it is becoming clear that interfaces also exist between the various processes described above. For instance, it is clear that induction of a heat shock response in tissue, involving primary induction of molecular chaperones, can have a major impact on situations of cell and tissue toxicity initiated by oxidative stress (Choi and Alam, 1996; Huot *et al.*, 1996; Marini *et al.*, 1996; Park *et al.*, 1998). Several studies now indicate that the prior induction of a classical heat shock response imparts considerable protection in both cells and the intact organism against ichemic injury (Andreeva *et al.*, 1997; Nakano *et al.*, 1997; Suzuki *et al.*, 1997). Indeed, it has been proposed that the induction of heat shock proteins may be intricately involved in the primary function of the state of fever seen in the tissue inflammation response to injury or infection (Lee *et al.*, 1995). This highlights a possible therapeutic use of heat shock stress. Thus, despite the present conceptual difficulties in the targeting of heat shock stress response, made none-the simpler by the evident variability of HSP expression in humans, the concept may prove very useful in disease management in the future.

Expanding on the theme of commonality, it is becoming apparent that many other biochemical components, particularly those involved in intracellular signal transduction and alteration to gene expression, are shared by the various stress responses discussed above. This is testament to the efficient, integrated manner in which biological systems have evolved adaptive stress responses to many stimuli which have occurred simultaneously during evolution.

CONCLUSION AND FUTURE TRENDS

The response of individual cells to chemical and/or physical insult seems pluripotent, driven by a limited number of rather fundamental biological needs. On the surface it seems that two basic options are open. Either the cell is to survive the insult outright and continue a defined function in the higher order of biological organization, or the cell is doomed to perish, hopefully to be replaced by new cells of the correct phenotype. Clearly, in terms of our present view of molecular and cellular events in toxicity, one further subtle option seems to be widely employed by cells, namely that of adaptive modification of cellular phenotype. This ensures advantageous changes to cellular phenotype capable of meeting the demands of continued insult and/or subsequent challenges. As this adaptation concept emerges, it is becoming clear that

delicate and dynamic lattice-works of biochemical processes are involved in cellular responses to stress during toxic insult. Having said this, the biological 'decision making' guiding the choice made in a particular cell between these options will certainly depend on the integration of a wide variety of intra-and extracellular influences.

In order to proceed conceptually and practically in this area of toxicology, we are now being required to take a rather holistic view of biochemistry and biology, away from that of our normal 'reductionist' approaches. However, the need to decipher complex patterns of biochemical alterations in cells, in association with the induction of toxicity and cellular stress, is currently being supported by some very rapid technical developments, particularly in the field of molecular biology. Thus, our knowledge of intracellular signal transduction mechanisms is accumulating rapidly. This is clearly exemplified by our present understanding of molecular events involved in directing necrotic and apoptotic changes in cells. Additionally, rapid developments in molecular biological tools is expanding our knowledge of the human genome, its organization and the regulation of expression of individual genes. Indeed, at present, a number of techniques exist which allow for the rapid 'array' of complex patterns of gene expression. These include differential display PCR (Liang and Pardee, 1997), serial analysis of gene expression (SAGE) (Velculescu *et al.*, 1995) and various solid-phase cDNA micro-array devices (Heller *et al.*, 1997). Thus, we are rapidly approaching a time where roboticized, chip-based screening of the entire cDNA expression library of a particular cell is a routine possibility. Similarly, rapid developments in two-dimensional protein separation, coupled to automated sequencing, so-called 'proteomics' (Fey *et al.*, 1997), is opening a portal to pattern recognition at the protein level. Combining these conceptual advancements and methodological possibilities will ensure that, by the turn of the century, we may be able to predict comfortably the outcome of toxic insult, be it adaptative survival, necrotic or apoptotic deletion or cell proliferation, based on the determination of distinctive biochemical 'fingerprints' of events, occurring at early time points in the cellular response to toxic insult.

REFERENCES

Alnemri, E. S., Livingston, D. J., Nicholson, D. W., Salvesen, G., Thornberry, N. A., Wong, W. W. and Yuan, J. (1996). Human ICE/CED-3 protease nomenclature. *Cell*, **87**, 171–178.

Ames, B. N., Profet, M. and Gold, L. S. (1990). Nature's chemicals and synthetic chemicals: comparative toxicology. *Proc. Natl. Acad. Sci. USA*, **87**, 7782–7786.

Andreeva, L, Motterlini, R. and Green, C. J. (1997). Cyclophilins are induced by hypoxia and heat stress in myogenic cells. *Biochem. Biophys. Res. Commun.*, **237**, 6–9.

Ankarcrona, M., Dypbukt, J. M., Bonfoco, E, Zhivotovsky, B., Orrenius, S., Lipton, S. A. and Nicotera, P. (1995). Glutamate-induced neuronal death: a succession of necrosis or apoptosis depending on mitochondrial function. *Neuron*, **15**, 961–973.

Archer, M. C. and Labuc, G. E. (1985). Nitrosamines. In Anders, M. W. (Ed.), *Bioactivation of Foreign Compounds*. Academic Press, New York, pp. 403–431.

Attardi, G. (1985). Animal mitochondrial DNA: an extreme example of economy. *Int. Rev. Cytol.*, **93**, 93–146.

Bartolone, J. B., Birge, R. B., Sparks, K, Cohen, S. D. and Khairallah, E. A. (1988). Immunochemical analysis of acetaminophen covalent binding to proteins. Partial characterization of the major acetaminophen-binding liver proteins. *Biochem. Pharmacol.*, **37**, 4763–4774.

Bellomo, G, Jewell, S. A. and Orrenius, S. (1982). The metabolism of menadione impairs the ability of rat liver mitochondria to take up and retain calcium. *J. Biol. Chem.*, **257**, 11558–11562.

Bellomo, G., Mirabelli, F., Richelmi, P. and Orrenius, S. (1983). Critical role of sulfhydryl group(s) in ATP-dependent Ca^{2+} sequestration by the plasma membrane fraction from rat liver. *FEBS Lett.*, **163**, 136–139.

Bellomo, G., Mirabelli, F., DiMonte, D., Richelmi, P., Thor, H., Orrenius, C. and Orrenius, S. (1987). Formation and reduction of glutathione–protein mixed disulfides during oxidative stress. A study with isolated hepatocytes and menadione (2-methyl-1,4-naphthoquinone). *Biochem. Pharmacol.*, **36**, 1313–1320.

Berezney, R., Mortillaro, M., Ma, H., Meng, C., Smarabandu, J., Wei, X., Somanthan, S., Liou, W. S., Pan, S. J. and Cheng, P. C. (1996). Connecting nuclear architecture and genomic function. *J. Cell. Biochem.*, **62**, 223–226.

Beynon, R. J. and Bond, J. S. (1986). Catabolism of intracellular protein: molecular aspects. *Am. J. Physiol.*, **251**, C141–C152.

Birnbaum, L. S. (1994). The mechanism of dioxin toxicity: relationship to risk assessment. *Environ. Health Perspect.*, **102**, 157–167.

Bolton, J. L. and Shen, L. (1996). *p*-Quinone methides are the major decomposition products of catechol estrogen *o*-quinones. *Carcinogenesis*, **17**, 925–929.

Brigelius, R. (1985). Mixed disulphides: biolgical functions and increase in oxidative stress. In Sies, H. (ed.), *Oxidative Stress*. Academic Press, London, pp. 243–272.

Brumell, J. H., Burkhardt, A. L., Bolen, J. B. and Grinstein, S. (1996). Endogenous reactive oxygen intermediates activate tyrosine kinases in human neutrophils. *J. Biol. Chem.*, **271**, 1455–1461.

Bruschi, S. A., West, K. A., Crabb, J. W., Gupta, R. S. and Stevens, J. L. (1993). Mitochondrial HSP 60 (P1 protein) and HSP70-like protein (mortalin) are major targets for modification during S-(1,1,2,2-tetrafluoroethyl)-1-cysteine-induced nephrotoxicity. *J. Biol. Chem.*, **268**, 23157–23161.

Chai, Y. C., Jung, C. H., Lii, C. K., Ashraf, S. S., Hendrich, S., Wolf, B., Sies, H. and Thomas, J. A. (1991). Identification of an abundant S-thiolated rat liver protein as carbonic anhydrase III; characterization of S-thiolation and dethiolation reactions. *Arch. Biochem. Biophys.*, **284**, 270–278.

Chen, Q., Jones, T. W. and Stevens, J. L. (1994). Early cellular events couple covalent binding of reactive metabolites to cell killing by nephrotoxic cysteine conjugates. *J. Cell Physiol.*, **161**, 293–302.

Choi, A. M. and Alam, J. (1996). Heme oxygenase-1: function, regulation, and implication of a novel stress-inducible protein in oxidant-induced lung injury. *Am. J. Resp. Cell Mol. Biol.*, **15**, 9–19.

Choi, D. J., Marino-Alessandri, D. J., Geacintov, N. E. and Scicchitano, D. A. (1994). Site specific benzo[a]pyrene diol epoxide–DNA adducts inhibit transcription elongation by bacteriophage T7 RNA polymerase. *Biochemistry*, **33**, 780–787.

Clark, R. S., Chen, J., Watkins, S. C., Kochanek, P. M., Chen, M., Stetler, R. A., Loeffert, J. E. and Graham, S. H. (1997). Apoptosis-suppressor gene bcl-2 expression after traumatic brain injury in rats. *J. Neurosci.*, **17**, 9172–9182.

Cohen, G., Farooqui, R. and Kesler, N. (1997). Parkinson disease: a new link between monoamine oxidase and mitochondrial electron flow. *Proc. Natl. Acad. Sci. USA*, **94**, 4890–4894.

Corcoran, G. B., Fix, L., Jones, D. P., Moslen, M. T., Nicotera, P., Oberhammer, F. A. and Buttyan, R. (1994). Apoptosis: molecular control point in toxicity. *Toxicol. Appl. Pharmacol.*, **128**, 169–181.

Cotgreave, I. A., Moldéus, P. and Orrenius, S. (1988) Host antioxidant defence against prooxidants. *Annu. Rev. Pharmacol. Toxicol.*, **28**, 189–213.

Cotgreave, I. A., Atzori, L. and Moldéus, P. (1989). Thiol–disulfide exchange: physiological and toxicological aspects. In Damani, L. A. (Ed.), *Sulphur Drugs and Related Chemicals*. Vol. 2B. Ellis Horwood, Chichester, pp. 101–119.

Cotgreave, I. A., Weis, M. and Moldéus, P. (1990). Glutathione and protein function. In Vina, J. (Ed.), *Glutathione: Metabolism and Physiological Function*. CRC Press, Boca Raton, FL, pp. 155–179.

Cotgreave, I. A. and Gerdes, R. (1998). Recent trends in glutathione biochemistry: glutathione protein interactions: a molecular link between oxidative stress and cell proliferation? *Biochem. Biophys. Res. Commun.*, **242**, 1–9.

Curran, T. (1992). Fos and Jun: oncogenic transcription factors. *Tohoku J. Exp. Med.*, **168**, 169–174.

Dahlin, D. C., Miwa, G. T., Lu, A. Y. and Nelson, S. D. (1984). N-Acetyl-*p*-benzoquinone imine: a cytochrome P-450-mediated oxidation product of acetaminophen. *Proc. Natl. Acad. Sci. USA* **81**, 1327–1331.

Darnay, B. G. and Aggarwal, B. B. (1997). Early events in TNF signaling: a story of associations and dissociations. *J. Leuk. Biol.*, **61**, 559–566.

Davis, D. A., Dorsey, K., Wingfield, P. T., Stahl, S. J., Kaufman, J., Fales, H. M. and Levine, R. L. (1996). Regulation of HIV-1 protease activity through cysteine modification. *Biochemistry*, **35**, 2482–2488.

Dawson, T. L., Gores, G. J., Nieminen, A. L., Herman, B. and Lemasters, J. J. (1993). Mitochondria as a source of reactive oxygen species during reductive stress in rat hepatocytes. *Am. J. Physiol.*, **264**, C961–C967.

Di Monte, D., Bellomo, G., Thor, H., Nicotera, P. and Orrenius, S. (1984). Menadione-induced cytotoxicity is associated with protein thiol oxidation and alteration in intracellular Ca^{2+} homeostasis. *Arch. Biochem. Biophys.*, **235**, 343–350.

Dypbukt, J. M., Ankarcrona, M., Burkitt, M., Sjöholm, A., Ström, K., Orrenius, S. and Nicotera, P. (1994). Different prooxidant levels stimulate growth, trigger apoptosis, or produce necrosis of insulin-secreting RINm5F cells. The role of intracellular polyamines. *J. Biol. Chem.*, **269**, 30553–30560.

Eguchi, Y., Shimizu, S. and Tsujimoto, Y. (1997). Intracellular ATP levels determine cell death fate by apoptosis or necrosis. *Cancer Res.*, **57**, 1835–1840.

Enari, M., Sakahira, H., Yokoyama, H., Okawa, K., Iwamatsu, A. and Nagata, S. (1998). A caspase-activated DNase that degrades DNA during apoptosis, and its inhibitor ICAD. *Nature*, **391**, 43–50.

Esterbauer, H. (1993). Cytotoxicity and genotoxicity of lipid-oxidation products. *Am. J. Clin. Nutr.* **57**, S779–S786.

Fadok, V. A., Voelker, D. R., Campbell, P. A., Cohen, J. J., Bratton, D. L. and Henson, P. M. (1992). Exposure of phosphatidylserine on the surface of apoptotic lymphocytes triggers specific recognition and removal by macrophages. *J. Immunol.*, **148**, 2207–2216.

Felsenfeld, G. and McGhee, J. D. (1986). Structure of the 30 nm chromatin fiber. *Cell*, **44**, 375–377.

Fernando, M. R., Nanri, H., Yoshitake, S., Nagata-Kuno, K. and Minakami, S. (1992). Thioredoxin regenerates proteins inactivated by oxidative stress in endothelial cells. *Eur. J. Biochem.*, **209**, 917–922.

Fey, S. J., Nawrocki, A., Larsen, M. R., Gorg, A., Roepstorff, P., Skews, G. N., Williams, R. and Larsen, P. M. (1997). Proteome analysis of *Saccharomyces cerevisiae*: a methodological outline. *Electrophoresis*, **18**, 1361–1372.

Floyd, R. A. (1990). Role of oxygen free radicals in carcinogenesis and brain ischemia. *FASEB J.*, **4**, 2587–2597.

Freedman, R. B., Hawkins, H. C. and MacLaughlin, S. H. (1995). Protein disulfide-isomerase. *Methods Enzymol.*, **251**, 397–406.

Freeman, B. C. and Morimoto, R. I. (1996). The human cytosolic molecular chaperones HSP90, HSP70 (HSC70) and hdj-1 have distict roles in recognition of non-native protein and protein refolding. *EMBO J.*, **15**, 2969–2979.

Geacintov, N., Cosman, M., Hingerty, B. E., Amin, S., Broyde, S. and Patel, D. (1997). NMR solution structures of stereomeric polycyclic aromatic carcinogen-DNA adducts: principles, patterns and diversity. *Chem. Res. Toxicol.*, **10**, 111–146.

Geierstanger, B. H. and Wemmer, D. E. (1995). Complexes of the minor groove of DNA. *Annu. Rev. Biomol. Struct.*, **24**, 463–493.

Gilbert, H. F. (1990). Molecular and cellular aspects of thiol–disulfide exchange. *Adv. Enzymol. Reat. Areas Mol. Biol.*, **63**, 69–172.

Gravina, S. A. and Mieyal, J. J. (1993). Thioltransferase is a specific glutathionyl mixed disulfide oxidoreductase. *Biochemistry*, **32**, 3368–3376.

Gray, M. W. (1989). Origin and evolution of mitochondrial DNA. *Annu. Rev. Cell. Biol.*, **5**, 25–50.

Grimm, L. M., Collison, M. W., Fisher, R. A. and Thomas, J. A. (1985). Protein mixed-disulfides in cardiac cells. *S*-Thiolation of soluble proteins in response to diamide. *Biochim. Biophys. Acta*, **844**, 50–54.

Guengerich, F. P. (1993). The 1992 Bernard B. Brodie Award Lecture. Bioactivation and detoxication of toxic and carcinogenic chemicals. *Drug Metab. Dispos.*, **21**, 1–6.

Halleck, M. M., Holbrook, N. J., Skinner, J., Liu, H. and Stevens, J. L. (1997a). The molecular response to reductive stress in LLC-PK1 renal epithelial cells: Coordinate transcriptional regulation of GADD 153 and grp78 genes by thiols. *Cell Stress Chaperones*, **2**, 31–40.

Halleck, M. M., Liu, H., North, J. and Stevens, J. L. (1997b). Reduction of *trans*-4,5-dihydroxy-1,2-dithiane by cellular oxidoreductases activates GADD153/chop and grp78 transcription and induces cellular tolerance in kidney epithelial cells. *J. Biol. Chem.*, **272**, 21760–21766.

Halliwell, B. and Gutteridge, J. M. C. (1989). *Free Radicals in Biology and Medicine*. Clarendon Press, Oxford.

Hampton, M. B., Zhivotovsky, B., Slater, A. F. G., Burgess, D. H. and Orrenius, S. (1998). Importance of the redox state of cytochrome *c* during caspase activation in cytosolic extracts. *Biochem. J.*, **329**, 95–99.

Heller, R. A., Schena, M., Chai, A., Shalon, D., Bedilion, T., Gilmore, J., Woolley, D. E. and Davis, R. W. (1997). Discovery and analysis of inflammatory disease-related genes using cDNA microarrays. *Proc. Natl. Acad. Sci. USA*, **94**, 2150–2155.

Hemminki, K., Paasivirta, J., Kurkirinne, T. and Virkki, L. (1980). Alkylation products of DNA bases by simple epoxides. *Chem.–Biol. Interact.*, **30**, 259–270.

Hiranruengchok, R. and Harris, C. (1995). Diamide-induced alterations of intracellular thiol status and the regulation of glucose metabolism in the developing rat conceptus *in vitro*. *Teratology*, **52**, 196–204.

Holmgren, A. and Åslund, F. (1995). Glutaredoxin. *Methods Enzymol.*, **252**, 199–208.

Huot, J., Houle, F., Spitz, D. R. and Landry, J. (1996). HSP27 phosphorylation-mediated resistance against actin fragmentation and cell death induced by oxidative stress. *Cancer Res.*, **56**, 273–279.

Iverson, S. L., Shen, L., Anlar, N. and Bolton, J. L. (1996). Bioactivation of estrone and its catechol metabolites to quinoid-glutathione conjugates in rat liver microsomes. *Chem. Res. Toxicol.*, **9**, 492–499.

Jernström, B. and Gräslund, A. (1994). Covalent binding of benzo[*a*]pyrene 7,8-dihydrodiol 9,10-epoxide to DNA: molecular structures, induced mutations and biological consequences. *Biophys. Chem.*, **49**, 185–199.

Jewell, S. A., Bellomo, G., Thor, H., Orrenius, S. and Smith, M. (1982). Bleb formation in hepatocytes during drug metabolism is caused by disturbances in thiol and calcium ion homeostasis. *Science*, **217**, 1257–1259.

Joyner, M. J. and Dietz, N. M. (1997). Nitric oxide and vasodilation in human limbs. *J. Appl. Physiol.*, **83**, 1785–1796.

Jung, C. H. and Thomas, J. A. (1996). *S*-Glutathiolated hepatocyte proteins and insulin disulfides as substrates for reduction by glutaredoxin, thioredoxin, protein disulfide isomerase, and glutathione. *Arch. Biochem. Biophys.*, **335**, 61–72.

Kamme, F. and Wieloch, T. (1996a). Induction of junD mRNA after transient forebrain ischemia in the rat. *Brain Res. Mol. Brain Res.*, **43**, 51–56.

Kamme, F. and Wieloch, T. (1996b). The effect of hypothermia on protein synthesis and the expression of immediate early genes following transient cerebral ischemia. *Adv. Neurol.*, **71**, 199–206.

Kanei-Ishii, C., Tanikawa, J. N., Akai, A. *et al.* (1997). Activation of heat shock transcription factor 3 by c-myb in the absence of cellular stress. *Science*, **277**, 246–248.

Kensler, T. W. (1997). Chemoprevention by inducers of carcinogen detoxication enzymes. *Environ. Health Perspect.*, **105**, 965–970.

Kharbanda, S., Pandey, P., Schofield, L., Israels, S., Roncinske, R., Yoshida, K., Bharti, A., Yuan, Z. M., Saxena, S., Weichselbaum, R., Nalin, C. and Kufe, D. (1997). Role for Bcl-xL as an inhibitor of cytosolic cytochrome *c* accumulation in DNA damage-induced apoptosis. *Proc. Natl. Acad. Sci. USA*, **94**, 6939–6942.

Kleman, M. I., Poellinger, L. and Gustafsson, J. Å. (1994). Regulation of dioxin receptor function by indolcarbazoles, receptor ligands of dietary origin. *J. Biol. Chem.*, **269**, 5137–5144.

Kluck, R. M., Bossy-Wetzel, E., Green, D. R. and Newmeyer, D. D. (1997a). The release of cytochrome *c* from mitochondria: a primary site for Bcl-2 regulation of apoptosis. *Science*, **275**, 1132–1136.

Kluck, R. M., Martin, S. J., Hoffman, B. M., Zhou, J. S., Green, D. R. and Newmeyer, D. D. (1997b) Cytochrome *c* activation of CPP32-like proteolysis plays a critical role in a *Xenopus* cell-free apoptosis system. *EMBO J.*, **16**, 4639–4649.

Koga, N., Inskeep, P. B., Harris, T. M. and Guengerich, F. P. (1986). *S*-[2-(*N*^{7}-Guanyl) ethyl]glutathione, the major DNA adduct formed from 1,2-dibromoethane. *Biochemistry*, **25**, 2192–2198.

Koob, M. and Dekant, W. (1991). Bioactivation of xenobiotics by formation of toxic glutathione conjugates. *Chem.–Biol. Interact.*, **77**, 107–136.

Kriek, E. and Westra, J. G. (1978). Metabolic activation of aromatic amines and amides and interactions with nucleic acids. In Grover, P. H. (Ed.), *Chemical Carcinogens and DNA*, Vol. II. CRC Press, Boca Raton, FL, pp. 1–28.

Krishna, T., Springall, D. R., Frew, A. J., Polak, J. M. and Holgate, S. T. (1996). Mediators of inflammation in response to air pollution: a focus on ozone and nitrogen dioxide. *J. R. Coll. Physicians London*, **30**, 61–66.

Lazebnik, Y. A., Cole, S., Cooke, C. A., Nelson, W. G. and Earnshaw, W. C. (1993). Nuclear events of apoptosis *in vitro* in cell-free mitotic extracts: a model system for analysis of the active phase of apoptosis. *J. Cell Biol.*, **123**, 7–22.

Lee, B. S., Chen, J., Angelidis, C., Jurivich, D. A. and Morimoto, R. I. (1995). Pharmacological modulation of heat shock factor 1 by antiinflammatory drugs results in protection against stress-induced cellular damage. *Proc. Natl. Acad. Sci. USA*, **92**, 7207–7211.

Leist, M. and Nicotera, P. (1997). The shape of cell death. *Biochem. Biophys. Res. Commun.*, **236**, 1–9.

Leist, M., Fava, E., Montecucco, C. and Nicotera, P. (1997a). Peroxynitrite and nitric oxide donors induce neuronal apoptosis by eliciting autocrine excitotoxicity. *Eur. J. Neurosci.*, **9**, 1488–1498.

Leist, M., Single, B., Castoldi, A. F., Kuhnle, S. and Nicotera, P. (1997b). Intracellular adenosine triphosphate (ATP) concentration: a switch in the decision between apoptosis and necrosis. *J. Exp. Med.*, **185**, 1481–1486.

Leppa, S. and Sistonen, L. (1997). Heat shock response: pathophysiological implications. *Ann. Med.*, **29**, 73–78.

Li, P., Nijhawan, D., Budihardjo, I., Srinivasula, S. M., Ahmad, M., Alnemri, E. S. and Wang, X. (1997). Cytochrome *c* and dATP-dependent formation of Apaf-1/Caspase-9 complex initiates an apoptotic protease cascade. *Cell*, **91**, 479–489.

Li, X., Johnson, D. C. and Rozman, K. K. (1997). 2,3,7,8-Tetrachlorodibenzo-*p*-dioxin (TCDD) increases release of leutinizing hormone and follicle-stimulating hormone from the pituitary of immature female rats *in vivo* and *in vitro*. *Toxicol. Appl. Pharmacol.*, **142**, 264–269.

Liang, P. and Pardee, A. B. (1997). Differential display. A general protocol. *Methods Mol. Biol.*, **85**, 3–11.

Liu, H., Lightfoot, R. and Stevens, J. L. (1996). Activation of heat shock factor by alkylating agents is triggered by glutathione depletion and oxidation of protein thiols. *J. Biol. Chem.*, **271**, 4805–4812.

Liu, H., Bowes, R. C., van de Water, B., Sillence, C., Nagelkerke, J. F. and Stevens, J. L. (1997). Endoplasmic reticulum chaperones GRP78 and calreticulin prevent oxidative stress, Ca^{2+} disturbances and cell death in renal epithelial cells. *J. Biol. Chem.*, **272**, 21751–21759.

Liu, X., Kim, N. C., Yang, J., Jemmerson, R. and Wang, X. (1996). Induction of apoptotic program in cell-free extracts: requirement for dATP and cytochrome *c*. *Cell*, **86**, 147–157.

Loechler, E. L. (1996). The role of adduct site-specific mutagenesis in understanding how carcinogen–DNA adducts cause mutations: perspective, prospects and problems. *Carcinogenesis*, **17**, 895–902.

Luger, K., Mäder, A. W., Richmond, R. K., Sargent, D. F. and Richmond, T. J. (1997). Crystal structure of the nucleosome core particle at 2.8 Å resolution. *Science*, **389**, 251–260.

Luo, M. F., Xu, G. T. and Cui, X. L. (1995). Further studies on the dynamic changes of glutathione and protein–thiol mixed disulfides in H$_2$O$_2$ induced cataract in rat lenses: distributions and effect of aging. *Curr. Eye Res.*, **14**, 951–958.

Maines, M. D. (1997). The heme oxygenase system: a regulator of second messenger gases. *Annu. Rev. Pharmacol. Toxicol.*, **37**, 517–554.

Marini, M., Frabetti, F., Musiani, D. and Franceschi, C. (1996). Oxygen radicals induce stress proteins and tolerance to oxidative stress. *Int. J. Radiat. Biol.*, **70**, 337–350.

McConkey, D. J., Hartzell, P., Nicotera, P. and Orrenius, S. (1989). Calcium-activated DNA fragmentation kills immature thymocytes. *FASEB J.*, **3**, 1843–1849.

McConkey, D. J., Zhivotovsky, B. and Orrenius, S. (1996). Apoptosis – molecular mechanisms and biomedical implications. *Mol. Aspects Med.*, **17**, 1–110.

McConkey, D. J. and Orrenius, S. (1997). The role of calcium in the regulation of apoptosis. *Biochem. Biophys. Res. Commun.*, **239**, 357–366.

McGhee, J. D. and Felsenfeld, G. (1980). Structure of nucleosome structure. *Annu. Rev. Biochem.*, **46**, 931–954.

Moore, G. A., O'Brien, P. J. and Orrenius, S. (1986). Menadione (2-methyl-1,4-naphthoquinone)-induced Ca^{2+} release from rat-liver mitochondria is caused by NAD(P)H oxidation. *Xenobiotica*, **16**, 873–882.

Moore, G. A., McConkey, D. J., Kass, G. E., O'Brien, P. J. and Orrenius, S. (1987a). 2,5-Di(*tert*-butyl)-1,4-benzohydroquinone: a novel inhibitor of liver microsomal Ca^{2+} sequestration. *FEBS Lett.*, **224**, 331–336.

Moore, G. A., Rossi, L., Nicotera, P., Orrenius, S. and O'Brien, P. J. (1987b). Quinone toxicity in hepatocytes: studies on mitochondrial Ca^{2+} release induced by benzoquinone derivatives. *Arch. Biochem. Biophys.*, **259**, 283–295.

Moriguchi, T., Seres, T., Ravichandran, V., Sasada, M. and Johnston, R. B., Jr. (1996). Diamide primes neutrophils for enhanced release of superoxide anion: relationship to *S*-thiolation of cellular proteins. *J. Leukocyte Biol.*, **60**, 191–198.

Morimoto, R. I., Kroeger, P. E. and Cotto, J. J. (1996). The transcriptional regulation of heat shock genes. A plethora of heat shock factors and regulatory conditions. *Exercise Sci.*, **77**, 139–163.

Nakagawa, Y., Moldéus, P. and Cotgreave, I. A. (1992). The *S*-thiolation of hepatocellular protein thiols during diquat metabolism. *Biochem. Pharmacol.*, **43**, 2519–2525.

Nakamura, H., Nakamura, K. and Yodoi, J. (1997). Redox regulation of cellular activation. *Annu. Rev. Immunol.*, **15**, 351–369.

Nakano, M., Mann, D. L. and Knowlton, A. A. (1997). Blocking the endogenous increase in HSP 72 increases susceptibility to hypoxia and reoxygenation in isolated adult feline cardiocytes. *Circulation*, **95**, 1523–1531.

Nellgard, B., Gustafson, I. and Wieloch, T. (1991). Lack of protection by the *N*-methyl-D-asparate receptor blocker dizocilpine (MK-801) after transient severe cerebral ischemia in the rat. *Anesthesiology*, **75**, 279–287.

Nicotera, P., Moore, M., Mirabelli, F., Bellomo, G. and Orrenius, S. (1985). Inhibition of hepatocyte plasma membrane Ca^{2+}-ATPase activity by menadione metabolism and its restoration by thiols. *FEBS Lett.*, **181**, 149–153.

Nicotera, P., Rundgren, M., Porubek, D. J., Cotgreave, I., Moldeus, P., Orrenius, S. and Nelson, S. D. (1989). On the role of Ca^{2+} in the toxicity of alkylating and oxidizing quinone imines in isolated hepatocytes. *Chem. Res. Toxicol.*, **2**, 46–50.

Orrenius, S. (1995). Apoptosis: molecular mechanisms and implications for human disease. *J. Int. Med.*, **237**, 529–536.

Orrenius, S., McConkey, D. J., Bellomo, G. and Nicotera, P. (1989). Role of Ca^{2+} in toxic cell killing. *Trends Pharmacol. Sci.*, **10**, 281–285.

Pang, Z. and Geddes, J. W. (1997). Mechanisms of cell death induced by the mitochondrial toxin 3-nitropropionic acid: acute excitotoxic necrosis and delayed apoptosis. *J. Neurosci.*, **17**, 3064–3073.

Park, E. M. and Thomas, J. A. (1989). The mechanisms of reduction of protein mixed disulfides (dethiolation) in cardiac tissue. *Arch. Biochem. Biophys.*, **274**, 47–54.

Park, Y. M., Han, M. Y., Blackburn, R. V. and Lee, Y. J. (1998). Overexpression of HSP25 reduces the level of TNF alpha-induced oxidative DNA damage biomarker, 8-hydroxy-2′-deoxyguanosine, in L929 cells. *J. Cell. Physiol.*, **174**, 27–34.

Parsadanian, A. S., Cheng, Y., Keller-Peck, C. R., Holtzman, D. M. and Snider, W. D. (1998). Bcl-xL is an antiapoptotic regulator for postnatal CNS neurons. *J. Neurosci.*, **18**, 1009–1019.

Payne, C. M., Bernstein, C. and Bernstein, H. (1995). Apoptosis overview emphasizing the role of oxidative stress, DNA damage and signal-transduction pathways. *Leukemia Lymphoma*, **19**, 43–93.

Pegg, A. E. (1984). Methylation of the O^6 position of guanine is the most likely initiating event in carcinogenesis by methylating agents. *Cancer Invest.*, **2**, 223–231.

Pelkonen, O. and Raunio, H. (1997). Metabolic activation of toxins: tissue-specific expression and metabolism in target organs. *Environ. Health Perspect.*, **105**, 767–774.

Persson, Å. E., Pontén, I., Cotgreave, I. and Jernström, B. (1996). Inhibitory effects on the DNA binding of AP-1 transcription factor to an AP-1 binding site modified by benzo[*a*]pyrene 7,8-dihydrodiol 9,10-epoxide diastereomers. *Carcinogenesis*, **17**, 1963–1969.

Petito, C. K., Torres-Munoz, J., Roberts, B., Olarte, J. P., Nowak, T. S., Jr. and Pulsinelli, W. A. (1997). DNA fragmentation follows delayed neuronal death in CA1 neurons exposed to transient global ischemia in the rat. *J. Cereb. Blood Flow Metab.*, **17**, 967–976.

Poellinger, L. (1996). Intracellular signal transmission via dioxin receptors. *Nord. Med.*, **111**, 45–48.

Pohjanvirta, R., Laitinen, J. T. and Vakkuri, O. (1996). Mechasnims by which 2,3,7,8-tetrachlorodibenzo-*p*-dioxin (TCDD) reduces circulating melatonin levels in the rat. *Toxicology*, **107**, 85–97.

Pratt, W. B. (1997). The role of HSP90-based chaperone system in signal transduction by nuclear receptors and receptors signalling via MAP kinase. *Annu. Rev. Pharmacol. Toxicol.*, **37**, 297–326.

Pruett, S. B., Ensley, D. K. and Crittenden, P. L. (1993). The role of chemical-induced stress responses in immunosuppression: a review of quantitative associations and cause–effect relationships between chemical-induced stress responses and immunosuppression. *J. Toxicol. Environ. Health.*, **39**, 163–192.

Pumford, N. R. and Halmes, N. C. (1997). Protein targets of xenobiotic reactive intermediates. *Annu. Rev. Pharmacol. Toxicol.*, **37**, 91–117.

Rabenstein, D. L. and Millis, K. K. (1995). Nuclear magnetic resonance study of the thioltransferase-catalyzed glutathione/glutathione disulfide interchange reaction. *Biochim. Biophys. Acta.*, **1249**, 29–36.

Raney, V. M., Harris, T. M. and Stone, M. P. (1993). DNA conformation mediates aflatoxin B1–DNA binding and the formation of guanine N7 adducts by aflatoxin B1 8, 9-*exo*-epoxide. *Chem. Res. Toxicol.*, **6**, 64–68.

Rando, R. R. (1996). Chemical biology of protein isoprenylation/methylation. *Biochim. Biophys. Acta*, **1300**, 5–16.

Ravichandran, V., Seres, T., Moriguchi, T., Thomas, J. A. and Johnston, R. B., Jr (1994). *S*-Thiolation of glyceraldehyde-3-phosphate dehydrogenase induced by the phagocytosis-associated respiratory burst in blood monocytes. *J. Biol. Chem.*, **269**, 25010–25015.

Rokutan, K., Johnston, R. B. and Kawai, K. (1994). Oxidative stress induces *S*-thiolation of specific proteins in cultured gastric mucosal cells. *Am. J. Physiol.*, **266**, G247–G254.

Ronai, Z. A., Lambert, M. E. and Weinstein, I. B. (1990). Inducible cellular responses to ultraviolet light irradiation and other mediators of DNA damage in mammalian cells. *Cell Biol. Toxicol.*, **6**, 105–126.

Rowan, S. and Fisher, D. E. (1997). Mechanisms of apoptotic cell death. *Leukemia*, **11**, 457–465.

Rundgren, M., Porubek, D. J., Harvison, P. J., Cotgreave, I. A., Moldéus, P. and Nelson, S. D. (1988). Comparative cytotoxic effects of *N*-acetyl-*p*-benzoquinone imine and two dimethylated analogues. *Mol. Pharmacol.*, **34**, 566–572.

Safe, S. H. and Sacharewsky, T. (1997). Organochlorine exposure and risk for breast cancer. *Prog. Clin. Biol. Res.*, **396**, 133–145.

Scarlett, J. L., Packer, M. A., Porteous, C. M. and Murphy, M. P. (1996). Alterations to glutathione and nicotinamide nucleotides during the mitochondrial permeability transition induced by peroxynitrite. *Biochem. Pharmacol.*, **52**, 1047–1055.

Schedl, P., Artavanis-Tsakonas, S., Steward, R., Gehring, W. J., Mirault, M. E., Goldschmidt-Clermont, M., Moran, L. and Tissieres, A. (1978). Two hybrid plasmids with *D. melanogaster* DNA sequences complementary to mRNA coding for the major heat shock protein. *Cell.*, **14**, 921–929.

Schlegel, J., Peters, I., Orrenius, S., Miller, D. K., Thornberry, N. A., Yamin, T. T. and Nicholson, D. W. (1996). CPP32/Apopain is a key interleukin 1J converting enzyme-like protease involved in Fas-mediated apoptosis. *J. Biol. Chem.*, **271**, 1841–1844.

Schuppe-Koistinen, I., Gerdes, R., Moldéus, P. and Cotgreave, I. A. (1994a). Studies on the reversibility of protein *S*-thiolation in human endothelial cells. *Arch. Biochem. Biophys.*, **315**, 226–234.

Schuppe-Koistinen, I., Moldéus, P., Bergman, T. and Cotgreave, I. A. (1994b). *S*-Thiolation of human endothelial cell glyceraldehyde-3-phosphate dehydrogenase after hydrogen peroxide treatment. *Eur. J. Biochem.*, **221**, 1033–1037.

Schuppe-Koistinen, I., Moldéus, P., Bergman, T. and Cotgreave, I. A. (1995). Reversible *S*-thiolation of human endothelial cell actin accompanies a structural rearrangement of the cytoskeleton. *Endothelium*, **3**, 301–308.

Schuur, A. G., Boekhorst, F. M., Brouwer, A. *et al.*, (1997). Extrathyroidal effects of 2,3,7,8-tetrachlorodibenzo-*p*-dioxin on thyroid hormone turnover in male Sprague Dawley rats. *Endocrinology*, **138**, 3727–3734.

Seres, T., Ravichandran, V., Moriguchi, T., Rokutan, K., Thomas, J. A. and Johnston, R. B. Jr (1996). Protein *S*-thiolation and dethiolation during the respiratory burst in human monocytes. A reversible post-translational modification withpotential for buffering the effects of oxidant stress. *J. Immunol.*, **156**, 1973–1980.

Singer, B. and Essigmann, J. M. (1991). Site-specific mutagenesis: retrospective and prospective. *Carcinogenesis*, **12**, 949–955.

Smith, M. T., Thor, H. and Orrenius, S. (1984). Detection and measurement of drug-induced oxygen radical formation. *Methods Enzymol.*, **105**, 505–510.

Sun, Y. and Oberley, L. W. (1996). Redox regulation of transcriptional activators. *Free Rad. Biol. Med.*, **21**, 335–348.

Suzuki, K., Sawa, Y., Kaneda, Y., Ichikawa, H., Shirakura, R. and Matsuda, H. (1997). *In vivo* gene transfection with heat shock protein 70 enhances myocardial tolerance to ischemia-reperfusion injury in rat. *J. Clin. Invest.*, **99**, 1645–1650.

Thomas, J. A., Poland, B. and Honzatko, R. (1995). Protein sulfhydryls and their role in the antioxidant function of protein *S*-thiolation. *Arch. Biochem. Biophys.*, **319**, 1–9.

Thornberry, N. A., Rano, T. A., Peterson, E. P., Rasper, D. M., Timkey, T., Garcia-Calvo, M., Houtzager, V. M., Nordstrom, P. A., Roy, S., Vaillancourt, J. P., Champman, K. T. and Nicholson, D. W. (1997). A combinatorial approach defines specificities of members of the caspase family and granzyme B. *J. Biol. Chem.*, **272**, 17907–17911.

Tobin, D., Nilsson, M. and Toftgard, R. (1996). Ras-independent activation of Rel-family transcription factors by UVB and TPA in cultured keratinocytes. *Oncogene*, **12**, 785–793.

Tobin, D., van Hogerlinden, M. and Toftgard, R. (1998). UVB-induced association of tumor necrosis factor (TNF) receptor

1/TNF receptor-associated factor-2 mediates activation of Rel proteins. *Proc. Natl. Acad. Sci. USA.*, **95**, 565–569.

Torchinski, Y. M. (1981). *Sulphur in Proteins*. Pergamon Press, Oxford, pp. 133–142.

Travers, A. A. (1987). DNA bending and nuclesome positioning. *Trends Biochem. Sci.*, **12**, 108–112.

Ursini, F., Maiorino, M. and Roveri, A. (1997). Phospholipid hydroperoxide glutathione peroxidase (PHGPx): more than an antioxidant enzyme? *Biomed. Environ. Sci.*, **10**, 327–332.

Van Bladeren, P. J. (1997). Influence of non-nutrient plant components on biotransformation enzymes. *Biomed. Pharmacother.*, **51**, 324–327.

Velculescu, V. E., Zhang, L., Vogelstein, B. and Kinzler, K. W. (1995). Serial analysis of gene expression. *Science*, **270**, 484–487.

Wallace, K. B., Eells, J. T., Madeira, V. M., Cortopassi, G. and Jones, D. P. (1997). Mitochondria-mediated cell injury. Symposium overview. *Fundam. Appl. Toxicol.*, **38**, 23–37.

Waring, M. J. (1986). Overview of the interaction between chemotherapeutic agents and DNA. *Drugs Exp. Clin. Res.*, **12**, 441–453.

Weis, M., Morgenstern, R., Cotgreave, I. A., Nelson, S. D. and Moldéus, P. (1992). *N*-Acetyl-*p*-benzoquinone imine-induced protein thiol modification in isolated rat hepatocytes. *Biochem. Pharmacol.*, **43**, 1493–1505.

Wilkinson, J. T. and Clapper, M. L. (1997). Detoxication enzymes and chemoprevention. *Proc. Soc. Exp. Biol. Med.*, **216**, 192–200.

Yang, J., Liu, X., Bhalla, K., Kim, C. N., Ibrado, A. M., Cai, J., Peng, T. -I., Jones, D. P. and Wang, X (1997). Prevention of apoptosis by Bcl-2: release of cytochrome *c* from mitochondria blocked. *Science*, **275**, 1129–1131.

Yang, X., Chang, H. Y., and Baltimore, D. (1998). Autoproteolytic activation of pro-caspase by oligomerization. *Mol. Cell.*, **1**, 319–325.

Yarosh, D. B. and Kripke, M. L. (1996). DNA repair and cytokines in antimutagenesis and anticarcinogenesis. *Mutat. Res.*, **350**, 255–60.

Ziegler, D. M. (1985). Role of reversible oxidation–reduction of enzyme thiols-disulfides inmetabolic regulation. *Annu. Rev. Biochem.*, **54**, 305–329.

Zhan, Y., Cleveland, J. L. and Stevens, J. L. (1997). A role for c-myc in chemically-induced renal cell death. *Mol. Cell Biol.*, **17**, 6755–6764.

Zhang, F. L. and Casey, P. J. (1996). Protein prenylation: molecular mechanisms and functional consequences. *Annu. Rev. Biochem.*, **65**, 241–269.

Zhivotovsky, B., Wade, D., Nicotera, P. and Orrenius, S. (1994). Role of nucleases in apoptosis. *Int. Arch. Allergy Immunol.*, **105**, 333–338.

Zhivotovsky, B., Burgess, D. H., Vanags, D. M. and Orrenius, S. (1997a). Involvement of cellular proteolytic machinery in apoptosis. *Biochem. Biophys. Res. Commun.*, **230**, 481–488.

Zhivotovsky, B., Gahm, A. and Orrenius, S. (1997b). Two different proteases are involved in the proteolysis of lamin during apoptosis. *Biochem. Biophys. Res. Commun.*, **233**, 96–101.

Zou, H., Henzel, W. J., Liu, X., Lutschg, A. and Wang, X. (1997). Apaf-1, a human protein homologous to *C. elegans* CED-4, participates in cytochrome *c*-dependent activation of caspase-3. *Cell.*, **90**, 405–413.

Chapter 9
Cell Death and Apoptosis

Sidhartha D. Ray

C O N T E N T S

INTRODUCTION

The study of the cellular reaction to injury is fundamental to the study of disease in all living systems. There is a basic similarity in such reactions whether the cell is that of an invertebrate, vertebrate or plant. Conceptually, this oversimplification has contributed to a better understanding of human disease. Among the many known cellular alterations in disease, cell death (irreversible loss of vital cellular functions and structure) is certainly the most drastic and one of the most frequently encountered and easily recognized. Cell death, a near equilibrium terminal end-stage, induced by severe physiological homeostatic perturbation, is a phenomenon ubiquitous in all biological organisms. This endpoint can be induced by ischaemia or hypoxia, drugs or chemicals, immune reactions (complement attack), microorganisms, high temperature or radiation and a variety of toxins. Historically, the first recognized mode of cell death was *necrosis*, a general term referring to a morphological stigmata of a cell that has committed to die. During this process, cells pass through a reversible phase, often followed, with explosive rapidity, by irreversible changes resulting from adverse stimuli. Mechanisms suggested to account for the irreversibility of necrotic changes include the release of lysosomal enzymes, activation of membrane-active proteases/phospholipases, gross impairment of ion homeostasis, generation of dangerous oxy-radicals or biological reactive intermediates (BRIs), a precipitous drop in the cellular energy status [depletion of intracellular cytoprotective agents, e.g. levels of antioxidants, ATP, glycogen or glutathione, and malfunctioning of cytoprotective enzymes, e.g. superoxide dismutase, catalase, peroxidase, glutathione peroxidase, poly(ADP-ribose) polymerase], and substantive insult to the integrity of genomic DNA beyond a critical point. Recent advances in our understanding of lethal injury, however, suggests that cell death may also occur via another distinct and dynamic process, i.e. *apoptosis*. Whereas necrosis is considered as the unprogrammed or accidental (unplanned) cell death resulting from adverse stimuli, apoptosis, regarded as the programmed or physiological (beneficial) form of cell death, can occur under both normal and adverse stimuli. Since details of necrotic cell death have been meticulously discussed in other chapters throughout this book, this chapter will primarily focus on drug and chemically induced apoptotic processes and their mechanisms of action.

When apoptosis (Ap oh' tosis or A 'poop tosis: Greek *apo*, meaning leaf, and *ptosis*, meaning falling off) was first described over a quarter of a century ago (Kerr *et al.*, 1972a), the terminologies describing these changes (councilman or acidophilic bodies in liver diseases, Klion and Schaffner, 1966; Child and Ruiz, 1968; civatte bodies in lichen planus, Montgomery, 1967; tingible bodies in lymphoid germinal centres, Nossal and Ada, 1971; basophilic or Benirschke granules characteristic of premenstrual endometrial glands, Ehrmann, 1969, etc.) were already in the perusal of scientists who coined, defined and differentiated 'apoptosis' from 'necrosis' based on changes in cellular ultrastructures (Kerr, 1969, 1971; Kerr *et al.*, 1972b). The naming of the process evolved from 'shrinkage necrosis' or 'coagulative necrosis' (early) exclusively on morphological grounds to 'apoptosis' (later) when it was found to play a role in regulating tissue morphogenesis and tissue size (see Majno and Jorris, 1995). The true importance of this unique cell death process was unknown until a recent upsurge in interest to unravel the mechanisms underlying this process. After a decade of dedicated efforts, it is now well understood that apoptosis is a very tightly regulated, energy-dependent, genetically programmed and evolutionarily conserved self-destruction process through which cells undergo organized suicide for beneficial purposes. In multicellular organisms, such beneficial functions include maintenance of optimal tissue growth and development and physiological activity (by a balance between proliferation, growth arrest and programmed cell death). Apoptotic cells, upon completion of their mission, execute a suicidal programme and form apoptotic bodies which are rapidly removed by the reticuloendothelial system (macrophages and phagocytes). Massive cell suicide by apoptosis usually does not lead to organ dysfunction as opposed to necrotic cell death. Another noteworthy attribute is the lack of involvement of inflammation during the progression of events. Although apoptosis and necrosis are diametrically opposed modes of cell death, many believe that they are parts of a continuum (Corcoran and Ray, 1992). Since PCD is often used synonymously with apoptosis, it is also very important to recognize the significance of the terms 'programmed cell death' (PCD) and 'apoptosis'. This chapter has used 'apoptosis' and 'programmed cell death' interchangeably.

Apoptosis is characterized by a series of well defined morphological changes (see **Figures 1–4**). Initially there is decrease or shrinkage in cell volume (cytoplasmic condensation), the generation of a pyknotic nucleus and condensation of the chromatin along the nuclear membrane. This is followed by loss of the nuclear membrane, fragmentation of the nuclear chromatin and subsequent formation of multiple fragments of condensed nuclear material along with cytoplasm, called apoptotic bodies. These may later appear on the cell surface as vesicles or blebs. The next stage is the phagocytosis of apoptotic bodies (by either neighbouring cells or phagocytes) preventing the release of cellular contents into the surrounding areas and avoiding an inflammatory response. The morphological changes associated with apoptosis contrast with those of necrosis, the alternative cell death process associated with pathological processes. Necrosis is an unprogrammed chaotic process characterized by cellular swelling and disintegration (intracellular structures loose volume and disintegrate rather than cellular shrinking) and the release of cellular contents that induce an inflammatory response in the surrounding tissue. The characteristics of apoptosis and necrosis are described in **Table 1** and **Figure 1**. In both PCD and apoptosis, it is believed that cells activate an intrinsic death programme and thus actively contribute to their own demise. Both PCD and apoptosis are gene directed and influenced by extrinsic and intrinsic signals **(Table 2)**. Therefore,

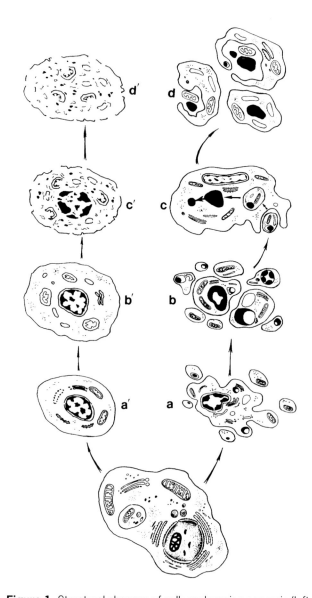

Figure 1 Structural changes of cells undergoing necrosis (left, a′–d′) and apoptosis (right a–d). Sequence of morphological changes in apoptosis are distinct from necrosis. In apoptosis the cells condense and shrink (a and b) rather than swell as in necrosis (a′ and b′). Typically in necrosis cell lysis precedes generalized swelling which progresses to disintegration of organelles including plasma membrane breakage (c′–d′). In contrast, cell–cell contacts, initially retained in necrosis, are broken down early in apoptosis, which is followed with explosive rapidity by specialized changes, e.g. loss of plasma membrane surface structures, condensation/compaction of cytoplasm coupled with condensation of heterochromatin, and its fragmentation. This phase is followed by migration of masses of condensed chromatin (chromatolysis) towards the periphery of the nuclear membrane. Chromatolysis usually involves activation of Ca^{2+} and Mg^{2+}-dependent endonuclease activity. Next, the condensed, membrane-bound fragments (apoptotic bodies) often containing intact cytoplasm (plus sometimes mitochondria) are characteristically seen to be phagocytosed by neighbouring cells or by phagocytes (c–d). Engulfed materials are usually internally digested to avert inflammation. Stages depicted as defined by Searle et al. (1982). Courtesy artwork of Tat Lam, MD, Kaiser Permanente, Woodland Hills, CA, USA.

Table 1 Distinguishing features of apoptosis (PCD: programmed cell death) and necrosis (unprogrammed or accidental cell death)

Characteristic	Apoptosis	Necrosis
1. Distribution	Affects individual cells scattered throughout a tissue	Affects massive and contiguous cells
2. Cellular morphology	Chromatin condensation and margination as large crescents to the nuclear membrane periphery, fragmentation in dense masses	Irregular clumping of chromatin, pyknosis or karyolysis; nucleolysis occasionally precedes collapse of nuclear membrane
	Cell volume decreases (compacts), organelles retain integrity, occasional swelling of organelles appear very late in the process; bleb positive late (organelles found in blebs)	Very early swelling of cell and intracellular organelles; cells lyse and every intracellular component appears chaotic, bleb positive (organelles not found in bleb)
	Membrane integrity retained, does not leak until late but loses specialized surface structures	Membrane collapses, loses integrity and lyse
3. DNA breakdown pattern (on agarose gels)	Internucleosomal cleavage, 'ladder-like' DNA fragmentation	Random DNA damage, appears as a 'smear' on gels
4. Duration of biochemical and morphological changes	Minutes to hours	Hours to days
5. Lysosomal enzyme release	Absent (clearly unknown)	Present (a battery of tissue-specific enzymes)
6. Transglutaminase activity	Increases	Remains unchanged
7. Cell fragmentation	Forms apoptotic bodies, contains fragments of nuclei plus intact organelles if any, e.g. mitochondria	No distinct bodies are formed, cells usually disintegrate
8. Cell removal	By phagocytosis (by phagocytes or neighbouring cells); receptor mediated	Cells rupture, contents are released
9. Exudative inflammatory changes	Absent	Present, sometimes extensive inflammation
10. Scar formation	Absent (organ dysfunction not reported)	Present (organ dysfunction reported)
11. Adhesion between cells and to basement membrane	Lost very early	Lost very late
12. Reversibility	Onset can be delayed but cannot be reversed after morphological changes develop	Can be blocked if detected early prior to point of no return in the total absence of plasma membrane damage
13. Overall regulation	Very tightly regulated (sometimes dependent on energy status, protein synthesis, gene transcription)	Not regulated, independent of energy status or protein synthesis or the gene transcription

although similar in all respects, programmed cell death occurs *in vivo*, whereas the others are apoptosis. The initiating signals are fundamentally similar. For example, cells exposed to ionizing radiation may undergo apoptosis, which is highly predictable in terms of the proportion of cells affected, but they are not programmed to die (unless they are exposed to radiation). Another programmed death example involves the ischaemic death of the endometrial lining of the uterus at the end of menstrual cycle **(Table 2)**. In addition, PCD can be affirmatively predicted in certain cells of the well known nematode *Caenorhabditis elegans*. *C. elegans* which matures as an adult hermaphrodite with 1090 cells of which 131 undergo programmed cell death (Ellis *et al.*, 1991). These PCD-designated cells at various locations automatically trigger suicidal death programmes at different but precisely defined times.

This finding led to the proposed scenario in which cells receiving death signals or lacking survival signals may turn on or off a genetic death programme regardless of the cause. Now, it has become clear, the regulatory mechanisms controlling apoptosis are as fundamental, and as complex, as those regulating cell proliferation. Based on the observations of the past two decades, the apoptotic response of a cell to a drug or toxin is determined at five distinct levels: (i) the stimulus (e.g. drug, chemical, concentration) and its bioavailability and metabolism; (ii) cellular defence mechanisms; (iii) signal transduction pathways; (iv) status of relevant oncogenes; and (v) intrinsic cellular susceptibility to apoptosis **(Table 2)**.

Table 2 Apoptosis or programmed cell death associated with physiological and pathological states

State or condition	Cells/organs involved
1. Normal cell turnover (in adult tissues)	Hepatocytes, adrenal cortex, intestinal crypt epithelium, spermatogonia, megakaryocytes, neutrophils
2. Embryogenesis/metamorphosis	Epithelial cell of small intestines; deletion of interdigital webs; regression of Mullerian ducts in males and Wolffian ducts in females; palate midline epithelium fusion; most neurons; pronephros, mesonephros and metanephros regression to form nephron and tubules; human tail regression; auditory vesicle invagination and detachment from ectoderm during the ear development; foetal periderm, intermediate epidermal cells and appendages during development and remodelling of skin
3. Thymocyte deletion	T-cell deletion during negative selection
4. Normal involutional processes	Uterine endometrium after menstrual cycle; mammary epithelium regression after lactation; hair follicles, ovarian follicular atresia, vaginal epithelial cells (stratum spinosum, stratum basalis) during late metoestrus and early dioestrus
5. Atrophic processes	Prostate changes after castration; adrenal cortex after ACTH depletion; kidney during hydronephrosis; thymus during glucocortocoid imbalance; pancreatic ductular obstruction
6. Immune-mediated cell killing	T-cell, killer cell and natural killer cells, allograft rejection, graft vs host disease, tumour necrosis factor-induced (TNF)
7. Cellular injury	Radiation, ischaemia, hyperthermia, calcium ionophores, many drugs and chemicals, toxins of plant and bacterial toxins, steroids, oxidants, carcinogens, anti-cancer agents
8. Viral diseases	Promoters: HIV (human immunodeficiency virus), human T-cell leukaemia virus, human papilloma virus, Parvo virus. Inhibitors: Herpes simplex, human cytomegalo virus, Epstein–Barr virus, vaccinia virus, cowpox virus, baculovirus, hepatitis B virus
9. Neurological diseases	Parkinson's disease, Alzheimer's disease, stroke, spinal muscular atrophy, HIV, encephalopathy, prions disease, Huntington's disease, amyotropic lateral sclerosis
10. Trophic factor withdrawal	Epidermal growth factor, insulin-like growth factor-I, oestrogen, IL-2, thrombin, nerve growth factor (NGF) and transforming growth factor dysregulation (TGFβ)
11. Others	Ageing, autoimmune disease, neoplasms, thermal stimuli (heat shock), drugs, chemicals

APOPTOSIS AND PROGRAMMED CELL DEATH: THEIR OCCURRENCE

Apoptosis is an operationally, morphologically and biochemically distinct form of cell death from necrosis (Kerr et al., 1972b; Wyllie, 1987). Owing to the multitude of signals and requisite cellular metabolic events which can lead to apoptosis, an enormous range of physiological and toxicological stimuli can practically initiate this death programme in numerous types of cells. It is clearly evident, however, that the induction of apoptosis in any given tissue is tightly regulated, so that the suicidal programme can only be induced by a particular tissue-specific signal. Alternatively, a signal that turns on the execution programme in one tissue may have very little apoptotic effect or even cause proliferation in another tissue. The wide range of cells that can undergo apoptosis in micro (well defined in vitro models) and macro (invertebrates, vertebrates and plants: in vivo models) environments suggests that practically each and every type of cell is potentially capable of executing terms and conditions of apoptosis. The tissue specificity of the induction of apoptosis and the molecular mechanism by which the apoptotic process occurs are poorly understood.

Cell death by apoptosis has been reported in plants (Basile et al., 1973; Wangenheim, 1987), nematodes (Yuan and Horvitz, 1990), insects (Lockshin and Williams, 1965), fish (Daoust et al., 1984), birds (Glucksmann, 1951; Hurle et al., 1977; Oppenheim 1985), amphibians (Searle et al., 1982) and mammals (Compton and Cidlowski, 1992). Regression of the tadpole tail during amphibian metamorphosis serves as one of the prime examples of ontogenic PCD, and perhaps is only rivalled by the cataclysms of insect metamorphosis (Lockshin, 1981; Bowen and Bowen, 1990). Tadpole tail fin collapse is followed by degradation of tail muscle, a spectacular event recorded by classical histopathologists. The mechanisms underlying this event have been unravelled by biochemists and cell biologists (Weber 1969, 1977; Fox 1987; Kerr et al., 1987). Another classic example of PCD is loss of cells at the interdigital zones during development in chickens, mice and humans (Bowen and Bowen, 1990). During embryological and foetal development of amphibia, chicken and mammals, experiments have confirmed that the peripheral innervation regulates the level of cell death (Levi-Montalcini and Brooker, 1960). Later, Levi-Montalcini and Aloe (1981) demonstrated that nerve growth factor (NGF) channelled via peripheral innervation plays a significant role in controlling the number of cells in developing neuronal ganglia, thus determining the final size of the ganglia. Enormous numbers of cells are deleted especially in the nervous system by apoptosis (Oppenheim, 1985; Clarke,

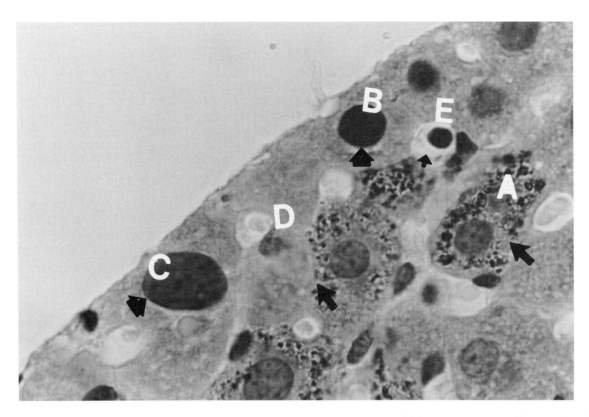

Figure 2   Light photomicrograph (×400) of paraffin-embedded mouse liver section PAS (periodic acid schiff reagent) ×1000, showing early ultrastructural changes typical of apoptosis induced by acetaminophen. The figure shows the presence of normal (A), apoptotic (B, C: various stages), and necrotic (D) hepatocytes (E: including shrinkage necrosis) following 500 mg kg^{-1} i.p. acetaminophen exposure for 6 h. The section exhibits the beginning of apoptotic changes, e.g. condensation of chromatin and enlargement of the nuclei (B, C). Nuclear alterations are evident in the near total absence of loss of volume regulation. Necrotic changes include nuclear and cytoplasmic damage with poor staining characteristics (D). A strongly PAS-positive glycogen-loaded normal hepatocyte shows normal nuclear morphology (A). Courtesy Yahya *et al.* (1995)

1990). In mammals, the secondary palate separating oral and nasal cavities develops by growth, rotation and fusion of left and right palatal shelves. The fusion of the shelves is mediated by decreased proliferation, increased adhesiveness and PCD of medial edge epithelial cells (Greene and Pratt, 1976; Pratt and Greene, 1976). During vertebrate sexual differentiation and maturation, the reproductive organs show spectacular changes which involve massive PCD. Despite the fact that both male and female embryos have the same reproductive rudiments, the Wolffian duct differentiates into epididymis and vas deferens whilst the Mullerian duct regresses in the male and the opposite occurs in the female; the Mullerian duct differentiates into the uterus in mammals or oviduct and shell gland in avian species. These events are directed by hormones, but cell removal occurs by apoptosis. All these observations indicate that 'apoptosis' or PCD is an equal and opposite force to mitosis (Kerr *et al.*, 1987). In certain tissues the cells survive until the organism dies while other cells are continually produced in self-renewing tissues, then differentiate to perform specific functions, and eventually die. Noted examples of these events are the life cycles of skin cells

(keratinocytes) and haematopoietic cells (Lord, 1979, 1986; Muel *et al.*, 1986; McCall and Cohen, 1991; Wangenheim, 1987). Prior to their destruction by PCD, these cells pass through a 'transit compartment' and a 'maturation compartment'. Many hormone and growth-factor sensitive tissues operate in a similar fashion and mimic the progression of events in order to maintain tissue homeostasis. Cells belonging to tissues and organs such as liver (Benedetti *et al.*, 1988a, b; Terada and Nakanuma, 1995), kidney (Glucksmann, 1951; Koseki *et al.*, 1992; Coles *et al.*, 1993), thymus (Compton and Cidlowski, 1986; Duke *et al.*, 1996), prostate (Kyprianou and Isaacs, 1988), ovary (Hopwood and Levison, 1976; Sandow *et al.*, 1979), uterus (Sandow *et al.*, 1979; Hopwood and Levison, 1976), adrenal cortex (Wyllie *et al.*, 1973), lymphoid cells (Koury and Bondurant, 1990; Williams *et al.*, 1990), nervous system (Glucksmann, 1951; Oppenheim 1991) and intestinal crypt cells (Milligan and Schwartz, 1996; see also Duke *et al.*, 1996) are vulnerable to apoptosis naturally or otherwise. Apoptotic death of immature thymocytes in our body is a classic example of PCD (Duke *et al.*, 1996).

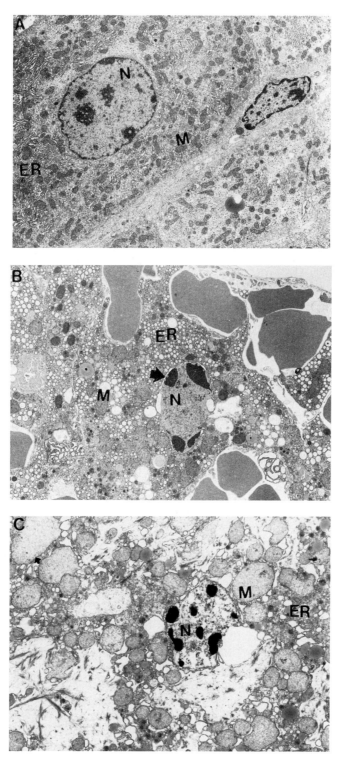

Figure 3 Acetaminophen (paracetamol)-induced hepatocellular apoptosis and necrosis. Electron photomicrographs from vehicle-treated (A) and 500 mg kg^{-1} i.p. acetaminophen-treated (B and C) liver sections at the end of 24 h period. The photomicrographs depict the architecture of a normal healthy hepatocyte (A), apoptotic hepatocyte (B) and a necrotic hepatocyte (C). However, this hepatocyte in acetaminophen-treated liver (B; × 8000) indicates characteristic features of apoptosis including some hypertrophied cytoplasmic changes. Note the condensation, fragmentation and margination of the heterochromatin in the absence of significant loss of mitochondrial volume. Remarkable necrotic changes (cytoplasmic and nuclear) are evident in section C (×8000). Compare the changes in volume in panels B and C with these in A. Note (in panel C) severe mitochondrial swelling and collapse of the mitochondrial boundary, nuclear damage and collapse of the nuclear membrane, and several other morphological aberrations of the cytoplasm in a necrotic cell. Scale; 1 μm = 8 mm at × 8000. M = mitochondria; N = nucleus; ER = endoplasmic reticulum. Source: Ray *et al.* (1996) with permission from the American Society of Pharmacology and Experimental Therapeutics.

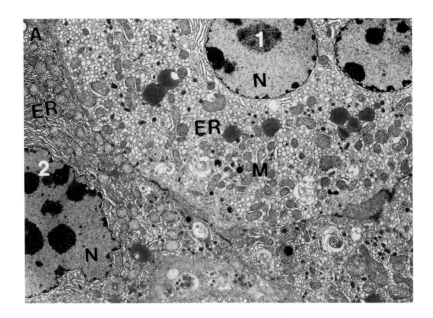

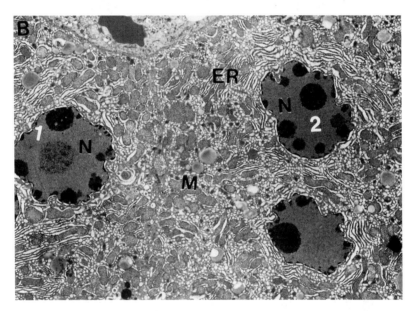

Figure 4 Time course of dimethylnitrosamine-induced hepatocellular apoptosis and necrosis. Electron photomicrographs from 100 mg kg^{-1} i.p. dimethylnitrosamine- treated (A–E) liver sections at the end of various hours (×8000). Note the sequence of apoptotic changes in hepatocytes. Four hours after the drug administration (note A1 and A2; ×8000), the hepatocytes begin to show chromatin condensation and fragmentation with no loss of mitochondrial volume except slightly hypertrophied cytoplasm. However, dimethylnitrosamine-treated liver (B; ×8000) indicates characteristic features of apoptosis including some hypertrophied cytoplasmic changes. Six hours of dimethylnitrosamine administration (B) clearly showed progress in apoptotic changes, i.e. margination of the fragmented nuclear heterochromatin towards the nuclear membrane periphery without any major mitochondrial or cytoplasmic changes. Endoplasmic reticulum appears normal. Section C (×12 000) demonstrates clear phagocytosis (P1) of apoptotic bodies and remnants by a macrophage in a 6 h dimethylnitrosamine-treated liver. Note the entire macrophage–apoptotic body complex is being attempted by another scavenger cell (super-phagocytosis: P2). Part D (×10 000) shows changes that are identical with those in B except additional ER damage coupled with accumulation of lipid droplets in the cytoplasmic area in the absence of loss of mitochondrial volume. Hypertrophied cytoplasm, along with condensation, fragmentation and margination of the heterochromatin are conspicuous at 12 h after dimethylnitrosamine exposure (D). Part E shows remarkable apoptotic and necrotic changes after 18 h of dimethylnitrosamine exposure. Necrotic changes (cytoplasmic and mitochondrial) with some of apoptotic morphology (condensed and fragmented chromatin) are evident in E. Compare the changes in volume regulation in A and B with those in E. Note severe plasma membrane, mitochondrial, cytoplasmic and ER damage including several other unidentifiable morphological aberrations of the cytoplasm of a puzzled hepatocyte (E1) in the neighbour of a normal hepatocyte (E2) Scale: 1 μm = 8mm at × 8000; 1 μm = 10mm at × 10 000; 1 μm = 12mm at × 12 000.M = mitochondria; N = nucleus; ER = endoplasmic reticulum; P1 = phagocytosis; P2 = super phagocytosis.

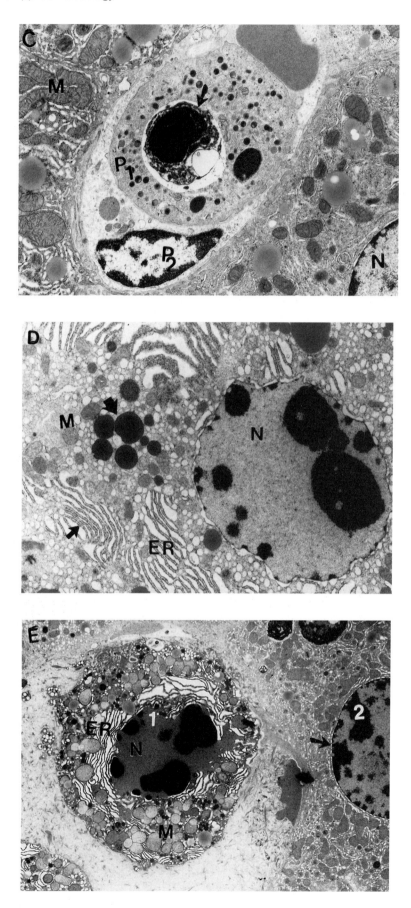

Figure 4 Cont.

MORPHOLOGY OF APOPTOSIS

After lingering on the edge of sceptical acceptance for a long time, apoptosis has broken its dormancy following confirmation of its highly characteristic and remarkably stereotyped morphological changes by light and electron microscopy. Although the most practicable and reliable way of unequivocally distinguishing between apoptosis and necrosis is by transmission electron microscopy, high-power ($\times$ 1000) brightfield microscopy has generated a lot of meaningful information in many studies (Ray et al., 1996). Pioneers of this method claim nuclear morphology to be the gold standard for distinguishing apoptotic from necrotic cells. Since this ongoing natural process in living systems can progress very quickly, within minutes to hours (Sanderson, 1976; Matter, 1979), and the cells are removed from the body extremely rapidly after the onset, it has been a cumbersome task to capture cells in various stages of this process for morphological analysis (Wyllie, 1987). Apoptotic cells die a clean death. The dead cells are eaten and digested by phagocytes with such speed and efficiency that their passing is histologically inconspicuous, whereas necrotic death is a messy and conspicuous death (Savill, 1994). However, under the influence of an inducing agent (*in vitro*) or in disease states (*in vivo*), abundant apoptotic cells can be found for discrete observations. A variety of stimuli (inducers) which can activate this process are listed in **Tables 3** and **4**. The time to onset of apoptosis after a lethal stimulus is variable but the changes are rapid. In apoptosis, coordinated changes occur in the nucleus, the cytoplasm and at the cell surface. *In vivo*, apoptosis usually affects single cells or small groups of cells in an asynchronous fashion and the entire process can be primarily divided into four steps.

Step I: **Cell shrinkage**. The earliest changes observed include the loss of cell junctions and other specialized plasma membrane structures such as microvilli. Simultaneously the cytoplasm becomes hypertrophied (see **Figure 4b**) and condenses and the entire cell shrinks. Unlike necrosis, an apoptotic cell lacks swelling but shrinks and pulls away from its neighbours without causing any disturbance to tissue architecture or function.

Step II: **Nuclear or chromatin condensation**. This is the most noticeable distinguishing feature of apoptosis. At this stage, chromatin condenses (coalesces) fragments into one or more large (or small) masses and migrates towards the periphery of the nuclear membrane. As the process continues, the nucleus breaks into several fragments. Under an electron microscope, these fragments appear very dense and dark in the near total absence or loss of volume regulation of organelles. The contraction of cytoplasmic volume is apparently associated with loss of intracellular fluid and ions (see some of the figures in this chapter which depict these stereotypic changes; **Figure 4**)

Step III: **Formation of apoptotic bodies**. The cell membrane transiently adopts a deeply convoluted outline and shows extensive surface blebbing. Subsequently, the cell breaks up into several membrane-bound smooth-surfaced apoptotic bodies that contain a variety of tightly compacted organelles and some nuclear fragments. These are designated apoptotic bodies.

Step IV: **Phagocytosis of apoptotic cells or bodies**. Apoptotic bodies vary greatly in size and shape. There is no limit to the number of apoptotic bodies formed from a single cell although the number may depend on the size of the cell. Apoptotic bodies are typically phagocytosed by 'professional phagocytes' (macrophages) or neighbouring cells serving as 'semiprofessional' phagocytes [glomerular mesangial cells (Savill et al., 1993); renal tubular cells (Savill, 1994); hepatocytes (Ray et al., 1996)]. These engulfing cells are typically members of reticuloendothelial system (mononuclear phagocytes, such as macrophages, phagocytes, etc.) but also can be any other normal or abnormal cell capable of phagocytosis (Wyllie et al., 1980). The endocytosed apoptotic masses are rapidly degraded within lysosomes and the adjacent cells migrate or proliferate to replace the space occupied by the recently deleted apoptotic cell (see **Figure 4C**).

Although apoptotic bodies provide a potent stimulus for phagocytosis, the mechanism of recognition of apoptotic bodies by the engulfing cell is not clearly understood. Apoptotic bodies rarely inhabit the extracellular space without some approaching or adhereing phagocytes. The recognition of apoptotic body by the phagocytic cells may involve a receptor-mediated process. Three different receptor-mediated phagocytoses, viz. macrophage lectins (carbohydrate receptor), vitronectin (thrombospondin) receptors and phosphatidylserine receptors, have been implicated (Savill et al., 1993). In lectin-mediated binding, an integrin–polypeptide type of molecular bridge, complemented with sugar–lectin interaction either directly or indirectly, is involved (Morris et al., 1984; Duvall et al., 1985; Arends and Wyllie, 1991). This theory is further supported by the observations that simple sugars (e.g. *N*-acetylglucosamine, *N*,*N*'-diacetylchitobiose, mannosamine) will block the recognition of apoptotic cells by macrophages (Duval et al., 1985; Savill et al., 1989). Loss of sialic acid from membrane glycoproteins would expose normally masked residues such as *N*-acetylglucosamine, *N*-acetylgalactosamine and galactose, rendering these available for interaction with macrophages lectins (Dini et al., 1992). Another type of recognition of apoptotic thymocytes by macrophages involves movement of phosphatidylserine from the inner to the outer surface of the apoptotic cell. Although this phospholipid is normally located on the inner surface of the plasma membrane, its movement to outer surface of apoptotic cells is facilitated by a decrease in aminophospholipid translocase, an enzyme which normally transports phosphatidylserine from the outside of

Table 3 Agents that induce apoptosis *in vivo*

Agent	Target organ	Reference
Acetaminophen (paracetamol)	Mouse liver	Ray *et al.* (1996)
Actinomycin D	Mouse gut crypt epithelial cell	Searle *et al.* (1982)
Benzene	Mouse femoral B/T-lymphocytes	Fariss *et al.* (1997)
Bleomycin	Mouse lung	Hagimoto *et al.* (1997)
Bromoethylamine 2-hydrobromide	Rat kidney	Gobe and Axelsen (1991)
Cadmium	Beagle kidney	Hamada *et al.* (1991)
Clodronate (bisphosphonates)	Mouse liver macrophage	Selander *et al.* (1996)
Colchicine, puromycin	Colonepithelial cells	Duncan and Heddle (1984)
Copper	Lamb	King and Bremner (1979)
Coumarin	Rat liver	Lake and Grasso (1996)
Cyanohydroxybutene	Rat pancreas	Wallig and Jeffery (1990)
Cycloheximide	Rat liver	Faa *et al.* (1994)
Cyclophosphamide	Rat germ cells/mouse tumours	Cai *et al.* (1997); Meyn *et al.* (1994)
Cyproterone acetate	Rat liver	Bursch *et al.* (1985; 1990)
Cytosine arabinoside	Mouse small intestine	Searle *et al.* (1982)
D-Galactosamine + lipipolysaccharide	Rat liver, kidney, thymus, spleen and lymph node	Morikawa *et al.* (1996)
Dimethylbenz[*a*]anthracene	Mouse thymus and Peyers patches	Burchiel *et al.* (1992)
1,2-Dimethylhydrazine	Mouse colon	Ijiri (1989)
1,2-Dimethylhydrazine + 1% orotic acid	Rat liver	Columbano *et al.* (1984)
Dimethylnitrosamine	Rat liver	Hirata *et al.* (1989); Pritchard and Butler (1989)
		Ray *et al.* (1992)
Doxorubicin	SHR kidney and intestine	Herman *et al.* (1997)
Enalapril (losartan and nifedipine)	SHR smooth muscle cell	deBlois *et al.* (1997)
Ethanol	Rat liver/SHR liver	Baroni *et al.* (1994); Manolas *et al.* (1997)
5-Fluorouracil	Rat thymus, spleen and ileum	Sakaguchi *et al.* (1994)
Furosemide (frusemide)	Mouse liver and kidneys	Strika *et al.* (1998)
FTY 720	Mouse lymphoid organs	Suzuki *et al.* (1997)
4-Hydroxynonenal (ozone)	Human lung cells	Hamilton *et al.* (1998)
4-Hydroxy non-2-enal (ozone)	Mouse lung	Kirichenko *et al.* (1996)
Indomethacin	Sheep ovary	Murdoch (1996)
Lead nitrate withdrawal	Rat liver	Fesus *et al.* (1987)
Lipopolysaccharide	Mouse liver, thymus	Zhang *et al.* (1993); Norimatsu *et al.* (1995)
Menadione	Rat kidney	Chiou *et al.* (1997)
Morphine	Mouse thymus	Fuchs and Pruett (1993)
Methylazoxymethanol	Mouse colon	Ijiri *et al.* (1989)
Methamphetamine	Rat thymus and spleen	Iwasa *et al.* (1996)
Methylmercury	Mouse cerebellum	Inouye *et al.* (1991)
Fe(III)-mitoxantrone	SHR kidney and intestine	Herman *et al.* (1997)

(Continued)

Table 3 *(Contd)*

Agent	Target organ	Reference
MPTP	Mouse brain	Hassouna *et al.* (1996)
Mitomycin C	Mouse testis	Nakagawa *et al.* (1997)
N-Methyl-*N*-nitrosourea	Mouse retina	Yuge *et al.* (1996); Hai *et al.* (1997)
OK-432 (5 Klinische Einheit)	Liver neutrophils	Shi *et al.* (1996a)
Ricin and abrin	Mouse lymphoid tissue	Griffiths *et al.* (1987)
Raw soya flour withdrawal (cholecystokinin)	Rat pancreas	Oates and Morgan (1986)
Silica (Min-U-Sil 5 silica)	Rat lung cells	Leigh *et al.* (1997)
Thioacetamide	Rat liver	Ledda-Columbano *et al.* (1991); Faa *et al.* (1992)
Thiobenzamide	Rat liver	Chieli *et al.* (1987)
T-2 toxin	Mouse thymus, liver and spleen	Ihara *et al.* (1997)
TPA (12-*O*-tetradecanoylphorbol 13-acetate)	Mouse brain, liver	Bagchi *et al.* (1998)
4-Vinylcyclohexene diepoxide	Rat ovaries	Springer *et al.* (1996)

Table 4 Agents that induce apoptosis *in vitro*

Agent	Cell	Reference
Acetaminophen (paracetamol)	Mouse hepatocytes	Shen *et al.* (1991, 1992)
Adriamycin	CML-lymphocytes	Anand *et al.* (1995)
Aphidicolin	CHO cells	Barry *et al.* (1990)
Arachidonic acid	Hep-G_2 cells	Chen *et al.* (1997)
Ara-C	Human myeloid leukaemia cells	Grant *et al.* (1994)
ATP	Thymocytes	Zheng *et al.* (1991)
Buthionine sulphoximine (BSO)	GT1-7 (neural cell)	Kane *et al.* (1993)
Bleomycin	Human hepatocytes/Hep-G_2	Galle *et al.* (1995)
Calphostin C	HL-60 cells (promyelocytic leukaemia)	Jarvis *et al.* (1994b)
Camptothecin	MLL cells	Kaufmann (1989)
C2-ceramide	U937 cells	Jarvis *et al.* (1994c); Verhej *et al.* (1996)
Chromium	CHO AA8 cells/macrophage J-774A.1 cells	Blankenship *et al.* (1994); Bagchi *et al.* (1998)
Cisplatin	CHO cells	Barry *et al.* (1990)
Colchicine	Rat hepatocytes	Tsukidate *et al.* (1993)
Doxorubicin (adriamycin)	Tumour cells	Skladanoski and Konopa (1993)
Etoposide	Mouse fibroblast (L929 cells)	Mizumoto *et al.* (1994)
Erythropoietin	Erythroid progenitor cells	Koury and Bondurant (1990)
5-Fluorodeoxyuridine	CHO cells	Barry *et al.* (1990)
Gossypol	HL-60 cells (promyelocytic leukaemia)	Jarvis *et al.* (1994b)
Hoechst 33258	Colon adenocarcinoma cells (HT-29-II)	Oberhammer *et al.* (1993)
Hydrogen peroxide	U 937 cells	Coppola *et al.* (1995)
Hydroxyurea	CML-lymphocytes	Anand *et al.* (1995)
Interleukin-1β	Pancreatic RIm5F cells	Ankarcrona *et al.* (1994)
Methotrexate	CHO cells	Barry *et al.* (1990)
Melphalan	HL60/U937 cells	Fernandes and Cotter (1994)
Mitomycin C	B-lineage lymphocytes	Potchinsky *et al.* (1995)
Okadaic acid	Normal rat kidney cell (NRK-52)	Davis *et al.* (1994)
	Rat hepatocyte, GH3 pituitary cell	Boe *et al.* (1991)
Sodium nitroprusside	RAW 264.7 macrophage cells	Messmer *et al.* (1995)
TCDD	Immature thymocytes	McConkey *et al.* (1988b)
Tributyltin	Thymocytes	Raffray *et al.* (1993)
Vinblastine	Rat hepatocytes	Tsukidate *et al.* (1993)
VP-16 (podophyllotoxin)	MOLT-4 cells	Catchpoole *et al.* (1995)

the plasma membrane to the inside, and/or an increase in scramblase, an enzyme that moves phospholipids in both directions (Fadok *et al.*, 1992, 1993). Another possibility is the exposure of the phosphatidylserine moiety on the apoptotic cell surface due to a loss of membrane symmetry. The third type of receptor, identified on the macrophage surface, is known to recognize apoptotic neutrophills by a mechanism involving vitronectin (one of the heterodimeric integrin molecules, $\alpha_v\beta_3$), CD_{36} and thrombospondin (Savill *et al.*, 1990, 1991) receptor complexes. Ellis *et al.*, (1991) have suggested the involvement of various genes (*ced-1, -2, -5, -6, -7, -8, -10*) in the corpse removal process (the roles of various genes are discussed elsewhere in this chapter).

This type of cell removal generally benefits the organism and does not threaten neighbouring cells or structures, because toxic contents of dying cells are digested internally, thus avoiding any inflammatory outcome. Apoptotic bodies are distinct membrane-encapsulated entities which can exclude vital dyes until they are degraded. Occasionally apoptotic bodies accidentally bypass phagocytosis and are released into the adjacent lumen. In such instances, apoptotic bodies demonstrate progressive dilation and degradation of the engulfed contents (e.g. mitochondria), in a process that has been called 'secondary necrosis' (see **Figure 2** in this chapter and Searle *et al.*, 1975).

BIOCHEMICAL CHANGES INVOLVED IN APOPTOSIS

Following the morphological classification of apoptosis, many fragmentary molecular and biochemical events were characterized mostly from studies on immature thymocytes *in vitro*. Since this is a very tightly regulated energy-dependent active process, cells succumbing to this phenomenon show orderly changes in an extremely timely fashion. Some of the key elements that predominantly orchestrate this beneficial form of death are Ca^{2+} and Mg^{2+} ions, DNA and the nuclear enzyme endonuclease. Wyllie (1980) and Cohen and Duke (1984) showed fairly convincingly that chromatin undergoes cleavage early during the killing of immature thymoctyes by glucocorticoids. Activation of a Ca^{2+}-sensitive endonuclease appears to be an obligatory step in the appearance of DNA cleavage (see **Figure 5**). These investigators highlighted the role that Ca^{2+} plays in the process and proposed that faltering Ca^{2+} regulation within the cell is needed for glucocorticoids to produce cell killing in this model. In a study that examined the killing of thymocytes by the immunotoxin 2,3,7,8-tetrachlorodibenzo-*p*-dioxin, Orrenius and co-workers concluded that this environmental chemical also promotes endonuclease-mediated DNA damage in a Ca^{2+}-dependent manner (McConkey *et al.*, 1988b). These discoveries raise a num-

ber of important questions. How do the mechanisms of acute cell killing gleaned from these *in vitro* models relate to cell death: (1) from other forms of cell insults, (2) in other cell types such as the hepatocyte and (3) under more realistic conditions such as in the living animal *in vivo*? Although most of these questions remain unanswered, leading laboratories throughout the world moved forward with apoptosis research using 'DNA ladder' as a yard-stick to diagnose drug- and chemically-induced apoptosis in a wide-range of model systems. Over time, this simple biochemical hallmark became so popular that its use resulted in a record number of publications for a decade (see **Figure 5**). In 1980, Wyllie showed that the morphological changes of apoptosis are associated with distinctive, double-strand cleavage of nuclear DNA (endonuclease-dependent) at the linker regions between nucleosomes. The resulting oligonucleosomal fragments can be demonstrated by agarose gel electrophoresis, where so called DNA ladder develops (see **Figure 5**). Necrosis, in contrast, is accompanied by random DNA degradation and digestion of histone, diffuse smear being seen in gels. Identification of this simple biochemical hallmark led to an explosion of investigations attempting to identify apoptogens by their ability to induce the DNA ladder. Few exceptions to this rule were noted during this period, leading to an appropriate conclusion that internucleosomal DNA cleavage cannot be used as the sole criterion for diagnosing apoptosis (Collins *et al.*, 1992). However, in the absence of any other dependable marker, demonstration of internucleosomal chromatin degradation continues to be a viable diagnostic aid particularly when morphological data are supplemented (Schwartzman and Cidlowski, 1993). This characteristic is reproducible in both *in vivo* and *in vitro* systems comprising normal or abnormal (cancer or leukaemia) cells. Since apoptotic and necrotic cells both share DNA as a common target, in most instances necrotic cells also show a DNA degradation pattern (smear-like pattern, haphazard, random or non-specifically degraded into a continuous spectrum of sizes on agarose gels). Apoptotic cells, on the other hand, invariably show a characteristic ladder-like pattern in almost all of the instances that have been studied (Huang *et al.*, 1997).

A rise in intracellular and/or intranuclear Ca^{2+} is a prerequisite for chromatin fragmentation since the enzyme responsible for cleaving DNA is Ca^{2+}- and Mg^{2+}-dependent. Calcium homeostasis seems to be under as careful regulation in the nucleus as elsewhere throughout the cell (Ray *et al.*, 1990, 1991a, b, 1993). The Ca^{2+} concentration gradient present between nucleus and cytoplasm (Williams *et al.*, 1988) implies the existence of structures that transport Ca^{2+} across the nuclear membrane. Skeletal muscle nuclei demonstrate Ca^{2+}-stimulated ATPase activity (Kulikova *et al.*, 1982). Nuclei isoiated from rat liver accumulate Ca^{2+} *in vitro* via an ATP- and calmodulin-dependent process and contain a constitutive endonuclease that responds to

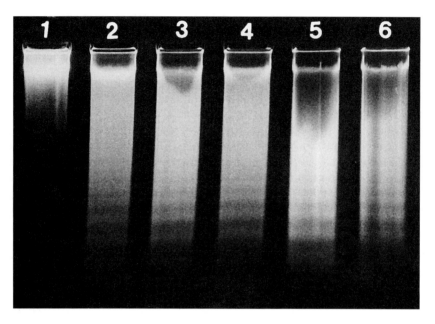

Figure 5 This ethidium bromide-stained agarose gel shows after-effects of acetaminophen (paracetamol) on the integrity of genomic DNA isolated from mouse liver. Electrophoretograms demonstrate the time course of acetaminophen (paracetamol)-induced DNA damage to hepatocellular genomic DNA (lane 1, vehicle-treated control; lanes 2, 3, 4, 5 and 6, situation 4, 6, 12, 18 and 24 h after 500 mg kg^{-1} acetaminophen treatment, respectively). This ethidium bromide-stained 1.4% agarose gel contains 10 μg of DNA per lane from acetaminophen-treated livers. Each lane contains DNA (10 μg per lane) from three animals at one time point (pooled DNA from three representative liver samples). Loss of large genomic DNA with concomitant appearance of a ladder-like fragmentation pattern typical of apoptosis was observed after 4 h following acetaminophen administration. Appearance of DNA ladder (lanes 2–6) is characteristic of Ca^{2+}/Mg^{2+}-dependent endonuclease activation. Severe loss of time-dependent large genomic DNA is evident in the acetaminophen-treated livers (see gradual loss of fluorescence intensity at the well). Courtesy Dhruva and Ray (1996); see also Ray *et al.* (1993).

pathophysiological Ca^{2+} concentrations in the submicromolar range by cleaving DNA into periodic intranucleosomal fragments (Jones *et al.*, 1989).

Considerable evidence now suggests that the role of Ca^{2+} is pivotal in the early stages of toxic injury leading to cell death (reviewed by Reed, 1990; Barry and Eastman, 1992; Corcoran and Ray, 1992; Trump and Berezesky, 1995). Accumulating evidence indicates that Ca^{2+} ion may be acting in a well known capacity as a principal intracellular messenger and it appears to convey the consequences of initial damage from diverse sites to one or more specific secondary loci that are critical for cell viability. In addition to Wyllie's (1980) experiments involving immature thymocytes, many laboratories reported that, in apoptosis, an elevated level of Ca^{2+} after a toxic insult was the 'cause' and endonuclease mediated DNA fragmentation leading to cell death was the 'effect' (Cohen and Duke, 1984; McConkey *et al.*, 1989, 1990a; Ray *et al.*, 1990). This cause-and-effect relationship was further verified by either exposing thymocytes to agents that elevate intracellular Ca^{2+} levels (e.g. glucocorticoids, calcium ionophores, radiation, 2,3,7,8-tetrachlorodibenzo-*p*-dioxin, tributyltin, natural killer cells or cytotoxic T-lymphocytes and anti-CD$_3$ antibody) or agents known to prevent intracellular Ca^{2+} accumulation (e.g. EGTA, verapamil, chlorproma-

zine, nifedipine, promethazine-HCl). Since protein synthesis is also important for mediating the influx of calcium, it is assumed, in the case of thymocytes, that the interaction of glucocorticoid with its plasma membrane receptor rapidly induces the synthesis of a protein which acts as a calcium pore (McConkey *et al.*, 1996). Subsequently it was unravelled that glucocorticoid-induced thymocyte apoptosis was sensitive to actinomycin D (inhibits RNA synthesis) and cycloheximide (inhibits protein synthesis) treatments whereas that induced by tributyltin was not. Further, endonuclease inhibitor, aurintricarboxylic acid and Zn^{2+} ion were shown to inhibit fragmentation of DNA in some model systems (Benchokroun *et al.*, 1995; Zalewski and Forbes, 1995). All of these effects suggest that, although not universal, apoptosis is an active process requiring RNA and protein synthesis especially for cell death to become irreversible. Studies demonstrating the necessity for *de novo* macromolecular synthesis for the execution of the cell death programme make the important distinction that toxic cell death (necrosis) does not require any such synthesis. Tributyltin-induced apoptosis provides a convincing example refuting the need for new macromolecular synthesis in apoptosis. Nickel, an agent that blocks non-voltage-dependent Ca^{2+} channels, blocks tributyltin-induced apoptosis, suggesting that tributyltin interacts directly with the plasma membrane of thymocytes to open Ca^{2+} channels, thus facilitating Ca^{2+} entry into the cell and bypassing the need for intracellular signalling and new protein synthesis. Pathways in which new protein synthesis or new gene expression are required for apoptosis after exposure to the stimulus may be referred to as induction pathways. Alternatively, apoptosis can result from inhibition of protein or messenger RNA synthesis, suggesting that a cell death pathway is constitutively expressed, yet kept in abeyance by short-lived inhibitors. Pathways that induce apoptosis by inhibiting protein synthesis are termed release pathways, and pathways that are not influenced by inhibition of protein synthesis, such as cytotoxic T-cell mediated apoptosis, may be termed transduction pathways (Patel and Gores, 1995). This body of thinking stresses the global role that ion regulation plays in continued cell vitality and emphasizes, in particular, the large number of regulatory systems that rely upon the actions of calcium ion.

The integrity of no single molecule appears to be as vital to the cell as that of DNA. Its safeguarding from any entity and perpetuation are among the most intricate and aggressively pursued goals of homeostatic regulatory controls. In the entire apoptosis literature, three distinct patterns of DNA fragmentation have so far been reported (Huang et al., 1997): (i) internucleosomal cleavage of genomic DNA (Wyllie et al., 1984); (ii) 30–50 kb large fragment cleavage (Roy et al., 1992); and (iii) single-stranded nicking (Ucker et al., 1992). The classic ladder-like pattern stems from DNA breakdown at the internucleosomal regions that generates fragments in 180–200 bp increments, finally yielding 3'-OH DNA termini. This type of fragmentation appears long before the onset of the stereotypic morphological changes and continues even after the removal of the death signal. The second type of DNA degradation appears after cleavage and involves fragmentation of a higher order structure of chromatin (700, 300, 50), known as a loop, into ca 50 kb portions that anchor to the nuclear matrix in the interloop or matrix attachment regions (MARS). Release of these ca 50 kb fragments is thought to result from cleavage in the MARS. The larger fragments appear to be intermediates in the process of DNA fragmentation that ultimately gives rise to DNA ladders. However, it is not clear whether the large fragments are produced by the activity of the enzymes responsible for forming the oligonucleosomal fragments, since concentrations of divalent cation requirements for their formation are different from those required by such enzymes. Future studies hopefully will determine whether this type of chromatin cleavage is universal, and is an irreversible commitment in all apoptotic cells, since a similar pattern of DNA fragmentation has also been found in necrotic cells (Sun et al., 1994; Bicknell and Cohen, 1995; Kataoka et al., 1995). The third type of fragmentation is single-stranded breaks in the core-histone-associated DNA and internucleosomal areas by Ca^{2+}-dependent endonuclease DNase-I (Peitsch et al., 1993). Addition of the enzyme to isolated nuclei, and other reconstituted systems, promotes the formation of DNA strand breaks which possess the same $5' - PO_4$ and $3' - OH$ end groups as those found in DNA fragments isolated from apoptotic cells. Two closely spaced single-stranded breaks on opposite strands of DNA may result in double-stranded DNA cleavage providing a super signal to apoptotic cascade but not a mechanism to explain chromatin cleavage. Huang et al., (1997) have reviewed the characteristics of candidate nucleases isolated from a variety of model systems. To date, DNase-I, DNase-II, NUC18, NUC40, NUC58, 27 kDa nuclease and a 37 kDa nuclease have been reported. Endonuclease activity in cells undergoing apoptosis can be regulated directly or indirectly by proto-oncogenes and tumour suppressor genes, such as c-myc, Ha-ras, bcl-2 and p-53 (Vanderbilt et al., 1982; Milligan and Schwartz, 1996; Huang et al., 1997), which have been discussed elsewhere in this chapter.

Transglutaminases, a family of Ca^{2+}-dependent enzymes, catalyse the formation of protein cross-links that are biologically irreversible. No enzyme capable of hydrolysing the cross-links formed by transglutaminases in substrate proteins have been found in vertebrates (Fesus et al., 1991). This cytosolic enzyme accumulates to high levels in some terminally differentiated cells and also in a number of cell types undergoing apoptosis both in vivo and in vitro. The enzyme is both induced and activated during apoptosis. Although the role of transglutaminase in apoptosis is poorly understood, it is likely that the cross-linking of proteins stabilizes the apoptotic bodies and prevents the leakage of intracellular constituents into the extracellular space (which can trigger inflammation). Intracellular activation of this enzyme can change adhesive properties (Byrd and Lichti, 1987; Nara et al., 1989) or may contribute to the altered cell surface properties of the apoptotic bodies (Fesus et al., 1991). Intriguingly, over-expression of the enzyme has been reported to activate apoptosis (Fesus et al., 1987; Knight et al., 1991).

Another group of thiol-containing and Ca^{2+}-dependent proteases, linked directly or indirectly to apoptosis, are calpains (Martin et al., 1995). Calpains, known as calcium-dependent and papain-like protease, occur in two forms (μ-calpain and m-calpain). m-Calpain and μ-calpain have identical regulatory subunits with distinct catalytic subunits, but the Ca^{2+} requirement is higher for activation of m-Calpain. Although their distribution is ubiquitous, calpains are non-lysosomal cytosolic modulatory proteases, and not digestive proteases occasionally localized at the plasma membrane. Calpain substrates include cytoskeletal proteins (actin-binding proteins, e.g. fodrin/spectrin, talin and filamin, and microtubule associated proteins), membrane proteins (growth factor receptors, e.g. EGF receptor; adhesion molecules, e.g. integrin and cadherin; ion transporters, e.g. Ca^{2+}-ATPase, and ion channels, e.g. Ca^{2+}-channel) and enzymes (kinases, e.g. PKC, calmodulin-dependent kinase; phosphatases, e.g. calcineurin, and phospholipases). Either directly or indirectly, calpains may influence cell shape, inactivate transcription factors (*c-fos* and *c-jun*) and jeopardize signal transduction pathways by attenuating PKC activity. Numerous Ca^{2+}-linked processes such as activation of the ICE family of proteases, protein kinase C, growth factor-dependent events and various signalling processes may be under the regulation of calpains (see Genetic Regulation of Apoptosis, later). Expression of calpains in apoptotic cells is a very early event occurring long before the onset of morphological changes. Activation of calpain is thought to play a role in glucocorticoid-induced thymocyte apoptosis and FAS/APO-1-mediated apoptosis of T-cell hybridomas (Squier *et al.*, 1994). Engagement of FAS/APO-1, a TNF-receptor superfamily member (in mammalian cells Fas/APO-1 is a CD 95) with specific antibodies, or upon exposure to its natural ligand, transduces an extremely rapid, synchronous and potent apoptotic signal to a variety of cell types (McConkey *et al.*, 1996). Since, calpains are Ca^{2+}-binding thiol (–SH) containing proteins, it has been suggested that their cleavage products may be involved in promoting some of the morphological features of apoptosis. Interestingly, in *C. elegans*, the products of the cell death genes *ced-3* and *ced-4* are a sulphydryl-containing protease and a Ca^{2+}-binding protein, respectively. There are numerous other Ca^{2+}-linked processes which are discussed elsewhere in this chapter.

Many different types of proteins that are either cleaved or selectively expressed during apoptosis include histone H1, topoisomerases I and II, lamins, U1-70 kDa and the nuclear enzyme poly(ADP-ribose)polymerase (Tanaka *et al.*, 1984; Kaufmann, 1989; Ray *et al.*, 1992; McConkey *et al.*, 1995). Among these proteins, poly(ADP-ribose) polymerase has gained the most attention. Activation of the DNA repair enzyme poly(ADP-ribose) polymerase (EC 2.4.2.30), considered another prominent biochemical event associated with apoptotic death, involves ribosylation of nuclear proteins (Marks and Fox, 1991). This process is mediated by the enzymes mono(ADP-ribosyl)transferase and poly(ADP-ribose)-synthetase and involves the transfer of ADP-ribose groups from NAD to protein acceptor sites and to existing ADP-ribose polymers. The ribosylation process facilitates the DNA-excision repair which antagonizes apoptotic processes. Massive activation of this enzyme leads to the lethal depletion of NAD, and indirectly ATP. Conversely, mild activation, often seen with submaximal injury, is associated with increased repair and decreased cytotoxicity or cytolethality. Therefore, some investigators have argued that depletion of NAD and ATP induced by DNA strand breakage is a critical event in apoptotic death (Carson *et al.*, 1986; Wielckens and Delfs, 1986). This ostensible antiapoptotic action of

poly(ADP-ribose) polymerase is substantiated by observations that poly(ADP-ribose) synthetase inhibitors such as nicotinamide and 3-aminobenzamide may either increase or decrease the sensitivity of apoptosis-inducing agents depending upon the concentration employed (Ray *et al.*, 1992; Yahya *et al.*, 1995). NAD, the poly(ADP-ribose) polymerase substrate, is also known to maintain cellular redox balance. Any gross shift in the physiological level of this component perturbs the tightly regulated myriad of metabolic functions coupled with cellular homeostasis, ultimately resulting in irreversible cytotoxicity. Likewise, ATP depletion leads to failure of ATP-dependent membrane pumps and results in the disturbance of cell's ionic equilibrium (e.g., Ca^{2+}), eventually causing activation of cytotoxic mechanisms involving proteases, phospholipases and endonucleases. In contrast to all these observations, H_2O_2, a potent necrogen which induces DNA strand breaks, is a powerful inducer of poly(ADP-ribose) polymerase in *in vitro* model systems. Hence both inhibition and activation of poly(ADP-ribose) synthetase may set the stage for endonucleases to proceed with their goals, either to complete or oppose the cell's final mission, i.e. apoptotic death (Nelipovich *et al.*, 1988; Ray *et al.*, 1992).

PROTEIN KINASES, SIGNALLING MECHANISMS AND APOPTOSIS

The past two decades have witnessed tremendous progress in understanding how extracellular signals are transduced across the plasma membrane and then transmitted within the cell to elicit specific physiological responses. Recently, intense interest has focused upon the potential involvement of diverse signalling processes in the regulation of apoptosis (McConkey *et al.*, 1990b). However, many elements of the signalling system(s) involved in the induction of apoptosis remain unknown. The signal generated by a stimulus must be transmitted to effector molecules that often lie in different subcellular compartments. Transduction pathways vary according to the trigger stimulus but two major areas of focus are cytosolic calcium and protein kinases. Participation of Ca^{2+}-/phospholipid-dependent protein kinase [protein kinase C (PKC)] in intracellular signalling processes has been demonstrated in many cell types. Physiologically, the activity of PKC is regulated upon its translocation from cytosol to the membrane, and it is at the plasma membrane that the enzyme is activated by its endogenous activator diacylglycerol. The breakdown of phosphatidylinositol triphosphate by phospholipase C results in the production of diacylglycerol, a second messenger cofactor that mediates activation of the PKC. Besides the reversible activation of PKC by Ca^{2+}, phospholipids, diacylglycerol, unsaturated fatty acids and phorbol esters, this enzyme is also irreversibly activated by limited proteolysis involving the intracellular protease calpain (see discussion elsewhere in this chapter). One of the pathways of the transmembrane signalling system operates through the activation of PKC, whereas the other signal system involves receptor-mediated activation of cAMP-dependent protein kinase. Information concerning a role for PKC in apoptosis mostly comes from studies with phorbol esters [12-O-tetradecanoylphorbol 13-acetate (TPA)]. These tumour promoters act by binding to the diacylglycerol-binding site on the enzyme and promote its activation. Ca^{2+} mobilization and the calmodulin-dependent regulatory system appear to work in concert with TPA (Kizaki *et al.*, 1989) involving the pathway of IL-2 gene expression. PKC-mediated phosphorylation of numerous protein substrates is associated with a wide range of biological effects, including stimulus secretion coupling, induction of cellular proliferation and differentiation, activation of nuclear transcription factors and cell surface receptors and tumour promotion. PKC is expressed in mammalian systems as a family of diverse serine–threonine kinases, consisting of at least nine isoforms differing in both substrate specificity and dependence upon Ca^{2+}. Mechanisms that explain the divergent actions of PKC are speculative at present. In haematopoietic cells, pharmacological agents that inhibit PKC activity, such as the isoquinolines, staurosporine and H7, inhibit the growth of both normal and leukaemic progenitors, suggesting the involvement of basal PKC activity in cell proliferation. In addition, PKC inhibitors block leukaemic cell differentiation in response to tumour-promoting phorboides. Since cell differentiation is associated with a loss of proliferative potential, these observations indicate that PKC inhibitors may exert pleitropic effects on haematopoietic cell behaviour. Efforts to define the role of PKC in the induction of apoptosis have been complicated by conflicting reports. For example, the observations that activation of PKC by exposure to PMA, either alone or in conjunction with Ca^{2+} ionophore, induces apoptosis in cells of lymphoid origin and that inhibition of PKC by exposure to H7 prevents glucocorticoid-induced apoptosis in murine thymocytes (McConkey *et al.*, 1995) suggest that PKC activation promotes this process. On the other hand, the ability of PMA to oppose steroid-induced apoptosis in thymic lymphocytes and to prevent growth factor-deprived haematopoietic cells from undergoing apoptotic cell death is instead consistent with an antagonistic influence (Jarvis *et al.*, 1994 a, b). Although most studies argue in favour of a role for PKC in apoptosis, future studies will pinpoint its specific contributory role in apoptosis.

Besides PKC, other kinases have been reported to be associated with apoptosis. Pl3 kinase [phosphatidylinositol(Pl) 3-kinase] is activated by different growth factors. Activation of Pl3 kinase leads to phosphorylation of AKT (Protein Kinase-B). Phosphorylated AKT induces phosphorylation of *bad* through certain kinase.

Phosphorylated *bad* remains inactive because it is squelched by 14-3-3 proteins and the cells survive. However, dephosphorylation of *bad* in the absense of phosphorylated AKT results in *bad* being dissociated from 14-3-3. The dissociated *bad* binds to *bcl-XL* releasing *bax*. This leads to apoptosis. AKT also phosphorylates procaspase-9, thereby inactivating caspase-9 mediated activation of caspase cascade (Rohn *et al.*, 1998; Cardone *et al.*, 1998).

Other important biochemical determinants of apoptosis include cAMP, ceramide and the redox status of a cell. The sphingomyelin pathway, initiated by hydrolysis of the phospholipid sphingomyelin in the cell membrane to generate the second messenger ceramide, is thought to mediate apoptosis in response to tumor necrosis factor-α (TNFα), to FAS ligand and to X-rays. Generation of ceramide (hydrolysis product of spingomyelin) through the spingmyelin pathway results in the induction of apoptosis in several cell lines. At least two specific intracellular targets for ceramide have been identified: (i) a membrane ceramide-activated protein kinase and (ii) a cytoplasmic ceramide-activated protein phosphatase. Ceramide promotes the formation and release of oligonucleosomal DNA fragments, produces corresponding loss of integrity of bulk DNA fragments and elicits the expression of the classical morphology of apoptosis. Interestingly, ceramide-related DNA damage consists exclusively of double-stranded breaks introduced into mature DNA, but not nascent DNA. Surprisingly, apoptosis is not initiated by diglyceride or other glycerophospholipid-derived messengers (e.g. Iysophosphatidylcholine, arachidonic acid or phosphatidic acid) in these cells (U937/HL60). However, a recent report claims that Hep-G$_2$ cells overexpressing P4502E1 undergo apoptosis upon exposure to arachidonic acid (Chen *et al.*, 1997). Similarly to ceramide, cAMP promotes palatal fusion which involves PCD of medial edge epithelial cells (Pratt and Martin, 1975). McConkey *et al.* (1990a) have reported that agents that elevate cAMP stimulate DNA fragmentation and apoptosis in thymocytes via activation of cAMP-dependent protein kinase A, whereas Edwards *et al.* (1991) have observed that analogues of cAMP inhibit apoptosis. This disparity may be due to the model system tested. Similarly to cAMP and ceramide, Ca^{2+} and other agents with a role in maintaining cellular redox status including antioxidants (e.g. vitamin C, vitamin E), ADP/ATP, NAD/NADH, NADP/NADPH, and GSH/GSSG ratios may influence apoptotic death by varied mechanisms. Fernandez *et al.* (1994) reported that marked GSH depletion enhances the cytotoxicity of alkylating agents (e.g. melphalan, chlorambucil), switching the programmed mode (apoptosis) to the unprogrammed mode (necrosis) of cell death, whereas Cotter and co-workers (Verhaegen *et al.*, 1995) claim that antioxidants including BHA inhibit apoptosis. Similarly, agents that deplete intracellular glutathione render cells more vulnerable to oxidative stress-induced apoptosis

(Zhong *et al.*, 1993). The redox potential of a cell is as critical as maintaining intracellular ion homeostasis or genomic integrity. An oxidative shift by ROS (reactive oxygen species) may modify the nature of the stimulatory signal, resulting in alteration of the direction of the programme (apoptosis/necrosis $\rightleftharpoons$ proliferation). Efficient activation of $NF_{\kappa}B$-dependent genes by TNF requires that a cell be in an oxidized state, suggesting that stimuli such as TNF and phorbol myristate acetate may exert only a limited response if the cell is not in an appropriate redox equilibrium (Israel *et al.*, 1992).

In this context, growing attention is now being devoted to mitochondrial functions during apoptosis. ROS, Ca^{2+}, MPT (mitochondrial permeability transition) and cyt-c (cytochrome *c*), are presumably all important for apoptosis. The first two entities, ROS and Ca^{2+}, are directly related under certain conditions. For example, ROS stimulate Ca^{2+} release from mitochondria, and when mitochondria cycles Ca^{2+} excessively their ROS production increases (Richter *et al.*, 1996). Mitochondria can initially protect the cell against toxic increases in Ca^{2+}; however, excess Ca^{2+} cycling may culminate in collapse of the $\Delta\psi$ (mitochondrial membrane potential), resulting in a variety of lethal molecular lesions. Similarly, TNF α stimulates ROS production by mitochondria, and the TNF α-induced apoptotic killing of few cell types is due to ROS-induced mitochondrial Ca^{2+} cycling since apoptosis is blocked by mitochondrial Ca^{2+} uptake inhibitors (Hennet *et al.*, 1993a, b). An important breakthrough in this direction, which provides a specific clue as to which mitochondrial parameter(s) may be important for the control of apoptosis, comes from the observation that the stabilization of $\Delta\psi$, either by overexpression of a death inhibitory gene (*bcl-2*) or by the ionophore nigericin, prevents apoptosis induced by TNFα. Many laboratories have reported that $\Delta\psi$, which is the driving force for mitochondrial ATP synthesis, decreases prior to DNA damage, and maintenance of $\Delta\psi$ prevents apoptosis (Shimizu *et al.*, 1996).

Ca^{2+}, oxidant chemicals and a range of other inducers (e.g. oxidative stress and alteration in cellular phosphorylation state) promote the onset of the mitochondrial permeability transition (MPT) in mitochondria. The MPT reflects the opening of a highly regulated pore within the inner mitochondrial membrane. Opening of high-conductance permeability transition pores causes the onset of the transition, leading to membrane depolarization, release of ions, uncoupling of oxidative phosphorylation, permeation of sucrose and other solutes of molecular weight less than 1500 and large amplitude mitochondrial swelling. Ca^{2+}, oxidant chemicals, Pi (inorganic phosphate), and membrane depolarization promote pore opening, whereas, Mg^{2+}, ADP, low pH and immunosuppressant cyclosporin-A favour the closed state. Oxidants, including doxorubicin, are the most thoroughly studied class of inducing agents. Doxorubicin interferes with the capacity of isolated cardiac mitochondria to accumulate and retain calcium, and it does this by selectively inducing the MPT, presumably via the free radical-mediated oxidation of critical protein thiols associated with the voltage-sensing element of the pore. Associated with this is an increased sensitivity to calcium-induced membrane depolarization and osmotic swelling. Mitochondrial osmotic swelling in response to pore formation may be responsible for the release of mitochondrial factors that are crucial in triggering the late stages of the apoptotic pathway. One such factor is cytochrome *c*, the release of which occurs in the absence of significant changes in $\Delta\psi$, suggesting a novel mechanism for cell death commitment. Cytochrome *c* from a variety of metazoan species, including the insect *Manduca sexta*, all function pro-apoptotically in *Xenopus* egg extracts. Thus, collectively, these studies indicate that loss of mitochondrial function may be an important pivotal point in modulating cellular energy status and influencing cell-death processes including apoptosis (Lemasters and Nieminen, 1998; Qian *et al.*, 1999).

GENETIC REGULATION OF APOPTOSIS

The concept of active cell death or PCD being a genetically encoded process has stimulated an intense search for the genes involved in the regulation of the cell-death programme. Although the active involvement of a number of proteins has been demonstrated in either the causation or prevention of apoptotic death, the precise molecular mechanism of apoptosis is still poorly understood. Three phases of cell death (induction, initiation and execution), however, appear to be involved in the progression of apoptosis. The induction phase corresponds to the initiation of the apoptotic signal which has a specific 'goal'. The stimuli may be composed of combinations of altered physiological signals, chemical or physical damage or lack of survival signals. The initiation of apoptotic response appears to involve a number of oncogenes and tumour suppressor genes with specific roles exclusively in cell death. However, their roles may be limited to a specific apoptotic system or systems as few, if any, of these play universal roles in all forms of cell death. This suggests that apoptosis is a result of the expression of specific genes whose products direct the process of cell death and account for its several characteristic features. Several genes (or gene products) participating in this process are listed in **Table 5a** and **5b**.

The maintenance of normal cell number in tissues (homeostasis) requires a delicate balance between the rate of cell division and the rate of cell death. When this balance favours the direction of increase in the rate of proliferation, a decrease in the rate of cell death, or both, it leads to benign or malignant tumours. Oncogenes positively influence cell proliferation and growth, whereas tumour suppressor genes (anti-oncogenes) act as negative regulators of growth. Since apoptosis

Table 5 Genes or gene product(s) involved in regulating apoptosis and programmed cell death

Gene or gene product	Influence on cell death/Putative mechanisms of action	References
Bcl-2	Inhibits/delays apoptosis, binds to *Bax and Bak*	(Vaux *et al.*, 1992; Hockenberry *et al.*, 1993; Hengartner and Horvitz, 1994)
Bcl-XL	Inhibits apoptosis; binds *Bax* and *Bak*	(Boise *et al.*, 1993)
A1	Inhibits apoptosis *Bcl-2* family member, early response gene, transcriptionally induced by GM-CSF	(Lin *et al.*, 1993)
Mcl-1	Inhibits apoptosis; *Bcl-2* family member	(Kozopas *et al.*, 1993; Reynolds *et al.*, 1994)
Ced-9	Anti-apoptotic, *C. elegans* major death inhibitor, homologous to *Bcl-2*	(Hengartner *et al.*, 1992; Hengartner and Horvitz, 1994)
BHRF-1	*Bcl-2* homolog that inhibits apoptosis, Epstein Barr Virus gene	(Marchini *et al.*, 1991)
ASFV HMWF5-HL	African Swine Fever Virus gene homologous to *Bcl-2*	(Neilan *et al.*, 1993)
Bad	Accelerates apoptosis, interacts with *Bcl-2* and *Bcl-XL*; can displace *Bax* from *Bcl-XL*	(Yang *et al.*, 1995)
Bak	Promotes or inhibits apoptosis; binds to *Bcl-2*, *Bcl-X*, and E1B 19K; sequence homology with *Bcl-2* within BH1 and BH2 regions	(Chittenden *et al.*, 1995; Farrow *et al.*, 1995; Keifer *et al.*, 1995)
Bax	Promotes apoptosis, binds to *Bcl-2*, *Bcl-XL*, E1B 19K	(Oltvai *et al.*, 1993)
Bcl-Xs	Promotes apoptosis, binds *Bcl-2*	(Boise *et al.*, 1993)
Nbk, Bik1	Apoptosis promoter, binds to *Bcl-2*, E1B 19K, *Bcl-XL*, and BHRF1, has only BH3 domain	(Boyd *et al.*, 1994)
Ced-3	*C. elegans* gene, apoptosis promoter	(Yuan *et al.*, 1993; Kumar *et al.*, 1994)
Ced-4	*C. elegans* gene, apoptosis promoter homologous to caspases and Apaf-1 in mammals	(Ellis and Horvitz, 1986; Yuan and Horvitz, 1990)
p35	Baculovirus gene, apoptosis inhibitor, binds to and inhibits caspases	(Bump *et al.*, 1995)
CrmA	Apoptosis inhibitor, cowpox viral protein, inhibits apoptosis induced by caspases	(Gagliardini *et al.*, 1994; Tewari *et al.*, 1995)
MORT-1/FADD	Apoptosis promoter, binds Fas; same as FADD	(Boldin *et al.*, 1995; Chinnaiyan *et al.*, 1995)
TRADD	Apoptosis promoter, binds TNFR-1	(Hsu *et al.*, 1995)
Reaper	Activator of programmed cell death in Drosophila, similarity to death domain of TNFR-1	(White *et al.*, 1994)
p53	Apoptosis promoter, tumour suppressor gene, transactivates *Bax* expression	(Younish-Rouch *et al.*, 1991; Miyashita *et al.*, 1994;)
C-myc	Apoptosis promoter, protooncogene, transcription factor	(Fanidi *et al.*, 1992; Evan *et al.*, 1992)
R-*ras*	Apoptosis promoter, binds *Bcl-2*	(Fernandez-Sarabia *et al.*, 1993; Wang *et al.*, 1995)
Rb	Involved during apoptosis, tumour suppressor	(Freeman *et al.*, 1994; deJong *et al.*, 1998)
C-fos	Upregulated during apoptosis, transcription factor, IER (immediate early response) genes	(Buttyan *et al.*, 1988; Janssen *et al.*, 1997)
C-Jun	Upregulated during apoptosis, IER gene, AP-1 group of transcription factors	(Estus *et al.*, 1994; Pandey and Wang, 1995; Walton *et al.*, 1998)
Hsp70	Involved during apoptosis, heat shock protein	(Buttyan *et al.*, 1988)
Sgp-2/TRPM-2	Involved during apoptosis, transfer lipids (?), complement inhibitor (?), include *clusterin* in this family	(Buttyan *et al.*, 1989)
cdk-4/cdk-5	Involved during apoptosis, cyclin dependent protein kinases	(Freeman *et al.*, 1994)
cyclin D1/cyclin D3	Involved during apoptosis, cell cycle regulator	(Freeman *et al.*, 1994; deJong *et al.*, 1998)
egr-1	Apoptosis promoter, transcription factor	(Liu *et al.*, 1998)
Rp-2/Rp-8	Apoptosis promoters, integral membrane protein (?) and DNA binding protein (?)	(Owens *et al.*, 1991)
Fas/APO1/CD95	Apoptosis promoter, members of TNF receptor superfamily	(Nagata and Golstein, 1995)
TNF-R1	Apoptosis promoter, cell surface receptor	(Cleveland and Ihle, 1995)
Dad-1	Apoptosis inhibitor	(Nakashima *et al.*, 1993)
Calpain	Accelerates apoptosis, induces proteolysis	(Squier and Cohen, 1997; Spinedi *et al.*, 1998)
Granzyme B	Apoptosis promoter, Serine protease, activates caspases, cytolytic to T cells	(Shi *et al.*, 1996; Trapani *et al.*, 1998)
Survival factors	Growth factors and cytokines such as IGF-1 and various interleukins that act to promote cell survival	(Raff 1992; Harrington *et al.*, 1994; O'Connor, 1998)
TGF-β	Apoptosis promoter, growth factor, may influence *Bcl-2* expression but not dependent upon *Bax* or *p53*	(Selvakumaran *et al.*, 1994; Buske *et al.*, 1997; Roberson *et al.*, 1997)

essentially counterbalances cell proliferation, genes involved in apoptosis may regulate growth. Cell-death research has primarily focused on 'death genes' and the 'survival genes'. Green and Cotter (1995) have classified 'death genes' as those that 'set up' conditions leading to apoptosis, for example by transducing signals, triggering other molecules and/or driving the cell cycle to a required point for exit into death pathway. Once apoptosis is 'set up', it presumably proceeds via the action of gene products that are common to all types of cell death.

The first anti-apoptotic gene to be clearly identified in humans was *bcl-2* (B-cell lymphoma-leukaemia-2 gene), cloned from the breakpoint of the t (14:18) translocation found in the majority of follicular lymphomas (Tsuji-moto *et al.*, 1984). The discovery of the *bcl-2* oncogene helped to stimulate recognition of the concept that gene products which modulate the susceptibility of certain cell types to apoptosis may play an important role in the process leading to malignant transformation. This is primarily due to the survival of cells in inappropriate physiological situations. In both pathological and physiological conditions, the *bcl-2* gene has emerged as a critical regulator of apoptosis. Although *bcl-2* is widespread in the developing embryo, in adults it is found only in the progenitor cells (Hockenbery *et al.*, 1991). *Bcl-2* expression is localized to mitochondrial, endoplasmic reticulum and nuclear membranes. The ability of *bcl-2* to extend cell survival by preventing cell death *in vivo* in different cell types and in response to different stimuli suggests that *bcl-2*, or *bcl-2*-like molecules, act at a central controlling point in the pathway to apoptotic cell death. Mice (knockout transgenic mice) which lack the *bcl-2* protein are normal at birth (possess impaired kidney development), but later progress to polycystic kidney disease and catastrophic postnatal immune function failure (Veis *et al.*, 1993). *In vivo*, *bcl-2* prevents many, but not all, forms of apoptotic death (Sentman *et al.*, 1991; Allsopp *et al.*, 1993; Cuende *et al.*, 1993). Cumulatively, all these observations suggest an important role for *bcl-2 in vivo*. Expression of the *bcl-2* protein has been shown directly to prevent apoptosis by enhancing cellular antioxidant capacity, possibly through scavenging reactive oxygen radicals (Kane *et al.*, 1993) or indirectly by counteracting oxidative stress (Hockenbery *et al.*, 1993a; Kane *et al.*, 1993). The other potential mechanisms of this gene include a role in intracellular calcium regulation, nuclear transport and control of signal transduction pathways (Reed, 1994). *Bcl-2* is no longer a single entity but one member of a growing multi-gene family. Included in this family are *bcl-x* (*bcl* − *x_L* and *bcl* − *x_S*), *mcl-1*, *bax*, *A1*, *bak*, *bad*, *bcl-w* and *Ced-9*. Viral homologues such as *BHRF1* (Epstein–Barr virus or EBV), *LMW5-HL* (African swine fever virus or AFSB) and *E1B 19K* (adenovirus) are also included. The transcripts of *bcl-x* are alternatively spliced to form *bcl* − *X_L* (designated as long form) and *bcl* − *X_S* (designated as short form). The former is a death inhibitor and the latter a

death inducer. *Bcl-x* is expressed widely during development (high levels are expressed in brain, kidney and thymus). *Bcl-2* and *bcl-x* complement each other in their functions. *Mcl-1* was cloned in a screen for genes with increased expression when a human myeloblastic leukaemia cell line was induced to differentiate by phorbol ester (Kozopas *et al.*, 1993). *Mcl-1* is considerably larger than *bcl-2*. *Mcl-1* is primarily membrane bound and its expression delays apoptosis induced by deregulated *c-myc* (Reynolds *et al.*, 1994). Another relative of *bcl-2*, *A1*, which was isolated from mouse bone marrow induced to proliferate with granulocyte macrophage colony-stimulating factor (GM-CSF), resembles an early response gene and is transcriptionally induced by GM-CSF (Lin *et al.*, 1993). The best evidence for a single apoptotic pathway comes from studies in the nematode *C. elegans*, in which genes whose functions appear to be required for all forms of developmental death have been identified (Ellis *et al.*, 1991). This invertebrate is well suited for the study of both normal and aberrant cell death at the cellular, genetic and molecular levels since this organism is essentially transparent throughout its life cycle, and individual nuclei can be readily visualized using differential interference contrast optics. There is no model system in which PCD is better understood. Among the genes involved, *Ced-3*, *Ced-4* and *Ced-9* have attracted the most attention. *Ced-3* and *Ced-4* enhance cell death by apoptosis, whereas *Ced-9* (*bcl-2*-like) opposes it. Mutation of any of these genes demonstrates opposite effects. Although *Ced-3* and *Ced-4* appear to have structural and functional homologues in mammalian cells, it is unlikely that a single pathway for apoptosis exists in mammals. Various genes and the roles they play, either *in vivo* or *in vitro*, are listed in **Table 5**.

Dismantling of cellular structures during apoptosis requires proteases. The involvement of proteases in apoptosis was implicated with the discovery of *Ced-3*. The first mammalian homolog of cysteine protease *Ced-3* was found to be ICE (interleukin-1β-converting enzyme). By now, 13 different cysteine proteases associated with apoptosis have been found and are called caspases (**Table 5a**) (Nicholson and Thornberry, 1997). The caspases have very high similarity in amino acid sequences, subunit structures, and substrate specificity. The caspases are synthesized as inactive pro-caspases (30 to 50 KD) with a pro-domain at the aminoterminus followed by the large subunit (~20 KD) and the small subunit (~10 KD) at the carboxyl terminus. Apoptotic signal leads to activation of caspases by proteolytic cleavage of procaspases either by autocatalysis or by active caspases. The two subunits (large and small) form heterodimer and the catalytic domain is shared by both the subunits. The caspases appear to be activated in cascades because the cleavage sites of proenzymes is the target of specific caspases. The initiator caspases are activated upon receiving apoptotic signal and they activate effector caspases. The effector caspases

Table 5a Various caspases involved in regulating apoptosis and programmed cell death

Caspase	Alternative name	Function in apoptosis
Caspase-1	ICE	
Caspase-2	ICH-1, Nedd-2 (mouse)	initiator/effector?
Caspase-3	CPP32, Yama, Apopain	effector
Caspase-4	TX, ICH-2, ICErel II	
Caspase-5	TY, ICErel III	
Caspase-6	Mch2	effector
Caspase-7	Mch3, CMH-1, ICE-LAP3	effector
Caspase-8	Mch5, MACHal, FLICE	initiator
Caspase-9	Mch6, ICE-LAP6	initiator?
Caspase-10		
Caspase-11		
Caspase-12		
Caspase-13		

in turn activate more initiator caspases by feed back regulation loop. This leads to amplification of caspase activation cascade. Activation of initiator caspases appear be regulated by interaction with different cofactors. However, not much is known about it. For example, activation of procaspase-8 and procaspase-9 require interaction with FADD (Fas activated death domain) and APAF-1 (mammalian homolog of Ced-4), respectively. The caspases are very specific proteases. They always cleave polypeptides only after aspartic acid residues. Different caspases recognize different target sequences which constitute at least four amino acids immediately aminoterminal to the aspartic acid residue. However, not all proteins with specific caspase target sequences are cleaved by the corresponding caspases. How caspases help kill the cell is not very well understood. About 40 different cellular proteins have been identified as targets of caspases. Although these proteins represent only a subset of the targets of caspases, they clearly indicate that caspases inactivate proteins associated with functions such as negative regulation of apoptosis (e.g., ICAD, bcl-2), building of cellular structures (e.g., lamins, gelsolin, focal adhesion kinase [FAK2], vimentin, fodrin), DNA repair (e.g., DNA-PKCs), mRNA splicing (e.g., U1-70K), and DNA replication (e.g., replication factor C) (see Thornberry et al., 1992; Wilson et al., 1994; Wang et al., 1994; Nicholson et al., 1995; Zhivotovsky et al., 1995; Faucheu et al., 1995) Overexpression of Ced-3 or ICE in mammalian cells induces apoptosis that is inhibitable by bcl-2. It is believed that the ICE family proteases may act on a very important DNA-repair enzyme, poly(ADP-ribose) polymerase (Lazebnik et al., 1994). Actin may also serve as a substrate for ICE; actin cleaved by an ICE loses its ability to polymerize and to inhibit deoxyribonuclease I activity, which may contribute to both the morphological changes and the DNA fragmentation observed during apoptosis. The other proteins which may undergo degradation during apoptotic death are phospholipase

A_2, PKC and cytoskeletal proteins such as fodrin and vimentin (McConkey et al., 1995).

Inhibitors of caspases were discovered by study of mode of prevention of apoptosis by viruses. By now, three different classes of inhibitors have been identified. They are p35, CrmA, and IAP. The p35 gene is expressed early in the infection of insect cells by the baculovirus. This early expression of p35 literally prevents cells from committing suicide. In the absence of p35 expression, the cells undergo apoptosis within a few hours after the infection. Expression of p35 in mammalian neural cells also inhibits apoptosis due to serum withdrawl, calcium ionophores and glucose withdrawal. The cowpox virus CrmA is a member of the serpin family of inhibitors. IAP is the only inhibitor to have mammalian homologs. It has been suggested that p35 antagonizes apoptosis by directly inhibiting pro-apoptotic cysteine proteases, i.e. the ICE family, in a fashion similar to that of cowpox CrmA (Bump et al., 1995).

The cellular protooncogene c-jun is an immediate early response gene (IER gene) known to participate in certain forms of apoptosis. It is a member of the leucine-zipper family and encodes with c-fos (which arises late in transcription). For example, c-jun is upregulated in human leukaemia cells undergoing apoptosis in response to diverse cytotoxic agents (ara-C, campothecin, VP-16), whereas it can block apoptosis in neoplastic lymphoid cells induced by growth factor deprivation. As a whole, c-fos and c-jun interact with APO-1 (Fas antigen) sites and regulate transcription and cell proliferation in addition to influencing PKC and apoptotic signalling pathways. Various studies have shown that environmental stresses can induce SAPK (stress-activated protein kinase) and JNK (jun-kinase) and SAPK/JNK signalling systems (Verheij et al., 1996), which involves sequential activation of the proteins MEKK1 (mitogen-activated protein kinase/extracellular signal regulated kinase kinase-1), SEK1 (stress-activated protein kinase/extracellular signal regulated kinase kinase-1) and c-jun (Pallardy et al., 1997). Ceramide production also leads to c-jun activation by the SAPK pathway and lead to ras activation (GTP binding protein/signal transduction). Specific inhibitors of ICE-like proteases can block apoptosis induced by ceramide, Fas ligand TNF_α and Reaper (Reaper is a Drosophila gene that codes for a protein consisting of a 65 amino acid minimal death domain). Interestingly, ceramide can activate mitogen-activated protein kinase (MAPKinase or MAPK), a family of serine/threonine kinases that are downstream of Raf-1 (serine/threonine kinases) in the ras pathway.

The FAS-L, FAS/APO-1 induced apoptotic process was briefly introduced in the calpain section of this chapter. These death domain proteins, FAS ligand (FAS-L) and TNFs (tumour necrosis factors), function as rapid inducers of cell death. The Fas/APO-1 belongs to the tumour necrosis factor (TNF) receptor superfamily which includes many death receptors besides FAS and TNFR. Upon interaction with death ligand, the death receptors can induce apoptosis in cells within minutes. The death receptors have a "death domain" in their cytoplasmic domains. Fas/APO-1/CD95 is associated with the regulation of immune response. Fas mediated apoptosis is involved in the following physiological conditions: elimination of activated mature T cells from peripheral blood at the end of an immune response; killing of target cells by cytotoxic T cells; and killing of inflammatory cells at the immune privileged sites. Fas ligand, like other TNF family members, is a homotrimeric molecule which binds to three Fas molecules, resulting in trimerization of Fas molecules. This leads to binding of the Fas activated death domain (FADD) protein to the death domain of Fas molecules through its own death domain. Anti-Fas antibody can also induce the same effect *in vitro*. The death effector domain (DED) of FADD recruits procaspase-8, which binds to the DED of FADD through its own DED by similar homophilic interaction, as in the case of Fas and FADD. This results in the activation of caspase-8 by autoproteolysis and the caspase cascade is activated, leading to cell death. Fas also transmits a death signal through binding of Daxx, instead of FADD, in the stress-activated JNK pathway.

TNF receptor (TNFR) is associated with both inflammatory and apoptotic response. Interaction of trimeric TNF with TNFR leads to the trimerization of TNFR molecules. This results in binding of the death domain of the TNFR-associated death domain (TRADD) protein to the death domain of TNFR. Binding of FADD to TRADD leads to apoptotic pathway through activation of caspase-8, as in the case of Fas and Fas ligand interaction. However, interaction of TRADD with TNFR-associated factor-2 (TRAF2) and receptor-interacting protein (RIP) leads to the activation of NF-kB or JNK/AP-1, which in turn leads to the induction of proinflammatory and immunomodulatory genes. Three different proteins, structurally unrelated, TRADD, FADD and RIP, were identified on the basis of their association with the cytoplasmic domains of TNF-R1 or FAS, and they also contain death domain motifs and apparently function in FAS-L-and TNF-induced cell death.

Another TNF family member, designated TNF-related apoptosis-inducing ligand (TRAIL), or alternatively APO-2, rapidly induces apoptosis in a wide variety of transformed cell lines of diverse origin (Nagata and Goldstein, 1995).

Another oncogene which was, long thought to play a critical role in life and death processes of cells is *c-myc*. The *c-myc* gene is the cellular homologue of the viral oncogene *v-myc*, and it plays a prominent role in carcinogenesis. The *c-myc* gene encodes nuclear phosphoprotein of approximately 60 kDa size, a member of the helix–loop–helix family of transcription factors abundant in proliferating cells. The expression of *c-myc* and cofactor

max appears transiently during castration-induced and post-lactation breast regression-induced apoptotic death of prostate and mammary cells, respectively (Buttyan *et al.*, 1988; Colombel *et al.*, 1992). In apoptotic cell death, the apparent role for *c-myc* was surprising and paradoxical because of its already recognized role in cell cycle progression and cell transformation. The *c-myc* level is higher in growing cells than in quiescent cells, indicating that expression of *c-myc* is necessary for cell proliferation. This is supported by the fact that its down regulation triggers growth arrest and differentiation. Chinese hamster ovary cells transfected with *c-myc* under the control of a heat-shock promoter undergo cell death associated with heat shock. Arends *et al.*, (1993) observed an increased rate of apoptotic death in fibroblasts that were transformed with the *myc* oncogene. Cells exhibiting dysregulated *c-myc* expression in the absence of adequate level of growth factors tend to undergo apoptosis, whereas in lymphocytes, antisense oligonucleotides to *c-myc* block certain forms of apoptosis (activation-induced) but not in others (steroid-induced). These events, together, may be interpreted as follows: growth arrest, *c-myc* off plus growth factors absent; population expansion, *c-myc* on plus growth factors present; and apoptosis, *c-myc* on plus growth factors absent. The *c-myc* protein has two distinct properties: (i) *myc* specifically binds to nucleotide sequences in DNA as a heterodimer with its cofactor max to regulate transcription; and (ii) *myc* can override the cell cycle block induced by *Rb-1* protein (Goodrich and Lee, 1992). In summary, the effect of *c-myc* depends on cell type and stimuli and is not needed for all forms of apoptosis. Inappropriate expression of *c-myc* may have evolved as a mechanism to prevent the development of neoplasia. This is particularly true for cells with dysregulated *c-myc* expression in situations where complementary growth factor-mediated signals were absent (Patel and Gores, 1995). However, the molecular mechanisms mediating these distinct and opposite functions of the *c-myc* protein remain unclear.

Considerable focus has fallen upon another gene, known as the guardian of the genome, associated with this suicidal process, namely *p53*. This suppressor gene codes for a 53 kDa protein that helps organisms cope with DNA damage by either stalling cell division or inducing cell death. This nuclear *p53* tumour suppressor gene is the most widely mutated gene in human tumourigenesis. Reintroduction of many mutants of this gene into transformed cells can induce either growth arrest (Harper *et al.*, 1993; Xiong *et al.*, 1993) or apoptosis (Yonish-Rouach *et al.*, 1991). The *p53* encodes a transcriptional activator whose targets may include genes that regulate genomic stability, cellular response to DNA damage and cell cycle progression. The *p53* gene product has been reported to function at both G1-S and G2-M checkpoints regulating cell cycle progression and induces cell-cycle arrest in response to DNA damage, allowing repair enzymes to function. It was appealing to think that *p53*-induced tumour suppression could arise through the activation of cell suicide that is irreversible, rather than through imposition of growth arrest as thought previously, which is inherently reversible. The consensus is that *p53* can induce growth arrest or apoptosis depending on the physiological circumstances or cell type, but that both activities are potentially involved in tumour suppression (White, 1996). Symonds *et al.* (1994) and Bardeesy *et al.* (1995) have demonstrated *p53*-mediated modulation of apoptosis in animal and human tumour models. *p53* accumulates and directs apoptosis in response to DNA damage in skin, thymocytes and intestinal epithelium. High levels of constitutive *c-myc* expression or exposure to chemotherapeutic agents elicits a *p53*-dependent apoptotic response. Since *p53* can function as a transcription factor, it may activate the transcription of death genes (*bax*) or repress the transcription of survival genes (*bcl-2*). Compared with the *p53*-expressing wild-type controls, tissues from *p53*-null mice show depressed *bax* expression and elevated *bcl-2* expression (Miyashita *et al.*, 1994).

All this experimental evidence suggests that up-regulation of *bax* transcription is a means by which *p53* induces apoptosis. *p53* contains three functional domains: an amino-terminal transcriptional activation domain, a central sequence-specific DNA binding domain and a carboxy-terminal oligomerization domain. The majority of the *p53* mutations sequenced from human tumours map within the sequence-specific DNA-binding domain and impair the ability of *p53* to bind DNA. *p53* has also been reported to induce Fas expression, which may represent an alternate, transcriptionally dependent means for *p53* to regulate apoptosis, in addition to induction of *bax*.

In summary, the participation of *p53* in apoptosis has important implications for the development of neoplastic disease. In tissues that are normally prone to *p53*-dependent apoptosis, inactivation of *p53* may promote tumour growth by allowing inappropriate cell survival following DNA damage. In other tissues, *p53* mutation may enhance the progression of neoplastic or pre-neoplastic lesions by eliminating an apoptotic programme that keeps tumour growth in check. Since *p53* also participates in a cell cycle checkpoint that arrests cell growth in response to DNA damage, several mechanisms may account for the high frequency of *p53* mutations occurring in human tumour.

In conclusion, genetic analysis of cell death has identified several key players required for the regulation and execution of cell-death pathway. More importantly, structurally related vertebrate genes that appear to play similar roles have been identified and characterized, indicating that the general framework of the cell-death mechanism has been conserved over the course of evolution. Depending upon the circumstances, cells may either oppose or follow the instructions of a single gene or several genes in a concerted fashion to follow or bypass the apoptotic pathway, whichever is beneficial for the organism (see review: Bredesen, 1995).

DRUG- AND CHEMICALLY INDUCED APOPTOSIS

It is an interesting paradox that life is dependent on cell death. Perturbations of normal life processes by toxic chemicals enable us to learn about the life processes themselves and represents an important aspect of toxicology. Life processes are highly dynamic, involving continuous turnover of cells, subcellular structures and biological molecules based upon opposing effects exemplified by death and regeneration, damage and repair, injury and compensation and degradation and resynthesis. Therefore, in order to define toxicity more precisely and to broaden the approach to mechanistic studies, the result of exposures to chemicals might be regarded as the product of divergent biological processes: injury on the one hand and compensation/repair on the other (Lotti, 1995).

Advances in our quest to understand lethal injury at the molecular level have built on discrete, novel observations. Each successive observation has stimulated a flurry of activity related to that biochemical or regulatory change and has led to heightened interest in the implicated subcellar organelle. Over time, attention has fallen on plasma membrane, cytoplasm, mitochondria, lyosomes and most other subcellular organelles. In considering the events described above, a most important stimulus for increased interest in the role of nucleus in lethal injury has come from the studies on programmed cell death. Hopefully, prior to the beginning of the millennium and beyond, research emphasis will continue to be placed upon cytoprotection and disease prevention strategies based on the knowledge gained from these mechanistic studies.

In the ever-increasing list of number of apoptogens, cancer chemotherapeutic agents, glucocorticoids and retinoids are the most extensively characterized (e.g. anti-metabolites, inhibitors of topoisomerase I and II and nucleoside analogues). Environmental contaminants such as dioxin, polychlorinated biphenyls (PCBs), polycyclic aromatic hydrocarbons (PAHs) and tributyltin are also capable of triggering apoptosis in relevant target tissues. Natural toxins capable of provoking apoptosis include ochratoxin-A, gliotoxin, diphtheria toxin, thapsigargin, staurosporine and genistin (McConkey *et al.*, 1995). From the plethora of accumulating reports it appears that most necrogens (drugs and chemicals capable of causing necrosis) are potential apoptogens (drugs and chemicals capable of inducing apoptosis), and vice versa. Likewise, most anti-necrogens are effective inhibitors of apoptosis and vice versa

(Ray *et al.*, 1996). Extensive studies on acetaminophen (paracetamol) offer some insights into these important but unresolved questions. It is known that acetaminophen directly alkylates genomic DNA both *in vivo* and *in vitro*, and that the analgesic produces genotoxic effects in a variety of test systems (Dybing *et al.*, 1984). These findings have now been extended to show that acetaminophen inhibits DNA synthesis and increases single strand breaks and sister chromatic exchanges of V79 Chinese hamster cells (Hongslo *et al.*, 1988). Although some of these events appear relatively late and may relate more to the carcinogenic rather than the hepatotoxic potential of acetaminophen, they are important in that they demonstrate the ability of acetaminophen to damage DNA directly or to inhibit systems that maintain DNA integrity. A series of publications by Ray and his collaborators indicated that acetaminophen-induced cell death *in vivo* (Ray *et al.*, 1990, 1991a, b, 1993) very closely resemble aspects of programmed cell death *in vitro*, particularly as described for the lymphoid cell model using immature thymocytes (Wyllie, 1980; Cohen and Duke, 1984). Classic apoptotic damage including Ca^{2+} accumulation, DNA fragmentation in the form of a ladder and decreased nuclear DNA recovery all appeared prior to extensive enzyme leakage [alanine aminotransferase (ALT)] into plasma and quantifiable liver damage in mice. The timing of these events suggested that faltering Ca^{2+} regulation throughout the cell, but particularly in the nucleus, leads to activation of an endonuclease very early during apoptosis, that has been described for thymocyte killing *in vitro* (Wyllie, 1980; Cohen and Duke, 1984). Shen *et al.* (1991, 1992) were able to reproduce these acetaminophen-induced *in vivo* effects in *in vitro* (cultured hepatocyte) model systems. It is now well established that a hepatotoxic dose of acetaminophen *in vivo* induces death of hepatocytes by apoptosis as well as necrosis (Alison and Sarraf, 1994; Ray *et al.*, 1996). Numerous cells undergoing apoptosis are found in the liver long after the progression of toxicity due to acetaminophen (even after 24 h of drug exposure). Since apoptotic cells are very rapidly removed from *in vivo* systems, the presence of a large number of this type of cells very late in the toxicosis may indicate two possibilities: (i) rapid onset of apoptosis in a large population of cells that cannot be quickly removed; or (ii) the efficiency of removal process slows down as the toxicosis progresses to a stage at which homeostatic chaos sets in (Ray *et al.*, 1996). Similarly, Prichard and Butler (1989) used dimethylnitrosamine (DMN: a powerful carcinogen and a potent hepato-, immuno- and nephrotoxin) as a model compound and demonstrated its potential to induce apoptosis in the liver *in vivo*. Later, Ray *et al.* (1992) unravelled some of the biochemical steps, e.g. Ca^{2+} dysregulation, involved in this DMN-induced death cascade, which were consistent with histochemical and ultrastructural changes of apoptosis observed by Prichard and Butler (1989). The biochemical changes involved in both DMN- and acetaminophen-induced apoptosis (Ray *et al.*, 1992, 1993) were similar and primarily involved intranuclear Ca^{2+}-mediated endonuclease-dependent fragmentation of genomic DNA. This observation was further substantiated by experiments with Ca^{2+}-channel blockers, e.g. verapamil and chlorpromazine, which prevented Ca^{2+} entry into the hepatocellular nucleus and protected DNA from the endonuclease attack, ultimately resulting in the prevention of hepatotoxicity and lethality (Ray *et al.*, 1993). In some of the *in vitro* experiments, aurintricarboxylic acid, an inhibitor of endonuclease and protein synthesis, was employed successfully to block DNA fragmentation and thus cells death (McConkey *et al.*, 1989; Shen *et al.*, 1992). Strika *et al.* (1998) used a loop diuretic, furosemide (frusemide), and showed that it can induce apoptosis in addition to necrosis in the mouse liver and kidney. Faa *et al.* (1994) used a translational inhibitor, cycloheximide, and demonstrated its potential to induce apoptosis in rat liver by electron microscopy. The ultrastructural changes observed in this study were classically apoptotic. Later, using transgenic liver cells (L_{37} SV_{40}), this apoptosis-inducing potential of cycloheximide was found to be due to growth factor deprivation (Bulera *et al.*, 1996).

The interaction of toxicants and apoptosis is complex and the mechanisms of interaction are likely to differ among different toxicants. The apoptosis-inducing potential of a variety of carcinogens has recently been addressed at great length. For many years, research with PAHs has focused on the ability of these common environmental chemicals to induce cell transformation. Many investigators share the notion that carcinogens antagonize (or alter) the apoptotic pathway and improve the chances of cell survival. In contrast, many carcinogens, including PAHs, are powerful inducers of apoptosis. PAHs are classic examples. Within the PAH chemical group, 7,12-dimethylbenz[*a*]anthracene (DMBA) is one of the most cytotoxic and immunosuppressive agents that has been studied. DMBA causes apoptotic death of cells in a variety of tissues *in vivo* and $A_{20.1}$ murine B-cell lymphoma *in vitro* (Burchiel *et al.*, 1992, 1993; Yamaguchi *et al.*, 1997). AhR (aryl hydrocarbon receptor)-mediated effects on Ca^{2+}-endonuclease possibly triggered the apoptotic events observed in these studies. The involvement of Ca^{2+}-endonuclease was also unequivocally demonstrated in TCDD (tetrachlorodibenzo-*p*-dioxin)-induced thymic cell apoptosis (McConkey *et al.*, 1988a). Fuchs and Pruett (1993) have demonstrated morphine-induced mouse thymocyte apoptosis *in vivo* but not *in vitro*, and suggest that both glucocorticoid and opiate receptors are involved in the process. The anti-tumour antibiotic mitomycin C, a DNA synthesis inhibitor, induces aspermatogenic cell apoptosis in mouse testis (Nakagawa *et al.*, 1997). Agents that induce apoptosis *in vivo* and *in vitro* are listed in **Tables 3** and **4**.

Numerous recent studies indicate that chemotherapeutic agents are capable of triggering apoptosis of both malignant and normal cells. Drugs as diverse as alkylating agents [*N*-(5,5-diacetoxypentyl)doxorubicin], DNA topoisomerase II inhibitors (fostriecin, etoposide, dactinomycin), DNA-intercalating compounds [1-(β-D-arabinofuranosyl)cytosine; Ara-C], DNA-binding compounds (actinomycin-D), DNA cross-linking agents (nitrogen mustard), protein phosphatase (1A, 2A) inhibitor (okadaic acid), PKC inhibitors (Ara-C, staurosporine, H7) and microtubule-disrupting agents (vinblastine, vincristine, colchicine, nocodazole) have all been demonstrated to be potent inducers of apoptosis although by different mechanisms (see **Tables 3–5**).

In recent years, another popular hepatotoxin, ethanol, has captured the attention of many researchers. Emerging data indicate that apoptotic death occurs in addition to necrotic death in several hepatobiliary diseases, including ethanol-induced liver injury, *in vivo* (Benedetti *et al.*, 1988a, b; Goldin *et al.*, 1993; Baroni *et al.*, 1994) and also in *in vitro* model systems (Chen *et al.*, 1997). Unlike acetaminophen and higher alcohols [C_3 (propan-2-ol) to C_8 (octanol)], however, one bolus dose of LD_{50} of ethanol fails to induce apoptosis in the rat liver. Higher alcohols (butanol, pentanol, hexanol and octanol) are potent inducers of apoptosis in the normal rat liver. Ray and co-workers also observed that spontaneously hypertensive rats were more sensitive to the apoptosis inducing potential of alcohols (Manolas *et al.*, 1997). Later, the same group showed that moderate ethanol exposure for 3 weeks (week 1, 3%; week 2, 4%; and week 3, 5%) followed by a low-level acetaminophen (300 or 400 mg kg^{-1}, i.p.) exposure dramatically potentiates the acetaminophen-induced apoptotic death rate of mouse liver cells *in vivo* (Ray, 1997). Although oxidative stress has been proposed to be a principal stimulus leading to apoptosis in this case (Kurose *et al.*, 1997), it is extremely difficult to pinpoint a definitive mechanistic conclusion for ethanol-induced apoptosis since the dose, duration, route of exposure and biosystems are diverse. Increased expression of *bcl-2* protein has recently been demonstrated in ethanol-exposed rat livers (Yacoub *et al.*, 1995). However, this increased *bcl-2* expression was found to be due to the presence of an excess number of inflammatory cells rather than an increase in expression of the gene in the liver cells. Similar observations were reported by Dhruva and Ray (1996), Dhruva *et al.* (1996) and Ray (1998) in acetaminophen-treated mouse livers, where they found no expression of *bcl-2* in the mouse livers. The fact that hepatocytes lack *bcl-2* altogether (Oberhammer *et al.*, 1992) and yet are subject to regulation by apoptosis suggests that *bcl-2*-independent mechanisms exist. Future studies with ethanol will elucidate its interaction at the organelle level (e.g. mitochondrial permeability transition or cytochrome *c* release) and/or at the genetic level (e.g. *bcl-2* regulation).

As a normal attribute of aerobic life, structural (cellular and subcellular structures), and functional (macromolecules, e.g. enzymes, DNA, proteins, carbohydrates) oxidative damage inflicted by ROS (reactive oxygen species: O_2^-, H_2O_2, $HO^{\bullet}$, etc.) has been called 'oxidative stress'. Buttke and Sandstrom (1994) have reviewed the role of oxidative stress in apoptosis. Many agents (either physical, e.g. ionizing/UV radiation, or chemical, e.g. redox cyclers) including anti-neoplastic agents are capable of provoking oxidative stress in addition to inducing apoptosis mediated by a variety of ROS (Buttke and Sandstrom, 1994; Pallardy *et al.*, 1997; Bagchi *et al.*, 1998). Evidence that oxidative stress can induce apoptosis came from studies in which apoptosis induced by ROS was inhibited by antioxidants. One such example is TNFα. Stimulation of the TNFα receptor escalates the intracellular production of ROS (increased mitochondrial superoxide anion production) which is linked to cell death, and interference of ROS production by *N*-acetylcysteine or a free radical scavenger, thioredoxin, prevents apoptotic cell death (Buttke and Sandstrom, 1994; Pallardy *et al.*, 1997). The Fas antigen, which is structurally related to the TNF receptor, also induces apoptosis when cross-linked with anti-Fas antibodies and its ability to induce apoptosis cell has been shown to be blocked by thioredoxin. Exogenous sources of ROS such as H_2O_2 and *tert*-butyl hydroperoxide induce apoptosis at doses below the necrogenic doses. Quinone compounds that undergo redox cycles and cause superoxide radical formation such as menadione or 2,3-dimethoxy-1,4-naphthoquinone provoke apoptosis (McConkey *et al.*, 1988b). Chronic inhibition of superoxide dismutase transcription or activity causes apoptotic death. Intracellular ROS may activate the genes responsible for apoptosis, conceivably through an oxidative stress-responsive nuclear transcription factor such as NF-κB (Sen and Packer, 1996).

In the past few years, another notorious ROS, nitric oxide (NO), has been the subject of intense debate in this field. NO orchestrates a number of useful and deleterious pathophysiological activities and is synthesized from molecular oxygen and the guanidino group of L-arginine by several isoforms of NOS (nitric oxide synthase: EC 1.14.13.39). NO is a messenger molecule which participates in drug-induced hepatotoxic reactions, relaxation of smooth muscle, neurotransmission and killing of tumour cells and bacteria. Recent evidence suggests that biochemical and toxicological effects of NO are mediated, in part, by $ONOO^-$ (peroxynitrite: a reaction product with superoxide anion, O_2^-). NO and $ONOO^-$ have both been shown to induce necrosis in many model systems (Ignarro, 1990; Nathan, 1992), however, their apoptogenic potential in murine macrophages, human epithelial cells and HL-60 cells is also remarkable (Messmer *et al.*, 1995; Sandoval *et al.*, 1997). Mechanisms proposed for NO toxicity include its interaction with protein thiol groups or iron sulphur proteins or by direct DNA damage. The genomic damage induced by radiation or by drugs such as etoposide, can result in apoptosis. NO may signal different forms of cell death depending on the type and/or the steady-state concentration of the NO redox species involved. A link between *p53* expression and NO synthesis dependence has been established (Memer *et al.*, 1994), although the connection between anti-death gene *bcl₂*, NO, and apoptosis remains open for investigation (Dhruva and Ray, 1996; Dhruva *et al.*, 1996). Similarly, the precise role of Kupffer cells, macrophages, neutrophils and phagocytes needs further scrutiny since they play a dominant role during NO-induced apoptosis *in vivo*.

Research has advanced our understanding of the molecular, cellular and systemic processes in the pathogenesis of diseases associated with exposure to environmental agents. Their potential to induce apoptosis is a very slowly but steadily emerging field, and it can be easily predicted that this branch of research will have a significant impact on the entire toxicology discipline in the upcoming millennium since newer toxicants are being routinely identified, characterized and added to the ever-growing list. Consequences of their exposure will provide the necessary momentum to explore the role of this beneficial form of death in their respective toxicities. Mounting evidence indicates that many of them are genotoxic and some of them are non-genotoxic. Among these, TCDD, TCE, DCE, CCl₄, CHCl₃, hexavalent chromium compounds, cadmium compounds, nickel compounds and tributyltins have been thoroughly investigated. Surprisingly, some of the historic compounds, e.g., ethylmethane sulfonate, CCl₄ and CHCl₃, lack the potential to induce apoptosis despite the observations that their toxicities are Ca^{2+} dependent (Long *et al.*, 1989; Ray and Fariss, 1994). In contrast, the other agents (e.g. DCE, TCE, TCDD) listed above are very efficient apoptosis inducers (Blankenship *et al.*, 1994; Costa, 1998). Besides TCDD (McConkey *et al.*, 1988b), mechanistically well defined examples from this category are tributyltin oxide [bis(tri-*n*-butyltin) oxide] and tributyltin-induced apoptotic death of immature thymocytes in culture (Raffray *et al.*, 1993). These investigators have demonstrated that tributyltin oxide, a potent but relatively non-specific agent, activates thymocyte apoptosis independent of protein synthesis and under conditions of severely compromised cellular energetics. This argues against the well received perception that apoptosis is a highly regulated intracellular event which is energy dependent and requires transcriptional and translational control. Unlike the oxide form of tributyltin, tributyltin chloride is a potent and rapid inducer of apoptosis *in vitro*; *in vivo* dibutyltin chloride seems to be much more potent in inducing thymic atrophy (Dobbelsteen *et al.*, 1997). However, future investigations may unravel the mysteries of these findings. Accumulating evidence also indicates that metals may either positively or negatively influence apoptotic processes. Some forms of metals,

e.g. calcium, magnesium, cadmium and chromium, favour apoptosis, whereas Zn^{2+} exerts an opposing role (Bagchi *et al.*, 1997). Unlike these, some metals exert an antagonistic influence on the action of metals, e.g. cadmium suppresses chromium-induced apoptosis (Shimada *et al.*, 1998). The roles which induce apoptosis of metals in toxicology are undergoing intense debate at this time.

Although the mechanisms of many anti-apoptotic agents such as cholesteryl hemisuccinate are unknown, the fact that dimethyl sulphoxide (a membrane-permeable solvent hydroxyl radical scavenger), thioredoxin (an intracellular thiol reducant), *o*-phenanthroline (hydroxyl radical formation blocker), *N*-(2-mercaptoethyl) propane-1,3-diamine (an inhibitor of membrane peroxidation) and the antioxidant vitamins C and E, as well as exogenous catalse, prevent apoptotic death in a variety of model systems (Buttke and Sandstrom, 1994) substantiate the role of ROS in apoptogenesis. Cholesteryl hemisuccinate prevents both of the forms of cell death induced by acetaminophen *in vivo* (Ray *et al.*, 1996). Many studies claim that agents that influence poly(ADP-ribose) polymerase activity, e.g. 3-aminobenzamide **(Figure 6)**, NAD, nicotinamide and caffeine and theophylline, depending upon the model system and concentration employed, either abrogate or escalate drug- or chemically induced programmed and unprogrammed cell death; however, the same agents interfere with the transmembrane signalling mechanisms if the model system is different, e.g. thymocytes (Ray *et al.*, 1992; McConkey *et al.*, 1995; Yahya *et al.*, 1995). The nitroso-containing free radical scavenger 5,5-dimethyl-1-pyrroline-*N*-oxide (DMPO) blocks methylprednisolone-induced apoptosis, and the Ca^{2+}-ATPase inhibitor thapsigargin, the Ca^{2+} chelator EGTA, the Zn^{2+} chelator N,N,N',N'-tetrakis(2-pyridylmethyl)ethylenediamine, Zn^{2+} salts (Bagchi *et al.*, 1997) and the topoisomerase II inhibitor etoposide block apoptosis in a variety of model systems under diverse conditions. The commonly used antioxidant BHA (butylated hydroxyanisole; frequently added as a preservative in foods), DTCs (dithiocarbamates), DETDTC (diethyl dithiocarbamate) and DMDTC (dimethyl dithiocarbamate) served as anti-apoptotic agents in radiation-induced leukaemic cells (Verhaegen *et al.*, 1995).

SUMMARY AND CONCLUSIONS

Apoptosis is a process of single-cell deletion requiring active participation of the cell in its own demise. It occurs during both physiological conditions, such as neural development, and pathological conditions (viz. acute myocardial infarction, ischaemia or stroke). It is morphologically distinct from necrosis and characteristically presents with cell shrinkage, dense fragmented chromatin and cellular budding with fragmentation. The process

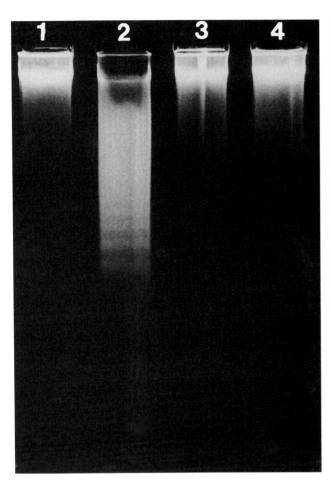

Figure 6 This ethidium bromide-stained agarose gel shows protection of acetaminophen-induced liver injury-associated DNA fragmentation by 3-aminobenzamide, a modulator of the DNA repair enzyme poly (ADP-ribose) polymerase activity. Male ICR mice were treated with acetaminophen (500 mg kg^{-1}, i.p.), followed by 3-aminobenzamide (400 mg kg^{-1} i.p.) 2 h later. This ethidium bromide-stained 1.4% agarose gel contains 10 μg of DNA per lane from variously treated livers. Severe loss of large genomic DNA is evident in the acetaminophen-treated livers (lane 2, see fluorescence intensity at the well). A ladder-like DNA fragmentation pattern reportedly diagnostic of apoptosis is also evident in the acetaminophen lane. However, a complete protection of DNA laddering (including absence of any loss) is clearly evident in the acetaminophen + 3-aminobenzamide group (lane 4). As expected, Control (lane 1, vehicle-treated) and 3-aminobenzamide (lane 3) treated livers demonstrated the absence of any chromatin cleavage or damage to the genomic DNA integrity to any extent. Whether this effect of 3-amino-benzamide is due to the mild activation of poly(ADP-ribose) poly-merase activity, or suppression of Ca^{2+}/Mg^{2+}-dependent endonuclease activity still remains obscure. Courtesy Dhruva and Ray (1996).

results in the formation of apoptotic bodies that are quickly phagocytosed by a variety of cells leaving the integrity of the tissue intact. In contrast to necrosis, apoptosis does not induce an inflammatory response. Apoptosis may be a result of an imbalance between the

activation of effector genes which promote cell death and repressor genes which enhance cell survival. Of these, Ca^{2+} ion regulation and several Ca^{2+}-dependent events have been investigated in depth; however, much of the evidence remains indirect and speculative. It is also not clear, when a particular cell turns on the death pro-gramme *in vivo* or *in vitro*, how the neighbouring cells react. Although in *in vivo* model systems the biochemical pathways for apoptosis are far from being understood, the TNFR superfamily, the caspases and the *bcl-2* gene products have been implicated in an effector role, and ceramide, reactive oxygen species, mitochondrial perme-ability transition and cellular energy status have been implicated as mediators. Cell cycle regulatory elements have gained considerable attention in recent years, and it is clear that apoptosis may require the action of several molecules that are normally involved in regulating cellu-lar proliferation. It is also evident that the mechanisms necessary for completing programmed cell death exist in every cell. Studies on the drug- and chemically induced apoptosis have been a noticeable marathon, in which *in vitro* model systems predominantly compete to interpret *in vivo* findings. The benefits of a comprehensive knowl-edge of cell death are not easily predicted but clearly stand to be immense.

What has propelled apoptosis into the forefront of basic research? This has been the identification of genes that control cell death and the appreciation of the role of apoptosis in development and disease. The efforts of many recognized leaders in toxicology to unravel the underlying mechanisms of drug- and chemically induced 'necrosis' and 'apoptosis' for the past two decades have yielded many fruitful observations; it is ironic that apop-tosis is a beneficial form of cell death. Most investigators associate programmed cell death with drug- and chemi-cally induced toxicity. Given that apoptosis is a benefi-cial form of cell death, then induction of apoptosis after a toxic assault should be beneficial. This should be regarded as a benefit rather than a loss, since loss of cells by apoptosis signals cells to divide. The concept that necrosis implicates a dissenting influence on any cellular organelle or cell as a whole, whereas apoptosis is confined, by and large, to alteration in the genomic material, is no longer valid. Instances have been reported where apoptosis has been observed either in the near total absence of genomic DNA digestion (Ucker *et al.*, 1992) or in the absence of a nucleus (Jacobson *et al.*, 1994). As it appears now, both of these processes para-doxically share almost similar intracellular mechanisms (e.g. oxidative stress, Ca^{2+} dysregulation, DNA frag-mentation, mitochondrial permeability transition, cellu-lar energy status, membrane potential fluctuations) to express their identities. Recently, Raffray and Cohen (1997) have elegantly addressed these concepts, and their opinion is that apoptosis and necrosis are essen-tially distinct modes with limited molecular and cell bio-logy overlaps, whereas mounting evidence suggests that apoptosis and necrosis could be viewed as parts of a cell death continuum (Wyllie, 1987; Corcoran and Ray, 1992; Ray and Raje, 1994; Tomei *et al.*, 1994; Ray *et al.*, 1996). Nevertheless, it is clear that several basic questions still remain to be answered.

The quest for commonalities among all drug- and chemically induced key cytotoxic mechanisms has met with limited success. From an operational standpoint, the killing of some cells can be viewed as occurring via direct means, whereas the killing of others takes place via indirect means. In toxicant-induced cell injury which ultimately results in cell death, changes that are responsible for cell death are joined and effectively concealed by a host of powerful but futile stimuli from a network of control systems that attempt to return the cell to homeostasis. While the control network strives to return to homeostasis, systems that are devoted to cellular repair and regeneration also become engaged through mechanisms that remain largely unidentified. Hence, it is apparent why most cell responses during lethal injury are believed to be unrelated to the ultimate cause of cell death. Only a select response or subset of responses is considered to be capable of producing permanent irreversible damage and the ultimate loss of viability.

The cell is the smallest autonomous unit of all living systems that has the capability to receive information from its environment, to transduce it according to the genetic information encoded in DNA and finally to put out appropriately processed signals into its environment in order to realize teleonomically designed organized functions (Ji, 1997). The information is transferred between the living cell and its environment through exchange of energy-driven biomolecules or inorganic ions, or both. Cell survival is normally mediated by factors in the extracellular environment, whereas genetic changes that constitutively activate intracellular survival pathways often occur in cancer. A number of disparate signals are capable of modulating apoptosis in different cells and in different contexts. Many of these signalling pathways, including components of the central apoptotic pathway, are evolutionarily conserved. The ultimate challenge may be to translate the knowledge gained from these signalling pathways into therapeutic strategies to improve the clinical outcome in the many diseases linked to disregulation of apoptosis.

The widespread involvement of apoptosis in diverse conditions gives rise to numerous hopes suggesting that targeting this response will lead to the development of novel therapeutic regimens. The presence of apoptotic machinery in tumours suggests that its induction could be used as a therapy. The ability to modify sensitivity to apoptosis through the regulatory pathways has clear implications for the treatment of malignancy. Potential strategies fall into three categories: direct induction of apoptosis by cytotoxic agents, enhancing vulnerability to apoptosis to increase the efficacy of other therapies and boosting the resistance of normal

cells to apoptosis (Bellamy *et al.*, 1995). Among these, direct antitumour therapy targeting apoptotic modulation may prove to be much less systemically toxic than standard chemotherapy and could also be used in an adjuvant manner, to increase the susceptibility of tumours at the time they are exposed to chemotherapy (Rudin and Thompson, 1997). The question of cause–effect in drug-induced apoptosis seems to be most crucial in order to appreciate the impact of apoptosis on chemotherapy and to position the protective action of death-inhibitory genes. The successful developments of agonists and antagonists of this process will provide a strong handle for an intervention of various regulatory pathways. Already, newly acquired knowledge concerning the regulation of apoptotic cell death is being applied clinically in the development of potentially useful prognostic indicators to predict disease progression and for the treatment of cancer. In the past decade, many insights have been made, primarily into the biochemistry of apoptosis and its regulation and initiation. Once the regulatory aspect of this cell-death process is clearly understood, specific therapies can be designed easily.

ACKNOWLEDGEMENTS

I am greatly indebted to Dr C. S. Reddy, School of Veterinary Medicine and Biomedical Sciences, University of Missouri, Columbia, and Dr. Vincent Reid of AMS College of Pharmacy for their time, invaluable help and critique during the preparation of this chapter. I also appreciate the encouragement and suggestions received from Dr R. R. Raje, and Dr Alex Gringauz of the Division of Pharmacology, Toxicology and Medicinal Chemistry of our institution. Constant help received from numerous graduate and undergraduate students (Ms S. Bogdanovic, A. Dobrogowska, V. Wong and Mr H. Parikh) during the preparation of this manuscript is acknowledged. Special thanks are due to Dr Nelu Jena, MIT, Cambridge, Massachussetts, for his input on the genetic regulation section of this chapter.

REFERENCES

Alison, M. R. and Sarraf, C. E. (1994). Liver cell death: patterns and mechanisms. *Gut*, **35**, 577–581.

Allsopp, T. E., Wyatt, S., Paterson, H. F. and Davies, A. M. (1993). The proto-oncogene bcl-2 can selectively rescue neurotrophic factor-dependent neurons from apoptosis. *Cell*, **73**, 295–307.

Anand, S., Verma, H., Kumar, L. and Singh, N. (1995). Induction of apoptosis in chronic myelogenous leukemia lymphocytes by hydroxyurea and adriamycin. *Cancer Lett.*, **88**, 101–105.

Ankarcrona, M., Dypbukt, J. M., Brune, B. and Nicotera, P. (1994). Interleukin-1 beta induced nitric oxide production activates apoptosis in pancreatic RINm5F cells. *Exp. Cell Res.*, **213**, 172–177.

Arends, M. J. and Wyllie, A. H. (1991). Apoptosis: mechanisms and role in pathology. *Int. Rev. Exp. Pathol.*, **32**, 223–254.

Arends, M. J., McGregor, A. H., Toft, N. J., Brown, E. J. and Wyllie, A. H. (1993). Susceptibility to apoptosis is differentially regulated by c-myc and mutated Ha-ras oncogenes and is associated with endonuclease availability. *Br. J. Cancer*, **68**, 1127–1133.

Bagchi, D., Vuchetich, P. J., Bagchi, M., Tran, M. X., Krohn, R. L., Ray, S. D. and Stohs, S. J. (1998). Protective effects of zinc salts on TPA-induced hepatic and brain lipid peroxidation, glutathione depletion, DNA damage and peritoneal macrophage activation in mice. *Gen. Pharmacol.*, **30**, 43–50.

Bagchi, D., Tran, M. X., Newton, S., Bagchi, M., Ray, S. D., Kuszynski, C. A. and Stohs, S. J. (1998). Chromium and cadmium induced oxidative stress and apoptosis in cultured J774A. 1 macrophage cells. *In Vitro and Mol. Toxicol.*, **11**, 171–181.

Bardeesy, N., Beckwith, J. B. and Pelletier, J. (1995). Clonal expansion and attenuated apoptosis in Wilm's tumors are associated with p53 gene mutations. *Cancer Res.*, **55**, 215–219.

Baroni, G. S., Marucci, L., Benedetti, A., Mancini, R., Jezequel, A. M. and Orlandi, F. (1994). Chronic ethanol feeding increases apoptosis and cell proliferation in rat liver. *J. Hepatol.*, **20**, 508–513.

Barry, M. A. and Eastman, A. (1992). Endonuclease activation during apoptosis: the role of cytosolic Ca^{2+} and pH. *Biochem. Biophys. Res. Commun.*, **186**, 782–792.

Barry, M. A., Behnke, C. A. and Eastman, A. (1990). Activation of programmed cell death (apoptosis) by cisplatin, other anticancer drugs, toxins and hyperthermia. *Biochem. Pharmacol.*, **40**, 2353–2362.

Basile, D. V., Wood, H. N. and Braun, A. C. (1973). Programming of cells for death under defined experimental conditions: relevance to the tumor problem. *Proc. Natl. Acad. Sci. USA*, **70**, 3055–3059.

Bellamy, C. O. C., Malcomson, R. D. G., Harrison, D. J. and Wyllie, A. H. (1995). Cell death in health and disease: the biology and regulation of apoptosis. *Can. Biol.*, **6**, 3–16.

Benchokroun, Y., Couprie, J. and Larsen, A. K. (1995). Aurintricarboxylic acid, a putative inhibitor of apoptosis, is a potent inhibitor of DNA topoisomerase II *in vitro* and in Chinese hamster fibrosarcoma cells. *Biochem. Pharmacol.*, **49**, 305–313.

Benedetti, A., Jezequel, A. M. and Orlandi, F. (1988a). Preferential distribution of apoptotic bodies in acinar zone 3 of normal human and rat liver. *J. Hepatol.*, **7**, 319–324.

Benedetti, A., Brunelli, E., Risicate, R., Cillufo, T., Jezequel, A. M. and Orlandi, F. (1988b). Subcellular changes and apoptosis induced by ethanol in rat liver. *J. Hepatol.*, **6**, 137–143.

Bicknell, G. R. and Cohen, G. M. (1995). Cleavage of DNA to large kilobase pair fragments occurs in some forms of necrosis as well as apoptosis. *Biochem. Biophys. Res. Commun.*, **207**, 40–47.

Blankenship, L. J., Manning, F. C., Orenstein, J. M. and Patierno, S. R. (1994). Apoptosis is the mode of cell death caused by carcinogenic chromium. *Toxicol. Appl. Pharmacol.*, **126**, 75–83.

Boe, R., Gjertsen, B. T., Vintermyr, O. K., Houge, G., Lanotte, M. and Doskeland, S. O. (1991). The protein phosphatase

inhibitor okadaic acid induces morphological changes typical of apoptosis in mammalian cells. *Exp. Cell Res.*, **195**, 237–246.

Boise, L. H., Gonzalez-Garcia, M., Postema, C. E., Ding, L., Lindsten, T., Turka, L. A., Mao, X., Nunez, G. and Thompson, C. B. (1993). Bcl-x, a bcl-2-related gene that functions as a dominant regulator of apoptotic cell death. *Cell*, **74**, 597–608.

Boldin, M. P., Varfolomeev, E. E., Pancer, Z., Mett, I. L., Camonis, J. H. and Wallach, D. (1995). A novel protein that interacts with the death domain of Fas/APO1 contains a sequence motif related to the death domain. *J. Biol. Chem.*, **270**, 7795–7798.

Bowen, I. D. and Bowen, S. (Eds) (1990). *Programmed Cell Death in Tumors and Tissues*. Chapman and Hall, London.

Boyd, J. M., Malstrom, S., Subramanian, T., Venkatesh, L. K., Schaeper, U., Elangovan, B., D'Sa-Eipper, C. and Chinnadurai, G. (1994). Adenovirus E1B 19kDa and Bcl-2 proteins interact with a common set of cellular proteins. *Cell*, **79**, 341–351.

Bredesen, D. E. (1995). Neural apoptosis. *Ann. Neurol.*, **38**, 839–851.

Bulera, S. J., Sattler, C. A. and Pitot, H. C. (1996). The translational inhibitor cycloheximide represses growth factor depletion-induced apoptosis in an alb-SV40T transgenic rat liver cell line. *Hepatology*, **23**, 1591–1601.

Bump, N. J., Hackett, M., Hugunin, M., Seshagiri, S., Brady, K., Chen, P., Ferenz, C., Franklin, S., Ghayur, T., Li, P., *et al.* (1995). Inhibition of ICE family proteases by baculovirus anti-apoptotic protein p35. *Science*, **269**, 1885–1888.

Burchiel, S. W., Davis, D. A. P., Ray, S. D., Archuleta, M. M., Thilstead, J. P. and Corcoran, G. B. (1992). DMBA-induced cytotoxicity in lymphoid and nonlymphoid organs of B6C3F1 mice: relation of cell death to target cell intracellular calcium and DNA damage. *Toxicol. Appl. Pharmacol.*, **113**, 126–132.

Burchiel, S. W., Davis, D. A. P., Ray, S. D. and Barton, S. L. (1993). DMBA induces programmed cell death (apoptosis) in the A20.1 murine B cell lymphoma. *Fundam. Appl. Toxicol.*, **21**, 120–124.

Bursch, W., Taper, H. S., Lauer, B. and Schulte-Herman, R. (1985). Quantitative histological and histochemical studies on the occurrence and stages of controled cell death (apoptosis) during regression of rat liver hyperplasia. *Virchows Arch. B Cell Pathol. Mol. Pathol.*, **50**, 153–166.

Bursch, W., Paffe, S., Putz, B., Barthel, G. and Schulte-Herman, R. (1990). Determination of the length of the histological stages of apoptosis in normal liver and in altered hepatic foci of rats. *Carcinogenesis*, **11**, 847–851.

Buske, C., Becker, D., Feuring-Buske, M., Hannig, H., Wulf, G., Schafer, C., Hiddemann, W. and Wormann, B. (1997). TGF-beta inhibits growth and induces apoptosis in leukemic B cell precursors. *Leukemia*, **11**, 386–392.

Buttke, T. M. and Sandstrom, P. A. (1994). Oxidative stress as a mediator of apoptosis. *Immunol. Today*, **15**, 7–10.

Buttyan, R., Zakeri, Z., Lockshin, R. and Wolgemuth, D. (1988). Cascade induction of c-fos, c-myc and heat shock 70K transcripts during repression of the rat ventral prostrate gland. *Mol. Endocrinol.*, **2**, 650–657.

Buttyan, R., Olsson, C. A., Pintar, J., Chang, C., Bandyk, M., Ng, P. Y. and Sawczuk, I. S. (1989). Induction of TRPM-2 gene in cells undergoing programmed cell death. *Mol. Cell. Biol.*, **9**, 3473–3481.

Byrd, J. C. and Lichti, U. (1987). Two types of transglutaminase in the P-12 pheochromocytoma cell line. Stimulation by sodium butyrate. *J. Biol. Chem.*, **246**, 11699–11705.

Cai, L., Hales, B. F. and Robaire, B. (1997). Induction of apoptosis in the germ cells of adult male rats after exposure to cyclophosphamide. *Biol. Reprod.*, **56**, 1490–1497.

Cardone, M. H., Roy, N., Stennicke, H. R., Salvesen, G. S., Franke, T. F., Stanbridge, E., Frisch, S. and Reed, J. C. (1998). Regulation of cell death protease caspase-9 by phosphorylation. *Science*, **282**, 1318–1321.

Carson, D. A., Seto, S., Wasson, D. B. and Carrera, C. J. (1986). DNA strand breaks, NAD metabolism, and programmed cell death. *Exp. Cell Res.*, **164**, 273–281.

Catchpoole, D. R. and Stewart, B. W. (1995). Formation of apoptotic bodies is associated with internucleosomal DNA fragmentation during drug-induced apoptosis. *Exp. Cell Res*, **216**, 169–177.

Chen, Q., Galleano, M. and Cedarbaum, A. I. (1997). Cytotoxicity and apoptosis produced by arachidonic acid in HepG2 cells overexpressing human cytochrome P4502E1. *J. Biol. Chem.*, **272**, 14532–14541.

Chieli, E., Saviozzi, M. and Malvaldi, G. (1987). Changes in the rat liver drug metabolizing system during a short thiobenzamide feeding cycle. *Arch. Toxicol.*, **61**, 150–154.

Child, P. and Ruiz, L. A. (1968). Acidophillic bodies: their chemical and physical nature in patients with bolivian hemorrhagic fever. *Arch. Pathol.*, **85**, 45–50.

Chinnaiyan, A. M., O'Rourke, K., Tewari, M. and Dixit, V. M. (1995). FADD, a novel death domain containing protein, interacts with the death domain of Fas and initiates apoptosis. *Cell*, **81**, 505–512.

Chiou, T. J., Zhang, J., Ferrans, V. J. and Tzeng, W. F. (1997). Cardiac and renal toxicity of menadione in rat. *Toxicology*, **124**, 193–202.

Chittenden, T., Harrington, E. A., O'Conner, R., Flemington, C., Lutz, R. J., Evan, G. I. and Guild, B. C. (1995). Induction of apoptosis by the bcl-2 homologue bak. *Nature*, **374**, 733–736.

Clarke, P. G. H. (1990). Developmental cell death: morphological diversity and multiple mechanisms. *Anat. Embryol.*, **181**, 195–213.

Cleveland, J. L. and Ihle, J. N. (1995). Contenders in FasL/TNF death signaling. *Cell*, **81**, 479–482.

Cohen, J. J. and Duke, R. C. (1984). Glucocorticoid activation of a calcium-dependent endonuclease in thymocyte nuclei leads to cell death. *J. Immunol.*, **132**, 38–42.

Coles, H. S. R., Burne, J. F., and Raff, M. C. (1993). Large-scale normal cell death in the developing rat kidney and its reduction by epidermal growth factor. *Development*, **118**, 777–784.

Collins, R. J., Harmon, B. V., Gobe, G. C. and Kerr, J. F. R. (1992). Internucleosomal DNA cleavage should not be the sole criterion for identifying apoptosis. *Int. J. Radiat. Biol.*, **61**, 451–453.

Colombel, M., Ng, C. A., Ng, P.-Y. and Buttyan, R. (1992). Hormone-regulated apoptosis results from re-entry of differentiated prostrate cells into a defective cell cycle. *Cancer Res.*, **52**, 4313–4319.

Columbano, A., Ledda-Columbano, G. M., Rao, P. M., Rajalakshmi, S. and Sarma, D. S. (1984). Occurrence of cell death

(apoptosis) in preneoplastic and neoplastic liver cells: a sequential study. *Am. J. Pathol.*, **116**, 441–446.

Compton, M. M. and Cidlowski, J. A. (1986). Rapid *in vivo* effects of glucocroticoids on the integrity of rat lymphocyte genomic deoxyribonucleic acid. *Endocrinology*, **118**, 38–45.

Compton, M. M. and Cidlowski, J. A. (1992). Thymocyte apoptosis. A model of programmed cell death. *Trends Endocrinol. Metab.*, **3**, 17–23.

Coppola, S., Nosseri, C., Maresca, V. and Ghibelli, L. (1995). Different basal NAD levels determine opposite effects of poly (ADP-ribosyl)polymerase inhibitors on H_2O_2-induced apoptosis. *Exp. Cell Res.*, **221**, 462–469.

Corcoran, G. B. and Ray, S. D. (1992). The role of the nucleus and other compartments in toxic cell death produced by alkylating hepatotoxicants. *Toxicol. Appl. Pharmacol.*, **113**, 167–83.

Costa, L. G. (1998). Signal transduction in environmental neurotoxicity. *Annu. Rev. Pharmacol. Toxicol.*, **38**, 21–43.

Cuende, E., Ales-Martinez, J. E., Ding, L., Gonzales-Garcia, M., Martinez-A, C. and Nunez, G. (1993). Programmed cell death by bcl-2-dependent and independent mechanisms in B lymphoma cells. *EMBO J.*, **12**, 1555–1560.

Daoust, P. Y., Wobeser, G. and Newstead, J. D. (1984). Acute pathological effects of inorganic mercury and copper in gills of rainbow trout. *Vet. Pathol.*, **21**, 93–101.

Davis, M. A., Smith, M. W., Chang, S. H. and Trump, B. F. (1994). Characterization of a renal epithelial cell model of apoptosis using okadaic acid and the NRK-52E cell line. *Toxicol. Pathol.*, **22**, 595–605.

deBlois, D., Tea, B. S., Than, V. D., Tremblay, J. and Hamet, P. (1997). Smooth muscle apoptosis during vascular regression in spontaneously-hypertensive rats. *Hypertension*, **29**, 340–349.

deJong, J. S., van Diest, P. J., Michalides, R. J., van der Valk, P., Meijer, C. J. and Baak, J. P. (1998). Correlation of cyclin D1 and Rb gene expression with apoptosis in invasive breast cancer. *Mol. Pathol.*, **51**, 30–34.

Dhruva, D. and Ray, S. D. (1996). Role of nitric oxide in acetaminophen-induced apoptosis and necrosis and its modulation by 3-aminobenzamide. *J. Toxicol. Clin. Toxicol.*, **34**, 575.

Dhruva, D., Sharma, S., Shleyfer, L., Raje, R. R. and Ray, S. D. (1996). Acetaminophen induced hepatocellular apoptosis *in vivo*: role of Ca^{2+}-activated nitric oxide pathway in the absence of bcl-2 expression. *Toxicologist*, **30**, 165.

Dini, L., Autuori, F., Lentini, A., Oliverio, S. and Piacentini, M. (1992). The clearance of apoptotic cells in the liver is mediated by the asiaglycoprotein receptor. *FEBS Lett.*, **296**, 174–178.

Dobbelsteen, D. J. V., Orrenius, S. and Slater, A. F. G. (1997). Environmental toxicants and apoptosis. In Ray, S. D. and Grant, S. (Eds), *Comments on Toxicology: Apoptosis*, Vol. 5. Gordon and Breach, New York, pp. 511–528.

Duke, R. C., Ojcius, D. M. and Young, J. D. (1996). Cell suicide in health and disease. *Sci. Am.*, December, 80–87.

Duncan, A. M. and Heddle, A. (1984). The frequency and distribution of apoptosis induced by three non-carcinogenic agents in mouse colonic crypts. *Can. Lett.*, **23**, 307–311.

Duvall, E., Wyllie, A. H. and Morris, R. G. (1985). Macrophage recognition of cells undergoing programmed cell death (apoptosis). *Immunology*, **56**, 351–358.

Dybing, E., Holme, J. A., Gordon, W. P., Soderlund, E. J., Dahlin, D. and Nelson, S. D. (1984). Genotoxicity studies with paracetamol. *Mutat. Res.*, **138**, 21–32.

Edwards, S. N., Buckmaster, A. E. and Tolkovsky, A. M. (1991). The death programme in cultured sympathetic neurons can be suppressed at the posttranslational level by nerve growth factor, cyclic AMP, and depolarization. *J. Neurochem.*, **57**, 2140–2143.

Ehrmann, R. L. (1969). Histologic dating of the endometrium. An invitational symposium. *J. Reprod. Med.*, **3**, 9–12.

Ellis, R. E. and Horvitz, H. R. (1986). Genetic control of programmed cell death in the nematode *C. elegans*. *Cell*, **44**, 817–829.

Ellis, R. E., Yuan, J. and Horvitz, H. R. (1991). Mechanisms and functions of cell death. *Annu. Rev. Cell Biol.*, **7**, 663–698.

Estus, S., Zaks, W. J., Freeman, R. S., Gruda, M., Bravo, R. and Johnson, E. M., Jr. (1994). Altered gene expression in neurons during programmed cell death: identification of c-jun as necessary for neuronal apoptosis. *J. Cell Biol.*, **127**, 1717–1727.

Evan, G. I. E., Wyllie, A. H., Gilbert, C. S., Littlewood, T. D., Land, H., Brooks, M., Waters, C. M., Penn, L. Z. and Hancock, D. C. (1992). Induction of apoptosis in fibroblasts by c-myc protein. *Cell*, **69**, 119–128.

Faa, G., Ambu, R., Congiu, T., Costa, V., Ledda-Columbano, G. M., Coni, P., Curto, M., Giacomi, L. and Columbano, A. (1992). Early ultrastructural changes during thioacetamide-induced apoptosis in rat liver. *J. Submicrosc. Cytol. Pathol.*, **24**, 417–424.

Faa, G., Ledda-Columbano, G. M., Ambu, R., Congiu, T., Coni, P., Riva, A. and Columbano, A. (1994). An electron microscopic study of apoptosis induced by cycloheximide in rat liver. *Liver*, **14**, 270–278.

Fadok, V. A., Voelker, D. R., Campbell, P. A., Cohen, J. J., Bratton, D. L. and Henson, P. M. (1992). Exposure of phosphatidylserine on the surface of apoptotic lymphocytes triggers specific recognition and removal by macrophages. *J. Immunol.*, **148**, 2207–2216.

Fadok, V. A., Laszlo, D. J., Noble, P. W., Weinstein, L., Riches, D. W. and Henson, P. M. (1993). Particle digestibility is required for induction of the phosphatidylserine recognition mechanism used by murine macrophage to phagocytose apoptotic cell. *J. Immunol.*, **151**, 4274–4285.

Fanidi, A., Harrington, E. A. and Evan, G. I. (1992). Cooperative interaction between c-myc and bcl-2 protooncogenes. *Nature*, **359**, 554–556.

Fariss, G. M., Robinson, S. N., Wong, B. A., Wong, V. A., Hahn, W. P. and Shah, R. (1997). Effects of benzene on splenic, thymic and femoral lymphocytes in mice. *Toxicology*, **118**, 137–148.

Farrow, S. N., White, J. H., Martinou, I., Raven, T., Pun, K. T., Grinham, C. J., Martinou, J. C. and Brown, R. (1995). Cloning of a bcl-2 homologue by interaction with adenovirus E1B 19K. *Nature*, **374**, 731–733.

Faucheu, C., Diu, A., Chan, A. W., Blanchet, A. M., Miossec, C., Herve, F., Collard-Dutilleul, V., Gu, Y., Aldape, R. A., Lippke, J. A., *et al.* (1995). A novel human protease similar to the interleukin-1 beta converting enzyme induces apoptosis in transfected cells. *EMBO J.*, **14**, 1914–1922.

Fernandes, R. S. and Cotter, T. G. (1994). Apoptosis or necrosis: intracellular levels of glutathione influence mode of cell death. *Biochem. Pharmacol.*, **48**, 675–681.

Fernandes-Alnemri, T., Litwack, G. and Alnemri, E. S. (1994). CPP32, a novel human apoptotic protein with homology to *Caenorhabditis elegans* cell death protein Ced-3 and mammalian interleukin-1 beta-converting enzyme. *J. Biol. Chem.*, **269**, 30761–30764.

Fernandez-Sarabia, M. J. and Bischoff, J. R. (1993). Bcl-2 associates with the ras-related protein R-ras p23. *Nature*, **366**, 274–275.

Fesus, L., Thomazy, V. and Falus, A. (1987). Induction and activation of tissue transglutaminase during programmed cell death. *FEBS Lett.*, **224**, 104–108.

Fesus, L., Davies, P. J. A. and Piacentini, M. (1991). Apoptosis: molecular mechanisms in programmed cell death. *Eur. J. Cell. Biol.*, **56**, 170–177.

Fox, H. (1973). Ultrastructure of tail degeneration in *Rana tempororia* larvae. *Fol. Morphol.*, **21**, 109–112.

Freeman, R. S., Estus, S. and Johnson, E. M., Jr. (1994). Analysis of cell cycle-related gene expression in postmitotic neurons: selective induction of cyclin D1 during programmed cell death. *Neuron*, **12**, 343–355.

Fuchs, B. A. and Pruett, S. B. (1993). Morphine induces apoptosis in murine thymocytes *in vivo* but not *in vitro*: involvement of both opiate and glucocorticoid receptors. *J. Pharmacol. Exp. Ther.*, **266**, 417–423.

Gagliardini, V., Fernandez, P. A., Lee, R. K., Drexler, H. C., Rotello, R. J., Fishman, M. C. and Yuan, J. (1994). Prevention of vertebrate neuronal death by the crmA gene. *Science*, **263**, 826–828.

Galle, P. R., Muller, M., Hagelstein, J., Hofman, W. J., Otto, G., Krammer, P. H. and Stremmel, W. (1995). Hepatoprotective effect of anti-APO-1/FAS F (AB′)$_2$-fragments in human liver cells. *Hepatology*, **22**, 229A.

Glucksmann, A. (1951). Cell death in normal vertebrate ontogeny. *Biol. Rev.*, **26**, 59–86.

Gobe, G. C. and Axelsen, R. A. (1991). The role of apoptosis in the development of renal cortical tubular atrophy associated with healed experimental renal papillary necrosis. *Pathology*, **23**, 213–223.

Goldin, R. D., Hunt, N. C., Clark, J. and Wickramasinghe, S. N. (1993). Apoptotic bodies in a murine model of alcoholic liver disease: reversibility of ethanol-induced changes. *J. Pathol.*, **171**, 73–76.

Goodrich, D. W. and Lee, W.-H. (1992). Abrogation by c-myc of G1 phase arrest induced by Rb protein but not by p53. *Nature*, **360**, 177–179.

Grant, S., Turner, A. J., Bartimole, T. M., Nelms, P. A., Joe, V. C. and Jarvis, W. D. (1994). Modulation of 1-[beta-D-arabinofuranosyl]cytosine-induced apoptosis in human myeloid leukemia cells by staurosporine and other pharmacological inhibitors of protein kinase C. *Oncol. Res.*, **6**, 87–99.

Green, D. R. and Cotter, T. G. (1995). Macromolecular synthesis, c-myc, and apoptosis. In Lavin, M. and Watters, D. (Eds), *Programmed Cell Death: the Cellular and Molecular Biology of Apoptosis*. Harwood Academic, Amsterdam, pp. 153–166.

Greene, R. M. and Pratt, R. M. (1976). Developmental aspects of secondary palate formation. *J. Embryol. Exp. Morphol.*, **36**, 225–245.

Griffiths, G. D., Leek, M. D. and Gee, D. J. (1987). The toxic plant proteins ricin and abrin induce apoptotic changes in mammalian lymphoid tissues and intestine. *J. Pathol.*, **151**, 221–229.

Hagimoto, N., Kuwano, K., Nomoto, Y., Kunitake, R. and Hara, N. (1997). Apoptosis and expression of Fas/Fas ligand m-RNA in bleomycin-induced pulmonary fibrosis in mice. *Am. J. Resp. Cell. Mol. Biol.*, **16**, 91–101.

Hai, H., Hardy, M. H., Black, W. D. and Goldberg, M. T. (1997). The *in vivo* effect of the tumor promoter 12-*O*-tetradecanoylphorbol-13-acetate on *N*-methyl-*N*-nitrosourea induced apoptosis in mouse hair follicles. *Fundam. Appl. Toxicol.*, **35**, 177–181.

Hamada, T., Nakano, S., Iwai, S., Tanimoto, A., Ariyoshi, K. and Koide, O. (1991). Pathological study on beagles after long-term oral administration of cadmium. *Toxicol. Pathol.*, **19**, 138–147.

Hamilton, R. F., Jr, Li, L., Eschenbacher, W. L., Szweda, L. and Holian, A. (1998). Potential involvement of 4-hydroxvnonenal in the response of human lung cells to ozone. *Am. J. Physiol.*, **274**, L8–L16.

Harrington, E. A., Bennett, M. R. and Evan, G. (1994). c-Myc-induced apoptosis in fibroblasts is inhibited by specific cytokines. *EMBO J.*, **13**, 3286–3295.

Harper, J. W., Adami, G. R., Wei, N., Keyomarsi, K. and Elledge, S. J. (1993). The p21 cdk interacting protein cip 1 is a potent inhibitor of G1 cyclin-dependent kinases. *Cell*, **75**, 805–816.

Hassouna, I., Wickert, H., Zimmermann, M. and Gillardon, F. (1996). Increase in bax expression in substantia niagra following 1-methyl-4-phenyl-1,2,3,6-tetrahydropyridine (MPTP) treatment of mice. *Neurosci. Lett.*, **204**, 85–88.

Hennet, T., Richter, C. and Peterhans, E. (1993a). Tumour necrosis factor-alpha induces superoxide anion generation in mitochondria of L929 cells. *Biochem. J.*, **289**, 587–592.

Hennet, T., Peterhans, E., Richter, C. and Bertoni, G. (1993b). Expression of Bcl-2 protein enhances the survival of mouse fibrosarcoid cells in tumor necrosis factor mediated cytotoxicity. *Cancer Res.*, **53**, 1456–1460.

Hengartner, M. O., Ellis, R. E. and Horvitz, H. R. (1992). *Caenorhabditis elegans* gene ced-9 protects cells from programmed cell death. *Nature*, **356**, 494–499.

Hengartner, M. O. and Horvitz, H. R. C. (1994). *C. elegans* cell survival gene ced-9 encodes a functional homolog of the mammalian proto-oncogene bcl-2. *Cell*, **76**, 665–676.

Herman, E. H., Zhang, J., Hasinoff, B. B., Clark, J. R., Jr. and Ferrans, V. J. (1997). Comparison of the structural changes induced by doxorubicin and mitoxanthrone in the heart, kidney and intestine and characterization of the Fe(III)–mitoxanthrone complex. *J. Mol. Cell. Cardiol.*, **29**, 2415–1430.

Hirata, K., Ogata, I., Ohta, Y. and Fujiwara, K. (1989). Hepatic sinusoidal cell destruction in the development of intravascular coagulation in acute liver failure of rats. *J. Pathol.*, **158**, 157–165.

Hockenbery, D. M., Zutter, M., Hickey, W., Nahm, M. and Korsmeyer, S. J. (1991). Bcl-2 protein is topographically restricted in tissues characterized by apoptotic cell death. *Proc. Natl. Acad. Sci. USA*, **88**, 6961–6965.

Hockenbery, D., Nunez, G., Milliman, C., Schreiber, R. D. and Korsmeyer, S. J. (1993a). Bcl-2 is an inner mitochondrial membrane protein that blocks programmed cell death. *Nature*, **348**, 334–336.

Hockenbery, D., Oltvai, Z., Yin, X.-M., Milliman, C. and Korsmeyer, S. J. (1993b). Bcl-2 functions in an antioxidant pathway in apoptosis. *Cell*, **75**, 241–251.

Hongslo, J. K., Christensen, T., Brunborg, G., Biornstad, C. and Holme, J. A. (1988). Genotoxic effects of paracetamol in V79 Chinese hamster cells. *Mutat. Res.*, **204**, 333–341.

Hopwood, D. and Levison, D. A. (1976). Atrophy and apoptosis in the cyclical human endometrium. *J. Pathol.*, **119**, 159–166.

Hsu, H., Xiong, J. and Goeddel, D. V. (1995). The TNF receptor 1-associated protein TRADD signals cell death and NF-kappa B activation. *Cell*, **81**, 495–504.

Huang, S. J., Hughes, F. M. and Cidlowski, J. A. (1997). Candidate nucleases responsible for genomic degradation during apoptosis. In Ray, S. D. and Grant, S. (Eds), *Comments on Toxicology*, Vol. **5**. Gordon and Breach, New York, pp. 555–569.

Hurle, J. M. (1988). Cell death in developing systems. *Meth. Achiev. Exp. Pathol.*, **13**, 55–86.

Hurle, J. M., Lafarga, M. and Ojeda, J. L. (1977). Cytological and cytochemical studies of the necrotic area of the bulbus of the chick embryo heart: phagocytosis by developing myocardial cells. *J. Embryol. Exp. Morphol.*, **41**, 161–173.

Ignarro, L. J. (1990). Biosynthesis and metabolism of endothelium-derived nitric oxide. *Annu. Rev. Pharmacol. Toxicol.*, **30**, 535–560.

Ihara, T., Sugamata, M., Sekijima, M., Okumura, H., Yoshino, N. and Ueno, Y. (1997). Apoptotic cellular damage in mice after T-2 toxin-induced acute toxicosis. *Nat. Toxins*, **5**, 141–145.

Ijiri, K. (1989). Apoptosis (cell death) induced in mouse bowel by 1,2-dimethylhydrazine, methylazoxymethanol acetate, and gamma-rays. *Cancer Res.*, **49**, 6342–6346.

Inouye, M., Kajiwara, Y. and Hirayama, K. (1991). Combined effects of low-level methylmercury and X-radiation on the developing mouse cerebellum. *J. Toxicol. Environ. Health*, **33**, 47–56.

Israel, N., Gougerot-Pocidalo, M. A., Aillet, F. and Virelizier, J. L. (1992). Redox status of cells influences constitutive or induced NFκB translocation and HIV long terminal repeat activity in human T and monocytic cell lines. *J. Immunol.*, **149**, 3386–3393.

Iwasa, M., Maeno, Y., Inoue, H., Koyama, H. and Matoba, R. (1996). Induction of apoptotic cell death in rat thymus and spleen after a bolus injection of methamphetamine. *Int. J. Legal Med.*, **109**, 23–28.

Jacobson, M. D., Burne, J. F. and Raff, M. C. (1994). Programmed cell death and bcl-2 protection in the absence of a nucleus. *EMBO J.*, **13**, 1899–1910.

Janssen, Y. M., Matalon, S. and Mossman, B. T. (1997). Differential induction of c-fos, c-jun, and apoptosis in lung epithelial cells exposed to ROS or RNS. *Am. J. Physiol.*, **273**, L789–L796.

Jarvis, W. D., Fornari, F. A., Browning, J. L., Gewirtz, D. A., Kolesnick, R. N. and Grant, S. (1994a). Attenuation of ceramide-induced apoptosis by diglyceride in human myeloid leukemia cells. *J. Biol. Chem.*, **269**, 31685–31692.

Jarvis, W. D., Turner, A. J., Povirk, L. F., Traylor, R. S. and Grant, S. (1994b). Induction of apoptotic DNA fragmentation and cell death in HL-60 human promyelocytic leukemia cells by pharmacological inhibitors of protein kinase C. *Cancer Res.*, **54**, 1707–1714.

Jarvis, W. D., Kolesnick, R. D., Fornari, F. A., Traylor, R. S., Gewirtz, D. A. and Grant, S. (1994c). Induction of apoptotic DNA damage and cell death by activation of the spingomyelin pathway. *Proc. Natl. Acad. Sci. USA (Cell Biol.)*, **91**, 73–77.

Ji, S. (1997). A cell linguistic analysis of apoptosis. In Ray, S. D. and Grant, S. (Eds.), *Comments on Toxicology: Apoptosis*. Harwood Academic/Gordon and Breach, Amsterdam.

Jones, D. P., McConkey, D. J., Nicotera, P. and Orrenius, S. (1989). Calcium-activated DNA fragmentation in rat liver nuclei. *J. Biol. Chem.*, **264**, 6398–6403.

Kane, D. J., Sarafin, T. A., Anton, R., Hahn, H., Gralla, E. B., Valentine, J. S., Ord, T. and Bredsen, D. E. (1993). Bcl-2 inhibition of neural death: decreased generation of reactive oxygen species. *Science*, **262**, 1274–1277.

Kataoka, A., Kubota, M., Wakazono, Y., Okuda, A., Bessho, R., Lin, Y. W., Usami, I., Akiyama, Y. and Furusho, K. (1995). *FEBS Lett.*, **364**, 264–267.

Kaufmann, S. H. (1989). Induction of endonucleolytic DNA cleavage in human acute myelogenous leukemia cells by etoposide, camptothecin, and other cytotoxic anticancer drugs: a cautionary note. *Cancer Res.*, **49**, 5870–5878.

Kerr, J. F. R. (1969). An electron microscope study of liver cell necrosis due to heliotrine. *J. Pathol.*, **97**, 557–562.

Kerr, J. F. R. (1971). Shrinkage necrosis: a distinct mode of cellular death. *J. Pathol.*, **105**, 13–22.

Kerr, J. F. R., Wyllie, A. H. and Currie, A. R. (1972a). Apoptosis: a basic biological phenomenon with wide ranging implications in tissue kinetics. *Br. J. Cancer*, **26**, 239–257.

Kerr, J. F. R., Harmon, B. V. and Searle, J. (1972b). An electron microscope study of cell deletion in the anuran tadpole tail during spontaneous metamorphosis with special reference to apoptosis of striated muscle fibres. *J. Cell. Sci.*, **14**, 571–585.

Kerr, J. F. R., Searle, J., Harmon, B. V. and Bishop, C. J. (1987). Apoptosis. In Potten, C. S. (Ed.), *Perspectives on Mammalian Cell Death*. Oxford University Press, Oxford, pp. 93–119.

Kiefer, M. C., Brauer, M. J., Powers, V. C., Wu, J. J., Umansky, S. R., Tomei, L. D. and Barr, P. J. (1995). Modulation of apoptosis by the widely distributed bcl-2 homologue bak. *Nature*, **374**, 736–739.

King, T. P. and Bremner, I. (1979). Autophagy and apoptosis in liver during the prehaemolytic phase of chronic copper poisoning in sheep. *J. Comp. Pathol.*, **89**, 515–530.

Kirichenko, A., Li, L., Morandi, M. T. and Holian, A. (1996). 4-Hydroxy-2-nonenal–protein adducts and apoptosis in murine lung cells after acute ozone exposure. *Toxicol. Appl. Pharmacol.*, **141**, 416–424.

Kizaki, H., Tadakuma, T., Odaka, C., Muramatsu, J. and Ishimura, Y. (1989). Activation of a suicide process of thymocytes through DNA fragmentation by calcium ionophores and phorbol esters. *J. Immunol.*, **143**, 1790–1794.

Klion, F. M. and Schaffner, F. (1966). The ultrastructure of acidophillic 'councilman-like' bodies in the liver. *Am. J. Pathol.*, **48**, 755–765.

Knight, C. R. L., Rees, R. C. and Griffin, M. (1991). Apoptosis: a potential role for cytosolic transglutaminase and its importance in tumor progression. *Biochim. Biophys. Acta*, **1096**, 312–318.

Koseki, C., Herzlinger, D. and Al-Awqati, Q. (1992). Apoptosis in metanephric development. *J. Cell. Biol.*, **119**, 1327–1333.

Koury, M. J. and Bondurant, M. C. (1990). Erythropoietin retards DNA breakdown and prevents programmed death in erythroid progenitor cells. *Science*, **248**, 378–381.

Kozopas, K. M., Yang, T., Buchan, H. L., Zhou, P. and Craig, R. W. (1993). MCL1, a gene expressed in programmed myeloid cell differentiation, has sequence similarity to Bcl-2. *Proc. Natl. Acad. Sci. USA*, **90**, 3516–3520.

Kulikova, O. G., Savostianov, G. A., Beliavsteva, L. M. and Razumovskaia, N. I. (1982). ATPase activity and ATP-dependent accumulation of Ca^{2+} in skeletal muscle nuclei. Effects of denervation and electrical stimulation. *Biokhimiya*, **47**, 1216–1221.

Kumar, S., Kinoshita, M., Noda, M., Copeland, N. G. and Jenkins, N. A. (1994). Induction of apoptosis by the mouse Nedd2 gene, which encodes a protein similar to the product of the *Caenorhabditis elegans* cell death gene ced-3 and the mammalian IL-1 beta converting enzyme. *Genes Dev.*, **8**, 1613–1626.

Kurose, I., Higuchi, H., Miura, S., Saito, H., Watanabe, N., *et al.* (1997). Oxidative stress-mediated apoptosis of hepatocytes exposed to acute ethanol intoxication. *Hepatology*, **25**, 368–378.

Kyprianou, N. and Isaacs, J. T. (1988). Activation of programmed cell death in the rat ventral prostrate after castration. *Endocrinology*, **122**, 552–562.

Lake, B. G. and Grasso, P. (1996). Comparison of the hepatotoxicity of coumarin in the rat, mouse and Syrian hamster: a dose and time–response study. *Fundam. Appl. Toxicol.*, **34**, 105–117.

Lazebnik, Y., Kaufmann, S. H., Desnoyers, S., Poirier, G. G. and Earnshaw, W. C. (1994). Cleavage of poly(ADP-ribose) polymerase by a proteinase with properties like ICE. *Nature*, **371**, 346–347.

Ledda-Columbano, G. M., Coni, P., Curto, M., Giacomini, L., Faa, G., Oliverio, S., Piacentini, M. and Columbano, A. (1991). Induction of two different modes of cell death, apoptosis and necrosis, in rat liver after a single dose of thioacetamide. *Am. J. Pathol.*, **139**, 1099–1109.

Leigh, J., Wang, H., Bonin, A., Peters, M. and Ruan, X. (1997). Silica-induced apoptosis in alveolar and granulomatous cells *in vivo*. *Environ. Health. Perspect.*, **105** (Suppl. 5), 1241–1245.

Lemasters, J. J. and Nieminen, A. L. (1998). Mitochondrial membrane permeability changes in necrotic and apoptotic cell death. *Toxicol. Sci.*, **42**, (*Toxicologist*, Suppl.) 232–233

Levi-Montalcini, R. and Brooker, B. (1960). Destruction of the sympathetic ganglia evoked by a protein isolated from mouse salivary glands. *Proc. Natl. Acad. Sci. USA*, **46**, 384–391.

Levi-Montalcini, R. and Aloe, L. (1981). Mechanisms of action of nerve cells in neonatal rodents, In Bowen, I. D. and Lockshin, R. A. (Eds), *Cell Death in Biology and Pathology*. Chapman and Hall, London, pp. 295–327.

Lin, E. Y., Orlofsky, A., Berger, M. S. and Prystowsky, M. B. (1993). Characterization of A1, a novel hemopoietic-specific early response gene with sequence similarity to bcl-2. *J. Immunol.*, **151**, 1979–1988.

Liu, C., Rangnekar, V. M., Adamson, E. and Mercola, D. (1998). Suppression of growth and transformation and induction of apoptosis by EGR-1. *Cancer Gene Ther.*, **5**, 3–28.

Lockshin, R. A. (1981). Cell death in metamorphosis. In Bowen, I. D. and Lockshin, R. A. (Eds), *Cell Death in Biology and Pathology*. Chapman and Hall, London, pp. 79–122.

Lockshin, R. A. and Williams, C. M. (1965). Programmed cell death: cytology of degeneration in the intersegmental muscles of the silkmoth. *J. Insect. Physiol.*, **11**, 123–133.

Long, R. M., Moore, L. and Schoenberg, D. R. (1989). Halocarbon hepatotoxicity is not initiated by Ca^{2+}-stimulated endonuclease activation. *Toxicol. Appl. Pharmacol.*, **97**, 350–359.

Lord, B. I. (1979). Proliferation regulation in haemopoiesis. In Lajtha, L. G. (Ed.), *Cellular Dynamics of Hemopoiesis, Clinics in Hematology*, Vol. 8. Saunders, Philadelphia, pp. 435–451.

Lord, B. I. (1986). Controls of the cell cycle. *Int. Radiat. Biol.*, **49**, 279–296.

Lotti, M. (1995). Injury and repair in neurotoxicology. In DeMatteis, F. and Smith, L. L. (Eds), *Molecular and Cellular Mechanisms of Toxicity*. CRC Press, Boca Raton, FL, pp. 19–34.

Majno, G. and Jorris, I. (1995). Apoptosis, oncosis, and necrosis: an overview of cell death. *Am. J. Pathol.*, **146**, 3–15.

Manolas, T., Wattamwar, A. and Ray, S. D. (1997). Induction of hepatocellular apoptosis by aliphatic alcohols in normal and spontaneously hypertensive stroke-prone rats. *Fundam. Appl. Toxicol. (Toxicologist*, Suppl.), **36**, 247.

Marchini, A., Tomkinson, B., Cohen, J. I. and Kieff, E. (1991). BHRF1, the Epstein–Barr virus gene with homology to bcl-2, is dispensible for B-lymphocyte transformation and virus replication. *J. Virol.*, **65**, 5991–6000.

Marks, D. I. and Fox, R. M. (1991). DNA damage, poly(ADP-ribosyl)ation and apoptotic cell death as a potential common pathway of cytotoxic drug action. *Biochem. Pharmacol.*, **42**, 1859–1867.

Martin, S. J., O'Brien, G. A., Nishioka, W. K., McGahon, A. J., Mahboubi, A., Saido, T. C. and Green, D. R. (1995). Proteolysis of fodrin (non-erythroid spectrin) during apoptosis. *J. Biol. Chem.*, **270**, 6425–6428.

Matter, A. (1979). Microcinematographic and electron microscopic analysis of target cell lysis induced by cytotoxic T lymphocytes. *Immunology*, **36**, 179–190.

McCall, C. A. and Cohen, J. J. (1991). Programmed cell death in terminally differentiating keratinocytes: role of endogenous nuclease. *J. Invest. Dermatol.*, **97**, 111–114.

McConkey, D. J., Hartzell, P., Nicotera, P., Wyllie, A. H. and Orrenius, S. (1988a). Stimulation of endogenous endonuclease activity in hepatocytes exposed to oxidative stress. *Toxicol. Lett.*, **42**, 123–130.

McConkey, D. J., Hartzell, P., Duddy, S. K., Hakasson, H. and Orrenius, S. (1988b). 2,3,7,8-Tetrachlorodibenzo-*p*-dioxin (TCDD) kills immature thymocytes by Ca^{2+}-mediated endonuclease activation. *Science*, **242**, 256–259.

McConkey, D. J., Nicotera, P., Hartzell, P., Bellomo, G., Wyllie, A. H. and Orrenius, S. (1989). Glucocorticoids activate a suicide process in thymocytes through an elevation of cytosolic Ca^{2+} concentration. *Arch. Biochem. Biophys*, **269**, 365–370.

McConkey, D. J., Orrenius, S. and Jondal, M. (1990a). Agents that elevate *cAMP* stimulate DNA fragmentation in thymocytes. *J. Immunol.*, **145**, 1227–1230.

McConkey, D. J., Orrenius, S. and Jondal, M. (1990b). Cellular signalling in programmed cell death (apoptosis). *Immunol. Today*, **11**, 120–121.

McConkey, D. J., Orrenius, S. and Jondal, M. (1995). Signal transduction in thymocyte apoptosis. In Lavin, M. and Watters, D. (Eds), *Programmed Cell Death: the Cellular and Molecular Biology of Apoptosis*. Harwood Academic Amsterdam, pp. 19–30.

McConkey, D. J., Zhivotovsky, B. and Orrenius, S. (1996). Apoptosis–molecular mechanisms and biomedical implications. *Mol. Aspects Med.*, **17**, 5–110.

Messmer, U. K., Ankarcrona, M., Nicotera, P. and Brune, B. (1994). p53 expression in nitric oxide-induced apoptosis. *FFBS Lett.*, **355**, 23–26.

Messmer, U. K., Lapetina, E. G. and Brune, B. (1995). Nitric oxide-induced apoptosis in RAW 264.7 macrophages is antagonized by protein kinase C-and protein kinase A-activating compounds. *Mol. Pharmacol.*, **47**, 757–765.

Meyn, R. E., Stephens, L. C., Hunter, N. R. and Milas, L. (1994). Induction of apoptosis in murine tumors by cyclophosphamide. *Cancer Chemother. Pharmacol.*, **33**, 410–414.

Milligan, C. E. and Schwartz, L. M. (1996). Programmed cell death during development of animals. In Holbrook, N. J., Martin, G. R. and Lockshin, R. A. (Eds), *Cellular Aging and Cell Death*. Wiley-Liss, New York, pp. 181–208.

Miyashita, T. and Reed, J. C. (1995). Tumor suppressor p53 is a direct transcriptional activator of the human bax gene. *Cell*, **80**, 293–299.

Miyashita, T., Krajewski, S., Krajewska, M., Wang, H. G., Lin, H. K., Liebermann, D. A., Hoffman, B. and Reed, J. C. (1994). Tumor suppressor p53 is a regulator of bcl-2 and bax gene expression *in vivo* and *in vitro*. *Oncogene*, **9**, 1799–1805.

Mizumoto, K., Rothman, R. J. and Farber, J. L. (1994). Programmed cell death (apoptosis) of mouse fibroblasts is induced by the topoisomerase II inhibitor etoposide. *Mol. Pharmacol.*, **46**, 890–895.

Montgomery, H. (1967). Lichen planus. In *Dermatopathology*, Vol. 1. Evanston, New York and Harper and Row, London, pp. 285–294.

Morikawa, A., Sigiyama, T., Kato, Y., Koide, N., Jiang, G. Z., Takahashi, K., Tamada, Y. and Yokochi, D. (1996). Apoptotic cell death in the response of D-galactosamine-sensitized mice to lipopolysaccharide as an experimental endotoxic shock model. *Infect. Immun.*, **64**, 734–738.

Morris, R. G., Hargreaves, A. D., Duvall, E. and Wyllie, A. H. (1984). Hormone-induced cell death: 2. surface changes in thymocytes undergoing apoptosis. *Am. J. Pathol.*, **115**, 426–436.

Muel, A. S., Chaudun, E., Courtois, Y., Modak, S. P. and Counis, M. F. (1986). Nuclear endogenous Ca_{2+}-dependent endodeoxyribonuclease in differentiating chick embryonic lens fibres. *J. Cell Physiol.*, **127**, 167–174.

Murdoch, W. J. (1996). Differential effects of indomethacin on the sheep ovary: prostaglandin biosynthesis, intracellular calcium, apoptosis, and ovulation. *Prostaglandins*, **52**, 497–506.

Nagata, S. and Goldstein, P. (1995). The Fas death factor. *Science*, **267**, 1449–1456.

Nakagawa, S., Nakamura, N., Fujioka, M. and Mori, C. (1997). Spermatogenic cell apoptosis induced by mitomycin-C in the mouse testis. *Toxicol. Appl. Pharmacol.*, **147**, 204–213.

Nakashima, T., Sekiguchi, T., Kuraoka, A., Fukushima, K., Shibata, Y., Komiyama, S. and Nishimoto, T. (1993). Molecular cloning of a human cDNA encoding a novel protein, DAD1, whose defect causes apoptotic cell death in hamster BHK21 cells. *Mol. Cell Biol.*, **13**, 6367–6374.

Nara, K., Nakanishi, K., Hagiwara, H., Wakita, K., Kojima, S. and Hirose, S. (1989). Retinol induced morphological changes of cultured bovine endothelial cells are accompanied by a marked increase in transglutaminase. *J. Biol. Chem.*, **264**, 19308–19312.

Nathan, C. (1992). Nitric oxide as a secretory product of mammalian cells. *FASEB J.*, **6**, 3051–3064.

Neilan, J. G., Lu, Z., Afonso, C. L., Kutish, G. F., Sussman, M. D. and Rock, D. L. (1993). An African swine fever virus gene with similarity to the proto-oncogene bcl-2 and the Epstein Barr virus gene BHRF1. *J. Virol.*, **67**, 4391–4394.

Nelipovich, P. A., Nikonova, L. V. and Umansky, S. R. (1988). Inhibition of poly(ADP-ribose) polymerase as a possible reason for activation of Ca^{2+} Mg-dependent endonuclease in thymocytes of irradiated rats. *Int. J. Radiat. Biol.*, **53**, 749–765.

Nicholson, D. W. and Thornberry, N. A. (1997). Caspases: killer proteases. *ITIBS*, **22**, 299–306.

Nicholson, D. W., Ali, A. and Thornberry, N. A. (1995). Identification and inhibition of the ICE/CED-3 protease necessary for mammalian apoptosis. *Nature*, **376**, 37–43.

Norimatsu, M., Ono, T., Aoki, A., Ohishi, K., Takahashi, T., Watanabe, G., Taya, K., Sasamoto, S. and Tamura, Y. (1995). Lipopolysaccharide-induced apoptosis in swine lymphocytes *in vivo*. *Infect. Immun.*, **63**, 1122–1126.

Nossal, G. J. V. and Ada, G. L. (1971). The functional anatomy of the lymphoid system. In *Antigens, Lymphoid Cells, and the Immune Response*. Academic Press, New York and London, 61–84.

Oates, P. S. and Morgan, R. G. (1986). Random or selective cell death during pancreatic involution following withdrawal of raw soya flour feeding in the rat. *Pathology*, **18**, 234–236.

Oberhammer, F. A., Pavelka, M., Sharma, S., Tiefenbaches, R., Purchio, A. F., Bursch, W. and Schulte-Herman, R. (1992). Induction of apoptosis in cultured hepatocytes and in regressing liver by transforming growth factor β1. *Proc. Natl. Acad. Sci. USA*, **89**, 5408–5412.

Oberhammer, F., Wilson, J. W., Dive, C., Morris, I. D., Hickman, J. A., Wakeling, A. E., Walker, P. R. and Sikorska, M. (1993). Apoptotic death in epithelial cells: cleavage of DNA to 300 and/or 50 kb fragments prior to or in the absence of internucleosomal fragmentation. *EMBO J.*, **12**, 3679–3684.

O'Connor, R. (1998). Survival factors and apoptosis. *Adv. Biochem. Eng. Biotechnol.*, **62**, 137–166.

Oltvai, Z. N., Milliman, C. L. and Korsmeyer, S. J. (1993). Bcl-2 heterodimerizes *in vivo* with a conserved homolog, bax, that accelerates programmed cell death. *Cell*, **74**, 609–619.

Oppenheim, R. W. (1985). Naturally occurring cell death during neural development. *Trends Neurosci.*, **8**, 487–493.

Oppenheim, R. W. (1991). Cell death during the development of the nervous system. *Annu. Rev. Neurosci.*, **14**, 453–501.

Owens, G. P., Hahn, W. E. and Cohen, J. J. (1991). Identification of m-RNAs associated with programmed cell death in immature thymocytes. *Mol. Cell Biol.*, **11**, 4177–4188.

Pallardy, M., Perrin-Wolf, M. and Biola, A. (1997). Cellular stress and apoptosis. *Toxicol. In Vitro*, **11**, 573–578.

Pandey, S. and Wang, E. (1995). Cells en route to apoptosis are characterized by the upregulation of c-fos, c-myc, c-jun, cdc2, and RB phosphorylation, resembling events of early cell-cycle traverse. *J. Cell. Biochem.*, **58**, 135–150.

Patel, T. and Gores, G. J. (1995). Apoptosis and hepatobiliary disease. *Hepatology*, **21**, 1725–1741.

Peitsch, M. C., Polzar, B., Stephan, H., Crompton, T., Robson, M., Mannherz, H. G. and Tschopp, J. (1993). Characterization of endogenous deoxyribonuclease involved in nuclear DNA degradation during apoptosis (programmed cell death). *EMBO J.*, **12**, 371–385.

Potchinsky, M. B., Muscarella, D. E., Hemendinger, R. A. and Bloom, S. E. (1995). Differential sensitivity of B-lineage lymphocytes compared to T-lineage lymphocytes to mitomycin-C-induced DNA damage involving cell cycle inhibition and apoptosis. *In Vitro Toxicol.*, **8**, 389–402.

Pratt, R. M. and Greene, R. M. (1976). Inhibition of palatal epithelial cell death by altered protein synthesis. *Dev. Biol.*, **54**, 135–145.

Pratt, R. M. and Martin, G. R. (1975). Epithelial cell death and cyclic AMP increase during palatal development. *Proc. Natl. Acad. Sci. USA*, **72**, 874–877.

Pritchard, D. J. and Butler, W. H. (1989). Apoptosis—the mechanisms of cell death in dimethylnitrosamine-induced hepatotoxicity. *J. Pathol.*, **158**, 253–260.

Quin, T., Herman, B. and Lemasters, J. J. (1999). The mitochondrial permeability transition mediates both necrotic and apoptotic death of hepatocytes exposed to Br-A23187. *Toxicol. Appl. Pharmacol.*, **154**, 117–125.

Raff, M. (1992). Social controls on cell survival and cell death. *Nature*, **356**, 397–400.

Raffray, M. and Cohen, G. M. (1997). Apoptosis and necrosis: a continuum or distinct modes of cell death. *Pharmacol. Ther.*, **75**, 153–177.

Raffray, M., McCarthy, D., Snowden, R. T. and Cohen, G. M. (1993). Apoptosis as a mechanism of tributyltin cytotoxicity to thymocytes: relationship of apoptotic markers to biochemical and cellular effects. *Toxicol. Appl. Pharmacol.*, **119**, 122–130.

Ray, S. D. (1997). Does ethanol potentiate acetaminophen-induced hepatocellular apoptosis? *Fundam. Appl. Toxicol.* (*Toxicologist*, Suppl.), **36**, 247.

Ray, S. D. (1998). Modulation of expression of bcl-2, bcl-XL and bcl-XS during acetaminophen-induced hepatocellular apoptosis. *Toxicol. Sci.* (*Toxicologist*, Suppl.), **42**, 190.

Ray, S. D. and Fariss, M. W. (1994). Role of cellular energy status in tocopheryl hemisuccinate cytoprotection against ethylmethanesulfonate-induced toxicity. *Arch. Biochem. Biophys.*, **311**, 180–190.

Ray, S. D. and Raje, R. R. (1994). Perplexed mouse hepatocytes *in vivo* show signs of both apoptosis and necrosis under the influence of acetaminophen and dimethylnitrosamine. *Presented at the Gordon Research Conference on Clinical and Experimental Cancer Chemotherapy, New Hampshire.*

Ray, S. D., Sorge, C. L., Raucy, J. L. and Corcoran, G. B. (1990). Early loss of large genomic DNA *in vivo* with accumulation of Ca^{2+} in the nucleus during acetaminophen-induced liver injury. *Toxicol. Appl. Pharmacol.*, **106**, 346–351.

Ray, S. D. and Corcoran, G. B. (1991a). Damage to the nucleus and acute cell death produced by alkylating hepatotoxins. In Ji, S. (Ed.), *Molecular Theories of Cell Life and Death*. Rutgers University Press, New Brunswick, NJ, Ch. 10, pp. 338–400.

Ray, S. D., Sorge, C. L., Tavacoli, A., Raucy, J. L. and Corcoran, G. B. (1991b). Extensive alteration of genomic DNA and rise in nuclear Ca^{2+} *in vivo* early after hepatotoxic acetaminophen overdose in mice. *Adv. Exp. Med. Biol.*, **238**, 699–705.

Ray, S. D., Sorge, C. L., Kamendulis, L. M. and Corcoran, G. B. (1992). Ca^{2+}-activated DNA fragmentation in dimethylnitrosamine-induced hepatic necrosis: effects of Ca^{2+} endonuclease and poly(ADP-ribose) polymearse inhibitors in mice. *J. Pharmacol. Exp. Ther.*, **263**, 2467–2471.

Ray, S. D., Kamendulis, L. M., Gurule, M. W., Yorkin, R. D. and Corcoran, G. B. (1993). Ca^{2+} antagonists inhibit DNA fragmentation and toxic cell death induced by acetaminophen. *FASEB J.*, **7**, 453–463.

Ray, S. D., Mumaw, V. R., Raje, R. R. and Fariss, M. W. (1996). Protection of acetaminophen induced hepatocellular apoptosis and necrosis by cholesteryl hemisuccinate pretreatment. *J. Pharmacol. Exp. Ther.*, **279**, 1470–1483.

Reed, D. J. (1990). Review of the current status of calcium and thiols in cellular injury. *Chem. Res. Toxicol.*, **3**, 495–502.

Reed, J. C. (1994). Bcl-2 and the regulation of programmed cell death. *J. Cell Biol.*, **124**, 1–6.

Reynolds, J. E., Yang, T., Qian, L. P., Jenkinson, J. D., Zhou, P., Eastman, A. and Craig. R. W. (1994). MCL-1, a member of the bcl-2 family, delays apoptosis induced by c-myc overexpression in Chinese hamster ovary cells. *Cancer Res.*, **54**, 6348–6352.

Richter, C., Schweizer, M., Cossarizza, A. and Franceschi, C. (1996). Control of apoptosis by the cellular ATP level. *FEBS Lett.*, **378**, 107–110.

Roberson, K. M., Penland, S. N., Padilla, G. M., Selvan, R. S., Kim, C. S., Fine, R. L. and Robertson, C. N. (1997). Fenretinide: induction of apoptosis and endogenous transforming growth factor beta in PC-3 prostate cancer cells. *Cell Growth Differ.*, **8**, 101–11.

Rohn, J. L., Hueber, A. O., McCarthy, N. J., Lyon, D., Navarro, P., Burgering, B. M. and Evan, G. I. (1998). The opposing roles of the AKT and *c-myc* signalling pathways in survival from CD95-mediated apoptosis. *Oncogene*, **17**, 2811–2818.

Roy, C., Brown, D. L., Little, J. E., Valentine, B. K., Walker, P. R., Sikorska, M., Leblanc, J. and Chaly, N. (1992). The topoisomerase II inhibitor teniposide (VM-26) induces apoptosis in unstimulated mature murine lymphocytes. *Exp. Cell Res.*, **200**, 416–424.

Rudin, C. M. and Thompson, C. B. (1997). Apoptosis and disease: regulation and clinical relevance of programmed cell death. *Annu. Rev. Med.*, **48**, 267–281.

Sakaguchi, Y., Sephens, L. C., Makino, M., Kaneko, T., Strebel, F. R., Danhauser, L. L., Jenkins, G. N. and Bull, J. M. (1994). Apoptosis in normal tissues induced by 5-fluorouracil: comparison between bolus injection and prolonged infusion. *Anticancer Res.*, **14**, 1489–1492.

Sanderson, C. J. (1976). The mechanism of thymus derived cell mediated cytotoxicity. Part 2. Morphological studies of cell deathby time lapse micro cinematography. *Proc. R. Soc. London, Ser. B, Biol. Sci.*, **192**, 224–255.

Sandoval, M., Zhang, X.-J., Liu, X., Mannick, E., Clark, D. A. and Miller, M. J. S. (1997). Peroxynitrite-induced apoptosis in T84 and RAW 264.7 cells: attenuation by *l*-ascorbic acid. *Free Rad. Biol. Med.*, **22**, 489–495.

Sandow, B. A., West, N. B., Norman, R. L. and Brenner, R. M. (1979). Hormonal control of apoptosis in hamster uterine luminal epithelium. *Am. J. Anat.*, **156**, 15–36.

Savill, J. S. (1994). Apoptosis and the kidney. *J. Am. Soc. Nephrol.*, **5**, 12–21.

Savill, J. S., Wyllie, A. H., Henson, J. E., Walport, M. J., Henson, P. M. and Haslett, C. (1989). Phagocytosis of aged human neutrophils by macrophages is mediated by a novel 'charge-sensitive' recognition mechanism. *J. Clin. Invest.*, **84**, 1518–1527.

Savill, J. S., Dransfield, I., Hogg, N. and Haslen, C. (1990). Vitronectin receptor–receptor mediated phagocytosis of cells undergoing apoptosis. *Nature*, **343**, 170–173.

Savill, J. S., Hogg, N. and Haslett, C. (1991). Macrophage vitronectin receptor, CD_{36} and thrombospondin cooperate in recognition of neutrophils undergoing programmed cell death. *Chest*, **99**, (Suppl. 3), 65 (Abstract).

Savill, J. S., Fadok, V., Hensen, P. and Haslett, C. (1993). Phagocyte recognition of cells undergoing apoptosis. *Immunol. Today*, **14**, 131–136.

Schwartzman, R. A. and Cidlowski, J. A. (1993). Apoptosis: the biochemistry and molecular biology of programmed cell death. *Endocrinol. Rev.*, **14**, 133–151.

Searle, J., Lawson, T. A., Abbot, P. J., Harmon, B. and Kerr, J. F. R. (1975). An electron microscope study of the mode of cell death induced by cancer-chemotherapeutic agents in populations of proliferating normal and neoplastic cells. *J. Pathol.*, **116**, 129–138.

Searle, J., Kerr, J. F. R. and Bishop, C. J. (1982). Necrosis and apoptosis: distinct modes of cell death with fundamentally different significance. *Pathol. Annu.*, **17**, 229–259.

Selander, K. S., Monkkonen, J., Karhukorpi, E. K., Harkonen, P., Hannuniemi, R. and Vaananen, H. K. (1996). Characteristics of clodronate-induced apoptosis in osteoclasts and macrophages. *Mol. Pharmacol.*, **50**, 1127–1138.

Selvakumaran, M., Lin, H. K., Miyashita, T., Wang, H. G., Krajewski, S., Reed, J. C., Hoffman, B. and Liebermann, D. (1994). Immediate early up-regulation of bax expression by p53 but not TGF beta 1: a paradigm for distinct apoptotic pathways. *Oncogene*, **9**, 1791–1798.

Sen, C. K. and Packer, L. (1996). Antioxidant and redox regulation of gene transcription. *FASEB J.*, **10**, 709–720.

Sentman, C. L., Shutter, J. R., Hockenbery, D., Kanagawa, O. and Korsmeyer, S. J. (1991). Bcl-2 inhibits multiple forms of apoptosis but not negative selection in thymocytes. *Cell*, **67**, 879–888.

Shen, W., Kamendulis, L. M., Ray, S. D. and Corcoran, G. B. (1991). Acetaminophen-induced cytotoxicity in cultured mouse hepatocytes: correlation of nuclear Ca^{2+} accumulation and early DNA fragmentation with cell death. *Toxicol. Appl. Pharmacol.*, **111**, 242–254.

Shen, W., Kamendulis, L. M., Ray, S. D. and Corcoran, G. B. (1992). Acetaminophen-induced cytotoxicity in cultured mouse hepatocytes: effects of Ca^{2+}-endonuclease, DNA repair, and glutathione depletion inhibitors on DNA fragmentation and cell death. *Toxicol. Appl. Pharmacol.* **112**, 32–40.

Shi, J., Fujieda, H., Kukubo, Y. and Wake, K. (1996a). Apoptosis of neutrophils and their elimination by Kupffer cells in rat liver. *Hepatology*, **24**, 1256–1263.

Shi, L., Chen, G., MacDonald, G., Bergeron, L., Li, H., Miura, M., Rotello, R. J., Miller, D. K., Li, P., Seshadri, T., Yuan, J. and Greenberg, A. H. (1996b). Activation of an interleukin 1 converting enzyme-dependent apoptosis pathways by granzyme B. *Proc. Natl. Acad. Sci. USA*, **93**, 11002–11007.

Shimada, H., Shiao, Y. H., Shibata, M. and Waalkes, M. P. (1998). Cadmium suppresses apoptosis induced by chromium. *J. Toxicol. Environ. Health*, **54**, 159–168.

Shimizu, S., Eguchi, Y., Kamiike, W., Waguri, S., Uchiyama, Y., Matsuda, H. and Tsujimoto, Y. (1996). Bcl-2 blocks loss of mitochondrial membrane potential while ICE inhibitors act at a different step during inhibition of death induced by respiratory chain inhibitors. *Oncogene*, **13**, 21–29.

Skladanowski, A. and Konopa, J. (1993). Adriamycin and daunomycin induce programmed cell death (apoptosis) in tumor cells. *Biochem. Pharmacol.*, **46**, 375–382.

Smith, S. B., Bora, N., McCool, D., Kutty, G., Wong, P., Kutty, R. K. and Wiggert, B. (1995). Photoreceptor cells in the vitilgo mouse die by apoptosis. TRPM-2/clusterin expression in increased in the neural retina and in the retinal pigment epithelium. *Invest. Opthalmol. Vis. Sci.*, **36**, 2193–2201.

Spinedi, A., Oliverio, S., Di Sano, F. and Piacentini, M. (1998). Calpain involvement in calphostin C-induced apoptosis. *Biochem. Pharmacol.*, **56**, 1489–1492.

Springer, L. N., McAsey, M. E., Flaws, J. A., Tilly, J. L., Sipes, I. G. and Hoyer, P. B. (1996). Involvement of apoptosis in 4-vinylcyclohexane diepoxide-induced ovotoxicity. *Toxicol. Appl. Pharmacol.*, **139**, 394–401.

Squier, M. K. and Cohen, J. J. (1997). Calpain, an upstream regulator of thymocyte apoptosis. *J. Immunol.*, **158**, 3690–3697.

Squier, M. K. T., Miller, A. C. K., Malkinson, A. M. and Cohen, J. J. (1994). Calpain activation in apoptosis. *J. Cell Physiol.*, **159**, 229–237.

Strika, S., Dobrogowska, A., Khander, A. and Ray, S. D. (1998). Furosemide induces apoptosis in the liver and kidneys *in vivo. Toxicol. Sci.* (*Toxicologist*, Suppl.), **42**, 357.

Sun, D. Y., Jiang, S., Zheng, L., Ojcius, D. M. and Young, J. D. (1994). Separate metabolic pathways leading to DNA fragmentation and apoptotic chromatin condensation. *J. Exp. Med.*, **179**, 559–568.

Suzuki, S., Li, X. K., Shinomiya, T., Enosawa, S., Amemiya, H., Amari, M. and Naoe, S. (1997). The *in vivo* induction of lymphocyte apoptosis in MRL-lpr/lpr mice treated with FTY720. *Clin. Exp. Immunol.*, **107**, 103–111.

Svegliati-Baroni, G., Marucci, L., Benedetti, A., Mancini, R., Jezequel, A.-M. and Orlandi, F. (1994). Chronic ethanol feeding increases apoptosis and cell proliferation in rat liver. *J. Hepatol.*, **20**, 508–513.

Symonds, H., Krall, L., Remington, L., Saenz-Robies, M., Lowe, S., Jacks, T. and Van Dyke, T. (1994). p53-Dependent apoptosis suppresses tumor growth and progression *in vivo. Cell*, **78**, 703–711.

Tanaka, Y., Yoshihara, K., Itaya, A., Kamiya, T. and Koide, S. S. (1984). Mechanism of the inhibition of Ca^{2+}, Mg^{2+}-dependent endonuclease of bull seminal plasma induced by ADP ribosylation. *J. Biol. Chem.*, **259**, 6579–6585.

Terada, T. and Nakanuma, Y. (1995). Detection of apoptosis and expression of apoptosis related proteins during human intrahepatic bile duct development. *Am. J. Pathol.*, **146**, 67–74.

Tewari, M., Quan, L. T., O'Rourke, K., Desnoyers, S., Zeng, Z., Beidler, D. R., Poirier, G. G., Salvesen, G. S. and Dixit, V. M. (1995). Yama/CPP32 beta, a mammalian homolog of CED-3, is a Crm-A-inhibitable protease that cleaves the death substrate poly (ADP-ribose) polymerase. *Cell*, **81**, 801–809.

Thornberry, N. A., Bull, H. G., Calaycay, I. R., Chapman, K. T., Howard, A. D., Kostura, M. J., Miller, D. K., Molineaux, S. M., Weidner, J. R. and Aunins, J. (1992). A novel heterodimeric cysteine protease is required for interleukin-1β processing in monocytes. *Nature*, **356**, 768–774.

Tomei, L. D., Cope, F. O. and Barr, P. J. (1994). Apoptosis: aging and phenotypic fidelity. In Tomei, L. D. and Cope, F. O. (Eds), *Apoptosis II: The Molecular Basis of Cell Death*, Cold Spring Harbor Laboratory Press, Cold Spring Harbor, NY, pp. 377–396.

Trapani, J. A., Jans, D. A., Jans, P. J., Smyth, M. J., Browne, K. A. and Sutton, V. R. (1998). Efficient nuclear targeting of granzyme B and the nuclear consequences of apoptosis induced by granzyme B and perforin are caspase-dependent, but cell death is caspase independent. *J. Biol. Chem.*, **273**, 27934–27938.

Trump, B. F. and Berezesky, I. (1995). Calcium-mediated cell injury and cell death. *FASEB J.*, **9**, 219–228.

Tsujimoto, Y., Finger, L. R., Tunis, J., Nowell, P. C. and Croce, C. M. (1984). Cloning of the chromosome breakpoint of neoplastic B cells with the t(14:18) chromosome translocation. *Science*, **226**, 1097–1099.

Tsukidate, K., Yamamoto, K., Snyder, J. W. and Farber, J. L. (1993). Microtubule antagonists activate programmed cell death (apoptosis) in cultured rat hepatocytes. *Am. J. Pathol.*, **143**, 918–925.

Ucker, D. S., Obermiller, P. S., Eckhart, W., Apgar, J. P., Berger, N. A. and Meyers, J. (1992). Genome digestion is a dispensable consequence of physiological cell death mediated by cytotoxic T lymphocytes. *Mol. Cell. Biol.*, **12**, 3060–3070.

Vanderbilt, J. N., Bloom, K. S. and Anderson, J. N. (1982). Endogenous nuclease. Properties and effects on transcribed genes in chromatin. *J. Biol. Chem.*, **257**, 13009–13107.

Vaux, D. L., Weissman, I. L. and Kim, S. K. (1992). Prevention of programmed cell death in *Caenorhabditis elegans* by human bcl-2. *Science*, **258**, 1955–1957.

Veis, D. J., Sorenson, C. M., Shutter, J. R. and Korsmeyer, S. J. (1993). Bcl-2 deficient mice demonstrate fulminant lymphoid apoptosis, polycystic kidneys, and hypopigmented hair. *Cell*, **75**, 229–240.

Verhaegen, S., McGowan, A. J., Brophy, A. R., Fernandes, R. S. and Cotter, T. G. (1995). Inhibition of apoptosis by antioxidants in the human HL-60 leukemia cell line. *Biochem. Pharmacol.*, **50**, 1021–1029.

Verheij, M., Bose, R., Lin, X. H., Yao, B., Jarvis, W. D., Grant, S., Birrer, M. J., Szabo, E., Zon, L. I., Kyriakis, J. M., Haimovitz-Friedman, A., Fuks, Z. and Kolesnick, R. N. (1996). Requirements for ceramide-initiated SAPK/JNK signalling in stress-induced apoptosis. *Nature*, **380**, 75–79.

Wallig, M. A. and Jeffery, E. H. (1990). Enhancement of pancreatic and hepatic glutathione levels in rats during cyanohydroxybutene intoxication. *Fundam. Appl. Toxicol.*, **14**, 144–159.

Walton, M., MacGibbon, G., Young, D., Sirimanne, E., Williams, C., Gluckman, P. and Dragunow, M. (1998). Do c-Jun, c-Fos, and amyloid precursor protein play a role in neuronal death or survival? *J. Neurosci. Res.*, **53**, 330–342.

Wang, H. G., Millan, J. A., Cox, A. D., Der, C. J., Rapp, U. R., Beck, T., Zha, H. and Reed, J. C. (1995). R-Ras promotes apoptosis caused by growth factor deprivation via a bcl-2 suppressible mechanism. *J. Cell Biol.*, **129**, 1103–1114.

Wang, L., Miura, M., Bergeron, L., Zhu, H. and Yuan, J. (1994). Ich-1, an Ice/ced-3-related gene, encodes both positive and negative regulators of programmed cell death. *Cell*, **78**, 739–750.

Wangenheim, K.-H. Von (1987). Cell death through differentiation. Potential immortality of somatic cells: a failure in control of differentiation. In Potten, C. S. (Ed.), *Perspectives on Mammalian Cell Death*. Oxford University Press, Oxford, pp. 129–159.

Weber, R. (1969). Tissues involution and lysosomal enzymes during anuran metamorphosis. In Dingle, J. T. and Fell, H. B. (Eds), *Lysosomes in Biology and Pathology*, Vol. 2. North-Holland, Amsterdam, pp. 437–461.

Weber, R. (1977). Biochemical characteristics of tail atrophy during anuran metamorphosis. *Colloq. Int. CNRS*, **266**, 137–146.

White, E. (1996). Life, death and the persuit of apoptosis. *Genes Dev.*, **10**, 1–15.

White, K., Grether, M. E., Abrams, J. M., Young, L., Farrell, K. and Steller, H. (1994). Genetic control of programmed cell death in *Drosophila*. *Science*, **264**, 677–683.

Wielckens, K. and Delfs, T. (1986). Glucocorticoid-induced cel death and poly(adenosine diphosphate (ADP)-ribosyl)ation: increased toxicity of dexamethasone on mouse S49.1 lymphoma cells with the poly(ADP-ribosyl)ation inhibitor benzamide. *Endocrinology*, **119**, 2383–2392.

Williams, D. A., Becker, P. L. and Fay, F. S. (1988). Regional changes in calcium underlying contraction of single smooth muscle cells. *Science*, **235**, 1644–1648.

Williams, G. T., Smith, C. A., Spooncer, E., Dexter, T. M. and Taylor, D. R. (1990). Haemopoietic colony stimulating factors promote cell survival by suppressing apoptosis. *Nature*, **343**, 76–79.

Williamson, R. (1970). Properties of rapidly labelled deoxyribonucleic acid fragments isolated from the cytoplasm of primary cultures of embryonic mouse liver cells. *J. Mol. Biol.*, **51**, 157–168.

Wilson, K. P., Black, J. F., Thomson, J. A., Kim, E. E., Griffith, J. P., Navia, M. A., Murcko, M. A., Chambers, S. P., Aldape, R. A., Raybuck, S. A. and Livingston, D. J. (1994). Structure and mechanism of interleukin-1β converting enzyme. *Nature*, **370**, 270–275.

Wyllie, A. H. (1980). Glucocorticoid-induced thymocyte apoptosis is associated with endogenous endonuclease activation. *Nature*, **284**, 555–556.

Wyllie, A. H. (1987). Apoptosis, cell death in tissue regulation. *J. Pathol.*, **153**, 313–316.

Wyllie, A. H., Kerr, J. F. and Currie, A. R. (1973). Cell death in the normal neonatal rat adrenal cortex. *J. Pathol.*, **111**, 255–261.

Wyllie, A. H., Kerr, J. F. R. and Currie, A. R. (1980). Cell death: the significance of apoptosis. *Int. Rev. Cytol.*, **68**, 251–306.

Wyllie, A. H., Morris, R. G., Smith, A. L. and Dunlop, D. (1984). Chromatin cleavage in apoptosis: association with condensed chromatin morphology and dependence on macromolecular synthesis. *J. Pathol.*, **142**, 67–77.

Xiong, Y., Hannon, G., Zhang, H., Casso, D., Kobayshi, R. and Beach, D. (1993). p21 is a universal inhibitor of cyclin kinases. *Nature*, **366**, 701–704.

Yacoub, L. K., Fogt, F., Griniuviene, B. and Nanji, A. A. (1995). Apoptosis and bcl-2 protein expression in experimental alcoholic liver disease in the rat. *Alc. Clin. Exp. Res.*, **19**, 854–859.

Yahya, S. M., Ray, S. D. and Raje, R. R. (1995). Abrogation of acetaminophen-induced hepatotoxicity by 3-aminobenzamide, a DNA repair modulator. *Fundam. Appl. Toxicol.* (*Toxicologist*), **15**, 133.

Yamaguchi, K., Matulka, R. A., Shneider, A. M., Toselli, P., Trombino, A. F., Yang, S., Hafer, L. J., Mann, K. K., Tao, X. J., Tilly, J. L., Near, R. I. and Sherr, D. H. (1997). Induction of pre-B cell apoptosis by 7, 12-dimethylbenz[*a*]anthracene in long-term primary murine bone marrow cultures. *Toxicol. Appl. Pharmacol.*, **147**, 192–203.

Yang, E., Zha, J., Jockel, J., Boise, L. H., Thompson, C. B. and Korsmeyer, S. J. (1995). Bad, a heterodimeric partner for bcl-XL and bcl-2, displaces bax and promotes cell death. *Cell*, **80**, 285–291.

Yonish-Rouach, E., Resnitzky, D., Lotem, J., Sachs, L., Kimchi, A. and Oren, M. (1991). Wild type p53 induces apoptosis of myeloid leukaemic cells that is inhibited by interleukin-6. *Nature*, **352**, 345–347.

Yuan, J. and Horvitz, H. R. (1990). The *Caenorhabditis elegans* genes *ced-3* and *ced-4* act cell autonomously to cause programmed cell death. *Dev. Biol.*, **138**, 33–41.

Yuan, J., Shaham, S., Ledoux, S., Ellis, H. M. and Horvitz, H. R. (1993). The *C. elegans* cell death gene ced-3 encodes a protein similar to mammalian interleukin-1 beta-converting enzyme. *Cell*, **75**, 641–652.

Yuge, K., Nambu, H., Senzaki, H., Nakao, I., Miki, H., Uyama, M. and Tsubura, A. (1996). N-Methyl-N-nitrosourea-induced photoreceptor apoptosis in the mouse retina. *In Vivo*, **10**, 483–488.

Zalewski, P. D. and Forbes, I. J. (1995). Intracellular zinc and the regulation of apoptosis. In Lavin, M. and Watters, D. (Eds), *Programmed Cell Death: the Cellular and Molecular Biology of Apoptosis*. Harwood Academic, Amsterdam, pp. 73–86.

Zhang, Y. H., Takahashi, K., Jiang, G. Z., Kwai, M., Fukada, M. and Yokochi, T. (1993). *In vivo* induction of apoptosis (programmed cell death) in mouse thymus by administration of lipopolysaccharide. *Infect. Immun.*, **61**, 5044–5048.

Zheng, L. M., Zychlinsky, A., Liu, C.-C., Ojcius, D. M. and Young, J. D. (1991). Extracellular ATP as a trigger for apoptosis or programmed cell death. *J. Cell. Biol.*, **112**, 279–288.

Zhivotovsky, B., Gahm, A., Ankarcrone, M., Nicotera, P. and Orrenius, S. (1995). Multiple proteases are involved in thymocyte apoptosis. *Exp. Cell Res.*, **221**, 404–412.

Zhong, L. T., Sarafian, T., Kane, D. J., Charles, A. C., Mah, S. P., Edwards, R. H. and Bredesen, D. E. (1993). Bcl-2 inhibits death of central neural cells induced by multiple agents. *Proc. Natl. Acad. Sci. USA*, **90**, 4533–4541.

FURTHER READING

Bowen, I. D. and Bowen, S. (1990). *Programmed Cell Death In Tumors and Tissues*. Chapman & Hall, London.

Holbrook, N. J., Martin, G. R. and Lockshin, R. A. (1996). *Cellular Aging and Cell Death*. Wiley-Liss, New York.

Lavin, M. and Watters, D. (1995). *Programmed Cell Death: the Cellular and Molecular Biology of Apoptosis*. Harwood Academic, Amsterdam.

Ray, S. D. and Grant, S. (Guest Eds) (1997). *Comments on Toxicology: Apoptosis (Special Issue)*. Harwood Academic/Gordon and Breach, Amsterdam.

McConkey, D. J., Zhivotovsky, B. and Orrenius, S. (1996). *Molecular Aspects of Medicine, Apoptosis: Molecular Mechanisms and Biomedical Implications*, Vol. 17.

Chapter 10

Pharmacogenetics and Toxicological Consequences of Human Drug Oxidation and Reduction

Hakam Hadidi, Cüneyt Güzey and Jeffrey R. Idle

CONTENTS

GENE–ENVIRONMENT INTERACTIONS IN A CHEMICAL UNIVERSE

Humans are exposed to perhaps two million discrete chemicals per day. Many of these are useful as sources of energy, as essential components of our internal biochemistry or as building blocks for new cell growth. Our exposure to anutrient chemicals, sometimes referred to as xenobiotics, is unavoidable. The food we eat, the air we breathe and the water we drink are all laced with numerous such chemicals, some man-made, others natural. Plants, for example, have evolved an impressive range of chemical defences and this is perhaps why we consume such a paltry number of the available plant species. That notwithstanding, chemicals such as alkaloids, terpenes and flavonoids are absorbed whenever we eat plants. The modern industrial era has witnessed an explosion of new chemical entities. These have found such uses as agrochemicals, pharmaceuticals, food additives, cosmetics and domestic products, and we are exposed to these intentionally, in addition to the myriad of unwanted chemical pollutants in water, air and the food chain. The chemical burden of modern life is maybe what separates us most from our forefathers.

The evolutionary pathway which has brought us from unicellular organisms to such a level of integrated biological sophistication has delivered not only complexity but also variety. The members of no other species of plant or animal display such broad interindividual variability. The advent of DNA fingerprinting alone has confirmed what we already knew innately, that no two persons are alike. Aspiring heterologous organ transplant recipients sometimes never find a donor organ which matches their MHC genotype. For *Homo sapiens*, this almost infinite diversity is the fruit of an evolutionary struggle as old as life itself, fuelled by the processes of natural selection, genetic drift and molecular drive. From the standpoint of our chemical environment, it has been argued (Gonzalez and Nebert, 1990) that molecular drive has been the process which has allowed animal populations to acquire novel variant genes that permit individuals to exploit new dietary sources of vegetation. The spread of such genes in the population could have assisted in adaptation to fresh toxic challenges from plants. Such increasingly diversified animal defences are then seen by Gonzalez and Nebert (1990) as triggering a co-evolution of plants by what they have termed 'animal-plant warfare', a rationale for the existence of a plethora of plant toxins and a multiplicity of mammalian defence systems.

Metabolism of xenobiotics is the principal means by which the animal rids itself of such chemicals. Not only does metabolism render the chemical intruder more water-soluble and readily excretable, but the toxic nature of the chemical is also frequently attenuated. This paradigm is sometimes inverted, whereby a seemingly innocuous chemical is converted to a toxic species by the processes of metabolism. In the context of animal–plant warfare, plants seem to have, by chance or design, evolved the ability to synthesize chemical Trojan horses. Only a full appreciation of the complexity of the xenobiotic metabolizing systems of animals and the extent to which genetic variability in these systems appears to have evolved can shed some light on animals' ability to detoxicate both direct-and indirect-acting chemical toxins.

OVERVIEW OF THE DRUG AND CHEMICAL METABOLIZING SYSTEMS

The guiding principles of xenobiotic metabolism were first laid down by Williams (1959), in which he envisioned a biphasic process comprising an initial phase (Phase I) which introduced or unmasked such chemical moieties as –OH, –NH$_2$, –COOH or –SH using the biochemical processes of oxidation, reduction and hydrolysis. This provides a chemical handhold for a series of synthetic (conjugation) reactions to occur during Phase II of the biotransformation process. Typical Phase II reactions involve the addition of sugars, amino acids, sulphate, methyl and acetyl groups. When taken together, Phase I and II reactions furnish a means to metabolize virtually all anutrient chemicals which enter the body. A list of the common enzymes is shown in **Table 1**. It is difficult to compute the exact number of human drug-metabolizing enzymes, but a crude estimate might be 200 distinct gene products. One group alone, the cytochrome P450 monooxygenases (CYPs), comprises a gene superfamily which, as of October 1995, comprised 481 genes from 85 eukaryote and 20 prokaryote species (Nelson *et al.*, 1996). *CYP* genes have been found in every species so far studied, but in many cases the gene products are concerned with the metabolism of endogenous substances such as steroids, fatty acids and ecosanoids. Insects, which have arguably a more intimate relationship with plants, are well endowed with *CYP* genes, *Anopheles albimanus* (a mosquito), *Drosophila melanogaster* and *Musca domestica* (the housefly) possessing at least 17, 17 and 16 *CYP* genes, respectively (Nelson, 1997). The occurrence of *CYP* genes in humans, together with some laboratory and domestic species, is given in **Table 2**. The prevalence of

these genes in the rat, mouse and rabbit, compared with the dog and non-human primate, probably is an artefact of the research focus to date. However, as of June 1997, 39 *CYP* genes had been sequenced from the human

Table 1 Overview of the drug and chemical metabolizing systems

Phase I enzymes

1. Oxygenases/dehydrogenases
   Cytochrome P450 monooxygenases (CYPs)
   Flavoprotein monooxygenases (FMOs)
   Dihydropyrimidine dehydrogenase (DPD)
   Alcohol dehydrogenases (ALHs)
   Aldehyde dehydrogenases (ALDHs)
   Aldehyde oxidases
   NAD(P)H:quinone oxidoreductase (NQO)

2. Reductases
   Nitroreductases
   Carbonylreductases
   Aldehyde reductases

3. Hydrolases
   Epoxide hydrolases
   Cholinesterases
   Arylesterases

Phase II enzymes

UDP-glucosyltransferases (UDPs)
Sulphotranferases
Glutathione *S*-transferases (GSTs)
N-Acetyltransferases (NATs)
Thiopurine methyltransferase (TPMT)
Catechol *O*-methyltransferase (COMT)
Imidazole *N*-methyltransferase
Acyl-CoA:amino acid *N*-acyltransferases
Kinases

Table 2 Species distribution of sequenced CYP genes and pseudogenes

Species	Number[a] of Sequenced CYP genes	Number[a] of Sequenced pseudogenes
Human	39	10
Laboratory animals		
Rat	60	4
Mouse	43	1
Rabbit	30	0
Hamster	15	0
Guinea pig	11	0
Dog	8	0
Baboon	3 fragments	0
Monkeys	8	0
Domestic animals		
Sheep	6	0
Goat	3	0
Pig	14	0
Cow	10	0
Horse	2	0

[a] As of 25 June 1997 (data from http://drnelson.utmem.edu/genesperspecies.html)

Table 3 Overview of human *CYP* genes, catalytic activities of the CYP proteins and evidence for genetic polymorphism

CYP gene	CYP activity	Genotypes	Phenotypes
CYP1A1	Benzo[*a*]pyrene epoxygenase	+	−
CYP1A2	Caffeine N^3-demethylase	−	+
CYP1B1 (adrenal cortex, breast)	17β-Oestradiol 4-hydroxylase 7, 12-Dimethylbenz[*a*]anthracene hydroxylase Aflatoxin B1 8,9-epoxygenase	−	−
CYP2A6	Coumarin 7-hydroxylase	+	+
CYP2A7	?	+	−
CYP2A13	?	−	−
CYP2B6	7-Ethoxycoumarin *O*-deethylase 6-Aminochrysene activation to mutagens 3-Methoxy-4-aminoazobenzene activation to mutagens	−	−
CYP2C8	Paclitaxel 6-hydroxylase Verapamil *O*-demethylase Arachidonic acid epoxygenase	−	−
CYP2C9	(*S*)-Warfarin 7-hydroxylase Tolbutamide 4-methylhydroxylase	+	−
CYP2C10	Tolbutamide 4-methylhydroxylase	−	−
CYP2C18	Verapamil *O*-demethylase	+	−
CYP2C19	Omeprazole 5-hydroxylase Mephenytoin 4′-hydroxylase	+	+
CYP2D6	Debrisoquine 4-hydroxylase Bufuralol 1′-hydroxylase Dextromethorphan *O*-demethylase	+	+
CYP2E1	Chlorzoxazone 6-hydroxylase Aniline 4-hydroxylase 1,1-Dichloroethene 2-hydroxylase	+	−
CYP2F1 (lung)	Ethoxycoumarin *O*-deethylase Styrene epoxygenase	−	−
CYP2J2 (heart, intestine, pancreas)	Arachidonic acid epoxygenase	−	−
CYP3A3	Benzoxazinorifampacin 30-hydroxylase Alprazolam 4-hydroxylase 4-Ipomeanol activation	−	−
CYP3A4	Testosterone 6β-hydroxylase Nifedipine dehydrogenase Alprazolam 4-hydroxylase Erythromycin *N*-demethylase 4-Ipomeanol activation Midazolam 1′-hydroxylase Midazolam 4-hydroxylase Oestrone 16α-hydroxylase Oestrone 2-hydroxylase Oestrone 4-hydroxylase	−	−
CYP3A5 (neutrophils, intestine, kidney)	Midazolam 1′-hydroxylase (> CYP3A4) Midazolam 4-hydroxylase (=CYP3A4)	−	−
CYP3A7 (endometrium, placenta, foetal liver)	?	−	−
CYP4A9	Lauric acid 12-hydroxylase (ω-hydroxylase)	−	−
CYP4A11	Lauric acid 12-hydroxylase (>CYP4A9)	−	−
CYP4B1	4-Ipomeanol activation	−	−

genome (Nelson, 1997). In approximate terms, 16 human CYPs are concerned only with endogenous metabolism, whilst 23 comprise a battery of isozymes with overlapping substrate specificities that can oxidize almost all anutrient chemicals entering the body. These 23 *CYP* genes, together with typical metabolic activities, are listed in **Table 3**. For a detailed account of the nomenclature system, evolution and organization of the *CYP* gene superfamily, see Nelson *et al*. (1996). Except where stated otherwise, these gene products are expressed in human liver. Certain of these *CYP* genes have been found to be genetically polymorphic, meaning that two or more different alleles exist at a particular *CYP* locus. Polymorphism in the CYP system was first detected phenotypically (Mahgoub *et al.*, 1977), before the advent of molecular biological methods such as cDNA cloning, sequencing and DNA amplification by the polymerase chain reaction (PCR). **Table 3** also shows for which loci multiple genotypes have been detected and for which functional phenotypes can be discerned. Only for three of the 23 genes (13%) are there visible phenotypes arising from detectable genotypes, the examples of *CYP2A6*, *CYP2C19* and *CYP2D6*. In one case, that of polymorphic caffeine N^3-demethylation, phenotypes have been observed, but to date DNA sequence differences have eluded detection. More commonly, as with *CYP1A1, CYP2A7, CYP2C9, CYP2C18* and *CYP2E1*, PCR methods detect more than one allele in the population, but a clear phenotypic difference has yet to emerge. The trend, however, is towards further disclosure of polymorphism.

OVERVIEW OF THE GENETIC POLYMORPHISMS IN CHEMICAL OXIDATION AND REDUCTION

Cytochrome P450 (CYP) polymorphisms

The CYP2D6 polymorphism

The independent discoveries, in London and Bonn, that the drugs debrisoquine (Mahgoub *et al.*, 1977) and sparteine (Eichelbaum *et al.*, 1979), respectively, displayed genetic polymorphism in their oxidative metabolism breathed life into the ailing subject of pharmacogenetics. The establishment that 5–10% of the population were unable to metabolize these two drugs, owing to their inheritance of the poor metabolizer (PM), rather than the common extensive metabolizer (EM), trait, helped rationalize observations a decade previously that one patient taking nortriptyline and one desmethylimipramine had steady-state plasma levels over five times higher than the modal value for the population of 66 patients (Hammer and Sjöqvist, 1967). Twin and family studies erroneously suggested that the metabolism of these antidepressant drugs was under polygenic, rather than monogenic, control. The debrisoquine hydroxylation defect was shown to be due to absent P450 activity in the liver (Davies *et al.*, 1981), leading to *in vitro* methods for the PM typing of human livers based upon attenuated activities such as bufuralol 1'-hydroxylase (Dayer *et al.*, 1982, 1984). The availability of PM livers from Switzerland, coupled with rabbit antibodies against rat P450 proteins prepared by Hardwick in the USA, led to the cloning and sequencing of the human P450db1 (now referred to as *CYP2D6*) cDNA and characterization of the basic genetic lesion by Gonzalez and colleagues at the

NIH, USA (Gonzalez *et al.*, 1988). The protein is referred to variously in the older literature as P-450buf1, P-450db1 and P-450IID6, before the introduction of the system of nomenclature used today (Nelson *et al.*, 1996). Many laboratories have described *CYP2D6* inactivating alleles, together with alleles which simply slow hydroxylation and also a somatic amplification of the *CYP2D6* gene, up to 13 copies. The only published consensus of *CYP2D6* alleles (Daly *et al.*, 1996) described two alleles with normal activity (*CYP2D6*1A* and *CYP2D6*1B*), five alleles conferring decreased activity (*CYP2D6*2*, *CYP2D6*9*, *CYP2D6*10A*, *CYP2D6*10B* and *CYP2D6*10C*), 16 completely inactivating alleles (*CYP2D6*3*, *CYP2D6*4A*, *CYP2D6*4B*, *CYP2D6*4C*, *CYP2D6*4D*, *CYP2D6*5 CYP2D6*6A*, *CYP2D6*6B*, *CYP2D6*7*, *CYP2D6*8*, *CYP2D6*11*, *CYP2D6*12*, *CYP2D6*13*, *CYP2D6*14*, *CYP2D6*15* and *CYP2D6*16*) and the amplified allele (*CYP2D6*2N*) which gives rise to increased metabolism and the phenotype known as ultrarapid metabolizer (UM). Accordingly, there are at least 24 *CYP2D6* alleles, each of which is now detectable by PCR. Routine PCR analysis in a clinical service setting in the authors' laboratory in Trondheim, forecasts the EM, PM and UM genotypes (see **Figure 1**) for patients with therapeutic difficulties, such as undetectable drug plasma levels and adverse drug reactions.

There now exists a long list of therapeutic agents which are CYP2D6 substrates. The list was added to significantly recently by a study of the interactions of amphetamine derivatives with CYP2D6 (Wu, D. *et al.*, 1997). This is given in **Table 4** and comprises 85 drugs, the majority of which are currently in clinical use. Many of these drugs act on either the central nervous system or the cardiovascular system, by modifying the behaviour of amine neurotransmitters, thus sharing chemical similarities. Although some rather complex computer-based models have been proposed for determining CYP2D6 substrate candidature *ab initio*, no simple theoretical method is available, to our knowledge. It is clinical or scientific intuition which has always taken the problem to the laboratory. Below we propose a simple means to predict new substrates for the CYP2D6 polymorphism. There are surely hundreds of, as yet untested, drugs and alkaloids which could be demonstrated experimentally to be CYP2D6 substrates, many of which may be of great toxicological significance. We stand today only on the tip of the iceberg.

Predicting new CYP2D6 substrates 'on paper'

Figure 2 is a cartoon of the predictive reasoning process. It predicts the correct outcome for 85/87 known CYP2D6 substrates listed in **Table 4**. It even predicts the somewhat bizarre example of procainamide *N*-hydroxylation (Lessard *et al.*, 1997), the only substantiated non-carbon oxidation mediated by CYP2D6. The

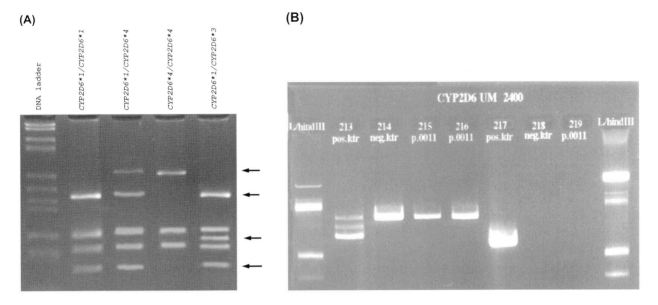

Figure 1 Detection of *CYP2D6* genotypes using the polymerase chain reaction (PCR) and gel electrophoresis. (A) The diagnostic fragments (marked with arrows) that permit detection of the *CYP2D6*1*, *CYP2D6*3* and *CYP2D6*4* alleles. Lane 4 (second from right) is from a phenotypic poor metabolizer (*CYP2D6*4/CYP2D6*4* genotype). (B) The diagnostic fragments that permit the detection of the *CYP2D6*2X2* allele which causes ultrarapid metabolism (UM phenotype). Lanes 2–5 and 6–8 derive from two different tests, one (lanes 2–5) which gives a PCR product when the *CYP2D6*2X2* allele is absent and the other (lanes 6–8) which gives a PCR product only when the *CYP2D6*2X2* allele is present.

Table 4 Drug substrates for the CYP2D6 polymorphism

Drug	Therapeutic group	Category[a]
Ajmaline	Antiarrhythmic	NR
Alprenolol	β-Blocker	ICU
Amiflamine	Antidepressant	ICU
Amiodarone	Antiarrhythmic	ICU
Amitriptyline	Antidepressant	ICU
Amphetamine	CNS symphathomimetic	ICU
Aprindine	Antiarrhythmic	ICU
Bufuralol	β-blocker	NR
Chlomipramine	Antidepressant	ICU
Chlorpheniramine	Antihistamine	ICU
Chlorpromazine	Antipsychotic	ICU
Chlorprotixen	Antipsychotic	ICU
Citalopram	Antidepressant	ICU
Clemastine	Antihistamine	ICU
Clozapine	Antipsychotic	ICU
Codeine	Analgesic	ICU
Debrisoquine	Antihypertensive	NLIU
Desmethylimipramine	Antidepressant	ICU
Dextromethorphan	Antitussive	ICU
Dihydrocodeine	Analgesic	ICU
Dimethindene	Antihistamine	ICU
Diphenhydramine	Antihistamine	ICU
Dixyrazin	Antipsychotic	ICU
Doxepine	Antidepressant	ICU
Encainide	Antiarrhythmic	NR
Ethylmorphine	Antitussive	ICU
Fenfluramine	Appetite suppressant	ICU
Flecainide	Antiarrhythmic	ICU

(Continued Over leaf)

Table 4 *(Contd)*

Drug	Therapeutic group	Category[a]
Fluoxetine	Antidepressant	ICU
Flupentixol	Antipsychotic	ICU
Fluphenazine	Antipsychotic	ICU
Folcodine	Antitussive	ICU
Granisetron	Antiemetic	ICU
Guanoxan	Antihypertensive	NLIU
Haloperidol	Antipsychotic	ICU
Hydrocodone	Antitussive	ICU
4-Hydroxyamphetamine	Psychedelic	ID
4-Hydroxymethamphetamine	Psychedelic	ID
Imipramine	Antidepressant	ICU
Indoramin	Antihypertensive	ICU
Loperamide	Antiperistaltic	ICU
Maprotiline	Antidepressant	ICU
MDA	Psychedelic	ID
MDMA ('Ecstasy')	Psychedelic	ID
Metaraminol	Cardiac stimulant	ICU
Methadone	Analgesic	ICU
Methamphetamine	Psychedelic	ID
2-Methoxyamphetamine	Psychedelic	ID
3-Methoxyamphetamine	Psychedelic	ID
4-Methoxyamphetamine	Psychedelic	ID
Methoxyphenamine	Bronchodilator	ICU
Methylphenidate	CNS sympathomimetic	ICU
Metoprolol	β-blocker	ICU
Mexilitine	Antiarrhythmic	ICU
Mianserine	Antidepressant	ICU
MMDA	Psychedelic	ID
MMDA-2	Psychedelic	ID
Nicotine	Tobacco replacement	ICU
Nortriptyline	Antidepressant	ICU
Noscapine	Antitussive	ICU
N-Propylajmaline	Antiarrhythmic	NR
Olanzapine	Antipsychotic	ICU
Ondansetron	Antiemetic	ICU
Oxprenolol	β-blocker	ICU
Paroxetine	Antidepressant	ICU
Perhexiline	Antianginal	NLIU
Periciazine	Antipsychotic	ICU
Perphenazine	Antipsychotic	ICU
Phenformin	Hypoglycaemic	NLIU
Pindolol	β-blocker	ICU
Procainamide	Antiarrhythmic	ICU
Prochlorperazine	Antipsychotic	ICU
Promethazine	Antihistamine	ICU
Propafenone	Antiarrhythmic	ICU
Propranolol	β-blocker	ICU
Respiridone	Antipsychotic	ICU
Sertraline	Antidepressant	ICU
Sparteine	Oxytotic	NLIU
Tamoxifen	Antiestrogen	ICU
Thioridazine	Antipsychotic	ICU
Timolol	β-blocker	ICU
2,4,6-TMA	Psychedelic	ID
3,4,5-TMA	Psychedelic	ID
Tramadol	Analgesic	ICU
Trimipramine	Antidepressant	ICU

(Continued)

Table 4 *(Contd)*

Drug	Therapeutic group	Category[a]
Tropisetron	Antiemetic	ICU
Zuclopentixol	Antipsychotic	ICU

[a] ID, illicit drug; ICU, in common usage; NLIU, no longer in use; NR, never registered.

two drugs which it fails to predict are perhexiline and nicotine. Cotinine formation from nicotine (the principal pathway of nicotine oxidation) does not fit the model, but the minor hydroxypyridine metabolites would fit the model. Recent studies show that nicotine is principally a CYP2A6 substrate (Messina *et al.*, 1997). Regarding perhexiline, its lack of fit to the model is unexplained, except to say that its metabolism in man is extremely slow compared with other CYP2D6 substrates.

Inspection of **Figure 2** shows that the quintessential requirement of the candidate drug is first to possess a basic nitrogen (a free lone pair of electrons, not one hybridized into an aromatic ring as occurs in the pyridine nitrogen, for example). Second, the molecule must possess an electron-withdrawing group, commonly an aromatic system, which should, third, be separated from the basic nitrogen by a two to four atom spacer. This 'separator' can be part of an alicyclic ring system and need not necessarily be aliphatic, or composed purely of carbon atoms. If these three criteria are met, then oxidation (in the form of aromatic hydroxylation, *O*-demethylation or even *N*-hydroxylation, as in the case of procainamide) occurs beyond the electron-withdraw-

ing group. **Figure 3** demonstrates four classical examples drawn from different therapeutic and chemical classes.

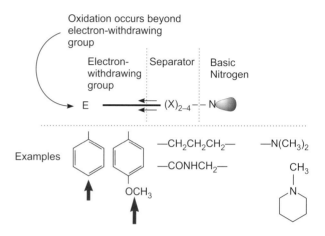

Figure 2 Simple predictive method for determining if a drug/chemical is a CYP2D6 substrate. The substance must have a basic nitrogen, separated from an electron-withdrawing group by a spacer of 2–4 atoms. Oxidation by CYP2D6 then occurs beyond the electron-withdrawing group. Examples of these moieties are given.

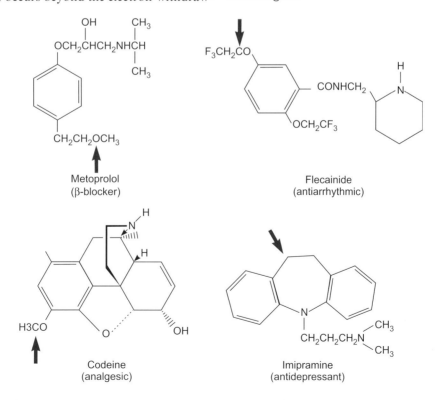

Figure 3 Examples of how the predictive method works using known CYP2D6 substrates from different drug classes. The arrow indicates the position of oxidation by CYP2D6.

Metoprolol has a secondary basic nitrogen, a three carbon spacer and a phenoxy electron-withdrawing group. *O*-Demethylation occurs beyond the electron-withdrawing group. Flecainide also has a secondary basic nitrogen, a three atom spacer (–CONHCH$_2$–) and a bis(trifluorethoxy)phenyl electron-withdrawing group. Oxidative *O*-dealkylation occurs at the least sterically hindered alkyl group. Codeine also has a secondary basic nitrogen and three possible spacers to the methoxyphenyl electron-withdrawing group, including the three carbon spacer which is β to the plane of the paper. Again, *O*-demethylation occurs beyond the electron-withdrawing group. Finally, imipramine has a tertiary basic nitrogen, a three carbon spacer to the second, only weakly basic nitrogen, whose lone pair of electrons is conjugated with the two aromatic rings in a single molecular orbital. Here again oxidation, in this case alicyclic (benzylic) hydroxylation, occurs beyond the electron-withdrawing group. This pattern is repeated throughout the known CYP2D6 substrates, with the two exceptions listed above. The reader is invited to peruse the pages of the Merck Index, for example, and select at will any number of candidate CYP2D6 substrates.

Toxicological consequences of the CYP2D6 polymorphism

The consequences of the existence of amplified alleles, alleles conferring reduced activity, together with inactivating alleles in a population are manifold. In the 11 years following the discovery of the CYP2D6 polymorphism by Mahgoub *et al.* (1977), this group at St Mary's Hospital Medical School, London, carried out over 17 000 phenotyping tests using debrisoquine. The range of metabolic ratios (MR, % dose as debrisoquine/% dose as 4-hydroxydebrisoquine in urine) was 0.01 to > 200, representing a range of metabolic activity from 0.5 to 99%, or 200-fold. There is no reason to suppose that other pure CYP2D6 substrates will show any less variability in the population. Experience shows that these urinary differences are reflected by a 3–10-fold difference in drug plasma levels between EMs and PMs (see Hall *et al.*, 1994 for a review). As a consequence, achieving the correct dose of a CYP2D6 substrate requires either stepwise dose escalation or, alternatively, what has been termed 'pharmacogenotyping' (Hall *et al.*, 1994). Inevitably, most physicians do neither of these things. Therefore, clinical use of CYP2D6 substrates is often associated with a high incidence of adverse drug reactions. For a list of typical clinical toxicities associated with this polymorphism, see Price Evans (1993) and Eichelbaum and Gross (1992).

Of perhaps greater toxicological importance is the impact of the CYP2D6 polymorphism on the metabolism of non-pharmaceutical chemical agents, chronic exposure to which might be associated with human disease. As has been mentioned, animal–plant warfare may have been the phenomenon by which a co-evolution of certain plants and animals occurred which would explain both the diversity of plant toxins against animals, such as the alkaloids, and the large number of *CYP* genes with gene products of broad and overlapping substrate specificities (Gonzalez and Nebert, 1990). Inspection of the chemistry of the alkaloids reveals that CYP2D6 should be able to metabolize a great number of them, according both to precedent (ajmaline, codeine, *N*-propylajmaline and sparteine in **Table 4** are all alkaloids) and to the predictive procedure outlined in the previous section.

For the purposes of illustration, we discuss here one group of alkaloids, the indole alkaloids. Indoles are found both in plants and animals. The amino acid tryptophan is an indole which gives rise in the body to a variety of indole metabolites, including tryptamine, 5-hydroxytryptamine (5-HT, serotonin) and *N*-acetyl-5-methoxytryptamine (melatonin). Recently, Benítez and his colleagues in Badajoz, Spain, reported a very interesting finding, that the endogenous brain amine tryptamine **(Figure 4)** is metabolized to tryptophol by CYP2D6 (Martínez *et al.*, 1997), a reaction traditionally believed to be carried out by monoamine oxidase (MAO). The implications that CYP2D6 has an endogenous substrate are not yet understood, but this promises to be a very important finding. The simplest of the indole alkaloids seem to act on the serotinergic system in the brain, which is so closely associated with mood and perception, and not surprisingly, many of these seem to have mood-and perception-altering properties. *N*, *N*-Dimethyltryptamine (DMT, **Figure 4**) is found in banana and pineapple and is a psychedelic substance (Strassman *et al.*, 1994), almost certainly the reason why it was commonplace in the youth culture of the 1960s to smoke banana skins. DMT is not active orally owing to its high first-pass metabolism in the liver, thought to be due to MAO activity. This must be reconsidered in the light of the discovery that the parent substance tryptamine is a CYP2D6 substrate. In both Amerindian and Asian cultures, it has long been known that the psychedelic properties of certain plants are radically enhanced by the co-administration of extracts of the leaves of *Banisteriopsis caapi* (a liana called locally 'Ayahuasca', the 'rope of death') or the seeds of *Peganum harmala*, which contain another group of indole alkaloids known as the β-carbolines. One of these, harmaline **(Figure 4)**, is thought to be an MAO inhibitor and for this reason promotes blood levels of ingested DMT. Harmaline, unlike the other β-carbolines harman, harmalol and harmine, is a candidate CYP2D6 substrate, predicted to undergo *O*-demethylation with CYP2D6 by the rule explained in the previous section. Presumably, therefore, *Banisteriopsis caapi* and *Peganum harmala* enhance the psychedelic effects of indole alkaloids by inhibiting CYP2D6, instead of, or in addition to, MAO. Finally, the species of grasses known as *Phalaris* contain both tryptamine-derived (5-methoxy-*N*, *N*-dimethyltryptamine, **Figure 4**) and

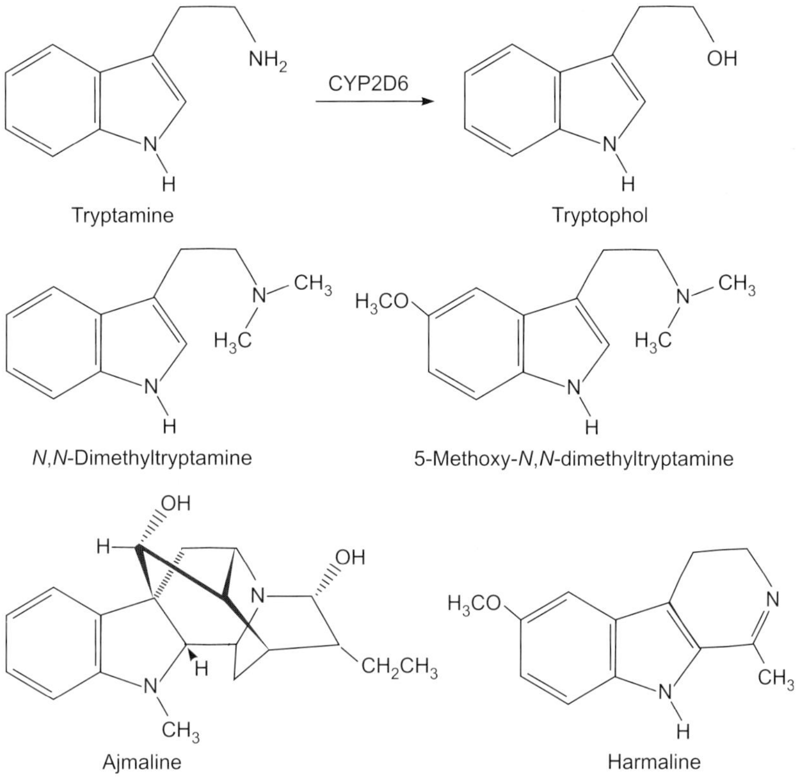

Figure 4 Naturally occurring CYP2D6 substrates, known or predicted. Examples include the biogenic amine tryptamine, the psychedelic indole alkaloids *N,N*-dimethyltryptamine (from banana) and 5-methoxy-*N,N*-dimethyltryptamine (from *Phalaris* spp.), the indole alkaloid ajmaline and the β-carboline alkaloid harmaline.

carboline alkaloids (Cheeke, 1995) which cause neurological symptoms such as 'staggers' and often death when consumed by sheep. The only xenobiotic metabolizing CYPs so far detected in sheep are CYP1A1 and CYP3A24 which would not, unlike a CYP2D isozyme, be expected to metabolize indole alkaloids. It is not known whether or not there exists a human counterpart to sheep 'staggers', but theoretically CYP2D6 PMs (5–10% of the population) could be at higher risk of the psychotropic effects of dietary indole alkaloids such as DMT.

Despite decades of research into the possible aetiology of the neurodegenerative disease Parkinson's disease (PD), relatively little is known about the mechanisms underlying cellular degeneration and the cause of the disease. In the late 1970s and early 1980s in California, serendipity produced a chemical model for PD. Young heroin addicts had been abusing a synthetic pethidine derivative called MPPP when a number of them presented with a parkinsonian illness. Langston *et al.* (1983) ultimately described seven cases in detail, which they showed had developed all the cardinal signs of PD owing to an impurity in the street drug MPPP called 1-methyl-4-phenyl-1,2,3,6-tetrahydropyridine (MPTP). The mechanism of the MPTP-induced lesion has been extensively studied and is known to involve metabolism of MPTP by MAO-B in glial cells or serotinergic neurones to a reactive metabolite MPP$^+$ (see Jenner, 1989). MPTP is also metabolized **(Figure 5)** both by a flavin-containing monooxygenase (FMO) to its *N*-oxide and by CYP2D6 (high affinity, $K_m = 48\,\mu M$) and CYP1A2 (low affinity, $K_m = 2882\,\mu M$) to the *N*-demethylated product (Coleman *et al.*, 1996). In addition, CYP2D6 has been shown to be expressed in the pigmented neurones of the substantia nigra (Gilham *et al.*, 1997), the target cell for MPTP. These new insights provide a plausible mechanism for the observation that both CYP2D6 and cigarette smoking (which induces CYP1A2 and also inhibits MAO-B (Fowler *et al.*, 1996)) may protect against PD. Molecular epidemiological studies have found both an excess of CYP2D6 PMs (odds ratio 2.54, 95% C.I. 1.51–4.28; Smith *et al.*, 1992) and of the *CYP2D6*4* allele (odds ratio 2.70, 95% C.I. 1.14–6.41; Armstrong *et al.*, 1992) (commonest inactivating allele in Caucasian populations) in Parkinson's disease, suggesting a neuroprotective effect of the active enzyme.

The earliest role suggested for CYP2D6 in chemical toxicity was in the occurrence of lung cancer. Using debrisoquine phenotyping, involving administration of a 10 mg tablet of the drug and collection of a 0–8 h urine as first described by Mahgoub *et al.* (1977), Hetzel *et al.* (1980) studied 106 British smokers who had been diagnosed with lung cancer and compared the findings with a historical population of 258 healthy British whites.

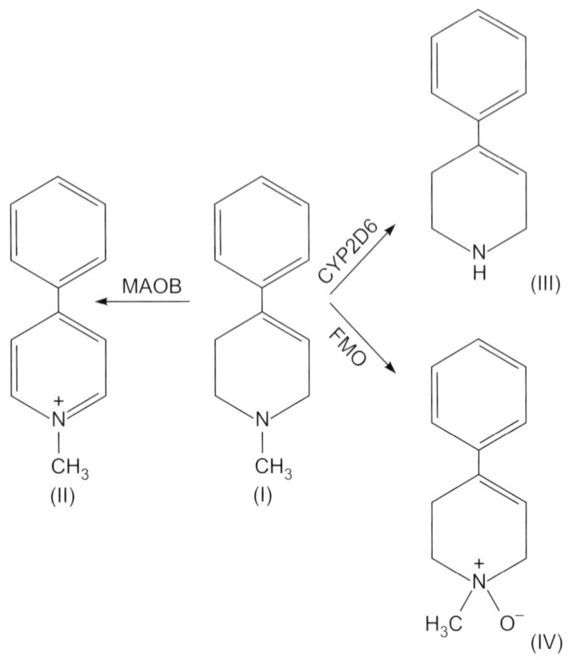

Figure 5 Activation and detoxication by polymorphic enzymes of the neurotoxin MPTP. (I) MPTP; (II) neurotoxic metabolite MPP$^+$, formed by monoamine oxidase B (MAOB); (III) N-demethylated metabolite formed by CYP2D6; (IV) N-oxide formed by a flavin-containing monooxygenase (FMO).

The incidence of PMs was 4–5-fold lower in the cancer group. This same group then performed a case-control study of 245 lung cancer cases and 234 age-, smoking history- and sex-matched controls with chronic obstructive pulmonary disease. Again, an under-representation (5.6-fold) of PMs was found in the cases (Ayesh *et al.*, 1984). These pioneering studies can be regarded amongst the first of their kind in the then emerging fields of biochemical and molecular epidemiology. Subsequently, after the molecular genetics of *CYP2D6* emerged (Gonzalez *et al.*, 1988), many investigators have surveyed the frequency of various *CYP2D6* alleles in lung cancer cases and controls. Not all have found a positive result and the issue of the role of CYP2D6 in lung cancer has remained highly controversial in recent years. The first independent study to carry out debrisoquine phenotyping in lung cancer was the study of Roots *et al.* (1988), who investigated 270 cases and 270 controls and found a reduced incidence (7.0% versus 11.1%) of PMs in the cases, which was not statistically significant ($P = 0.067$). Using a PCR-based assay, Wolf *et al.* (1992) found no difference between the proportion of PMs in 361 lung cancer cases and a control group. In contrast, a study in Finland (Hirvonen *et al.*, 1993) found 1/106 cases and 7/122 controls ($P = 0.05$) to be PM using a restriction fragment length polymorphism (RFLP) non-PCR method. A study of 218 Norwegian cases and 289 controls, using a combination of PCR and RFLP analyses, found no significant differences between cases

and controls in *CYP2D6* allele frequency (Tefre *et al.*, 1994). A PCR-based study of the occurrence of *CYP2D6*1*, *CYP2D6*3* and *CYP2D6*4* alleles in a Slovene case-control study (200 cases, 107 controls) found a significant decrease in the number of genotypically PMs in the cases (2.5%) compared with controls (6.5%), consistent with the original phenotyping studies. Underlining the importance of cell type, a French study (Stucker *et al.*, 1995) found in 301 cases and 310 controls a significantly higher number of genotypic PMs in adenocarcinoma of the lung. In a study looking at the interaction of *CYP2D6* genotype and tobacco exposure, Bouchardy *et al.* (1996) found in 128 cases and 157 controls that *CYP2D6* was a risk factor only amongst heavy smokers. One of the minor controversies in the field has surrounded the role of the *CYP2D6*9* allele, associated with decreased but not absent activity. Originally, in 89 Spanish cases and 98 controls, Agúndez *et al.* (1994) reported a sixfold increase in the *CYP2D6*9* allele in the cases. Subsequent studies in France (249 cases and 265 controls, Legrand *et al.*, 1996) and the USA (98 incident cases and 110 controls, Shaw *et al.*, 1997) have failed to reproduce this finding. The largest case-control study to date has been a cooperative effort between Los Angeles and Newcastle, UK. These investigators recruited 341 incident cases and 710 population controls of both Caucasian and African-American origin. *CYP2D6*1*, *CYP2D6*3*, *CYP2D6*4*, *CYP2D6*5* and *CYP2D6*16* alleles were determined in each subject (London *et al.*, 1997). This study did not confirm the association between CYP2D6 genotype and lung cancer, but did make a new and interesting finding: when the *CYP2D6*2X2* allele (two copies of the active gene on one chromosome, without an inactivating allele on the other) was determined in cases and controls, a significant odds ratio of 3.61 (95% C.I. 1.08–11.7) was found for these genotypic ultra-rapid metabolizers (UM), compared with subjects with inactivating alleles. In summary, the epidemiological data, both metabolic and molecular, are inconsistent. Part of the problem is thought to be biases which are not corrected for by the investigators, together with laboratory testing of insufficient power to avoid misclassification bias. However, there are some mechanistic data which support a role for *CYP2D6* in lung, and perhaps other, cancers. The tobacco-specific nitrosamine 4-(methylnitrosamino)-1-(3-pyridyl)-1-butanone, known as NNK, is found in mainstream cigarette smoke at between 0.02 and 0.8 μg per cigarette (IARC, 1985). NNK has multiple metabolites, but it is the pathway that leads to DNA adducts which is of greatest interest **(Figure 6)**. Crespi *et al.* (1991) showed that heterologously expressed *CYP2D6* cDNA in a human lymphoblastoid cell line could activate NNK, although other isozymes such as CYP2A6, CYP2E1 and CYP1A2 are also involved. This provides a plausibility to the epidemiological question regarding whether or not *CYP2D6* genotypes are associate with lung cancer. The use of

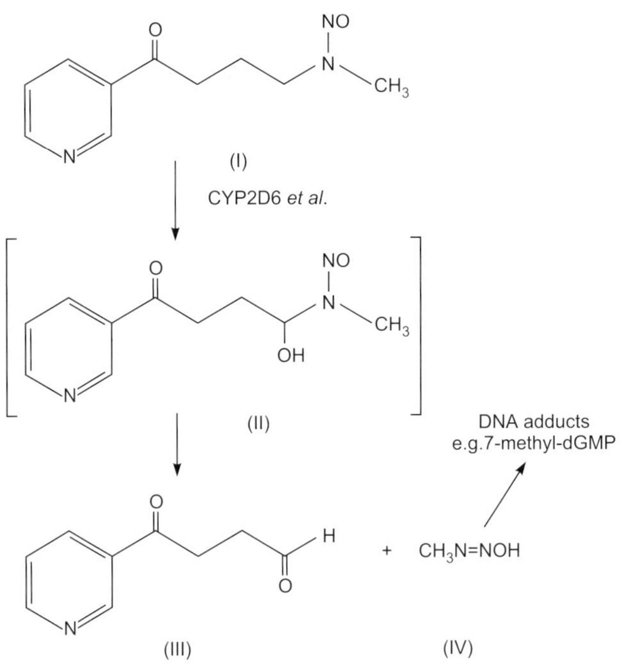

Figure 6 Activation of NNK (I) by CYP2D6 and other CYP isozymes forming the α-hydroxy intermediate (II). Decomposition leads to an aldehyde (III) and the proximate mutagen diazomethane (IV).

biomarkers such as carcinogen–DNA and carcinogen–protein adducts is commonly used to attempt to evaluate the exposure of individuals to chemical mutagens and carcinogens. One popular area has been the determination of 4-aminobiphenyl–haemoglobin adducts by tandem mass spectrometry. Weston *et al.* (1991) showed that there was no relationship between this type of adduct and debrisoquine metabolism. However, the same laboratory has demonstrated that the adduct formed by NNK and other *N*-nitrosamines, 7-methyl-2′-deoxyguanosine-3′-monophosphate (7-methyl-dGMP), was associated with *CYP2D6* genotype, especially in persons with low serum cotinine (primary metabolite of nicotine, often employed as a marker of nicotine exposure) concentrations. One of the interpretations of these data is that the adducts arise from a non-tobacco source. Nevertheless, the authors concluded that 'genetic polymorphisms are predictive of carcinogen–DNA adduct levels and would thus be predictive of an individual's lifetime response to carcinogen exposure'. It seems that there exist strong *a priori* reasons for believing in a role for CYP2D6 in lung cancer and that what are required are better designed and controlled epidemiological studies.

The toxicological significance of CYP2D6 can be summarized as follows:

1. The polymorphism is important in understanding the origins of inappropriate plasma levels of 85 drugs. This can lead to both over-response, including excess-

ive pharmacological response and alternative toxic responses, and under-response. There is a 200-fold variation in metabolic capacity in the population, largely due to multiallelism at the *CYP2D6* locus. At least 24 alleles can now be detected by PCR.

2. The polymorphism may have important consequences for the functioning of the central nervous system. The brain amine tryptamine is a substrate for CYP2D6. Dietary substances, especially alkaloids from plants, whose candidature as CYP2D6 substrates can now be determined using a simple set of rules, may have long-term consequences for PMs who are unable to metabolize them. Neither these consequences nor the full range of CYP2D6 substrates from the environment are yet appreciated, but we strongly suspect that our knowledge base is currently very limited.

3. The CYP2D6 polymorphism is certainly important in the toxicity of the neurotoxin MPTP and there is evidence that it may have a role in idiopathic Parkinson's disease. Because the environmental causative agent(s) are not yet known, the full potential of this neurotoxin-metabolizing enzyme has yet to emerge.

4. The CYP2D6 polymorphism has a role in individual risk of lung cancer, perhaps from smoking or some other environmental cause. Both epidemiological studies and mechanistic investigations support this contention.

5. There is likely to exist a number of other gene–environment scenarios where CYP2D6 will play some role in determining individual susceptibility to disease. As we learn that more and more diseases are neither purely genetic nor environmental in origin, but are due to a toxic environmental insult on the cell or the genome, then where chemicals of a basic nature, such as dietary alkaloids, are involved, CYP2D6, this highly polymorphic human gene, will surely be a candidate in the disease diathesis.

The CYP2C19 polymorphism

This was the second of the CYP polymorphisms to be uncovered. As with the CYP2D6 polymorphism (see Idle, 1988), its discovery arose from a chance observation in a single human volunteer taking part in a metabolic study (Küpfer *et al.*, 1979). Küpfer and his colleagues in Nashville, USA, were concerned with the stereoselective hydroxylation of the anticonvulsant drug mephenytoin. Using pseudoracemic mephenytoin, with differentially radiolabelled enantiomers, they were monitoring, in a panel of volunteers, the metabolic pathways of (*R*)- and (*S*)-mephenytoin, as shown in **Figure 7**. Investigation of the family of a single volunteer who had complained of excessive sedation led to the discovery of the (*S*)-mephenytoin 4′-hydroxylation polymorphism (Küpfer *et al.*, 1979). A full account of the background to this polymorphism can be found in Wilkinson *et al.* (1992). The (*R*)-enantiomer appears not to undergo

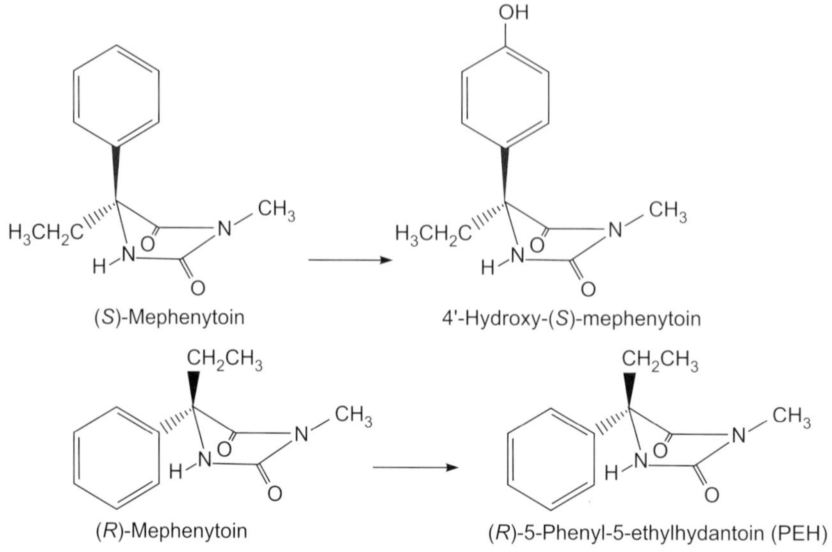

Figure 7 Enantioselective metabolism of mephenytoin. (S)-Mephenytoin is 4'-hydroxylated by polymorphic CYP2C19 and (R)-mephenytoin is not a CYP2C19 substrate and undergoes N-demethylation.

4'-hydroxylation by the same enzyme which metabolizes the (S)-enantiomer, preferring to be metabolized by N-demethylation to (R)-5-phenyl-5-ethylhydantoin (see Wilkinson *et al.*, 1992; **Figure 7**). The biochemical basis of this polymorphism was found to reside in CYP2C19 (Wrighton *et al.*, 1993; Goldstein *et al.*, 1994). Two separate inactivating alleles give rise to the PM phenotype, which is found in 2–5% of Caucasians and 13–23% of Orientals (see Wilkinson *et al.*, 1992). The most common variant allele (*CYP2C19m1*, now called *CYP2C19*2*, Daly *et al.*, 1996) is a G to A substitution in exon 5 causing aberrant splicing (de Morais *et al.*, 1994a) and comprises 75–85% of variant alleles in Caucasians and Orientals. A second variant allele (*CYP2C19m2*, now called *CYP2C19*3*, Daly *et al.*, 1996) arises from a G to A mutation in exon 4 which causes a premature stop codon and a truncated protein (de Morais *et al.*, 1994b). This allele is extremely rare in Caucasians but accounts for the remaining 20% of variant alleles in Orientals. The allele conferring the EM phenotype is now known as *CYP2C19*1* and no longer as 'wild-type', a phrase which is now discouraged (Daly *et al.*, 1996). The three alleles *CYP2C19*1*, *CYP2C19*2* and *CYP2C19*3* can all be detected by simple PCR methodology (de Morais *et al.*, 1994a,b). Several other minor alleles have now been detected (J. Goldstein, personal communication).

The range of substrates for the CYP2C19 polymorphism is by no means as long as that for the CYP2D6 polymorphism, although 30 years ago, when hydantoin and barbiturate drugs were more popular in therapeutics, the list would have been more extensive. Nevertheless, there are a number of historical and commonly used drugs which are metabolized by the polymorphic CYP2C19 isozyme and therefore subject to polymorph-

ism, particularly in Oriental populations. **Figure 8** gives the chemical structures of the known CYP2C19 substrates and, where the compound possesses an unsaturated ring and/or a chiral centre, the three-dimensional structure has been drawn to give some semblance of the stereoselective nature of the CYP2C19-mediated oxidation. The minor metabolite of (S)-mephenytoin, resulting from N-demethylation, (S)-PEH, also known as nirvanol (another anticonvulsant like mephenytoin), itself undergoes 4'-hydroxylation by CYP2C19. Likewise, the two barbiturates (R)-mephobarbitone and (R)-hexobarbitone undergo 4'-and 3'-hydroxylation, respectively, by CYP2C19. Interestingly, although the popular anticonvulsant drug phenytoin is not a CYP2C19 substrate, its N^1-methyl analogue is. This compound, whilst not chiral, is however pro-chiral, meaning that the two apparently identical phenyl rings (see **Figure 8**) can be hydroxylated to produce chiral 4'-hydroxy metabolites. Hydroxylation of only the ring leading to (R)-4-hydroxy-N^1-methylphenytoin, and not the (S)-enantiomeric metabolite, is performed by CYP2C19. Thus, hydroxylation of the (S)-enantiomers of hydantoins and the (R)-enantiomers of barbiturates are the reactions of CYP2C19. The reader will note from a comparison of the structures of (S)-mephenytoin **(Figure 7)** and the (R)-enantiomers of the barbiturates **(Figure 8)** that the moiety which is hydroxylated by CYP2C19 has the same orientation in space with respect to the N-methyl group within the ring. The nomenclature of absolute configuration is such that, when a carbonyl group is added to a five-membered hydantoin ring to yield a six-membered barbiturate ring, the absolute configuration is reversed; therefore, (S)-mephenytoin, on addition of a carbonyl group, becomes (R)-mephobarbitone.

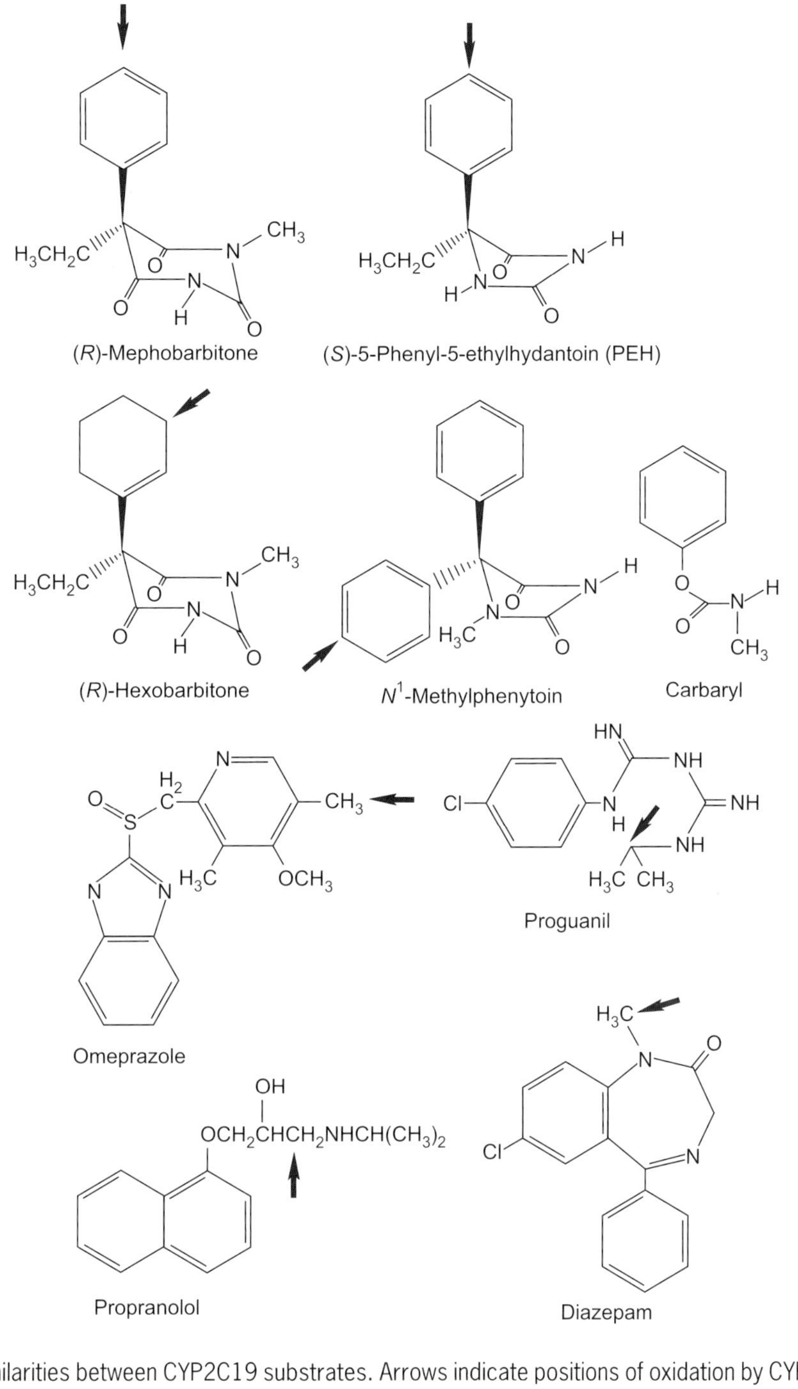

Figure 8 Structural similarities between CYP2C19 substrates. Arrows indicate positions of oxidation by CYP2C19.

Carbaryl is a so-called contact insecticide. It found domestic use for the eradication of cockroaches, for example. Its chemical structure **(Figure 8)** resembles a fragment of a molecule of mephenytoin or mephobarbitone. Although we are unaware of any published literature on the metabolism of carbaryl by CYP2C19, the Nashville group did study a patient who showed marked toxicity on exposure to trivial amounts of carbaryl in the home and who was found to be a poor metabolizer of mephenytoin (A. Küpfer, personal communication).

Figure 8 also depicts the structures of four non-hydantoin/non-barbiturate substrates of CYP2C19. A more extensive discourse can be found in Wilkinson *et al.* (1992). It is important to point out that the 5'-methyl hydroxylation of omeprazole is mediated by CYP2C19. Omeprazole, a proton-pump inhibitor used to treat gastric and duodenal ulcers and related conditions exacerbated by gastric acid secretion, is currently the world's top selling prescription drug. For the same dose, PMs receive over 10 times the systemic dose as EMs (see Andersson *et al.*, 1992). Proguanil is an antimalarial drug which is metabolized by CYP2C19 to an active metabolite known as cycloguanil, a ring-closed metabolite presumably formed via hydroxylation in the ω-1 position of the biguanide side-chain, as shown by the arrow in **Figure 8**. Propranolol, the archetypal non-selective β-blocker, is mainly metabolized by CYP2D6. However, a minor metabolite is 1-naphthoxylactic acid, which is produced by CYP2C19 presumably by N-dealkylation as shown in **Figure 8**. Finally, the once popular benzodiazepine hypnotic and tranquillizer diazepam (Valium) has many of the characteristics of a CYP2C19 substrate, but also many anomalies (see Wilkinson *et al.*, 1992). Its N-demethylation, plus the further metabolism of the desmethyl compound, both appear to be mediated by CYP2C19.

In summary, therefore, a handful of commonly used drugs, especially omeprazole, are metabolized by CYP2C19. The insecticide carbaryl may also be a substrate. CYP2C19 does not seem to play a role in the

metabolic activation of any known carcinogens or participate in the detoxication of harmful chemicals. There are three known alleles which can be detected by PCR and the global heterogeneity in these alleles can explain interethnic differences in the metabolism and disposition of omeprazole. The toxicological significance of this polymorphism has yet to emerge.

The CYP2C9 polymorphism

This polymorphism is a true example of 'reverse pharmacogenetics'. Unlike the CYP2D6 and CYP2C19 polymorphisms, which were discovered on the basis of an unexpected reaction (phenotype) in a single subject, CYP2C9 variability first emerged at the DNA (genotype) level. There was one early clue with the pharmacokinetics of the hypoglycaemic sulphonylurea drug tolbutamide **(Figure 9)**, whose methyl hydroxylation is

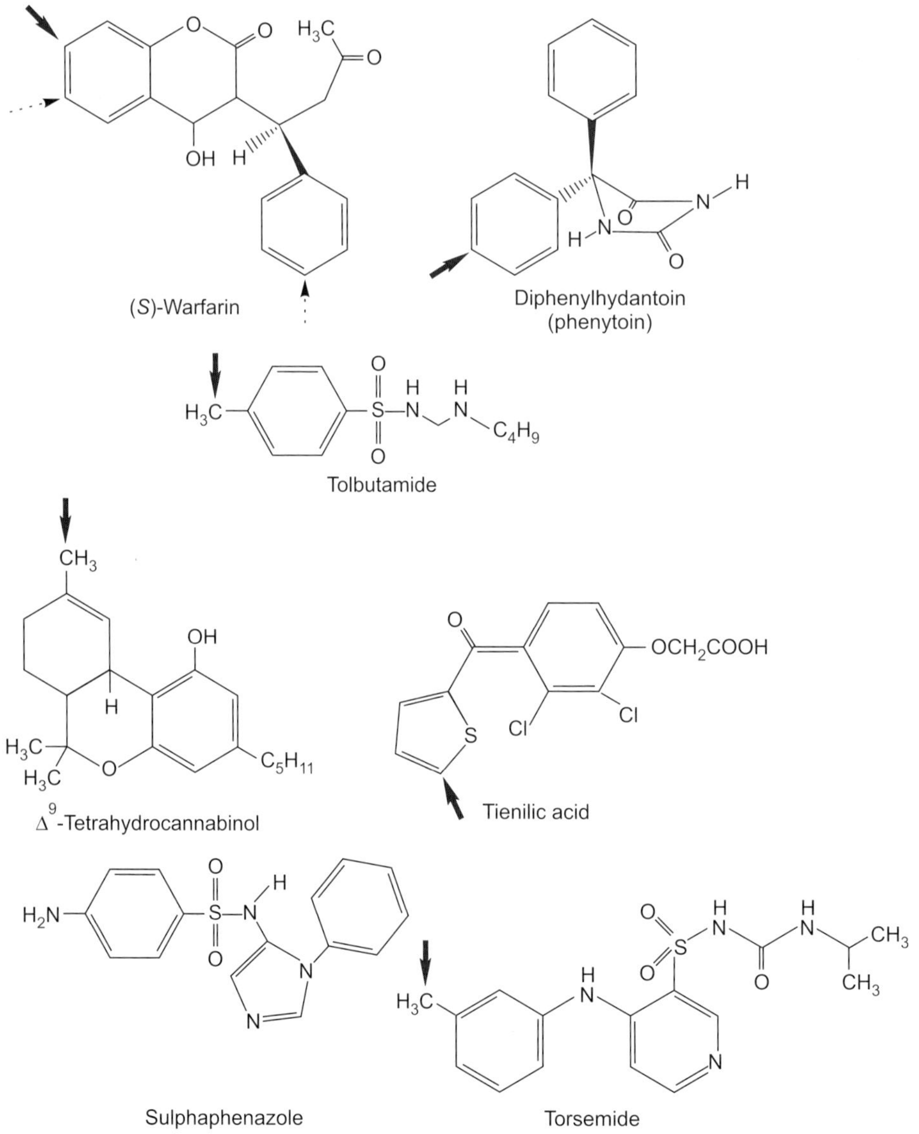

Figure 9 Chemical structures of CYP2C9 substrates. Arrows indicate positions of oxidation by CYP2C9.

the rate-limiting step in the drug's elimination from plasma. In 1979, Scott and Poffenbarger suggested that the first-order elimination rate constant (K_{el}) for tolbutamide was trimodally distributed in the population. Unfortunately, these observations were never confirmed. Once it was established that tolbutamide was not metabolized by CYP2C19 (see Wilkinson et al., 1992), but rather by a closely related isozyme, there was a suspicion that this new isozyme might display genetic polymorphism. The answers were to come from molecular biology. The major contribution to the characterization of the CYP2C subfamily genes **(Table 3)** has come from three laboratories in the USA, those of Goldstein, Guengerich and Gonzalez, all of which cloned and sequenced *CYP2C9* and related cDNAs (see Goldstein and de Morais (1994) for a review).

Because of the number *of CYP2C9* cDNAs which had been cloned in several laboratories, it was not long before variant alleles emerged, although their function was only speculative. One variant cDNA, which bore a Arg144Cys substitution (substitution of cysteine for arginine in the 144th amino acid of the peptide) was expressed heterologously in HepG2 cells and tested for its ability to hydroxylate (*S*)-warfarin **(Figure 9)** by Rettie et al. (1994). The estimated V_{max}/K_m ratio for (*S*)-warfarin 7-hydroxylation (the principal metabolic pathway for this enantiomer, see **Figure 9**) was reduced 5.6-fold for the Cys-144 allele compared with the Arg-144 allele (referred to as *CYP2C9*2* and *CYP2C9*1*, respectively, Daly et al., 1996). A second *CYP2C9* polymorphism involving an isoleucine to leucine conversion at position 359 (Ile359-Leu) has been studied in some detail with respect to tolbutamide, phenytoin and (*S*)-warfarin hydroxylations **(Figure 9)**. The isoleucine variant is considered to be part of *CYP2C9*1*, whilst the leucine variant is named *CYP2C9*3* (Daly et al., 1996). At present therefore, we know of one allele of high activity (*CYP2C9*1*) and two which effect reduced turnover of (*S*)-warfarin 7-hydroxylation (*CYP2C9*2* and *CYP2C9*3*). These alleles are readily detected by PCR methods.

Evidence for a functional CYP2C9 polymorphism comes from the study of patients administered warfarin by mouth as an anticoagulant. Pharmaceutical warfarin is racemic, but it is generally considered that the (*S*)-enantiomer is about three times more potent than the (*R*)-enantiomer, despite its higher plasma clearance (Choonara et al., 1986). In a study in Newcastle, UK (Furuya et al., 1995), DNA from 94 patients attending anticoagulation clinics in the city in two consecutive weeks was investigated for the presence of the *CYP2C9*1* and *CYP2C9*2* alleles by PCR. The presence of the *CYP2C9*3* allele was not determined. A 20% lower weekly warfarin dose was required for those patients who had one *CYP2C9*2* allele, compared with *CYP2C9*1* homozygotes. No patient was homozygous for the *CYP2C9*2* allele. This study gave the first signs that CYP2C9 polymorphism might be important for

dose adjustment with warfarin, a drug normally requiring dose titration and repeated determinations of blood clotting parameters.

It appears that the *CYP2C9*3* allele may also be important in avoiding warfarin toxicity, which can be fatal if unrecognized. Steward et al. (1997) reported a single 66-year-old male patient who was administered 10 mg of racemic warfarin in hospital after a myocardial infarction, followed by a further 10 mg the following day. Instead of a target value of 2–3, the patient's International Normalised Ratio (INR), the common and standardized measurement of retardation of blood clotting, reached a maximum value of 9.7, requiring reversal of anticoagulation with vitamin K. In order to reach a target INR of 2–3, the dose of warfarin was reduced to 1 mg every second day, one-twentieth of the original dose. In addition, the patient's plasma warfarin (*S*)/(*R*)-enantiomer ratio was determined. Because (*S*)-warfarin is metabolized faster than (*R*)-warfarin, the normal values for this ratio are 0.3–0.9, after reaching steady state on 4–8 mg of warfarin per day (Steward et al., 1997). The toxic patient, even after 5 months of therapy on only 0.5 mg per day, had a plasma warfarin (*S*)/(*R*)-enantiomer ratio of 3.9, demonstrating that he had a gross impairment in (*S*)-warfarin metabolism. The patient was genotyped as a *CYP2C9*3/CYP2C9*3* homozygote using DNA sequencing, the low-activity Leu-359 variant. Clearly, such PCR-based testing is of value in avoiding near-fatal or fatal warfarin toxicity and is in routine clinical use in this context in the authors' laboratory in Trondheim.

Other drugs which are CYP2C9 substrates **(Figure 9)** include the two diuretic agents tienilic acid and torsemide, the former of which caused a number of fatal cases of autoimmune hepatitis. Whether or not these patients were one particular genotype is not known. Δ^9-Tetrahydrocannabinol (THC) is the principal psychoactive component of hashish and marijuana and the synthetic material is now available in several countries as an appetite stimulant, for example in AIDS patients, and as an antiemetic drug for cancer patients. Unpublished reports of HPLC analyses of urine from marijuana users in Switzerland contain the observation that about one in ten samples has a 'missing' cannabinoid metabolite. This must surely be due to the CYP2C9 polymorphism, since the principal component THC is a CYP2C9 substrate. Such genetic polymorphism may be important in modulating the effects of both prescribed and illicit use of cannabis derivatives.

One group of drugs is closely associated with CYP2C9 metabolism, the non-steroidal anti-inflammatory drugs (NSAIDs). The structures of some known CYP2C9 substrates are shown in **Figure 10**. Both adverse drug reactions and drug–drug interactions are commonplace with this group of drugs. Research is urgently required to evaluate the importance or otherwise of the common polymorphism in CYP2C9 on complications of therapy with NSAIDs.

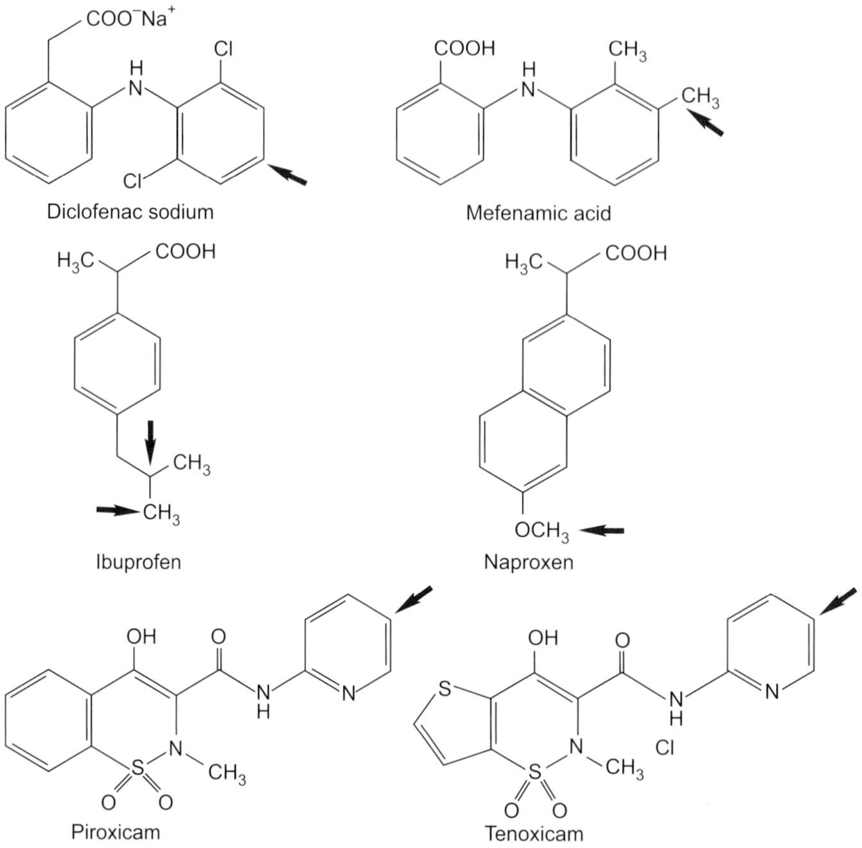

Figure 10 Chemical structures of some non-steroidal anti-inflammatory drugs which are CYP2C9 substrates. Arrows indicate positions of oxidation by CYP2C9.

In summary, CYP2C9 has at least three alleles, two of which are associated with impairment of metabolism. These alleles are detectable using PCR methodologies. Areas of toxicological significance for this polymorphism include anticoagulant therapy with oral warfarin, social and medical uses of cannabis products, together with the non-steroidal anti-inflammatory drugs. Because this polymorphism has only recently surfaced, the broader toxicological significance is not yet known but, because many of the substrates for CYP2C9 have a narrow margin of safety (phenytoin, warfarin and NSAIDs), it is likely that many examples of clinical relevance will emerge.

The CYP2A6 polymorphism

The classical substrate for CYP2A6 is the ubiquitous environmental contaminant coumarin (2*H*-1-benzo-pyran-2-one, **Figure 11**). This pleasantly sweet-smelling plant and fungal metabolite is used extensively as an additive in perfumes, detergents, hair products, cosmetics and toothpaste, for example (Egan *et al.*, 1990). It is also present in many green vegetables, making exposure to human populations unavoidable. It has been used as a pharmaceutical agent, particularly in lymphoedema,

at doses of 400–800 mg per day (Mortimer, 1997), 100–1000 times the background environmental exposure (Hadidi *et al.*, 1998). Coumarin is metabolized in humans by 7-hydroxylation **(Figure 11)**, which accounts for 60–95% of the dose excreted in urine (Cholerton *et al.*, 1992; Rautio *et al.*, 1992) and this reaction is mediated purely by CYP2A6. In a panel of monoclonal antibodies against human P450s, only anti-CYP2A6 inhibited coumarin 7-hydroxylation, and then remarkably with 100% inhibition (H. Gelboin, personal communication). This confirms earlier work using heterologously expressed human P450 cDNAs which showed that CYP2A6 (then called CYP2A3) is the only cytochrome performing this reaction (Yamano *et al.*, 1990). Coumarin is hepatotoxic to rats (see Lake, 1984). The covalent binding of coumarin metabolites to cellular macromolecules appears to be a function of the 3-hydroxylation pathway **(Figure 11)**, the dominant pathway in the rat, but generally considered to be of trivial importance in humans (Lake *et al.*, 1992). The cloning and characterization of a battery of human *CYP2A* genes and pseudogenes on chromosome 19 (Fernandez-Salguero *et al.*, 1995b) have permitted new experimental strategies for the study of coumarin metabolism and its variability. Two variant alleles have been described (Fernandez-Salguero *et al.*,

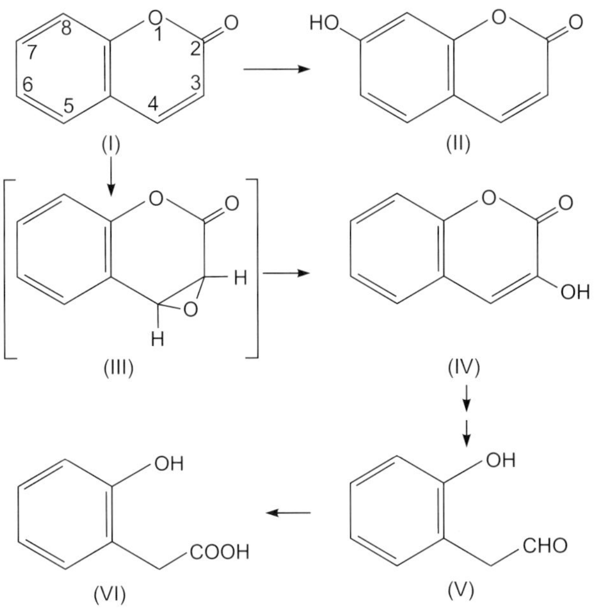

Figure 11 Alternative pathways of coumarin metabolism. Coumarin (I) is hydroxylated predominantly in humans by CYP2A6 to 7-hydroxycoumarin (II). Alternatively, and in the rat, coumarin is hydroxylated by a non-CYP2A6 isozyme to 3-hydroxycoumarin (IV) [possibly via an unstable 3,4-epoxide (III)] and then ring opening occurs to yield the proximate hepatotoxin 2-hydroxyphenylacetaldehyde (V) and the urinary excretion product 2-hydroxyphenylacetic acid (VI).

1995a) which abolish CYP2A6 activity. These were termed v1 and v2, but are now correctly referred to as *CYP2A6*2* and *CYP2A6*3*, respectively (Daly *et al.*, 1996), with the active allele called *CYP2A6*1*. These alleles can be detected using a nested PCR strategy in which the entire *CYP2A6* gene is first amplified using long-PCR, this to avoid priming sequences from the highly homologous *CYP2A* genes and pseudogenes, such as *CYP2A7* and *CYP2A13*. The *CYP2A6*2* allele causes a single amino acid substitution (Leu160His) in the peptide, abolishing catalytic activity.

The effect of this mutation has been studied in a single family in which it was identified by metabolic studies, after the administration of 2 mg of coumarin by mouth, that there existed a subject with no detectable coumarin 7-hydroxylation (Hadidi *et al.*, 1997). Subsequently, this individual was found to be a *CYP2A6*2* homozygote and had therefore inherited the ability to make only the inactive peptide containing the His-160 residue. We wished to know whether or not this metabolic 'block' altered the overall pattern of coumarin metabolism in this subject. Using a selected-ion monitoring gas chromatographic–mass spectrometric (SIM-GCMS) method we had developed, we screened the urine of this subject for the alternative potential metabolites, 2-hydroxyphenylacetic acid (2OHPAA, see **Figure 11**), 2-hydroxyphenylethanol (a potential reduced metabolite of the toxic intermediate 2-hydroxyphenylacetaldehyde, **Figure 11**),

coumaranone (ring-closed 2OHPAA) and 4-hydroxycoumarin. This subject, remarkably, excreted 50% of the administered dose as 2OHPAA, showing that coumarin had been metabolized down the putative hepatotoxic pathway thought to be unimportant in humans, but the key to hepatotoxicity in the rat. It appears, therefore, that the risk assessment for exposure of humans to this rat hepatotoxin, based upon a qualitative difference in coumarin metabolism between rat and human, may not be valid. It appears that the CYP2A6 polymorphism may switch the pattern of metabolism away from detoxication to toxicity in a proportion of individuals who are homozygous for the variant alleles. We next asked the question of how frequent aberrant coumarin metabolism was in the population; 103 Jordanian volunteers were administered an oral dose of 2 mg of coumarin and 0–8 h urine samples were analysed for coumarin metabolites by SIM-GCMS. Unfortunately, no DNA was available from this population but, nevertheless, 3/103 persons excreted 43–70% of the dose as 2OHPAA and statistical analysis of the population suggested the presence of two distinct phenotypes, one with low 7-hydroxylation/high 3-hydroxylation (8/103, 7.8%) and the other with high 7-hydroxylation/low 3-hydroxylation (95/103, 92.2%) (Hadidi *et al.*, 1998). Values for the subject from the previous family study (Hadidi *et al.*, 1997) fell in the middle of the values for the eight low 7-hydroxylators, confirming that this phenotype is not uncommon. In summary, there may exist a coumarin hepatotoxicity hypersusceptible subgroup in the population, identifiable by PCR-based methods which determine *CYP2A6* genotype. It is not prudent to make human risk assessments based upon the metabolic behaviour of the majority of the population without taking account of genetic susceptibility.

Other known substrates of CYP2A6 are shown in **Figure 12**. Thiotepa, an anticancer cytostatic drug, undergoes oxidative desulphuration in human liver microsomes catalysed by CYP2A6 (Höfer and Idle, 1996). This may have important consequences for the outcome of chemotherapy with thiotepa. Probably the most important CYP2A6 substrate discovered to date is nicotine. The metabolism of (*S*)-nicotine is almost totally performed by CYP2A6 (Messina *et al.*, 1997). The polymorphism of CYP2A6 has enormous implications for both the pharmacology and toxicology of nicotine. Clearly, slow metabolizers of nicotine would be less able to tolerate doses of nicotine. This might be one factor contributing to smoking behaviour. Since nicotine and the tobacco-specific nitrosamine NNK (see **Figure 6**) are both, to a greater or lesser extent, metabolized by CYP2A6, then the CYP2A6 poor metabolizer might consume less nicotine by using less tobacco product. He/she would then be consuming less NNK and, as a bonus, have an enzyme system less capable of activating NNK to DNA methylating species. Apart from NNK, the other procarcinogens aflatoxin B$_1$,

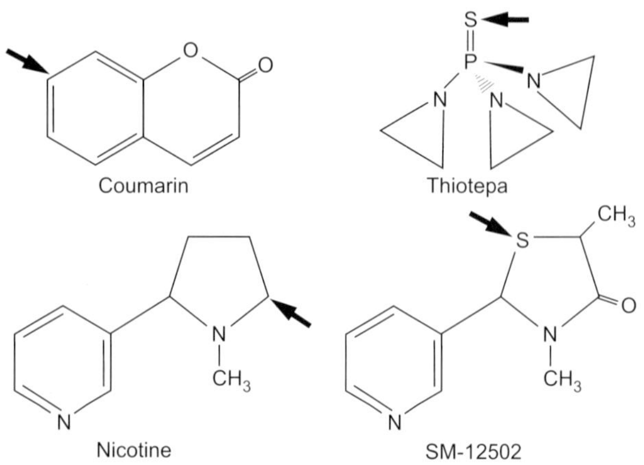

Figure 12 Chemical structures of some CYP2A6 substrates. Arrows indicate positions of oxidation by CYP2A6.

hexamethylphosphoramide and nitrosodimethylamine are all metabolized by CYP2A6 (see Messina et al., 1997). This new polymorphism, detectable both by molecular methods (Fernandez-Salguero et al., 1995) or by a coumarin test (Hadidi et al., 1997, 1998), might have profound implications for chemically induced cancers. As with CYP2D6, carefully designed and executed molecular epidemiological studies are urgently required.

Flavin-containing monooxygenase (FMO) polymorphisms

The flavin-containing monooxygenases (FMOs) are a second family of monooxygenases, unrelated to the cytochromes P450 (CYPs), found in the endoplasmic reticulum of cells. These enzymes catalyse largely the N-,P-,S- and Se-oxidation of a wide range of dietary compounds, drugs and pesticides which contain a polarizable electron-rich soft nucleophilic centre as the site of oxygenation (Ziegler, 1993). Biochemically, it is possible to distinguish between oxidations mediated in vitro by FMOs or CYPs owing to the differential heat inactivation of FMO activity, in the absence of NADPH, and the inhibition of CYP activity by carbon monoxide and N-benzylimidazole (Grothusen et al., 1996). Despite the plethora of probe drugs for the evaluation of CYP activity in vivo, there have been few compounds suitable for assessing FMO activity in vivo, including in animals. Recently, it has been proposed (Damani and Nnane, 1996) that ethyl methyl sulphide and trimethylamine might be suitable for this purpose, at least in rats.

Like CYPs, FMOs are also a multigene family of enzymes which display pronounced species, gender and tissue specificity and which comprise (at present) five principal subfamilies, FMO1, FMO2, FMO3, FMO4 and FMO5 (Lawton et al., 1994). In humans, each FMO gene displays a characteristic developmental and organ-specific pattern of expression (Phillips et al., 1995; Dolphin et al., 1996). FMO1 is expressed only in the adult human kidney, but in foetal liver and kidney. Other species, such as pig and rabbit, have abundant hepatic FMO1 expression. FMO2 is expressed only in lung. FMO3 is expressed mainly in the liver where FMO3 is the predominant hepatic isozyme, but not in all persons (see below). FMO4 seems to be expressed in both foetus and adult in only small amounts in the liver, lung and kidney. FMO5 is expressed in adult liver and lung. In mouse liver the situation is somewhat different. Murine hepatic FMO1 expression is 2–3 times higher in female mice than in males. FMO3 expression is similar to FMO1 expression in females but undetectable in male mice. FMO5 expression is similar in both sexes. FMO2 and FMO4 transcription was not detected in either male or female mouse liver. The gender differences were identical in CD-1, Swiss–Webster, C57BL/6 and DBA/2 strains (Falls et al., 1995).

One organ which has attracted special interest regarding FMO activity is the brain. In 1988, Chiba et al. demonstrated that the Parkinson's disease-inducing neurotoxin 1-methyl-4-phenyl-1,2,3,6-tetrahydropyridine (MPTP; see **Figure 5**) is detoxicated in mouse liver 32 times faster by FMO than by CYP activities. Using the oxidation of NADPH in the presence of the FMO model substrates N, N-dimethylaniline and methimazole and the antidepressant drugs imipramine and fluoxetine, Bhamre et al. (1993) showed activity for all four substrates in rat brain microsomes. N-Oxidation of imipramine was inhibited by 43% by an antibody raised against rabbit lung FMO. These authors concluded that the FMO-mediated metabolism of antidepressant drugs in the brain was 'of profound pharmacological significance'. The same authors then showed that both human brain microsomes and an FMO purified from human brain could form imipramine N-oxide and that the co-oxidation of NADPH gave an erroneously high estimates of FMO activity compared with the rates of formation of imipramine N-oxide (Bhagwat et al., 1996). The FMO protein was located predominantly in the neuronal cell bodies of magnocellular reticular nuclei, colliculi and substantia nigra (Bhamre et al., 1995). Parallel investigations in Japan complement the Indian studies. Kawaji et al. (1994, 1995, 1997) showed that microsomes from rat brain, particularly the olfactory bulb, contain FMO-mediated benzydamine N-oxidation activity which is partially inhibited (30%) by rabbit anti-rat FMO antiserum, that partially purified rat brain FMO could N-oxidize the neurotoxins MPTP, 1,2,3,4-tetrahydroisoquinoline (TIQ) and N-methyl-TIQ (NMTIQ) and that the FMO isozyme present in the brains of rat, mouse, hamster and guinea pig is different from that from rabbit brain and likely not to be FMO4. However, using a PCR technique, Blake et al. (1996) amplified a cDNA fragment of FMO4 from total rabbit brain mRNA and concluded that this gene is the only

FMO gene expressed in rabbit brain and at low levels only. The role of FMO isoforms in the human brain in protecting against the neurotoxicity of MPTP and other neurotoxins remains unclear and whether or not polymorphisms of FMOs could be risk factors in conditions such as Parkinson's disease is unknown.

It is of interest to consider briefly the range of substrates for FMO and the degree of selectivity of these substrates for particular FMO isoforms, for this colours our view of the potential toxicological significance of genetic polymorphisms in the FMO gene family. The burden of experience with FMO-mediated metabolism has been gained *in vitro* and with preparations from laboratory animals. Many investigators have traditionally not sought to measure the product of the drug meta

bolic reaction, but rather the co-oxidation of NADPH. This, as was discussed earlier, can lead to erroneously high turnover numbers. The range of substrates used in such an *in vitro* study is typically that employed by Itoh *et al.* (1997). A cloned mouse *FMO1* cDNA expressed in yeast was shown to carry out thiobenzamide *S*-oxidation and to oxidize NADPH during the *N*-oxidation of *N*, *N*-dimethylaniline, *N,N*-dimethylhydrazine, imipramine, nicotine, trimethylamine and TIQ (see above), as well as the *S*-oxidation of chlorpromazine, thioacetamide and thiourea. The chemical structures of typical FMO substrates are given in **Figure 13**. Oxidation occurs at either the nitrogen or the sulphur centre in all these substrates. There is considerable substrate specificity displayed by the FMO isozymes. This is ably illustrated by the example of the *S*-oxidation of the nephrotoxic *S*-alkylcysteine conjugates, as shown in **Figure 14**. Ripp *et al.* (1997) have shown that cDNA-expressed rabbit FMO isoforms each displays a distinct pattern of *S*-oxidation of these closely related cysteine derivatives.

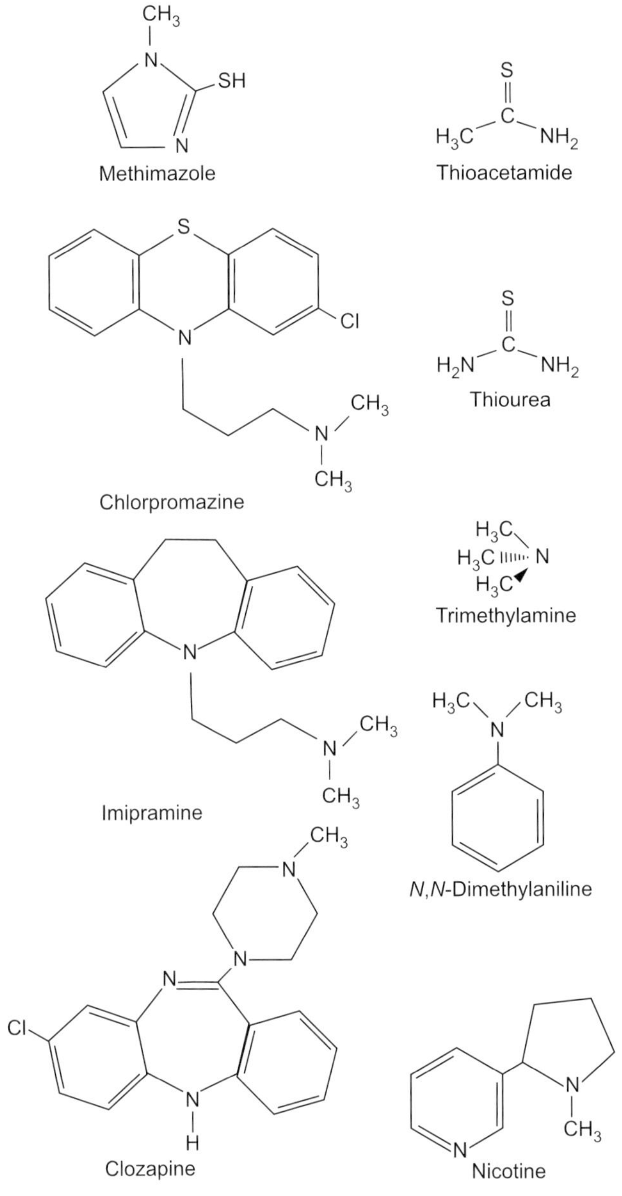

Figure 13 Chemical structures of some flavin-containing monooxygenase (FMO) substrates. Oxidation occurs at nitrogen or sulphur centres.

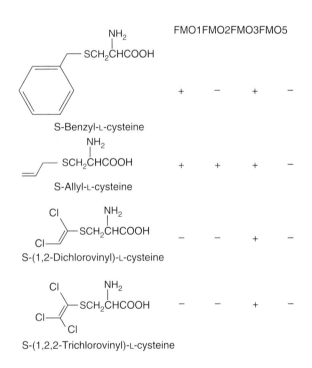

Figure 14 Differential metabolism of related *S*-alkylcysteines by flavin-containing monooxygenase (FMO) isozymes.

The FMO3 polymorphism

Of the human FMO isozymes, FMO3 is the only one so far known to display genetic polymorphism, but the phenomenon is of considerable interest because it underlies an inborn error of metabolism known as the 'fish-odour syndrome'. The story began with fishy smelling hens' eggs. It had been observed (Pearson *et al.*, 1978) that a diet of 10% rapeseed meal fed to laying hens (*Gallus domesticus*) exacerbated fatty liver-haemorrhagic syndrome (FLHS), which was thought to be the underlying cause of the production of fishy smelling eggs by these hens. These investigators also noted that the rapeseed-fed hens developed thyroid hypertrophy which correlated with the trimethylamine content of the tainted eggs. They concluded that rapeseed meal goitrogens might be a secondary cause of trimethylamine-containing eggs. In addition, the hepatic trimethylamine oxidase activity was also reduced. These goitrogens comprise a group of chemicals known as glucosinolates, about 10 of the 100 known phytochemical examples of which are found in *Brassica* species, including *Brassica campestris*, the rapeseed plant (Stoewsand, 1995). Although not demonstrated to our knowledge, the inhibition of the metabolism in hen liver of malodorous and volatile trimethylamine (TMA) to its non-odorous N-oxide metabolite (TMAO) is surely effected by glucosinolates or their aglycone metabolites. One such glucosinolate, sinigrin (1-thio-β-D-glucopyronosyl-1-N-(sulphoxy)-3-butenimidate) produces many breakdown products, including dimethyl disulphide and allyl isothiocyanate. *S*-Methylcysteine sulphoxide is also present in large amounts in rapeseed and these or related compounds are almost certainly responsible for inhibition of TMA N-oxidation.

It soon became apparent that domestic fowl harboured constitutive variations in TMA metabolism to TMAO which were clearly genetic in origin. The TMA oxidase activity exhibited two phenotypes, 'low' and 'high' (normal). One-day-old chicks showed a sevenfold difference in enzyme activity between phenotypes, which increased to 26-fold at 22 days (Pearson and Butler, 1983). Learning of these studies in hens, Smith at St Mary's Hospital Medical School, London, made the intellectual jump from the chicken to man. He was aware that a very few cases of human subjects had been reported who excreted TMA in excessive amounts in their urine, breath and sweat and had been labelled as sufferers of a 'fish-odour syndrome' (Humbert *et al.*, 1970). He mused if this condition could be due to an inherited deficiency in TMA N-oxidation, as it was in hens. He bade one of us (J. R. I.) to set up an assay for TMA and TMAO in urine and from there the pharmacogenetics of FMO3 began, taking over 10 years to reach a satisfactory conclusion.

The St Mary's group first reported that fish-odour syndrome was an inborn error of TMA N-oxidation (Al-Waiz *et al.*, 1987a) with population-based studies (Al-Waiz *et al.*, 1987b) and investigations in families (Al-Waiz *et al.*, 1988). In a UK population of 169, two persons were found with partially reduced TMAO urinary excretion, but without the signs and symptoms of fish-odour syndrome. They fitted the criteria for heterozygosity, as determined by a challenge with oral TMA.HCl, equivalent to a dose of 600 mg of TMA (Al-Waiz *et al.*, 1989). It is possible to estimate that the prevalence of fish-odour syndrome in the UK might

therefore be about 35 persons per million population. This contrasts with a study in Jordan which detected 8/82 subjects who could fit the criteria for trimethylaminuria carriers and gives a calculated prevalence of the syndrome of about two persons per thousand population (Hadidi *et al.*, 1995). It was shown, using isotopically labelled TMA and TMAO, that oral TMA administration leads to almost quantitative urinary excretion of TMAO (Al-Waiz *et al.*, 1987c) but that, after administration of TMAO by mouth, the dose is first reduced to TMA, presumably in the gut, before being reoxidized to TMA prior to urinary excretion. This process was termed 'metabolic retroversion' (Al-Waiz *et al.*, 1987d). There occurred a sudden resurgence of interest in trimethylaminuria. Gut and Conney (1991) demonstrated that TMA N-oxidation was carried out by FMO, not a cytochrome P450. New methods were developed to detect simultaneously in urine TMA and TMAO, of particular interest being a proton NMR spectroscopic method which can analyse urine directly and detect new cases (Abeling *et al.*, 1995; Maschke *et al.*, 1997). Also of interest is the exacerbation of trimethylamine odours in women during menstruation (Zhang *et al.*, 1996) and that bacterial vaginosis, with its attendant fishy smelling vaginal discharge, is also related to a woman's ability to N-oxidize TMA (Sardas *et al.*, 1996).

Of the FMO isozymes, Dolphin *et al.* (1997a) identified FMO3 as the most likely candidate for the basis of fish-odour syndrome. These workers identified a single amino acid change (Pro153Leu), arising from a C $\rightarrow$ T transition in exon 4 of the *FMO3* gene, which completely abolishes TMA N-oxidation and which cosegregates with fish-odour syndrome in a family pedigree (Dolphin *et al.*, 1997b). It is therefore now possible to detect the disease and its carriers using a simple PCR method, although it is likely that other mutations in *FMO3* could also cause the condition.

Toxicological consequences of the FMO3 polymorphism

The fish-odour syndrome is in itself a distressing condition which can lead to clinical depression and even suicide (see Ayesh *et al.*, 1993, for an overview). There is evidence that the FMO3 polymorphism might play a role in organic disease causation. It appears that TMAO can promote the formation of disulphide bridges between cysteine or homocysteine residues (Brzezinski and Zundel, 1993). What endogenous function TMAO could serve is at present purely speculative. Although fish muscle is able to convert TMAO directly to dimethylamine (DMA) (Parkin and Hultin, 1982), the precursor of the chemical mutagen and carcinogen N-nitrosodimethylamine (NDMA), of greater interest is the dealkylation of TMA to DMA and formaldehyde in the human body. Presumably, persons with a reduced FMO3 capacity and therefore a higher TMA body burden could form greater amounts of toxic NDMA. In chemical studies it is possible to form NDMA directly from either TMA or TMAO by nitrosation with nitrite (Ohshima and Kawabata, 1978). To our knowledge, the hypothesis that FMO3 polymorphism may contribute to the risk of certain tumours has not been addressed. The availability of molecular tools for *FMO3* allele detection should make the task a straightforward one.

Dihydropyrimidine dehydrogenase (DPD) polymorphism

Dihydropyrimidine dehydrogenase (DPD) is the initial and rate-limiting enzyme in the catabolism of uracil and thymidine and the only pathway for the synthesis of *β*-alanine. The excretion of large amounts of uracil, thymine and 5-hydroxymethyluracil in the urine, consequent upon DPD deficiency, has become known as 'hereditary thymine-uraciluria' (Berger *et al.*, 1984). This condition is associated with developmental delay in affected children and sometimes even autism, convulsions or psychomotor retardation (see OMIM entry 274270; Online Mendelian Inheritance in Man, http://www.hgmp.mrc.ac.uk/omim/index.html).

DPD deficiency is also one of the clinically most important pharmacogenetic polymorphisms because of its role in precipitating severe toxicity in patients administered the anticancer drug 5-fluorouracil (5-FU). The clinical problem first emerged via a case report of a 27-year-old woman who suffered an unexpected severe reaction to 5-FU when given only a relatively small dose. Her symptoms included stomatitis, leucopaenia, thrombocytopaenia, alopecia, diarrhoea, fever, marked weight loss and cerebellar ataxia, with neurological symptoms which progressed to semicoma (Tuchman *et al.*, 1985). DPD deficiency is an autosomal recessive phenotype which can be determined from the DPD activity of peripheral lymphocytes (Johnson *et al.*, 1997a). The enzyme is predominantly hepatic and is localised exclusively in the cytosol (van Kuilenburg *et al.*, 1997). The expression levels of DPD in lymphocytes can be determined by Western immunoblotting methods which correlate well with the enzyme activity in those same cells determined using radiolabelled uracil and TLC separation of metabolites (Fernandez-Salguero *et al.*, 1995a). Lymphocytic DPD activity in the population shows considerable variation, even amongst persons unaffected by the deficiency, with an 8.4-fold variation in enzyme activity reported (McMurrough and McLeod, 1996). The molecular basis of the DPD deficiency has been elucidated (Meinsma *et al.*, 1995) and appears to be due to a loss of 165 nucleotides in the mRNA spanning a complete exon in the *DPYD* gene and arising from a G → A point mutation at the 5′-splicing site consensus sequence (GT → AT), which causes skipping of the complete exon prior

to the mutation during transcription of the *DPYD* gene (Wei *et al.*, 1996). Accordingly, the defect can now be detected using PCR-based methods. A number of other missense mutations have since been described, including Arg235Trp and Cys29Arg, both of which in an *E. coli* expression system lack DPD activity. An Arg886His mutation retained 25% residual activity under the same conditions (Vreken *et al.*, 1997). Recently, the DPD gene has been shown to be 150 kb in length, with 23 exons (Johnson *et al.*, 1997b).

Toxicological consequences of the DPD polymorphism

Chemotherapy with 5-FU is commonplace. It is used alone or in combination in the adjuvant treatment of breast and gastrointestinal cancer and in the palliative treatment of inoperable tumours of the gastrointestinal tract, breast, head and neck, liver, genito-urinary system and pancreas (Diasio and Harris, 1989). Heterozygotes for DPD deficiency, who can comprise up to 3% of cancer patients, are at increased risk of unusually severe, and often fatal, adverse reactions to the drug. Patients require supportive care and there is some evidence that administration of thymidine may reverse the neurological symptoms such as encephalopathy and coma (Morrison *et al.*, 1997). Whilst systemic toxicity is certainly determined by DPD phenotype, it is becoming clear that DPD expression within the tumour itself may be the basis of the chemotherapeutic response to 5-FU (Milano and Etienne, 1994, 1996). It would seem even more prudent that *DPYD* genotype (or DPD phenotype) be determined on all patients scheduled for 5-FU single-agent or combination chemotherapy, in order to maximize therapeutic response and avoid unwanted life-threatening toxicity. However, if a dose reduction strategy is employed in the *DPYD* heterozygotes (who presumably have less DPD enzyme expressed in their tumour also), then these patients will possibly not respond to 5-FU treatment. Perhaps genetic screening for the DPD polymorphism will ultimately guide the choice of chemotherapeutic agent used.

Alcohol dehydrogenase (ADH) polymorphisms

The alcohol dehydrogenases (ADHs) have been reviewed in detail by Agarwal and Goedde (1992) and by Price Evans (1993). This section will consider only a few important points. ADH is the principal enzyme metabolizing ethanol in humans and also converts a wide range of substituted alcohols to their corresponding aldehydes or ketones. Most work has centred around the metabolism of ethanol by ADH and its consequences for human health. That alcohol metabolism was a pharmacogenetic phenomenon has, as stated by Price Evans (1993), only comparatively recently been recognized. It is worth repeating the quotation of von Wartburg (1980) as cited by Price Evans (1993):

'Pharmacogenetic phenomena are the expression of pre-existing inborn differences among individuals which become apparent upon exposure of the body to drugs. If alcohol is considered to be a drug and the differences in biological sensitivity have a genetic origin they may be called pharmacogenetic'.

There are at least five distinct gene loci which code for human ADH. Eight different 40 kDa subunit types, α, β_1, β_2, β_3, γ_1, γ_2, π and χ, associate into homo-and heterodimers which yield the various phenotypic enzymes of 80 kDa. The subunit combinations and the classification of ADH genes, alleles and phenotypes are beyond the scope of this chapter and the reader is referred to Agarwal and Goedde (1992). However, it is important to note here that a variant enzyme arising from the *ADH2* gene, known commonly as 'atypical ADH' is of intense interest with respect to ethanol metabolism, for it has a higher K_m for ethanol and the cofactor NAD^+ and also a higher V_{max} for ethanol. The atypical phenotype is common in certain populations and less common in others and has been speculated to be the cause of ethnic differences in ethanol tolerability (see Agarwal and Goedde, 1992). The frequency of the atypical phenotype is highest amongst Japanese (85–98%) and Chinese (89–92%) and low amongst Swiss (20%), English (5–10%), Germans (9–14%), black Americans (< 10%), white Americans (< 5%) and Brazilians (2.8%), whilst being undetectable in Asian Indians and American Indians (Sioux, Navajo, Pueblo).

The understanding of the molecular genetics of ADHs has caused a quantum leap in the quantity and quality of studies on this enzyme system. This has enabled the number of *ADH* genes to be clarified, expanding the number from the original cluster of five genes (*ADH1–ADH5*) on 4q21–q25 to seven, by the additional cloning of *ADH6* (Yasunami *et al.*, 1991) and *ADH7* (Yokoyama *et al.*, 1994, 1995). PCR-based methods have rapidly evolved to identify variant allels at the polymorphic *ADH2* and *ADH3* loci (see Groppi *et al.*, 1990; Suzuki *et al.*, 1994; Wall *et al.*, 1997).

ADHs can metabolize multiple substrates, including many endogenous compounds. For example, retinol oxidation to retinoic acid via retinal is mediated by various ADHs, including ADH7 (Satre *et al.*, 1994). Certain steroids and bile acids appear to be metabolized by ADHs, for example 3β-hydroxy-5β-steroids (see Agarwal and Goedde, 1992). Serotonin (5-hydroxytryptamine) is metabolized to 5-hydroxytryptophol and then via the aldehyde to 5-hydroxyindol-3-ylacetic acid, which is excreted in urine unchanged and as conjugates with glycine, glutamine and glucuronic acid. Helander *et*

al. (1994) have examined the effect of polymorphisms in *ADH2*, *ADH3* and *ALDH2* on the pattern of serotonin metabolites in both Swedish and Chinese subjects. No genetic effects were observed, nor was there an ethnic difference. The range of ADH substrates includes primary and secondary aliphatic alcohols, diols, cyclic and aromatic alcohols and ω-hydroxy-fatty acids. All ADHs seem to metabolize primary alcohols efficiently, but ADH1 oxidizes secondary alcohols much more efficiently than either ADH2 or ADH3.

Toxicological consequences of ADH polymorphism

The acute reactions to ethanol ingestion which are manifested by the metabolite of ADH, acetaldehyde (ethanal), may be related to ADH polymorphism, since they occur much more frequently in oriental populations, but the picture is complicated by polymorphism in the aldehyde dehydrogenases (ALDHs) which further metabolize acetaldehyde (see below). Until the development of genotyping methods requiring only genomic DNA and not a liver biopsy specimen, it was more difficult to design investigations to answer the questions regarding the genetics of alcohol toxicity and alcoholism. These new technologies have found particular utility in the study of oriental populations. Thomasson *et al.* (1991) genotyped a cohort of alcoholic and non-alcoholic Chinese men in Taiwan, for polymorphisms at the *ADH2*, *ADH3* and *ALDH2* loci. The frequency of the *ADH2*2*, *ADH3*1* and *ALDH2*2* alleles was significantly lower in the alcoholics, suggesting that genetic variation at these loci influences alcohol tolerability, drinking habits and thus the development of alcoholism. In contrast, a study in 82 UK subjects undergoing treatment for alcohol-related problems showed no differences in allele frequency at these same three loci (Gilder *et al.*, 1993). Perhaps the small sample size and the difference in allele frequency between Caucasian and Chinese populations combined to render the study of insufficient power to detect such a difference. A more recent study in Taiwanese Chinese subjects (Luu *et al.*, 1995), which genotyped 273 male subjects for polymorphism at these three loci, found 143 individuals who were homozygous for both *ADH2*2* and *ADH3*1* alleles. Eight of these subjects were also homozygous for the *ALDH2*2* allele. On administration of 0.2 g/kg body weight of ethanol, *ALDH*2* homozygotes reported more pronounced subjective effects of alcohol (palpitation, facial warming, dizziness and 'effects of alcohol'), concomitant with higher plasma acetaldehyde levels, both peak and AUC (area under the curve). Alcoholic liver disease may also have a similar genetic component. In a further Taiwanese study, 27 cases of alcohol-related cirrhosis were compared with healthy controls, 29 cases of viral hepatitis and 30 cases of gastric and duodenal ulcer unrelated to alcohol. The *ADH2*2* allele (57%), *ADH3*1* allele (78%)

and *ALDH2*2* allele (9%) were significantly lower in the alcoholic cirrhotic patients than any of the other three groups (Chao *et al.*, 1994), again suggesting that these alleles cause aversion to alcohol and therefore 'protect' against its toxic effects.

The genetics of alcohol toxicity are further complicated by the fact that not only are ADH2, ADH3 and ALDH2 involved in the metabolism of ethanol, but also the ethanol-inducible cytochrome P450 CYP2E1. Although no functional (phenotypic) polymorphism of CYP2E1 has been established, there does exist polymorphism within the 5'-region of the *CYP2E1* gene (see **Table 3**) which can be detected by digestion of the PCR product with either *Dra*I or *Rsa*I. In healthy Taiwanese, the frequency of the two *Dra*I alleles is 79% and 21% and that of the *Rsa*I alleles is 82% and 18%, with all persons exhibiting the *Rsa*I minor allele always having the minor *Dra*I allele, but not *vice versa* (Hildesheim *et al.*, 1995). In a Japanese study, the odds ratios in alcoholic liver disease for *ALDH2*2* homozygosity and homozygosity for the *CYP2E1 Rsa*I minor allele were 4.6 and 4.0, respectively (Yamauchi *et al.*, 1995). All of these genes (*ADH2, ADH3, ALDH2* and *CYP2E1*) have been screened for polymorphism in Taiwanese alcoholics. The study concludes that the *ALDH2*1* allele is the most important gene affecting predisposition to alcohol, whilst *ADH2*2* may influence susceptibility to acute alcoholic pancreatitis (Chao *et al.*, 1997). The differences in *CYP2E1* genotypes reported in Japanese were not observed by these Taiwanese investigators.

Many epidemiological studies have shown that moderate alcohol consumption protects against coronary disease. A mechanism involving ADH has been proposed (Bello *et al.*, 1994). Apparently, an ADH isozyme is expressed in blood vessels, as demonstrated by both immunoblotting of vascular homogenates, immunohistochemistry on blood vessel sections and PCR with a human aortic cDNA library. The authors proposed that reduction of NAD^+ to NADH in vessel walls by the ADH-mediated metabolism of ethanol could provide a reducing environment which protects against lipid peroxidation and subsequent atherosclerosis. It is not known whether or not this putative process is influenced by the genetics of ADH.

The role of ADH in the toxicity of other alcohols is clear. Methanol, 2-propanol, ethylene glycol and 1,2-propanediol all lead to poisoning when ingested and the toxic pathways involve ADH (Agarwal and Goedde, 1992). The role of ADH polymorphism in these toxicities is unclear. The cardiac glycosides digoxin, digitoxin and gitoxin are all metabolized by hepatic ADH to their corresponding 3-oxo derivatives. This forms the basis of an important potential drug-drug interaction between cardiac glycosides and ethanol, which could have toxicological consequences (Agarwal and Goedde, 1992).

Aldehyde dehydrogenase (ALDH) polymorphisms

The aldehyde dehydrogenase (ALDH) polymorphisms have been reviewed by Goedde and Agarwal (1992). ALDH is a homotetrameric enzyme comprising subunits of about 54 kDa each. There exist at least seven discrete isozymes, ALDH1–ALDH7, with the major human hepatic forms being ALDH1 and ALDH2. The high-affinity enzyme is ALDH2, which is localized in mitochondria, whilst the lower affinity ALDH1, ALDH3 and ALDH4 are found in the cytosol (see Weber, 1997, for a review). Like ADHs, the cofactor is also NAD^+ and both ALDH1 and ALDH2 have K_m values in the μM range for acetaldehyde and propionaldehyde oxidation, whilst ALDH3 and ALDH4 have values in the mM range (Goedde and Agarwal, 1992). Accordingly, hepatic ALDH1 and ALDH2 are sometimes referred to as 'true' aldehyde dehydrogenases (Weber, 1997). ALDH3 is found in stomach and does not metabolize small aliphatic aldehydes such as formaldehyde and acetaldehyde, but rather has activity towards aromatic aldehydes such as furan-2-al (furfural) and benzaldehyde. High ALDH3 activity has also been detected in the cornea (Goedde and Agarwal, 1992).

Molecular biology has expanded our knowledge of the ALDHs enormously. For example, Hsu *et al.* (1994a) have sequenced an *ALDH6* cDNA from human salivary gland and Hsu *et al.* (1994b) have cloned an *ALDH7* cDNA from human kidney which is also expressed in the lung. Hsu and Chang (1996) cloned an *ALDH8* cDNA, possibly a pseudogene, expressed only in the salivary gland. The main interest in ALDH polymorphism has been with ALDH2 because of its role in the overall hepatic metabolism of alcohol and the part played by polymorphism in alcohol-related diseases. Genetic variation in ALDH2 is commonplace amongst oriental populations, with about 50% of Chinese and Japanese post-mortem livers lacking this isozyme. In 12 Caucasian and Negroid populations studied, comprising over 1400 subjects, no ALDH2-deficient persons were detected (see Goedde and Agarwal, 1992). The oriental deficiency is due to a Lys487Glu substitution arising from a single G→A transition in exon 12 which can be detected by PCR (Tu and Israel, 1993; Dandre *et al.*, 1995).

Toxicological consequences of ALDH polymorphism

Work surrounding *ALDH2* polymorphism and alcohol-related disease has often been closely linked with the *ALDH2* and *ALDH3* genes (see earlier) and will not be discussed further here. Of additional interest is the role of ALDH in the metabolism of, and clinical response to, the widely used cytostatic drug cyclophosphamide. Some years ago we showed that the inactivation of cyclophosphamide, by conversion of its aldophosphamide metabolite to carboxyphosphamide, is widely variable in adult cancer patients (Hadidi *et al.*, 1988). Furthermore, we proposed the existence of two phenotypes, 'high carboxylators' and 'low carboxylators'. The low carboxylators comprised about 36% of the cancer patient group. We subsequently replicated this finding in a group of adult Turkish cancer patients, where the low carboxylator phenotype was about 24% of the group (Boddy *et al.*, 1992). The same polymorphic pattern was also seen in children treated with cyclophosphamide (Tasso *et al.*, 1992). Although the biochemical and molecular basis of these findings has never been investigated, it appears likely that ALDH1 may be involved, for it is this isozyme which is responsible for the inactivation of cyclophosphamide, by the same pathway, in cyclophosphamide-resistant tumour cells (Moreb *et al.*, 1996) and for the systemic metabolism of aldophosphamide in erythrocytes (Dockham *et al.*, 1997). These findings are consistent with case reports of individual subjects lacking erythrocytic ALDH1 or hepatic cytosolic ALDH1 (see Goedde and Agarwal, 1992). However, no common genetic polymorphism of *ALDH1*, which could explain the variability in cyclophosphamide metabolism, has ever been described, although genetic variants of *ALDH1* have been described (Yoshida and Chen, 1989) which might be associated with alcohol flushing (Yoshida, 1994). Inherited electrophoretic variants of ALDH1 in rat liver cytosol have recently been described (Negoro *et al.*, 1997). Genetic variation in cytotoxic drug detoxication would be important to establish. Cancer chemotherapy is one of the most important areas to which pharmacogenetics can contribute.

Aldehyde oxidase (AO) polymorphisms

Aldehyde oxidase (AO) is a molybdenum hydroxylase closely related to xanthine oxidase and xanthine dehydrogenase which catalyses the transfer of water-derived oxygen into a broad range of *N*-heterocycles and aldehydes (Beedham, 1998). Unlike other oxidoreductases, AO requires no NAD$^+$ or NADP$^+$ cofactors. AO is found in the cytosol, predominantly in the liver. The name is somewhat of a misnomer because many of the substrates are not aldehydes, but rather insertion of oxygen occurs in the heterocycle at an electron-deficient carbon adjacent to a nitrogen atom, yielding a lactam. **Figure 15** shows some typical reactions mediated by AO. In addition to the oxidation of aldehydes such as indol-3-ylmethanal to their corresponding acids, AO can insert oxygen α to the N in such substrates as nicotine $\Delta^{1'(5')}$-iminium ion (the intermediate metabolite of nicotine in the CYP2A6-mediated formation of cotinine; Gorrod, 1993) and 5-fluoropyrimidin-2-one (a pro-drug of the cytostatic antimetabolite 5-fluorouracil; Guo *et al.*,

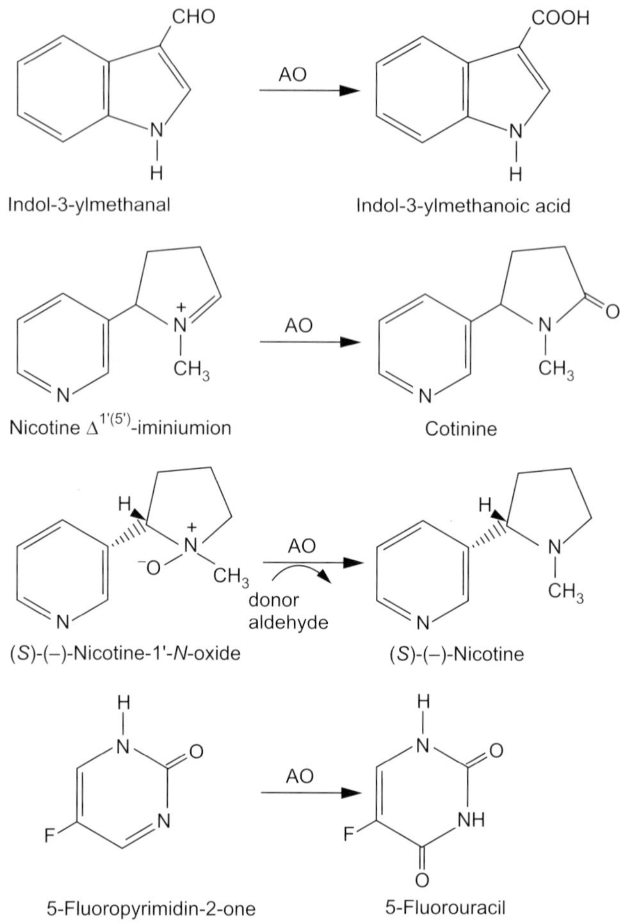

Figure 15 Metabolic reactions mediated by aldehyde oxidases (AO).

1995). In addition, AO can function as a reductase of a wide variety of substrates such as *N*-oxides (Kitamura and Tatsumi, 1984), *S*-oxides (Yoshihara and Tatsumi, 1990), azoaromatic compounds (Stoddart and Levine, 1992) and nitroaromatic compounds (Bauer and Howard, 1991), together with epoxides (Hirao *et al.*, 1994). The reduction of the *N*-oxide of (*S*)-nicotine is also shown in **Figure 15**. The reductive properties of AO seem to be restricted to *in vitro* experiments with lowered oxygen tension and the reaction appears to require the presence of an electron donor such as an aldehyde. In other words, AO may, as a consequence of aldehyde oxidation, reduce 'bystander' substrates, in the way that other oxidoreductases will reduce NAD$^+$ to NADH. The physiological relevance of such reductions by AO is dubious.

There occur marked species differences in hepatic AO activity (see Beedham, 1998), with rat and dog liver having low or negligible activity, baboon liver being highly active and marmoset and guinea pig having the closest spectrum of activities to human liver with a range of substrates (Beedham *et al.*, 1987). These inter-species differences in AO activity can lead to qualitative differences in the comparative metabolism of a drug. Consider the antiglaucoma drug brimonidine, for example, where the 2-oxo, 3-oxo and 2,3-dioxo metabolites predominate in liver fractions from rat, rabbit, monkey and human, but dog liver converts brimonidine to its $4', 5'$-dehydro metabolite and a ring-opened guanidino metabolite, with no oxo metabolites (Acheampong *et al.*, 1996). Moreover, the new antiherpes agent famciclovir is a prodrug of the active metabolite penciclovir, the final stage of the conversion from the intermediate metabolite 6-deoxypenciclovir to penciclovir being mediated by AO from rat, guinea pig and human liver (Rashidi *et al.*, 1997). However, some Sprague–Dawley rats, designated as 'AO-inactive' (compared with others which were designated 'AO-active'), did not carry out the *in vitro* oxidation of the penciclovir precursors, despite possessing high activity of the related molybdenum hydroxylase xanthine oxidase. This pharmacogenetic approach has revealed that the activation of famciclovir is exclusively carried out by AO (Rashidi *et al.*, 1997). Such qualitative intra-species variation in AO activity has been noted elsewhere, particularly in rat and mouse inbred strains. For example, examination of AO activity in 25 Sprague–Dawley rat livers revealed no detectable oxidation of either phenanthridine or phthalazine in 15 (60%) of them (Beedham, 1998). The genetic or molecular bases of these observations are not known. However, a study by Sugihara *et al.* (1995) found a 63.5-fold difference between two strains of rat with respect to benzaldehyde oxidation, which paralleled differences in AO protein content of hepatic cytosols determined by immunoblotting. Genetically determined electrophoretic variants of AO have been observed in the livers of inbred mouse strains (Holmes, 1985), whereby the existence of two AO mouse genes *Aox-1* and *Aox-2*, closely linked on mouse chromosome 1, was proposed (Holmes, 1980). A null *Aox-1* allele and a high-activity *Aox-2* allele have been described and used to map these genes (Holmes *et al.*, 1981). At least four alleles at the Aox-2 locus have been described (Mather *et al.*, 1983). Both the murine AO isozymes are hepatic, with Aox-1 being the predominant form.

It appears that AO is not restricted to the liver and also seems to be co-expressed with xanthine oxidase, another molybdenum hydroxylase. Immunohistochemical staining for AO in rat tissues showed a distribution of the enzyme in renal tubules, oesophageal, gastric, intestinal and bronchial epithelia, together with hepatic cytoplasm (Moriwaki *et al.*, 1996). Using the more specific technique of *in situ* hybridization with a labelled cDNA probe, Bendotti *et al.* (1997) have demonstrated that the murine AO gene is expressed in the epithelium of the choroid plexus and in the large motor neurons of the facial, motor trigemini and hypoglossus nerves and in the motor neurons of the anterior horns of the spinal chord. This investigation was performed because AO is a candidate gene for a familial motor neuron disease called amyo-

trophic lateral sclerosis (ALS), a progressive, adult-onset, neurodegenerative disorder characterized by the death of large motor neurons from the cerebral cortex, brainstem and spinal cord, one of the genes for which (*ALS1*) maps to the region 21q21–21q22.1 (Figlewicz *et al.*, 1994). Only about 10% of ALS is familial and in the majority of families the mode of inheritance is autosomal dominant (Figlewicz *et al.*, 1994). However, the *ALS1* gene has been shown to be Cu/Zn-binding superoxide dismutase (*SOD1*), a cytosolic metalloenzyme which converts toxic $O_2^{-\bullet}$ to O_2 and H_2O_2 (Rosen *et al.*, 1993). ALS is a highly heterogeneous disease with multiple mutations in the *SOD1* gene associated with it (see Siddique and Hentati, 1995, for a review) and a fraction of the families in which the disease displays autosomal recessive inheritance. This so-called recessive familial ALS (RFALS or FALS-AR) has been mapped to chromosome 2q33, the location of the human AO gene and it is suggested strongly, owing to the lack of recombination between FALS-AR and a polymorphic marker (*D2S116*) only 280 kb from the AO gene, that AO is a candidate for FALS-AR (Berger *et al.*, 1995). Drug metabolism has not, to our knowledge, been investigated in FALS-AR patients with AO deficiency. Finally, AO deficiency can occur due to a rare molybdenum cofactor deficiency which affects not only AO but also sulphite oxidase and xanthine oxidase activities and presents soon after birth with developmental delay and seizures (Aukett *et al.*, 1988; OMIM Entry 252150).

Progress towards the cloning and characterization of AO genes has been relatively slow but has been catalysed by the interest in the devastating disease ALS discussed above. Complete sequences of two cDNAs from maize have been acquired, encoding proteins of around 146 kDa (Sekimoto *et al.*, 1997). A bovine liver AO cDNA has also been cloned, with a deduced peptide of 147 kDa (Calzi *et al.*, 1995). A complete sequence of a human cDNA remains elusive.

Aldehyde oxidase polymorphism is poised to be characterized at the molecular level and to explain the functional polymorphism in the rat reported by Beedham (1998) and the wide inter-species differences in AO activities. Aldehyde oxidase is an enzyme with considerable toxicological importance, for it metabolizes a broad range of potentially toxic chemicals and drugs, including the metabolic activation of anticancer and antiviral drugs (see above). It is also an important component of nicotine metabolism to cotinine and may well be responsible for a high turnover of acetaldehyde in the hepatic cytosol after alcohol consumption, especially since it does not require NAD^+ cofactor for this purpose (C. Beedham, personal communication). This often overlooked enzyme may play a quintessential role in alcohol-induced hepatotoxicity because it has been shown that AO is not only capable of metabolizing the acetaldehyde produced by ALH-mediated metabolism of ethanol in the liver, but can also oxidize the resultant NADH with high affinity ($K_{\mathrm{m}} = 28\,\mu$M), yielding reactive oxygen species plus NAD$^+$ (Mira *et al.*, 1995). The NAD$^+$ may then be re-used by ALH to generate further acetaldehyde from ethanol, whilst the reactive oxygen species could contribute to hepatocellular toxicity via lipid peroxidation. Clearly, any genetic polymorphism in AO could have an impact on alcohol toxicity, nicotine pharmacokinetics, and the outcome of therapy with a range of new prodrugs designed specifically to be activated in the liver. This will be a very fruitful area for future research.

NAD(P)H:quinone oxidoreductase (NQO) polymorphisms

NAD(P)H:quinone oxidoreductase (NQO) is a cytosolic enzyme that was formerly known as DT-diaphorase and catalyses the two-electron reduction of quinones to hydroquinones, using either NADH or NADPH as electron donors (Lind *et al.*, 1990). Other substrates include quinone imines and azo dyes. It is generally believed that NQO protects cells against the toxic effects of oxidative stress and redox cycling that result from the generation of free radicals and active oxygen species as a consequence of metabolism by single-electron reducing enzymes such as NADPH:cytochrome P450 reductase (Monks *et al.*, 1992). It is thought that these ubiquitous enzymes are encoded by four genes, two of which, *NQO1* (Robertson *et al.*, 1986; Williams *et al.*, 1986; Jaiswal *et al.*, 1988; Bayney *et al.*, 1989; Shaw *et al.*, 1991) and *NQO2* (Jaiswal *et al.*, 1990) have been cloned and characterized. The regulation of *NQO1* transcription is complex and involves both the cytosolic Ah receptor, together with AP1 elements and the Fos and Jun proteins (Jaiswal, 1994). Thus many external stimuli are able to induce the transcription of *NQO1*. *NQO1* expression is also some 20–50-fold increased in hepatocellular carcinoma compared with surrounding liver tissue (Cresteil and Jaiswal, 1991). It seems likely that the reductive metabolic activation of the antitumour drug mitomycin C occurs at the level of the tumour by NQO1 (Traver *et al.*, 1992), thus displaying some degree of selective toxicity. Cell lines derived from gastric and colon carcinomas which do not have NQO1 activity are resistant to mitomycin C, whilst those with activity are sensitive. When a resistant cell line was transfected with an expression vector containing *NQO1*, a 5–10-fold increase in sensitivity to mitomycin C was observed, paralleling the increase in NQO1 activity (Mikami *et al.*, 1996). Three quinone-containing antitumour drugs are shown in **Figure 16**. Both mitomycin C and diaziquone (AZQ) are activated to alkylating species by quinone reduction to the corresponding hydroquinone which, in turn, facilitates activation of the aziridine groups (DeVita *et al.*, 1997). Doxorubicin (adriamycin), the archetypal anthracycline antitumour agent, causes both acute and chronic

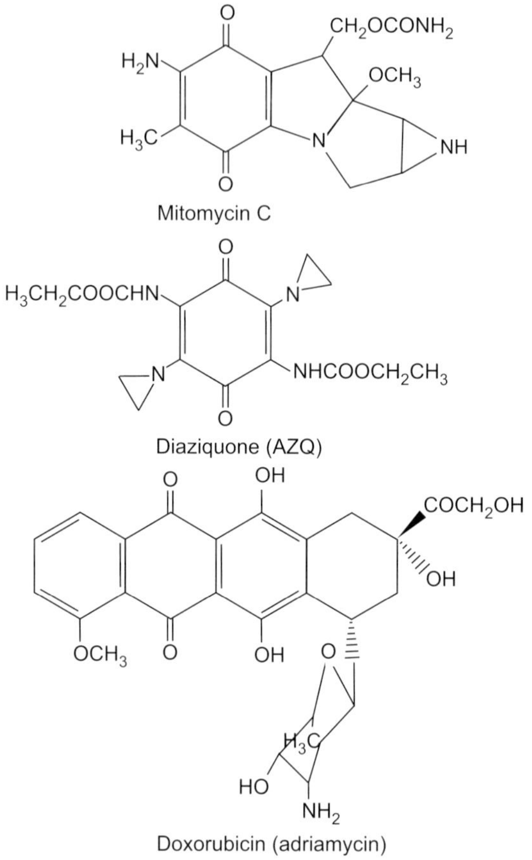

Figure 16 Some anticancer drugs which metabolized by NAD(P)H:quinone oxidoreductase 1 (NQO1).

cardiac toxicity through a mechanism involving quinone reduction (DeVita *et al.*, 1997). The haemopoietic toxicity of benzene involves hydroxylation of benzene by CYP2E1, followed by activation by bone marrow myeloperoxidases to reactive quinones, which, in turn, can be detoxicated by NAD(P)H:quinone oxidoreductase (Ross, 1996). The genotoxic nitroaromatic compound 4-nitroquinoline 1-oxide is toxic to HepG2 cells, but this toxicity is considerably elevated when NQO1 activity is inhibited using dicoumarol (Hasspieler *et al.*, 1997). NQO1 is therefore an enzyme of considerable interest in the detoxication of reactive quinone metabolites of xenobiotics and in the bioactivation of certain anticancer drugs. Genetic variation in NQO1 activity would clearly be of importance (see below).

The *NQO2* cDNA was cloned by Jaiswal and colleagues from a human liver cDNA library and found to be 54% and 49% similar to *NQO1* at the nucleotide and deduced peptide sequence levels, respectively (Jaiswal *et al.*, 1990a). Genomic sequences revealed that sizes and sequences of exons 3–6 are highly conserved between *NQO1* and *NQO2* (Jaiswal, 1994b). Unlike NQO1, which is expressed in every human tissue examined, NQO2 was found to be expressed in only heart, brain, lung, liver and skeletal muscle (Jaiswal, 1994). Recently, another interesting difference has been reported. NQO2 uses dihydronicotinamide riboside (NRH), rather than NAD(P)H, as an electron donor (Wu, K. *et al.*, 1997). It can also catalyse four-electron reductions and catalyses the nitroreduction of the cytotoxic compound 5-(aziridin-1-yl)-2,4-dinitrobenzamide 3000 times faster than NQO1. It is resistant to inhibitors of NQO1, such as dicoumarol and phenindione, but is strongly inhibited by the flavone quercetin, with a K_i, with respect to NRH, of 21 nM. NQO2 is therefore an NRH-dependent oxidoreductase which catalyses two- and four-electron reductions (Wu, K. *et al.*, 1997).

A genetic polymorphism in *NQO1* has been described, arising from a C→T substitution at nucleotide 609 and causing a Pro187Ser substitution (Jaiswal *et al.*, 1988; Jaiswal, 1991). Kuehl *et al.* (1995) showed that this allele was present in about 50% of Canadians with 8.5% being homozygous deficient. Subsequently, Traver *et al.* (1997) have demonstrated that the Ser-187 cDNA expressed in *E. coli* had only 2% of the activity of the Pro-187 cDNA. These authors also estimated the frequency of the homozygous Ser-187 genotype (deficient phenotype) to be 7%.

Toxicological consequences of NQO1 polymorphism

In a case-control study in China of occupational benzene poisoning resulting in haematotoxicity, Rothman *et al.* (1997) studied the combined effects of the NQO1 Pro187Ser substitution and increased CYP2E1 activity, the latter determined from the pharmacokinetics of the CYP2E1 substrate chlorozoxazone. CYP2E1 activity is seen as exacerbating, and NQO1 activity as ameliorating, benzene myelotoxicity (see above). Subjects with a rapid chlorzoxazone 6-hydroxylation combined with homozygosity for the *NQO1 Ser-187* allele had a 7.6-fold (95% C.I. 1.8–31.2) increased risk of benzene toxicity compared with slow chlorzoxazone 6-hydroxylation combined with either homozygosity or heterozygosity for the *NQO1 Pro-187* allele (Rothman *et al.*, 1997). Interestingly, the *CYP2E1 Rsa*I polymorphism (see above) was not associated with risk of benzene toxicity and therefore presumably does not predict CYP2E1 activity with respect to either benzene or chlorzoxazone metabolism. In this regard, the study is a triumph of phenotyping over genotyping, with respect to CYP2E1.

Rosvold *et al.* (1995) studied the NQO1 polymorphism in 150 American lung cancer cases and two reference populations, finding a weak association between the variant *NQO1* allele and lung cancer when a French control population was employed ($\chi^2 = 5.52$, $P < 0.019$). This difference disappeared when a local control group was substituted for the French controls. Wiencke *et al.* (1997) studied 177 lung cancer cases and 297 community controls, of which 222/474 were Mexican-Americans and 252/474 were African-Americans. The cases overall were more commonly homozygous for the *NQO1 Pro-187* allele (odds ratio 1.79, $P = 0.002$). In addition, African-Americans had a twofold higher frequency of the commoner *Pro-187* allele ($P < 0.001$). These authors concluded that the *NQO1* polymorphism may be a significant risk factor for lung cancer in some ethnic minorities, although the data from this study are hard to explain in terms of a carcinogenic mechanism. Schulz *et al.* (1997) have examined the proposition that the *NQO1* polymorphism is a risk factor in urological malignancies. They studied 260 control DNAs, together with 131 patients with renal cell carcinoma and 99 with urothelial carcinoma. In the German control population, 4/250 (1.6%) persons were homozygous for the *Ser-187* allele. The rarer allele occurred more frequently in the cancer groups, with odds ratios (homozygous *Ser-187 versus* other genotypes) of 1.7 and 3.6 for renal cell carcinoma and urothelial carcinoma, respectively. This interesting finding, consistent with the detoxicating role of NQO1, is in stark contrast to the American lung cancer study of Wiencke *et al.* (1997). Future investigations of the *NQO1* polymorphism are likely to yield interesting findings and provide further insights into mechanisms of chemically induced disease.

Aldo–keto reductase (AKR) polymorphisms

The aldo–keto reductases represent a large superfamily of enzymes, widely distributed throughout the phyla and their tissues. Whilst these enzymes contain many members capable of metabolizing the aldehyde and ketone moieties of drugs and other xenobiotics, there are also a number of enzymes in this class whose primary role appears to lie in the interconversion of steroids and prostaglandins. In general, the steroid-metabolizing enzymes are named after the back reaction, *i.e.* as dehydrogenases, rather than reductases, suggesting that their role is to form ketones from secondary alcohols of steroids. To the casual reader of the pertinent literature this can be confusing. Therefore, the various hydroxysteroid dehydrogenases, for example 20β-hydroxysteroid dehydrogenase (EC 1.1.1.53), are in fact aldo–keto reductases, akin to carbonyl reductase (EC 1.1.1.184), aldehyde reductase (EC 1.1.1.2) and aldose reductase (EC 1.1.1.21). Yet more confusing is the fact that the prostaglandin-metabolizing enzymes in this group are called 'synthases', for example prostaglandin F synthase, which reduces PGH2 to PGF2 and PGD2 to 9α, 11β-PGF2 (Watanabe *et al.*, 1991). As with other gene superfamilies, the aldo–keto reductases form a single group owing to sequence alignment and homology, rather than substrate specificity. When performing aldehyde and ketone reduction these enzymes utilize NADPH and, for the back reaction, as in the case of some of the hydroxysteroid dehydrogenases, they are NADP$^+$-dependent.

The advent of *in vitro* drug metabolism studies in the 1960s saw the first investigation of the cofactor requirements for aromatic and aliphatic ketone reduction. It was soon concluded that NADPH was required, in contrast to 'liver alcohol dehydrogenase' (LAD), which was NAD[+]-dependent. Scientists working at Eli Lilly in the USA were charged with working out the rodent and human metabolism of their new antidiabetic drug acetohexamide which had been awarded a patent in 1962. McMahon and his colleagues established the metabolic pattern of acetohexamide (McMahon *et al.*, 1965), observing that the principal biotransformation of this acetophenone derivative was to the corresponding alcohol. This led to the first mechanistic study of ketone reduction, establishing the dependence upon NADPH (Culp and McMahon, 1968). This group further clarified the structure–activity relationships of their rabbit kidney cortex ketone reductase (Hermann *et al.*, 1969). As more and more substrates were studied *in vitro*, it became apparent that activity resided in both the cytosolic and microsomal fractions of many tissues. In addition, compounds were uncovered which would inhibit the reduction of one ketone but not another. Gradually, a crude classification of the aldo–keto reductases grew up, based upon the biochemical criteria of differential inhibition and induction of activities, which permitted the differentiation of aldehyde reductase and ketone reductase activities. The literature is now large, diffuse and still somewhat confusing regarding the exact nature and number of the discrete aldo–keto reductases. However,

gene technology has undoubtedly revealed most of our current knowledge about the organization of this superfamily. One of the consequences of this has been the gradual recognition (Lee *et al.*, 1993) that the abundant and soluble structural proteins of the eye lens, the crystallins, which endow this tissue with its refractive properties, have been recruited from the oxidoreductase enzymes. The mechanism is believed to be a modification of gene expression without prior gene duplication (Lee *et al.*, 1993). Interestingly, η-crystallin, which in elephant shrew lenses comprises 25% of total protein, is identical with cytoplasmic aldehyde dehydrogenase. In frog lenses, ρ-crystallin is a member of the aldo–keto reductases and ϕ-crystallin from guinea pig and camel lenses is related to alcohol dehydrogenases (Lee *et al.*, 1993). The crystallins bind NADPH and have retained enzymatic activities.

Some characteristics of cloned aldo–keto reductases are given in **Table 5**. To us they appear to segregate into two groups, those with molecular weights of 35–37 kDa and those of 26–30 kDa. All the carbonyl reductases fall in this latter group. Many of these cloned enzymes derive from sex hormone-responsive tissues such as ovary, testis, placenta and breast, where they may be intimately concerned with steroid hormone interconversions. Others derive from the liver or lung where their role may be more one of xenobiotic detoxication. The number of exogenous aldehydes and ketones, both aromatic and aliphatic, which are substrates for the aldo–keto reductases is huge and includes a number of important

Table 5 Characteristics of some cloned aldo–keto reductases

Enzyme activity	M_R (Da)	Amino acids	Species	Tissue	Reference
High molecular weight forms (35–37 kDa)					
17β-HSD[a]	37 055	323	Mouse	Liver	Deyashiki *et al.* (1995)
20α-HSD	37 000	323	Rat	Ovary	Miura *et al.* (1994)
20α-HSD	37 000	–	Human	Corpus luteum	Albarracin *et al.* (1994)
PGF synthase[b]	36 000	–	Ox	Lung	Watanabe *et al.* (1991)
Aldo–keto reductase	35 000	–	Chinese hamster	Ovary (CHO cells)	Hyndman *et al.* (1997)
Aldose reductase	–	316	Human	Placenta	Bohren *et al.* (1989)
Aldehyde reductase	–	325	Human	Liver/placenta	Bohren *et al.* (1989)
ρ-Crystallin	–	324	Bullfrog	Eye lens	Lu *et al.* (1995)
Low molecular weight forms (26–30 kDa)					
20β-HSD	–	289	Pig	Testis	Tanaka *et al.* (1992)
Carbonyl reductase (tetrameric)	25 985	244	Pig	Lung	Nakanishi *et al.* (1993)
Carbonyl reductase	27 000	244	Mouse	Lung/adipocyte	Nakanishi *et al.* (1995)
Carbonyl reductase (inducible)	–	277	Rat	Ovary/testis	Aoki *et al.* (1997)
Carbonyl reductase (non-inducible)	–	276	Rat	Ovary/testis	Aoki *et al.* (1997)
Carbonyl reductase	30 375	277	Human	Breast (MCF-7 cells)	Forrest *et al.* (1990)
Carbonyl reductase	30 375	277	Human	Placenta	Wermuth *et al.* (1988)
Sepiapterin reductase	28 047	261	Human	Liver	Ichinose *et al.* (1991)

[a] HSD means Hydroxysteroid dehydrogenase; [b] PGF means Prostaglandin F

drugs such as warfarin, haloperidol, progesterone, oestradiol and daunorubicin. In this last case, the cytotoxic properties of the drug are ameliorated by reduction of the ketone in the aliphatic side-chain to an alcohol called daunorubicinol.

No information exists at present regarding allelomorphism of the aldo–keto reductases, perhaps because they have been cloned comparatively recently. Nevertheless, several attempts have been made, largely in Kalow's laboratory in Toronto, to uncover functional polymorphism in ketone reduction *in vitro*. Wong *et al.* (1993) studied 4-nitroacetophenone reduction in the cytosol from 17 human livers. At low substrate concentration (50 μM), a unimodal distribution of activities was observed, but at a concentration of 500 μM a non-normal distribution was obtained. Three out of 17 livers showed abnormally low activity of the high-affinity form of carbonyl reductase. A study of 11 human livers in Japan reported contrary findings (Iwata *et al.*, 1993). These workers employed four different substrates, 4-nitrobenzaldehyde, 4-nitroacetophenone, 4-benzoylpyridine and 13, 14-dihydro-15-ketoprostaglandin F2α. The standard deviations were modest (17–59%), not indicative of significant variation between livers in any of the reduction pathways. It must be said that the number of subjects in both these studies was small and that rarely, if ever, has a genetic polymorphism been uncovered by such *in vitro* methods. More recently, Rady-Pentek *et al.* (1997) investigated the ketone reduction of 13, 14-dihydro-15-ketoprostaglandin E1 in 37 human livers and in erythrocytes from a further 29 subjects. Enzymic activity in lysed erythrocytes varied only twofold between the 29 subjects, but in the 37 liver samples there was a 10-fold variation with a non-normal distribution. There exist strong signs, therefore, that this aldo–keto reductase may display genetic polymorphism.

When genetic polymorphism of aldo–keto reductases is properly established, as seems very likely in the short-term, there will be many clinical and toxicological implications. Many xenobiotic substrates, both aldehydes and ketones, for this superfamily of enzymes exist, which can be both detoxicated and metabolically activated by these enzymes. In addition, a plethora of steroids and prostaglandins undergo ketone reduction and therefore genetic polymorphism in these pathways may have profound effects on infection, immunity, inflammation, neoplasia and disease susceptibility. This is an important focus of development in this field.

ACKNOWLEDGEMENTS

We thank our colleagues in the Department of Medical Genetics, Regional Hospital, Trondheim, for their forbearance during the writing of this chapter. We are grateful to Eva Svaasand for providing the gels in **Figure 1**. The advice of Drs Frank Gonzalez (Bethesda), Christine Beedham (Bradford) and Anil Jaiswal (Houston) and Professor Adrian Küpfer (Berne) is much appreciated.

REFERENCES

Abeling, N. G., van Gennip, A. H., Bakker, H. D., Heerschap, A., Engelke, U. and Wevers, R. A. (1995). Diagnosis of a new case of trimethylaminuria using direct proton NMR spectroscopy of urine. *J. Inherit. Metab. Dis.*, **18**, 182–184.

Acheampong, A. A., Chien, D. S., Lam, S., Vekich, S., Breau, A., Usansky, J., Harcourt, D., Munk, S. A., Nguyen, H., Garst, M. and Tang-Liu, D. (1996). Characterization of brimonidine metabolism with rat, rabbit, dog, monkey and human liver fractions and rabbit liver aldehyde oxidase. *Xenobiotica*, **26**, 1035–1055.

Agarwal, D. P. and Goedde, H. W. (1992). Pharmacogenetics of alcohol dehydrogenase. In Kalow, W. (Ed.), *Pharmacogenetics of Drug Metabolism*. Pergamon Press, New York, pp. 263–280.

Agúndez, J. A, Martinez, C., Ladero, J. M., Ledesma, M. C., Ramos, J. M., Martin, R., Rodrigez, A., Gara, C. and Benitez, J. (1994). Debrisoquine oxidation genotype and susceptibility to lung cancer. *Clin. Pharmacol. Ther.*, **55**, 10–14.

Albarracin, C. T., Parmer, T. G., Duan, W. R., Nelson, S. E. and Gibori, G. (1994). Identification of a major prolactin-regulated protein as 20 alpha-hydroxysteroid dehydrogenase: coordinate regulation of its activity, protein content, and messenger ribonucleic acid expression. *Endocrinology*, **134**, 2453–2460.

Al-Waiz, M., Ayesh, R., Mitchell, S. C., Idle, J. R. and Smith, R. L. (1987a). Trimethylaminuria (fish-odour syndrome): an inborn error of oxidative metabolism. *Lancet*, **i**, 634–635.

Al-Waiz, M., Ayesh, R., Mitchell, S. C., Idle, J. R. and Smith, R. L. (1987b). A genetic polymorphism of the *N*-oxidation of trimethylamine in humans. *Clin. Pharmacol. Ther.*, **42**, 588–594.

Al-Waiz, M., Mitchell, S. C., Idle, J. R. and Smith, R. L. (1987c). The metabolism of ^{14}C labelled trimethylamine and its *N*-oxide in man. *Xenobiotica*, **17**, 551–558.

Al-Waiz, M., Ayesh, R., Mitchell, S. C., Idle, J. R. and Smith, R. L. (1987d). Disclosure of the metabolic retroversion of trimethylamine *N*-oxide in humans: a pharmacogenetic approach. *Clin. Pharmacol. Ther.*, **42**, 608–612.

Al-Waiz, M., Ayesh, R., Mitchell, S. C., Idle, J. R. and Smith, R. L. (1988). Trimethylaminuria ('fish-odour syndrome'): a study of an affected family. *Clin. Sci.*, **74**, 231–236.

Al-Waiz, M., Ayesh, R., Mitchell, S. C., Idle, J. R. and Smith, R. L. (1989). Trimethylaminuria: the detection of carriers using a trimethylamine load test. *J. Inherit. Metab. Dis.*, **12**, 80–85.

Andersson, T., Regårdh, C.-G., Lou, Y.-C., Zhang, Y., Dahl, M.-L. and Bertilsson, L. (1992). Polymorphic hydroxylation of *S*-mephenytoin and omeprazole in Caucasian and Chinese subjects. *Pharmacogenetics*, **2**, 25–31.

Aoki, H., Okada, T., Mizutani, T., Numata, Y., Minegishi, T. and Miyamoto, K. (1997). Identification of two closely related genes, inducible and noninducible carbonyl reductases in the rat ovary. *Biochem. Biophys. Res. Commun.*, **230**, 518–523.

Armstrong, M., Daly A. K., Cholerton, S., Bateman, D. N., Idle, J. R. (1992). Mutant debrisoquine hydroxylation genes in Parkinson's disease. *Lancet*, **339**, 1017–1018.

Aukett, A., Bennett, M. J. and Hosking, G. P. (1988). Molybdenum co-factor deficiency: an easily missed inborn error of metabolism. *Dev. Med. Child Neurol.*, **30**, 531–535.

Ayesh, R., Idle, J. R., Ritchie, J. C., Crothers, M. J. and Hetzel, M. R. (1984). Metabolic oxidation phenotypes as markers for susceptibility to lung cancer. *Nature*, **311**, 169–170.

Ayesh, R., Mitchell, S. C., Zhang, A. and Smith R. L. (1993). The fish odour syndrome: biochemical, familial, and clinical aspects. *Br. Med. J.*, **307**, 655–657.

Bauer, S. L. and Howard, P. C. (1991). Kinetics and cofactor requirements for the nitroreductive metabolism of 1-nitropyrine and 3-nitrofluoranthrene by rabbit liver aldehyde oxidase. *Carcinogenesis*, **12**, 1545–1549.

Bayney, R. M., Morton, M. R., Favreau, L. V. and Pickett, C. B. (1989). Rat liver NAD(P)H:quinone oxidoreductase: regulation of quinone reductase gene expression by planar aromatic compounds and determination of the exon structure of the quinone reductase structural gene. *J. Biol. Chem.*, **264**, 21793–21797.

Beedham, C. (1998). Oxidation of carbon via molybdenum hydroxylases. In *Drug Metabolism: Towards the Next Millennium*. In press.

Beedham, C., Bruce, S. E., Critchley, D. J., Al-Tayib, Y. and Rance, D. J. (1987). Species variation in hepatic aldehyde oxidase activity. *Eur. J. Drug Metab. Pharmacokinet.*, **12**, 307–310.

Bello, A. T., Bora, N. S., Lange, L. G. and Bora, P. S. (1994). Cardioprotective effects of alcohol: mediation by human vascular alcohol dehydrogenase. *Biochem. Biophys. Res. Commun. Sep 30*, **203**(3), 1858–1864.

Bendotti, C., Prosperini, E., Kurosaki, M., Garattini, E. and Terao, M. (1997). Selective localization of mouse aldehyde oxidase mRNA in the choroid plexus and motor neurons. *Neuroreport*, **8**, 2343–2349.

Berger, R., Stoker-de Vries, S. A., Wadman, S. K., Duran, M., Beemer, F. A., de Bree, P. K., Weits-Binnerts, J. J., Penders, T. J. and van der Woude, J. K. (1984). Dihydropyrimidine dehydrogenase deficiency leading to thymine-uraciluria: an inborn error of pyrimidine metabolism. *Clin. Chim. Acta*, **141**, 227–234.

Berger, R., Mezey, E., Clancy, KP, Harta, G., Wright, R. M., Repine, J. E., Brown, R. H., Brownstein, M. and Patterson, D. (1995). Analysis of aldehyde oxidase and xanthine dehydrogenase/oxidase as possible candidate genes for autosomal recessive familial amyotrophic lateral sclerosis. *Somat. Cell Mol. Genet.*, **21**, 121–131.

Bhagwat, S. V., Bharme, S., Boyd, M. R. and Ravindranath, V. (1996). Cerebral metabolism of imipramine and a purified flavin-containing monooxygenase from human brain. *Neuropsychopharmacology*, **15**, 133–142.

Bhamre, S., Bhagwat, S. V., Shankar, S. K., Williams, D. E. and Ravindranath, V. (1993). Cerebral flavin-containing monooxygenase-mediated metabolism of antidepressants in brain: immunochemical properties and immunocytochemical localization. *J. Pharmacol. Exp. Ther.*, **267**, 555–559.

Bhamre, S., Bhagwat, S. V., Shankar, S. K., Boyd, M. R. and Ravindranath, V. (1995). Flavin-containing monooxygenase mediated metabolism of psychoactive drugs by human brain microsomes. *Brain Res.*, **672**, 276–280.

Blake, B. L., Philpot, R. M., Levi, P. E. and Hodgson, E. (1996). Xenobiotic biotransforming enzymes in the central nervous system: an isoform of flavin-containing monooxygenase (FMO4) is expressed in rabbit brain. *Chem.–Biol. Interact.*, **99**, 253–261.

Boddy, A. V., Furtun, Y., Sardas, S., Sardas, O. and Idle, J. R. (1992). Individual variation in the activation and inactivation metabolic pathways of cyclophosphamide. *J. Natl. Cancer Inst.*, **84**, 1744–1748.

Bohren, K. M., Bullock, B., Wermuth, B. and Gabbay, K. H. (1989). The aldo–keto reductase superfamily. cDNAs and deduced amino acid sequences of human aldehyde and aldose reductases. *J. Biol. Chem.*, **264**, 9547–9551.

Bouchardy, C., Benhamou, S. and Dayer, P. (1996). The effect of tobacco on lung cancer risk depends on CYP2D6 activity. *Cancer Res.*, **56**, 251–253.

Brzezinski, B. and Zundel, G. (1993). Formation of disulphide bonds in the reaction of SH group-containing amino acids with trimethylamine N-oxide. A regulatory mechanism in proteins. *FEBS Lett.*, **333**, 331–333.

Calzi, M. L., Raviolo, C., Ghibaudi, E., de Gioia, L., Salmona, M., Cazzaniga, G., Kurosaki, M., Terao, M. and Garattini, E. (1995). Purification, cDNA cloning, and tissue distribution of bovine liver aldehyde oxidase. *J. Biol. Chem.*, **270**, 31037–31045.

Chao, Y. C., Liou, S. R., Chung, Y. Y., Tang, H. S., Hsu, C. T., Li, T. K. and Yin, S. J. (1994). Polymorphism of alcohol and aldehyde dehydrogenase genes and alcoholic cirrhosis in Chinese patients. *Hepatology*, **19**, 360–366.

Chao, Y. C., Young, T. H., Tang, H. S. and Hsu, C. T. (1997). Alcoholism and alcoholic organ damage and genetic polymorphisms of alcohol metabolizing enzymes in Chinese patients. *Hepatology*, **25**, 112–117.

Cheeke, P. R. (1995). Endogenous toxins and mycotoxins in forage grasses and their effects on livestock. *J. Anim. Sci.*, **73**, 909–918.

Chiba, K., Kubota, E., Miyakawa, T., Kato, Y. and Ishizaki, T. (1988). Characterization of hepatic microsomal metabolism as an *in vivo* detoxication pathway of 1-methyl-4-phenyl-1,2,3,6-tetrahydropyridine in mice. *J. Pharmacol. Exp. Ther.*, **246**, 1108–1115.

Cholerton, S., Idle, M. E., Vas, A., Gonzalez, F. J. and Idle, J. R. (1992). Comparison of a novel thin-layer chromatographic–fluorescence detection method with a spectrofluorometric method for the determination of 7-hydroxycoumarin in human urine. *J. Chromatogr. Biomed. Appl.*, **575**, 325–330.

Choonara, I. A., Cholerton, S., Haynes, B. P., Breckenridge, A. M. and Park, BK. (1986). Stereoselective interaction between the *R*-enantiomer of warfarin and cimetidine. *Br. J. Clin. Pharmacol.*, **21**, 271–277.

Coleman, T., Ellis, S. W., Martin, I. J., Lennard, M. S. and Tucker, G. T. (1996). 1-Methyl-4-phenyl-1,2,3,6-tetrahydropyridine (MPTP) is N-demethylated by cytochromes P450 2D6, 1A2 and 3A4—Implications for susceptibility to Parkinson's disease. *J. Pharmacol. Exp. Ther.*, **277**, 685–690.

Crespi, C. L., Gonzalez, F. J., Steimel, D. T., Turner, T. R., Gelboin, H. V., Penman, B. W. and Langenbach, R. (1991). A tobacco smoke-derived nitrosamine, 4-(methylnitrosamino)-1-(3-pyridyl)-1-butanone, is activated by multiple human cytochrome P450s including the polymorphic cytochrome P4502D6. *Carcinogenesis*, **12**, 1197–1201.

Cresteil, T. and Jaiswal, A. K. (1991). High levels of expression of NAD(P)H:quinone oxidoreductase (*NQO1*) gene in tumor cells compared to normal cells of the same origin. *Biochem. Pharmacol.*, **42**, 1021–1027.

Culp, H. W. and McMahon, R. E. (1968). Reductase for aromatic aldehydes and ketones. The partial purification and properties of a reduced triphosphopyridine nucleotide-dependent reductase from rabbit kidney cortex. *J. Biol. Chem.*, **243**, 848–852.

Daly, A. K., Brockmöller, J., Broly, F., Eichelbaum, M., Evans, W. E., Gonzalez, F. J., Huang, J.-D., Idle, J. R., Ingelman-Sundberg, M., Ishizaki, T., Jacqz-Agrain, E., Mayer, U. A., Nebert, D. W., Steen, V. M., Wolf, C. R. and Zanger, U. M. (1996). Nomenclature for human *CYP2D6* alleles. *Pharmacogenetics*, **6**, 193–201.

Damani, L. A. and Nnane, I. P. (1996). The assessment of flavin-containing monooxygenase activity in intact animals. *Drug Metab. Drug Interact.*, **13**, 1–28.

Dandre, F., Cassaigne, A. and Iron, A. (1995). The frequency of the mitochondrial aldehyde dehydrogenase I2 (atypical) allele in Caucasian, Oriental and African black populations determined by the restriction profile of PCR-amplified DNA. *Mol. Cell. Probes*, **9**, 189–193.

Davies, D. S., Kahn, G. C., Murray, S., Brodie, M. J. and Boobis, A. R. (1981). Evidence for an enzymatic defect in the 4-hydroxylation of debrisoquine by human liver. *Br. J. Clin. Pharmacol.*, **11**, 89–91.

Dayer, P., Balant. L., Courvoisier, F., Küpfer, A., Kubli, A., Gorgia, A. and Fabre, J. (1982). The genetic control of bufuralol metabolism in man. *Eur. J. Drug Metab. Pharmacokinet.*, **7**, 73–77.

Dayer, P., Gasser, R., Gut, J., Krombach, T., Robertz, G.-M., Eichelbaum, M. and Mayer U. A. (1984). Characterisation of a common genetic defect of cytochrome P450 function (debrisoquine–sparteine type polymorphism)—Increased Michaelis constant (K_m) and loss of stereoselectivity of bufuralol 1′-hydroxylation in poor metabolisers. *Biochem. Biophys. Res. Commun.*, **125**, 374–379.

de Morais, S. M. F., Wilkinson, G. R., Blaisdell, J., Meyer, U. A., Nakamura, K. and Goldstein, J. A. (1994a). The major genetic defect responsible for the polymorphism of *S*-mephenytoin in humans. *J. Biol. Chem.*, **269**, 15419–15422.

de Morais, S. M. F., Wilkinson, G. R., Blaisdell, J., Nakamura, K., Meyer, U. A. and Goldstein, J. A. (1994b). Identification of a new genetic defect responsible for the polymorphism of *S*-mephenytoin metabolism in Japanese. *Mol. Pharmacol.*, **46**, 594–598.

DeVita, V. T., Jr, Hellman, S. and Rosenberg, S. A. (1997). *Cancer. Principles and Practice of Oncology*, 5th edn. Lippincott-Raven, Philadelphia.

Deyashiki, Y., Ohshima, K., Nakanishi, M, Sato, K., Matsuura, K. and Hara, A. (1995). Molecular cloning and characterization of mouse estradiol 17 beta-dehydrogenase (A-specific), a member of the aldoketoreductase family. *J. Biol. Chem.*, **270**, 10461–10467.

Diasio, R. B. and Harris, B. E. (1989). Clinical pharmacology of 5-fluorouracil. *Clin. Pharmacokinet.*, **16**, 215–237.

Dockham, P. A., Sreerama, L. and Sladek, N. E. (1997). Relative contribution of human erythrocyte aldehyde dehydrogenase to the systemic detoxification of the oxazaphosphorines. *Drug Metab. Dispos.*, **25**, 1436–1441.

Dolphin, C. T., Cullingford, T. E., Shephard, E. A., Smith, R. L. and Phillips, I. A. (1996). Differential developmental and tissue-specific regulation of the flavin-containing monooxygenase family of man, FMO1, FMO3, and FMO4. *Eur. J. Biochem.*, **235**, 683–689.

Dolphin, C. T., Riley, J. H., Smith, R. L., Shephard, E. A. and Phillips, I. A. (1997a) Structural organization of the human flavin-containing monooxygenase 3 gene (*FMO3*), the favored candidate for fish-odor syndrome, determined directly from genomic DNA. *Genomics*, **46**, 260–267.

Dolphin, C. T., Janmohamed, A., Smith, R. L., Shephard, E. A. and Phillips, I. A. (1997b). Missense mutation in flavin-containing monooxygenase 3 gene, *FMO3*, underlies fish-odour syndrome. *Nature Genet.*, **17**, 491–494.

Dolzan, V., Rudolf, Z. and Breskva, K. (1995). Human *CYP2D6* gene polymorphism in Slovene cancer patients and healthy controls. *Carcinogenesis*, **16**, 2675–2678.

Egan, D., O'Kennedy, R., Mora, E., Cox, D., Prosser, E. and Thornes, R. D. (1990). The pharmacology, metabolism, analysis, and applications of coumarin and coumarin-related compounds. *Drug Metab. Rev.*, **22**, 503–529.

Eichelbaum, M. and Gross, A. S. (1990). The genetic polymorphism of debrisoquine/spartaine metabolism-chemical aspects. *Pharmacol. Thes*, **46** (3), 337–394.

Eichelbaum, M., Spannbrucker, N., Steinke, B. and Dengler H. J. (1979). Defective *N*-oxidation of sparteine in man: a new pharmacogenetic defect. *Eur. J. Clin. Pharmacol.*, **16**, 183–187.

Falls, J. G., Blake, B. L., Cao, Y., Levi, P. E. and Hodgson, E. (1995). Gender differences in hepatic expression of flavin-containing monooxygenase isoforms (FMO1, FMO3, and FMO5) in mice. *J. Biochem. Toxicol.*, **10**, 171–177.

Fernandez-Salguero, P., Gonzalez, F. J., Etienne, M. C., Milano, G. and Kimura, S. (1995a). Correlation between catalytic activity and protein content for the polymorphically expressed dihydropyrimidine dehydrogenase in human lymphocytes. *Biochem. Pharmacol.*, **50**, 1015–1020.

Fernandez-Salguero, P., Hoffman, S. M. G., Cholerton, S., Mohrenweiser, H., Raunio, H., Rautio, A., Huang, J.-D., Evans, W. E., Idle, J. R. and Gonzalez, F. J. (1995b). A genetic polymorphism in coumarin 7-hydroxylation: sequence of the human CYP2A genes and identification of variant *CYP2A6* alleles. *Am. J. Hum. Genet.*, **57**, 651–660.

Figlewicz, D. A., McInnis, M. G., Goto, J., Haines, J. L., Warren, A. C., Krizus, A., Khodr, N., Brown, R. H., Jr, McKenna-Yasek, D., Antonarakis, S. E. *et al.* (1994). Identification of flanking markers for the familial amyotrophic lateral sclerosis gene *ALS1* on chromosome 21. *J. Neurol. Sci.*, **124**, Suppl, 90–95.

Finuya, H., Fernandez-Salguero, P., Gregory, W., Taber, H., Steward, A., Gonzales, F. J. and Idle, J. (1995). Genetic polymorphism of CYP2C9 and its effect on warfarin maintenance dose requirement in patients undergoing anticoagulation therapy. *Pharmacogenetics*, **5**, 389–392.

Forrest, G. L., Akman, S., Krutzik, S., Paxton, R. J., Sparkes, R. S., Doroshow, J., Felsted, R. L., Glover, C. J., Mohandas, T., Bachur, N. R. (1990). Induction of a human carbonyl reductase gene located on chromosome 21. *Biochim. Biophys. Acta*, **1048**, 149–155.

Fowler, J. S., Volkow, N. D., Wang, G. J., Pappas, N., Logan, J., Macgregor, R., Alexoff, D., Shea, C., Schlyer, D., Wolf,

A. P., Warner, D., Zezulkova, I. and Cilento, R. (1996). Inhibition of monoamine oxidase B in the brains of smokers. *Nature*, **379**, 733–736.

Gilder, F. J., Hodgkinson, S. and Murray, R. M. (1993). ADH and ALDH genotype profiles in Caucasians with alcohol-related problems and controls. *Addiction*, **88**, 383–388.

Gilham, D. E., Cairns, W., Paine, M. J., Modi, S., Poulsom, R., Roberts, G. C. and Wolf, C. R. (1997). Metabolism of MPTP by cytochrome P4502D6 and the demonstration of 2D6 mRNA in human foetal and adult brain by *in situ* hybridisation. *Xenobiotica*, **27**, 111–125.

Goedde, H. W. and Agarwal, D. P. (1992). Pharmacogenetics of aldehyde dehydrogenase. In Kalow, W. (Ed.), *Pharmacogenetics of Drug Metabolism*. Pergamon Press, New York, pp. 281–311.

Goldstein, J. A. and de Morais, S. M. F. (1994). Biochemistry and molecular biology of the human CYP2C subfamily. *Pharmacogenetics*, **4**, 285–299.

Goldstein, J. A., Faletto, M. B., Romkes-Sparks, M., Sullivan, T., Kitareewan, S., Raucy, J. L., Lasker, H. M. and Ghanayem, B. L. (1994). Evidence that CYP2C19 is the major (*S*)-mephenytoin 4′-hydroxylase in humans. *Biochemistry*, **33**, 1743–1752.

Gonzalez, F. J. and Nebert, D. W. (1990). Evolution of the P450 gene superfamily: animal-plant 'warfare', molecular drive and human genetic differences in drug oxidation. *Trends Genet.*, **6**, 182–186.

Gonzalez, F. J., Skoda, R. C., Kimura, S., Umeno, M., Zanger, U. M., Nebert, D. W., Gelboin, H. V., Hardwick, J. P. and Mayer, U. A. (1988). Characterisation of the common genetic defect in humans deficient in debrisoquine metabolism. *Nature*, **331**, 442–446.

Gorrod, J. W. (1993). The mammalian metabolism of nicotine: an overview. In Gorrod, J. W. and Wahren, J. (Eds), *Nicotine and Related Alkaloids. Absorption, Distribution, Metabolism and Excretion*. Chapman and Hall, London, pp. 31–43.

Groppi, A., Begueret J. and Iron, A. (1990). Improved methods for genotype determination of human alcohol dehydrogenase (ADH) at *ADH2* and *ADH3* loci using polymerase chain reaction-directed mutagenesis. *Clin. Chem.*, **36**, 1765–1768.

Grothusen, A., Hardt, J., Brautigam, L., Lang, D and Bocker, R. (1996). A convenient method to discriminate between cytochrome P450 enzymes and flavin-containing mono-oxygenases in human liver microsomes. *Arch. Toxicol.*, **71**, 64–71.

Guo, X., Lerner-Tung, M., Chen, H. X., Chang, C. N., Zhu, J. L., Chang, C. P., Pizzorno, G., Lin, T. S. and Cheng, Y. C. (1995). 5-Fluoro-2-pyrimidinone, a liver aldehyde oxidase-activated prodrug of 5-fluorouracil. *Biochem. Pharmacol.*, **49**, 1111–1116.

Gut, I. and Conney, A. H. (1991). The FAD-containing mono-oxygenase-catalysed *N*-oxidation and demethylation of trimethylamine in rat liver microsomes. *Drug Metab. Drug Interact.*, **9**, 201–208.

Hadidi, A.-H. F. A., Coulter, C. E. A. and Idle, J. R. (1988). Phenotypically deficient urinary elimination of carboxyphosphamide after cyclophosphamide administration to cancer patients. *Cancer Res.*, **48**, 5167–5171.

Hadidi, H. F., Cholerton, S., Atkinson, S., Irshaid, Y. M., Rawashdeh, N. M. and Idle, J. R. (1995). *Br. J. Clin. Pharmacol.*, **39**, 179–181.

Hadidi, H., Zahlsen, K., Idle, J. R. and Cholerton, S. (1997). A single amino acid substitution (Leu160His) in cytochrome P450 CYP2A6 causes switching from 7-hydroxylation to 3-hydroxylation of coumarin. *Food Chem. Toxicol.*, **35**, 903–907.

Hadidi, H., Irshaid, Y., Cholerton, S., Zahlsen, K. and Idle J. R. (1998). Variability of coumarin 7- and 3-hydroxylation in a Jordanian population: first evidence for a functional polymorphism of cytochrome P450 CYP2A6. *Eur. J. Clin. Pharmacol.*, **54**, 437–441.

Hall, M. C. S., Gregory, W. L. and Idle, J. R. (1994). Pharmacogenetics: can the therapeutic key objective be accomplished? In Seymour, C. A. and Weetman, R. A. (Eds.), *Horizons in Medicine*. Vol 5. Blackwell, London, pp. 79–91.

Hammer, W. and Sjöqvist F. (1967). Plasma levels of monomethylated tricyclic antidepressants during treatment with imipramine-like compounds. *Life Sci.*, **6**, 1895–1903.

Hasspieler, B. M., Haffner, G. D. and Adeli, K. (1997). Roles of DT diaphorase in the genotoxicity of nitroaromatic compounds in human and fish cell lines. *J. Toxicol. Environ. Health*, **52**, 137–148.

Helander, A., Walzer, C., Beck, O., Balant, L., Borg, S. and von Wartburg, J. P. (1994). Influence of genetic variation in alcohol and aldehyde dehydrogenase on serotonin metabolism. *Life Sci.*, **55**, 359–366.

Hermann, R. B., Culp, H. W., McMahon, R. E. and Marsh, M. M. (1969). Structure–activity relationships among substrates for a rabbit kidney reductase. Quantum chemical calculation of substituent parameters. *J. Med. Chem.*, **12**, 749–754.

Hetzel, M. R., Law, M., Keele, E. E., Sloan, T. P., Idle J. R. and Smith, R. L. (1980). Is there a genetic component in bronchial carcinoma in smokers? *Thorax*, **35**, 709.

Hildesheim, A., Chen, C.-J., Caporaso, N. E., Chen, Y.-J., Hoover, R. N., Hsu, M.-M., Levine, P. H., Chen, I.-H., Chen, J.-Y., Yang, C.-S., Daly, A. K. and Idle, J. R. (1995). Cytochrome P4502E1 genetic polymorphisms and risk of nasopharygeal carcinoma: results from a case-control study conducted in Taiwan. *Cancer Epidemiol. Biomarkers Prev.*, **4**, 607–610.

Hirao, Y., Kitamura, S. and Tatsumi, K. (1994). Epoxide reductase activity of mammalian liver cytosols and aldehyde oxidase. *Carcinogenesis*, **15**, 739–743.

Hirvonen, A., Husgavel-Pursiainen, K., Anttila, S., Karjalainen, A., Pelkonen, O. and Vainio, H. (1993). PCR-based *CYP2D6* genotyping for Finnish lung cancer patients. *Pharmacogenetics*, **3**, 19–27.

Höfer, C. C. and Idle, J. R. (1996). Oxidative desulfuration of thiotepa to tepa is mediated by CYP2A6 in man and by CYP2E1 in the rat. Abstract. Norwegian Biochemical Society Winter Meeting, Geilo, January, 1996.

Holmes, R. S. (1980). Genetic regulation of alcohol dehydrogenase, aldehyde dehydrogenase and aldehyde oxidase isozymes in the mouse. *Adv. Exp. Med. Biol.*, **132**, 57–66.

Holmes, R. S. (1985). Genetic variants of enzymes of alcohol and aldehyde metabolism. *Alcohol Clin. Exp. Res.*, **9**, 535–538.

Holmes, R. S., Leijten, L. R. and Duley, J. A. (1981). Liver aldehyde oxidase and xanthine oxidase genetics in the mouse. *Anim. Blood Groups Biochem. Genet.*, **12**, 193–199.

Hsu, L. C. and Chang, W. C. (1996). Sequencing and expression of the human ALDH8 encoding a new member of the aldehyde dehydrogenase family. *Gene*, **174**, 319–322.

Hsu, L. C., Chang, W. C., Hiraoka, L. and Hsieh, C. L. (1994a). Molecular cloning, genomic organization, and chromosomal localization of an additional human aldehyde dehydrogenase gene, *ALDH6*. *Genomics*, **24**, 333–341.

Hsu, L. C., Chang, W. C. and Yoshida, A. (1994b). Cloning of a cDNA encoding human *ALDH7*, a new member of the aldehyde dehydrogenase family. *Gene*, **151**, 285–289.

Humbert, J. R., Hammond, K. B., Hathaway, K. E., Marcoux, J. G. and O'Brien, D. (1970). Trimethylaminuria: the fish odour syndrome. *Lancet*, **ii**, 770–771.

Hyndman, D. J., Takenoshita, R., Vera, N. L., Pang, S. C. and Flynn, T. G. (1997). Cloning, sequencing, and enzymic activity of an inducible aldo–keto reductase from Chinese hamster ovary cells. *J. Biol. Chem.*, **272**, 13286–13291.

IARC (1985). *IARC Monographs on the Evaluation of the Carcinogenic Risk of Chemicals to Humans*, Vol. **37**. IARC, Lyon, pp. 209–223.

Ichinose, H., Katoh, S., Sueoka, T., Titani, K., Fujita, K. and Nagatsu, T. (1991). Cloning and sequencing of cDNA encoding human sepiapterin reductase—an enzyme involved in tetrahydrobiopterin biosynthesis. *Biochem. Biophys. Res. Commun.*, **179**, 183–189.

Idle, J. R. (1988) Enigmatic variations, *Nature*, **331**, 391–392.

Itoh, K., Nakamura, K., Kimura, T., Itoh, S. and Kamataki, T. (1997). Molecular cloning of mouse liver flavin-containing monooxygenase (FMO1) cDNA and characterization of the expression product: metabolism of the neurotoxin, 1,2,3,4-tetrahydroisoquinoline (TIQ). *J. Toxicol. Sci.*, **22**, 45–56.

Iwata, N., Inazu, N., Hara, S., Yanase, T., Kano, S., Endo, T., Kuriiwa, F., Sato, Y. and Satoh, T. (1993). Interindividual variability of carbonyl reductase levels in human livers. *Biochem. Pharmacol.*, **45**, 1711–1714.

Jaiswal, A. K. (1991). Human NAD(P)H: quinone oxidoreductase (NQOI) gene structure and induction by dioxin. *Biochemistry*, **30**, 10647–10653.

Jaiswal, A. K. (1994a). Human NAD(P)H:quinone oxidoreductase 2. Gene structure, activity, and tissue-specific expression. *J. Biol. Chem.*, **269**, 14502–14508.

Jaiswal, A. K. (1994b). Jun and Fos regulation of NAD(P)H:-quinone oxidoreductase gene expression. *Pharmacogenetics*, **4**, 1–10.

Jaiswal, A. K., McBride, O. W., Adesnik, M. and Nebert, D. W. (1988). Human dioxin-inducible cytosolic NAD(P)H:quinone oxidoreductase. *J. Biol. Chem.*, **263**, 13572–13578.

Jaiswal, A. K., Burnett, P., Adesnik, M. and McBride, O. W. (1990). Nucleotide and deduced amino acid sequence of a human cDNA (NQO₂) corresponding to a second member of the NAD(P)H:quinone oxidoreductase gene family. Extensive polymorphism at the NQO_2 gene locus on chromosome 6. *Biochemistry*, **29**, 1899–1906.

Jenner, P. (1989). MPTP-induced parkinsonism: the relevance to idiopathic Parkinson's disease. In Quinn, N. P. and Jenner, P. (Eds), *Disorders of Movement. Clinical, Pharmacological and Physiological Aspects*. Academic Press, London, pp. 157–175.

Johnson, M. R., Yan, J., Shao, L., Albin, N. and Diasio, R. B. (1997a) Semi-automated radioassay for determination of dihydropyrimidine dehydrogenase (DPD) activity. Screening cancer patients for DPD deficiency, a condition associated with 5-fluorouracil toxicity. *J. Chromatogr. B*, **696**, 183–191.

Johnson, M. R., Wang, K., Tillmanns, S., Albin, N. and Diasio, R. B. (1997b). Structural organization of the human dihydropyrimidine dehydrogenase gene. *Cancer Res.*, **57**, 1660–1663.

Kato, S., Bowman, E. D., Harrington, A. M., Blomeke, B. and Shields, P. G. (1995). Human lung carcinogen-DNA adduct levels mediated by genetic polymorphisms *in vivo*. *J. Natl. Cancer Inst.*, **87**, 902–907.

Kawaji, A, Ohara, K. and Takabatake, E. (1994). Determination of flavin-containing monooxygenase activity in rat brain microsomes with benzylamine *N*-oxidation. *Biol. Pharm. Bull.*, **17**, 603–606.

Kawaji, A., Miki, T. and Takabatake, E. (1995). Partial purification and substrate specificity of flavin-containing monooxygenase from rat brain microsomes. *Biol. Pharm. Bull.*, **18**, 1657–1659.

Kawaji, A., Isobe, M. and Takabatake, E. (1997). Differences in enzymatic properties of flavin-containing monooxygenase in brain microsomes of rat, mouse, hamster, guinea pig and rabbit. *Biol. Pharm. Bull.*, **20**, 917–919.

Kitamura, S. and Tatsumi, K. (1984). Reduction of tertiary amine *N*-oxides by liver preparations: function of aldehyde oxidase as a major *N*-oxide reductase. *Biochem. Biophys. Res. Commun.*, **121**, 749–754.

Kuehl, B. L., Paterson, J. W. E., Peacock, J. W., Paterson, M. C. and Rauth, A. M. (1995). Presence of a heterozygous substitution and its relationship to DT-diaphorase activity. *Br. J. Cancer*, **72**, 555–561.

Küpfer, A., Desmond, P., Schenker, S. and Branch, R. A. (1979). Family study of a genetically determined deficiency of mephenytoin hydroxylation in man. *Pharmacologist*, **21**, 173.

Lake, B. G. (1984). Investigations into the mechanisms of coumarin-induced hepatotoxicity in the rat. *Arch. Toxicol.*, Suppl 7, 16–29.

Lake, B. G., Gaudin, H., Price, R. J. and Walters, D. G. (1992). Metabolism of (3-¹⁴C)coumarin to polar and covalently bound products by hepatic microsomes from the rat, Syrian hamster, gerbil and humans. *Food Chem. Toxicol.*, **30**, 105–115.

Langston, J. W., Ballard, P., Tetrud, J. W. and Irwin, I. (1983). Chronic Parkinsonism in humans due to a product of meperidine-analog synthesis. *Science*, **219**, 979–980.

Lawton, M. P., Cashman, J. R., Crestiel, T., Dolphin, C. T., Elfarra, A. A., Hines, R. N., Hodgson, E., Kimura, T., Ozols, J., Phillips, I. R., Philpot, R. M., Poulsen, L. L., Rettie, A. E., Shephard, E. A., Williams, D. E. and Ziegler, D. M. (1994). A nomenclature for the mammalian flavin-containing monooxygenase gene family based on amino acid sequence identities. *Arch. Biochem. Biophys.*, **308**, 254–257.

Lee, D. C., Gonzalez, P., Rao, P. V., Zigler, J. S. Jr. and Wistow, G. J. (1993). Carbonyl-metabolising enzymes and their relatives recruited as structural proteins in the eye lens. *Adv. Exp. Med. Biol.*, **328**, 159–168.

Legrand, M., Stucker, I., Marez, D., Sabbagh, N., Lo-Guidice, J. M. and Broly, F. (1996). Influence of a mutation reducing the catalytic activity of the cytochrome P450 CYP2D6 on lung cancer susceptibility. *Carcinogenesis*, **17**, 2267–2269.

Lessard, E., Fortin, A., Belanger, P. M., Beaune, P., Hamelin, B. A. and Turgeon, J. (1997). Role of CYP2D6 in the *N*-hydroxylation of procainamide. *Pharmacogenetics*, **7**, 381–390.

Lind, C., Cadenas, E., Hochstein, P. and Ernster, L. (1990). DT-diaphorase: purification, properties and function. *Methods Enzymol.*, **186**, 287–301.

London, S. J., Daly, A. K., Leathart, J. B., Navidi, W. C., Carpenter, C. C. and Idle, J. R. (1997). Genetic polymorphism of CYP2D6 and lung cancer risk in African-Americans and Caucasians in Los Angeles County. *Carcinogenesis*, **18**, 1203–1214.

Lu, S. F., Pan, F. M. and Chiou, S. H. (1995). Sequence analysis of frog rho-crystallin by cDNA cloning and sequencing: a member of the aldo–keto reductase family. *Biochem. Biophys. Res. Commun.*, **214**, 1079–1088.

Luu, S. U., Wang, M. F., Lin, D. L., Kao, M. H., Chen, M. L., Chiang, C. H., Pai, L. and Yin, S. J. (1995). Ethanol and acetaldehyde metabolism in Chinese with different aldehyde dehydrogenase-2 genotypes. *Proc. Natl. Sci. Counc. Repub. China B*, **19**, 129–136.

Mahgoub, A., Idle, J. R., Dring, L. G., Lancaster, R. and Smith, R. L. (1977). Polymorphic hydroxylation of debrisoquine in man. *Lancet*, **ii**, 584–586.

Martínez, C., Agúndez, J. A. G., Gervasine, G., Martín, R. and Benítez, J. (1997) Tryptamine: a possible endogenous substrate for CYP2D6. *Pharmacogenetics*, **7**, 85–93.

Maschke, S., Wahl, A., Azaroual, N., Boulet, O., Crunelle, V., Imbenotte, M., Foulard, M., Vermeersch, G. and Lhermitte, M. (1997). H-NMR analysis of trimethylamine in urine for the diagnosis of fish-odour syndrome. *Clin. Chim. Acta*, **263**, 139–146.

Mather, P. B., Duley, J. A. and Holmes, R. S. (1983). Aldehyde oxidase and alcohol dehydrogenase genetics in the mouse. New alleles for *Aox-2* and *Adh-3* loci. *Anim. Blood Groups Biochem. Genet.*, **14**, 279–286.

McMahon, R. E., Marshall, F. J. and Culp, H. W. (1965). The nature of the metabolites of acetohexamide in the rat and in the human. *J. Pharmacol. Exp. Ther.*, **149**, 272–279.

McMurrough, J. and McLeod, H. L. (1996). Analysis of the dihydropyrimidine dehydrogenase polymorphism in a British population. *Br. J. Clin. Pharmacol.*, **41**, 425–427.

Meinsma, R., Fernandez-Salguero, P., van Kuilenburg, A. B., van Gennip, A. H. and Gonzalez, F. J. (1995). Human polymorphism in drug metabolism: mutation in the dihydropyrimidine dehydrogenase gene results in exon skipping and thymine uraciluria. *DNA Cell Biol.*, **14**, 1–6.

Messina, E. S., Tyndale, R. and Sellers, E. M. (1997). A major role for CYP2A6 in nicotine *C*-oxidation by human liver microsomes. *J. Pharmacol. Exp. Ther.*, **282**, 1608–1614.

Mikami, K., Naito, M., Tomida, A., Yamada, M., Sirakusa, T. and Tsuruo, T. (1996). DT-diaphorase as a critical determinant of sensitivity to mitomycin C in human colon and gastric carcinoma cell lines. *Cancer Res.*, **56**, 2823–2826.

Milano, G. and Etienne, M. C. (1994). Dihydropyrimidine dehydrogenase (DPD) and clinical pharmacology of 5-fluorouracil (review). *Anticancer Res.*, **14**, 2295–2297.

Milano, G. and Etienne, M. C. (1996). Individualizing therapy with 5-fluorouracil related to dihydropyrimidine dehydrogenase: theory and limits. *Ther. Drug Monit.*, **18**, 335–340.

Mira, L., Maia, L., Barreira, L. and Manso, C. F. (1995). Evidence for free radical generation due to NADH oxidation by aldehyde oxidase during ethanol metabolism. *Arch. Biochem. Biophys.*, **318**, 53–58.

Miura, R., Shiota, K., Noda, K., Yagi, S., Ogawa, T. and Takahashi, M. (1994). Molecular cloning of cDNA for rat ovarian 20 alpha-hydroxysteroid dehydrogenase (HSD1). *Biochem. J.*, **299**, 561–567.

Monks, T. J., Hanzlik, R. P., Cohen, G. M., Ross, D. and Graham, D. G. (1992). Quinone chemistry and toxicity. *Toxicol. Appl. Pharmacol.*, **112**, 2–16.

Moreb, J., Schweder, M., Suresh, A. and Zucali, J. R. (1996). Overexpression of the human aldehyde dehydrogenase class I results in increased resistance to 4-hydroperoxycyclophosphamide. *Cancer Gene Ther.*, **3**, 24–30.

Moriwaki, Y., Yamamoto, T., Yamaguchi, K., Takahashi, S. and Higashino, K. (1996). Immunohistochemical localization of aldehyde and xanthine oxidase in rat tissues using polyclonal antibodies. *Histochem. Cell Biol.*, **105**, 71–79.

Morrison, G. B., Bastian, A., Dela Rosa, T., Diasio, R. B. and Takimoto, C. H. (1997). Dihydropyrimidine dehydrogenase deficiency: a pharmacogenetic defect causing severe adverse reactions to 5-fluorouracil-based chemotherapy. *Oncol. Nurs. Forum*, **24**, 83–88.

Mortimer, P. S. (1997) Therapy approaches for lymphedema. *Angiography*, **48**, 87–91.

Nakanishi, M., Deyashiki, Y., Nakayama, T., Sato, K. and Hara, A. (1993). Cloning and sequence analysis of a cDNA encoding tetrameric carbonyl reductase of pig lung. *Biochem. Biophys. Res. Commun.*, **194**, 1311–1316.

Nakanishi, M., Deyashiki, Y., Ohshima, K. and Hara, A. (1995). Cloning, expression and tissue distribution of mouse tetrameric carbonyl reductase. Identity with an adipocyte 27-kDa protein. *Eur. J. Biochem.*, **228**, 381–387.

Negoro, M., Hatake, K., Taniguchi, T., Ouchi, H., Minami, T. and Hishida, S. (1997). Liver cytosolic aldehyde dehydrogenase (ALDH1) polymorphism and its inheritance in Wistar rats. *Nihon Arukoru Yakubutsu Igakkai Zasshi*, **32**, 182–188.

Nelson, D. R. (1997). http://drnelson.utmem.edu/genesperspecies.html

Nelson, D. R., Koymans L., Kamataki, T., Stegeman, J. J., Feyereisen, R., Waxman D. J., Waterman M. R., Gotoh, O., Coon, M. J., Estabrook, R. W., Gunsalus I. C. and Nebert, D. W. (1996). P450 superfamily: update on new sequences, gene mapping, accession numbers and nomenclature. *Pharmacogenetics*, **6**, 1–42.

Ohshima, H. and Kawabata, T. (1978). Mechanism of *N*-nitrosodimethylamine formation from trimethylamine and trimethylaminoxide. *IARC Sci. Pub.*, **19**, 143–153.

Parkin, K. L. and Hultin, H. O. (1982). Fish muscle microsomes catalyze the conversion of trimethylamine oxide to dimethylamine and formaldehyde. *FEBS Lett.*, **139**, 61–64.

Pearson, A. W. and Butler, E. J. (1983). Effects of selective breeding and age on the ability of the domestic fowl (*Gallus domesticus*) to oxidise trimethylamine. *Comp. Biochem. Physiol. C*, **76**, 67–74.

Pearson, A. W., Butler, E. J., Curtis, R. F., Fenwick, G. R., Hobson-Frohock, A., Land, D. G. and Hall, S. A. (1978). Effects of rapeseed meal on laying hens (*Gallus domesticus*) in relation to fatty liver-haemorrhagic syndrome and egg taint. *Res. Vet. Sci.*, **25**, 307–313.

Phillips, I. R., Dolphin, C. T., Clair, P., Hadley, M. R., Hutt, A. J., McCombie, R. R., Smith, R. L. and Shephard, E. A. (1995). The molecular biology of the flavin-containing monooxygenases of man. *Chem.–Biol. Interact.*, **96**, 17–32.

Price Evans, D. A. (1993). *Genetic Factors in Drug Therapy*. Cambridge University Press, Cambridge.

Rady-Pentek, P., Mueller, R., Tang, B. K. and Kalow, W. (1997). Interindividual variation in the enzymatic 15-keto-reduction of 13, 14-dihydro-15-keto-prostaglandin E1 in human liver and in human erythrocytes. *Eur. J. Clin Pharmacol.*, **52**, 147–153.

Rashidi, M. R., Smith, J. A., Clarke, S. E. and Beedham, C. (1997). *In vitro* oxidation of famciclovir and 6-deoxypenciclovir by aldehyde oxidase from human, guinea pig, rabbit, and rat liver. *Drug Metab. Dispos.*, **25**, 805–813.

Rautio, A., Kraul, H., Kojo, A., Salmela, E. and Pelkonen, O. (1992). Individual variability of coumarin 7-hydroxylation in healthy volunteers. *Pharmacogenetics*, **2**, 227–233.

Rettie, A. E., Wienkers, L. C., Gonzalez, F. J., Trager, W. F. and Korzekwa, K. R. (1994). Impaired (*S*)-warfarin metabolism catalysed by the R144C allelic variant of *CYP2C9*. *Pharmacogenetics*, **4**, 39–42.

Ripp, S. L., Overby, L. H., Philpot, R. M. and Elfarra, A. A. (1997). Oxidation of cysteine *S*-conjugates by rabbit liver microsomes and cDNA-expressed flavin-containing monooxygenases: studies with *S*-(1,2-dichlorovinyl)-L-cysteine, *S*-(1,2,2-trichlorovinyl)-L-cysteine, *S*-allyl-L-cysteine, and *S*-benzyl-L-cysteine. *Mol. Pharmaol.*, **51**, 507–515.

Robertson, J. A., Chen, H. C. and Nebert, D. W. (1986). NAD(P)H:menadione oxidoreductase: novel purification of enzyme, cDNA and complete amino acid sequence and gene regulation. *J. Biol. Chem.*, **261**, 15794–15799.

Roots, I., Drakoulis, N., Ploch, M., Heinemeyer, G., Loddenkemper, R., Minks, T., Nitz, M., Otte, F. and Koch, M. (1988) Debrisoquine hydroxylation phenotype, acetylation phenotype, and ABO blood groups as genetic host factors of lung cancer. *Klin. Wochenschr.*, **66**, Suppl. 11, 87–97.

Rosen, D. R., Siddique, T., Patterson, D., Figlewicz, D. A., Sapp, P., Hentati, A., Donaldson, D., Goto, J., O'Regan, J. P., Deng, H. X. *et al.*, (1993). Mutations in Cu/Zn superoxide dismutase gene are associated with familial amyotrophic lateral sclerosis. *Nature*, **362**, 59–62.

Ross, D. (1996). Metabolic basis of benzene toxicity. *Eur. J. Haematol.*, **60**, Suppl., 111–118.

Rosvold, E. A., McGlynn, K. A., Lustbader, E. D. Buetow, K. H. (1995). Identification of an NAD(P)H:quinone oxidoreductase polymorphism and its association with lung cancer and smoking. *Pharmacogenetics*, **5**, 199–206.

Rothman, N., Smith, M. T., Hayes, R. B., Traver, R. D., Hoener, B., Campleman, S., Li, G. L., Dosemeci, M., Linet, M., Zhang, L., Xi, L., Wacholder, S., Lu, W., Meyer, K. B., Titenko-Holland, N., Stuart, J. T., Yin, S. and Ross, D. (1997). Benzene poisoning, a risk factor for haematological malignancy, is associated with the NQO1 609C→T mutation and rapid fractional excretion of chlorzoxazone. *Cancer Res.*, **57**, 2839–2842.

Sardas, S., Akyol, D., Green, R. L., Mellon, T., Gokmen, O. and Cholerton, S. (1996). Trimethylamine *N*-oxidation in Turkish women with bacterial vaginosis. *Pharmacogenetics*, **6**, 459–463.

Satre, M. A., Zgombic-Knight, M. and Duester, G. (1994). The complete structure of human class IV alcohol dehydrogenase (retinol dehydrogenase) determined from the *ADH7* gene. *J. Biol. Chem.*, **269**, 15606–15612.

Schulz, W. A., Krummeck, A., Rösinger, I., Eickelmann, P., Neuhaus, C., Ebert, T., Schmitz-Dräger, B. J. and Sies, H. (1997). Increased frequency of a null allele for NAD(P)H:-quinone oxidoreductase in patients with urological malignancies. *Pharmacogenetics*, **7**, 235–239.

Scott, J. and Poffenbarger, P. L. (1979). Pharmacogenetics of tolbutamide metabolism in humans. *Diabetes*, **28**, 41–51.

Sekimoto, H., Seo, M., Dohmae, N., Takio, K., Kamiya, Y. and Koshiba, T. (1997). Cloning and molecular characterization of plant aldehyde oxidase. *J. Biol. Chem.*, **272**, 15280–15285.

Shaw, G. L., Weiffenbach, B., Falk, R. T., Frame, J. N., Issaq, H. J., Moir, D. T. and Caporaso, N. (1997). Frequency of the variant allele *CYP2D6(C)* among North American Caucasian lung cancer patients and controls. *Lung Cancer*, **17**, 61–68.

Shaw, P. M., Reiss, A., Adesnik, M., Nebert, D. W., Schembri, J. and Jaiswal, A. K. (1991). The human dioxin-inducible NAD(P)H:quinone oxidoreductase cDNA-encoded protein expressed in COSI Cells is identical to diaphorase 4. *Eur. J. Biochem.*, **195**, 171–176.

Siddique, T. and Hentati, A. (1995). Familial amyotrophic lateral sclerosis. *Clin. Neurosci.*, **3**, 338–347.

Smith, C. A., Gough, A. C., Leigh, P. N., Summers, B. A., Harding, A. E., Maraganore, D. M., Sturman, S. G., Shapira, A. H., Williams, A. C., Wolf, C. R. (1992). Debrisoquine hydroxylase gene polymorphism and susceptibility to Parkinson's disease. *Lancet*, **339**, 1375–1377.

Steward, D. J., Haining, R. L., Henne, K. R., Davis, G., Rushmore, T. H., Trager, W. F. and Rettie, A. E. (1997). Genetic association between sensitivity to warfarin and expression of *CYP2C9*3*. *Pharmacogenetics*, 7, 361–367.

Stoddart, A. M. and Levine, W. G. (1992). Azoreductase activity by purified rabbit liver aldehyde oxidase. *Biochem. Pharmacol.*, **43**, 2227–2235.

Stoewsand, G. S. (1995). Bioactive organosulfur phytochemicals in *Brassica oleracea* vegetables—a review. *Food Chem. Toxicol.*, **33**, 537–543.

Strassman, R. J., Qualls, C. R., Uhlenhuth, E. H. and Kellner, R. (1994). Dose–response study of *N*, *N*-dimethyltryptamine in humans. II. Subjective effects and preliminary results of a new rating scale. *Arch. Gen. Psychiatry*, **51**, 98–108.

Stucker, I., Cosme, J., Laurent, P., Cenee, S., Beaune, P., Bignon, J., Depierre, A., Milleron, B. and Hemon, D. (1995). *CYP2D6* genotype and lung cancer risk according to histologic type and tobacco exposure. *Carcinogenesis*, **16**, 2759–2764.

Sugihara, K., Kitamura, S. and Tatsumi, K. (1995). Strain differences of liver aldehyde oxidase activity in rats. *Biochem. Mol. Biol. Int.*, **37**, 861–869.

Suzuki, K., Uchida, A., Mizoi, Y. and Fukunaga, T. (1994). A study on *ADH2* and *ALDH2* genotyping by PCR-RFLP and SSCP analyses with description of allele and genotype frequencies in Japanese, Finn and Lapp populations. *Alcohol Alcoholism*, **29**, Suppl. 1, 21–27.

Tanaka, M., Ohno, S., Adachi, S., Nakajin, S., Shinoda, M. and Nagahama, Y. (1992). Pig testicular 20 beta-hydroxysteroid dehydrogenase exhibits carbonyl reductase-like structure and activity. cDNA cloning of pig testicular 20 beta-hydroxysteroid dehydrogenase. *J. Biol. Chem.*, **267**, 13451–13455.

Tasso, M. J., Boddy, A. V., Price, L., Wyllie, R. A., Pearson, A. D. J. and Idle, J. R. (1992). Pharmacokinetics and metabolism of cyclophosphamide in paediatric patients. *Cancer Chemother. Pharmacol.*, **30**, 207–211.

Tefre, T., Daly, A. K., Armstrong, M., Leathart, J. B., Idle, J. R., Brøgger A. and Børresen, A. L. (1994). Genotyping of the *CYP2D6* gene in Norwegian lung cancer patients and controls. *Pharmacogenetics*, **4**, 47–57.

Thomasson, H. R., Edenberg, H. J., Crabb, D. W., Mai, X. L., Jerome, R. E., Li, T. K., Wang, S. P., Lin, Y. T., Lu, R. B. and

Yin, S. J. (1991). Alcohol and aldehyde dehydrogenase genotypes and alcoholism in Chinese men. *Am. J. Hum. Genet.*, **48**, 677–681.

Traver, R. D., Horikoshi, T., Danenberg, K. D., Stadlbauer, T. H., Danenberg, P. V., Ross, D. and Gibson, N. W. (1992). NAD(P)H:quinone oxidoreductase gene expression in human colon carcinoma cells: characterization of a mutation which modulates DT-diaphorase activity and mitomycin sensitivity. *Cancer Res*, **52** (4), 797–802.

Traver, R. D., Siegel, D., Beall, H. D., Phillips, R. M., Gibson, N. W., Franklin, W. A. and Ross, D. (1997). Characterization of a polymorphism in NAD(P)H:quinone oxidoreductase (DT-diaphorase). *Br. J. Cancer*, **75**, 69–75.

Tu, G. C. and Israel, Y. (1993). A new approach for the rapid detection of common and atypical aldehyde dehydrogenase alleles. *Eur. J. Clin. Chem. Clin. Biochem.*, **31**, 591–594.

Tuchman, M., Stoeckeler, J. S., Kiang, D. T., O'Dea, R. F., Ramnaraine, M. L. and Mirkin, B. L. (1985). Familial pyrimidinemia and pyrimidinuria associated with severe fluorouracil toxicity. *N. Engl. J. Med.*, **313**, 245–249.

van Kuilenburg, A. B., van Lenthe, H., Wanders, R. J. and van Gennip, A. H. (1997). Subcellular localization of dihydropyrimidine dehydrogenase. *Biol. Chem.*, **378**, 1047–1053.

von Wartburg, J. P. (1980). Alcohol metabolism and alcoholism—pharmacogenetic considerations. *Acta Psychiatr. Scand.*, **286**, 179–188.

Vreken, P., van Kuilenburg, A. B., Meinsma, R. and van Gennip, A. H. (1997). Dihydropyrimidine dehydrogenase (DPD) deficiency: identification and expression of missense mutations C29R, R886H and R235W. *Hum. Genet.*, **101**, 333–338.

Wall, T. L., Garcia-Andrade, C., Thomasson, H. R., Carr, L. G. and Ehlers, C. L. (1997). Alcohol dehydrogenase polymorphisms in Native Americans: identification of the *ADH2*3* allele. *Alcohol Alcoholism*, **32**, 129–132.

Watanabe, K., Fujii, Y., Ohkubo, H., Kuramitsu, S., Kagamiyama, H., Nakanishi, S. and Hayaishi, O. (1991). Expression of bovine lung prostaglandin F synthase in *Escherichia coli*. *Biochem. Biophys. Res. Commun.*, **181**, 272–278.

Weber, W. W. (1997). *Pharmacogenetics*. Oxford University Press, New York.

Wei, X., McLeod, H. L., McMurrough, J., Gonzalez, F. J. and Fernandez-Salguero, P. (1996). Molecular basis of the human dihydropyrimidine dehydrogenase deficiency and 5-fluorouracil toxicity. *J. Clin. Invest.*, **98**, 610–615.

Wermuth, B., Bohren, K. M., Heinemann, G., von Wartburg, J. P. and Gabbay, K. H. (1988). Human carbonyl reductase. Nucleotide sequence analysis of a cDNA and amino acid sequence of the encoded protein. *J. Biol. Chem.*, **263**, 16185–16188.

Weston, A., Caporaso, N. E., Taghizadeh, K., Hoover, R. N., Tannenbaum, S. R., Skipper, P. L., Resau, J. H., Trump, B. F. and Harris, C. C. (1991). Measurement of 4-aminobiphenyl–hemoglobin adducts in lung cancer cases and controls. *Cancer Res.*, **51**, 5219–5223.

Wienke, J. K., Spitz, M. R., McMillan, A. and Kelsey, K. T. (1997). Lung cancer in Mexican-Americans and African-Americans is associated with the wild-type genotype of the NAD(P)H:quinone oxidoreductase polymorphism. *Cancer Epidemiol. Biomarkers Prev.*, **6**, 87–92.

Wilkinson, G. R., Guengerich, F. P. and Branch, R. A. (1992). Genetic polymorphism of *S*-mephenytoin hydroxylation. In Kalow, W. (ed.), *Pharmacogenetics of Drug Metabolism*. Pergamon Press, New York, pp. 657–685.

Williams, J. B., Lu, A. Y. H., Cameron, R. G. and Pickett, C. B. (1986). Rat liver NAD(P):quinone reductase. *J. Biol. Chem.*, **261**, 5524–5528.

Williams, R. T. (1959). *Detoxication Mechanisms*, 2nd edn. Chapman and Hall, London.

Wolf, C. R., Smith, C. A., Gough, A. C., Moss, J. E., Vallis, K. A., Howard, G., Carey, F. J., Mills, K., McNee, W., Carmichael, J. *et al.* (1992), Relationship between the debrisoquine hydroxylase polymorphism and cancer susceptibility. *Carcinogenesis*, **13**, 1035–1038.

Wong, J. M., Kalow, W., Kadar, D., Takamatsu, Y. and Inaba, T. (1993). Carbonyl (phenone) reductase in human liver: interindividual variability. *Pharmacogenetics*, **3**, 110–115.

Wrighton, S. A., Stevens, J. C., Becker, B. W. and Vanden-Branden, M. (1993). Isolation and characterization of human liver cytochrome P450 2C19: correlation between 2C19 and *S*-mephenytoin 4′-hydroxylation. *Arch. Biochem. Biophys.*, **306**, 240–245.

Wu, D., Otton, S. V., Inaba, T., Kalow, W. and Sellers, E. M. (1997). Interactions of amphetamine analogs with human liver CYP2D6. *Biochem. Pharmacol.*, **53**, 1605–1612.

Wu, K., Knox, R., Sun, X. Z., Joseph, P., Jaiswal, A. K., Zhang, D., Deng, P. S. and Chen, S. (1997). Catalytic properties of NAD(P)H:quinone oxidoreductase-2 (NQO2), a dihydronicotinamide riboside dependent oxidoreductase. *Arch. Biochem. Biophys.*, **347**, 221–228.

Yamano, S., Tatsuno, J. and Gonzalez, F. J. (1990). The *CYP2A3* gene catalyses coumarin 7-hydroxylation in human liver microsomes. *Biochemistry*, **29**, 1322–1329.

Yamauchi, M., Maezawa, Y., Mizuhara, Y., Ohata, M., Hirakawa, J., Nakajima, H. and Toda, G. (1995). Polymorphisms in alcohol metabolizing enzyme genes and alcoholic cirrhosis in Japanese patients: a mutivariate analysis. *Hepatology*, **22**, 1136–1142.

Yasunami, M., Chen, C. S. and Yoshida, A. (1991). A human alcohol dehydrogenase gene (ADH6) encoding an additional class of enzyme. *Proc. Natl. Acad. Sci. USA*, **88**, 7610–7614.

Yokoyama, H., Baraona, E. and Lieber, C. S. (1994). Molecular cloning of human class IV alcohol dehydrogenase cDNA. *Biochem. Biophys. Res. Commun.*, **203**, 219–224.

Yokoyama, H., Baraona, E. and Lieber, C. S. (1995). Comparison of *ADH7* gene structure in Caucasian and Japanese subjects. *Biochem. Biophys. Res. Commun.*, **212**, 875–878.

Yoshida, A. (1994). Genetic polymorphisms of alcohol metabolizing enzymes related to alcohol sensitivity and alcoholic diseases. *Alcohol Alcoholism*, **29**, 693–696.

Yoshida, A. and Chen, S. H. (1989). Restriction fragment length polymorphism of human aldehyde dehydrogenase 1 and aldehyde dehydrogenase 2 loci. *Hum. Genet.*, **83**, 204.

Yoshihara, S. and Tatsumi, K. (1990). Metabolism of diphenyl sulfoxide in perfused guinea pig liver. Involvement of aldehyde oxidase as a sulfoxide reductase. *Drug Metab. Dispos.*, **18**, 876–881.

Zhang, A. Q., Mitchell, S. C. and Smith, R. L. (1996). Exacerbation of symptoms of fish-odour syndrome during menstruation. *Lancet*, **348**, 1740–1741.

Ziegler, D. M. (1993). Recent studies on the structure and function of multisubstrate flavin-containing monooxygenases. *Annu. Rev. Biochem. Toxicol.*, **33**, 179–199.

Chapter 11
Circadian Toxicology

Patricia A. Wood, David W. Lincoln, II, Imran Imam and William J. M. Hrushesky

C O N T E N T S

INTRODUCTION

Biological Rhythms

Endogenous biological rhythms are those rhythms that exist even in situations where the organism is isolated from all zeitgebers (time-givers), such as sunlight, timing of meals and other inputs. The existence of these rhythms has been demonstrated in experiments in which people were carefully observed during summer time in the arctic, or in specialized temporal isolation units, or were required to stay awake for 24 h and to eat a constant snack every hour (Arendt et al., 1989). There are three general categories of endogenous biological rhythms; ultradian frequency (less than 24 h), circadian rhythms (approximately 20–28 h), and those with infradian frequency (longer than 24 h).

The biological rhythms most commonly studied are the circadian rhythms. These rhythms are about 24 h in duration. The basis for the circadian clock is genetic in nature and is then continually modified, within certain limits, by environmental input. Circadian rhythms, which confer stability, exist amongst all creatures in the plant and animal kingdoms and in the natural environment and they are continuously reinforced by cyclical, about 24 h, changes in all aspects of the environment. All events of cellular action and organismic physiology are tightly organized within each day. Circadian rhythms prominently affect drug toxicity through the temporal organization of drug pharmacokinetics, including drug absorption, distribution, metabolism, excretion, and by the temporal organization of tissue susceptibility patterns (circadian chronopharmacodynamics) (**Figure 1**). Circadian organization of processes affecting all aspects of toxicology is the focus of this chapter. This review will be limited to the circadian frequency owing to the large amount of research done on circadian rhythms as com-

pared with the other biological rhythms. Other rhythms do, however, exist of lower and higher frequencies and have additional predictable toxicological effects.

Potentially relevant ultradian rhythms include brain electroencepholographic activity (EEG), heart and respiratory rates, rhythm in blood pressure, rapid eye movements of sleep (REM), and pulsatile secretion of hormones. Infradian rhythms of note include circaseptan rhythms, which are usually about 7 (5–10) days in length and have been demonstrated in unicellular organisms, insects, rodents and humans. Menstrual cycles are usually about 28 (20–36) days in duration and originate from a rhythmic pattern of the brain hypothalamus and various hormones that determine relative fertility by temporally organizing the ovarian cycles of mammals. Interestingly, another term, circatrigintan (30 days) or circavigintan (20 days), may be technically more appropriately used since rhythms of these durations have been shown to exist in other biological aspects in males and pre-and post-menopausal women (Haus and Touitou, 1992). Finally, circannual or seasonal rhythms are composed of about year-long rhythms. These rhythms have not been studied as extensively because of the time it takes to complete such experiments. Some interesting data have nonetheless emerged. For example, seasonal patterns of detection and death from breast cancer that differ between pre- and post-menopausal women are provocative. Prominent seasonal availability of xenobiotic and even industrial toxicants gives one pause to dismiss seasonal toxicology. This topic, however, must be left for another time.

Importance of Biological Rhythms

Biological rhythms are toxicologically important because they have a positive or negative effect upon all measures of normal physiological function and health of the individual. Problems associated with the circadian clock 'getting out of phase' with the environment include symptoms of jet lag, and those invariably associated with shift work. For example, someone working a night shift might be more susceptible to occupational toxin-associated asthma or respiratory problems since the lungs are more vulnerable to bronchospasm at night. In addition, another potentially important consequence of the existence of biological rhythms is the time of day variant damage to normal tissue resulting from drug exposure. Most drugs and toxins properly studied have demonstrated circadian stage-dependent toxicities. These circadian toxicological differences may be irrelevant for drugs with large therapeutic indices, but they are relevant for all drugs with less than perfect toxic–therapeutic ratios. Therefore, specific drugs given at one time of the day will be reproducibly more toxic than if they are given at another time of the day. This knowledge has led to the discovery of new therapeutic approaches based upon optimal drug timing within the day (chronotherapy).

This chapter focuses upon how circadian rhythms affect the mechanisms responsible for drug toxicity and efficacy, as well as adverse outcome from environmental toxins, in addition to describing different classes of drugs and toxins that exhibit circadian toxicity patterns. For ease of comparison among different types of studies and animal models, and for greater clarity of translation of rodent findings to those in humans, time of day (circadian time) is referenced to the sleep or activity phases of the host rather than light and dark or day and night. This serves to eliminate confusion that otherwise invariably arises, since some of the experimental animal models (e.g. rodents) are nocturnally active and others (e.g. humans) are diurnally active. Extreme care must be taken when reading the literature since many of the original rodent studies refer to certain results in the 'night' or the time of darkness for human beings, which is actually the activity phase of the rodent.

MECHANISMS BY WHICH CIRCADIAN RHYTHMS AFFECT TOXICOLOGY

Circadian Toxin Availability or Exposure

Circadian differences in the availability, and hence exposure, to different levels of toxins and carcinogens can play a major role in generating a time of day dependence to toxicological outcome. Examples include daily variations in ultraviolet light, radon concentrations, airborne particulates and other toxins. These are discussed below under specific toxin classes. This diurnal exposure rhythm may be entirely responsible for circadian toxicology or this may then add to the two other general cate-

gories of mechanisms responsible for circadian toxicology rhythms. These include daily rhythms in toxin metabolism and resultant circadian pharmacokinetics, and toxin tissue susceptibility and resultant circadian pharmacodynamics.

Circadian Pharmacokinetics

Circadian pharmacokinetics is the study of the daily rhythms in drug pharmacokinetics generated by the differential absorption, distribution, metabolism and excretion of drugs as a function of the time within the circadian cycle the drug is administered. The importance of these rhythms is supported by a large body of data for plants, insects, animals and humans for a wide variety of drugs and toxins. Factors such as the daily rhythms in organ blood flow and function, as well as rhythms in the activities of specific metabolic pathways, are major determinants of the circadian pharmacokinetics for each individual drug or toxin.

Absorption

Circadian patterns of drug/toxin absorption result from a combination of circadian differences in cutaneous gastric and intestinal physiology. Therefore, circadian patterns in gastro-intestinal pH, motility, digestive secretions, intestinal blood flow and membrane permeability each cause non-trivial and reproducible circadian variation in drug absorption (Bruguerolle, 1992). Clinical and experimental studies have shown that drug absorption is dependent upon the time of day of administration. Other exogenous factors such as food intake, posture (affects blood flow) and galenic (construction of pill) considerations must also be taken into account since they each affect drug absorption. Blood flow, for example, is rate limiting to drug diffusion. When food is present, drugs pass more quickly through the membranes, probably because the lipophilic drugs may be absorbed more readily in the presence of fatty foods. In studies with slow-release forms of theophylline, large circadian changes in its absorption occur for different galenic formulations (Smolensky, 1989). However, when these three factors are controlled, a circadian variation still remains in the absorption of many drugs which indicates that the efficiency of absorption of drugs still has an endogenous circadian component.

For example, in studies done in man, where the effects of posture and food were controlled, lorazepam and triazolam were found to be more quickly absorbed in the morning (Bruguerolle et al., 1984; Smith et al., 1986). Similar results were found for propranolol absorption (Langner and Lemmer, 1988). Lipophilic drugs tend to be absorbed faster in the morning than in the evening. From studies in mice with acetaminophen (paracetamol),

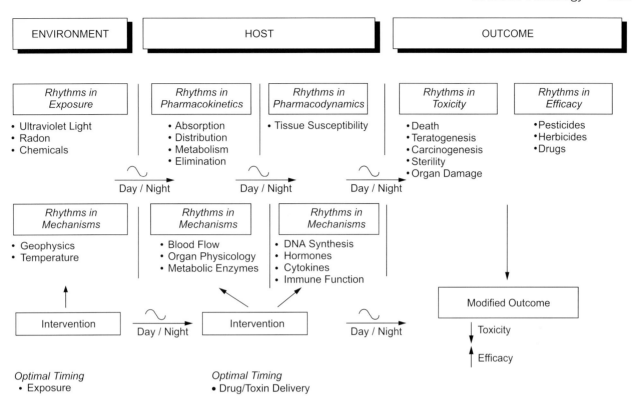

Figure 1 Impact of circadian rhythms upon the outcome from toxin or drug exposure. Circadian rhythms in the environment and in the host can result in a time of day dependence of toxicity and efficacy. Environmental circadian rhythms in toxin availability or exposure to various agents occur as a result of geophysical and temperature cycles. Host circadian rhythms in toxin or drug pharmacokinetics and pharmacodynamics each contribute to time of day-dependent outcome resulting from the underlying circadian coordination of tissue function as listed. The final outcome is a circadian variation (50%–10-fold) in toxicity and efficacy. Opportunities to intervene or utilize this time structure are also shown. By using optimal circadian timing of exposure and/or drug or toxin delivery, toxicity can be reduced and efficacy often improved. This approach is especially advantageous for agents with narrow toxic–therapeutic ratios and important to the economics of utilizing less of an expensive chemical or drug for the same desired effect.

antipyrine, furosemide (frusemide), hydrochlorothiazide, indomethacin and phenylbutazone, it was concluded that circadian variations in the absorption of these drugs depend greatly upon their solubility (Belanger *et al.*, 1981). Water-soluble drugs, such as antipyrine, did not show a large circadian absorption variation. However, drugs that were lipid soluble showed a circadian variation, being more rapidly absorbed at the beginning of the daily activity span. In another study with carbamazepine, it was found that circadian variations in absorption remain even when the effect of intake of food is controlled (Bruguerolle *et al.*, 1981). A clinical study of childhood acute lymphocytic leukaemia found the durations of disease remission and the likelihood of survival were each significantly greater when oral maintenance chemotherapy with 6-mercaptopurine (6-MP) was administered in the evening hours rather than in the morning (Rivard *et al.*, 1985). In this case the difference may, at least in part, be attributed to improved absorption of the drug at that time of the day (Pinkerton *et al.*, 1980; Riccardo *et al.*, 1986), but the susceptibility of leukaemia cells to 6-MP may also vary with time of day.

Distribution

Protein Binding

Once the drug/toxin has been absorbed, it is transported to its target tissue sites and its elimination sites. One way in which this is done is by binding to plasma proteins such as serum albumin, α_1-acid glycoprotein, globulins and lipoproteins. This phenomenon is important because the unbound drug is its active form. Therefore, circadian variations in the amount or efficiency of plasma protein binding can have an effect upon the amount of functional drug available. Different factors can influence drug/toxin protein binding, such as temperature, pH, physicochemical properties of the drug/toxin and plasma concentration of the carrier protein (Bruguerolle, 1992). Each of these factors can have its own distinct circadian rhythms and thereby uniquely affect the circadian pattern of distribution. Large circadian variations have been shown in humans and rats in plasma protein binding of wide range of drugs. Carbamazepine has its lowest free level (or highest protein binding) late in a rat's daily activity span, with the highest level of free carbamazepine at the time of day when the concentration of circulating albumin was the lowest (Bruguerolle et al., 1980; Bruguerolle, 1989). Relevant clinical studies have also been performed (Bruguerolle, 1989). In humans, the lowest free levels (highest protein binding) of diazepam (Naranjo et al., 1980) and carbamazepine (Riva et al., 1984) were found following morning ingestion. The lowest protein binding for phenytoin and valproic acid occur when these drugs, are given in the daily late rest period (Patel et al., 1982; Lockard et al., 1985). Cisplatin, containing a heavy metal and an important anticancer drug, is most thoroughly protein bound following afternoon administration (Hecquet and Bonneterre, 1984) whereas lidocaine (lignocaine) is most highly protein bound when given during the late activity phase (Bruguerolle, 1989).

The serum concentrations of other plasma proteins that bind drugs vary throughout each day (Bruguerolle, 1989). The serum concentration of orosomucoid, prealbumin, transferrin, haptoglobin and α_1-antitrypsin are highest around the middle of the daily activity period. It is interesting that in cancer patients, most of the proteins may not display clear circadian variation and that for the two proteins that do, their circadian phase may not be normal. It has been documented for α_1-acid glycoprotein that circadian variations exist in healthy subjects, but an ultradian (12 h) rhythm may predominate in some cancer patients (Bruguerolle, 1992). Finally, the clinical significance of these circadian differences in plasma protein concentration and binding are most relevant to drugs or toxins which are highly protein bound.

Red Cell Binding

In addition, drug/toxin transport can occur by their binding to red blood cells. In general, lipophilic materials pass into blood cells more rapidly than hydrophilic materials. For two drugs, lidocaine (Bruguerolle and Jadot, 1983) and indomethacin (Bruguerolle, 1989), data suggest significant circadian variations in drug binding to red blood cells. Circadian variation with respect to drug permeability of the blood–brain barrier is of interest, but very few data exist. In one study, a circadian variation in valproic acid concentration in the cerebrospinal fluid of monkeys was clearly documented (Lockard et al., 1985).

Blood Flow Patterns

Significant circadian variations in blood flow to the organs of drug elimination (liver, kidney, lung) exist in both humans and experimental animals. These physical circadian rhythms can obviously affect drug metabolism. In an experiment where the subjects were fasting and lying in a supine position, maximum hepatic blood flow was determined to occur with a profound circadian rhythm peaking at the early activity phase (Lemmer and Nold, 1991). This rhythm is bound to have significant effects upon the catabolism or excretion of drugs that are largely extracted by the liver such as lidocaine and propranolol (Bruguerolle, 1992). Correlatively, plasma clearance of drugs varies throughout the day. In man midazolam, a benzodiazepine, has a higher plasma clearance rate following administration early in the daily activity phase (Klotz and Ziegler, 1982). In rats, propranolol plasma clearance is higher at the end of the daily activity span, and its clearance depends markedly upon the liver blood flow (Lemmer, 1981). Circadian variation of blood flow to the kidneys has also been documented, with a lower renal blood flow occurring late in the daily activity span and during the daily sleep span (Koopman et al., 1985). Similarly, drugs with high renal extraction ratios can demonstrate circadian clearance rates based largely upon circadian differences in renal blood flow.

Metabolism

Metabolism of drugs and toxins includes processes such as oxidation, reduction, hydrolysis and conjugation reactions (Belanger, 1987). These reactions have been divided into two categories, called phase I and phase II reactions. Phase I reactions include oxidation, reduction and hydrolysis and are so grouped because they convert drugs into more polar metabolites which can be excreted readily by the kidney. Phase I reactions usually produce inactive or less active metabolites of the parent toxin or drug, but can sometimes liberate more active compounds. Phase II reactions are conjugations in which an endogenous substrate, such as glucuronate or sulphate, is added to the parent drug. The majority of this type of metabolism takes place within the liver owing to its large size and massive proportionate blood flow; however, these processes can also occur in other organs such as the lungs and kidney. The majority of hepatic metabolic reactions and the level of many enzyme activities vary reproducibly throughout each day (Belanger and Labrecque, 1989).

Oxidation–Reduction P450 Systems

In drug metabolism, oxidation–reduction reactions are among the most important to drug disposition since they are often rate-limiting to the relevant metabolic process (Belanger and Labrecque, 1989). These reactions take place in the monooxygenase system, which is a multicomponent electron transport system, present primarily in the smooth endoplasmic reticulum, composed of two predominant protein families, cytochrome P450s and their reductases, such as cytochrome c reductase, and a phospholipid fraction consisting mostly of phosphatidylcholine. Cytochrome P450s represent a population of different haemoproteins having distinct substrate specificity and unique responses to inducers and inhibitors (Belanger, 1987). At least 12 distinct cytochrome P450 isoenzymes have been isolated from rat liver (Waxman, 1986). A comprehensive review and biochemical organization of the circadian time structure of the cytochrome P450 system and its different isoenzymes have been presented (Belanger *et al.*, 1987). Cytochrome P450 daily rhythms are most often biphasic, with two times each day for peak and valley reaction kinetics (Haen and Golly, 1986). In general, with some exceptions, hepatic microsomal oxidase activities in rodents are highest during the daily activity span and lowest during the daily rest period. This circadian variation in oxidase activity is often responsible for meaningful differences in drug activity. For example, hexobarbital, a hypnotic drug, is eliminated from the body by the oxidation reactions that occur in the liver. Maximal hexobarbital oxidase activity (early daily sleep phase) is linked with minimal hypnotic effect, and that minimal oxidase activity (mid-activity) is linked to maximal hypnotic effect (Cooper and Brodie, 1955). The inducibility of the cytochrome P450 system is also circadian time dependent. For example, dichlorophenoxypropionic acid induces ethylmorphine *N*-demethylase activity and shortens hexobarbital sleeping time only at the times of day when the underlying circadian rhythms of these endpoints were at their lowest daily levels and not at other times of day (Clausing *et al.*, 1991). The activity of the enzyme that hydroxylates cholesterol (hepatic cytochrome P450 CYP7) is also circadian variant, as is the inducibility of this enzyme by cholestyramine (Brassil *et al.*, 1995). The major contribution to inter-individual variation of human hepatic epoxidase activity is endogenous (e.g. circadian) and exogenous (inducer exposure and timing) rather than genetic polymorphisms (Wolff and Strecker, 1992). One practical consequence of this chronobiology is that statins work much better in lowering cholesterol when they are given at bedtime compared to other times of day.

The GSH/GSSG Cycle

Another major biochemical pathway for drug metabolism in the liver is the glutathione-mediated oxidation/reduction cycle. Also known as the GSH/GSSG cycle, this metabolic cycle has a critical role in the detoxification of many compounds, especially xenobiotic toxins. The reduced form of GSH removes and neutralizes peroxides and other oxygen radicals produced directly by toxins or by various other enzyme systems and forms adducts with reactive intermediates of drugs or toxic agents. For these reasons, depleted GSH states are associated with susceptibility to cell death, tissue necrosis and resultant toxicity, because reactive drug and oxygen intermediates are left unchecked. Different drugs such as 1,1-dichloroethylene (Jaeger *et al.*, 1973), allyl alcohol (Hanson and Anders, 1978), chloroform (Lavigne *et al.*, 1983; Belanger *et al.*, 1988) and acetaminophen (Schnell *et al.*, 1983, 1984) and anticancer agents such as doxorubicin and mitomycin C are more toxic if low concentrations of GSH are present. GSH concentrations show clear high-amplitude circadian variations in both rodent and human tissues. According to Belanger and co-workers, there is a striking cross-species agreement between

various studies with respect to times of day for peak and trough concentrations of GSH (Belanger and Labrecque, 1989). Maximum concentrations were usually found early in the daily activity span, while the minimum concentrations were found to occur about 12 h later. These rhythms are, to some extent, experimentally manipulable. Pretreating mice with adrenocorticotropin, either 4 or 24 h before administration of doxorubicin, raised tissue GSH concentration to the maximum daily concentration. This allowed for each time of day of doxorubicin administration to result in toxicity similar to that usually seen with the time of day of lowest toxicity (Haus *et al.*, 1980; Lévi *et al.*, 1981). These findings suggest the possibility that tissue GSH balance could conceivably be coordinated, in part, by the circadian pattern of adrenal corticosteroid secretion.

Hydrolysis and Glucuronidation

Circadian studies of hydrolysis and glucuronidation reactions are more limited than oxidative reactions. These are important reactions that are catalysed by enzymes located throughout the body. In rats, glucuronidation is higher during daily activity, and sulphation is twice as efficient during daily sleep (Belanger *et al.*, 1985). In a clinical study, acetaminophen, which is eliminated by these pathways, has a 15% longer plasma half-life when given at (0600 h) early activity than at (1400 h) mid-activity (Shivley and Vesell, 1975). A similar circadian pattern has been documented in the rat (Belanger *et al.*, 1987). This time of day, mid-activity, correlates with the time of day when humans and animals are consuming the majority of their daily food intake, which also is when enzyme activities for metabolism and detoxification of absorbed nutrients and toxicants are greatest, an obvious biological economy relevant to the prevention of dietary poisoning.

Elimination

Biliary Excretion

The final step in drug pharmacokinetics is drug elimination. Most drugs are eliminated by the kidneys, but the liver and lungs are other important routes for drug elimination. Biliary excretion is an important elimination route for many xenobiotics (Smith, 1973; Garrett, 1978; Levine, 1983) The rate and extent of biliary excretion of agents such as bile acids, phospholipids and cholesterol metabolites depend upon the flow and composition of the bile (Belanger and Labrecque, 1992). A circadian variation in the biliary excretion of dibromosulphthalein, a dye, which is only cleared by the bile is 25% higher at midnight than noon (Vonk *et al.*, 1978).

Renal Excretion

The major elimination route for drugs is through the kidneys. Renal elimination is affected by the circadian differences in renal blood flow and glomerular filtration rate, pH and renal tubular function. Exogenous factors affect renal elimination such as posture, food and fluid intake, activity and sleep. It is a well established fact that urinary flow has a profound and stable circadian rhythm, peaking in the afternoon, with a daily nadir in the middle of the night (Cambar *et al.*, 1992a). In accord with studies of animals, the daily peak in renal function occurs during the daily activity span. Circadian pH variations that occur in the renal tubules and are reflected by urinary pH are highly relevant to circadian drug elimination. Large pH changes from across three orders of magnitude routinely occur during each day, with the low values, high proton concentrations occurring in sleep, and high values, low proton concentrations occurring during the daytime (Robertson *et al.*, 1977). Urinary pH determines the ionized or non-ionized state of a molecule and thus controls its tendency to precipitate or remain in solution and be either excreted or reabsorbed (Cambar *et al.*, 1992a). Therefore, excretion of a drug will increase if it is ionized, and reabsorption of a drug will increase if it is non-ionized. For this reason, it is assumed that increased acidity of the nocturnal urine allows for excretion of basic drugs and diminishes the excretion of acidic forms of a drug (Waterhouse and Minors, 1989).

Renal elimination of a drug is also determined by both the rate of filtration from the bloodstream and subsequent rate of reabsorption of the drug in the tubules (Aherne, 1989). The glomerular filtration rate has been well documented to vary with circadian time. It is maximum during the activity cycle and minimum during the sleep cycle (Koopman *et al.*, 1985). One reason for this is the circadian rhythm in arterial blood pressure (Hermida *et al.*, 1993), which co-varies with the concentration of atrial natriuretic peptide which modifies many aspects of renal tubular function. The circadian variation of the glomerular filtration rate has been correlated in humans with the highest removal rate of water-soluble drugs during the day (Aherne, 1989). Finally, circadian variations in urinary excretion and concentration of the anticancer drug cisplatin have been correlated with circadian dependent drug-induced kidney damage (Lévi, 1982). This drug is more efficiently eliminated by the kidney at the time of day associated with its highest nephrotoxicity, owing to the presence of higher concentrations of the drug in the kidney tubules in the early morning hours around daily awakening. These renal rhythms are routinely responsible for several-fold, time of day-dependent differences, in drug elimination by the kidney.

Pulmonary Drug Excretion

Few data exist with respect to circadian variation in elimination of drugs from the lungs. However, the lungs do have circadian patterns in blood flow, pulmonary vascular resistance, airway tone, bronchial responsiveness, receptor function, endogenous catecholamines and cholinergic reflex mechanisms (Barnes, 1989). The circadian pattern of asthma exacerbations is obviously nocturnal with heightened airway reactivity at this time of day. Therefore, theophylline chronotherapy has been designed to deliver more of this toxic drug when it is needed (night) and less when it is not (day).

Tissue Susceptibility Patterns

The manner in which many anticancer drugs work and in which many toxins damage cells and tissues is by attacking proliferating cells. For this reason, cells that divide more frequently are often damaged to a greater extent. Tumour cells are often, thereby, susceptible to these cancer drugs by reason of their higher proliferative capacity. However, many of the toxic side-effects that cancer patients suffer is due to the fact that anticancer drugs also attack host cells that are rapidly proliferating in normal tissues, such as the bone marrow, gastro-intestinal tract, hair follicles, skin and gonads. Tissue cytokinetics are tightly coordinated throughout each day. DNA synthesis and mitotic rates vary throughout the day in several different tissues of the gastro-intestinal tract in animals (Scheving *et al.*, 1978, 1994; Qui *et al.*, 1994) and in humans in both fed and fasted conditions (Buchi *et al.*, 1991). Similarly, DNA synthesis, mitotic rate and the number of stem cells and differentiated progenitor cells residing in the marrow vary throughout the day in mice (Stoney *et al.*, 1975; Moskalik, 1976; Aardal and Laerum, 1983; Wood *et al.*, 1998a) and in humans (Smaaland *et al.*, 1992). This coordination of tissue DNA synthesis (S phase) may also be the basis for circadian differences in the activities of important S phase-regulated enzymes such as thymidylate synthase, thymidine kinase and dihydrofolate reductase, which are critical for the action of some of the major categories of successful antiproliferative cancer drugs (Wood *et al.*, 1998b; Zhang *et al.*, 1993; Ohdo *et al.*, 1997a).

Other circadian rhythms are responsible for circadian susceptibility of a tissue to a given toxin or therapeutic insult. Such rhythms include rhythms in serum steroid hormone concentrations and protein growth factors which modulate cellular function, and thereby organ susceptibility. Circadian differences in both cellular and humoral immunity and immune cell numbers and functions have been well described. These underlying rhythms are also undoubtedly important if a toxin or drug acts through deleterious effects upon the immune system.

More limited studies have shown that tumours in animals and humans actually do maintain some circadian physiologic and proliferative coordination. Rhythms in tumour blood flow (Hori *et al.*, 1992) and DNA synthesis and mitotic rates have been shown in animal and human tumours (Klevecz and Braly, 1987; Smaaland *et al.*, 1993; Hrushesky *et al.*, 1998).

CIRCADIAN TOXICOLOGY BY TOXIN CLASS

Many preclinical and clinical data exist that demonstrate that outcome following exposure to a wide range of toxins is dependent upon the circadian time of exposure. In general, this may result from either a rhythmic circadian variation in the environmental exposure or rhythms in the bio-availability of a toxin that is physically equally available throughout each day, or from circadian variation in the susceptibility of specific target tissues of the exposed organism (e.g. plant, insect, mammal) to the toxin throughout the day, and/or to the summation of these circadian time structures (**Figure 1**). For example, fatal poisoning cases referred to hospitals in one study were more common between 1 pm and 1 am, probably reflecting both environmental/social rhythms impinging upon host susceptibility rhythms (Ghazi-Khansari and Oreizi, 1995). In this section, effects of circadian rhythms upon toxicology are discussed according to the type or class of toxin and/or therapeutic drug. This approach is often useful, since common mechanisms for a given toxin class may exist which may then, in practice, allow manipulation of the host or environment to modulate toxicological outcome and may lead to a better understanding of the biochemical and pathological mechanisms involved in circadian toxicology patterns of the specific agent.

Hepatotoxicology

The liver is an important site for the metabolism of many natural and synthetic toxins, as well as therapeutic drugs. As discussed above, many of the factors which determine the extent of hepatic metabolism vary predictably with circadian time. These include, among others, hepatic blood flow, activity of virtually all hepatic enzyme systems (e.g. cytochromes, hydroxylases, conjugases) and concentrations of essential cofactors (e.g. glutathione, folate, B_{12}, melatonin or fat-soluble vitamins or naturally available dietary antioxidants). The liver is also the target for a wide range of toxic compounds. The toxicity of many hepatotoxins varies with the time of day of exposure. These data exist for toxins, and potential carcinogens, such as 1,1-dichloroethylene, chloroform, and carbon tetrachloride, and also for potentially toxic drugs such as thioacetamide, and acetaminophen. Chloroform-induced hepatotoxicity is greater when mice are exposed during early activity phase of their circadian cycle with more severe pathological changes and greater depression of glutathione levels observed then (Lavigne et al., 1983; Desgagne et al., 1988) Greater toxicity is seen during exposure to thioacetamide during the activity phase of rats (Lawrence and Beesley, 1988). A similar circadian susceptibility pattern has also been reported

for carbon tetrachloride-induced liver toxicity in rats (Bruckner et al., 1984). Large regular diurnal variations in hepatic reduced and total glutathione concentrations have been correlated with the circadian rhythm in hepatic and lethal toxicity seen following 1, 1-dichloroethylene inhalation (Jaeger et al., 1973) and acetaminophen ingestion with few serious side-effects if these agents are administered during the early sleep phase of the circadian cycle (Schnell et al., 1983).

Heavy Metal Toxicology

Circadian rhythms in heavy metal toxicology have been described for mercury (Cal, 1983), cadmium (Cambar et al., 1983) and several derivatives of platinum (Lévi et al., 1982). Cal (1983) showed that nephrotoxicity and the renal concentration of mercury are greatest when rats are given mercuric chloride in the middle of the usual daily sleep span. Mercury, cadmium and the platinum derivatives (e.g. cisplatin) exhibit a similar circadian dependence with respect to heavy metal-induced renal toxicity and lethal toxicity (Cambar et al., 1992b). The renal concentration of the metals appears to depend upon at least three circadian rhythmic factors, the glomerular filtration rate (GFR), the plasma concentration of the metal and the reabsorptive capacity of the renal tubules at the time of day of heavy metal exposure. GFR is highest in the middle of the daily activity phase. Tubular metal reabsorption is most efficient towards the end of daily sleep and near daily awakening when heavy metal kidney damage is most severe and the urinary excretion of the metal is highest. Other factors also play a role in kidney defence systems such as the circadian availability of kidney tubular sulphydryl groups and GSH.

The platinum derivatives, which are used as anticancer agents, will be further discussed in the anticancer drug section. Studies in non-mammalian species such as rainbow trout also document time of day susceptibility patterns to heavy metals such as zinc (MacLeay and Munro, 1979).

Hydrocarbon Toxicology

Human exposure studies to monoaromatic hydrocarbons, such as benzene, have documented twofold higher levels of exposure during the daytime compared with the night (Leung and Harrison, 1998). Benzene-induced depression in rat lymphocyte counts is most profound when the benzene is administered in the late sleep to early activity phase. The level of liver microsomal benzene hydroxylase activity is highest at this time of day. The survival time of exposed animals was shortest when high doses of benzene were given during the late sleep/early activity phase of rats (Starek et al., 1989).

Continuous darkness or illumination schedules can modulate the circadian patterns of its subacute lethality. The pattern of relevant metabolic enzyme activity indicates that these particular susceptibility rhythms are tightly tied to the sleep, wake, meal timing and light–dark cycles.

Carcinogenicity and Teratogenicity

A limited amount of data exists with respect to the effects of circadian timing of toxin exposure upon carcinogenesis and teratogenesis. Several classes of chemotherapy drugs are known carcinogens and teratogens. The majority of circadian chemotherapy drug studies have rather focused upon acute toxicity and antitumour efficacy (see below), with many fewer studies focusing upon carcinogenicity or teratogenicity of these agents (Sauerbier, 1992).

Teratogenicity of Cytoxic Agents

The teratogenicity of the chemotherapy drugs 5-fluorouracil (5-FU) (Sauerbier, 1986a), hydroxyurea (Clayton et al., 1975) and cyclophosphamide (Schmidt, 1978; Sauerbier, 1981) has been shown to vary with the time of day of administration in pregnant rodents. No circadian-dependent embryotoxic effect was seen with cytosine arabinoside (Ara-C); however, only two times of day were examined and key circadian test stages may well have been omitted (Endo et al., 1987). The time of day of greatest lethal toxicity was in the early sleep for hydroxyurea and cyclophosphamide and in the middle of the sleep phase for 5-FU. These particular drugs are most toxic during the S phase of the cell cycle, so circadian coordination of tissue DNA synthesis could, in part, contribute to the observed differences in their toxicology. The circadian time structure of the foetus with respect to DNA synthesis has not been well studied. However, maternal drug anabolism (5-FU) and catabolism (cyclophosphamide), primarily by the liver, may also contribute to these teratogenicity circadian rhythms. The embryotoxicity of a nitrogen mustard was greatest with administration during early activity (Sauerbier, 1981).

Teratogenicity of Anticonvulsants, Corticoids and Alcohol

Circadian timing of the anticonvulsant drug valproic acid has been reported to affect the degree of embryotoxicity and the degree of toxicity to pregnant and non-pregnant mice, with similar time of day patterns to the adult and embryo. This circadian rhythmicity was not explained by simple differences in plasma or tissue drug concentrations, implying that the rhythm might be more related to the circadian pattern in sensitivity of the dam and the embryo to valproic acid (Ohdo et al., 1995, 1996). Other studies have documented circadian-dependent teratogenesis of dexamethasone with a greater incidence of cleft palates when given in the activity phase of rodents at a time when corticosterone levels were low (Sauerbier, 1986b). Circadian variation in the susceptibility of foetal tissues to ethanol has been well documented, with the greatest effects on embryos and pups with maternal exposure during the early and mid-daily activity phases (Sturtevant and Garber, 1985; Sauerbier, 1987). Some of the potential contributing factors may be the circadian variation in blood ethanol levels related to circadian-dependent metabolism of ethanol (Sturtevant and Garber, 1986; Sauerbier, 1987). Circadian rhythms in placental function and placental blood flow and their responses to ethanol may undoubtedly contribute (Walker et al., 1977; Walsh et al., 1984).

Bladder and Skin Carcinogenicity

The carcinogenicity of a given compound in the urinary bladder has been reported to be directly and indirectly influenced by the diurnal variations in several different physiological (e.g. bladder distention, urine volume) and biochemical (urine pH, chemical and protein constituents) parameters of the urine and bladder circadian physiology (Cohen, 1995). The efficiency of chemical carcinogenesis in the skin varies with the circadian time of application of methynitrosourea (Iversen and Iversen, 1995) and methylcholanthrene (Iversen et al., 1970; Iversen and Iversen, 1976) and dimethylbenze[a]anthracene (Frei and Ritchie, 1964), with the highest tumour yield and shortest latency duration associated with skin painting during the daily activity phase of mice. The fraction of cells in the skin undergoing DNA synthesis and the rate of DNA synthesis are each highly rhythmic throughout each day, with the highest values occurring during the activity phase of mice (Frei and Ritchie, 1964; Tvermyr, 1972). In vitro studies have shown that cells in the late G_1 and S phase of the cell cycle are maximally sensitive to carcinogen-induced transformation by some carcinogens (Marquardt, 1974). This time of day corresponds to when in the day a greater proportion of cells in the epidermis are more susceptible to certain carcinogenic effects (e.g. cells undergoing DNA synthesis) and to the daily timing of the peak incidence of circadian-dependent carcinogenesis in the skin. In vivo studies have also demonstrated the association or importance of tissue DNA synthesis for carcinogen-induced tumorigenesis (Nagasawa et al., 1976).

Hepatic and Gastrointestinal Carcinogenesis

The mechanism of the circadian dependence of carcinogen action varies with the type of carcinogen, depending upon whether the toxin is first metabolized and then acts indirectly or whether it acts directly upon cells. Hepatocarcinogenesis induced by diethylnitrosamine is reported to be influenced by the lighting schedule, with increased tumour size and incidence when rats are housed in continuous illumination compared with 12 h of alternating light and dark (Depres et al., 1997). Circadian timing of another hepatocarcinogen was reported to cause a greater amount of DNA strand breaks when administered in the daily activity phase of rats (Ziliani et al., 1984). Carcinogenesis in the intestine by N-methyl-N-nitrosourea is also dependent upon the circadian time of toxin exposure, with the highest intestinal tumour rates with administration during mid-sleep. This is the time of day of overall highest lethality with this same toxin (Beland et al., 1988). Other authors have described the effects of the circadian time of carcinogen administration upon outcome (Anisimov and Zhukova, 1994).

The daily rhythms in environmental availability of potential carcinogens are obviously important in studies of mammals outside the laboratory setting, including environmental exposures that occur during normal daily living activities and occupational exposure. This is discussed in other sections with regard to potential carcinogens such as hydrocarbons and radon and the daily variations in ultraviolet light.

Pesticide Toxicology

Insecticides

Circadian susceptibility rhythms of insects to radiation (Haverty and Ware, 1970), to narcosis-inducing agents (e.g. ether, chloroform, carbon tetrachloride) (Nowosielski et al., 1964) and to a number of different pesticides have been demonstrated in a variety of adult insects and in some larval stages. High-amplitude circadian susceptibility patterns (e.g. knockdown or mortality end-points) in insects to pesticides have been described in the grandis beetle to parathion-methyl (Cole and Adkisson, 1964), house flies and madeira cockroaches to pyrethrum (Sullivan et al., 1970), house flies to dieldrin and malathion (Frudden and Wellso, 1968; Shipp and Otten, 1976), American cockroach to dichlorvos (Eesa et al., 1987), mosquito larvae to chlorpyrifos (Dursban) (Roberts et al., 1974) and locust larvae to dieldrin (Onyeocha and Fuzeau-Braesch, 1991), to mention just a few. Many of these studies show increased susceptibility of the insect to the toxin during the spans for crepuscullarly active insects of early dark and early dawn; however, the exact timing of each agent varies somewhat and there are some exceptions, such as increased insect (house fly and cockroach) sensitivity to pyrethrum which occurs in the mid-afternoon. Therefore, the same concentration of an insecticide toxin can result in very different toxicology or degree of efficacy in many different types of insects simply depending upon when in the day it is applied. Optimal timing of application of these toxins can potentially diminish the amount of pesticide needed, and at the same time increase its relative efficacy with both economic benefits if less toxin or fewer applications are needed and benefits with respect to decreased potential pesticide exposure to mammalian hosts and environmental exposure to human beings.

With respect to occupational exposure, circadian susceptibility rhythms in mammals to organophosphate pesticides have been well described (Mayersbach, 1974; Fatranska et al., 1978). The pesticides studied have variable target organs for toxicity and variable modes of detoxification or metabolism. Therefore, as would be expected because of the distinct circadian time structures of each of the relevant metabolic pathways, the most toxic time of day (LD_{50} analysis) in rats for administration differs for fenitrothion, dichlorvos and paraoxon (E 600). Interestingly, there was a lack of a prominent circadian susceptibility to methyl parathion lethality in these studies, further indicating the necessity for the careful circadian study of each individual pesticide.

Herbicides

Circadian variation in the sensitivity patterns of plants to various agents has also been studied. Studies in cotton seedlings showed that the degree of damage imparted by three herbicides (fluazifop, acifluorfen, bentazone) was greatest during the middle of the daily dark span (Rikin and Anderson, 1990). The defence mechanisms of plants, such as glutathione levels, are known to be lower in the dark period and this may contribute to the observed effects (Setsuo and Patterson, 1988). In cotton seedlings, the degree and length of stimulation of ethylene biosynthesis by application of ethylene (a plant hormone) are also much greater when administered at the beginning of the dark period (Rikin and Anderson, 1990).

Endotoxin/TNF Toxicology

Microbial agents such as bacterial or viral toxins have demonstrated circadian-dependent patterns in their toxicities. In two studies in mice, the lethal toxicity resulting from endotoxin administration varied markedly with the circadian time of administration, with the most toxic time being during the late sleep phase (Halberg et al., 1960; Elliot et al., 1991) Since the toxicity of endotoxin is, in part, mediated by tumour necrosis factor (TNF), it is consistent that the TNF-induced mortality rates are also dependent upon the time of day of TNF administration, with greatest toxicity seen in late sleep (Hrushesky et al., 1994).

Radiation Toxicology

Radon

Diurnal fluctuations in radon levels due to occupational exposure (Merrill and Akbar-Kanzadeh, 1998) and household and outdoor exposure (Sheets, 1992; Porstendorfer et al., 1994) to radon-producing materials have been well documented. These circadian rhythms co-vary either directly or inversely with atmospheric temperature. They are highly dependent upon the airflow conditions in the tested dwellings. Occupational levels and outdoor levels are highest in the early morning hours, being influenced by the ubiquitous biometeorological circadian patterns in wind speed and direction and humidity.

Gamma Irradiation

Investigation of the circadian aspects of radiation exposure can be considered in both therapeutic terms (e.g. cancer therapeutic agent) or as an environmental hazard. The importance of cell proliferation and differentiation to radiation effects was first noted in 1906 by Bergonie and Tribondeau, who formulated the theory upon which radiotherapy of cancer is based. This theory states that the sensitivity of cells to irradiation is directly proportional to their reproductive activity and inversely proportional to their degree of differentiation. Experimentally, less differentiated tissue cells are more radiosensitive, as are cells in the G_2–M phase of the cell cycle, while more differentiated cells and those in the G_1–S phase of the cell cycle are more radioresistant.

Circadian Radiosensitivity of Normal Tissues

One might therefore predict that the toxicity of radiation to a particular tissue or organ would be circadian time dependent, since the percentage of proliferating and thereby mitotic cells in a large number of tissues varies substantially and reproducibly throughout each day due the number of stem cells and differentiated cells in some tissues (e.g. bone marrow). A 2–3-fold circadian difference exists in the number of marrow multipotential stem cells, as determined by in vitro multipotential CFU-GEMM colonies (Wood et al., 1998a) or by in vivo spleen colony formation (CFU-S) (Stoney et al., 1975; Aardal and Laerum, 1983; Sletvold and Laerum, 1988) with a clear daily maximum during the early sleep phase of each circadian cycle. This time of day (late activity/early sleep) with the highest number of marrow multipotential cells is also the time of day when whole-body irradiation results in the greatest depression of marrow cell numbers (Haus et al., 1974b) and the lowest number of surviving endogenous spleen cell colonies (Uneo, 1968; Vacek and Rotkovska, 1970), and likewise when in the day the greatest radiation-induced lethality occurs (Pizzarello et al.,

1963; Pizzarello et al., 1964; Halberg, 1975). This is also the time of day associated with the highest mitotic index of the bulk of bone marrow cells (Pizzarello and Witcofski, 1970).

The radiosensitivity of the mouse small intestine varies with the time of day of irradiation. During the middle of the activity phase, the crypt cells of the intestine are most severely reduced, as measured by crypt survival, which is the time of day associated with the highest daily crypt mitotic activity (Hendry, 1975). The number of early apoptotic cells in the intestine following radiation is highest following treatment in the early sleep phase (Ijiri and Potten, 1990). The differences in the rhythm of these two responses to radiation might possibly reflect separate effects on two different cell populations.

Circadian Radiosensitivity of Cancer

The circadian susceptibility of tumours to radiation has not been thoroughly investigated but could potentially be utilized to improve the efficacy of this cancer treatment. In one study, tumour-bearing mice survived longer when radiation was given during the middle of the daily activity span (Fochem et al., 1967). This is also the time of day when tumour blood flow is the highest (Hori et al., 1992), which is one of the important variables for optimal radiation tumour response.

Circadian Susceptibility to Radiation-induced Cancer

Tumour induction by radiation treatment is a known medical complication of this therapy. The incidence of lung adenomas and adenocarcinomas following thoracic radiation was reported by one group to be higher when it was given during the activity phase of mice (Hashimoto et al., 1994). However, another study found a higher lung tumour incidence following radiation during the middle of the sleep phase of mice (Endoh et al., 1987). Both of these studies suffered the shortcoming of examining only two times of day for treatment timing, which is inadequate to define circadian rhythms meaningfully and clearly. More complete studies are essential.

Therapeutic Drug Toxic–Therapeutic Ratio

Anticancer Drug Toxic–Therapeutic Index

Metal-based Compounds
Metal-based compounds for treating cancer are usually platinum-based compounds, such as cisplatin, carboplatin and oxaliplatin. The last two compounds are known bone marrow toxins. Cisplatin causes neurotoxicity in

addition to renal toxicity since it is entirely excreted by the kidneys. These compounds are thought to work against tumours by cross-linking DNA and ultimately causing strand breaks. It has been hypothesized that the optimal time to administer cisplatin is during the second half of the daily activity span since this is also when the plasma filtration rate of the kidneys is the fastest. This prediction was confirmed by a study that demonstrated optimal timing of cisplatin to be during the early evening for humans (Hrushesky *et al.*, 1982). Animal studies with oxaliplatin and carboplatin also indicate that the safest time to administer these drugs is during the evening (Boughattas *et al.*, 1990). Optimal timing for each of these drugs seems to be the same, and the benefit of administration at the optimal time of day is substantial protection of kidney, neural tissue, bone marrow and gastro-intestinal mucosa.

Antimetabolites

Antimetabolites are agents which have similar chemical structures to physiological metabolic intermediates. They function as substrate analogues derailing important enzymatic reactions. These drugs are the most widely used in cancer treatment, and act by competitive inhibition of intracellular metabolism essential for cell division. We shall discuss 5-fluorouracil (5-FU), fluorodeoxyuridine (FUdR), cytosine arabinoside (Ara-C), methotrexate and purine analogues.

Fluoropyrimidines

The two commonly used fluoropyrimidine antimetabolites are 5-FU and FUdR. The anabolism of these drugs, which causes activation of the drug, can occur from different pathways which can be catalysed by various enzymes such as uridine phosphorylase, orotate phosphoribosyltransferase, thymidine phosphorylase, thymidine kinase, uridine kinase, nucleotide monophosphate and diphosphate kinases, and ribonucleotide reductase. The activity levels of the majority of these anabolic enzymes show large circadian variations and have been reviewed by Zhang and Diasio (1994). Similarly, the catabolism of these drugs by dihydropyrimidine dehydrogenase (DPD) and its circadian rhythm were also reviewed. Studies with FUdR have been performed on mice, rats and humans. Overall the results have shown that FUdR is most safely given and may be more effective against cancer when it is given during the latter part of the daily activity cycle and the first half of the daily sleep span (von Roemeling and Hrushesky, 1990). Studies with 5-FU have shown similar results to FUdR, in that it is least toxic between late activity and early sleep (Peters *et al.*, 1987; Wood *et al.*, 1995). Clinical studies have also shown decreased toxicity and improved tumour responses with optimally timed 5-FU-based chemotherapy (Lévi *et al.*, 1997) and decreased toxicity and increased dose intensity with circadian-timed FUdR therapy (Hrushesky *et al.*, 1990).

Cytosine Arabinoside

Ara-C differs from other natural nucleosides by having an arabinose sugar moiety instead of a ribose or deoxyribose. Ara-C is metabolized in a similar manner, in that activation requires anabolism and elimination requires catabolism. However, data do not exist to indicate whether there are circadian patterns in these enzyme activities. Ara-C works by inhibiting DNA synthesis, inhibiting DNA repair and being incorporated into subsequently malfunctioning nucleic acids. Experiments have clearly shown, however, that the toxicity and efficacy of Ara-C are each markedly dependent upon when in the day it is administered. Mice receiving an equal single dose of Ara-C at one of six equispaced times of the day showed the lowest death rate when the drug was given during the daily sleep span (Cardoso *et al.*, 1970). The antitumour efficacy of Ara-C was studied in mice treated with sinusoidal administration, meaning that they received the highest treatment dose when the host toxicity was the lowest, and the lowest dose when the toxicity was the highest, or with a constant dosage of Ara-C. The survival rate resulting from the antitumour activity of Ara-C in mice treated in the sinusoidal case was five times greater than that seen with a fixed concentration of Ara-C (Scheving *et al.*, 1976). The sinusoid responsible for the best outcome also peaked during the daily sleep span, demonstrating that toxicity would be diminished at the same time efficacy was enhanced by optimal circadian Ara-C timing.

Methrotrexate

Methotrexate is another antimetabolite used extensively in cancer treatment. In rats, methotrexate is least toxic when given around mid-activity and most toxic during late activity phase or early rest phase (English *et al.*, 1982). Another study confirmed this same pattern of toxicity and also correlated the toxicity pattern with circadian differences in methotrexate pharmacokinetics and with the susceptibility pattern (e.g. fraction of cells in S phase) of the bone marrow (Ohdo *et al.*, 1997a).

6-MP and 6-TG

Purine analogues are synthetic analogues of the naturally occurring purines adenine and guanine. They function by becoming incorporated into subsequently malfunctioning DNA. The two such drugs used widely for cancer chemotherapy are 6-mercaptopurine (6-MP) and 6-thioguanine (6-TG). In one study a fivefold greater risk of relapse by children suffering from acute lyphoblastic leukaemia was observed in those given 6-MP in the morning compared with those who took the drug in the evening (Rivard *et al.*, 1985).

Antibiotic Anticancer Drugs

Antibiotic agents are metabolized in the liver for both activation and elimination. The toxicities of these agents are often due to the generation of toxic free radicals such as hydroxyl or superoxide anions. Since the glutathione cycle is largely responsible for detoxification of these toxic anions, the toxicity of these cytotoxic antibiotics depends largely upon the circadian pattern of glutathionine in the target tissues. Actinomycin D is used to treat rhabdomyosarcoma and Wilms tumour in children, and works by binding double-stranded DNA, which causes anticancer activity and toxicity (Zhang and Diasio, 1994). Daunorubicin is used in treating acute leukaemias and doxorubicin is used for treating many different kinds of solid tumours. Different studies have shown that an optimal timing of administration exists for different antibiotics.

In clinical studies, cancer patients were administered doxorubicin and cisplatin 12 h apart; however, some received doxorubicin in the morning and cisplatin in the night, while the others received doxorubicin in the night and cisplatin in the morning. From these data it was determined that the optimal timing to reduce doxorubicin toxicity is in the morning and cisplatin in the evening. These results were predicted by circadian studies in rodents (Hrushesky, 1985; Hrushesky et al., 1987b, 1989b). Studies in mice with other drugs in this class such as daunorubicin and epirubicin indicated that optimal tolerance of the drug was during the sleep span (Davies et al., 1974; Sothern et al., 1981; Langevin et al., 1987).

Other Cancer Drugs

Many other cancer treatment drugs exist that have demonstrated a circadian pattern with respect to toxicity. For example, cyclophosphamide is known to be least toxic when given after daily rising (Hans et al., 1974a; Cardoso et al., 1978; Hacker et al., 1983). Ifosfamide has showed least toxicity when given late in the activity phase (Snyder et al., 1981). Of the plant alkaloid class of drugs, vincristine has been found to be least toxic in early activity, vinblastine in mid-activity, vinorelbine in late activity and etoposide in late sleep (Halberg et al., 1977; Lévi et al., 1985; Mormont et al., 1986; Tampellini et al., 1995). New drugs such as docetaxel and irinotecan also show circadian-dependent toxicity and antitumour efficacy (Ohdo et al., 1997b; Tampellini et al., 1998). The particularly narrow therapeutic index of anticancer drugs demands that their circadian toxic–therapeutic ratio patterns be explored in order to control and diminish drug toxicity better.

Bronchodilator Toxic–Therapeutic Index

Bronchial Chrono-physiology

Perhaps the most prominently circadian of all diseases is asthma, which affects one out of every 20 people worldwide. Asthma is a contraction of the smooth muscle surrounding the airways that makes it excruciatingly difficult to breathe. The great majority of asthma attacks take place between two and six o'clock in the morning. That circadian pattern is caused by the concurrence of many normal physiological processes.

Airway size and breathing patterns change rhythmically throughout the day in both healthy people and asthmatics. Generally the airways are open widest during the day. There is a rhythmic reduction in the airflow after midnight, and particularly between the critical hours of two and six in the morning. Those normal fluctuations can become extreme in response to both internal and external stimuli: allergens in the sleeping room, the supine posture and mucus retention during sleep, the cooling of the airway caused by breathing through the mouth, and circadian patterns in muscle and sympathetic nervous tone and in the circulation of cortisol, histamine and the hormone epinephrine (adrenaline).

Bronchial Chrono-pathology

The so-called chronopathology of asthma suggests that drug treatments should be designed to anticipate the temporal onset of an attack. One of the most successful kinds of chronotherapy yet developed is the bronchodilator preparation for nocturnal asthma. Many such drugs are on the market, each one absorbed, metabolized and excreted differently, depending on when it is ingested. The optimal once-a-day bronchodilator must make its active ingredient most available between the critical hours of two and six in the morning. Hence an evening dose should delay delivery for between 4 and 6 h, and a morning dose should do so for between 16 and 18 h.

Bronchodilators

The two most commonly used asthma drugs are theophylline and β-agonist bronchodilators. In the past they have been given on a equal dose, equal time treatment schedule throughout the day. This kind of treatment pattern has assumed that the risk of asthma attacks is equal throughout the 24 h of a day, and that the pharmacokinetics and bioactivities of these drugs are constant throughout each day. None of these assumptions is valid. Many studies have shown that symptoms for most asthma patients worsen in the night (Smolensky, 1989). One of the treatments for asthma has been to administer theophylline as a one-time dose treatment in the night, when the patient is most susceptible to asthma attacks. From several studies it has been reported that patient airway status and sleep quality are improved with this approach (Smolensky, 1989). With respect to β-agonist tablets, it was been shown that when terbutaline was given in unequal doses, with more given in the night than the morning, that patients showed greater improvements (Smolensky, 1989). The literature on bronchosensitivity to a wide range of agents is extensive and beyond the scope of this review.

Anti-allergy Drugs

The drugs used to control allergy symptoms, including antihistamines and decongestants, represent one of the largest and most profitable pharmaceutical markets in the world. A great deal of effort, time and money has been spent developing such drugs, with an eye towards diminishing their sedative or stimulatory side-effects. It does not take a genius, however, to realize that antihistamines, which generally act as sedatives, are better taken in the evening, and that decongestants, which exert a stimulatory effect, should be used during the day and be avoided at night. Aside from that kind of logical treatment, other less obvious and even surprising circadian differences in drug absorption, excretion, metabolism and effectiveness have recently become clear. Allergic reactions are cued by the overzealous response of the body's primordial defence against invasion, the inflammatory reaction. When a person is exposed to an allergen, be it dust, pollen or a particular food, the bloodstream sends a crowd of circulating white blood cells to the site of contact. There they proceed to react with and engulf the foreign agent. Some of those white cells, the basophils, release histamines, chemicals that increase local blood flow, cause leaks in small blood vessels and spark a flood of more white cells. The result is swelling, pain, itchiness, burning and redness. This response can serve as the take-off point for either allergy or exaggerated inflammation. Inflammation can also trigger an aberrant immune response against normal tissues. Both the immune system and the inflammatory response are orchestrated primarily by circadian rhythms in the release and action of glucocorticoids, steroid hormones made in the adrenal gland. Glucocorticoids, especially cortisol, promote the manufacture of glucose out of protein and fat stored in the body. Their intense release, along with the release of epinephrine (adrenaline), is part of the flight-or-fight response to times of heightened, short-term stress (a mugging, say, or a job interview). Glucocorticoids also regulate and, if present in excess, depress the immune system, which may explain why people are more susceptible to illness when they are under stress and why the hormones, especially cortisol, turn out to be valuable in reducing the redness, pain and burning of inflammation. Cortisol concentration in the blood is highest in the morning, around five or six o'clock; as expected, the inflammatory reaction is weakest at that time. However, in the evening, when the blood concentration of cortisol is lowest, inflammatory activity is at its strongest. The daily waxing and waning of cortisol concentration has broad implications for the timing of virtually any anti-inflammatory agent. That profoundly stable rhythm may also be responsible, at least in part, for the circadian coordination of all the body's defence networks and even the daily pattern of cell division—in other words, for the renewal of almost all bodily tissues.

Anti-inflammatory Agent Toxic–Therapeutic Ratio

Inflammatory Chrono-pathology
Arthritis, an all too common inflammatory disease of the joints, also runs on a biological clock. The condition comes in two major varieties. In rheumatoid arthritis a disordered immune system attacks components of the joint. Non-rheumatic arthritis includes a wide range of degenerative diseases. Some of them are associated with the formation of crystal deposits in the joints; others are set off by wear and tear, trauma or infection. Various forms of rheumatoid arthritis affect millions of people, whereas non-rheumatic arthritis to some extent affects most people who live past the age of 40. For generations physicians have differentiated between the two kinds of arthritis according to the circadian patterns of their symptoms. In rheumatoid arthritis the joints are most stiff, swollen, hot and painful when one arises; they 'work themselves out' as the day progresses. In contrast, in non-rheumatic arthritis, such as osteoarthritis, the redness, pain and swelling build throughout the day and are relieved only by a good night's rest. By timing the medication and optimizing the relation between dose and time of day, one can better control the symptoms and reduce the side-effects of drugs.

Anit-inflammatory Drugs
Arthritis is often treated with NSAIDs (non-steroidal anti-inflammatory drugs), among which are aspirin and ibuprofen. Depending on the release characteristics of the specific preparation, NSAIDs can best be taken at one time of day or another. An NSAID taken in the evening that hits its peak of release within 4–10 h after ingestion would best treat rheumatic diseases. A once-a-day preparation taken at bedtime for osteoarthritis, however, should peak the following afternoon, between 14 and 20 h later. In addition to symptom patterns, many other considerations relate to the construction of an optimized pill—one that, taken at a certain time of day, provides the highest levels of its active ingredient when it is needed and the lowest levels when it is least needed and most damaging. The absorption of a standard drug preparation in the gut also depends on when the drug is taken. Sodium salicylate, for instance, which is prescribed for osteoarthritis, is absorbed relatively slowly in the morning; ketoprofen, prescribed for the same condition, is absorbed quickly in the morning. Sometimes NSAIDs are not enough. For the most severe cases of rheumatoid arthritis, physicians typically prescribe steroids. This is because steroids are hormones that occur naturally in the body, their side-effects, including weight gain, thinning bones, diabetes, mania, high blood pressure, suppression of the adrenal gland and increased risk of infection, can be diminished if the hormones' usual circadian rhythms are mimicked, taking advantage of the body's capacity to neutralize their toxic effects. The patient takes most of each day's dose on arising or takes a larger morning dose every other day.

Cardiovascular Drug Toxic–Therapeutic Ratio

Cardiac Chrono-pathology

Only recently has it come to be understood that cardiovascular disease, the number-one killer of adults, is heavily influenced by circadian rhythms in pulse rate, blood pressure, the tendency of blood to clot, the interactions between blood cells and the walls of the blood vessels, and important interactions in the part of the nervous system that controls involuntary functions. Consider angina pectoris, a chest pain caused when the heart muscle does not receive enough oxygen. Oxygen is carried to the heart by the blood through the coronary arteries. A partial blockage of those arteries may prevent some area of the heart muscle from getting enough blood, an ongoing condition known as myocardial ischaemia; this ischaemia can be silent or it can manifest itself as angina. The timing of ischaemia during the day makes it clear that getting oxygen to the heart muscle is sensitive to circadian rhythms, and so those rhythms are potentially highly relevant to coronary artery disease. Several large studies have shown that ischaemia is much more frequent and severe in the 4–6 h after people arise in the morning than it is at other times of day. Whatever its precise cause, this finding has obvious implications for the development of anti-anginal drug-delivery systems. Several large studies have demonstrated that myocardial infarctions (heart attacks) strike twice as often in the morning as they do during the rest of the day. Like angina, heart attacks result from a lack of blood, and hence of oxygen, in the heart muscle. The condition can arise from a variety of problems inside the blood vessels, and one of the most significant of these problems is high blood pressure (hypertension).

Chronobiology of Hypertension

Blood pressure is strongly circadian; thus transient hypertension in response to daily stresses may not be as ominous as blood pressure that is abnormally elevated at a time of day when it is usually much lower. The main problem with hypertension is that it gives an unhealthy battering to the walls of the blood vessels. This raises the likelihood that the vessels will be damaged, giving rise to a blood clot and causing a heart attack or a stroke. Another threat to the blood vessels is intensified shear stress, the pulling or tearing force exerted on the vessel wall by the flow of blood cells. Shear stress relates in complicated ways to blood pressure, to the rate of blood flow and to the diameter of the blood vessel. The most prominent increase in shear stress takes place, again, when one gets up in the morning: when one stands upright after lying down for a long while, the nervous system cues an increase in blood pressure and a change in blood flow, as well as a constriction of the blood vessels. The shear stress and change in blood pressure ultimately damage the vessel walls.

Chronophysiology of Blood Clotting

The third important factor in the evolution of heart disease is an unfortunate side-effect of the body's mechanisms for controlling bleeding. When a small wound opens in the skin, the blood cells known as platelets clump together at the site of the injury. However, blood vessels damaged by hypertension or shear stress also appear wounded to the platelets, and so large numbers of platelets can aggregate inside the blood vessels and eventually set off a chain reaction that can block the passage of the blood. Platelets tend to be stickier in the morning than they are at other times of day; hence it is safer to shave in the morning than at night. The tendency is associated with increased levels of catecholamines, stress hormones released when a person assumes an upright posture. Any drug that might suppress the morning surge in stress hormones should reduce the tendency of arterial platelets to clump together. Also, drugs that directly interfere with platelet function should be given in such a way that most of their activity takes place in the morning. Another important factor in the control of bleeding is fibrinogen, the main clotting protein in the blood. The concentrations of fibrinogen in blood plasma peak in the morning and then plunge into an evening trough. In normal circumstances blood clots are constantly dissolved by fibrinolysis, a process whereby the crucial clotting proteins are absorbed by the body. Fibrinolytic activity has a prominent circadian rhythm, with a morning trough and a nocturnal peak, which helps account for the inverse pattern of fibrinogen concentration. Any strategy for interrupting the cascade of events leading to a heart attack would do well to account for all the foregoing circadian dynamics. In the morning the heart's need for oxygen should be decreased; small doses of anticoagulants should be prescribed; blockers of the effects of stress hormones must be administered to counteract the tendency of damaged blood vessels feeding the heart muscle to contract and thereby decrease the flow of oxygen; and blood pressure, which tends to leap after one awakens, must be modulated.

Neuroleptic and Psychotropic Drugs

Neuroleptic and psychotropic drug effects vary with their circadian time of administration. Chlorpromazine has different bioactivities based on the timing of and dosage received. Peak sedative effects were observed in the middle of the sleep phase at low dosage [2.5 mg (kg body weight)$^{-1}$], but moved forward in time as the dosage increased, shifting its peak efficacy to the early activity phase of daily activity at a dose of 20 mg (kg body weight)$^{-1}$ (Nagayama and Takahashi, 1989). Studies in humans with diazepam, amitriptyline and haloperidol demonstrated better absorption rates in the morning than the evening (Nakano, 1989). However, some drugs show different optimal timings for different effects. For example, chlorpromazine has the best sedative effect at night (sleep phase), while the best antipsychotic effect occurs upon rising (activity phase). In addition, this drug is most toxic at bedtime (Nagayama and Takahashi, 1989). Finally, in a study treating 34 schizophrenic patients with timiperone, the best improvement was observed in those patients who received it in the evening (Nagayama and Takahashi, 1989). In general, in order to determine the optimal circadian time for a neuroleptic, the time structure of the pathology, in addition to drug pharmacology and pharmacodynamics, must each be carefully considered. The toxicology of neuroleptics is responsible for tens of thousands of hopitalizations and thousands of US deaths annually.

Peptides and Proteins

Protein and peptide growth factors such as erythropoietin (EPO), interleukin-1 (IL-1), interleukin-2 (IL-2), interferons and tumour necrosis factor, each have unique circadian patterns of toxicity and/or therapeutic efficacy. EPO differentially expands marrow erythroid progenitors depending on the circadian time of administration and progenitor cell harvesting (Wood *et al.*, 1998a). IL-1, which is important in the inflammatory response and regulation of hematopoiesis, body temperature and sleep, has its highest level in the serum, and greatest production rate by monocytes at the late activity phase (Zabel *et al.*, 1990). Tumour necrosis factor-alpha (TNF), which modulates the symptoms of rheumatoid arthritis and is used in antitumour treatment, has a prominent circadian pattern of its potentially lethal toxicity. Toxicities include shock-like syndromes, capillary leakage, myelotoxicity and neurotoxicity and death, which have also limited TNF's clinical utility. In mice, up to ninefold differences were found in TNF-induced mortality rates depending solely upon the time of day of administration of TNF. The greatest toxicity is observed when this peptide is injected just prior to usual awakening (Hrushesky *et al.*, 1994). IL-2 also shows great circadian differences in toxicity, with the least toxicity and highest anti-tumour associated survival rates when high-dose IL-2 was given during the late activity phase (Lévi *et al.*, 1992) and greater desired immune cell effects when low-dose IL-2 was given in the activity phase (von Roemeling *et al.*, 1990). Studies with recombinant IFN-α or IFN-γ administered subcutaneously daily in mice indicated that the circadian time of administration is responsible for large differences in the degree of myelotoxicity (Koren and Fleischmann, 1993a,b), fever induction, plasma pharmacokinetics and antiviral activity (Koyanagi *et al.*, 1997). The efficacy of the myeloid growth factor granulocyte colony-stimulating factor (G-CSF) to raise peripheral blood neutrophil counts is by far greatest when administered to mice during late activity to early sleep phase rather than at other times of day (Wood *et al.*, 1993; Ohdo *et al.*, 1998) The antitumor efficacy of TNF, interferons and IL-2 in rodents can be

markedly enhanced by optimal circadian timing of these proteins (Hrushesky *et al.*, 1987a, 1992; Kemeny et al., 1992; Koren *et al.*, 1993).

Other Drugs

Studies of drug-induced lethality in rodents have demonstrated circadian-dependent toxicity for cardiac drugs such as ouabain, propranolol and procainamide, addictive substances such as ethanol and nicotine, local anaesthetics such as lidocaine (lignocaine), sedatives such as diazepam, and antibiotics such as gentamycin. The circadian dependence of sublethal acute toxicities has also been described for many of these same drugs (Cambar *et al.*, 1992b).

CONCLUSIONS

Implications of Circadian Toxicology

Toxicity Testing and Drug Development

Circadian Variability of Results
Circadian time structure is not routinely considered in toxicity drug testing in human or preclinical (usually rodent) models. If fact, much testing is not even fixed to the same time of day, which invariably adds unnecessary variability to test results. For example, methods for population screening for genetic heterogeneity in the ability of individuals to metabolize certain chemicals have been established and utilized in studies of cancer susceptibility. However, results of these tests at different centres have not always reproduced one another. One very interesting and relevant study showed that the rate of debrisoquine metabolism (screening method for slow or fast metabolic phenotyping) varied with the time of day of administration of the test substance. It was concluded that fixing the time of day of testing can greatly improve testing accuracy as evidenced by the circadian variation in debrisoquine metabolic rate and hence phenotyping (Shaw *et al.*, 1990).

Systematic Errors
Another major area of misunderstanding of circadian time structure and drug toxicology screening is the use of preclinical rodent systems to assess toxicology which then is extrapolated to humans. Nearly all rodent (rat, mouse) testing is conducted during the time when the animal lights are on for the convenience of human experimenters. Being nocturnally active, this means that rodents are actually being treated or tested during their usual daily sleep phase, yet the results obtained are applied to Phase I studies of humans performed in their activity phase, exactly the opposite circadian phase. Since lethality and other end-points can vary anywhere from 50% to 10-fold depending on the time of day,

misleading conclusions will necessarily be drawn from these study paradigms. This systematic error results routinely in promising new drugs unnecessarily and wastefully being excluded from the drug development process simply because of circadian stage-dependent toxicities that would be avoided simply by optimal circadian timing in Phase I and Phase II studies that knock drugs out of the pipeline.

Timing of Toxic Occupational Exposures

It has been shown earlier that the human body is more susceptible to certain agents at different times. It is very likely that agents that normally do not bother people during the day at a factory might cause more of a problem in the night. Given daily rhythms in some environmental levels of toxins, avoidance of exposure by considering circadian time is one approach. Using toxins at times of day when they are more efficacious (e.g. insecticides for plants, herbicides for plants, chemotherapy drugs for patients) might allow the dose used to be decreased for an equal effect. This could result in less exposure to the worker, the environment and other hosts, or the cancer patient to the unwanted and toxic, teratogenic or carcinogenic effects of such compounds. In addition, disturbances in circadian rhythms comparable to continuous jet lag and in some shift workers cause ill effects on performance and increased accident rates.

Cancer Chronotherapy

An important implication of circadian rhythms in toxicity and efficacy is that they can be used to an advantage in a new field called chronotherapy. The data underlying this new field suggest that certain drugs have an optimal time for administration with respect to reduced toxicity, and greatest anti-tumour or other desired effect. If this information is properly utilized, not only will the patient suffer less from the toxicity of the drug but also a much better therapeutic effect will occur. This chronotherapeutic concept is also being applied in other disease states such as chronotherapy in asthma, arthritis, ulcer disease, heart disease and depression (Hrushesky, 1994).

Other Rhythms

Circadian rhythms are not the only rhythms which modulate the outcome following drug or toxin exposure. Other cycles such as the fertility cycle (menstrual in humans, oestrous in rodents) and seasonal (circannual) cycles markedly and reproducibly alter toxicity profiles. These additional rhythms and other factors, such as sex, can further reproducibly and predictably modulate the pattern or the extent of circadian-dependent toxicology of some compounds.

Fertility Cycle Toxicology

The lethality and subsequent reproductive toxicity in survivors given a high dose of the anticancer drug 5-fluorouracil varies with the fertility cycle stage, with greatest toxicity during oestrus (Hrushesky et al., 1999). Cyclophosphamide-induced bladder damage also varies with the fertility cycle stage, again with the greatest toxicity during oestrus (Bon et al., 1997). The toxicity and antitumour efficacy of 5-fluorouracil in tumour-bearing mice varies with the stage of the fertility cycle of administration (Wood and Hrushesky, 1997). Carcinogen induction of breast tumours is known to vary with the oestrous cycle phase of carcinogen administration. For N-methyl-N-nitrosourea-induced breast tumours, higher tumour rates and numbers and shorter latency times are seen when rats are treated in pro-oestrus and oestrus (Lindsey et al., 1981; Ratko and Beattie, 1995). Similar results were found with 7,12-dimethylbenz[a]anthracene (DMBA)-induced mammary tumours, with greater tumour numbers when given in pro-oestrus than in di-oestrus (Nagasawa et al., 1976). The incidence of mammary tumours following DMBA is known to depend upon the density of terminal end-buds and ductuals and their DNA labeling indexes (Nagasawa et al., 1976; Russo and Russo, 1978) The mitotic index and percentage of cells undergoing DNA synthesis in the breast vary predictably throughout the fertility cycle (Bresciani, 1968; Purnell and Kopen, 1976).

Surgical cure rates of breast cancer appear to vary with the time within the mammalian fertility cycle when the surgery is performed. In one experiment, a significant difference was noted in the successful treatment of mice with breast cancer depending upon when in the fertility cycle the surgery took place. Twice as many mice were cured of a breast cancer when the surgery was performed at a time near the surge in follicle-stimulating hormone (FSH) and luteinizing hormone (LH) and when progesterone was rising (Ratajczak et al., 1988). Mice in this stage of the fertility cycle also have higher levels of natural killer cell activity and splenocyte interleukin-2 production (Hrushesky et al., 1988). Retrospective human clinical data also support the benefit of optimal timing of surgical resection during the menstrual cycle. In 10 studies of more than 2500 young women, the 10 year survival rate was enhanced by 30% when the resection of primary breast cancers was performed in the 7–10 days immediately following the FSH and LH surge, near and following putative ovulation (Hrushesky et al., 1989a; Hagen and Hrushesky, 1998). If this chronobiology is as it appears, some 12 000–15 000 young American women whose breast cancers are, by chance, extirpated at an inopportune menstrual cycle stage are unnecessarily sentenced to death each and every year.

Seasonal Rhythms

A number of studies have documented the outcome following toxin or drug exposure varies throughout the year (Cambar *et al.*, 1992b). A few select examples include the seasonal degree of acute toxicity from radiation (Fochem *et al.*, 1967), phenobarbital (phenobarbitone) (Bruguerolle *et al.*, 1988), several types of chemotherapy drugs (Lévi *et al.*, 1987), mercuric chloride (Cal *et al.*, 1986) and in the number of carcinogen-induced DNA strand breaks in the liver (Ziliani *et al.*, 1984). Again, seasonal rhythms in toxicology outcome can arise through several mechanisms, including circannual rhythms in toxin availability/exposure such as radon (Merrill and Akbar-Kanzadeh, 1998) or airborne methylarsenic compounds (Mukai *et al.*, 1986), as well as circannual rhythms in tissue function such as bone marrow progenitor numbers, amount of DNA synthesis in bone marrow and rectal mucosa (Aardal, 1984; Sothern *et al.*, 1995), reproductive function and other physiological processes. Seasonality to the occurrence/detection of several types of cancer has also been reported (Cohen *et al.*, 1983). Increasing evidence supports a genetic and inherited basis for a circannual time keeping or clock which is then modified by environmental clues, analogous to circadian time keeping system.

In summary, considering toxicology in the absence of proper triangulation within the biological time structure of living animals is uneconomical, misleading and unwise.

ACKNOWLEDGMENTS

This work was supported by ACS CDA, NIH BRSG S07RR05394–29 (P. A. W.) and NIH RO1 CA31635, RO1 CA50749 (W. J. M. H), Office of Research and Development, Medical Research Service, Department of Veterans Affairs (P. A. W., W. J. M. H.).

REFERENCES

Aardal, N. P. (1984). *Exp. Hematol.*, **12**, 61–67.

Aardal, N. P. and Laerum, O. D. (1983). *Exp. Hematol.*, **11**, 792–801.

Aherne, G. (1989). In Arendt, J., Minors, D. and Waterhouse, J. (Eds), *Biological Rhythms in Clinical Practice.*, Butterworth, London, pp. 8–19.

Anisimov, V. and Zhukova, O. (1994). *Eksp. Onkol.*, **16**, 123–127.

Arendt, J., Minors, D. and Waterhouse, J. (1989). In Arendt, J., Minors, D. and Waterhouse, J. (Eds), *Biological Rhythms in Clinical Practice*. Butterworth, London, pp. 3–7.

Barnes, P. (1989). In Arendt, J., Minors, D. and Waterhouse, J. (Eds), *Biological Rhythms in Clinical Practice*. Butterworth, London, pp. 71–82.

Beland, F., Dooley, K., Sheldon, W. and Delongchamp, R. (1988). *J. Natl. Cancer Inst.*, **80**, 325–330.

Belanger, P. (1987). *Annu. Revi. Chronopharmacol.*, **4**, 1–46.

Belanger, M. P. and Labrecque, G. (1989). In Lemmer, B. (Ed.), *Chronopharmacology: Cellular and Biochemical Interactions.* pp. 15–34. Dekker, New York.

Belanger, P. and Labrecque, G. (1992). In Touitou, Y. and Haus, E. (Eds), *Biologic Rhythms in Clinical and Laboratory Medicine*. Springer, New York, pp. 403–409.

Belanger, P. Labrecque, G. and Dore, F. (1981). *Int. J. Chronobiol.*, **7**, 208–215.

Belanger, P. M., Lalande, M., Labrecque, G. and Dore, F. M. (1985). *Drug Metab. Dispos.*, **13**, 386–389.

Belanger, P., Lalande, M., Dore, F. and Labrecque, G. (1987). *J. Pharmacokinet. Biopharm.*, **15**, 133–143.

Belanger, P., Desgagne, M. and Boutet, M. (1988). *Annu. Rev. Chronopharmacol.*, **5**, 235–238.

Bon, K., Lanteri-Minet, M., Menetrey, D. and Berkley, K. (1997). *Pain*, **73**, 423–429.

Boughattas, A. N., Fournier, C., Hecquet, B., Lemaigre, G., Roulon, A., Reinberg, A., Mathé, G. and Lévi, F. (1990). *Annu. Rev. Chronopharmacol.*, **7**, 231–234.

Brassil, P., Edwards, R. and Davies, D. (1995). *Biochem. Pharmacol.*, **50**, 311–316.

Bresciani, F. (1968). *Cell Tissue Kinet.*, **1**, 51–63.

Bruckner, J., Luthra, R., Lakatua, D. and Sackett-Lunden, L. (1984). *Annu. Rev. Chronopharmacol.*, **1**, 373–376.

Bruguerolle, B. (1989). In Lemmer, B. (Ed.), *Chronopharmacology: Cellular and Biochemical Interactions*. Markel Dekker, New York, pp. 3–13.

Bruguerolle, B. (1992). In Touitou, Y. and Haus, E. (Eds), *Biologic Rhythms in Clinical and Laboratory Medicine* Springer, New York, pp. 113–137.

Bruguerolle, B., and Jadot, G. (1983). *Chronobiologia*, **10**, 295–297.

Bruguerolle, B., Valli, M., Jadot, G., Bouyard, L. and Bouyard, P. (1980). *Comm. 14th Rencontres Internationale Chimie Therapie Marseille.*

Bruguerolle, B., Valli, M., Jadot, G., Bouyard, L. and Bouyard, P. (1981). *Eur. J. Drug Metab. Pharmacokinet.*, **6**, 189–194.

Bruguerolle, B., Bouvenot, G. and Bartolin, R. (1984). *Annu. Rev. Chronopharmacol.*, **1**, 21–24. Pergamon Press, New York.

Bruguerolle, B., Prat, M., Douylliez, C. and Dorfman, P. (1988). *Fundam. Clin. Pharmacol.*, **2**, 301–304.

Buchi, K. N., Moore, J. G., Hrushesky, W. J. M., Sothern, R. B. and Rubin, N. H. (1991). *Gastroenterology*, **101**, 410–415.

Cal, J. (1983). *DEA de Nutrition*. University of Bordeaux, Bordeaux.

Cal, J. C., Dorian, C. and Cambar, J. (1986). *Annu. Rev. Chronopharmacolo.*, **3**, 143–176.

Cambar, J., Cal, J., Desmouliere, A. and Guillemain, J. (1983). *C. R. Acad. Sci.*, **296**, 949–952.

Cambar, J., Cal, J. and Tranchot, J. (1992a). In Touitou, Y. and Haus, E. (Eds), *Biologic Rhythms in Clinical and Laboratory Medicine*. Springer, New York, pp. 470–482.

Cambar, J., L'Azou, B. and Cal, J. (1992b). In Touitou, Y. and Haus, E. (Eds), *Biologic Rhythms in Clinical and Laboratory Medicine*. Springer, New York, pp. 138–150.

Cardoso, S. S., Scheving, L. E. and Halberg, F. (1970). *Pharmacologist*, **12**, 302.

Cardoso, S. S., Avery, T., Venditti, J. M. and Goldin, A. (1978). *Eur. J. Cancer*, **14**, 949–954.

Clausing, P., Gericke, S. and Dressel, U. (1991). *J. Exp. Anim. Sci.*, **34**, 153–157.

Clayton, D., Mullen, A. and Barnett, C. (1975). *Chronobiologia*, **2**, 210–217.

Cohen, P., Wax, Y. and Modan, B. (1983). *Cancer Res.*, **43**, 892–896.

Cohen, S. (1995). *Food Chem. Toxicol.*, **33**, 715–730.

Cole, C. and Adkisson, P. (1964). *Science*, **144**, 1148–1149.

Cooper, J. and Brodie, R. (1955). *J. Pharmacol. Exp. Ther.*, **114**, 409–417.

Davies, G., MacDonald, J. and Halberg, F. (1974). *Lancet*, **i**, 779.

Depres, P., Laustrat, B., Reynes, M. and Levi, F. (1997). *Proc. Am. Assoc. Cancer Res.*, **38**, 584.

Desgagne, M., Boutet, M. and Belanger, P. (1988). *Annu. Rev. Chronopharmacol.*, **5**, 235–238.

Eesa, N., Cutkomp, L., Cornelissen, G. and Halberg, F. (1987). *Adv. Chronobiol.*, Part A, 265–279.

Elliot, G. T., Welty, D. and Kuo, Y. D. (1991). *J. Immunol.*, **10**, 69–74.

Endo, A., Saki, N. and Ohwada, K. (1987). *Teratogenesis*, **7**, 475–482.

Endoh, D., Suzuki, A., Kuwabara, M., Satoh, H. and Sato, F. (1987). *J. Radiat. Res.*, **28**, 186–189.

English, J., Aherne, G. W. and Marks, V. (1982). *Cancer Chemother. Pharmacol.*, **9**, 114–117.

Fatranska, M., Vargova, M., Rosival, L., Batora, V., Nemeth, S. and Janekova, D. (1978). *Chronobiologia*, **5**, 39–44.

Fochem, K., Michalica, W. and Picha, E. (1967). *Strahlentherapie*, **133**, 256–261.

Frei, J. and Ritchie, A. (1964). *J. Natl. Cancer Inst.*, **32**, 1213–1220.

Frudden, L. and Wellso, S. (1968). *J. Econ. Entomol.*, **61**, 1692–1694.

Garrett, E. (1978). *Int. J. Clin. Pharmacol.*, **16**, 155–172.

Ghazi-Khansari, M. and Oreizi, S. (1995). *Vet. Hum. Toxicol.*, **37**, 449–452.

Hacker, M. P., Ershler, W. B., Newman, R. A. and Fagan, M. A. (1983). *Chronobiologia*, **10**, 301–306.

Haen, E. and Golly, I. (1986). *Annu. Rev. Chronopharmacol.*, **3**, 357–360.

Hagen, A. and Hrushesky, W. (1998). *Am. J. Surg.*, **104**, 245–261.

Halberg, F. (1975). *Indian J. Cancer*, **12**, 1–20.

Halberg, F., Johnson, E. A., Brown, B. W. and Bittner, J. J. (1960). *Proc. Soc. Exp. Biol. Med.*, **103**, 142–144.

Halberg, F., Gupta, B., Haus, E., Halberg, E., Deka, A., Nelson, W., Sothern, R., Cornellissen, G., Lee, J., Lakuta, D., Scheving, L. E. and Burns, E. R. (1977). In *Proceedings of the 14th International Congress of Therapeutics*. L'Expansion Scientifique Française, Paris, pp. 151–196.

Hashimoto, N., Endoh, D., Kumbara, M., Satoh, H. and Sato, F. (1994). *J. Vet. Med. Sci.*, **56**, 493-498.

Hanson, S. and Anders, M. (1978). *Toxicol. Lett.*, **1**, 301–305.

Haus, E. and Touitou, Y. (1992). In Touitou, Y. and Haus, E. (Eds), *Biologic Rhythms in Clinical and Laboratory Medicine*, Springer, New York, pp. 6–34.

Haus, E., Fernandes, G., Kuhl, J. F. W., Yunis, E. J., Lee, J. P. and Halberg, F. (1974a). *Chronobiologia*, **1**, 270–277.

Haus, E., Halberg, F. and Loken, M. K. (1974b). In Scheving, L. E., Halberg, F. and Pauly, J. E. (Eds), *Chronobiology*. pp. 115–122. Iaku Shoin, Tokyo.

Haus, E., Halberg, F., Sothern, R. B., Lakatua, D., Scheving, L. E., Sanchez, A., Sanchez, E., Melby, J., Wilson, T., Brown, H., Berg, H., Levi, F., Culley, D., Halberg, E., Hrushesky, W. J. M. and Pauly, J. E. (1980). *Chronobiologia*, **7**, 211.

Haverty, M. and Ware, G. (1970). *J. Econ. Entomol.*, **63**, 1296–1300.

Hecquet, B. and Bonneterre, J. (1984). *Annu. Rev. Chronopharmacol.*, **1**, 115–118.

Hendry, J. (1975). *Br. J. Radiol.*, **48**, 312–314.

Hermida, R. C., Ayeda, D. E., Fernandez, J. R. and Major, A. (1993). *Biomed. Instrum. Technol.*, **27**, 235–243.

Hori, K., Suzuki, M., Tanda, S., Saito, S., Shinozaki, M. and Zhang, Q. H. (1992). *Cancer Res.*, **52**, 912–916.

Hrushesky, W. J. M. (1985). *Science*, **228**, 73–75.

Hrushesky, W. (1994). *Sciences*, **34**, 32–37.

Hrushesky, W. J. M., Lévi, F., Halberg, F. and Kennedy, B. J. (1982). *Cancer Res.*, **42**, 945–949.

Hrushesky, W. J. M., Langevin, T., Nygaard, S., Young, J. and Roemeling, R. (1987a). Presented at the International Conference on Tumor Necrosis Factor and Related Cytokines, Heidelberg.

Hrushesky, W. J. M., Roemeling, R. V., Wood, P. A., Langevin, T. R., Lange, P. and Fraley, E. (1987b). *J. Clin. Oncol.*, **5**, 450–455.

Hrushesky, W. J. M., Gruber, S. A., Sothern, R. B., Hoffman, R. A., Lakatua, D., Carlson, A., Cerra, F. and Simmons, R. L. (1988). *J. Natl. Cancer Inst.*, **80**, 1232–1237.

Hrushesky, W. J. M., Bluming, A. Z., Gruber, S. A. and Sothern, R. B. (1989a). *Lancet*, **ii**, 949–952.

Hrushesky, W. J. M., von Roemeling, R. and Sothern, B. (1989b). In Lemmer, B. (Ed.), *Chronopharmacology: Cellular and Biochemical Interactions*. Marcel Dekker, New York, pp. 439–473.

Hrushesky, W. J. M., von Roemeling, R., Lanning, R. M. and Rabatin, J. T. (1990). *J. Clin. Oncol.*, **8**, 1504–1513.

Hrushesky, W. J. M., Sánchez, S., Wood, P. A., Martynowicz, M., Wighton, T., Lobo, S. and Vyzula, R. (1992). *Proceedings, American Association for Cancer Research*, **33**, 300.

Hrushesky, W. J. M., Langevin, T., Kim, Y. J. and Wood, P. A. (1994). *J. Exp. Med.*, **180**, 1059–1065.

Hrushesky, W., Lannin, D. and Haus, E. (1998). *J. Natl. Cancer Inst.*, **90**, 1480–1484.

Hrushesky, W., Vyzula, R. and Wood, P. (1999). *Reprod. Toxicol.*, submitted.

Ijiri, K. and Potten, C. (1990). *Int. J. Radiat. Biol.*, **58**, 165–175.

Iversen, O. and Iversen, U. (1976). *Acta Pathol. Microbiol. Scand. A*, **84**, 406–414.

Iversen, O. and Iversen, U. (1995). *In Vivo*, **9**, 117–132.

Iversen, U., Iverson, O., Hennings, H. and Bjerknes, R. (1970). *J. Natl. Cancer Inst.*, **45**, 269–276.

Jaeger, R. J., Conolly, R. B. and Murphy, S. D. (1973). *Res. Commun. Chem. Pathol. Pharmacol.*, **6**, 465.

Kemeny, M., Alava, G. and Oliver, J. (1992). *J. Immunother.*, **12**, 219–223.

Klevecz, R. R. and Braly, P. S. (1987). *Chronobiol. Int.*, **4**, 513–523.

Klotz, U. and Ziegler, G. (1982). *Clin. Pharmacol. Ther.*, **32**, 107–112.

Koopman, M. G., Krediet, R. T. and Arisz, L. (1985). *Neth. J. Med.*, **28**, 416–423.

Koren, S. and Fleischmann, W. R. (1993a). *Exp. Hematol.*, **21**, 552–559.

Koren, S. and Fleischmann, W. R. (1993b). *J. Interferon Res.*, **13**, 187–194.

Koren, S., Whorton, E. J. and Fleischmann, W. J. (1993). *J. Natl. Cancer Inst.*, **85**, 1927–1932.

Koyanagi, S., Ohdo, S., Yukawa, E. and Higuchi, S. (1997). *J. Pharmacol. Exp. Ther.*, **283**, 259–264.

Langevin, A. M., Koren, G., Soldin, S. and Greenberg, M. (1987). *Lancet*, **ii**, 505–506.

Langner, B. and Lemmer, B. (1988). *Annu. Rev. Chronopharmacol.*, **5**, 335–338.

Lavigne, J., Belanger, P., Dore, F. and Labrecque, G. (1983). *Toxicology*, **26**, 267–273.

Lawrence, G. and Beesley, A. (1988). *Drug Metab. Drug Interact.*, **6**, 359–370.

Lemmer, B. (1981). *Naunyn Schmiedebergs Arch. Pharmacol.*, **316**, R60.

Lemmer, B. and Nold, G. (1991). *Br. J. Pharmacol.*, **32**, 627–629.

Leung, P. and Harrison, R. (1998). *Occup. Environ. Med.*, **55**, 249–257.

Lévi, F. (1982). Thesis, Université Paris VI.

Lévi, F., Hrushesky, W. J. M., Holtzman, J., Halberg, G., Sanchez, S. and Kennedy, B. J. (1981). *Int. J. Chonobiol.*, **7**, 277.

Lévi, F. A., Hrushesky, W. J. M., Blomquist, C. H., Lakuta, D. J., Haus, E., Halberg, F. and Kennedy, B. J. (1982). *Cancer Res.*, **42**, 950–955.

Lévi, F., Mechkouri, M., Roulon, A., Bailleul, F., Horvath, C., Reinberg, A. and Mathé, G. (1985). *Cancer Treat. Rep.*, **69**, 1443–1445.

Lévi, F., Boughattas, N. A. and Blazsek, I. (1987). *Annu. Rev. Chronopharmacol.*, **4**, 283–331.

Lévi, F., Bourin, P., Pages, N., Mechkouri, M., Lemaigre, G., Auzeby, A., Touitoi, Y., *et al.* (1992). *Proc. Am. Assoc. Cancer Res.*, **33**, 329.

Lévi, F., Zidani, R. and Misset, J.-L. (1997). *Lancet*, **360**, 681–686.

Kennedy, B. J. (1982). *Cancer Res.*, **42**, 950–955.

Levine, W. (1983). In J. C. and Jacoby, W. (Eds), *Biological Basis of Detoxification*. Academic Press, New York, pp. 251.

Lindsey, W., Gupta, T. and Beattie, C. (1981). *Cancer Res.*, **41**, 3857–3862.

Lockard, J., Viswanathan, C. and Levy, R. (1985). *Life Sci.*, **36**, 1281–1285.

MacLeay, D. and Munro, J. (1979). *Bull. Environ. Contam. Toxicol.*, **23**, 552–557.

Marquardt, H. (1974). *Cancer Res.*, **34**, 1612–1615.

Mayersbach, H. (1974). In Scheving, L., Halbert, F. and Pauly, J. (Eds), *Chronobiology*. Iaku Shoin, Tokyo, pp. 191–196.

Merrill, E. and Akbar-Kanzadeh, F. (1998). *Health Phys.*, **74**, 568–573.

Mormont, M. C., Berestka, J., Mushiya, T., Langevin, T., von Roemeling, R., Rabatin, J., Sothern, R. and Hrushesky, W. J. M. (1986). *Annu. Rev. Chronopharmacol.*, **3**, 187–190.

Moskalik, K. G. (1976). *Bull. Exp. Biol. (USSR)*, **81**, 741–743.

Mukai, H., Ambe, Y., Muku, T., Takeshita, K. and Fukuma, T. (1986). *Nature*, **324**, 239–241.

Nagasawa, H., Yanai, R. and Taniguchi, H. (1976). *Cancer Res.*, **36**, 2223–2226.

Nagayama, H. and Takahashi, R. (1989). In Lemmer, B. (Ed.), *Chronopharmocology: Cellular and Biochemical Interactions*. Marcel Dekker, New York, pp. 255–265.

Nakano, S. (1989). In Lemmer, B. (Ed.), *Chronopharmacology: Cellular and Biochemical Interactions*. Marcel Dekker, New York, pp. 267–280.

Naranjo, C., Sellers, E., Giles, H. and Abel, J. (1980). *Br. J. Clin. Pharmacol.*, **9**, 265–272.

Nowosielski, J., Patton, R. and Naegele, J. (1964). *J. Cell. Comp. Physiol.*, **63**, 393–398.

Ohdo, S., Arata, N., Furukubo, T., Yukawa, E., Higuchi, S. and Nakano, S. (1998). *J. Pharmacol. Exp. Ther.*, **285**, 242–246.

Ohdo, S., Watanabe, H., Ogawa, N., Yoshiyama, Y. and Sugiyama, T. (1995). *Eur. J. Pharmacol.*, **293**, 281–285.

Ohdo, S., Watanabe, H., Ogawa, N., Yoshiyama, Y. and Sugiyama, T. (1996). *Jpn. J. Pharmacol.*, **70**, 253–258.

Ohdo, S., Inoue, K., Yukawa, E., Higuchi, S., Nakano, S. and Ogawa, N. (1997a). *Jpn. J. Pharmacol.*, **75**, 283–290.

Ohdo, S., Makinosumi, T., Ishizaki, T., Yukawa, E., Higuchi, S., Nakano, S. and Ogawa, N. (1997b). *J. Pharmacol. Exp. Ther.*, **283**, 1383–1388.

Onyeocha, F. and Fuzeau-Braesch, S. (1991). *Chronobiol. Int.*, **8**, 103–109.

Patel, I., Venkataramanan, R., Levy, R., Viswanathan, C. and Ojemann, L. (1982). *Epilepsia*, **32**, 282–290.

Peters, G. J., Van Dijk, J., Nadal, J. C., Van Groeningen, C. J., Lankelman, J. and Pinedo, H. M. (1987). *In Vivo*, **1**, 112–118.

Pinkerton, C. R., Welshman, S. G., Glasgow, J. F. T. and Bridges, J. M. (1980). *Lancet*, **ii**, 944–945.

Pizzarello, D. J. and Witcofski, R. L. (1970). *Radiology*, **97**, 165–167.

Pizzarello, D. J., Witcofski, R. L. and Lyons, E. A. (1963). *Science*, **139**, 349.

Pizzarello, D. J., Isaak, D. and Chua, K. E. (1964). *Science*, **145**, 286–291.

Porstendorfer, J., Butterweck, G. and Reineking, A. (1994). *Health Phys.*, **67**, 283–287.

Purnell, D. M. and Kopen, P. (1976). *Anat. Rec.*, **186**, 39–48.

Qui, J., Roberts, S. and Potten, C. (1994). *Epith. Cell. Biol.*, **3**, 137–148.

Ratajczak, H. V., Sothern, R. B. and Hrushesky, W. J. M. (1988). *J. Exp. Med.*, **168**, 73–83.

Ratko, T. and Beattie, C. (1995). *Cancer Res.*, **45**, 3042–3047.

Riccardo, R., Balis, F. M., Ferrara, P., Lasorella, A., Poplack, D. G. and Mastrangelo, R. (1986). *Pediatr. Hematol. Oncol.*, **3**, 319–324.

Rikin, A. and Anderson, J. (1990). In Hayes, D., Pauly, J. and Reiter, R. (Eds), *Chronobiology: Its Role in Clinical Medicine, General Biology, and Agriculture, Part B*. Wiley-Liss, New York, pp. 895–903.

Riva, R., Albani, F., Ambrosetto, G., Contin, M., Cortelli, P., Perucca, E. and Baruzzi, A. (1984). *Epilepsia*, **25**, 476–481.

Rivard, G., Infante-Rivard, C., Hoyoux, C. and Champagne, J. (1985). *Lancet*, **ii**, 1264–1266.

Roberts, D., Smolensky, M., Hsi, B. and Scanlon, J. (1974). In Scheving, L. E., Halbery, F. and Pauly, J. E. (Eds.), *Chronobiology*, pp. 612–616. Iaku Shoin Ltd, Tokyo.

Robertson, W., Hodgkinson, A. and Marshall, D. (1977). *Clin. Chim. Acta*, **80**, 347–353.

Russo, J. and Russo, I. (1978). *J. Natl. Cancer Inst.*, **61**, 1451–1457.

Sauerbier, I. (1981). *Prog. Clin. Biol. Res.*, **59C**, 143–149.

Sauerbier, I. (1986a). *Chronobiol. Int.*, **3**, 161–164.

Sauerbier, I. (1986b). *Drug Chem. Toxicol.*, **9**, 25–31.

Sauerbier, I. (1987). *Am. J. Anat.*, **178**, 170–174.

Sauerbier, I. (1992). In Touitou, Y. and Haus, E. (Eds), *Biologic Rhythms in Clinical and Laboratory Medicine*. Springer, Berlin, pp. 151–157.

Scheving, L. E., Haus, E., Kuhl, J. F. W., Pauly, J. E., Halberg, F. and Cardoso, S. S. (1976). *Cancer Res.*, **36**, 113–117.

Scheving, L. E., Burns, E. R., Pauli, J. E. and Tsai, T. H. (1978). *Anat. Rec.*, **191**, 479–486.

Scheving, L., Feures, R., Tsai, T. and Scheving, L. (1994). In Hrushesky, W. (Ed.), *Circadian Cancer Therapy*. CRC Press, Boca Raton, FL, pp. 19–40.

Schmidt, R. (1978). *Biol. Rundsch.*, **16**, 243–248.

Schnell, R., Bozigian, H., Davies, M., Merrick, B. and Johnson, K. (1983). *Toxicol. Appl. Pharmacol.*, **71**, 353–361.

Schnell, R., Bozigian, H., Davies, M., Merrick, B., Park, K. and McMillan, D. (1984). *Pharmacology*, **29**, 149–157.

Setsuo, K. and Patterson, B. (1988). *Hort. Sci.*, **23**, 713–714.

Shaw, G., Falk, R., Caporaso, N., Issaq, H., Kase, R., Fox, S. and Tucker, M. (1990). *J. Natl. Cancer Inst.*, **82**, 1573–1575.

Sheets, R. (1992). *J. Air Waste Manage. Assoc.*, **42**, 457–459.

Shipp, E. and Otten, J. (1976). *Entomol. Exp. Appl.*, **19**, 163–171.

Shivley, C. A. and Vesell, E. S. (1975). *Clin. Pharmacol. Ther.*, **18**, 413–424.

Sletvold, O. and Laerum, O. D. (1988). *Eur. J. Haematol.*, **41**, 230–236.

Smaaland, R., Laerum, O., Sothern, R., Sletvold, O., Bjerknes, R. and Lote, K. (1992). *Blood*, **79**, 2281–2287.

Smaaland, R., Lote, K., Sothern, R. B. and Laerum, O. D. (1993). *Cancer Res.*, **53**, 3129–3138.

Smith, R. (1973). *The Excretory Function of the Bile*. Chapman and Hall, London.

Smith, R., Kroboth, P. and Phillips, J. (1986). *J. Clin. Pharmacol.*, **26**, 120–124.

Smolensky, M. (1989). In Lemmer, B. (Ed.), *Chronopharmocology: Cellular and Biochemical Interactions*. Marcel Dekker, New York, pp. 65–113.

Snyder, N. K., Smolensky, M. and Hsi, B. P. (1981). *Chronobiologia*, **8**, 33–44.

Sothern, R., Halberg, F., Zinneman, H. and Kennedy, B. (1981). *Chronopharmacology and Chronotherapeutics*. Florida A&M University Foundation, Tallahassee, FL.

Sothern, R., Smaaland, R. and Moore, J. (1995). *FASEB J.*, **9**, 397–403.

Starek, A., Oginski, A., Rutenfranz, J. and Pokorski, J. (1989). *Pol. J. Occup. Med.*, **2**, 186–191.

Stoney, P. J., Halberg, F. and Simpson, H. W. (1975). *Chronobiologia*, **2**, 319–324.

Sturtevant, R. and Garber, S. (1985). *Anat. Rec.*, **211**, 187.

Sturtevant, R. and Garber, S. (1986). *Annu. Rev. Chronopharmacol.*, **4**, 47–76.

Sullivan, W., Crawley, B., Hayes, D., Rosenthal, J. and Halberg, F. (1970). *J. Econ. Entomol.*, **63**, 159–163.

Tampellini, M., Filipski, E. and Levi, F. (1995). *Chronobiol. Int.*, **12**, 195–198.

Tampellini, M., Filipski, E., Liu, X., Lemaigre, G., Li, X., Vrignaud, P., Francois, E., Bissery, M. and Levi, F. (1998). *Cancer Res.*, **58**, 3896–3904.

Tvermyr, E. (1972). *Virchows Arch. B*, **11**, 43–52.

Uneo, Y. (1968). *Int. J. Radiat. Biol.*, **14**, 307–312.

Vacek, A. and Rotkovska, D. (1970). *Strahlentherapie*, **140**, 302–306.

von Roemeling, R., DeMaria, L., Salzer, M., Connerty, M., Wood, P., Portuese, E., Sánchez de la Peña, S., DeConti, G., Chikkappa, G., Pasquale, D., Ferro, T. and Hrushesky, W. (1990). *Annu. Rev. Chronopharmacol.*, **7**, 173–176.

von Roemeling, R. and Hrushesky, W. J. M. (1990). *J. Natl. Cancer Inst.*, **82**, 386–393.

Vonk, R., Scholtens, E. and Strubbe, J. (1978). *Clin. Sci. Mol. Med.*, **55**, 399–406.

Walker, A., Oakes, G., McLanghlin, M., Ehrenkranz, R., Chez, R. and Alling, D. (1977). *Gynecol. Invest.*, **8**, 288–298.

Walsh, S., Ducsay, C. and Novy, M. (1984). *Am. J. Obstet. Gynecol.*, **150**, 745–753.

Waterhouse, J. M. and Minors, D. S. (1989). In Lemmer, B. (Ed.), *Chronopharmacology: Cellular and Biochemical Interactions*. Marcel Dekker, New York, pp. 35–50.

Waxman, D. (1986). In Montellano, P. O. D. (Ed.), *Cytochrome P-450: Structure, Mechanism, and Biochemistry*. Plenum Press, London, pp. 525–540.

Wolff, T. and Strecker, M. (1992). *Exp. Toxicol. Pathol.*, **44**, 263–271.

Wood, P. and Hrushesky, W. (1997). *Proc. AACR*, **38**, 475.

Wood, P., Hrushesky, W. and Klevecz, R. (1998a). *Exp Hematol*, **26**, 523–533.

Wood, P., Lincoln, D. and Hrushesky, W. (1998b). *Proc AACR*, **39**, 469.

Wood, P. A., Vyzula, R. and Hrushesky, W. J. M. (1993). *J. Infus. Chemother.*, **3**, 89–95.

Wood, P. A., Peace, D., Torosoff, M., Vyzula, R. and Hrushesky, W. J. M. (1995). *J. Invest. Med.*, **43**, 371A.

Zabel, P., Horst, H., Kreiber, C. and Schlaak, M. (1990). *Klin. Wochenschr.*, **68**, 1217–1221.

Zhang, R. and Diasio, R. (1994). In Hrushesky, W. (Ed.), *Circadian Cancer Therapy*. CRC Press, Boca Raton, FL, pp. 61–103.

Zhang, R., Lu, Z., Liu, T., Soong, S. and Diasio, R. (1993). *Cancer Res.*, **53**, 2816–2822.

Ziliani, S., Presta, M., Mazzocchi, C., Mazzoleni, G., Calovini, D. and Ragnotti, G. (1984). *Cancer Lett.*, **23**, 245–251.

FURTHER READING

Arendt, J., Minors, D. and Waterhouse, J. (Eds) (1989). *Biological Rhythms in Clinical Practice*. Butterworth, London.

Hrushesky, W. J. M. (Ed.) (1994). *Circadian Cancer Therapy*. CRC Press, Boca Raton, FL.

Lemmer, B. (Ed.) (1989). *Chronopharmacology: Cellular and Biochemical Interactions*. Marcel Dekker, New York.

Touitou, Y. and Haus, E. (Eds) (1992). *Biologic Rhythms in Clinical and Laboratory Medicine*. Springer, New York.

Wood, P. and Hrushesky, W. (1996). *Crit. Rev. Eukaryot. Gene Express.*, **6**, 299–343.

Wood, P. A. (1995). *J. Infus. Chemother.*, **5**, 20–23.

Chapter 12

Interspecies Differences in Xenobiotic Metabolizing Enzymes and Their Importance for Interspecies Extrapolation of Toxicity

Jan Georg Hengstler and Franz Oesch

C O N T E N T S

INTRODUCTION

Extrapolation from laboratory animals to man represents one of the most complex challenges to the toxicologist. For this purpose, species differences in uptake, distribution, metabolism, site of action, elimination and accumulation must be taken into account. For the experimental toxicologist, the occurrence of differences between animal species in the metabolism of xenobiotics probably represents the most frequent reason for interspecies differences, being responsible for qualitative and quantitative differences in toxic effects.

Ideally, species which metabolize the respective test substance in the same way as man should be used for toxicological tests. Generally this ideal is not attainable. However, it should be possible to identify the species with the metabolism for a specific compound closest to man. For this purpose, isolated hepatocytes have been used successfully, since a good correlation between the metabolism of a xenobiotic *in vivo* and in isolated hepatocytes of the same species *in vitro* has been observed (Oesch and Diener, 1995). Since the introduction of the two-step collagenase isolation technique, primary hepatocytes *in vitro* have been widely used in toxicity tests. One major obstacle for this procedure, the limited availability of human hepatocytes, has been overcome by adequate cryopreservation techniques (Diener *et al.*, 1994; Steinberg *et al.*, 1998). Thus, a reasonable interspecies extrapolation from animals to humans and safety assessment can be performed in most cases if we have (i) an adequate understanding of the metabolism and mechanism of toxicity of a given compound, (ii) data on its metabolism and toxicity (e.g. on DNA adducts or unscheduled DNA synthesis) in primary hepatocytes of humans and relevant laboratory animal species and (iii) toxicity data including carcinogenicity studies in these species. In this chapter this will be demonstrated for heterocyclic amines, polycyclic aromatic hydrocarbons, aflatoxin B$_1$ and the anticancer drug tamoxifen. In contrast, the cardiac glycoside digitoxin will be discussed as an example where interspecies differences are mainly due to differences in pharmacodynamics and not to metabolism.

It should be considered that there are examples where interspecies differences in toxicity are a consequence of differences in target mechanisms, for instance the $\alpha2_\mu$-globulin nephropathy, which has been recognized as a male rat-specific problem, and for peroxisome proliferation and associated hepatocarcinogenesis, which is a phenomenon in rats and mice (Caldwell, 1992). However, keeping the exceptions in mind, the mechanisms of toxicity are similar in animals and man for the majority of substances.

HETEROCYCLIC AMINES

Today at least 20 different heterocyclic amines have been isolated from cooked foods, primarily fish, chicken, and pork, and several additional heterocyclic amines have been reported, but their structures have not been elucidated (Adamson *et al.*, 1996). The formation of heterocyclic amines results from the reaction of creatine in muscle meats with amino acids at customary cooking temperatures. Since all known heterocyclic amines have planar structures, they are able to intercalate into GC pair rich stretches of DNA. 2-Amino-3-methylimidazo[4,5-*f*]quinoline (IQ), 2-amino-3,8-dimethylimidazo[4,5-*f*]quinoxaline (MeIQx) and 2-amino-1-methyl-6-phenylimidazo[4,5-*b*]pyridine (PhIP) represent three of the most prevalent heterocyclic amines found in the Western diet.

A principal route of metabolic activation of heterocyclic amines includes *N*-oxidation to hydroxylamines, primarily by CYP 1A2 but also by other CYP isoforms, their subsequent *O*-esterification by acetyltransferase or sulphotransferase to reactive ester intermediates, which can spontaneously lose acetate or sulphate to form a nitrenium ion that can covalently bind to DNA **(Figure 1)**. Hydroxylation of exocyclic amino groups of heterocyclic amines is believed to be an initial activation step, whereas ring hydroxylation and subsequent hydroxylations are predominantly detoxification pathways (Buonarati and Felton, 1990). Some metabolites of heterocyclic amines, e.g. *N*-hydroxy-PhIP or *N*-acetoxy-PhIP, can be transported from the liver to extrahepatic tissues (Kadlubar *et al.*, 1995). In addition, glucuronides derived from heterocyclic amines are secreted into the bile, owing to their relatively high molecular weight. In the colon, the heterocyclic hydroxylamines may then be released from the conjugates due to the action of bacterial glucuronidases. In contrast to the original *not* hydroxylated heterocyclic amines, the hydroxylamines represent good substrates for NAT2, which is expressed in relatively high levels in colon epithelial cells. This mechanism may explain the colon-specific carcinogenic effect of some heterocyclic amines.

Large interspecies differences in metabolism, mutagenicity and carcinogenicity of heterocyclic amines have been observed. To date, 10 heterocyclic amines, including IQ, MeIQx and PhIP, have been shown to be carcinogenic in rats and mice (Adamson *et al.*, 1996). In addition, IQ has been shown to be a potent hepatocarcinogen in cynomolgus monkeys, whereas MeIQx lacks the potency of IQ to induce hepatocellular carcinoma after a 5-year dosing period (Snyderwine *et al.*, 1997). The carcinogenicity of PhIP in the cynomolgus monkey is not yet known. To examine interspecies differences, liver microsomes from cynomolgus monkeys, rats and humans were added to *Salmonella typhimurium* TA 98 in the Ames test as an activating system (Davis *et al.*, 1993). Differences between species were most pronounced when MeIQx was tested. Incubations with 0.5 μg of MeIQx resulted in 1243 ± 48, 1070 ± 75, 695 ± 35 and 129 ± 19 revertant colonies per plate for human, male rat, female rat and cynomolgus monkey microsomes, respectively

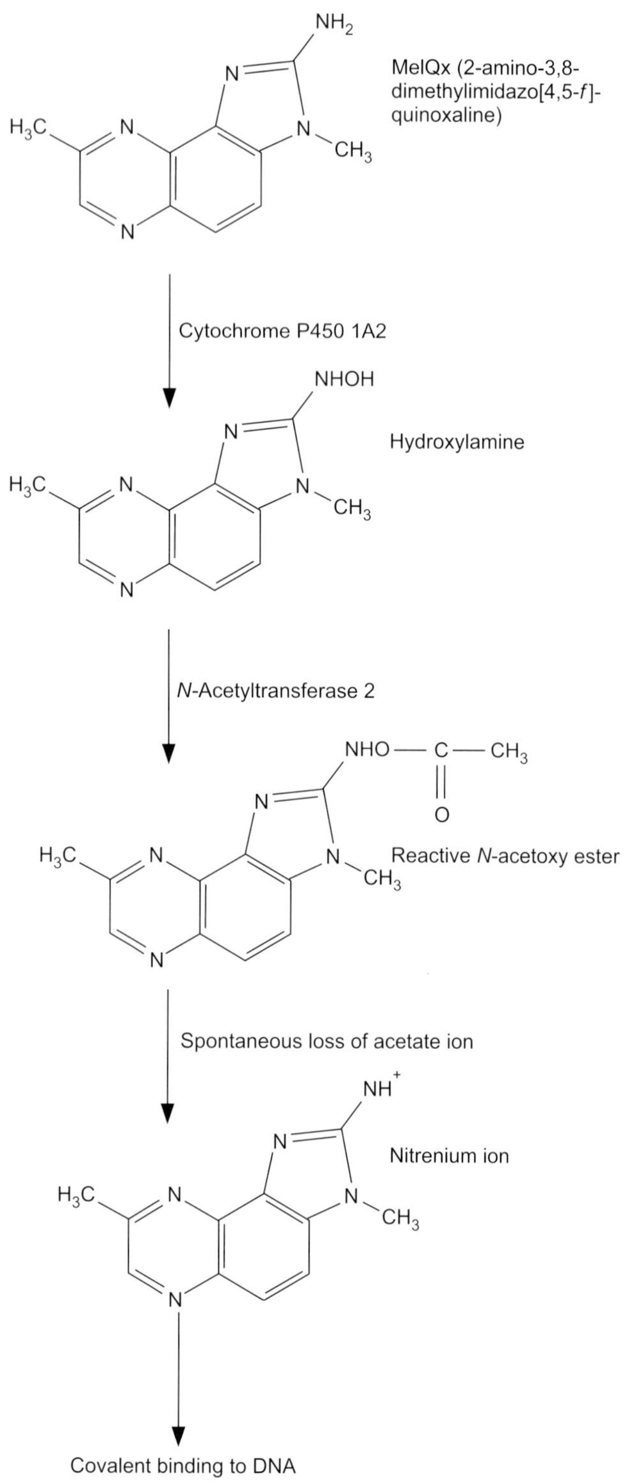

Figure 1 Metabolic activation of MeIQx (2-amino-3,8-dimethylimidazo[4,5-*f*]quinoxaline) by cytochrome P450 1A2 and *N*-acetyltransferase 2.

(Figure 2). Similarly, DNA adducts after oral application of MeIQx were highest in male rats, followed by female rats, and were much lower in cynomolgus monkeys (Davis *et al.*, 1993). Both rats and humans have constitutive levels of hepatic CYP 1A2 (Sesardic *et al.*, 1989,

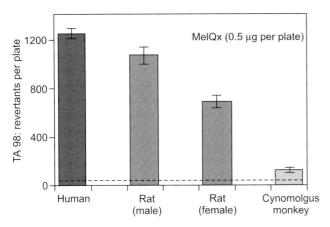

Figure 2 Activation of 2-amino-3,8-dimethylimidazo[4,5-*f*]qui-noxaline (MeIQx) to a bacterial mutagen by microsomes from humans, male and female rats and cynomolgus monkeys (untreated animals). The line gives the number of spontaneous TA 98 revertants. Source: Davis *et al.* (1993).

1990), whereas cynomolgus monkeys do not (Sadrieh and Snyderwine, 1995). The results suggest that lack of constitutive CYP 1A2 expression in cynomolgus monkeys is responsible for the low capacity to activate MeIQx, which protects this species from genotoxicity and carcinogenicity due to MeIQx. In contrast to the cynomolgus monkey, the marmoset monkey shows constitutive hepatic expression of CYP 1A2 similar to that in human liver (Edwards *et al.*, 1994). Liver microsomes from the marmoset monkey activated MeIQx to a bacterial mutagen to a similar extent as human liver microsomes (Edwards *et al.*, 1994). Hence the marmoset is a more suitable model than the cynomolgus monkey for carcinogenicity studies with MeIQx.

Comparing human and rat CYP 1A2 it was suggested that the rat enzyme is catalytically less efficient than the human enzyme in activating MeIQx via *N*-hydroxylation (review: Boobis *et al.*, 1996). In addition, the almost exclusive *N*-hydroxylation of MeIQx by human liver microsomes in contrast to the competing detoxicating ring hydroxylation reactions by rat liver microsomes (Turesky *et al.*, 1988; Alexander *et al.*, 1989) may explain the higher efficiency of human microsomes to activate MeIQx to mutagenic metabolites.

The higher capacity of male compared with female rat liver microsomes to activate MeIQx to mutagenic metabolites might be explained by CYP-male, an isoform which exists in male but not in female rats (Yamazoe *et al.*, 1988; Davis *et al.*, 1993). The difference between male and female rats cannot be explained by CYP 1A2, since about twofold higher levels of CYP 1A2 have been observed in female than male rats (Yamazoe *et al.*, 1988).

For IQ, a completely different constellation compared with MeIQx has been reported. The *N*-hydroxylation of IQ appears to be carried out largely by hepatic CYP 3A4 and/or CYP 2C9/10 (Snyderwine *et al.*, 1997). Vice versa,

CYP 3A4 and CYP 2C9/10 were unable to *N*-hydroxylate MeIQx.

Western blot analysis showed that cynomolgus monkey hepatic microsomes constitutively express CYP isoforms immunologically related to the human CYP 3A, CYP 2C and very low levels of CYP 1A1 (Sadrieh and Snyderwine, 1995). CYP 3A constitutes about 20% of the total hepatic CYP in cynomolgus monkeys and is at least 90% homologous to human CYP 3A4 (Ohmori *et al.*, 1993). This may explain why the mutagenic activation of IQ by human and cynomolgus liver microsomes is very similar, with only slightly higher numbers of TA 98 revertants per plate for human microsomes (Davis *et al.*, 1993). The differences in CYP isoenzymes involved in initial activation of MeIQx and IQ have also been confirmed by differential induction of cytochrome P450 (Sadrieh and Snyderwine, 1995): treatment of cynomolgus monkeys with rifampicin induced hepatic microsomal proteins related to human CYP 3A and CYP 2C and was accompanied by a threefold increase in the mutagenic activation of IQ, without any alterations in the mutagnic activation of MeIQx. In addition, human recombinant CYP 3A4 and CYP 2C9 were shown to activate mutagenically IQ but not MeIQx (Aoyama *et al.*, 1990). Treatment of cynomolgus monkeys with TCDD significantly increased mutagenic activation of both MeIQx and IQ, consistent with an induction of CYP 1A isozymes, suggesting that TCDD-inducible CYP 1A enzymes *N*-hydroxylate both substrates without selectivity.

In an extensive study considering phase I and II metabolism, species differences in the bioactivation of PhIP between human, rat and mouse were examined (Lin *et al.*, 1995). Human hepatic microsomes had the highest capacity to catalyse the initial activation step to *N*-hydroxy-PhIP that was 1.8-and 1.4-fold higher than in rats and mice, respectively. In addition, the ratio of the activating *N*-hydroxylation to the detoxifying ring hydroxylation resulting in 4'-hydroxy-PhIP was 97:1 for human hepatic microsomes, which was much greater than that of rat (33:1) or mouse (1.7:1). The high ratio of *N*-to 4'-hydroxylation by human microsomes may be due to the extremely low CYP 1A1 expression in human liver, which is the principal enzyme responsible for the formation of 4'-hydroxy-PhIP in rodents (Wallin *et al.*, 1990). To examine the role of acetyltransferase and sulfotransferase, calf thymus DNA was incubated together with [³H]*N*-hydroxy-PhIP and liver cytosol with and without addition of the cofactors acetyl CoA and 3'-phosphoadenosine-5'-phosphosulphate (PAPS). Subsequently PhIP-DNA binding was determined. Acetyl coenzyme A-dependent DNA binding of *N*-hydroxy-PhIP was similar to that in human rapid acetylators, but was 2.6-fold higher than that in human slow acetylators. *O*-Acetyltransferase activity for PhIP was lowest in mice, which was only 11% of that in rats and 12 and 29% of that in human rapid and slow acetylators, respectively. In contrast, mouse hepatic cytosols exhibited the highest sulphotransferase activity for PhIP activation, which was 4.9-and 2.3-fold higher than that in rats and humans, respectively. PhIP–DNA binding was increased significantly by GST inhibitors (triethyltin bromide for human and triphenyltin chloride for rodent glutathione S-transferases) for human and rat cytosols, but not for mouse cytosols.

In conclusion, humans may be more susceptible to the carcinogenic effect of heterocyclic amines than monkeys, rats or mice. Some individuals, namely those with high CYP 1A2 and 3A4 activities and the rapid acetylator phenotype, can be expected to have an especially high risk. The polymorphism of NAT2 further complicates the complex situation of heterocyclic amines (review: Hengstler et al., 1998). The rapid acetylator phenotype, assessed by the rate of orally given sulphamethazine, a substrate specific to NAT2, was shown to be associated with colorectal cancer (odds ratio, 1.8; 95% CI, 1.0–3.3; number of patients, 110) (Roberts-Thomson et al., 1996). In this study, the highest risk was observed in the youngest tertile (<64 years) of patients (odds ratio, 8.9; 95% CI, 2.6–30.4) and increased with increasing intake of meat in rapid, but not in slow, acetylators. In addition, the risk of colorectal cancer was higher for individuals consuming well done cooked meat, which is known to contain higher levels of heterocyclic amines, compared with individuals usually eating less well done meat (Schiffmann and Felton, 1990; Gerhardsson de Verdier et al., 1991; Lang et al., 1994). Although these studies did not directly measure the intake of heterocyclic amines, the total constellation suggests that heterocyclic amines consumed with meat contribute to human carcinogenesis.

In addition to rapid acetylation, rapid metabolizers of CYP 1A2 are also expected to have a higher risk of heterocyclic amine-induced colon cancer. It is known that cigarette smoking (and other hydrocarbon-containing mixtures) induce CYP 1A2 in human liver (Boobis et al., 1996). Hence it should be expected that for individuals who regularly eat meat, cigarette smoking represents a risk factor for colon cancer. At first glance it seems intriguing that epidemiological studies suggest the opposite (Giovannuci et al., 1994). Although smoking itself is a positive risk factor, smokers eating meat were at reduced risk of colorectal cancer compared with non-smokers with a similar meat consumption. However, this is not the only report showing that cigarette smoking, although representing a risk factor itself, may provide protection from additional genotoxic exposures, e.g. N-nitrosodiethanolamine or ethylene oxide (Oesch et al., 1994). It was speculated that cigarette smoking, besides increasing CYP 1A2 levels, leads to reduced genotoxicity of these compounds through parallel induction of glutathione S-transferase A1-1 (GST A1), which may serve to detoxify heterocyclic amines in the colon (Boobis et al., 1996). Indeed, it was shown that GST A1 could be induced in human hepatocytes, but inducibility was observed only in a subgroup of individuals (Morel et

al., 1993; Schrenk et al., 1995). Whether this reflects interindividual variation in protection against heterocyclic amines still has to be examined.

Since heterocyclic amines most probably contribute to human carcinogenesis, strategies to minimize their intake and genotoxicity should be considered. In this context, it seems important that heterocyclic amines induce their own activation in humans (Sinha et al., 1994). In non-smokers, consumption of pan-fried meat cooked at high temperature (250 °C) for 7 days (which was shown to contain MeIQx, PhIP and DiMeIQx) significantly increased CYP 1A2 activity, whereas meat cooked at only 100 °C did not. In addition, chronic treatment of cynomolgus monkeys with IQ (10 mg kg^{-1}) increased the capacity of liver microsomes to activate MeIQx to a bacterial mutagen (Sadrieh and Snyderwine, 1995). Indeed, at a substrate concentration of 5 μg of MeIQx, microsomes from IQ-treated versus control monkeys caused 430 versus 40 revertants per plate, respectively. Thus, it might reduce heterocyclic amine genotoxicity if meat consumption were followed by a period without meat consumption to avoid having the next heterocyclic amine exposure when CYP 1A2 is still induced. In addition, exposure to heterocyclic amines might be reduced by cooking meat at low temperature (about 100 °C) and eating beef cooked medium instead of well done. Some further methods to minimize the consumption of heterocyclic amines (Adamson et al., 1996)—the use of microwaves, wraping meat or fish in aluminium foil to prevent contact with an open flame, using bacon grease sparingly for cooking, removing the meat juice and blackend parts of meat—are mentioned for completeness, but are inacceptable from a gourmet's point of view.

AFLATOXIN B$_1$

Aflatoxin B$_1$ (AFB1) is one of the most potent hepatocarcinogens known. It represents a liver cell type-specific toxin, since it induces the formation of tumours developing from parenchymal and bile duct epithelial cells but not from Kupffer or endothelial cells in a variety of animal species (Steinberg et al., 1996). AFB1 has been identified as a human carcinogen based on data from epidemiological studies of hepatocellular cancer in AFB1-exposed populations (Wild et al., 1993). In addition, the risk for developing hepatocellular cancer was multiplicative in individuals with both AFB1 exposure and chronic infection with hepatitis B.

Striking interspecies variation in susceptibility to AFB1 carcinogenesis has been observed, with rats representing the most sensitive and mice the most resistant species, refractory to dietary levels three orders of magnitude higher than rats (Busby and Wogan, 1984). TD$_{50}$ values (statistical estimate of the dose required to result in 50% incidence of tumours) from lifetime feeding studies were 1.3, 5.8 and > 70 μg AFB1 (kg body weight)$^{-1}$ day^{-1} in male Fischer rats, male Wistar rats and male C57BL mice, respectively (review: Wild et al., 1996). In another study, susceptibilities of male Fischer rats and male Syrian golden hamsters were compared. Fisher rats treated with 1 mg AFB1 kg^{-1} day^{-1} (5 days/week for 6 weeks) all developed hepatocellular cancer during 46 weeks, whereas only one hamster (treated with 2 mg kg^{-1} day^{-1}, 5 days per week for 6 weeks) developed a hepatocellular carcinoma after 78 weeks.

The level of DNA adducts in livers of AFB1-treated animals was at least qualitatively associated with species-specific susceptibility to AFB1 hepatocarcinogenesis (Wild et al., 1996). The level of AFB1–DNA adducts in liver decreased in the order rat $\geqslant$ guinea pig > hamster > mouse, suggesting that guinea pigs—for which to our knowledge no carcinogenicity studies are available—are more susceptible than mice and hamsters and almost as sensitive as rats (Wild et al., 1996). These data are consistent with those from other studies, which reported that AFB1–DNA adduct levels in rats were 1.5-fold higher than in guinea pigs (Ueno et al., 1980), 3-fold higher than in hamsters (Garner and Wright, 1975; Lotlikar et al., 1984) and between 40- and 600-fold higher than in mice (Lutz et al., 1980; Croy and Wogan, 1981).

Hence for risk assessment of humans one would ideally want to measure AFB1–N^7-guanine adducts in the DNA of hepatocytes, the target cell for carcinogensis. However, there have been few such measurements in human liver, because of difficulties in obtaining tissue samples, including samples from appropriate control subjects. As an alternative, determination of AFB1–albumin adducts (expressed as pg AFB1–lysine equivalent per mg albumin) in peripheral blood has been established (Wild et al., 1996). AFB1–albumin adducts in peripheral blood have been shown to be a reliable marker of AFB1–DNA adducts in the liver of rodents and to be at least qualitatively associated with species susceptibility to AFB1 hepatocarcinogenesis of rats, hamsters and mice (Wild et al., 1996). The level of AFB1–albumin adduct formed as a function of a single dose of AFB1 in rodents was compared with data for humans from The Gambia and southern China with an estimated exposure of about 850 ng AFB1 (kg body weight)$^{-1}$ day^{-1}. This cross-species comparison resulted in values for Sprague–Dawley, Fischer and Wistar rats of between 0.3 and 0.5 pg AFB1–lysine equivalent (mg albumin)$^{-1}$ (μg AFB1)$^{-1}$ (kg body weight)$^{-1}$ and values of < 0.025 for the mouse, whereas 1.56 was estimated for exposed humans (Figure 3). This suggests that a given exposure in humans results in even higher adduct levels than in rats, whereby rats already represent a species with high susceptibility to AFB1 carcinogenesis. However, cross-species extrapolation was made on a μg basis. In most instances (e.g. in clinical practice of cytostatic drug application), the use of body surface is considered to be a more appropriate basis. If the cross-species

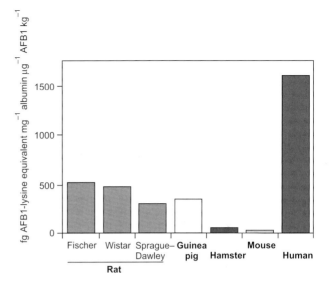

Figure 3 Interspecies comparison of aflatoxin B$_1$–albumin adducts (expressed as fg AFB$_1$–lysine equivalent mg^{-1} albumin) in rodents and humans for a given intake of aflatoxin B$_1$. Source: Wild et al. (1996).

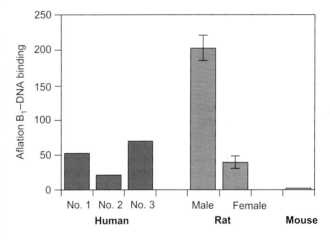

Figure 4 Amount of [^{3}H]aflatoxin B$_1$ bound to DNA isolated from cultured primary hepatocytes from human, rat (Sprague–Dawley) and mouse (CD-1 Swiss) after exposure to 200 nM aflatoxin B$_1$ for 24 h. Source: Cole et al. (1988).

comparison in **Figure 3** is made on the basis of surface area, using a mean surface area of 1.6 m^2 for humans (60 kg) and 0.02 m^2 for rats (100 g), the adduct range for rats is 0.06–0.07 pg AFB1–lysine equivalent (mg albumin)$^{-1}$ (μg aflatoxin)$^{-1}$ (m surface area)$^{-2}$, whereas the value for humans is 0.04. Hence the susceptibility of humans seems to be similar to that of rats, which means that humans have to be considered as a species with relatively high sensitivity to AFB1. This is in agreement with another study, which compared DNA binding of [^{3}H]AFB1 to DNA of primary hepatocytes of humans, rats and mice (Cole et al., 1988). Similar DNA binding was observed in hepatocytes of humans and

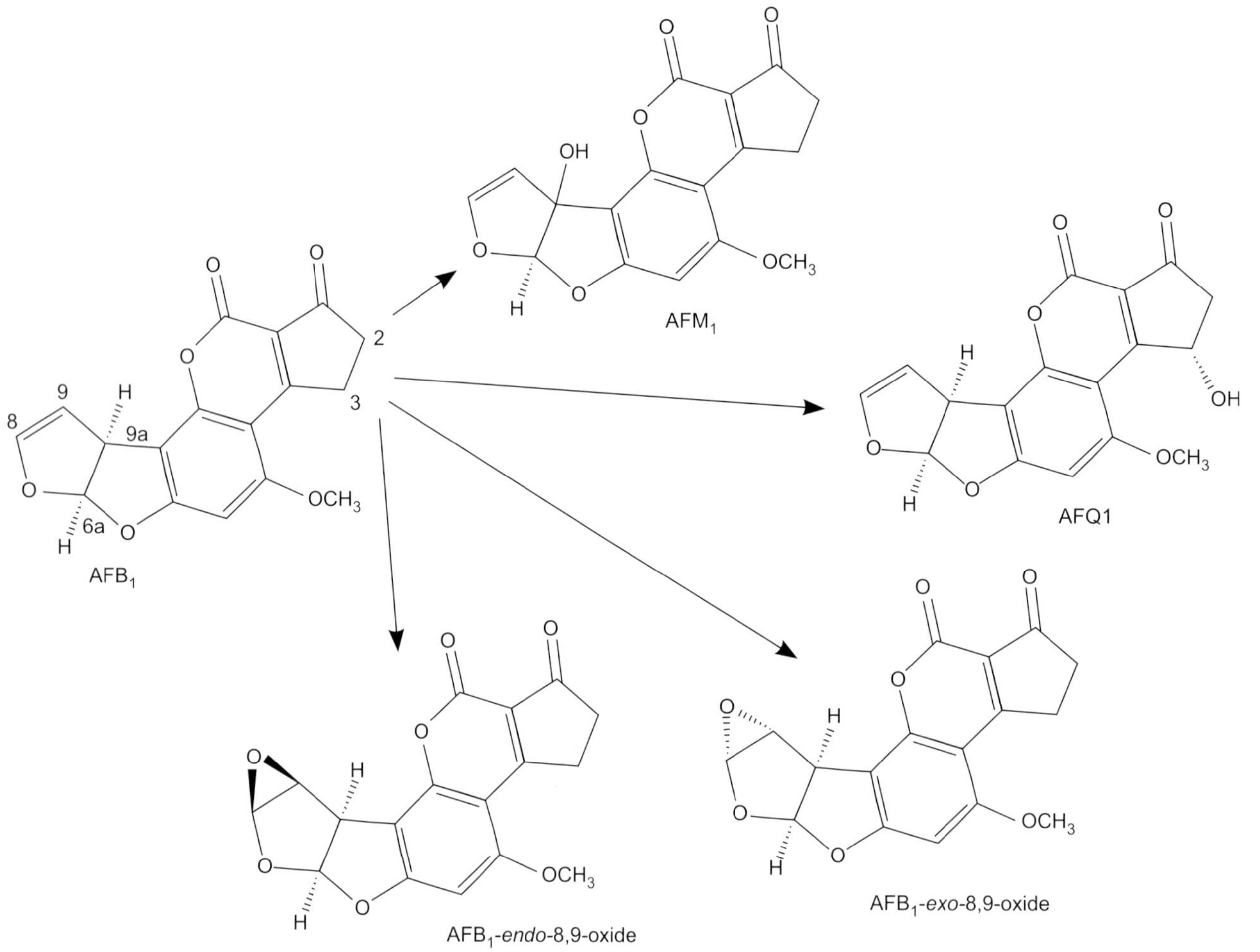

Figure 5 Phase I metabolism of aflatoxin B_1 (AFB1). Source: Guengerich (1996).

female rats, whereas DNA binding in hepatocytes of mice was much lower **(Figure 4)**. The constellation of mice representing the most resistant and rats a relatively susceptible species for AFB1 genotoxicity was also confirmed by the determination of chromosomal aberration and micronuclei in bone marrow (Anwar *et al.*, 1994). In addition, induction of unscheduled DNA synthesis (UDS) by AFB1 in primary hepatocyte cultures was strongest for human hepatocytes, whereby also rat (male Fischer-344) hepatocyte cultures yielded a dose-related increase in UDS, which was almost as strong as for human hepatocytes, whereas mouse hepatocyte cultures were the least responsive to AFB1 exposure (Steinmetz *et al.*, 1988). Hepatocyte cultures from male cynomolgus monkeys yielded a similarly weak response as mouse hepatocytes. This may be due to the lack of constitutive CYP 1A2 expression, which, similarly to the constellation observed for some heterocyclic amines, renders the cynomolgus monkey an inadequate species for extrapolation of human risk.

Numerous studies were performed to examine whether interspecies variation in susceptibility to AFB1 carcinogenesis and AFB1 adducts can be explained by interspecies differences in metabolism. Phase I metabolism of AFB1 by mammalian liver microsomes results in four main metabolites **(Figure 5)**. The AFB1-*exo*-8, 9-oxide represents the most relevant metabolite, which forms DNA adducts, almost exclusively at N-7 of guanine, much more efficiently than the AFB1-*endo*-8,9-oxide (Guengerich, 1996). AFM1 and AFQ1 are considered to be detoxication products. AFQ1 is the predominant product produced by microsomes of humans and monkeys (Ramsdell and Eaton, 1990), whereas the main metabolite formed by rat and mouse microsomes is AFB1-8,9-epoxide. In addition, mouse and rat microsomes caused at least twofold higher rates of AFB1-8,9-epoxide formation, suggesting that toxification of AFB1 by phase I metabolism is more efficient by rodent than human liver microsomes. This was confirmed by a study which examined the induction of sister chromatid exchanges (SCEs) by AFB1 in human mononuclear leucocytes, with addition of human, rat and mouse liver microsomes as a metabolizing system (Wilson *et al.*, 1997). Mouse liver microsomes activated AFB1 to a greater extent than either rat or human liver microsomes, although the differences were moderate **(Figure 6)**. In

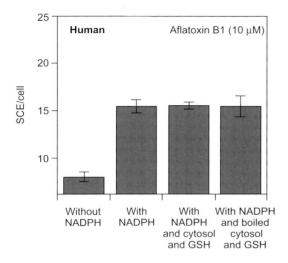

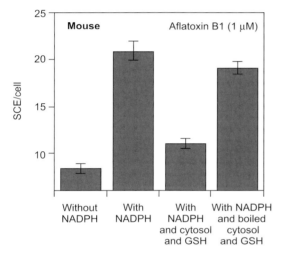

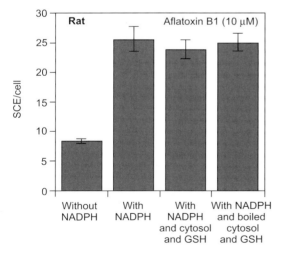

Figure 6 Effect of phase I and phase II metabolism on aflatoxin B$_1$ genotoxicity determined by sister chromatid exchange (SCE) induction. Venous blood from a human donor was incubated with aflatoxin B$_1$ (1 or 10 μM) in the presence of mouse, rat or human liver microsomes (with and without NADPH) in the absence or presence of mouse, rat or human liver cytosol with reduced glutathione (2.5 mM). The human individual examined in this experiment was positive for glutathione S-transferase M1. Source: Wilson *et al.* (1997).

humans interindividual differences in the potential of liver microsomes to bioactivate AFB1 to an SCE-inducing metabolite were observed, which significantly correlated with CYP 1A2 activity of the liver, as determined by tacrine 1-hydroxylation (Wilson *et al.*, 1997). In addition to CYP 1A2, CYP 3A4 can also activate AFB1 in human liver. However, different kinetic characteristics were reported, with a relatively low K_m for CYP 1A2 compared with the relatively high K_m for CYP 3A4, the main cytochrome P450 in human liver (Gallagher *et al.*, 1994). Thus, at the low AFB1 concentrations expected in human liver *in vivo*, metabolic activation is expected to be catalysed predominantly by CYP 1A2 in most individuals (Gallagher *et al.*, 1994; Buetler *et al.*, 1996). However, after high exposures to AFB1 and humans with low levels of CYP 1A2 and high levels of CYP 3A4, significant amounts of AFB1 might be converted to AFB1-8,9-epoxide also by CYP 3A4.

If the above-mentioned incubations of human mononuclear blood cells with AFB1 and liver microsomes were performed in the presence of mouse, rat or human liver cytosol plus reduced glutathione (at a concentration of 2.5 mM, which is high enough to allow GST activity, whereas almost no GST activity was present in the microsomal incubations due to dilution of the cofactor) the rate of SCE induction was reduced by almost 90% by mouse cytosol, whereas cytosol of human and rat showed no significant effect **(Figure 6)**. This suggests that efficient conjugation with glutathione confers resistance to mice, but not to humans or rats. Indeed, hepatic GST-mediated conjugation of microsomally generated AFB1-8,9-epoxide was 7080, 930 and 140 pmol min^{-1} mg^{-1} cytosolic protein for the mouse, hamster and rat, respectively, whereas GST-mediated conjugation by human liver cytosol was below the detection limit (Slone *et al.*, 1995). The high activity of AFB1 conjugation by mouse liver cytosol is due to a constitutively expressed α-class GST isoform (mYc) with an extremely high activity to AFB1-8,9-epoxide (Quinn *et al.*, 1990; Ramsdell and Eaton, 1990; Hayes *et al.*, 1991; Buetler *et al.*, 1992; Slone *et al.*, 1995). A homologous GST isoform (Yc2) with high activity towards AFB1-8,9-epoxide was observed to be inducible in rats by antioxidants such as ethoxyquin, and it is responsible for much of the chemoprotective effects of a variety of natural dietary compounds that act via the antioxidant response element (Eaton and Gallagher, 1994). However, this particular form of GST is expressed constitutively only at very low levels in rats. In contrast to mouse GSTs, human α-class GSTs exhibit relatively little activity towards AFB1-8,9-epoxide (Slone *et al.*, 1995). In conclusion, phase I metabolism provides a greater extent of AFB1 activation in mice than humans and rats. However, an extra-efficient GSH conjugation of AFB1-8,9-epoxide by GST mYc confers resistance to mice, whereas humans and uninduced male rats represent species with high susceptibility to AFB1 hepatocarcino-genesis, owing to the lack of a similarly effective phase II detoxification pathway as for mice.

In addition to the differences between species in covalent binding of AFB1 to liver DNA, **Figure 4** shows a 5–6-fold greater binding of [^{3}H]AFB1 to DNA from male than female hepatocytes (Cole *et al.*, 1988). Similarly, binding of AFB1 *in vivo* was shown to be greater in male than female rats (Gurtoo and Motycka, 1976) and liver microsomes from males were about three times more active than microsomes from females in metabolizing AFB1 to DNA-binding metabolites. In addition, male rats are more susceptible than female rats to the hepatocarcinogenic effects of AFB1 (Eaton and Gallagher, 1994). This sex difference in susceptibility might be explained by the lack of expression of CYP 3A2 in female rats and by an approximately 10-fold greater expression of GST Yc2 in livers of adult female rats compared with adult male rats, whereby the latter constitutively express only very low levels of GST Yc2 (Hayes *et al.*, 1994; Buetler *et al.*, 1996). Interestingly the frequency of hepatocellular carcinoma in AFB1-exposed individuals in Thailand has been shown to be greater for men than for women (Shank *et al.*, 1972; Peers and Linsell, 1977). This might be due to the fact that CYP 1A2 activity determined by caffeine metabolism is significantly lower in women than in men, as reported by Rasmussen and Brosen (1996). It might be of relevance that among women, those taking oral contraceptives have lower CYP 1A2 activities (Horn *et al.*, 1995). In addition, nulliparous women had lower CYP 1A2 activities than parous women. Since activation of AFB1 by human liver microsomes significantly correlated with the CYP 1A2 phenotype (Wilson *et al.*, 1997), it might be worth examining whether oral contraceptives, besides their well known protection against ovarian cancer, also protect AFB1-exposed women from hepatocellular cancer.

Oltipraz, an antischistosomal agent, has been shown to protect rats from the hepatocarcinogenic effect of AFB1 (Bolton *et al.*, 1993). Based on the anticarcinogenic effect of oltipraz in rats, phase II clinical trials have been initiated in the Qidong region in China, where individuals are highly exposed to AFB1. Most probably the rat is protected against AFB1-induced hepatocarcinogenesis by oltipraz treatment, because this compound induces GSTs including GST Yc2-Yc2, which possesses an especially high conjugating activity for AFB1-8,9-epoxide (Buetler *et al.*, 1996). However, there is no evidence to date suggesting the existence of a human GST isozyme with an AFB1-8, 9-epoxide-conjugating activity, relevant to the *in vivo* situation. For this reason, clinical trials with oltipraz as a protecting agent against hepatocarcinogenesis have been criticized (Buetler *et al.*, 1996). Although this argumentation may be correct for GSTs, oltipraz was reported to inhibit AFB1 activation by decreasing CYP 1A2 and CYP 3A4 activities in cultured primary human hepatocytes (Langouet *et al.*, 1995;

Morel *et al.*, 1997). In addition, oltipraz inhibited human recombinant CYP 1A2 and 3A4. Thus, humans may also be protected by oltipraz (although to our knowledge this has not yet been confirmed by the still ongoing clinical studies), whereby chemoprotection of humans may be due to an inhibition of an activation of AFB1, in contrast to rats, which seem to be protected by an induction of GST-mediated detoxication of the active AFB1-8, 9-epoxide.

BENZO[*a*]PYRENE

The role of polycyclic aromatic hydrocarbons in induction of human lung and skin cancer (review: Luch and Platt, 1996) has often been discussed and will not be repeated here. However, interspecies extrapolation invites another hypothesis that environmental exposure to benzo[*a*]pyrene contributes significantly to human breast cancer. Despite an increasing incidence of human breast cancer, its aetiology remains unknown. Several polycyclic aromatic hydrocarbons, including benzo[*a*]pyrene and 7,12-dimethylbenz[*a*]anthracene (DMBA), have been shown to induce mammary tumours in rodents (Dao, 1964; Huggins, 1979). While DMBA is a potent mammary carcinogen is rats, benzo[*a*]pyrene exhibits a lower but still significant carcinogenic activity. To extrapolate to human risk, culture techniques with human and rat mammary epithelial cells, isolated by collagenase digestion, were established (Moore *et al.*, 1987a). In these assays mammary epithelial cells activate putative procarcinogens and mutations are quantitated in co-cultured V79 cells (Gould *et al.*, 1986). In the human mammary cell co-culture system, benzo[*a*]pyrene was much more effective in the induction of mutations than in the rat system under comparable conditions. In contrast, rat mammary epithelial cells were more effective in activating DMBA compared with the human mammary epithelial cell system. Studies on the level of total DNA binding in human and rat mammary epithelial cells showed that human cells bound more benzo[*a*]pyrene than DMBA to DNA, whereas the opposite pattern was found in rat cells (Moore *et al.*, 1987a). DMBA adduct profiles in human and rat mammary cells were qualitatively identical, although total adduct levels in rat cells were significantly higher than in human cells (Moore *et al.*, 1987a). The predominant adduct in human and rat cells results from the binding of *syn*-7, 12-dimethylbenz[*a*]anthracene-3, 4-dihydrodiol-1, 2-epoxide to deoxyadenosine, an adduct which has been shown to be associated with mouse skin carcinogenesis (DiGiovanni *et al.*, 1979). In contrast to DMBA, examination of DNA binding of benzo[*a*]pyrene to human and rat mammary epithelial cells revealed qualitative (and quantitative) differences (Moore *et al.*, 1987b). In human mammary epithelial cells (+)-*anti*-BPDE–deoxyguanosine was the major DNA adduct formed after benzo[a]pyrene treatment (Moore et al., 1987b). However, this adduct was detectable only in very small amounts in rat mammary epithelial cells and other investigators (Phillips et al., 1985) did not detect formation of the (+)-anti-BPDE–deoxyguanosine adduct in rat mammary epithelial cells. These data are in agreement with another study, which demonstrated a positive UDS response in human mammary epithelial cells after incubation with benzo[a]pyrene but not with DMBA (Eldridge et al., 1992).

If the hypothesis that environmental benzo[a]pyrene exposure contributes to human breast cancer is true, benzo[a]pyrene-specific DNA adducts would be expected to be present in human breast tissue. To examine this hypothesis, 87 surgical specimens of normal breast tissue from breast cancer patients and breast tissue from 29 non-cancer patients undergoing reduction mammoplasty were examined by ^{32}P-postlabelling (Li et al., 1996). The total adduct levels in cancer patients (mean: $97.4/10^9$ nucleotides) was significantly higher than in the non-cancer controls (mean: $18.1/10^9$ nucleotides). In addition, a benzo[a]pyrene-like DNA adduct was observed in 36 of the breast cancer patients, 27 of whom were non-smokers, whereas this adduct was absent in all of the non-cancer control tissues (Li et al., 1996).

In conclusion, the data support the hypothesis that environmental exposure to benzo[a]pyrene, in addition to cigarette smoking, contributes to breast cancer and that humans are more susceptible to benzo[a]pyrene-induced mammary carcinogenesis than rodents.

Several studies examined bioactivation of benzo[a]-pyrene mediated by liver microsomes of several species and tried to obtain a correlation between the extent of activation by various animal species and particular enzyme activities. Using microsomes from untreated male Sprague–Dawley rats, benzo[a]pyrene induced a maximum increase in Salmonella typhimurium TA 1537 revertants in the Ames test (plate incorporation assay) of only 1.7-fold compared with spontaneous TA 1537 revertants (Oesch et al., 1977). In contrast, microsomes from untreated male C3H mice caused a ca 20-fold increase in TA 1537 revertants under comparable conditions. As an explanation for the species-specific mutagenic response, the ratios of cytochrome P450-dependent benzo[a]pyrene monooxygenase/microsomal epoxide hydrolase have been suggested (Oesch et al., 1977; Oesch, 1980). C3H mice have been shown to have high levels of monooxygenase [850 ± 54 pmol 3-OH-benzo[a]-pyrene fluorescent equivalents min^{-1} (mg protein)$^{-1}$], but low levels of microsomal epoxide hydrolase [1.0 ± 0.1 nmol styrene glycol min^{-1} (mg protein)$^{-1}$] (Oesch et al., 1977). The opposite has been shown to be true for Sprague–Dawley rats, which exhibit relatively low monooxygenase activities [410 ± 32 pmol 3-OH-benzo[a]pyrene fluorescent equivalents min^{-1} (mg protein)$^{-1}$] but relatively high activities of epoxide hydrolase [7.2 ± 0.2 nmol styrene glycol min^{-1} (mg protein)$^{-1}$].

Further evidence of a causal link between these enzyme patterns and the mutagenic effect was given by the use of two different types of epoxide hydrolase inhibitors, namely 1,1,1-trichloropropene 2,3-oxide and cyclohexene oxide. Indeed, inhibition of epoxide hydrolase in untreated Sprague–Dawley rat liver microsomes led to a strong increase of the mutagenic effect of benzo[a]pyrene. In addition, the use of microsomes from male Sprague–Dawley rats pretreated with 10 mg kg^{-1} of 3-methylcholanthrene, which increased benzo[a]pyrene monooxygenase activities about fourfold, led to a much stronger increase in benzo[a]pyrene-induced TA 1537 revertants than liver microsomes from untreated rats. After phenobarbital induction of mice and rats, the differences in enzyme patterns (epoxide hydrolase and benzo[a]pyrene monooxygenase) were much smaller than was the case between untreated rats and mice. Accordingly, the differences in liver microsomes of both species in bioactivation of benzo[a]pyrene to a mutagenic species were much less (Oesch et al., 1977). One more interspecies difference, which is associated with the ratio of benzo[a]pyrene monooxygenase to microsomal epoxide hydrolase, was observed between Sprague–Dawley rats and Beagle dogs (Oesch, 1980). Since humans have much higher epoxide hydrolase activities than mice and even moderately higher activities than rats (using benzo[a]pyrene-4,5-oxide as a substrate) (**Table 1**), interspecies extrapolation would suggest that humans are less susceptible to benzo[a]pyrene than mice and probably also rats (Oesch, 1980). However, it has become clear that the simple ratio of monooxygenase to epoxide hydrolase can explain interspecies or sex differences only in a small number of cases. For instance, the sex difference of C3HeB/FeJ × A/J mice, where benzo[a]-pyrene efficiently induces liver tumours in male but not in female animals, cannot be explained by differences in epoxide hydrolase activity (Glatt and Oesch, 1987). In addition, activities and inducibilities of monooxygenase and glutathione S-transferase (toward benzo[a]pyrene and benzo[a]pyrene 4,5-oxide) were similar between males and females. Liver microsomes from male and female animals activated benzo[a]pyrene to a bacterial mutagen to a similar extent, showing that the sex difference cannot be explained merely by phase I metabolism, or by comparison of the mentioned enzyme activities using diagnostic substrates. The described species difference between mice and rat liver microsomes in benzo[a]-pyrene activation to a bacterial mutagen was not confirmed by another group (Phillipson and Ioannides, 1989). However, different animal strains (male albino CDI mice and male Wistar albino rats) and a different Salmonella typhimurium tester strain (TA 100) was used. An interesting conclusion from this study is that hamster liver microsomes are more efficient than liver microsomes from mouse, rat, pig and man in activating several polycyclic aromatic hydrocarbons to bacterial mutagens (Phillipson and Ioannides, 1989). While this was true for

Table 1 Epoxide hydrolase activity in liver microsomes from various species

Species, strain	No. of individuals	Sex	Activity [nmol diol (mg protein)$^{-1}$ min^{-1}]		
			HEOM[a]	Styrene 7,8-oxide	Benzo[a]pyrene 4,5-oxide
Mouse					
C3H/HeJ	6	Male	0.81	0.73	1.5
A7J	6	Male	0.93	1.30	2.1
C3HeB/FeJ × A/J	6	Male	0.97	1.97	1.8
C57BL/6J	6	Male	0.94	1.10	2.0
C3HeB/FeJ	6	Male	1.10	0.97	1.6
C57BL/6J × C3HeB/FeJ	6	Male	1.10	0.93	1.8
Rat					
Sprague – Dawley	6	Male	3.0	6.4	6.1
Fischer	3	Male	nt[b]	3.2	2.4
DA	3	Male	nt	8.8	6.1
Syrian hamster	9	Male	nt	35.9	11.7
Chinese hamster	4	Male	nt	4.1	4.1
	4	Female	nt	5.9	nt
Guinea pig	4	Male	15	12	18
Dog (beagle)	3	Male	nt	14.9	14.7
Human	26	Male and Female	nt	nt	9.8 ± 5.0[c]

a 1,2,3,4,9,9-Hexachloro-6,7-epoxy-1,4,4a,5,6,7,8a-octahydro-1,4-methanonaphthalene.
b nt, Not tested.
c Mean ± standard deviation.

benzo[a]pyrene, 3-methylcholanthrene, dibenzo[a,i]pyrene, benzo[a]anthracene and dibenz[a,h]anthracene, an exception of the rule was observed for 7,12-dimethylbenz[a]anthracene. The latter substance was activated most efficiently by human liver microsomes.

Comparative ^{32}P-postlabelling analysis of benzo[a]pyrene adducts to purified DNA in the presence of liver microsomes of hamster, mice, rabbits, rat and humans showed large quantitative and qualitative interspecies differences (Roggenband et al., 1993). With hamster liver microsomes the highest total adduct level was obtained (158 ± 34 adducts/10[8] nucleotides), followed by liver microsomes from rabbits (106 ± 37 adducts/10[8] nucleotides), Wag/MBL rats (24.3 ± 10.2 adducts/10[8] nucleotides), BALB/c mice (22.0 ± 7.2 adducts/10[8] nucleotides), Wistar rats (7.6 ± 0.6 adducts/10[8] nucleotides) and humans (range for four individuals: 2.9–4.6 adducts/10[8] nucleotides). The authors compared the low level of adducts obtained with human liver microsomes with the low content of total P450 per mg microsomal protein in human liver microsomes (**Table 2**). (Roggenband et al., 1993). The total adduct levels were in the same range as those observed with rat and mouse liver when related to the amount of cytochrome P450 during incubation. However, in the examined species no correlation of adduct levels with EROD activity (used as diagnostic substrate for those cytochromes P450 which contribute most to benzo[a]pyrene oxidative metabolism) in non-induced liver microsomes was obtained.

Table 2 Total amount of cytochrome P450 in humans and male rats, mice, hamsters and rabbits (mean ± standard deviation)

Species	Cytochrome P-450 [nmol (mg microsomal protein)$^{-1}$
Human	
Individual No. 1	0.13 ± 0.03
Individual No. 2	0.15 ± 0.00
Individual No. 3	0.15 ± 0.02
Individual No. 4	0.13 ± 0.01
Rat	
Wistar	0.74 ± 0.16
Wag/MBL	0.71 ± 0.02
Mouse	
BALB/c	0.73 ± 0.13
Hamster	
Syrian Golden	0.63 ± 0.04
Rabbit	
New Zealand White	0.38 ± 0.12

Source: Roggenband et al. (1993).

In conclusion, the hamster, which also exhibits the highest P450 content, generally exhibits a higher capacity than other animals and man for activating polycyclic aromatic hydrocarbons to mutagens, which corresponds to the well known cancer susceptibility of the hamster to this group of chemical carcinogens (Phillipson and Ioannides, 1989). However, much remains to be elucidated for a more comprehensive and more detailed analysis of species differences in benzo[a] pyrene-metabolizing enzymes and isoenzymes and their relationship to species differences in the susceptibility to cytotoxic and carcinogenic action of the compound.

2,3,7,8-TETRACHLORODIBENZO-*p*-DIOXIN (TCDD) AND RELATED COMPOUNDS

TCDD, a combustion product of chlorine-containing wastes and a contaminant in certain organohalogen compounds, such as the herbicide 2,4,5-trichlorophenol, represents a prototype of several halogenated aromatic compounds. TCDD has received considerable attention owing to its presence as a trace contaminant in food (especially in fish and meat), water and soil and its extremely high acute toxicity to some experimental animals, e.g. guinea pigs (LD_{50} 1 $\mu g\,kg^{-1}$) (McConnell *et al.*, 1978).

Most but not all of the toxicological effects of TCDD and other halogenated aromatic hydrocarbons are mediated by the aryl hydrocarbon receptor (review: Hankinson *et al.*, 1996). The aryl hydrocarbon receptor protein evolved about 450 million years ago, early in vertebrate evolution. Ligands for the aryl hydrocarbon receptor, particularly TCDD, cause several toxic effects, including cancer, progressive weight loss, toxicity to the immune system, foetal toxicity, birth defects, dysregulation of endocrine (thyroid, androgen, oestrogen and growth factor) homeostasis and decreases in male and female reproductive performance. TCDD has proved to be the most potent tumour promoter analysed and also acts as a complete carcinogen. Unlike polycyclic aromatic hydrocarbons or heterocyclic amines, TCDD is not activated to a mutagen and does not bind to DNA.

The unligated aryl hydrocarbon receptor is located in the cytoplasm, where it is associated with two molecules of the 90 kDa heat shock protein and another protein of about 43 kDa (review: Hankinson *et al.*, 1996). This complex is termed the unligated aryl hydrocarbon receptor complex. After binding of TCDD or other ligands, the aryl hydrocarbon receptor is released from the 90 kDa heat shock proteins and the 43 kDa protein and associates with the hydrocarbon receptor nuclear translocator protein (ARNT) **(Figure 7)**. The latter complex binds to specific recognition motifs of DNA [termed dioxin-responsive element which has a consensus sequence of T(T/A)GCGTG upstream of the CYP 1A1 gene, resulting in enhanced transcription]. Genes which have been shown to exhibit increased transcription rates by this mechanism include CYP 1A1, 1A2 and 1B1, the glutathione *S*-transferase subunit GSTYa, the UDP-glucuronosyltransferase UGT 1*O6, the aldehyde dehydrogenase ALDH3c and the NAD(P)H:quinone reductase NQO_1.

Contrary to what its name suggests, ARNT is not involved in translocating the aryl hydrocarbon receptor to the nucleus, since TCDD induced nuclear translocation of the liganded aryl hydrocarbon receptor also in ARNT-deficient mouse Hepa-1 cells (review: Hankinson *et al.*, 1996). Nevertheless, ARNT is essential for DNA binding of the aryl hydrocarbon receptor.

Recently, aryl hydrocarbon receptor knockout mice were generated (Fernandez-Salguero *et al.*, 1995). Almost half of the knockout mice (Ahr −/−) died shortly after birth, whereas survivors were fertile, but showed deficiencies in liver function (50% reduction in size; decrease in retinoic acid metabolism; decreased CYP 1A2 levels) and in the immune system (Fernandez-Salguero *et al.*, 1996; Andreola *et al.*, 1997). The aryl hydrocarbon receptor-deficient mice are relatively resistent to doses of TCDD (2000 $\mu g\,kg^{-1}$) 10-fold higher than those found to induce severe toxicity in littermates expressing a functional aryl hydrocarbon receptor (Fernandez-Salguera *et al.*, 1996). However, at higher doses of TCDD the aryl hydrocarbon receptor deficient mice displayed single cell necrosis and vasculitis in their livers and lungs, showing the existance of aryl

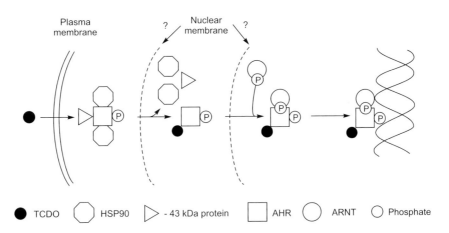

Figure 7 Transformation of the aryl hydrocarbon receptor. The lack of resolution as to where the 300 kDa complex dissociates is indicated by two alternative positions for the nuclear membrane. Source: Hankinson *et al.* (1996).

hydrocarbon receptor-independent pathways of TCDD-induced toxicity.

Homozygous knockout mice for the aryl hydrocarbon nuclear translocator (ARNT) died *in utero* between 9.5 and 10.5 days of gestation (Kozak *et al.*, 1997). The primary cause of lethality was failure of the embryo to vascularize and form the spongiotrophoblast. This is in agreement with the known role of ARNT in induction of angiogenesis.

Extremely large interspecies differences in TCDD-induced toxicity are known. The guinea pig is the most TCDD-susceptible mammal known, with an LD_{50} in the range 1–2 μg TCDD kg^{-1} (Schwetz *et al.*, 1973). In contrast, the hamster is the most TCDD-resistant species concerning acute toxicity with an $LD_{50} > 3000\ \mu$g kg^{-1} (Olson *et al.*, 1980).

Exposure to TCDD during pregnancy causes prenatal mortality in all mammals examined (Peterson *et al.*, 1993). The rank order of susceptibility from the most to the least sensitive species was reported to be monkey = guinea pig > rabbit = rat = hamster > mouse **(Table 3)**. Adult hamsters are about three orders of magnitude more resistant than adult guinea pigs. However, the difference in prenatal mortality between these species was only about one order of magnitude. Interpretation of the prenatal mortality data is complex, since species-specific differences in the most sensitive periods during pregnancy have to be considered, which will not be discussed in this review. In most laboratory mammals, gestational exposure to TCDD caused a common pattern of foetotoxic responses. These common responses include decreased foetal growth, subcutaneous oedema and thymic hypoplasia. In addition to these common effects, highly species-specific malformations have been described. Examples of TCDD effects that occur only in a single susceptible species are cleft palate formation in the mouse, intestinal haemorrhage in the rat and the formation of extra ribs in the rabbit (Peterson *et al.*, 1993).

Table 3 Interspecies differences in prenatal toxicity and toxicity to adult female animals (maternal toxicity) of 2,3,7,8-tetrachlorodibenzo-*p*-dioxin

Species	Cumulative dose (μg kg^{-1})	
	Maternal toxicity[a]	Prenatal toxicity[b]
Rhesus monkey	1	1
Guinea pig (Hartley)	1.5	1.5
Rabbit (New Zealand)	2.5	2.5
Rat (Wistar)	10	5
Rat (Sprague – Dawley)	5	20
Hamster (Syrian Golden)	> 3000	18
Mouse (CD-1)	2000	1000

a Decreased body weight gain or marked oedema compared with controls.
b Cumulative doses are given which caused at least a twofold increase in the percentage of absorptions plus late gestational deaths over controls.
Source: Peterson *et al.* (1993).

TCDD acts as a complete carcinogen in chronic animal studies with doses as low as 0.001 μg kg^{-1} day^{-1} in rats (Huff *et al.*, 1991). In rats, neoplasms in the lung, oral/nasal cavity, thyroid, adrenal glands and liver were observed. In mice, TCDD induced neoplasms in the liver, subcutaneous tissue, thyroid gland and thymic lymphomas. In hamsters, squamous cell carcinomas of the facial skin were obserced after intraperitoneal and subcutaneous injections of relatively high doses of TCDD (total dose 600 μg kg^{-1}). Based on these data, carcinogenesis is one of the primary concerns associated with human exposures to TCDD. The majority of scientists suggested that humans appear to be less susceptible than most laboratory animals to the carcinogenic effects of TCDD (review: Hays *et al.*, 1997). However, others suggested that humans respond similarly to rodents. Recently, the TCDD-related carcinogenic response in rats was compared to that in humans (Hays *et al.*, 1997). For this purpose the internal biological dose, measured as blood lipid or adipose tissue TCDD levels, were determined for rats and humans (NIOSH cohort) exposed to TCDD. Although the workers exposed to TCDD (NIOSH cohort) experienced internal exposures similar to or higher than those in rats treated with TCDD, rats exhibited a greater tumour response. At comparable peak serum lipid TCDD levels (about 7000 ppt), the tumour response in rats was more than ninefold greater than the human response. It should be considered that the average AUC for TCDD in the NIOSH cohort was about 1000-fold greater than the average background in the general population. It was concluded that humans are less susceptible to TCDD-induced carcinogenesis than rats and that human exposure to background levels of TCDD (about 5 ppt serum lipid) is not likely to cause an incremental cancer risk (Hays *et al.*, 1997).

Although the interspecies differences of TCDD toxicity are more than three orders of magnitude, little is known about the mechanisms responsible for these differences. It seems probable that a universal mechanism, which determines TCDD susceptibility, does not exist. Possibly the basic mechanism responsible for specific effects differs between species.

However, some differences in TCDD susceptibility have been shown to be due to differences in the affinity of the aryl hydrocarbon receptor to bind ligands, such as TCDD (Gielen *et al.*, 1972; Poland *et al.*, 1994), although this explanation seems to be limited to some mouse strains. The murine Ah locus was originally defined as a difference in susceptibility of mouse strains to polycyclic aromatic hydrocarbons. Later it was shown to encode the aryl hydrocarbon receptor, which binds planar aromatic ligands and mediates most of their effects. For instance, C57BL/6 mice treated with 3-methylcholanthrene show an induction of CYP1A1, whereas DBA/2 mice fail to respond. Administration of TCDD induces CYP 1A1 activity in both mouse strains; however, a larger dose is required for DBA/2 mice. Genetic crosses and backcrosses between these mouse strains showed that responsiveness is inherited as an autosomal dominant trait. The allele associated with responsiveness was termed Ah[b], whereas the non-responsive allele was termed Ah[d]. The latter allele expresses a protein with diminished binding affinity for ligands, resulting in a diminished sensitivity to TCDD (Gielen et al., 1972; Poland and Glover, 1980; Poland et al., 1994). The cDNAs of four murine aryl hydrocarbon alleles have been cloned and sequenced (Poland et al., 1994). Three alleles with the higher ligand binding affinity (Ah[b−1], Ah[b−2] and Ah[b−3]), which differ only by a few point mutations and one allele, with the low binding affinity (Ah[d]) have been described. The latter allele is most appropriately compared with the Ah[b−2] allele, both of which express proteins of the same size (ca 104 kDa) that differ in only two amino acids. The lower ligand affinity of the Ah[d] receptor has been shown to be caused by an alanine → valine substitution at position 375 of the Ah[b−2] receptor. In similar genetic crosses also other effects of TCDD, such as thymic atrophy (Poland and Glover, 1980), hepatic porphyria (Jones and Sweeney, 1980) and immunosuppressive effects (Vecchi et al., 1983) have been shown to segregate with the Ah locus. In addition, developmental toxicity was related to the Ah locus in mice (review: Peterson et al., 1993). In five mouse strains with low-affinity receptors there was only a 0–3% incidence of cleft palate formation, whereas four of five strains with high-affinity aryl hydrocarbon receptors developed a ⩾50% incidence (Poland and Glover, 1980). However, one strain with the high-affinity receptor was resistant, showing that alternative mechanisms protecting from developmental toxicity must exist.

Although the data show convincingly that the affinity of the aryl hydrocarbon receptor segregates with TCDD susceptibility, it seems impossible to extrapolate interspecies toxicity by receptor affinity. The time course of association of [³H]TCDD with hepatic cytosol from hamsters, mice, rats, gerbillinae and guinea pigs showed significant interspecies differences (Nakai et al., 1994). However, their rank order of affinity did not correlate with the rank ordering of their toxic potency. In another study, both binding of [³H]TCDD to cytosol and TCDD-induced binding of the aryl hydrocarbon receptor to the dioxin responsive element (determined by gel retardation analysis) were compared for various species (**Table 4**) (Bank et al., 1992). These experiments indicate that the TCDD-resistant hamster shows a similar [³H]TCDD binding to cytosolic protein as the sensitive guinea pig (**Table 4**). On the other hand, binding to the dioxin-responsive element was greater for the guinea pig than hamster. However, the relatively small difference between hamsters and guinea pigs is unlikely to explain the large interspecies differences shown in **Table 3**. An additional argument against the thesis that aryl hydrocarbon receptor affinity determines TCDD

Table 4 Interspecies differences in specific binding of [³H]TCDD to hepatic cytosol and binding of transformed aryl hydrocarbon receptor to the dioxin-responsive element cannot sufficiently explain interspecies differences in toxicity shown in Table 3

Species	Binding of [³H]TCDD to hepatic cytosol [fmol (mg protein)$^{-1}$]	Binding to the dioxin responsive element (relative amount)
Human LS180 cells	260.0 ± 3.0	+++
Guinea pig (Hartley)	43.2 ± 4.5	++++
Rabbit (New Zealand)	75.1 ± 3.5	+++
Rat (Sprague–Dawley)	51.0 ± 2.0	+++
Hamster (Syrian Golden)	50.4 ± 5.4	++
Mouse (C57BL/6N)	41.2 ± 1.7	+
Chicken	41.3 ± 2.3	+
Rainbow trout	5.1 ± 2.6	−

Source: Bank et al. (1992).

susceptibility as a common mechanism was given by a study comparing Han/Wistar with Long–Evans rats (Rozman, 1989). The LD$_{50}$ of Han/Wistar rats was > 300 μg TCDD kg^{-1}, compared with only 12 μg TCDD kg^{-1} for Long–Evans rats. This interstrain difference in TCDD toxicity did not match the receptor binding affinity, which was almost identical in both strains.

A typical sign of acute TCDD intoxication is the wasting syndrome, which is defined as decreased feed intake and body weight decrease. In Sprague–Dawley rats TCDD has been shown to inhibit gluconeogenesis. It has been suggested that the progressive hypoglycaemia observed in TCDD-treated rats causes the wasting syndrome (Rozman, 1989; Weber et al., 1991). However, in another study plasma glucose remained unaltered in TCDD-treated hamsters and also in guinea pigs (Unkila et al., 1995). In addition, no decrease in gluconeogenesis due to suppression of phosphoenolpyruvate carboxykinase was observed in TCDD-treated guinea pigs. Hence dysregulation of glucose homeostasis and inhibition of gluconeogenesis cannot constitute a general mechanism for the wasting syndrome (Unkila et al., 1995). As another thesis to explain the mechanism of the wasting syndrome, a TCDD-induced increase of tryptophan in the plasma has been suggested, based on the observation that in susceptible Long–Evans rats TCDD caused a dose-dependent increase in free tryptophan in the plasma, whereas TCDD-resistant Han/Wistar rats did not exhibit these changes (Unkila et al., 1994). It was suggested that increased tryptophan levels in the brain might mediate TCDD anorexia. However, treatment of guinea pigs with doses of TCDD, which caused wasting syndrome, did not affect brain tryptophan as well as plasma total and free tryptophan (Unkila et al., 1995). Hence it seems probable that the mechanism responsible for the wasting syndrome, in spite of similar clinical symptoms, differs between species.

Recently, it was suggested that the adipose tissue serves as a protective reservoir against the toxic effects of TCDD (Geyer *et al.*, 1997). In the adipose tissue, persistent lipophilic compounds, such as TCDD, may accumulate, so that only a small fraction of the incorporated dose can reach the target organs and exert their toxic effects. A relationship between the oral 30-day LD_{50} ($\mu g\ kg^{-1}$) of TCDD in different mammalian species and their total body fat content (TBF%) was reported: $LD_{50} = 6.03 \times 10^{-4} \times (TBF\%)^{5.30}$ (Geyer *et al.*, 1997). This equation obviously suggests 'survival of the fattest'. It would predict an LD_{50} of about 6000 $\mu g\ kg^{-1}$ for an adult man of 70 kg body weight. However, human newborns and embryos would be much more sensitive. However, several aspects which could be concluded from the body fat model still have to be confirmed. For instance, despite a similar TCDD exposure, some individuals develop chloracne, whereas others do not. It would be interesting to examine whether this difference in susceptibility is associated with differences in body fat contents.

In addition, species variation in TCDD susceptibility could be due to some more physiological characteristics including pharmacokinetics and metabolism. A pharmacokinetic analysis of the relationship between the external dose of TCDD and resulting TCDD concentrations in liver and adipose tissue of humans, rats and mice showed a variation by as much as 700–fold. It is known that at the same external doses, the internal concentration increases with increase in body weight, an effect which is not specific to TCDD. Thus, at the same external dose (calculated for 100 pg TCDD kg^{-1} day^{-1} by Lawrence and Gobas, 1997), the internal concentration of TCDD in the organism will be about sevenfold higher for humans than mice and fourfold higher than for rats, owing to the smaller elimination rate constant in humans.

Marked interspecies differences have also been described for TCDD metabolism, which renders TCDD more water soluble and increases excretion. Primary hepatocytes from untreated rats, having an LD_{50} 25-fold greater than guinea pigs, metabolized TCDD 2.8-fold faster then primary hepatocytes from untreated guinea pigs (Wroblewski and Olson, 1985). Pretreatment with TCDD (5 $\mu g\ kg^{-1}$ i.p.) 72 h prior to hepatocyte isolation increased the metabolic rate of TCDD 3.2-fold for rats, whereas no increase was observed in guinea pigs, resulting in ninefold greater metabolic rates of treated rats versus treated guinea pigs. Hence constitutive TCDD metabolism as well as the species-specific ability of TCDD to induce its own rate of metabolism may contribute to the varying susceptibility of species to TCDD.

TAMOXIFEN

The non-steroidal antioestrogen tamoxifen is used in the treatment of pre- and postmenopausal women suffering from breast cancer. Besides its species-specific genotoxic effects, tamoxifen exhibits large interspecies differences in oestrogenic/antioestrogenic effects. The drug is a full oestrogen in the mouse, a partial oestrogen/antioestrogen in humans and rats and an antioestrogen in the chick (Jordan and Robinson, 1987). Tamoxifen induced hepatocellular carcinomas in male and female rats after oral application and also acted as a promoting agent in a two-stage model of carcinogenesis in rat liver initiated by diethylnitrosamine followed by partial hepatectomy (reviews: Tannenbaum, 1997; Wogan, 1997). However, in mice tamoxifen did not induce malignancies when administered according to dosing protocols effective in causing carcinomas in rat liver (Wogan, 1997). In contrast, tamoxifen protected against oestrogen-induced hepatocarcinogenesis in hamsters (Coe *et al.*, 1992).

An unusual species-specific effect of oestrogens, such as ethinyloestradiol, diethylstilboestrol and zeranol, on the liver of Chinese and Armenian hamsters is known, inducing both hepatotoxicity and hepatocarcinogenesis. Administration of tamoxifen simultaneously with ethinyloestradiol, diethylstilboestrol or zeranol abrogated the induction of hepatotoxicity and hepatic neoplasia in hamsters. This effect is in contrast to the carcinogenic and tumour-promoting activity of tamoxifen in rats, but can be explained on the premise that tamoxifen competitively blocks oestrogen binding to the receptor, which seems to be a necessary prerequisite for oestrogen-induced hepatocarcinogenesis in the hamster.

Several studies have shown that tamoxifen is activated to a DNA-binding metabolite by a combination of phase I and phase II metabolism. The cytochrome P450-catalysed hydroxylation of tamoxifen to give α-hydroxytamoxifen and subsequent conjugation with sulphate or acetate giving a good leaving group may be the major carcinogenic pathway for tamoxifen (Ramakrishna *et al.*, 1997; Wogan, 1997). The important role of α-hydroxylation of tamoxifen has been shown by comparing the formation of DNA adducts in rat hepatocytes by tamoxifen and α-hydroxytamoxifen by ^{32}P-postlabelling (Phillips *et al.*, 1996). Incubation with α-hydroxytamoxifen resulted in up to 63-fold higher levels of adducts compared with equimolar concentrations of tamoxifen. The importance of phase II metabolism has been shown by comparing tamoxifen with α-sulphate-*cis*-tamoxifen and α-acetoxytamoxifen for adduct formation in calf thymus DNA (Dasaradhi and Shibutani, 1997). The formation of tamoxifen DNA adducts induced by α-sulphate-*cis*-tamoxifen and α-acetoxytamoxifen was 1100- and 1600-fold higher, respectively, than that of α-hydroxytamoxifen.

However, *in vivo* the role of phase II metabolism for tamoxifen genotoxicity seems to be complex: the sulphotransferase inhibitor 2,6-dichloro-4-nitrophenol significantly reduced the formation of a group of less polar adducts (termed group II adducts) by tamoxifen in female Sprague–Dawley rats (Randerath *et al.*, 1994b), consistant with the proposal that α-hydroxylation of the ethyl group of tamoxifen followed by sulphate conjugation represents a mechanism of tamoxifen activation. On the other hand 2,6-dichloro-4-nitrophenol had no effect on the formation of a group of more polar tamoxifen adducts (termed group I adducts). Application of the phenolic metabolite 4-hydroxytamoxifen exclusively caused the formation of the latter group I adducts. Co-administration of pentachlorophenol, another sulphotransferase inhibitor, led to an 11-fold enhancement of group I adduct formation, whereas group II adducts were suppressed sixfold. A possible explanation of these results might be that sulphotransferase catalyses both activating and inactivating reactions, whereby α-hydroxytamoxifen is activated (leading to group II adducts) and 4-hydroxytamoxifen (leading to group I adducts) is deactivated via the stable polar sulphate (Randerath et al., 1994a, b).

Another mechanism which has been suggested to be responsible for tamoxifen–DNA binding is a combination of α-hydroxylation and 4-hydroxylation to give a quinone methide structure, binding to DNA at the α-carbon of tamoxifen (review: Tannenbaum, 1997).

Although the mechanisms and interspecies differences of tamoxifen metabolism are not clear in detail, several studies have been performed which show major differences between humans, rats and mice with respect to tamoxifen metabolism and DNA adduct formation and clearly indicate that rats are orders of magnitude more susceptible than humans to tamoxifen genotoxicity. The pattern of the main metabolites obtained with human liver microsomes resembles qualitatively that of rat liver microsomes. However, the amount of hydroxylated tamoxifen metabolites was much lower by human than rat and mouse liver microsomes (Mani et al., 1993; Lim et al., 1994; review: Tannenbaum, 1997). Especially the lower capacity of human liver microsomes to produce 4-hydroxy- and α-hydroxytamoxifen, which may be further activated by sulphonation or acetylation, seems to be of relevance **(Table 5)**. In addition, after incubation of primary hepatocyte cultures of humans, rats and mice about 50-fold lower concentrations of α-hydroxytamoxifen were determined in the culture medium of human than rat and mouse hepatocytes (Phillips et al., 1996).

The lower capacity of human liver microsomes to metabolize tamoxifen is reflected by a smaller extent of DNA adduct formation. Incubation of primary hepatocytes with 10 μM tamoxifen caused 90 adducts/10^8 nucleotides in rat and 15 adducts/10^8 nucleotides in mouse hepatocytes, whereas no significant increase of adducts was detected in human hepatocytes with a detection limit for the assay of 4 adducts/10^{10} nucleotides (Phillips et al., 1996). Incubation of human hepatocytes with α-hydroxytamoxifen resulted in a detectable increase in DNA adducts, but a 300-fold higher increase was observed for rat hepatocytes treated under the same

Table 5 Interspecies differences in metabolism of tamoxifen between humans, rats and mice

Metabolite	Rank order of formation
4-Hydroxy	Mouse > rat > human
α-Hydroxy	Mouse = rat >>> human
N-Oxide	Mouse >>> rat > human
N-Desmethyl	Mouse > rat = human

Source: Tannenbaum (1997).

conditions (Phillips et al., 1996). In addition, no increase in total DNA adducts in DNA extracted from the livers of seven women treated with 20 mg of tamoxifen once or twice daily was observed compared with adduct levels in untreated women and the adduct patterns from treated women were different from that observed in DNA of tamoxifen-treated rats (Martin et al., 1995).

In addition to the liver, tamoxifen was shown to induce DNA adducts in rat endometrium (Pathak et al., 1996). A single DNA adduct was induced in the endometrium of rats treated with 20 mg kg^{-1} of tamoxifen for 7 days. However, tamoxifen did not induce DNA adducts in the endometrium of women ($n = 18$) treated with 10–40 mg of tamoxifen for 3–108 months (Carmichael et al., 1996). In addition, tamoxifen did not induce a significant increase in DNA adducts in white blood cells of breast cancer patients (Phillips et al., 1996).

These data clearly show major differences between humans and rodents with respect to tamoxifen bioactivation and DNA adduct formation, with humans being several orders of magnitude less susceptible.

DIGITOXIN

For more than 200 years, the cardiac glycoside digitoxin has been used clinically in the treatment of congestive heart failure. In rats, cytochrome P450 3A has been reported to be an important determinant of digitoxin toxicity (Eberhart, 1991). CYP 3A cleaves the two sugar residues of digitoxin to give digitoxigenin bisdigitoxide and digitoxigenin monodigitoxide, the latter being conjugated by UDP-glucuronosyltransferase (Hazelton and Klaassen, 1988). Induction of CYP 3A by treatment of rats with pregnenolone-16α-carbonitrile and dexamethasone decreased digitoxin toxicity. In addition, the constitutive levels of CYP 3A (measured as testosterone 6β-hydroxylase activity) are greater in male than female rats, which is responsible for the higher toxicity of digitoxin in female (LD$_{50}$ 8.9 mg kg^{-1} i.v.) versus male (LD$_{50}$ 15.4 mg kg^{-1} i.v.) rats (Scott et al., 1971). This might suggest that extrapolation of digitoxin toxicity between different species may be performed by comparing CYP 3A levels. Indeed, an excellent correlation between LD$_{50}$ and liver microsomal CYP 3A activity (measured as testosterone 6β-hydroxylase activity) was obtained for several mammalian species, suggesting that the susceptibility of mammals to digitoxin is inversely related to the activity of liver microsomal CYP 3A (Eberhard, 1991). For humans (22 different individuals including 14 males and eight females), 6β-hydroxylation of testosterone ranged from 1.2 to 13.8 nmol mg^{-1} min^{-1}. Thus, if the animal data could be extrapolated to man, extremely large interindividual differences in toxicity ranging over 3–4 orders of magnitude should be expected. However, the rate of (inactivating) digitoxin metabolism (formation of the main metabolite digitoxigenin bisdigitoxide) and total metabolism did not correlate with differences in digitoxin toxicity of the examined species. Similarly, 6β-hydroxylation of testosterone was not correlated with total digitoxin oxidation in these species (Eberhart, 1991). Hence the correlation between digitoxin toxicity and CYP 3A acticity is either fortuitous or due to yet unknown reasons.

Most of the evidence indicates that species differences in digitoxin toxicity are due to species differences of the Na$^+$/K$^+$-ATPase. The Na$^+$/K$^+$-ATPase from cell lines of resistant species (e.g. mouse and hamster) was inhibited at much higher concentrations of digitoxin compared with sensitive species, such as human and monkey (Gupta *et al.*, 1986). Hence the role of oxidative digitoxin metabolism in species differences of toxicity remains unclear, but is probably of minor importance.

REFERENCES

Adamson, R. H., Thorgeirsson, U. P. and Sugimura, T. (1996). Extrapolation of heterocyclic amine carcinogenesis data from rodents and nonhuman primates to humans. *Arch. Toxicol., Suppl.*, **18**, 303–318.

Alexander, J., Wallin, H., Home, J. A. and Becher, G. (1989). 4-(2-Amino-1-methylimidazo[4,5-b]pyrid-6-yl)phenyl sulfate—a major metabolite of the food mutagen 2-amino-1-methyl-6-phenylimidazo[4,5-b]pyridine (PhIP) in the rat. *Carcinogenesis*, **10**, 1543–1547.

Andreola, F., Fernandez-Salguero, P. M., Chiantore, M. V., Petkovich, M. P., Gonzalez, F. J. and De-Luca, L. M. (1997). Aryl hydrocarbon receptor knockout mice (AHR−/−) exhibit liver retinoid accumulation and reduced retinoic acid metabolism. *Cancer Res.*, **57**, 2835–2838.

Anwar, W. A., Khalil, M. M. and Wild, C. P. (1994). Micronuclei, chromosomal aberrations and aflatoxin-albumin adducts in experimental animals after exposure to aflatoxin B1. *Mutat. Res.*, **322**, 61–67.

Aoyama, T., Gelboin, H. V. and Gonzalez, F. J. (1990). Mutagenic activation of 2-amino-3-methylimidazo [4,5-f]quinoline by complementary DNA-expressed human liver P-450. *Cancer Res.*, **50**, 2060–2063.

Bank, P. A., Yao, E. F., Phelps, C. L., Harper, P. A. and Denison, M. S. (1992). Species-specific binding of transformed Ah receptor to a dioxin responsive transcriptional enhancer. *Eur. J. Biochem.*, **228**, 85–94.

Bolton, M. G., Munoz, A., Jacobson, L. P., Groopman, J. D., Maxuitenko, Y. Y., Roebuck, B. D. and Kensler, T. W. (1993). Transient intervention with oltipraz protects against aflatoxin-induced hepatic tumorigenesis. *Cancer Res.*, **53**, 3499–3504.

Boobis, A. R., Gooderham, N. J., Edwards, R. J., Murray, S., Lynch, A. M., Yadollahi-Farsani, M. and Davies, D. S. (1996). Enzymic and interindividual differences in the human metabolism of heterocyclic amines. *Arch. Toxicol., Suppl.*, **18**, 286–302.

Buetler, T. M., Slone, D. and Eaton, D. L. (1992). Comparison of the aflatoxin B$_1$-8,9-epoxide conjugating activities of two bacterially expressed alpha class glutathione *S*-transferase isozymes from mouse and rat. *Biochem. Biophys. Res. Commun.*, **188**, 597–603.

Buetler, T. M., Bammler, T. K., Hayes, J. D. and Eaton, D. L. (1996). Oltipraz-mediated changes in aflatoxin B$_1$ biotransformation in rat liver: implications for human chemointervention. *Cancer Res.*, **56**, 2306–2313.

Buonarati, M. and Felton, J. S. (1990). Activation of 2-amino-1-methyl-6-phenylimidazo[4,5-b]pyridine (PhIP) to mutagenic metabolites. *Carcinogenesis*, **11**, 1133–1138.

Busby, W. F. and Wogan, G. N. (1984). Aflatoxins. In: Searle, C. E. (Ed.), *Chemical Carcinogens*, Vol. 2. American Chemical Society Monograph 182, American Chemical Society, Washington, DC, pp. 945–1136.

Caldwell, J. (1992). Problems and opportunities in toxicity testing arising from species differences in xenobiotic metabolism. *Toxicol. Lett.*, **64/65**, 651–659.

Carmichael, P. L., Ugwumadu, A. H. N., Neven, P., *et al.* (1996). Lack of genotoxicity of tamoxifen in human endometrium. *Cancer Res.*, **56**, 1475–1479.

Coe, J. E., Ishak, K. G., Ward, J. M., *et al.*, (1992). Tamoxifen prevents induction of hepatic neoplasms by zeranol, an estrogenic food contaminant. *Proc. Natl. Acad. Sci. USA*, **89**, 1085–1089.

Cole, K. E., Jones, T. W., Lipsky, M. M., Trump, B. F. and Hsu, I. C. (1988). *In vitro* binding of aflatoxin B$_1$ and 2-acetylaminofluorene to rat, mouse and human hepatocyte DNA: the relationship of DNA binding to carcinogenicity. *Carcinogenesis*, **9**, 711–716.

Croy, R. G. and Wogan, G. N. (1981). Quantitative comparison of covalent aflatoxin–DNA adducts formed in rat and mouse livers and kidneys. *J. Natl. Cancer Inst.*, **66**, 761–768.

Dao, T. L. (1964). Carcinogenesis of mammary gland in rat. *Prog. Exp. Tumor Res.*, **5**, 157–216.

Dasaradhi, L. and Shibutani, S. (1997). Identification of tamoxifen adducts formed by alpha-sulfate tamoxifen and alpha-acetoxytamoxifen. *Chem. Res. Toxicol.*, **10**, 189–196.

Davis, C. D., Adamson, R. H. and Snyderwine, E. G. (1993). Studies on the mutagenic activation of heterocyclic amines by cynomolgus monkey, rat and human microsomes show that cynomolgus monkeys have a low capacity to N-oxidize the quinoxaline-type heterocyclic amines. *Cancer Lett.*, **73**, 95–104.

Diener, B., Traiser, M., Arand, M., Leissner, J., Witzsch, U., Hohenfellner, R., Fändrich, F., Vogel, I., Utesch, D. and Oesch, F. (1994). Xenobiotic metabolizing enzyme activities in isolated and cryopreserved human liver parenchymal cells. *Toxicol. In vitro*, **8**, 1161–1166.

DiGiovanni, J., Romson, J. R., Linville, D. and Juchau, M. R. (1979). Covalent binding of polycyclic aromatic hydrocarbons to adenine correlates with tumorigenesis in mouse skin. *Cancer Lett.*, **7**, 39–53.

Eaton, D. L. and Gallagher, E. P. (1994). Mechanism of aflatoxin carcinogenesis. *Annu. Rev. Pharmacol. Toxicol.*, **34**, 135–172.

Eberhard, D. C. (1991). Species differences in the toxicity and cytochrome P450 IIIA-dependent metabolism of digitoxin. *Mol. Pharmacol.*, **40**, 859–867.

Edwards, R. J., Murray, B. P., Murray, S., Schultz, T., Neubert, D., Gant, T. W., Thorgeirsson, S. S., Boobis, A. R. and Davies, D. S. (1994). Contribution of CYP 1A1 and CYP 1A2 to the activation of heterocyclic amines in monkeys and human. *Carcinogenesis*, **15**, 829–836.

Eldridge, S. R., Gould, M. N. and Butterworth, B. E. (1992). Genotoxicity of environmental agents in human mammary epithelial cells. *Cancer Res.*, **52**, 5617–5621.

Fernandez-Salguero, P., Pineau, T., Hilbert, D. M., McPhail, T., Lee, S. S., Kimura, S., Nebert, D. W., Rudikoff, S., Ward, J. M. and Gonzalez, F. J. (1995). Immune system impairment and hepatic fibrosis in mice lacking the dioxin-binding Ah receptor. *Science*, **268**, 722–726.

Fernandez-Salguero, P. M., Hilbert, D. M., Rudikoff, S., Ward, J. M. and Gonzalez, F. J. (1996). Aryl-hydrocarbon receptor-deficient mice are resistant to 2,3,7,8-tetrachlorodibenzo-*p*-dioxin-induced toxicity. *Toxicol. Appl. Pharmacol.*, **140**, 173–179.

Gallagher, E. P., Wienkers, L. C., Stapleton, P. L., Kunze, K. L. and Eaton, D. L. (1994). Role of human microsomal and human complementary DNA-expressed cytochrome P450 1A2 and cytochrome P450 3A4 in the bioactivation of aflatoxin B$_1$. *Cancer Res.*, **54**, 101–108.

Garner, R. C. and Wright, C. M. (1975). Binding of [^{14}C]aflatoxin B$_1$ to cellular macromolecules in the rat and hamster. *Chem.–Biol. Interact.*, **11**, 123–131.

Gerhardsson de Verdier, M., Hagman, U., Peters, R. K., Steineck, G. and Overvik, E. (1991). Meat cooking methods and colorectal cancer: a case-referent study in Stockholm. *Int. J. Cancer*, **49**, 520–525.

Geyer, H. J., Schramm, K.-W., Scheunert, I., Schughart, K., Buters, J., Wurst, W., Greim, H., Kluge, R., Steinberg, C. E. W., Kettrup, A., Madhukar, B., Olson, J. R. and Gallo, M. A. (1997). Considerations on genetic and environmental factors that contribute to resistance or sensitivity of mammals including humans to toxicity of 2,3,7,8-tetrachlorodibenzo-*p*-dioxin (TCDD) and related compounds. *Ecotoxicol. Environ. Saf.*, **36**, 213–230.

Gielen, J. E., Goujon, F. M. and Nebert, D. W. (1972). Genetic regulation of aryl hydrocarbon hydroxylase induction. II. Simple Mendelian expression in mouse tissues *in vivo*. *J. Biol. Chem.*, **247**, 1125–1137.

Giovannucci, E., Rimm, E. B., Stampfer, M. J., Colditz, G. A., Ascherio, A. and Willett, W. C. (1994). Intake of fat, meat and fiber in relation to risk of colon cancer in men. *Cancer Res.*, **54**, 2390–2397.

Glatt, H. R. and Oesch, F. (1987). Species differences in enzymes controlling reactive epoxides. *Arch. Toxicol., Suppl.*, **10**, 111–124.

Gould, M. N., Grau, D. R., Seidman, L. A. and Moore, C. J. (1986). Interspecies comparison of human and rat mammary epithelial cell-mediated mutagenesis by polycyclic aromatic hydrocarbons. *Cancer Res.*, **46**, 4942–4945.

Guengerich, F. P. (1996). Metabolic control of carcinogens. In Hengstler, J. G. and Oesch, F. (Eds), *Control Mechanisms of Carcinogens*. Publishing House of the Editors, Mainz, pp. 12–35.

Gupta, R. S., Chopra, A. and Stetsko, D. K. (1986). Cellular basis for the species differences in sensitivity to cardiac glycosides (digitalis). *J. Cell Physiol.*, **127**, 197–206.

Gurtoo, H. L. and Motycka, L. (1976). Effect of sex differences on the *in vitro* and *in vivo* metabolism of aflatoxin B$_1$ by the rat. *Cancer Res.*, **36**, 4663–4671.

Hankinson, O., Bacsi, S. G., Fukunaga, B. N., Kozak, K. R., McNulty, S. E., Minehart, E., Probst, M. R., Reisz-Porszasz, S., Sun, W. and Zhang, J. (1996). Role of the aryl hydrocarbon receptor in carcinogenesis. In Hengstler, J. G. and Oesch, F. (Eds), *Control Mechanisms of Carcinogenesis*. Publishing House of the Editors, Mainz, pp. 36–45.

Hayes, J. D., Judah, D. J., McLellan, L. I., Kerr, L. A., Peacock, S. D. and Neal, G. E. (1991). Ethoxyquin-induced resistance to aflatoxin B1 in the rat is associated with the expression of a novel alpha-class glutathione S-transferase subunit Yc2, which possesses high catalytic activity for aflatoxin B1-8,9-epoxide. *Biochem. J.*, **279**, 385–398.

Hayes, J. D., Nguyen, T., Judah, D. J., Petersson, D. G. and Neal, G. E. (1994). Cloning of cDNAs from fetal rat liver encoding glutathione S-transferase Yc polypeptides: the Yc2 subunit is expressed in adult rat liver resistant to the hepatocarcinogen aflatoxin B$_1$. *J. Biol. Chem.*, **269**, 20707–20717.

Hays, S. M., Aylward, L. L., Karch, N. J. and Paustenbach, D. J. (1997). The relative susceptibility of animals and humans to the carcinogenic hazard posed by exposure to 2,3,7,8-tetrachlorodibenzo-*p*-dioxin: an analysis using standard and internal measures of dose. *Chemosphere*, **34**, 1507–1522.

Hazelton, G. A. and Klaassen, C. D. (1988). UDP-glucuronosyltransferase activity toward digitoxigenin-monodigitoxide. Differences in activation and induction properties in rat and mouse liver. *Drug Metab. Dispos.*, **16**, 30–36.

Hengstler, J. G., Arand, M., Herrero, M. E., and Oesch, F. (1998). Polymorphisms of *N*-acetyltransferases, glutathione *S*-transferases, microsomal epoxide hydrolase and sulfotransferases: influence on cancer susceptibility. In Schwab, M. (Ed.), *Genes and Environment*. Springer, New York, pp. 47–85.

Horn, E. P., Tucker, M. A., Lambert, G., Silverman, D., Zametkin, D., Sinha, R., Hartge, T., Landi, M. T. and Caporaso, N. E. (1995). A study of gender-based cytochrome P4501A2 variability: a possible mechanism for the male excess of bladder cancer. *Cancer Epidemiol. Biomarkers Prev.*, **4**, 529–533.

Huff, J. E., Salmon, A. G., Hooper, N. K. and Zeise, L. (1991). Long-term carcinogeresis studies on 2,3,7,8-tetrachlorodibenzo-*p*-dioxin and hexachlorodibenzo-*p*-dioxins. *Cell. Biol. Toxicol.*, **7**, 67–94.

Huggins, C. B. (1979). *Experimental Leukemia and Mammary Cancer*. University of Chicago Press, Chicago, Chapt. 6, pp. 73–99.

Jones, K. G. and Sweeney, G. D. (1980). Dependence of the porphyrogenic effect of 2,3,7,8-tetrachlorodibenzo-*p*-dioxin upon inheritance of aryl hydrocarbon hydroxylase responsiveness. *Toxicol. Appl. Pharmacol.*, **53**, 42.

Jordan, V. C. and Robinson, S. P. (1987). Species-specific pharmacology of antiestrogens: role of metabolism. *Fed. Proc.*, **46**, 1870–1874.

Kadlubar, F., Kaderlik, R. K., Mulder, G. J., Lin, D., Butler, M. A., Teitel, C. H., Minchin, R. F., Ilett, K. F., Friesen, M. D., Bartsch, H., et al. (1995). Metabolic activation and DNA adduct detection of PhIP in dogs, rats, and humans in relation to urinary bladder and colon carcinogenesis. In Proceedings of the 23rd Princess Takamatsu Cancer Research Symposium. Princeton Science Publishers, Princeton, NJ, pp. 207–213.

Kozak, K. R., Abbott, B. and Hankinson, O. (1997). ARNT-deficient mice and placental differentiation. Dev. Biol., 191, 287–305.

Lang, N. P., Butler, M. A., Massengill, J., Lawson, M., Stotts, R. C., Hauer-Jensen, M. and Kadlubar, F. F. (1994). Rapid metabolic phenotypes for acetyltransferase and cytochrome P4501A2 and putative exposure to food-borne heterocyclic amines increase the risk for colorectal cancer or polyps. Cancer Epidemiol. Biomarkers Prev., 3, 675–682.

Langouet, S., Coles, B., Morel, F., Becquemont, L., Beaune, P., Guengerich, F. P., Ketterer, B. and Guillouzo, A. (1995). Inhibition of CYP1A2 and CYP3A4 by oltipraz results in reduction of aflatoxin B1 metabolism in human hepatocytes in primary culture. Cancer Res., 55, 5574–5579.

Lawrence, G. S. and Gobas, F. A. (1997). A pharmacokinetic analysis of interspecies extrapolation in dioxin risk assessment. Chemosphere, 35, 427–452.

Li, D., Wang, M., Dhingra, K. and Hittelman, W. N. (1996). Aromatic DNA adducts in adjacent tissues of breast cancer patients: clues to breast cancer etiology. Cancer Res., 56, 287–293.

Lim, C. K., Yuan, Z.-X., Lamb, J. H., et al. (1994). A comparative study of tamoxifen metabolism in female rat, mouse and human liver microsomes. Carcinogenesis, 15, 589–593.

Lin, D.-X., Lang, N. P. and Kadlubar, F. F. (1995). Species differences in the biotransformation of the food-borne carcinogen 2-amino-1-methyl-6-phenylimidazo[4,5-b]pyridine by hepatic microsomes and cytosols from humans, rats, and mice. Drug Metab. Dispos., 23, 518–524.

Lotlikar, P. D., Jhee, E. C., Insetta, S. M. and Clearfield, M. S. (1984). Modulation of microsome-mediated aflatoxin B$_1$ binding to exogenous and endogenous DNA by cytosolic glutathione S-transferase in rat liver. Carcinogenesis, 5, 269–276.

Luch, A. and Platt, K. L. (1996). Metabolism, DNA-interaction and mutagenesis: fundamental events in carcinogenesis by polycyclic aromatic hydrocarbons. In Hengstler, J. G. and Oesch, F. (Eds), Control Mechanisms of Carcinogenesis. Publishing House of the Editors, Mainz, pp. 66–97.

Lutz, W. K., Jaggi, W., Luthy, J., Sagelsdorff, P. and Schlatter, C. (1980). In vivo covalent binding of aflatoxin B$_1$ and aflatoxin M$_1$ to liver DNA of rat, mouse and pig. Chem.–Biol. Interact., 32, 249–250.

Mani, C., Gelboin, H. V., Park, S. S., et al. (1993). Metabolism of the antimammary cancer antiestrogenic agent tamoxifen. I. Cytochrome P-450-catalyzed N-demethylation and 4-hydroxylation. Drug Metab. Dispos., 21, 645–656.

Martin, E. K., Rich, K. J., White, I. N. H., et al. (1995). ^{32}P-postlabelled DNA adducts in liver obtained from women treated with tamoxifen. Carcinogenesis, 16, 1651–1654.

McConnell, E. E., Moore, J. A., Haseman, J. K. and Harris, M. W. (1978). The comparative toxicity of chlorinated dibenzo-p-dioxin in mice and guinea pigs. Toxicol. Appl. Pharmacol., 44, 335–356.

Moore, C. J., Eldridge, S. R., Tricomi, W. A. and Gould, M. N. (1987a). Quantitation of benzo[a]pyrene and 7,12-dimethyl-benz[a]anthracene binding to nuclear macromolecules in human and rat mammary epithelial cells. Cancer Res., 47, 2609–2613.

Moore, C. J., Pruess-Schwartz, D., Mauthe, R. J., Gould, M. N. and Baird, W. M. (1987b). Interspecies differences in the major DNA adducts formed from benzo[a]pyrene but not 7,12-dimethylbenz[a]anthracene in rat and human mammary cell cultures. Cancer Res., 47, 4402–4406.

Morel, F., Fardel, O., Meyer, D. J., Langouet, S., Gilmore, K. S., Meunier, B., Tu, C. P., Kensler, T. W., Ketterer, B. and Guillouzo, A. (1993). Preferential increase of glutathione S-transferase class alpha transcripts in cultured human hepatocytes by phenobarbital, 3-methylcholanthrene, and dithiolethiones. Cancer Res., 53, 231–234.

Morel, F., Langouet, S., Maheo, K. and Guillouzo, A. (1997). The use of primary hepatocyte cultures for the evaluation of chemoprotective agents. Cell Biol. Toxicol., 13, 323–329.

Nakai, J. S., Winhall, M. J. and Bunce, N. J. (1994). Comparative kinetic study of the binding between 2,3,7,8-tetrachlorodibenzo-p-dioxin and related ligands with the hepatic Ah receptors from several rodent species. J. Biochem. Toxicol., 9, 199–209.

Oesch, F. (1980). Species differences in activating and inactivating enzymes related to in vitro mutagenicity mediated by tissue preparations from these species. Arch. Toxicol., Suppl., 3, 179–194.

Oesch, F. and Diener, B. (1995). Cell systems for use in studies on the relationship between foreign compound metabolism and toxicity. Pharmacol. Toxicol., 76, 325–327.

Oesch, F., Raphael, D., Schwind, H. and Glatt, H. R. (1977). Species differences in activating and inactivating enzymes related to the control of mutagenic metabolites. Arch. Toxicol., 39, 97–108.

Oesch, F., Hengstler, J. G. and Fuchs, J. (1994). Cigarette smoking protects mononuclear blood cells of carcinogen exposed workers from additional work-exposure induced DNA single strand breaks. Mutat. Res., 321, 175–185.

Ohmori, S., Horie, T., Guengerich, F. P., Kiuchi, M. and Kitada, M. (1993). Purification and characterization of two forms of hepatic microsomal cytochrome P450 from untreated cynomolgus monkeys. Arch. Biochem. Biophys., 305, 405–413.

Olson, J. R., Holscher, M. A. and Neal, R. A. (1980). Toxicity of 2,3,7,8-tetrachlorodibenzo-p-dioxin in the golden Syrian hamster. Toxicol. Appl. Pharmacol., 55, 67–78.

Pathak, D. N., Pongraez, K. and Bodell, W. J. (1996). Uterine peroxidase activation of tamoxifen metabolites to form DNA adducts: comparison with the adducts formed in the uterus of Sprague-Dawley rats treated with tamoxifen. Proc. Am. Assoc. Cancer Res., 37, 119.

Peers, F. G. and Linsell, C. A. (1977). Dietary aflatoxins and human primary liver cancer. Ann. Nutr. Aliment., 31, 1005–1018.

Peterson, R. E., Theobald, H. M. and Kimmel, G. L. (1993). Developmental and reproductive toxicity of dioxins and related compounds: cross-species comparisons. Crit. Rev. Toxicol., 23, 283–335.

Phillips, D. H., Hewer, A. and Grover, P. L. (1985). Aberrant activation of benzo[a]pyrene in cultured rat mammary cells *in vitro* and following direct application in rat mammary glands *in vivo. Cancer Res.*, **45**, 4167–4174.

Phillips, D. H., Carmichael, P. L., Hewer, A., Cole, K. J., Hardcastle, I. R., Poon, G. K., Keogh, A. and Strain, A. J. (1996). Activation of tamoxifen and its metabolite alpha-hydroxytamoxifen to DNA-binding products: comparisons between human, rat and mouse hepatocytes. *Carcinogenesis*, **17**, 89–94.

Phillipson, C. E. and Ioannides, C. (1989). Metabolic activation of polycyclic aromatic hydrocarbons to mutagens in the Ames test by various animal species including man. *Mutat. Res.*, **211**, 147–151.

Poland, A. and Glover, E. (1980). 2,3,7,8-Tetrachlorodibenzo-*p*-dioxin: segregation of toxicity with the Ah locus. *Mol. Pharmacol.*, **17**, 86.

Poland, A., Palen, D. and Glover, E. (1994). Analysis of the four alleles of the murine aryl hydrocarbon receptor. *Mol. Pharmacol.*, **46**, 915–921.

Quinn, B. A., Crane, T. L., Kocal, T. E., Best, S. J., Cameron, R. G., Rushmore, T. H., Faber, E. and Hayes, M. A. (1990). Protective activity of different hepatic cytosolic glutathione S-transferases against DNA-binding metabolites of aflatoxin B$_1$. *Toxicol. Appl. Pharmacol.*, **105**, 351–363.

Ramakrishna, K. V., Fan, P. W., Boyer, C. S., Dalvie, D. and Bolton, J. L. (1997). Oxo substituents markedly alter the phase II metabolism of alpha-hydroxybutenylbenzenes: models probing the bioactivation mechanisms of tamoxifen. *Chem. Res. Toxicol.*, **10**, 887–894.

Ramsdell, H. S. and Eaton, D. L. (1990). Species susceptibility to aflatoxin B$_1$ carcinogenesis: comparative kinetics of microsomal biotransformation. *Cancer Res.*, **50**, 615–620.

Randerath, K., Bi, J., Mabon, N., Sriram, P. and Moorthy, B. (1994a). Strong intensification of mouse hepatic tamoxifen DNA adduct formation by pretreatment with the sulfotransferase inhibitor and ubiquitous environmental pollutant pentachlorophenol. *Carcinogenesis*, **15**, 797–800.

Randerath, K., Moorthy, B., Mabon, N. and Sriram, P. (1994b). Tamoxifen: evidence by ^{32}P-postlabeling and use of metabolic inhibitors for two distinct pathways leading to mouse DNA adduct formation and identification of 4-hydroxytamoxifen as a proximate metabolite. *Carcinogenesis*, **15**, 2087–2094.

Rasmussen, B. B. and Brosen, K. (1996). Determination of urinary metabolities of caffeine for the assessment of cytochrome P450 1A2, xanthine oxidase, and N-acetyltransferase activity in humans. *Ther. Drug Monit.*, **18**, 254–262.

Roberts-Thomson, I. C., Ryan, P., Khoo, K. K., Hart, W. J., McMichael, A. J. and Butler, R. N. (1996). Diet, acetylator phenotype, and risk of colorectal neoplasia. *Lancet*, **347**, 1372–1374.

Roggenband, R., Wolterbeek, A. P. M., Rutten, A. A. J. J. L. and Baan, R. A. (1993). Comparative ^{32}P-postlabeling analysis of benzo[*a*]pyrene-DNA adducts *in vitro* upon activation of benzo[*a*]pyrene by human, rabbit and rodent liver microsomes. *Carcinogenesis*, **14**, 1945–1950.

Rozman, K. (1989). A critical review on the mechanisms of toxicity of 2,3,7,8-tetrachlorodibenzo-*p*-dioxin. Implications for human safety assessment. *Dermatosen Beruf Umwelt*, **38**, 95–95.

Sadrieh, N. and Snyderwine, E. G. (1995). Cytochromes P450 in cynomolgus monkeys mutagenically activate 2-amino-3-methylimidazo[4,5-*f*]quinoline (IQ) but not 2-amino-3,8-dimethylimidazo[4,5-*f*]quinoxaline (MeIQx). *Carcinogenesis*, **16**, 1549–1455.

Schiffmann, M. H. and Felton, J. S. (1990). Fried foods and the risk of colon cancer. *Am. J. Epidemiol.*, **131**, 376–378.

Schrenk, D., Stuven, T., Goh, G., Viebahn, R. and Bock, K. W. (1995). Induction of CYP1A and glutathione S-transferase activities by 2,3,7,8-tetrachlorodibenzo-*p*-dioxin in human hepatocyte cultures. *Carcinogenesis*, **16**, 943–946.

Schwetz, B., Norris, J., Sparschu, G., Rowe, V., Gehring, P., Emerson, J. and Gerbig, C. (1973). Toxicology of chlorinated dibenzo-*p*-dioxins. *Environ. Health Perspect.*, **5**, 87–99.

Scott, W. J., Beliles, R. P. and Silverman, H. I. (1971). The comparative acute toxicity of two cardiac glycosides in adult and newborn rats. *Toxicol. Appl. Pharmacol.*, **20**, 599–601.

Sesardic, D., Boobis, A. R., Edwards, R. J. and Davies, D. S. (1989). A form of cytochrome P450 in man, orthologous to form d in the rat catalyzes the O-deethylation of phenacetin and is inducible by cigarette smoking. *Br. J. Clin. Pharmacol.*, **26**, 363–372.

Sesardic, D., Cole, K. J., Edwards, R. J., Davies, D. S., Thomas, P. E., Levin, W. and Boobis, A. R. (1990). The inducibility and catalytic activity of cytochromes P450c (P4501A1) and P450d (P4501A2) in rat tissues. *Biochem. Pharmacol.*, **39**, 499–506.

Shank, R. C., Bhamarapravati, N., Gordon, J. E. and Wogan, G. N. (1972). Dietary aflatoxins and human liver cancer. IV. Incidence of primary liver cancer in two municipal populations in Thailand. *Food Cosmet. Toxicol.*, **10**, 171–179.

Sinha, R., Rothman, N., Brown, E. D., Mark, S. D., Hoover, R. N., Caporaso, N. E., Levander, O. A., Knize, M. G., Lang, N. P. and Kadlubar, F. F. (1994). Pan-fried meat containing high levels of heterocyclic aromatic amines but low levels of polycyclic aromatic hydrocarbons induces cytochrome P450 1A2 activity in humans. *Cancer Res.*, **54**, 6154–6159.

Slone, D. H., Gallagher, E. P., Ramsdell, H. S., Rettie, A. E., Stapleton, P. L., Berlad, L. G. and Eaton, D. L. (1995). Human variability in hepatic glutathione S-transferase-mediated conjugation of aflatoxin B$_1$-epoxide and other chemicals. *Pharmacogenetics*, **5**, 224–233.

Snyderwine, E. G., Turesky, R. J., Turteltaub, K. W., Davis, C. D., Sadrieh, N., Schut, H. A., Nagao, M., Sugimura, T., Thorgeirsson, U. P., Adamson, R. H. and Thorgeirsson, S. S. (1997). Metabolism of food-derived heterocyclic amines in nonhuman primates. *Mutat. Res.*, **376**, 203–210.

Steinberg, P., Jennings, G. S., Schlemper, B. and Oesch, F. (1996). Molecular mechanisms underlying the liver cell-type specific toxicity of Aflatoxin B$_1$. In Hengstler, J. G. and Oesch, F. (Eds), *Control Mechanisms of Carcinogenesis*. Publishing House of the Editors, Mainz, pp. 135–147.

Steinberg, P., Biefang, K., Kiulies, S., Fischer, T., Platt, K. L., Oesch, F., Böttger, T. and Hengstler, J. G. (1998). Drug metabolizing capacity of cryopreserved human, rat and mouse liver parenchymal cells held in suspension. Submitted.

Steinmetz, K. L., Green, C. E., Bakke, J. P., Spak, D. K. and Mirsalis, J. C. (1988). Induction of unscheduled DNA synthesis in primary cultures of rat, mouse, hamster, and human hepatocytes. *Mutat. Res.*, **206**, 91–102.

Tannenbaum, S. R. (1997). Comparative metabolism of tamoxifen and DNA adduct formation and *in vitro* studies on genotoxicity. *Semin. Oncol.*, **24**, Suppl. I, pp. S1-81–S1-86.

Turesky, R. J., Aeschbacher, H. U., Würzner, H. P., Skipper, P. L. and Tannenbaum, S. R. (1988). Major routes of metabolism of the food-borne carcinogen 2-amino-3,8-dimethylimidazo [4,5-*f*]quinoxaline in the rat. *Carcinogenesis*, **9**, 1043–1048.

Ueno, I., Friedman, L. and Stone, C. L. (1980). Species difference in the binding of aflatoxin B1 to hepatic macromolecules. *Toxicol. Appl. Pharmacol.*, **52**, 177–180.

Unkila, M., Pohjanvirta, R., MacDonald, E. and Tuomistro, J. (1994). Characterization of 2,3,7,8-tetrachlorodibenzo-*p*-dioxin (TCDD)-induced brain serotonin metabolism in the rat. *Eur. J. Pharmacol.*, **270**, 157–166.

Unkila, M., Ruotsalainen, M., Pohjanvirta, R., Viluksela, M., MacDonald, E., Tuomistro, J., Rozman, K. and Tuomisto, J. (1995). Effect of 2,3,7,8-tetrachlorodibenzo-*p*-dioxin (TCDD) on tryptophan and glucose homeostasis in most TCDD-susceptible and the most TCDD-resistant species, guinea pigs and hamsters. *Arch. Toxicol.*, **69**, 677–683.

Vecchi, A., Sironi, M., Antonia, M., Recchia, C. M. and Garattini, S. (1983). Immunosuppressive effects of 2,3,7,8-tetrachlorodibenzo-*p*-dioxin in strains of mice with different susceptibility. *Proc. Natl. Acad. Sci. USA*, **87**, 6917.

Wallin, H., Milkalsen, A., Guengerich, F. P., Ingelman-Sundberg, M., Solberg, K. E., Rossland, O. J. and Alexander, J. (1990). Differential rates of metabolic activation and detoxication of the food mutagen 2-amino-1-methyl-6-phenylimidazo[4,5-*b*]pyridine by different cytochrome P450 enzymes. *Carcinogenesis*, **11**, 489–492.

Weber, L. D. W., Lebofsky, M., Stahl, B. U., Gorski, J. R., *et al.* (1991). Reduced activities of key enzymes of gluconeogenesis as a possible cause of acute toxicity of 2,3,7,8-tetrachlorodibenzo-*p*-dioxin (TCDD) in rats. *Toxicology*, **66**, 133.

Wild, C. P., Jansen, A. M., Cova, L. and Montesano, R. (1993). Molecular dosimetry of aflatoxin exposure: contribution to understanding the multifactorial etiopathogenesis of primary hepatocellular carcinoma with particular reference to hepatitis B virus. *Environ. Health Perspect.*, **99**, 115–122.

Wild, C. P., Hasegawa, R., Barraud, L., Chutimataewin, S., Chapot, B., Nobuyuki, I. and Montesano, R. (1996). Aflatoxin-albumin adducts: a basis for comparative carcinogenesis between animals and humans. *Cancer Epidemiol. Biomarkers Prev.*, **5**, 179–189.

Wilson, A. S., Williams, D. P., Davis, C. D., Tingle, M. D. and Park, B. K. (1997). Bioactivation and inactivation of aflatoxin B$_1$ by human, mouse and rat liver preparations: effect on SCE in human mononuclear leucocytes. *Mutat. Res.*, **373**, 257–264.

Wogan, G. N. (1997). Review of the toxicology of tamoxifen. *Semin. Oncol.*, **24**, S1-87–S1-97.

Wroblewski, V. J. and Olson, J. R. (1985). Hepatic metabolism of 2,3,7,8-tetrachlorodibenzo-*p*-dioxin (TCDD) in the rat and guinea pig. *Toxicol. Appl. Pharmacol.*, **81**, 231–240.

Yamazoe, Y., Abu-Zeid, M., Manabe, S., Toyama, S. and Kato, R. (1988). Metabolic activation of a protein pyrolysate promutagen 2-amino-3,8-dimethylimidazo[4,5-*f*]quinoxaline by rat liver microsomes and purified cytochrome P450. *Carcinogenesis*, **9**, 105–109.

Chapter 13

Statistics for Toxicology

Peter N. Lee and David Lovell

CONTENTS

INTRODUCTION

This chapter concerns statistical aspects of the design, conduct, analysis and interpretation of toxicological data. It is intended mainly for the reader not qualified in statistics and is more concerned with principles than with techniques. A major concern of this chapter is with the typical long-term rat or mouse carcinogenicity study, particular attention being given to the appropriate treatment of pathological data on the incidence of tumours and non-neoplastic findings, though many of the principles and methods described apply much more widely in toxicology. The chapter ends with a section referring to additional reading which may be helpful when analysing not only pathology, but also a range of other types of toxicological data.

ROLE OF THE STATISTICIAN

Having read this chapter and the references, the pathologist or toxicologist should be in a good position to be able to carry out appropriate analyses in a number of standard situations. However, it is still important that an expert statistician be available for advice and assistance, even if only to confirm quickly that what has been done is sensible. All too frequently, where a statistician is not involved at any stage, reports and papers end up with conclusions that are invalid because the statistics have been carried out wrongly.

Although a statistician may carry out the statistical analysis, it is vital that the pathologist or toxicologist and the statistician have regular discussions. The pathologist or toxicologist should make it clear what questions are to be answered and, where relevant, describe how different variables interrelate biologically. The statistician should ensure that the pathologist or toxicologist fully understands why the selected methods of analysis have been chosen and what any output means. The pathologist or toxicologist should be reluctant to accept reports from the statistician consisting of hundreds of pages of computer-produced statistical tables where the vast majority of the output is irrelevant to the questions of interest.

SOME GENERAL PRINCIPLES

Bias and Chance

Any toxicological study aims to determine whether a treatment elicits a response. An observed difference in response between a treated and control group need not necessarily be a result of treatment. There are, in principle, two other possible explanations—*bias*, or systematic differences other than treatment between the groups, and *chance*, or random differences. A major objective of both experimental design and analysis is to try to avoid bias. Wherever possible, treated and control groups to be compared should be alike in respect of all other factors. Where differences remain, these should be corrected for in the statistical analysis. Chance cannot be wholly excluded, since identically treated animals will not respond identically. While even the most extreme difference might in theory be due to chance, a proper statistical analysis will allow the experimenter to assess this possibility. The smaller the probability of a 'false positive', the more confident the experimenter can be that the effect is real. Good experimental design improves the chance of picking up a true effect with confidence by maximizing the ratio between 'signal' and 'noise'.

Hypothesis Testing and Probability (p) Values

A relationship of treatment to some toxicological end-point is often stated to be 'statistically significant ($p < 0.05$)'. What does this really mean? A number of points have to be made. *First*, statistical significance need not necessarily imply biological importance, if the end-point under study is not relevant to the animal's well-being. *Second*, the statement will usually be based only on the data from the study in question and will not take into account prior knowledge. In some situations, e.g. when one or two of a very rare tumour type are seen in treated animals, statistical significance may not be achieved but the finding may be biologically extremely important, especially if a similar treatment was previously found to elicit a similar response. *Third*, the p value does not describe the probability that a true effect of treatment exists. Rather, it describes the probability of the observed response, or one more extreme, occurring on the assumption that treatment actually had no effect whatsoever. A p value that is not significant is consistent with a treatment having no effect but is also consistent with a treatment having a small effect, not detected with sufficient certainty in this study. *Fourth*, there are two types of p value. A 'one-tailed (or one-sided) p value' is the probability of getting by chance a treatment effect in a specified direction as great as or greater than that observed. A 'two-tailed p value' is the probability of getting, by chance alone, a treatment difference in either direction which is as great as or greater than that observed. By convention p values are assumed to be two-tailed unless the contrary is stated. Where, which is unusual, one can rule out in advance the possibility of a treatment effect except in one direction, a one-tailed p value should be used. Often, however, two-tailed tests are to be preferred, and it is certainly not recommended to use one-tailed tests and *not* report large differences in the other direction. In any event, it is important to make it absolutely clear whether one- or two-tailed tests have been used.

It is a great mistake, when presenting results of statistical analyses, to mark, as do some laboratories, results simply as significant or not significant at one defined probability level (usually $p < 0.05$). This poor practice does not allow the reader any real chance to judge whether or not the effect is a true one. Some statisticians present the actual p value for every comparison made.

While this gives precise information, it can make it difficult to assimilate results from many variables. One practice we recommend is to mark p values routinely using plus signs to indicate positive differences (and minus signs to indicate negative differences) as follows: $+++$ $p < 0.001$, $++$ $0.001 \leqslant p < 0.01$, $+$ $0.01 \leqslant p < 0.05$, $(+)$ $0.05 \leqslant p < 0.1$. This highlights significant results more clearly and also allows the reader to judge the whole range from 'virtually certain treatment effect' to 'some suspicion'. Note that using two-tailed tests, bracketed plus signs indicate findings that would be significant at the conventional $p < 0.05$ level using one-tailed tests but are not significant at this level using two-tailed tests. In interpreting p values it is important to realize they are only an aid to judgement to be used in conjunction with other available information. One might validly consider a $p < 0.01$ increase as chance when it was unexpected, occurred only at a low dose level with no such effect seen at higher doses, and was evident in only one subset of the data. In contrast, a $p < 0.05$ increase might be convincing if it occurred in the top dose and was for an end-point one might have expected to be increased from known properties of the chemical or closely related chemicals.

Multiple Comparisons

When a p value is stated to be < 0.05, this implies that, for that particular test, the difference could have occurred by chance less than 1 time in 20. Toxicological studies frequently involve making treatment–control comparisons for large numbers of variables and, in some situations, also for various subsets of animals. Some statisticians worry that the larger the number of tests the greater is the chance of picking up statistically significant findings that do not represent true treatment effects. For this reason, an alternative 'multiple comparisons' procedure has been proposed in which, if the treatment was totally without effect, then 19 times out of 20 *all* the tests should show non-significance when testing at the 95% confidence level. Automatic use of this approach cannot be recommended. Not only does it make it much more difficult to pick up any real effects, but also there is something inherently unsatisfactory about a situation where the relationship between a treatment and a particular response depends arbitrarily on which other responses happened to be investigated at the same time. It is accepted that in any study involving multiple end-points there will inevitably be a grey area between those showing highly significant effects and those showing no significant effects, where there is a problem distinguishing chance and true effects. However, changing the methodology so that the grey areas all come up as non-significant can hardly be the answer.

Estimating the Size of the Effect

It should be clearly understood that a *p* value does not give direct information about the size of any effect that has occurred. A compound may elicit an increase in response by a given amount, but whether a study finds this increase to be statistically significant will depend on the size of the study and the variability of the data. In a small study, a large and important effect may be missed, especially if the end-point is imprecisely measured. In a large study, on the other hand, a small and unimportant effect may emerge as statistically significant.

Hypothesis testing tells us whether an observed increase can or cannot be reasonably attributed to chance, but not how large it is. Although much statistical theory relates to hypothesis testing, current trends in medical statistics are towards confidence interval estimation with differences between test and control groups expressed in the form of a best estimate, coupled with the 95% confidence interval (CI). Thus, if one states that treatment increases response by an estimated 10 units (95% CI 3–17 units), this would imply that there is a 95% chance that the indicated interval includes the true difference. If the lower 95% confidence limit exceeds zero, this implies the increase is statistically significant at $p < 0.05$ using a two-tailed test. One can also calculate, for example, 99% or 99.9% confidence limits, corresponding to testing for significance at $p < 0.01$ or $p < 0.001$.

In screening studies of standard design, the tendency has been to concentrate mainly on hypothesis testing. However, presentation of the results in the form of estimates with confidence intervals can be a useful adjunct for some analyses, and is very important in studies aimed specifically at quantifying the size of an effect.

GOOD LABORATORY PRACTICE AND QUALITY ASSURANCE

Before going on to discuss specific considerations relating to the design, conduct and analysis of toxicological studies, it is important to refer to the concept of studies being performed to Good Laboratory Practice (GLP) with the inclusion of a formal Quality Assurance (QA) component. This aspect has been a response to examples of poor and in some cases fraudulent practice in studies in the past. GLP compliance requires written description of the experimental protocol and the development of Standard Operating Procedures (SOPs) which govern how procedures are carried out. Specific attention is given to the collection and maintenance of the integrity of the raw data collected in a study. Quality Assurance Personnel responsible for monitoring studies for GLP compliance are likely to require evidence that the study was conducted according to the defined protocol and that any statistical analyses and reporting of the data were carried out as described in the study protocol. Evidence will be needed that any statistical package used had previously been validated to ensure that it was providing appropriate results. GLP is now a central feature of standard toxicological tests carried out for regulatory purposes. Its influence and importance are likely to increase and the development of the related concept Good Scientific Practice (GSP) for use in more basic experimental studies is now in progress.

EXPERIMENTAL DESIGN AND CONDUCT

Issues relating to experimental design and conduct are considered in detail in Chapter 3 of Gart *et al.* (1986) and in Lee (1993), and will be discussed only briefly here. In many cases, the experimental design is governed in part by regulatory requirement and little input of a statistical nature is either feasible or needed.

There are ten facets of any study which may affect its ability to detect an effect of a treatment. The first six concern minimizing the role of chance and the last four relate to avoidance of bias.

Choice of Species and Strain

Ideally, the responses of interest should be rare in untreated control animals but should be reasonably readily evoked by appropriate treatments. Some species or specific strains, perhaps because of inappropriate diets (Roe, 1989), have high background tumour incidences which make increases both difficult to detect and difficult to interpret when detected.

Dose Levels

This is a very important and controversial area. In screening studies aimed at hazard identification it is normal, in order to avoid requiring huge numbers of animals, to test at dose levels higher than those to which man will be exposed, but not so high that marked toxicity occurs. A range of doses is usually tested to guard against the possibility of a misjudgement of an appropriate high dose and that the metabolic pathways at the high doses differ markedly from those at lower doses and, perhaps, to ensure no large effects occur at dose levels in the range to be used by man. In studies aimed more at risk estimation, more and lower doses may be tested to obtain fuller information on the shape of the dose–response curve.

Number of Animals

This is obviously an important determinant of the precision of the findings. The calculation of the appropriate number depends on: (1) the critical difference, i.e. the size of the effect it is desired to detect; (2) the false positive rate, i.e. the probability of an effect being detected when none exists (equivalent to the 'α level' or 'Type I error'); (3) the false negative rate, i.e. the probability of no effect being detected when one of exactly the critical size exists (equivalent to the 'β level' or 'Type II error'); and (4) some measure of the variability in the material.

Tables relating numbers of animals required to obtain values of critical size, α and β are given in Lee (1993) and software (nQUERY ADVISOR) is also available for this purpose. As a rule of thumb, to reduce the critical difference by a factor n for a given α and β, the number of animals required will have to be increased by a factor n^2.

Duration of the Experiment

It is obviously important not to terminate the study too early for fatal conditions, which are normally strongly age-related. Less obviously, going on for too long in a study can be a mistake, partly because the last few weeks or months may produce relatively few extra data at a disproportionate cost, and partly because diseases of extreme old age may obscure the detection of tumours and other conditions of more interest. For non-fatal conditions, the ideal is to sacrifice the animals when the average prevalence is around 50%.

Accuracy of Determinations

This is of obvious importance. Although GLP and advances in technology have improved the situation here, there is an ever-present need for those taking part in the study to be diligent.

Stratification

To detect a treatment difference with accuracy, it is important that the groups being compared are as homogeneous as possible with respect to other known causes of the response. In particular, suppose that there is another known important cause of the response for which the animals vary, so that the animals are a mixture of hyper- and hypo-responders from this cause. If the treated group has a higher proportion of hyper-responders it will tend to have a higher response even if treatment has no effect. Even if the proportion of hyper-responders is the same as in the controls, it will be more difficult to detect an effect of treatment because of the increased between-animal variability.

Given that this other factor is known, it will be sensible to take it into account in both the design and analysis of the study. In the design, it can be used as a 'blocking factor' so that animals at each level are allocated equally (or in the correct proportion) to control and treated groups. In the analysis, the factor should be treated as a stratifying variable, with separate treatment–control comparisons made at each level, and the comparisons combined for an overall test of difference. This is discussed later, where we refer to the factorial design as one example of the more complex designs that can be used to investigate the separate effect of multiple treatments.

Randomization

Random allocation of animals to treatment groups is a prerequisite of good experimental design. If not carried out, one can never be sure whether treatment–control differences are due to treatment or to 'confounding' by other relevant factors. The ability to randomize easily is a major advantage animal experiments have over epidemiology.

While randomization eliminates bias (at least in expectation), simple randomization of all animals may not be the optimal technique for producing a sensitive test. If there is another major source of variation (e.g. sex or batch of animals), it will be better to carry out stratified randomization (i.e. carry out separate randomizations within each level of the stratifying variable).

The need for randomization applies not only to the allocation of the animals to the treatment, but also to anything that can materially affect the recorded response. The same random number that is used to apply animals to treatment group can be used to determine cage position, order of weighing, order of bleeding for clinical chemistry, order of sacrifice at termination, and so on.

Adequacy of Control Group

While historical control data can, on occasion, be useful, a properly designed study demands that a relevant concurrent control group be included with which results for the test group can be compared. The principle that like should be compared with like, apart from treatment, demands that control animals should be randomized from the same source as treatment animals. Careful consideration should also be given to the appropriateness of the control group. Thus, in an experiment involving treatment of a compound in a solvent, it would often be inappropriate to include only an untreated control group, as any differences observed could only be attributed to the treatment–solvent combination. To determine the specific effects of the compound, a comparison group given the solvent only, by the same route of administration, would be required.

Animal Placement

It is not always generally realized that the position of the animal in the room in which it is kept may affect the animal's response. An example is the strong relationship between incidence of retinal atrophy in albino rats and closeness to the lighting source. Systematic differences in cage position should be avoided, preferably via randomization.

Data Recording

Two distinct sources of systematic bias may occur in data recording. One is that awareness of treatment may, consciously or subconsciously, affect the values recorded by the measurer. This can be avoided by organizing data recording so that observations are made blind. The second is that there is a systematic shift in the standard of measurement with time, coupled with a tendency for different groups to be measured at different time points. This is particularly important when a pathologist grades a lesion for severity and when the control and high-dose animals are read before the intermediate-dose animals. In some situations it may be necessary to reread all the slides blind and in random order to be sure that 'diagnostic drift' is avoided.

Valid analysis cannot be conducted unless one can distinguish animals which were examined and did not have the relevant response and animals which were not examined. It can also be important clearly to identify why data are missing.

STATISTICAL ANALYSIS—GENERAL CONSIDERATIONS

Introduction

In the next section different techniques that might generally be applied to different types of toxicological data are summarized. Before doing so, a number of points are worthy of discussion. Some are quite general, while others relate more specifically to problems in dealing with data from pathological investigations.

Variables to be Analysed

Although some pathologists still regard their discipline as providing qualitative rather than quantitative data, it is abundantly clear that pathology, when applied to routine screening of animal toxicity and carcinogenicity studies, has to be quantitative to at least some degree so that statistical statements can be made about possible treatment effects. Inevitably, there will be some descriptive

text which will not be appropriate for statistical analysis. However, the main objective of the pathologist should be to provide information on the presence or absence (with severity grade or size where appropriate) of a list of conditions, consistently recorded from animal to animal by well defined criteria, which can be validly used in a statistical assessment.

Given that statistical analysis is worth doing and data are available that would be analysed, should one then analyse all the end-points recorded? Some arguments have been put forward against analysing all the end-points studied, none of which really holds water.

One argument is that some end-points are not of interest. Perhaps the study is essentially a carcinogenicity study, so that non-neoplastic end-points are not considered to be 'background pathology' and almost *per se* unrelated to treatment. In our view, this is illogical. If the pathologist has gone to the trouble of recording the data, then surely, in general, they ought to be analysed; otherwise, why record them in the first place? After all, the costs of the statistical analysis are much less than those of doing the study and the pathology. While one might justify failure to analyse non-neoplastic data where tumour analysis has already shown that the compound is clearly carcinogenic and no longer of market potential, the general rule ought to be to analyse everything that has been specifically investigated.

Another argument put forward against doing multiple analyses is that it may yield many chance significant *p* values that have to be 'explained away'. This seems to us a poor reason for not exploring the data fully. A detailed look at the data can only aid interpretation, provided that one is not hide-bound by the false argument that statistical significance necessarily equates with biological importance and definitely indicates a true effect of treatment.

Another reason not to analyse might be that visual inspection of summary tables reveals no suspicion of an effect for some end-point. This seems to be, in this age of rapid and efficient computer programs, totally the wrong way to organize things. If the data are held on a computer, it is much better and quicker to do the actual analysis than to do the inevitably subjective, unreliable and slow pre-screening process. In any case, where there are substantial differences in survival between groups, it is very difficult to form a reliable view by inspection of non-age-adjusted frequencies on whether an effect might or might not have occured.

A final, more valid, reason is that some end-points occur only very rarely. One should, however, be clear what 'very rarely' is. For a typical study with a control and three dose groups of equal size, one would get a significant trend statistic if all three cases occurred at the top dose level or in the control group (two-tailed $p \approx 0.03$), so a total of three cases will normally be enough for statistical analysis. End-points occurring once or twice only are not worth analysing formally, although, if only seen in the top dose group, they may be worth noting in the report. This is especially true if they are lesions that are rarely reported.

Combination of Pathological Conditions

There are four main situations where one might consider combining pathological conditions in a statistical analysis.

The first is when essentially the same pathological condition has been recorded under two or more different names or even under the same name in different places. Here failure to combine these conditions in the analysis may severely limit the chances of detecting a true treatment effect. It should be noted, however, that grouping together conditions which are actually different may also result in the masking of a true treatment effect, particularly if the treatment has a very specific effect.

The second is when separately recorded pathological conditions form successive steps on the pathway of the same process. The most important example of this is for the incidence of related types of malignant tumour, benign tumour, and focal hyperplasia. It will normally be appropriate to carry out analyses of (1) incidence of malignant tumour, (2) incidence of benign or malignant tumour and, where appropriate, (3) incidence of focal hyperplasia, benign or malignant tumour. It will not normally be appropriate to carry out analyses of benign tumour incidence only or of the incidence of hyperplasia only.

The third situation for combining is when the same pathological condition appears in different organs as a result of the same underlying process. Examples of this are the multicentric tumours (such as myeloid leukaemia, reticulum cell sarcoma and lymphosarcoma) or certain non-neoplastic conditions (such as arteritis/peri-arteritis and amyloid degeneration). Here analysis will normally be carried out only of incidence at any site, although in some situations site-specific analyses might be worth carrying out.

The final situation where an analysis of combined pathological conditions is normal is for analyses of overall incidence of malignant tumour at any site, of benign or malignant tumour at any site or of multiple tumour incidence. While analyses of tumour incidence at specific sites are normally more meaningful, since treatments often affect only a few specific sites, these additional analyses are usually required to guard against the possibility that treatment had some weak but general tumour-enhancing effect not otherwise evident.

In some situations, one might also envisage analyses of other combinations of specific tumours, such as tumours at related sites (e.g. endocrine organs if the compound had a hormonal effect) or of similar histological type.

Taking Severity into Account

The same line of argument that suggests that if the pathologist records data they should be analysed, also suggests that if the pathologist chooses to grade a condition for severity, the grade should be taken into account in the analysis. There are two ways to carry out analysis when the grade has to be taken into account. In one, analyses are carried out not only of whether or not the animal has a condition, but also of whether or not the condition is at least grade 2, at least grade 3, etc. In the other approach, non-parametric (rank) methods are used. The latter approach is more powerful, as it uses all the information in one analysis, although the output may not be so easily understood by those without some statistical training.

Note that the analyses based on grade can be carried out only if grading has been consistently applied throughout. If a condition has been scored only as present/absent for some animals, but has been graded for others, it is not possible to carry out graded analyses unless the pathologist is willing to go back and grade the specific animals showing the condition.

Using Simple Methods which Avoid Complex Assumptions

Different methods for statistical analysis can vary considerably in their complexity and in the number of assumptions they make. Although the use of statistical models has its place, more so for effect estimation that for hypothesis testing, and more so in studies of complex design than in those of simple design, there are advantages in using, wherever possible, statistical methods that are simple, robust and make as few assumptions as possible. There are three reasons for this. First, such methods are more generally understandable to the toxicologist. Second, there are hardly ever extensive enough data in practice to validate any given formal model fully. Third, even if a particular model were known to be appropriate, the loss of efficiency in using appropriate simpler methods is often only very small.

The methods we advocate for routine use for the analysis of tumour incidence tend, therefore, not to be based on the use of formal parametric statistical models. For example, when studying the relationship of treatment to incidence of a pathological condition and wishing to adjust for other factors (in particular, age at death) that might otherwise bias the comparison, methods involving 'stratification' are recommended, rather than a multiple regression approach or time-to-tumour models. Analysis of variance (ANOVA) methods can be useful in the case of continuously distributed data for estimating treatment effects. However, they involve underlying assumptions (normally distributed variables, variability equal in each group). If these assumptions are violated, non-parametric methods based on the rank of observations, rather than their actual value, may be preferable for hypothesis testing.

Using All the Data

Often information is available about the relationship between treatment and a condition of interest for groups of animals differing systematically in respect of some other factor. Obvious examples are males and females, differing times of sacrifice, and differing secondary treatments. While it will be necessary, in general, to look at the relationship within levels of this other factor, it will also generally be advisable to try to come to some assessment of the relationship over all levels of the other factors combined. There are some situations where the effect of treatment varies markedly by level of the other factor, and where a combined inference is not sensible, but in far more situations this is not the case, and using all the data in one analysis allows a more powerful test of the relationship under study. Some scientists consider that conclusions for males and females should always be drawn separately, but there are strong statistical arguments for a joint analysis.

Combining, Pooling and Stratification

Suppose, in a hypothetical study of a toxic agent which induces tumours that do not shorten the lives of tumour-bearing animals, the data regarding the number of animals with tumour out of number examined are as follows:

	Control	Exposed	Combined
Early deaths	1/20 (5%)	18/90 (20%)	19/110 (17%)
Late deaths	24/80 (30%)	7/10 (70%)	31/90 (34%)
Total	25/100 (25%)	25/100 (25%)	50/200 (25%)

It can be seen that if the time of death is ignored and the *pooled* data are studied, the incidence of tumours is the same in each group, resulting in the *false* conclusion that treatment had no effect. Looking within each time of death, however, an increased incidence in the exposed group can be seen. An appropriate statistical method would *combine* a measure of difference between the groups based on the early deaths and a measure of difference based on the late deaths, and conclude *correctly* that incidence, after adjustment for time of death, is greater in the exposed groups.

In this example, time of death is the 'stratifying variable', with two strata—early deaths and late deaths. The essence of the methodology is to make comparisons only within strata (so that one is always comparing like with like except in respect of treatment) and then to combine the differences over strata. Stratification can be used to

adjust for any variable, or indeed combinations of variables.

Some studies are of factorial design, in which combinations of treatments are tested. The simplest such design is one in which four equal sized groups of animals receive (1) no treatment, (2) treatment A only, (3) treatment B only and (4) treatments A and B. If one is prepared to assume that any effects of the two treatments are independent, one can use stratification to enable more powerful tests to be conducted of the possible individual treatment effects. Thus, to test for effects of treatment A for example, one conducts comparisons in two strata, the first consisting of groups 1 and 2 not given treatment B and the second consisting of groups 3 and 4 given treatment B. Combination of results from the two strata is based on twice as many animals, and is therefore markedly more likely to detect possible effects of treatment A than is a simple comparison of groups 1 and 2. There is also the possibility of identifying interactions, such as synergism and antagonism, between the two treatments.

Multiple Control Groups

In some routine long-term screening studies, the study design involves five groups of (usually) 50 animals of each sex, three of which are treated with successive doses of a compound and two of which are untreated controls. Assuming that there is no systematic difference between the control groups (e.g. the second control group in a different room or from a different batch of animals), it will be normal to carry out the main analyses with the control groups treated as a single group of 100 animals. It will usually be a sensible preliminary precaution to carry out additional analyses comparing incidences in the two control groups.

Trend Analysis, Low-dose Extrapolation and NOEL Estimation

While comparisons of individual treated groups with the control group are important, a more powerful test of a possible effect of treatment will be to carry out a test for a dose-related trend. This is because most true effects of treatment tend to result in a response which increases (or decreases) with increasing dose, and because trend tests take into account all the data in a single analysis. In interpreting the results of trend tests, it should be noted that a significant trend does not necessarily imply an increased risk at lower doses. Nor, conversely, does a lack of increase at lower doses necessarily indicate evidence of a threshold (i.e. a dose below which no increase occurs).

Note that testing for trend is seen as a more sensitive way of picking up a possible treatment effect than simple pairwise comparisons of treated and control groups. Attempting to estimate the magnitude of effects at low doses, typically below the lowest positive dose tested in the study, is a much more complex procedure, and is heavily dependent on the assumed functional form of the dose–response relationship.

Such low dose extrapolation is typically only conducted for tumours believed to be caused by a genotoxic effect which some, but by no means all, scientists believe has no threshold. For other types of tumours and for many non-neoplastic end-points a threshold is generally considered likely to exist. While the precise threshold cannot be estimated directly from data at a limited number of dose levels, a no observed effect level (NOEL) can be estimated by finding the highest dose level at which there is no significant increase in effects.

Need for Age Adjustment

Where there are marked differences in survival between treated groups, it is widely recognized that there is a need for an age adjustment (i.e. an adjustment for age at death or onset). This is illustrated in the example above, where, because of the greater number of deaths occurring early in the treated group, the true effect of treatment disappears if no adjustment is made. Thus, a major purpose of age adjustment is to avoid bias.

It is not so generally recognized, however, that, even where there are no survival differences, age adjustment can increase the power to detect between-group differences. This is illustrated in the example below:

	Control	Exposed
Early deaths	0/20	0/20
Middle deaths	1/10	9/10
Late deaths	20/20	20/20
Total	21/50	29/50

Here treatment results in a somewhat earlier onset of a condition which occurs eventually in all animals. Failure to age-adjust will result in a comparison of 29/50 with 21/50, which is not statistically significant. Age adjustment will essentially ignore the early and late deaths, which contribute no comparative statistical information, and be based on the comparison of 9/10 with 1/10, which is statistically significant. Here age adjustment sharpens the contrast, rather than avoiding bias, by avoiding diluting data capable of detecting treatment effects with data that are of little or no value for this purpose.

Need to Take Context of Observation into Account

It is now widely recognized that age adjustment cannot properly be carried out unless the context of observation is taken into account. There are three relevant contexts, the first two relating to the situation where the condition is only observed at death (e.g. an internal tumour) and the third where it can be observed in life (e.g. a skin tumour).

In the first context the condition is assumed to have caused the death of the animal, i.e. to be *fatal*. Here the incidence rate for a time interval and a group is calculated by

> (number of animals dying in the interval because of the lesion)/(number of animals alive at the start of the interval).

In the second context, the animal is assumed to have died of another cause, i.e. the condition is *incidental*. Here the rate is calculated by

> (number of animals dying in the interval with the lesion)/(total number of animals dying in the interval).

In the third context, where the condition is *visible*, the rate is calculated by

> (number of animals getting the condition in the interval)/(number of animals without the condition at the start of the interval).

A problem with the method of Peto *et al.* (1980), which takes context of observation into account, is that some pathologists are unwilling or feel unable to decide whether, in any given case, a condition is fatal or incidental. A number of points should be made here.

First, where there are marked survival differences, it may not be possible to conclude reliably whether a treatment is beneficial or harmful unless such a decision is made. This is well illustrated by the example in Peto *et al.* (1980), where assuming all pituitary tumours were fatal resulted in the (false) conclusion that *N*-nitrosodimethylamine (NDMA) was carcinogenic, while assuming they were all incidental resulted in the (false) conclusion that NDMA was protective. Using, correctly, the pathologist's best opinion as to which were, and which were not, likely to be fatal, resulted in an analysis which (correctly) concluded NDMA had no effect. If the pathologist, in this case, had been unwilling to make a judgement as to fatality, believing it to be unreliable, no conclusion could have been reached. This state of affairs would, however, be a fact of life, and *not* a position reached because an inappropriate statistical method was being used.

Although it will normally be a good routine for the pathologist to ascribe 'factors contributory to death' for each animal that was not part of a scheduled sacrifice, it is in fact not strictly necessary to determine the context of observation for all conditions at the outset. An alternative strategy is to analyse under differing assumptions: (1) no cases fatal, (2) all cases occurring in decedents fatal and (3) all cases of same defined severity occurring in decedents fatal, with, under each assumption, other cases incidental.

If the conclusion turns out the same under each assumption, or if the pathologist can say, on general grounds, that one assumption is likely to be a close approximation to the truth, it may not be necessary to know the context of observation for the condition in question for each individual animal. Using the alternative strategy might result in a saving of the pathologist's time by only having to make a judgement for a limited number of conditions where the conclusion seems to hang on correct knowledge of the context of observation.

Finally, it should be noted that, although many non-neoplastic conditions observed at death are never causes of death, it is, in principle, as necessary to know the context of observation for non-neoplastic conditions as it is for tumours.

Experimental and Observational Units

In many situations, the animal is both the 'experimental unit' and the 'observational unit', but this is not always so. For determining treatment effects by the methods of the next section, it is important that each experimental unit provides only one item of data for analysis, as the methods all assume that individual data items are statistically independent. In many feeding studies, where the cage is assigned to a treatment, it is the cage, rather than the animal, that is the experimental unit. In histopathology, observations for a tissue are often based on multiple sections per animal, so that the section is the observational unit. Multiple observations per experimental unit should be combined in some suitable way into an overall average for that unit before analysis.

Missing Data

In many types of analysis, animals with missing data are simply removed from the analysis. There are, however, some situations where this can be an inappropriate thing to do. One situation is when carrying out an analysis of a condition that is assumed to have caused the death of the animal. Although an animal dying at week 83 for which the section was unavailable for microscopic examination cannot contribute to the group comparison at week 83, one knows that it did not die because of any condition in previous weeks, so it should contribute to the denominator of the calculations in all previous weeks.

Another situation is when histopathological examination of a tissue is not carried out unless an abnormality is seen at post mortem. In such an experiment one might have the following data for that tissue:

Control group: 50 animals, 2 abnormal at post mortem, 2 examined microscopically, 2 with tumour of specific type.

Treated group: 50 animals, 15 abnormal at post mortem, 15 examined microscopically, 14 with tumour of specific type.

Ignoring animals with no microscopic sections, one would compare $2/2 = 100\%$ with $14/15 = 93\%$ and conclude treatment non-significantly decreased incidence. This is likely to be a false conclusion, and it would be better here to compare the percentages of animals which had a post mortem abnormality which turned out to be a tumour, i.e. $2/50 = 4\%$ with $14/50 = 28\%$. Unless some aspect of treatment made tumours much easier to detect at post mortem, one could then conclude that treatment did have an effect on tumour incidence.

Particular care has to be taken in studies where the procedures for histopathological examination vary by group. In a number of studies conducted in recent years, the protocol demands full microscopic examination of a given tissue list in decedents in all groups, and in terminally killed controls in high-dose animals. In other animals, terminally killed low- and mid-dose animals, microscopic examination of a tissue is only conducted if the tissue is found to be abnormal at post mortem. Such a protocol is designed to save money, but leads to difficulty in comparing the treatment groups validly. Suppose, for example, responses in terminally killed animals are 8/20 in the controls, 3/3 (with 17 unexamined) in the low-dose and 5/6 (with 14 unexamined) in the mid-dose animals. Is one supposed to conclude that treatment at the low- and mid-doses increased response, based on a comparison of the proportions examined microscopically (40%, 100% and 83%), or that it decreased response, based on the proportion of animals in the group (40%, 15% and 25%)? It could well be that treatment had no effect but some small tumours were missed at post mortem. In this situation, a valid comparison can only be achieved by ignoring the low- and mid-dose groups when carrying out the comparison for the age stratum 'terminal kill'. This, of course, seems wasteful of data, but these are data that cannot be usefully used owing to the inappropriate protocol.

Use of Historical Control Data

In some situations, particularly where incidences are low, the results from a single study may suggest an effect of treatment on tumour incidence but be unable to demonstrate it conclusively. The possibility of comparing results in the treated groups with those of control groups from other studies is then often raised. Thus, a non-significant incidence of 2 cases out of 50 in a treated group may seem much more significant if no cases have been seen in, say, 1000 animals representing controls from 20 similar studies. Conversely, a significant incidence of 5 cases out of 50 in a treated group as compared with 0 out of 50 in the study controls may seem far less convincing if many other control groups had incidences around 5 out of 50.

While not understating the importance of looking at historical control data, it must be emphasized that there are a number of reasons why variation between study may be greater than variation within study. Differences in diet, in duration of the study, in intercurrent mortality and in who the study pathologist is may all contribute. Statistical techniques that ignore this and carry out simple statistical tests of treatment incidence against a pooled control incidence may well give results that are seriously in error, and are likely to overstate statistical significance considerably. Appropriate tests allow for the possibility of this extra-binomial variation (Tarone, 1982; Gart et al., 1986).

STATISTICAL ANALYSIS—SUMMARY OF APPROPRIATE METHODS

Types of Response Variable

Responses measured in toxicological studies can normally be classified into one of the following three types:

(1) Presence/absence: a condition either occurs or it does not.
(2) Ranked: a condition may be present at various discrete levels.
(3) Continuous: a condition may take any value, at least within a given range.

Strictly, each type of response requires a different sort of statistical technique. Methods for presence/absence data can be used for ranked or continuous data by defining a cut-off point above which is deemed present, but this is rather wasteful of data. Methods for ranked data can also be used for analysing continuous data, and probably should be if one is not confident about the assumptions of normality and homogeneity of variance underlying the standard parametric methods used such as ANOVA.

Types of Comparison

There are basically three different types of comparison between groups. The first is the *pairwise comparison*, in which the responses in two different groups, usually a treated group and the control group, are compared. The second, only applicable to studies with more than two treatment groups, is the test for *heterogeneity*, which tests whether, taken as a whole, there is significant evidence of departure from the (null) hypothesis that the groups do not differ in their effect. The third, applicable only to studies with more than two treatment groups in which the different groups represent different doses of the same compound, is the test for a *dose-related trend*.

Recommended Methods for Between-animal Comparisons

The methods recommended are as follows, references only being given to the less well known tests.

Presence/absence data

Individual group comparisons	Fisher's exact test	Unstratified data
	2×2 corrected chi-squared test	Stratified or unstratified data
Heterogeneity (of k groups)	$2 \times k$ chi-squared test	Stratified or unstratified data
Dose-related trend	Exact trend test	Unstratified data
	Cochran–Armitage trend test	Stratified or unstratified data

Where context of observation has to be taken into account, the Peto/IARC test is appropriate for individual group comparisons, heterogeneity or dose-related trend.

Ranked data

Individual group comparisons	Mann–Whitney U test	Unstratified data
	Fry and Lee (1988) test	Stratified data
Heterogeneity	Kruskal–Wallis one-way ANOVA	Unstratified data
	Fry and Lee (1988) test	Stratified data
Dose-related trend	Marascuilo and McSweeney (1967) test	Unstratified data
	Fry and Lee (1988) test	Stratified data

Continuous data

Test for homogeneity of variance	Bartlett test	Unstratified data

If the data show appreciable heterogeneity of variance, consider transformation by logarithms and/or square roots. Alternatively, use the methods for ranked data.

Individual group comparisons	Student's t-test or least significant difference test	Unstratified data
Heterogeneity	One-way ANOVA	Unstratified data

Dose-related trend	Linear regression	Unstratified data analysis

Analysis of continuous data to correct for sources of potential bias is not normally carried out by methods involving stratification, but by the methods of analysis of covariance, multiple regression and linear models. These, and more complex ANOVA methods required for factorial designs, probably need discussion with a statistician.

Other Statistical Methods

The methods described in the previous subsection have concentrated on the common experimental situation where interest is centred on evidence of variation between groups in respect of a single variable, with the possible confounding effect of other variables taken account of by stratification. There are a number of different situations, considered briefly below, where alternative statistical techniques are required.

Relationships Between Two Variables

For presence/absence data, relationships between two variables can be studied by Fisher's exact test or a corrected chi-squared test. For ranked and continuous data, the correlation coefficients of, respectively, Spearman and Pearson can be used. Techniques are also available for determining whether these relationships differ for different treatment groups.

Multivariate Methods

Situations involving the interrelationship of a large number of variables normally require the advice of a professional statistician, and involve such methods as multiple regression, discriminant and factor analysis.

Multiple Observations on the Same Animal

In long-term studies, it is common to make similar measurements, e.g. of body weight on the same animal at different stages of the study. To look for evidence of a between-group difference in changes in responses over a given period, the preferred technique is analysis of covariance, where differences in mean values at the second time-point are studied after adjustment for values observed at the first time-point. Alternatively, parametric growth curves may be fitted and the groups compared in respect of these parameters, but such techniques tend to be complex.

Paired Data

Sometimes studies consist of pairs of animals, each pair of animals being similar in respect of important potential confounding variables, e.g. litter, and differing only in respect of treatment. It is important to take the pairing into account for analysis. Appropriate techniques to use are the sign test or McNemar's test for presence/absence data, the Wilcoxon matched-pair signed-ranks test for ranked data, and the matched-pair t-test for continuous data. Considerable care is needed to ensure that the appropriate paired or unpaired test is used. A common error in analysis is to use a paired test on unpaired data or vice versa.

LD$_{50}$

Some toxicological studies calculate the dose of a substance at which 50% of the animals respond. This is known as the LD$_{50}$ when the response is death (LD = lethal dose) and more generally as the median-effective dose. The classical technique to calculate the LD$_{50}$ from data consisting of the percentage responding at each of a range of dose levels is known as probit analysis. Sequential methods which require fewer animals are increasingly being applied to reduce the number of animals used in this controversial and unpopular toxicological test.

SOFTWARE

The recommended methods for between-animal comparisons are all available in the comprehensive computer program for data entry, reporting and statistical analysis of pathological data ROELEE 84. The GLIM program (Baker and Nelder, 1978) is also useful for carrying out the methods of multiple regression and linear models. Various other standard statistical packages, such as GENSTAT, MINITAB, SAS, S-PLUS, SPSS and SYSTAT, include many of the techniques described here. With the advent of much more powerful computers, there has been a tendency in many situations to move from the formerly used approximate asymptotic statistical tests to exact randomization tests. STAT-XACT facilitates many such tests while ROELEE 84 includes an exact version of the Peto *et al.* (1980) test. nQUERY ADVISOR is helpful for determining appropriate group sizes when designing a study.

RECOMMENDED READING

Lee (1993) provides a simple text, aimed at toxicologists and including worked examples, for many of the methods we recommend. Peto *et al.* (1980) describes and justifies the most commonly used test for comparison of age-adjusted tumour incidences taking context of observation into account. Gart *et al.* (1986) is a more detailed text, aimed more at statisticians, describing methods of analysis of carcinogenicity data, while Krewski and Franklin (1991) is an extensive textbook covering a wide range of issues relating to statistics in toxicology. For those concerned with estimation of effect rather than with determining statistical significance, Gardner and Altman (1989) gives details of how to calculate confidence limits for many tests. Gad and Weil (1982) also contains useful material on other types of data, such as body and organ weights, clinical chemistry, haematology, reproduction, teratology, dominant lethal assay and mutagenesis. Kirkland (1989) provides an overview of the statistical issues and methods used in genetic toxicology and mutagenicity studies.

REFERENCES

Baker, R. J. and Nelder, J. A. (1978). *Generalised Linear Interactive Modelling*. Release 3. Numerical Algorithms Group, Oxford.

Fry, J. S. and Lee, P. N. (1988). Stratified rank tests. *Appl. Stat.*, **37**, 264–266.

Gad, S. C. and Weil, C. S. (1982). Statistics for toxicologists. In Hayes, A. W. (Ed.), *Principles and Methods of Toxicology*, Raven Press, New York, pp. 147–175.

Gardner, M. J. and Altman, D. G. (1989). *Statistics with Confidence. Confidence Intervals and Statistical Guidelines*. British Medical Journal, London.

Gart, J. J., Krewski, D., Lee, P. N., Tarone, R. E. and Wahrendorf, J. (1986). *Statistical Methods in Cancer Research, Vol. III: The Design and Analysis of Long-term Animal Experiments*. IARC Scientific Publications No. 79. IARC, Lyon.

Kirkland, D. J. (1989). *UK Environmental Mutagen Society Subcommittee on Guidelines for Mutagenicity Testing, Part III*. Cambridge University Press, Cambridge.

Krewski, D. and Franklin, C. (1991). *Statistics in Toxicology*, Gordon and Breach, New York.

Lee, P. N. (1993). Statistics. In Anderson, D. and Conning, D. M. (Eds), *Experimental Toxicology: the Basic Issues*, 2nd edn. Royal Society of Chemistry, London, pp. 405–441.

Marascuilo, L. A. and McSweeney, M. (1967). Nonparametric post hoc comparisons for trend. *Psychol. Bull.*, **67**, 401–412.

Peto, R., Pike, M. C., Day, N. E., Gray, R. G., Lee, P. N., Parish, S., Peto, J., Richards, S. and Wahrendorf, J., (1980). Guidelines for simple, sensitive significance tests for carcinogenic effects in long-term animal experiments. In *Long-term and Short-term Screening Assays for Carcinogens: a Critical Appraisal*. IARC Monographs on the Evaluation of the Carcinogenic Risk of Chemicals to Humans, Supplement 2. IARC, Lyon, pp. 311–426.

Roe, F. J. C. (1989). What is wrong with the way we test chemicals for carcinogenic activity? In Dayan, A. D. and Price, A. J. (Eds), *Advances in Applied Toxicology*. Taylor and Francis, London, pp. 1–77.

Tarone, R. E. (1982). The use of historical control information in testing for a trend in proportions. *Biometrics*, **37**, 79–85.

SOFTWARE ADDRESSES

GENSTAT 5	The Numerical Algorithms Group Ltd, Wilkinson Road, Jordan Hill House, Oxford OX2 8DR, UK
GLIM 5	The Numerical Algorithms Group Ltd, Wilkinson Road, Jordan Hill House, Oxford OX2 8DR, UK
MINITAB	Minitab Inc., 3081 Enterprise Drive, State College, PA 16801–3008, USA
nQUERY ADVISOR	Statistical Solutions, 60 State Street, Ste. 700, Boston, MA 02109, USA
ROELEE84	P. N. Lee Statistics and Computing Ltd, 17 Cedar Road, Sutton, Surrey SM2 5DA, UK
S-PLUS	StatSci Europe, Osney House, Mill Street, Oxford OX2 0JX, UK
SAS	SAS Institute Inc., SAS Campus Drive, Cary, NC 27513, USA
SPSS	SPSS UK Ltd, London House, 243–253 Lower Mortlake Road, Richmond TW9 2LL, UK
STATXACT	Cytel Statistical Software, 675 Massachusetts Avenue, Cambridge, MA 02139, USA
SYSTAT	Clecom Software Specialists, The Computer Algebra Centre, The Research Park, Vincent Drive, Edgbaston, Birmingham B15 2SQ, UK

Chapter 14
Toxicology of Chemical Mixtures

Flemming R. Cassee, Jürgen Sühnel, John P. Groten and Victor. J. Feron

CONTENTS

INTRODUCTION

The majority of studies to assess the toxicity of chemicals deal with exposures to single compounds. In reality, however, humans are exposed to complex and ever-changing mixtures of compounds in the food, water and beverages they ingest, the air they breathe, the consumer products they use and the surfaces they touch (Sexton *et al.*, 1995). Despite the growing interest in investigating chemical mixtures (Calabrese, 1991; Krishnan and Brodeur, 1991; Mumtaz *et al.*, 1993; Yang, 1994a; Cassee *et al.*, 1998), it is generally uncertain how the combined toxicity should be taken into account in a standard setting for the individual chemicals, or how the toxicity of chemical mixtures should be assessed. National and international guidelines for exposure limits not infrequently suggest the use of simple 'dose addition' models for evaluating the hazard of a chemical mixture, not taking into account the mode of action of the individual chemicals. Obviously, such an approach might greatly overestimate the risk in the case of chemicals that act by mechanisms for which the dose additivity assumption is invalid. One of the most distinct examples are the essential nutrients (vitamins, trace elements, essential amino and fatty acids), with their relatively small margins of safety between the dose that is required and the lowest toxic dose (Feron, 1997); simultaneous consumption of these nutrients at their recommended intake levels would turn out to be an unhealthy custom if the toxicity of this mixture were to be assessed on the basis of the 'dose addition' concept (similar joint action). If chemicals in a mixture are known to have simple dissimilar modes of action, recent studies have shown that they do not constitute an evidently increased hazard compared with that of exposure to the individual chemicals, provided that the exposure level of the chemicals in the mixture is at most equal to their own no observed adverse effect level (Feron *et al.*, 1995a, b). The health risk of such mixtures is fully determined by the health risk associated with the 'most risky chemical' in the mixture, provided that the risk quotients of the other compounds in the mixture do not exceed unity.

Another important issue is the use of the correct parameter for summation of the effects of the individual compounds. An illustrative example is the addition of water to ethanol. In that case not the volume but the weight ought to be used. The use of the appropriate parameters and evaluation models is of paramount importance in predicting the hazard of a mixture relative to that of its constituents. If chemicals in a mixture interact with one another, more than additive or less than additive effects may occur.

A further important aspect of toxicity studies with mixtures is the exponential multiplication of the number of test groups with increasing numbers of chemicals in a mixture: to test all combinations (in a complete experimental design) at only one dose level of each chemical in a mixture consisting of three, four or five chemicals, $8(2^3)$, $16(2^4)$ or $32(2^5)$ experimental groups (including a control group), respectively, would be required.

The use of more than one dose level will also increase the number of test groups significantly: testing of a mixture with three chemicals at two dose levels requires $27 (3^3)$ test groups. Studies of this kind become impracticable from a pragmatic, an economical and often also an ethical point of view.

We will discuss in this chapter the terminology and concepts to describe combined and interactive effects of chemicals. Special attention will be paid to methods for the evaluation of the effects of simple (defined) or complex mixtures, including the utilization of effective statistical designs that can reduce the number of test groups. To illustrate the complexity of mixture toxicology on the one hand, and to offer pragmatic approaches for dealing with safety aspects of mixtures on the other, a number of real-life examples will be discussed in some detail.

TERMINOLOGY AND CONCEPTS OF THE TOXICOLOGY OF CHEMICAL MIXTURES

There is widespread disagreement over the terminology, definitions and models for the evaluation of interactions (Berenbaum, 1989; Gebhart, 1992; Miaskowski and Levine, 1992; Suzuki, 1994; Greco *et al.*, 1995). Despite several attempts to standardize the terminology for assessing the effects of mixtures in relation to their constituents, a consistent language for this complex and challenging area of toxicology is still lacking (Simmons, 1995). The usual approach is to calculate from the effects of single agents what is expected for the combination effect in the case of 'no interaction', whatever this means. Regardless of the model applied, deviations of the observed effect from the expected effect is often called an 'interaction'. It is therefore recommended to define clearly each term and concept used in publications.

The study of combined action or interaction of chemicals involves the challenge of how to characterize antagonistic, additive or synergistic action. Understanding the terminology that describes the combined or interactive effect of agents in terms of the mechanisms of action is of crucial importance. The international Study Group on Combination Effects has made attempts to come up with uniform definitions of, for example, synergism, potentiation and antagonism and ways to characterize these types of effects (Pöch and Herzig, 1997).

Three basic concepts for the description of the toxicological action of constituents of a mixture were defined by Bliss (1939) and are still valid over half a century later.

Simple similar action

Simple similar action, also known as 'simple joint action', 'Loewe additivity' or 'concentration/dose addition', is a non-interactive process, which means that the chemicals in the mixture do not affect the toxicity of one another. Each of the chemicals in the mixture contributes to the toxicity of the mixture in proportion to its dose, expressed as a percentage of the dose of that chemical alone which would be required to obtain the given effect of the mixture. All chemicals of concern in a mixture act in the same way, by the same mechanism and differ only in their potencies. This form of action also serves as the basis for the use of 'toxic equivalency factors'. Similar joint action allows us to describe the additive effect mathematically using the summation of the doses of the individual compounds in a mixture after adjustment for the differences in potencies. This method is often assumed to be only valid for linear and/or monotonous dose–response/effect curves (Steel and Peckham, 1979; Kodell and Pounds, 1991).

Simple dissimilar action

In simple dissimilar action, also referred to as 'simple independent action' (Finney, 1942), 'independent joint action', 'effect addition', or 'response addition', the agents of a mixture do not affect each other's toxic effect. The mode of action and possibly, but not necessarily, the nature and site of action differ among the constituents of the mixture. There can be some confusion with respect to the difference between *effect* and *response*. The term *effect* addition should be used to refer to an average effect of a mixture on a group and is a *qualitative* measure. *Response* addition is referred to if each individual of a population has a certain tolerance to each of the chemicals of a mixture and will only exhibit a response to a toxicant if the concentration exceeds the tolerance dose. In this case the number of responders will be given rather than the mean effect. Thus, by definition, response addition is determined by summing the *quantal* responses of the animals to each toxicant in a mixture. Three different theories have been developed for response additivity depending on the correlation of susceptibility of subjects to toxic agents:

(i) *Complete positive correlation*: individuals most susceptible to one toxicant are also most susceptible to the other. The toxicity of the mixtures will be determined by the chemical with the highest toxic concentration and the proportion of individuals responding to the mixture will be equal to the response to the most toxic agent in a mixture:

$$P_{\text{mixture A,B}} = P_A \text{ if toxicityA} \geqslant B \qquad (1)$$

Thus, if doses of two chemicals A and B result in 20 and 30% deaths, respectively, the mixture of AB will result in 30% deaths.

(ii) *Complete negative correlation*: individuals most susceptible to one toxicant are least susceptible to the other. The percentage *P* of the individuals responding to the mixture will be equal to the sum of the response to each of the components of the mixture:

$$P_{\text{mixture A,B}} = P_A + P_B \leqslant 1 \qquad (2)$$

Thus, if the doses of two chemicals A and B result in 20 and 30% deaths, respectively, the mixture of AB will result in 50% deaths.

(iii) *No correlation*: the proportion of individuals responding to the mixture will be equal to the sum of the proportion of individuals responding to the response to each of the toxicants taking into account that those individuals that respond to constituent A cannot also react to B:

$$P_{\text{mixture A,B}} = P_A + P_B(1 - P_A) = P_A + P_B - P_A P_B. \qquad (3)$$

This is better referred to as Bliss independence. If the doses of two chemicals A and B result in 20 and 30% deaths, respectively, the mixture of AB will result in $(0.2 + 0.3 - 0.2 \times 0.3) = 0.44 = 44\%$ deaths. Note that although this type of correlation seems similar to *complete negative correlation*, the difference is that in this case an individual can respond to both agents A and B but not to both at the same time.

Finally, it should be mentioned that the term response addition is often used for case (ii) only. Moreover, Berenbaum (1989) has provided arguments that the difference between combinations of agents with similar and dissimilar mechanisms of action is not revealed by different dose–response curves.

Interactions

All deviations from the former two concepts are defined as 'interactions'. The term 'interaction' describes the combined effect between two chemicals resulting in a stronger effect (synergism, potentiation, supra-additivity) or weaker effect (antagonism, sub-additivity, inhibition) than expected on the basis of additivity. The term 'interaction' should not be viewed in the physiological sense as describing biological interference for a target or receptor, but as an empirical description to characterize departure from additivity. The mechanism behind the 'interactions' may be of physico-chemical and/or biological nature and an interaction might occur in the exposure phase, in the toxicokinetic phase (processes of uptake, distribution, metabolism and excretion) or, in the toxicodynamic phase (effects of chemicals on the receptor, cellular target or organ) or/and be due to chemical and physical reactions.

In the environment and in food, physical or chemical reactions between two or more chemicals can result in new compounds with a different toxic potential compared with the original compounds. A well known example is the formation of carcinogenic nitrosamines from nitrite and secondary amines in an acidic environment such as the stomach.

The most obvious cases for more or less than additive effects in the toxicokinetic phase are enzyme induction and/or inhibition, since metabolism is an important determinant of toxicity (either reactive intermediates are formed—activation—or the toxic agent is removed—detoxification). Compounds that influence the amount of biotransformation enzymes can have large effects on the biotransformation (and thus on the toxicity) of other chemicals.

For a mixture of compounds with the same target receptor but with (different) non-linear dose–effect relationships, mathematical or physiological (toxicodynamic) modelling can be applied to describe the combined action. The joint action between two chemicals can, for instance, be described by Michaelis–Menten kinetics. In general, this will result in a phenomenon such as 'competitive agonism', 'competitive inhibition' or 'non-competitive inhibition'. In the case of allosteric enzymes, Michaelis–Menten kinetics are too limited, although it is still possible to model the joined action of substrates. In these cases the type of interaction can also be considered as a special case of similar joint action (dose-addition).

All three basic principles of joint action are theoretical. In reality, however, one will most likely have to deal with these concepts at the same time, especially when mixtures consist of more than two compounds and when the targets (individuals rather than cells) are more complex. The first educated guess to predict whether compounds behave in a dose or effect additive way will be based on the (toxicological) knowledge of the individual compounds or classes of compounds. From this starting point on, one might speculate on how the compounds will behave in a mixture in acute, single-dose experiments. However, the more realistically the mixture study is designed (i.e. repeated doses at low exposure levels), the more complex is the list of toxicokinetic and dynamic end-points that one has to account for, and as a result the prediction will be very speculative. The only way for the toxicologist to describe the combined action of the compounds in the mixture is to perform experimental studies comparing the effect of the mixture with that of the individual compounds. The quintessence is to perform a study with a minimum number of test groups resulting in the maximum amount of information on the effects of both the individual compounds and all combinations of the chemicals.

METHODS FOR MIXTURE STUDIES

Mixtures can roughly be divided into simple and complex mixtures (Feron *et al.*, 1995a, b; Fay and Feron, 1996). To study the toxicology of mixtures successfully, it is essential to understand the basic concepts of the combined action and interaction of chemicals (Mumtaz *et al.*, 1994), and to distinguish between whole mixture analysis (top-down approach) and component interaction analysis (bottom-up approach) (Yang *et al.*, 1995). A complex mixture is defined as a mixture that consists of, say, more than 10 chemicals and of which the quantitative and qualitative composition in not (fully) known. Clear examples are ambient particulate matter, tobacco smoke and welding fumes. A simple mixture is defined as a mixture that consists of a relatively small number of chemicals and the composition of which is qualitatively and quantitatively known, for example certain medicines, solvents in paint and pesticide cocktails.

In the past decade, a number of approaches has been presented to evaluate the effect of a mixture compared with its components (Henschler *et al.*, 1996). Ultimately, all chemicals in a mixture need to be identified. Subsequently, the toxicological information from the existing literature should be obtained or the toxicity of each of the constituents should be determined. On the basis of the mechanism of action and the individual dose–effect equations, one can try to predict the joint effect of chemicals in a mixture. However, all this information is often not available and additional testing should resolve the uncertainties.

To obtain toxicological information on mixtures with a limited number of test groups, various test scenarios can be used. The study design will largely depend on the number of compounds in a mixture and on the question of whether it is desirable to assess all possible interactions between chemicals in a mixture. Several experimental designs can be used to accomplish toxicological information on mixtures with a restricted number of test groups. Preferably mixtures should be tested both at effective (often relatively high) dose levels and at low (realistic) dose levels. One pragmatic approach is to test the toxicity of the whole mixture without assessing the type of interactions. By making appropriate dilutions of the mixture, a mixture–effect relationship can be obtained

Interactive effects between two or three compounds can be identified by physiologically based toxicokinetic modelling, isobolographic or dose–effect surface analysis or comparison of dose–effect curves.

Interactive effects of compounds in mixtures with more than three components can be best ascertained with the help of statistical designs such as (fractionated) factorial designs, ray designs, or dose–effect surface analysis.

Whole mixtures

The simplest way to study the effects of mixtures is to compare the effect of a mixture with the effects of all its constituents at comparable concentrations and duration of exposure at one dose level without testing all possible combinations of chemicals. Although this approach requires a minimum number of experimental groups ($n + 1$, the number of compounds in a mixture plus the mixture itself) and the design of these studies is chosen to reflect the net effect of all compounds in the mixture, it will not be possible to describe the effect of the mixture in terms of synergism, potentiation, antagonism, etc., if there are no dose–effect curves for each of the individual compounds. For example, if two chemicals A and B have dose–effect relationships with different slopes ($A > B$) and agent A inhibits the action of agent B, one can understand that the effect of agent B at low dose levels cannot be predicted from the information on the effect at high dose levels.

The so-called top-down approach is mostly chosen in order to limit the number of test groups and identification of possible interactive effects of the chemicals in

relation to the effects of individual chemicals is not or cannot be taken into account. This strategy has been used to assess the combined toxicity of undefined (drinking water, coke oven emission, cigarette smoke) and defined chemical mixtures (nephrotoxicants, pesticides, carcinogens and fertilizers). The question of whether high to low-dose extrapolation is allowed remains to be resolved.

A bottom-up approach is virtually impossible for complex mixtures. For some mixtures such as workplace, ambient or chemical waste site atmospheres, whole mixture analysis seems to be impracticable and meaningless. In these cases, a selection of priority chemicals or groups of chemicals has been recommended for hazard identification (Feron *et al.*, 1995a; Fay and Feron, 1996).

Interactive Effects Between Small Numbers of Compounds

To study interactive effects between two or three compounds physiologically based toxicokinetic modelling, isobolographic or dose–effect surface analysis are used. Physiologically based toxicokinetic modelling would be especially useful for interactions in the toxicokinetic phase—note that despite similar biotransformation pathways, the mechanism to activate toxicants might be different or toxicants might be influencing each others' biotransformation through induction or inhibition.

Isobolographic and dose–effect surface analysis are most suitable for (and limited to) situations where the *target* is the same for a limited number of compounds, thus where possible interaction takes place in the toxicodynamic phase.

Physiologically Based Toxicokinetic Modelling

In the risk assessment of xenobiotics, adequate human data are often not available. The current practice is to extrapolate the risk for man, using animal studies combined with arbitrary safety factors. However, for many compounds, their metabolism is the major determinant of the risk and for several hazardous substances a considerable insight into the role of metabolism in toxic reactions has become available from laboratory experiments. In principle, the *in vivo* human metabolism can be predicted using *in vitro* enzyme kinetics, and thus may be compared with *in vitro* and *in vivo* data from animal studies. In several cases, experiments with microsomal fractions and hepatocytes have been shown to predict accurately the *in vivo* velocity of metabolism, for a single metabolic pathway. Such data may be applied in physiologically based toxicokinetic modelling. This technique has been reviewed extensively. Several physiologically based toxicokinetic models have recently become available which offer the possibility of incorporating the interferences between two compounds in the same metabolic pathways.

Ploemen *et al.* (1997) presented a strategy to combine physiologically based toxicokinetic modelling with human *in vitro* metabolic data, to explore the relative and overall contributions of critical metabolic pathways *in vivo* in man. Four distinct steps can be recognized in this strategy. First, the principal isoenzymes involved in the metabolism and their rate of catalysis are determined *in vitro*. Second, the rate is scaled up to the rate per milligram of subcellular fractions (cytosol and microsomes). After validation of the prediction at this second level, the rate is expressed per gram of whole liver for the relevant metabolic routes (third phase). These values are then used to calculate the ratio of these pathways at 'fixed' liver concentrations. In the fourth step, the metabolic parameters are integrated in a physiologically based toxicokinetic model to predict the relative contribution of the metabolic pathways *in vivo*.

This shows exactly the extent to which physiologically based toxicokinetic models may be used in combination toxicology. First, one of the components of the mixture is regarded as the 'prime toxicant', the effect of which is modified by the other compounds. Effects of induction or inhibition of specific biotransformation isozymes may then be incorporated in the model and the effects determined and compared with the differences that occur in any event because of already existing individual differences. Effects of competition between chemicals in a mixture for the same biotransformation enzymes can also be incorporated by translating the effects into effects on the Michaelis–Menten parameters which are then introduced into the model. An example of using a physiological model based on an artificial data set **(Table 1)** is given in **Figure 1**. Using the individual concentration–effect data and assuming that these are compounds that all act on the same receptor, the equilibration constant and the maximum effect can be calculated. Using equations for competitive agonism, the effect of all possible mixtures can be predicted. For instance, Cassee *et al.* (1996a) studied sensory irritation of mixtures of formaldehyde (FRM), acrolein (ACR) and acetaldehyde (ACE) as measured by the decrease in breathing frequency of rats. For the mixtures the predicted values were compared with the observed values using both the model for effect addition (adding the expected effects of single aldehydes based on the individual dose–effect equations) and a mechanistic model for competitive agonism represented by

where D_{mix} is the decrease in breathing frequency of a mixture of FRM, ACR and ACE, D_{max} and K are the maximum decrease in breathing frequency and the dissociation constant for each compound, respectively,

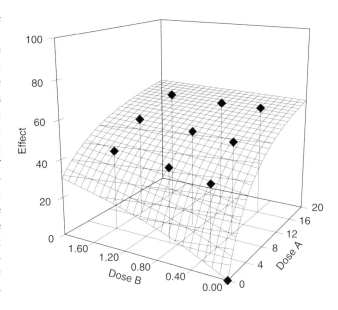

Figure 1 An example of two chemicals acting on the same target receptor. Using data for compounds A and B from **Table 1** and Michaelis–Menten kinetics for competitive agonism, the observed effects (in %) can be accurately predicted as shown by the surface through the data points.

and [FRM], [ACR] and [ACE] are the concentrations of FRM, ACR and ACE, respectively.

The results of this study allow the conclusions that (a) sensory irritation in rats exposed to mixtures of irritant aldehydes is more severe than that caused by each of the aldehydes separately and (b) the decrease in breathing frequency caused by mixtures of these aldehydes is predicted better by using a mechanistic model for competitive agonism between the three chemicals than by using effect addition. Thus, this indicates that these compounds act in a dose-additive manner and support the idea that the application of the commonly used effect additivity rule would have overestimated the predicted effect of mixtures of sensory irritants.

Isoboles

An isobole (Loewe and Muischnek, 1926; Gessner, 1988) is a contour line that represents equi-effective quantities of two agents or their mixtures. The theoretical line of additivity is the straight line connecting the individual doses of each of the single agents that produce the fixed effect alone **(Figure 2)**. The method is used for a graphical representation to establish whether two chemicals act according to the dose-additivity criteria (similar mode of action). It requires tedious experimental determinations of the effects of a number of mixtures and it

$$D_{mix} = \frac{D_{FRM, max} \cdot K_{ACR} \cdot K_{ACE} \cdot [FRM] + D_{ACR, max} \cdot K_{FRM} \cdot K_{ACE} \cdot [ACR] + D_{ACE, max} \cdot K_{FRM} \cdot K_{ACR}[ACE]}{K_{FRM} \cdot K_{ACR} \cdot K_{ACE} + K_{ACR} \cdot K_{ACE} \cdot [FRM] + K_{FRM} \cdot K_{ACE} \cdot [ACR] + K_{FRM} \cdot K_{ACR} \cdot [ACE]} \qquad (4)$$

Table 1 Artificial dataset showing effects of individual chemicals A, B and C and effects of mixtures of A and B and of A, B and C (a dose of 0 does not produce an effect in either single chemical or mixture exposures)

Effects of individual chemicals				Effects of mixtures of A and B			Effects of mixtures of A, B and C			
Dose A	Dose B	Dose C	Effect (%)	Dose A	Dose B	Effect (%)	Dose A	Dose B	Dose C	Effect (%)
0.5			6	4	0.4	35	0.5	0.2	400	18
1			11	9	0.4	49	0.5	0.6	400	24
2			20	16	0.4	59	0.5	1.2	400	30
4			32	4	0.9	39	0.5	0.2	1200	32
6			40	9	0.9	51	0.5	0.6	1200	35
8			46	16	0.9	59	0.5	1.2	1200	40
10			50	4	1.6	42	0.5	0.2	3600	57
20			62	9	1.6	53	0.5	0.6	3600	58
	2		30	16	1.6	60	0.5	1.2	3600	60
	4		43				1.5	0.2	400	26
	8		55				1.5	0.6	400	30
	12		60				1.5	1.2	400	35
	16		63				1.5	0.2	1200	37
	20		65				1.5	0.6	1200	40
	40		70				1.5	1.2	1200	43
		125	3				1.5	0.2	3600	59
		250	7				1.5	0.6	3600	60
		500	13				1.5	1.2	3600	61
		1000	23				4.5	0.2	400	40
		1500	31				4.5	0.6	400	42
		2500	45				4.5	1.2	400	45
		3500	55				4.5	0.2	1200	47
		5000	66				4.5	0.6	1200	49
		8000	80				4.5	1.2	1200	51
							4.5	0.2	3600	63
							4.5	0.6	3600	64
							4.5	1.2	3600	64

generally assumes parallel dose–effect curves (positive correlation coefficient of 1). When all equi-effect concentrations are connected by a downward concave line, the effect of the combinations is more than additive, and a concave upward curve indicates a less than additive effect. Such conclusions depend strongly on the accuracy of estimated intercepts of the theoretical isobole with the axis (representing the dose of one of the compounds of the mixture inducing the desired effect level). In many cases large standard deviations of these intercepts do not allow a reliable conclusion concerning the deviation from additivity. Dose-additivity isoboles are described by the equation

$$I = \sum_n d_n / D_n \qquad (5)$$

where d_n are the doses of agents in a mixture and D_n are the doses of the individual agents producing the same effects as the mixture. For binary mixtures, Equation 5 describes a straight line (isobole) joining D_A and D_B and passing trough (d_a, d_b). For values of I equal to, smaller than or larger than 1, the mixture shows zero interaction, synergy or antagonism using dose-addition, respectively. Even if a heterogeneous combination is considered, in which agent A produces an effect and B does not, this equation is valid. In this case D_B is considered to be infinite and the equation is reduced to one term only. The maginitude of I will depend on the ratio of the concentrations of the constituents of the mixture (**Figure 3**) and thus will not result in one value of I for a specific mixture. This means that the interaction may be dose-dependent. It is widely assumed that Equation 5 is only valid in the case of simple similar joint action (agents with similar-shaped CEC but different potencies). Berenbaum (1989) has provided arguments, however, that this equation and thus the dose-additivity criterion, in general, for defining zero interaction can be applied to all cases independent of the shapes of the dose–response curves and of the underlying mechanism. This controversy continues to exist and is one of the reasons for the confusion in the field of combination-action assessment. In addition, the statistical basis for testing whether or not a specific I deviates from 1 (additivity) is very complex.

Steel and Peckham (1979) modified the isobole approach by suggesting the construction of an additivity envelope, where the borders are set by using either effect or dose addition. This can be used if two chemicals are expected to have some kind of joint action, but the mechanism is not fully understood or the effect of the mixture is a combination of both dose and effect addition. The relative position of the effect point in a plot will be indicative for the kind of additivity. The boundaries of the envelope are found by using mode I and II addition. Mode I addition, also referred to as heteroadditivity (Kodell and Pounds, 1991), is the simplest form of effect addition and is described by

$$E(d_1, d_2) = E(d_1) + E(d_2) \qquad (6)$$

where d_1 and d_2 represent the doses of two compounds each resulting in an effect E that can be summed to give $E(d_1, d_2)$, the fixed effect due to exposure to the mixture.

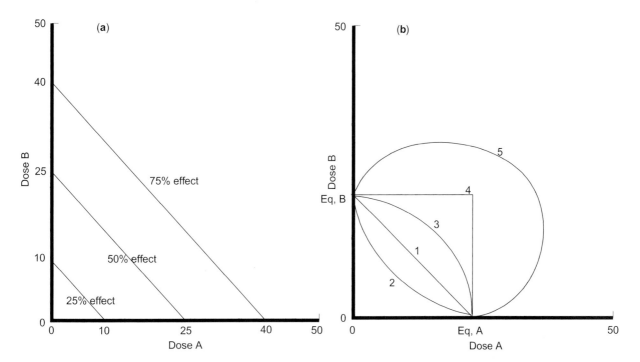

Figure 2 Isoboles of two compounds. On the axes are the doses of A and B that produce an equal effect (for instance, a 50% reduction of cell survival). 3(a) Isoboles for different effect levels; (b) isoboles indicating different types of (inter)action: 1 = dose-additivity; 2 = synergism; 3 = partial addition; 4 = no addition; 5 = antagonism.

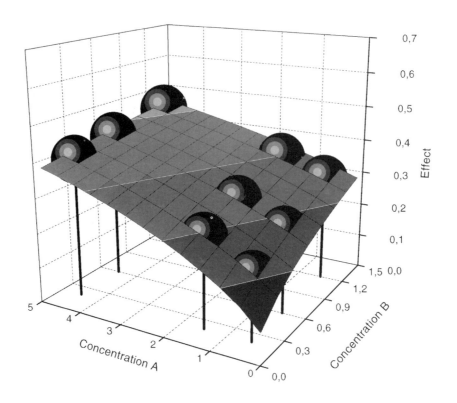

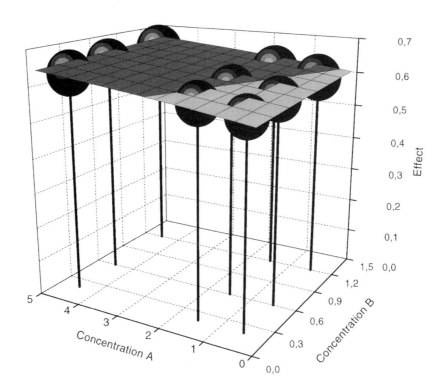

Figure 3 Zero interaction response surfaces for the combination of three agents A, B and C, according to the dose-additivity criterion (Equation 2) derived from single-agent data in **Table 1** keeping the dose of agent C fixed at (a) 400 and (b) 3600 compared with the combination data in **Table 1** (solid spheres). The single-agent dose–response curves were determined using the Hill equation $E(d) = d^{\mu}/(d^{\mu} + a^{\mu})$. The parameters obtained are as follows: A, $a = 10.26587 \pm 0.31563$, $\mu = 0.83392 \pm 0.02836$, $\chi^2 = 0.00016$; B, $a = 6.62456 \pm 0.35694$, $\mu = 0.72518 \pm 0.04156$, $\chi^2 = 0.00053$; and C, $a = 2417.78604 \pm 330.384$, $\mu = 1.07252 \pm 0.19068$, $\chi^2 = 0.00715$. The equation for calculating the zero interaction dose–response surface is given in Sühnel (1992).

Mode II addition or isoadditivity (Kodell and Pounds, 1991) represents the general form of the concentration additivity concept. In this case a dose d_1 will result in an effect E_1 and the second agent will add up with a complementary dose of d_1 to result in $E(d_1, d_2)$ **(Figure 2)**. Kodell and Pounds (1991) provided a mathematical equation for mode I:

$$E[d_1(d_2 - p_2 d_1)] = E(p_2 d_1) = E(d_2) \quad (7)$$

where p_2 is defined as the relative potency factor of agent 2. However, when the dose–response curves are non-linear and cannot be linearized by biologically sensible transformation, there is no obvious way to determine a potency factor.

Although isoboles are very illustrative representations of combined action or interactions, the use of isobolograms has a number of drawbacks. For instance, equi-effective doses of each of the constituents of the mixtures have to be known very precisely: large standard deviations make the observed effects plotted in the isobologram difficult to interpret. As a consequence, extensive studies must be carried out with the individual compounds. Moreover, the huge number of valuable data is not fully exploited in this method and there is no easy statistical basis for a conclusion to be drawn from the isobologram. Although a graphical presentation is illustrative, it is obvious that an isobole analysis can only be done at clear effect levels and their graphical nature limits the number of agents to be evaluated in a mixture to three. To overcome this problem, a system of parallel coordinate axes representing hyperdimensional figures are proposed to overcome this problem to some extent and permit the ready visualization and characterization of interaction effects with a polynomial model (Gennings *et al.*, 1990).

Effect or Response Surface Analysis

Conceptually less easy to interpret, but much easier to perform, are response-surface analyses. The response-or effect-surface methodology will yield a statistically based mathematical relationship between the doses of each of the agents of a mixture and the effect parameter (Greco *et al.*, 1995). One of the simplest expressions for a three-compound mixture is

$$E = \alpha + \beta_1 d_1 + \beta_2 d_2 + \beta_3 d_3 + \gamma_1 d_1 d_2$$
$$+ \gamma_2 d_1 d_3 + \gamma_3 d_2 d_3 + \delta_1 d_1 d_2 d_3 \quad (8)$$

where d_n represents the dose of a chemical in the mixture. By means of a t-test and the standard error of a coefficient, the p value for the regression coefficient can be estimated. The p value measures the probability of observing the value of the coefficient or a more extreme value given that the null hypothesis (the coefficient is zero) is true. In the case of significant interaction terms, these coefficients should always be interpreted with the responding main effects. The coefficient α represents the control situation (e.g. 100% viability) and the constants β are associated with the main effect of each of the compounds. The coefficients γ and δ are indications of two- and three-factor interactions, respectively. In this example, for viability a positive value of γ or δ (in association with a negative value for β) indicates a less than additive effect due to an interaction between two (or three) compounds of the mixture. Zero values of γ or δ suggest the absence of a particular interaction. The advantage of this method is that it includes all data points obtained and it does not require dose–effect equations for all individual chemicals of the mixture *per se*. If the equation is extended by quadratic or even more complex terms, then this simple interpretation is no longer correct.

A different response surface approach is that the combined action will be assessed using the information from single-agent dose–response relations. This information can be used to calculate a zero interaction response surface according to the criterion one prefers (dose addition, independence, etc.). Next, experimental data can be compared with the calculated effects and a significant deviation from the calculated effects indicates an interaction according to the criterion adopted for defining zero interaction (Sühnel, 1992, 1996). This approach is illustrated in **Figure 2** using the dataset of **Table 1** for two fixed concentrations of agent C. The approach avoids the difficulties which may occur when determining a relatively large number of parameters of a response surface (Equation 8) from experimental combination effects by a regression technique. It requires information on single-agent dose–response relations, however. Non-linear regression calculations for single-agent dose–response relations are easier than for response surfaces. On the other hand, the method cannot predict any interactive combination effects. However, it has conceptual advantages because widely used experimental designs such as the dose variation of one agent in the presence of a fixed amount of another one or a simultaneous variation of various doses keeping the dose ratio fixed, represent cross-sections through the response surface.

Knowing that at relatively high exposure levels saturation and competition will play a major role in the establishment of the combined effect, one should avoid working at high effect levels in this type of analysis. Instead, we recommend choosing a concentration range not exceeding an (arbitrary) 50% effect level, or even less, since at present there is an increasing awareness that in the field of (combination) toxicology it would be more interesting to investigate the effects of mixtures at no-effect levels or minimal-effect levels of the individual constituents.

Comparison of Individual Dose–Response Curves

Comparison of dose–response curves (DRCs) of an agent in the absence and presence of a second agent has been proposed by Pöch *et al.* (1990a, b). For this purpose, the corresponding theoretical DRCs for dose-additive and independent combinations have to be constructed in order to compare the observed combined response with the expected response. An independent effect can be calculated with the equation

$$E_{AB} = E_A + E_B - (E_A E_B) \qquad (9)$$

with the assumption that there is no correlation between the chemicals in the mixture, as mentioned earlier (Equation 3) and is valid for the fractional effect.

Independent DRCs are shifted upwards **(Figure 3)**. For calculation and construction of the additive DRC, the equi-effective dose $d_{A,equi}$ of compound A resulting in the same effect as d_B is estimated. Under the assumption that additive combinations of compound B must behave like $d_{A,equi}$, the same effect is expected in additive combinations at the applied doses of $d_A - d_{A,equi}$ **(Figure 3)**. All additive DRCs of A + B reach the same maximum as the maximum of DRC$_A$, provided that the effect of B is smaller than A$_{max}$. However, in the case of competitive agonism, the effect of B does not affect the effect of A + B at higher doses of A. Considerably fewer data are then needed to describe the combined effects using this evaluation method compared with isobolographic evaluations. Although this method is easier and more

straightforward than the isobole method, it still requires complete DRCs of compound A in the presence and absence of a fixed effective concentration of compound B. The method including a statistical interpretation is restricted to binary mixtures and has been presented for both dose-frequency and 'quantitative' curves (Pöch, 1993; Dawson and Pöch, 1997; Holzmann *et al.*, 1997). In the latter case, the number of experimental data points above or below, respectively, the theoretical curves (median values) are compared with total $n/2$ 'expected'. As an alternative, 95% confidence intervals of experimental and theoretical effects are compared graphically (Holzmann *et al.*, 1997).

Combination Index (CI) and Hazard Index (HI)

Chou and Talalay (1984) proposed judging the occurrence of additivity, antagonism and synergism using a so called combination index (CI). The approach distinguishes chemicals with the same (similar joint action) and different (independent) mechanisms of action:

$$CI = \frac{D_1}{D(x)_1} + \frac{D_2}{D(x)_2} + \alpha \frac{D_1 D_2}{D(x)_1 D(x)_2} \qquad (10)$$

where $D(x)_n$ is the dose of chemical n that will result in $x\%$ effect if dosed as single compound and D_n is the dose of chemical n in the mixture that will result in $x\%$ effect; $\alpha = 0$ for chemicals with independent joint action (mutually exclusive agents) and $\alpha = 1$ for chemicals that influence each others' mechanisms of action (mutually non-exclusive agents). Note that Equation (10) is identical with the isobole Equation (5) for $\alpha = 0$ and bears a resemblance to Equation (9) for $\alpha = 1$. The following conclusions can be drawn from the CI values of a mixture:

CI = 1 no interaction
CI > 1 antagonism
CI < 1 synergism

It should be noted that Equation (10) was derived from mass-action considerations. It represents a further derivation of the isobole Equation (5).

The HI as put forward in the US EPA mixture guidelines should be regarded as an approximation of the risk posed by exposure to the mixture. The HI method is based on the assumption of dose additivity (similar joint action) and is therefore only valid under the condition that the compounds in the mixture induce the same toxic effect, via the same mode of action. In this approach, the hazard quotients are calculated for individual compounds and the quotients for each compound in the mixture are then added. The 'hazard index' (US EPA, 1986) can be calculated from the equation

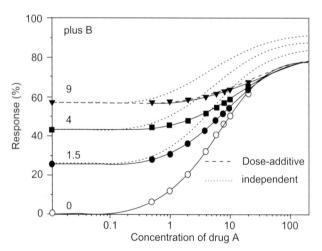

Figure 4 Dose–response curve (DRC) of A alone (open symbols) and in the presence of fixed doses of B (closed symbols) as indicated. In addition to experimental sigmoidal curves (solid lines), theoretical curves for dose-additivity and independence are also shown. Note that experimental DRCs of A in the presence of B match dose-additive curves. DRCs were constructed with SigmaPlot (Jandel/SPSS) by means of user-defined worksheets and program files (Pöch *et al.*, 1997). Data obtained from Table 1.

$$HI = \frac{D_1}{RfD_1} + \frac{D_2}{RfD_2} + \cdots + \frac{D_n}{RfD_n} \qquad (11)$$

where D is the level of exposure and RfD is some defined limit exposure value (reference dose). If HI in this equation exceeds unity, the concern is the same as if an individual chemical exposure exceeded its acceptable level by the same proportion. In case of independent joint action the HI will be that of the agent with the highest quotient. Thus, in a three-compound mixture ABC with exposure levels of A = 4, B = 0.25 and C = 192 and DLs of A = 40, B = 0.5 and C = 320, the HIs are 0.1, 0.5 and 0.6 for the individual chemicals, respectively. In the case of dissimilar joint action, the HI of the mixture ABC will be 0.6, whereas with similar joint action the HI of the mixture would be 1.2. If the hazard index is greater than 1, there might be an increased risk of exposure to this mixture. It will often be impossible to obtain sufficient and adequate toxicological information on each of the compounds in a mixture to make these calculations. Hence data on interaction are not included in this approach.

The HI can be classified according to **Table 2**.

A different approach, originally published by Mumtaz and Durkin (1992), takes into account both synergistic and antagonistic interations in the derivation of the HI. In this approach a weight-of-evidence (WOE) classification is followed to estimate the joint actions (additivity, antagonism and synergism) for binary mixtures of chemicals based on information about the individual compounds:

$$HI_{WOE} = HI \times UF_{WOE} \qquad (6)$$

Where UF stands for the uncertainty factor and the WOE for using an interaction factor (additivity = 0; synergism = +; antagonism = −). In this WOE approach, several 'weighing factors' are taken into account in the final classification, such as the mechanistic understanding of the binary interactions, the demonstration of toxicity, and additional uncertainty factors, i.e. modifiers of interactions, such as route of exposure and *in vitro* data. The better the data set on the individual compounds is, the more precisely the joint action can be predicted.

Table 2 Terminology used to classify an effect of a mixture using the hazard index

HI	Effect
< 0	Antagonism
0	No-dose addition (complete positive correlation)
0–1	Partial addition
1	Dose-addition
> 1	More than dose-additive (synergy, potentiation)

Interactive effects between many compounds

Any time a mixture consists of more than two compounds, many two- or three-factor interactions may occur. If all these factors are carefully thought about in an experimental set-up, the number of possible test combinations increases exponentially with increasing number of compounds in a mixture. Likewise, the number of experimental groups will also increase with increase in the number of doses of each compound. Both ethical and practical reasons force researchers to lower the number of experimental groups. A number of statistical designs are available to evaluate the effects of mixtures compared with those of their constituents, for instance, ray, central composite and factorial designs (Box *et al.*, 1978; Svengaard and Hertzberg, 1994; Gennings, 1996; Schoen, 1996; Simmons and Gennings, 1996). One way to detect interactive effects, i.e. non-additive effects, between more than two chemicals in a chemical mixture is to use factorial designs. The use of factorial designs, in which n chemicals are studied at x dose levels (xn treatment groups), has been suggested by the US EPA as one of the valuable statistical approaches for risk assessment of chemical mixtures. Full factorial designs, however, lead to very costly experiments, and even if only two dose levels are used, it is already virtually impossible to perform complete, conventional toxicity tests using 2^n test groups to identify interactions between all chemicals of interest. One way to deal with this problem is to use fractionated factorial designs (Groten *et al.*, 1996, 1997). Fractionated designs still identify most of the interactions between the compounds and determine which compounds are important in causing effects and have the advantage that the number of test groups is manageable. Fractional factorial designs have been shown to be an efficient, i.e. cost-effective, approach to identify interactive effects between trace elements and the cadmium accumulation in the body, to determine structure–activity relationships for halogenated aliphatic hydrocarbons and to determine interactions between drugs and contaminants in food.

If the risk assessor does not attempt to model the complete dose–response surface of the mixture, another approach might be followed in which the interest is focused on the departure from additivity of the mixture as a whole, rather than on the identification of specific interactions. This approach, suggested by Berenbaum (1989), utilizes single chemical dose–response information in addition to the observed responses induced by the particular combinations of interest. Clearly, the advantage offered by such an approach becomes apparent upon comparing the number of experimental groups employed in its application with that required by the use of factorial designs. Apart from this limitation, the strength of the (fractionated) factorial approach is the possibility of formulating a more accurate hypothesis as to most of the relevant or critical interactions, and to show which compounds are important in the particular mixture in terms of hazard identification.

If whole response surfaces are to be studied for several chemicals at the same time, factorial designs are too complex in structure. In these cases, other designs such as the Box–Behnken designs or Central Composite designs can be useful to study deviations from additivity as a first start. These designs should be applied to determine an optimum effect and to perform in a cost-effective way response-surface analyses. As a follow-up after this first screening, a factorial design can be applied to verify interactions between selected compounds (Schoen, 1996).

EXAMPLES

To study successfully the toxicology of mixtures and to assess properly their potential health risks, it is essential to understand the basic concepts of combined action and interaction of chemicals, and to distinguish between whole mixture analysis (top-down approach) and component interaction analysis (bottom-up approach). In our view, it is equally important to make a clear distinction between simple and complex chemical mixtures. A *simple* mixture is defined as a mixture that consists of a relatively small number of chemicals, say 10 or less, the composition of which is qualitatively and quantitatively known; examples are a cocktail of pesticides, a combination of medicines or a group of irritating aldehydes. A *complex* mixture is defined as a mixture that consists of tens, hundreds or thousands of chemicals, of which the composition is qualitatively and quantitatively not fully known; examples are welding fumes, a workplace atmosphere, environmental tobacco smoke, drinking water or a new food product. It is self-evident that a bottom-up approach for studying the toxicology of complex mixtures is virtually impossible, implying that the top-down approach is the option left. For some complex mixtures the top-down approach may be appropriate; for others, such as the atmosphere at a hazardous waste site or a workplace atmosphere, whole mixture analysis seems to be impracticable and meaningless.

As a rule, exposure to mixtures of chemicals at (low) non-toxic doses of the individual chemicals in the mixture is of no health concern, and the probability of increased health hazard due to additivity or potentiating interaction seems to be very small, since the dose of chemicals to which humans are exposed is *generally* much lower than the 'no observed adverse effect level' (NOAEL). Exceptions to these rules may be mixtures of chemicals with a similar mode of action or with evidence of potentiating interaction, and mixtures with no or very

small MOS such as carcinogens, the outdoor air (a mixture with as major constituents PM2.5, ozone, nitrogen dioxide and sulphur dioxide) and food additives or nutrients. To trace such exceptional mixtures is one of the priorities of the mixture toxicologist.

This section briefly reviews a few examples from the real world.

Carcinogens

The principles of hazard identification and risk assessment of mixtures of carcinogens have been elegantly discussed by Hasegawa *et al.* (1994) and Portier and Sherman (1994). In this section, some major characteristics of the safety evaluation of mixtures of carcinogens will be highlighted in a narrative way.

The multistage model of chemical carcinogenesis, now widely accepted as a theoretical basis of carcinogenesis, assumes at least initiation, expansion, promotion and progression. Each of these steps can be affected in a dose-related manner at different rates by the different carcinogens in a mixture, the existence of a threshold dose level for promoters and epigenetic carcinogens being a feature of considerable importance.

When the mechanism of carcinogenesis is essentially similar for the various carcinogens in a mixture, the cancer response will be additive. In case of dissimilar (independent) mechanisms of carcinogenesis, the cancer response of the mixture may vary from equal to the strongest individual response (in case of fully positive correlation of susceptibility) to equal to the sum of the individual responses (in case of fully negative correlation of susceptibility). Hence the response to combined exposure to complete carcinogens (with initiating and promoting activity) with non-interactive mode of actions will generally follow the rules of response additivity, as has been demonstrated for combinations of carcinogenic nitrosamines (Hasegawa *et al.*, 1994).

Synergistic (or antagonistic) interactions between (incomplete) carcinogens in a mixture may involve effects on bioavailability or metabolic activation/detoxification of a carcinogen, effects on DNA repair processes or proliferation of cells with DNA damage and effects on hormonal or immunological conditions. Such interactive effects may particularly occur after exposure to genotoxic and non-genotoxic (epigenetic carcinogens or promoters) carcinogens with often widely varying modes of action. The existence of a threshold for promoting or inhibiting activity leads to a true no-effect level for such activity, indicating the importance of dose for (predicting) the type and degree of interaction between such carcinogens. As a consequence, low-dose extrapolation as a crucial step in risk assessment may be very precarious for mixtures of such types of carcinogens. Synergism (but also antagonism) occurring at relatively high exposure levels may not occur at all at (much) lower levels, as is exemplified by the following recently published study. Straight-run kerosene and straight-run gas oils containing low levels of carcinogenic polycyclic aromatic hydrocarbons were examined for carcinogenicity in a 2-year mouse skin study. These petroleum middle distillates produced severe skin irritation and increased the skin tumour response when tested undiluted. However, when diluted (same total dose) the irritant effects were reduced and no significant increase in the number of skin tumours was observed. These data indicate that these distillates do not represent a skin cancer hazard to humans as long as prolonged skin irritation is avoided. Risk assessment based on the findings with the undiluted distillates alone might have resulted in a completely different but erroneous conclusion (Priston *et al.*, 1997).

Air pollutants

Air pollution is a variable complex mixture of chemicals that consists of gases, vapours and aerosols. Exposure to these chemicals is hard to avoid. The diversity of environments where exposure might occur and the number of pollutants that may be present pose a challenge in investigating the health effects of air pollutants. The toxicity of these mixtures is not only determined by the adverse effects of the single compounds but also by interactions between two or more chemicals of the mixture. We have to face the problem that air pollution is a continuously varying complex mixture with its numerous possible combined actions.

Air pollution is not only a problem for man outside or in the workplace—indoor air pollution may be just as effective and sometimes can cause even more problems than outdoor pollution. Since exposure concentrations of air pollution are often relatively low, the possibility of a cumulative chemical exposure should not be discounted. Inhaling one pollutant may not make one sick, but the chances of one's health suffering are much greater on exposure to more chemicals.

Although it is often not possible to identify all chemicals within the complex mixture of air pollutants, a useful approach can be to identify specific air (categories of) contaminants such as aldehydes, PM10, ozone and polycyclic aromatic hydrocarbons. However, to establish causal relationships between air pollution and adverse health effects, specific agents still need to be identified.

By studying chemical–chemical interactions in the toxicology of air pollutants, it was shown that the untoward effect of certain oxidants may be enhanced in the presence of other pollutants. Damage to the alveolar zone by the antioxidant butylated hydroxytoluene (BHT) can be greatly enhanced by subsequent exposure to oxygen concentrations which, otherwise, would have little if any demonstrable effect. The synergistic interaction between BHT and oxygen results in interstitial pulmonary fibrosis.

Synergistic interactions between either ozone or nitrogen dioxide and relative high levels of aerosols of sulphuric acid or ammonium bisulphate have been reported and were seen as increases in alveolar macrophages and fibroblasts, increased collagen synthesis and total protein contents in lavage fluid, and a more than additive increase in lipid peroxidation in the lung (Gelzleichter *et al.*, 1992). In most of these cases exposure levels were used that exceeded reality and whether these additive and synergistic effects found at high levels are predictive for joint action at lower levels (preferably around the NOAEL) has not yet been fully established.

Considerable attention has been paid to the joint action of aldehydes. Aldehydes constitute a group of relatively reactive organic compounds that are omnipresent in the environment as a result of incomplete combustion or pyrolysis of organic materials such as fuels, polymers, food and tobacco (Feron *et al.*, 1991).

Combined exposure of rats to formaldehyde and acrolein has been reported to result in significantly higher yields of DNA–protein cross-links in nasal epithelium than exposure to formaldehyde alone, most probably because of inhibition of the oxidative metabolism of formaldehyde due to glutathione depletion by acrolein (Lam *et al.*, 1985). Toxicity studies with mixtures of aldehydes showed that histopathological changes and cell proliferation of the nasal epithelium by mixtures of formaldehyde, acetaldehyde and acrolein appeared to be more severe and more extensive, both in the respiratory and the olfactory epithelium, than those observed after exposure to the individual aldehydes at comparable exposure levels (Cassee *et al.*, 1996b). However, the prediction of joint action of these aldehydes at NOAELs of the individual chemicals seemed not to be possible. Therefore, overall these studies indicate that combined exposure to aldehydes with the same target organ (nose), and exerting the same type of adverse effect (nasal irritation), but with partly different target sites, is not associated with increased nose irritation as compared with exposure to the individual chemicals.

Mixtures of aerosols and gases

Recent epidemiological studies have associated particulate matter (PM) with health effects such as increased daily mortality and hospital admissions, exacerbation of asthma, increase in respiratory symptoms and lung function decline (Roemer *et al.*, 1993; Dockery and Pope, 1994, and the large number of references cited therein; Hoek and Brunekreef 1993). The levels of PM at which these effects are observed are significantly lower than those previously thought to protect human health. Since PM is a complex mixture and the current standard is to a large extent based on information from studies using single chemical aerosols, more than additive effects of chemicals in the mixture of PM or with gaseous components in air pollution cannot be excluded. For instance, the combination of ozone and acid aerols have been shown to have the potential to act synergistically (Last *et al.*, 1986; Warren *et al.*, 1986). However, at present there is scant toxicological information on PM. Several approaches have been put forward based on different hypotheses. Obviously, it is not possible to identify the critical chemicals in these complex mixtures by testing the toxicity using advanced statistical designs and experimental set-ups using artificially generated aerosols only. Real-world aerosols from locations dominated by different emission sources such as rural versus urban versus industrialized areas might be useful in identifying those aerosols that are causally related to the observed adverse health effects. It is obvious that such complex mixtures cannot easily be tested in an experimental set-up. Several factors should be taken into account. For instance, particulate air pollution cannot be characterized only by its chemical composition and mass concentration but also by its physical properties such as particle number, concentration and particle surface area. It is noteworthy that this latter aspect means that large changes in the numbers of the ultrafine particles in the ambient aerosol will be reflected only marginally in changes in, e.g., the PM10 mass concentration. In general, pulmonary deposition is dependent on the particle size, favouring smaller ($< 0.2\mu$m) particles being deposited in the alveolar region and larger (1–10 μm) particles being deposited in the upper respiratory tract. This means that an extremely toxic particle larger than 10μm has a very small chance of reaching the (lower) airways. In addition to these different dose measures, the dosimetry of PM is also highly dependent on host responsiveness. Differences in airway function can greatly influence the ultimate effect. It has been estimated that in compromised airways the deposition pattern of particles is changed compared with healthy airways. Owing to increased minute ventilation, the total deposition may also be enhanced and shifted towards the alveolar region. Consequently, compromised airways may have a greater probability of interaction of PM with potential targets of PM toxicity, and thus an increased chance of adverse effects.

Large safety factors have been applied to set exposure limits for indoor air pollutants. However, for both PM and ozone, these margins of safety are small and special attention should be paid to the tracing of hazardous combinations within PM but also between PM and other air pollutants. Owing to recent epidemiological studies in which serious health effects were associated with PM without a sound toxicological explanation, much effort is being put into elucidating the toxicological mechanisms underlying these effects. The complexity of PM forces investigators to use study designs that can identify possible interactions of critical components of these mixtures or with gaseous compounds of air pollution.

Threshold levels for combined or interactive effects of chemicals and the underlying mechanisms described in experimental animals are not clearly defined, so their relevance to humans chronically exposed to low levels of these chemicals remains unclear. As to how far the results of animal studies at high dose levels predict the potential health hazard in humans exposed to (much) lower (no-effect) concentrations of the individual chemicals is not clear. Undoubtedly, studies on combinations of air pollutants using more realistic concentrations including levels around the NOEL are needed.

Food

Food is an extremely complex and variable chemical mixture estimated to consist of several hundred thousand chemicals. Clearly, in principle food chemicals may exhibit joint similar or joint dissimilar action, leading to non-interactive combined effects, and may also interact with one another, altering the degree and maybe also the nature of the potential toxic effects of individual food chemicals. How likely is it that such adverse combined or interactive effects will occur?

- Nutrients
- Non-nutritive naturally occurring components
- Man-made contaminants
- Additives

Thorough toxicological studies and examinations are necessary for additives and man-made chemicals that may contaminate food such as pesticides, veterinary drugs and chemicals from food packaging materials. Health-based (toxicologically based) limit values are recommended by national and international committees, usually applying large safety factors of 100 or more (Feron, 1997). The food-oriented additives are preferably as inert as possible towards the body, which explains their relatively large margin of safety (MOS). Potentiating interaction is expected to be only of minor importance in view of the low intake levels of non-nutritive food components. In contrast, nutrients have often small MOS between Recommended Daily Allowances (RDAs) and the minimum toxic dose, e.g. 15 for vitamin A, 10 for zinc, 5 for sodium, 5 for vitamin D, 2 for manganese and 1.4 for fat (Feskens, 1997). There is still a knowledge gap regarding the toxicity of the vast majority of natural food chemicals (Van Genderen, 1997).

The category of food chemicals of greatest health concern is therefore the (essential) nutrients. Nutritional imbalance may result in deficiencies but also in exceeding the MOS. Nutrients are reactive, body-oriented chemicals. For the mixture toxicologist the priority category of food chemicals would seem to be the nutrients with their body orientation and small MOS. However, the mixture of nutrients is necessary for growth, maintenance and reproduction of humans, and when in balance the mixture as such is a prerequisite rather than a threat to human health; in fact, a balanced mixture of nutrients (a balanced diet) is the pre-eminent medicine of life. On the other hand, because of the importance of nutrients for life, the nutritionist has to be on the alert for interactions of non-nutritive and even non-food chemicals with nutrients, leading to nutritional deficiencies (there are many examples of such interactions), while the food toxicologist should always consider the possibility of potentiating interactions between non-nutritive or non-food chemicals (e.g. drugs) and nutrients. The mixture of nutrients is an example to illustrate that application of the dose-addition — (as a default concept) — to mixtures of chemicals that act by mechanisms would overestimate the health risks of such mixtures.

Aquatic environments

Starting with the concept of simple similar action, Könemann (1981) has shown that the toxicity of a large number of chemicals could be predicted by concentration addition. Toxicity experiments with guppies have been conducted, using six mixtures of 3–50 chemicals. Groups of chemicals that could be described by a good structure–activity relationship (QSAR) probably have the same mode of action. Equitoxic mixtures of 50 selected lipophilic organics without a specific mode of action resulted in death with these fish. A 50% death rate (LC_{50}) was found for mixtures in which each of the individual chemicals was mixed at one-fiftieth of its own LC_{50}. Similar results were found for mixtures of chlorophenols.

CONCLUSION

From a public health point of view, it is most relevant to answer the question of whether or not chemicals in a mixture interact in a way that results in a reduced or increased overall response as compared with the sum of the responses to the individual chemicals in the mixture. Approaches for identifying the type of effect and interaction of chemicals of mixtures rely heavily on some form of additivity model. Three concepts are defined: similar mode of action, dissimilar mode of action and interaction. Interactions of chemicals can take place during several phases (the environment, in the toxicokinetic or toxicodynamic phase) or due to physico-chemical reaction between chemicals. Although the additivity models are mathematically simple, they require assumptions about the mode of action. For a real understanding of an interaction, information on the mechanism is quintessential. Nevertheless, it may happen that a separate

definition of interaction for each new mechanism is needed. Furthermore, very often mechanisms have to be modified over the years, which may possibly result in revised definitions of interaction. This means that mechanistic definitions of interaction alone do not resolve all problems. The advantage of empirical approaches such as the dose-additivity and the independence approach is that in a certain sense they also contain some very basic 'mechanistic' information. Hence the most promising approach will probably be a combination of empirical and mechanistic approaches.

Overall, the potential adverse health effects of exposure to (mixtures of) chemicals at realistic exposure levels should be a primary research topic of toxicologists in the near future, focusing on mechanisms of action and the development of pragmatic approaches to assess interaction data.

ACKNOWLEDGEMENTS

We express our gratitude to Professor Dr Gerald Pöch and Professor Dr P. J. van Bladeren for their contributions.

REFERENCES

Berenbaum, M. C. (1989). What is synergy? *Pharmacol. Rev.*, **41**, 93–141.

Bliss, C. I. (1939). The toxicity of poisons applied jointly. *Ann. Appl. Biol.*, **26**, 585–615.

Box, G. E. P., Hunter, W. G. and Hunter, J. S. (1978). *Statistics for Experimenters*. Wiley, New York, p. 653.

Calabrese, E. J. (1991). *Multiple Chemical Interactions*. Lewis Publishers, Chelsea, MI, p. 704.

Cassee, F. R., Arts, J. H. E., Groten, J. P. and Feron, V. J. (1996a). Sensory irritation to mixtures of formaldehyde, acrolein, and acetaldehyde in rats. *Arch. Toxicol.*, **70**, 329–337.

Cassee, F. R., Groten, J. P. and Feron, V. J. (1996b). Changes in the nasal epithelium of rats exposed by inhalation to mixtures of formaldehyde, acetaldehyde and acrolein. *Fundam. Appl. Toxicol.* **29**, 208–218.

Cassee, F. R., Groten, J. P., Van Bladeren, P. J. and Feron, V. J. (1998). Toxicological evaluation and risk assessment of chemical mixtures. *Crit. Rev. Toxicol.*, **28**(1), 73–101.

Chou, T.-C. and Talalay, P. (1984). Quantitative analysis of dose–effect relationships: the combined effects of multiple drugs or enzyme inhibitors. *Adv. Enzyme Regul.*, **22**, 27–55.

Dawson, D. A. and Pöch, G. (1997). A method for evaluating mechanistic aspects of chemical mixture toxicity. *Toxicol. Methods*, submitted.

Dockery, D. W. and Pope, C. A., III (1994). Acute respiratory effects of particulate air pollution. *Annu. Rev. Publi. Health*, **15**, 107–132.

Fay, R. M. and Feron, V. J. (1996). Complex mixtures: hazard identification and risk assessment. *Food Chem. Toxicol.*, **34**, 1175–1176.

Feron, V. J. (1997). Introduction to adverse effects of food and nutrition. In de Vries, J. (Ed.), *Food Safety and Toxicity*. CRC Press, Boca Raton, FL, pp. 111–120.

Feron, V. J., Til, H. P., de Vrijer, F., Woutersen, R. A., Cassee, F. R. and Van Bladeren, P. J. (1991). Aldehydes: occurrence, carcinogenic potential, mechanism of action and risk assessment. *Mutat. Res.*, **259**, 363–385.

Feron, V. J., Groten, J. P., Jonker, D., Cassee, F. R. and Van Bladeren, P. J. (1995a). Risk assessment of simple (defined) mixtures of chemicals. In Burgat-Sacaze, V., Descotes, J., Gaussens, P. and Leslie, G. B. (Eds), *Toxicology and Air Pollution: Risk Assessment*. Faculté de Médicine et de Pharmacie, Université de Bourgogne, Dijon, pp. 31–42.

Feron, V. J., Groten, J. P., Jonker, D., Cassee, F. R. and Van Bladeren, P. J. (1995b). Toxicology of chemical mixtures: challenges for today and the future. *Toxicology*, **105**, 415–428.

Feskens, E. J. M. (1997). Introduction to risk assessment. In de Vries, J. (Ed.), *Food Safety and Toxicity*. CRC Press, Boca Raton, Fh., pp. 215–228.

Finney, D. J. (1942). The analysis of toxicity tests on mixtures of poisons. *Annals Appl. Biol.*, **29**, 82–94.

Gebhart, G. F. (1992). Comments on the isobole method for analysis of drug interactions [Letter]. *Pain.*, **51**, 381–388.

Gelzleichter, T. R., Witschi, K. and Last, J. A. (1992). Synergistic interaction of nitrogen dioxide and ozone on rat lungs: acute responses. *Toxicol. Appl. Pharmacol.*, **116**, 1–9.

Gennings, C. (1996). Economical designs for detecting and characterizing departure from additivity in mixtures of many chemicals. *Food. Chem. Toxicol.*, **34**, 1053–1058.

Gennings, C., Dawson, K. S., Carter, W. H. and Myers, R. H. (1990). Interpreting plots of a multidimensional dose–response surface in a parallel coordinate system. *Biometrics*, **46**, 719–735.

Gessner, P. K. (1988). A straightforward method for the study of drug interactions: an isobolographic analysis primer. *J. Am. Coll. Toxicol.*, **7**, 987–1012.

Greco, W. R., Bravo, G. and Parsons, J. C. (1995). The search for synergy: a critical review from a response surface perspective. *Pharmacol. Rev.*, **47**, 332–385.

Groten, J. P., Schoen, E. D. and Feron, V. J. (1996). Use of factorial designs in combination toxicity studies. *Food Chem. Toxicol.*, **34**, 1083–1089.

Groten, J. P., Schoen, E. D., van Bladeren, P. J., Kuper, C. F., van Zorge, J. A. and Feron, V. J. (1997). Subacute toxicity of a combination of nine chemicals in rats: detecting interactive effects with a two level factorial design. *Fundam. Appl. Toxicol.*, **36**, 15–29.

Hasegawa, R., Takayama, S. and Ito, N. (1994). Effects of low level exposure to multiple carcinogens in combination. In R. S. H. Yang (Ed.), *Toxicology of Mixtures*. Academic Press, San Diego, pp. 361–382.

Henschler, D., Bolt, H. M., Jonker, D., Pieters, M. N. and Groten, J. P. (1996). Experimental designs and risk assessment in combination toxicology: panel discussion. *Food Chem. Toxicol.*, **34**, 1183–1185.

Hoek, G. and Brunekreef, B. (1993). Acute effects of a winter air pollution episode on pulmonary function and respiratory symptoms of children. *Arch. Environ. Health*, **48**, 328–335.

Holzmann, S., Dittrich, P. and Pöch, G. (1997). Computerized construction of dose–response curves of vasorelaxing agents. *J. Exp. Clin. Cardiol.*, submitted.

Kodell, R. L. and Pounds, J. G. (1991). Assessing the toxicity of mixtures of chemicals. In Krewski, D. and Franklin, C. (Eds), *Statistics in Toxicology*. Gordon and Breach, New York, pp. 559–591.

Könemann, H. (1981). Fish toxicity tests with mixtures of more than two chemicals: a proposal for a quantitative approach and experimental. *Toxicology*, **19**, 229–238.

Krishnan, K. and Brodeur, J. (1991). Toxicological consequences of combined exposure to environmental pollutants. *Arch. Complex Environ. Stud.* **3**, 1–104.

Lam, C. W., Casanova, M. and Heck, H.d'A. (1985). Depletion of nasal glutathione by acrolein and enhancement of formaldehyde induced DNA protein cross linking by simultaneous exposure to acrolein. *Arch. Toxicol.*, **58**, 67–71.

Last, J. A., Guth, D. J. and Warren, D. L. (1986). Synergistic interaction of ozone and respirable aerosols on rat lungs. I. Importance of aerosol acidity. *Toxicology*, **39**, 247–257.

Loewe, S. and Muischnek, H. (1926). Über Kombinationswirkungen. *Arch. Exp. Pathol. Pharmakol*, **114**, 313–326.

Miaskowski, C. and Levine, J. D. (1992). Comments on the evaluation of drug interactions using isobolographic analysis and analysis of variance. *Pain*, **49**, 383–387.

Mumtaz, M. M. and Durkin, P. R. (1992). A weight-of-evidence approach for assessing interactions in chemical mixtures. *Toxicol. Ind. Health.*, **8**, 377–406.

Mumtaz, M. M., Sipes, I. G., Clewell, H. J. and Yang, R. S. H. (1993). Risk assessment of chemical mixtures: biologic and toxicologic issues. *Fundam. Appl. Toxicol.*, **21**, 258–269.

Mumtaz, M. M., DeRosa, C. T. and Durkin, P. R. (1994). Approaches and challenges in risk assessments of chemical mixtures. In Yang, R. S. H. (Ed.), *Toxicology of Chemical Mixtures*. Academic Press, San Diego, pp. 565–598.

Ploemen, J. H. T. M., Wormhoudt, L. W., Haenen, G. R. M. M., Oudshoorn, M. J., Commandeur, J. N. M., Vermeulen, N. P. E., de Waziers, I., Beaune, P. H., Watabe, T. and van Bladeren P. J. (1997). The use of human *in vitro* metabolic parameters to explore the risk of hazardous compounds: the case of ethylene dibromide. *Toxicol Appl. Pharmacol.*, **143**, 56–69.

Pöch, G. (1993). *Combined Effects of Drugs and Toxic Agents. Modern Evaluation in Theory and Practice*. Springer, New York.

Pöch, G. and Dittrich, P. (1996). Convenient construction of dose-response curves and its application to toxicology. *Toxicol. Lett. Suppl 1/88*, 106.

Pöch, G., Dittrich, P., and Holzmann, S. (1990a). Evaluation of combined effects in dose–response studies by statistical comparison with additive and independent interactions. *J. Pharmacol. Methods*, **24**, 311–325.

Pöch, G. Dittrich, P., Reiffenstein, R. J., Lenk, W. and Schuster, A. (1990b). Evaluation of experimental combined toxicity by use of dose-frequency curves: comparison with theoretical additivity as well as independence. *Can. J. Physiol. Pharmacol.*, **68**, 1338–1345.

Pöch, G. and Herziq, S. (1997). Study design and evaluation of combined effects of drugs and toxic agents: recommendations. Personel communication.

Pöch, G., Holzmann, S. and Baer, H.-P. (1997). Convenient calculation of experimental and theoretical dose–response curves of combinations. *Res. Discov.*, **1**, 4–5.

Portier, C. J. and Sherman, C. D. (1994). Potential effects of chemical mixtures on the carcinogenic process within the context of the mathematical multistage model. In Yang, R. S. H. (Ed.), *Toxicology of Mixtures*. Academic Press, San Diego, pp. 665–686.

Priston, R. A. J., Nessel, C. S., Cruzan, G., Hageman, R., McKee, R. H., Riley, A. J. and Simpson, B. J. (1997). Effect of irritation on mouse skin carcinogenicity of petroleum middle distillates. *Human and Experimental Toxicology*, **16**(7), 417.

Roemer, W., Hoek, G. and Brunekreef, B. (1993). Effect of ambient winter air pollution on respiratory health of children with chronic respiratory symptoms. *Am. Rev. Respir. Dis.*, **147**, 118–124.

Schoen, E. D. (1996). Statistical designs in combination toxicology: a matter of choice. *Food Chem. Toxicol.*, **34**, 1059–1065.

Sexton, K., Beck, B. D., Bingham, E., Brain, J. D., DeMarini, D. M., Hertzberg, R. C., O'Flaherty, E. J. and Pounds, J. G. (1995). Chemical mixtures from a public health perspective: the importance of research for informed decision making. *Toxicology*, **105**, 429–441.

Simmons, J. E. (1995). Chemical mixtures: challenge for toxicology and risk assessment. *Toxicology*, **105**, ISS 2–3, 111–119

Simmons, J. E. and Gennings, C. (1996). Experimental designs, statistics and interpretation. *Food Chem. Toxicol.*, **34**, 1169–1171.

Steel, G. G. and M. J. Peckham (1979). Exploitable mechanisms in combined radiotherapy–chemotherapy: the concept of additivity. *Int. J. Radiat. Oncol. Biol. Phys.*, **5**, 85–91.

Sühnel, J. (1992). Zero interaction response surfaces, interaction functions and difference response surfaces for combinations of biologically active agents. *Arzneim.-Forsch.*, **42**, 1251–1258.

Sühnel, J. (1996). Zero interaction response surfaces for combined-action assessment. *Food Chem. Toxicol*, **34**, 1151–1153.

Suzuki, S. (1994). The synergistic action of mixed irradiation with high-LET and low-LET radiation. *Radiat. Res.*, **138**, 297–301.

Svengaard, D. J. and Hertzberg, R. C. (1994). Statistical methods for toxicological evaluation. In Yang, R. S. H. (Ed.), *Toxicology of Chemical Mixtures*. Academic Press, San Diego, pp. 599–642.

US EPA (1986). Guidelines for the health risk assessment of chemical mixtures. *Fed. Regist.*, **51**, 34014–34025.

Van Genderen, H. (1997). Toxicology of mixtures in the light of food safety. In de Vries, J. (Ed.), *Food Safety and Toxicity*. CRC Press, Boca Raton, FL, pp. 177–182.

Warren, D. L., Guth, D. J. and Last, J. A. (1986). Synergistic interaction of ozone and respirable aerosols on rat lungs. II. Synergy between ammonium sulfate aerosol and various concentrations of ozone. *Toxicol. Appl. Pharmacol.*, **84**, 470–479.

Yang, R. S. H. (1994a). Introduction to the toxicology of chemical mixtures. In Yang, R. S. H. (Ed.), *Toxicology of Chemical Mixtures*. Academic Press, San Diego, pp. 1–10.

Yang, R. S. H. (1994b). *Toxicology of Chemical Mixtures*. Academic Press, San Diego.

Yang, R. S. H., El-Masri, H. A., Constan, A. A. and Tessari, J. D. (1995) The application of physiologically based pharmacokinetic/pharmacokinetic (PBPK/PD) modeling for exploring risk assessment approaches of chemical mixtures *Toxicol. Lett.*, **79**, 193–200.

PART TWO
TECHNIQUES

Chapter 15
The Design of Toxicological Studies

Alan J. Paine and T. C. Marrs

C O N T E N T S

INTRODUCTION

There is no fundamental difference in the approach to experimental design in toxicology from that used in other scientific disciplines and mechanistic toxicology experiments are much like any other biological studies. In regulatory toxicology, by contrast, experimental design may be constrained by a number of factors, but even here, considerations such as the statistical power of the study are as important as in any other biological science. Moreover, the aim of regulatory toxicology is frequently to predict what will happen in a large, usually human, population, using smallish groups of animals. To compensate for the disparate group sizes, the dose used in the experimental animals is often much larger than that to which the humans are exposed, raising problems of overloading detoxication systems.

As toxicology has matured over the last 40 years, the design of studies for regulatory purposes has become increasing prescribed by national or international regulatory bodies. A noteworthy feature of regulatory toxicology studies is the desire of the toxicologist to elicit no-effect levels (NELs), no observed effect levels (NOELs) or no observed adverse effect levels (NOAELs) at least for end-points other than genotoxicity and carcinogenicity. NELs and NOAELs are, in fact, thresholds and the reason for the wish to establish them is that the existence of a threshold and its measurement enable the regulator to set acceptable human exposure figures, using some sort of safety factor in the extrapolation from animals to humans. These exposure figures may be acceptable daily intakes (ADIs) for chemicals in food or acceptable operator exposure levels (AOELs) for chemicals in the workplace. Almost always, there is no theoretical basis for the factors used in extrapolation from animal to man: the 100-fold safety factor used is based upon tradition and represents an empirical approach that has stood the test of time. It is often said that of this 100-fold safety factor, 10 is for interspecies differences and 10 for intraspecies differences; again, this is empirical (see Calabrese, 1983).

THE DOSE–RESPONSE RELATIONSHIP

The relationship between the degree of response and amount of chemical administered is the most fundamental and pervasive concept in toxicology. It also generates a vocabulary with which the student of toxicology needs to become familiar. The typical sigmoidal curve obtained by plotting response against administered dose is shown in **Figure 1A**. **Figure 1B** shows the normal Gaussian distribution that lethality exhibits. The data used to construct this histogram are the same as those used to generate the sigmoidal curve but the bars represent the percentage of animals that die at each dose minus the percentage that died at the lower dose. One can very clearly see that only a few animals responded at the lowest dose and only a small number responded at the highest dose. Larger numbers of animals responded to doses intermediate between these two extremes, and the maximum frequency of response occurred in the middle portion of the dose range. These curves can be transformed

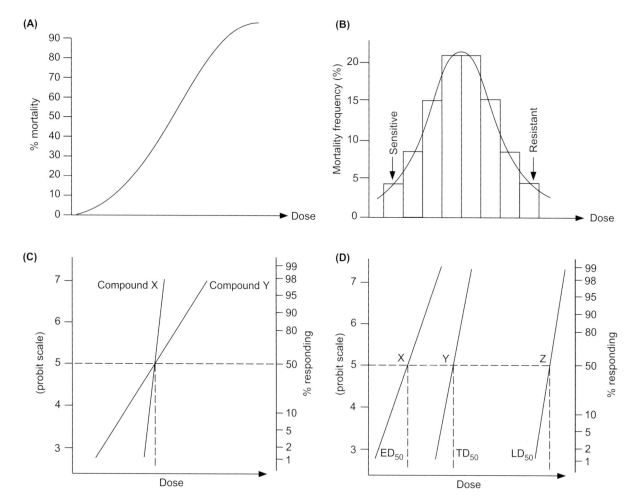

Figure 1 Typical dose–response curves. **(A)** Percentage mortality plotted against the log of the dose. **(B)** Mortality frequency plotted against log dose. **(C)** Comparison of the toxicities of two compounds X and Y. Although they have the same LD_{50} the slope shows compound X to be more potent than compound Y at high doses. **(D)** Comparison of the dose–response cures for efficacy (X), toxicity (Y) and lethality (Z).

into a more manageable straight line **(Figure 1C)** by probit analysis and the median lethal dose (LD_{50}) or for that matter the lethal dose for any percentage of the population (e.g. LD_{10}) can then easily be determined.

The LD_{50} value in its simplest form is the dose of a compound that causes 50% mortality in a population. A more precise definition is the statistically derived single dose that can be expected to cause death in 50% of the animals under the specific conditions of the test. Thus, the LD_{50} value of a compound is not a mathematical constant but is a statistical term that describes the lethal response to a compound in a particular population under some discrete set of experimental conditions (e.g. age, general health and diet of the population). Although the numerical value of the LD_{50} has been used to classify and compare toxicity among chemicals, it must be remembered that lethality is only one of many indices in assessing toxicity and that there are several other possible variables that can be measured, such as time to death or non-lethal end-points.

The slope of the log dose–response curve is perhaps as important in risk assessment as the numerical value of the LD_{50}, because more insight into the intrinsic toxic characteristics of a compound is available. For example, a steep slope may indicate rapid onset of action or faster absorption. A larger margin of safety may be predicted when a compound has a flat slope, i.e. a large increase in dose produces only a small increase in response. With the slope it is often possible to extrapolate the response to a low dose, for example, LD_1. Knowing the slope is especially important when comparing a series of compounds. For example, two compounds may have identical LD_{50} values but different slopes indicating quite different toxicological characteristics **(Figure 1C)**. The LD_{50} is not equivalent to toxicity, as chemicals can induce irreversible damage to physiological, biochemical, immunological, neurological or anatomical systems and, depending on the severity and extent of the disturbance, the animal may survive the toxic response. These non-lethal adverse effects are undesirable and must be taken into account in the risk assessment of a chemical. Such non-lethal responses often follow a dose–response curve, and the term 'toxic dose' (TD) or more commonly 'effective dose' (ED) is used to describe these **(Figure 1D)**. The term 'median effective dose' (ED_{50}) is often used in the standardization of biologically active compounds, such as drugs, and has a similar meaning to LD_{50} except that it is designed to examine non-lethal parameters such as pharmacological response or other non-lethal adverse effects. The ratio LD_{50}/ED_{50} defines the therapeutic index (TI) of a drug. The higher the index, the greater is the margin of safety with a drug, in that a large difference exists between the amount of a compound predicted to kill 50% of the animals and the amount predicted to elicit a particular response in 50% of the animals. The TI gives an even greater estimate of safety when the LD_1 or TD_1 is compared with the ED_{99}. What is being aimed for in the development of a pharmaceutical is a safety factor of 100–200–fold between the pharmacological and toxicological responses.

DURATION OF TOXICITY STUDIES

From the point of view of duration, three types of study have become mandatory in the safety evaluation of a chemical. These are as follows.

Acute studies demonstrate the adverse effects occuring within a short time, usually up to 14 days, following administration of a single dose of a substance or multiple doses given within 24 h. *Repeated-dose (subacute/subchronic) studies*. The definition of subchronic toxicity is confusing, as opinions differ as to the length of exposure that constitutes a subacute study. However, their purpose is the same—namely to demonstrate adverse effects occuring as a result of repeated daily doses of a chemical for part, not exceeding 10%, of the life-span of an animal. Thus, 14, 21 and 28 day studies in rats are generally referred to as 'subacute' studies, while 90 day studies constitute 'subchronic' tests. Significant findings that appear only after more than 6 months are uncommon, so that the toxic potential (excluding tumorigenicity) can probably be adequately assessed by a study of 6 months duration (Lumley *et al.*, 1992). *Chronic studies* are those carried out over the whole or a considerable proportion of an animal's lifespan. There is some disagreement over the description of 1 year studies in the larger laboratory species.

When these types of toxicity studies are translated into terms of human exposure, acute toxicity represents life-threatening crises of accidental catastrophes, overdoses or suicidal attempts. Subchronic/subacute toxicity represents frequent exposure to certain workplace and domestic chemicals, food additives, therapeutic agents or environmental pollutants at lower dose levels relative to accidental exposure. Chronic toxicity represents the daily ingestion of additives or agricultural residues in food.

ANIMAL HUSBANDRY AND OBSERVATIONS

The most important facet of any toxicological experiment is the condition of the test animals. Accordingly, all toxicity studies should be conducted in a controlled environment, which for rats means a temperature of $22 \pm 3°C$ with adequate ventilation (i.e. 10 changes of air per hour), relative humidity between 30 and 70% and a 12 h light/dark cycle. The diet and quality of drinking water should be standardized and maintained throughout the experiment, and this should be carried out to Good Laboratory Practice standards (see chapter 21) to ensure reproducibility/validity of data. It should be noted that factors such as whether rodents are housed individually or in groups may profoundly affect endpoints such as tumor occurrence and survival (Haseman *et al.*, 1994). Moreover, diet and nutrition can also seriously affect various outcomes of toxicology studies depending on the duration of the study and the species and strain of animal; dietary restriction tends to reduce weight gain, but increase longevity and resistance to tumor induction in rodent long-term feeding studies (Tucker, 1979, 1987; Lansdown and Conning, 1990). The survival of some strains of rats, e.g. Sprague–Dawley and F344, has been declining, and dietary restriction may increase longevity (Dixit and Kacew, 1997). Diets made unsavory by the addition of unpalatable test compound may have a similar effect, as well as decreasing weight gain by comparison with the controls.

Healthy young adult animals should be used, which means a body weight of 15–16 g for mice, 150–250 g for rats, 350–450 g for guinea pigs and 2–3 kg for rabbits. Upon receipt, the animals should be allowed to acclimatize to the conditions of the animal room for at least a week prior to dosing. During this period the animals should be individually and uniquely identified by tattooing or ear marking. Then all animals with health problems or body weights differing by more than 20% from the mean body weight should be discarded and the remaining animals randomized, to ensure a homogeneous population, to the different dose groups.

For acute oral toxicity studies a minimum of 10 animals, 5 male and 5 female, has been recommended in most regulatory guidelines. Therefore, rats and mice can be housed by sex and dose group according to current regulations concerning animal experimentation. Larger animals should be caged individually. For the determination of acute dermal and acute inhalation toxicities, 5 animals per dose level and sex are again sufficient, but these should be housed singly to prevent oral ingestion of the test substance by preening. Practical details of dosing by oral, dermal and inhalation routes are provided by Hayes (1982).

After dosing, observations should be made at frequent intervals in order to determine the onset of adverse effects, time to death or time to recovery. A mortality check should also be frequent enough to minimize unnecessary loss of animals due to autolysis or cannibalism. The observations should include any changes in the skin colour (e.g. cyanosis due to cardiac insufficiency), fur (e.g. piloerection due to disturbance of the autonomic nervous system), eyes (e.g. lachrymation indicating autonomic disturbances) and nostrils (e.g. discharge may indicate pulmonary oedema). Other pharmacotoxic signs such as tremor, convulsions, salivation, diarrhoea, lethargy, sleepiness and morbidity, should be recorded in order to obtain the maximum amount of information from the experiment. Necropsies must be performed on animals that are moribund, found dead or killed at the end of the experiment. At necropsy changes in size, colour or texture of the major organs should be recorded and, if noted, tissues should be preserved in an appropriate fixative for histopathological examination. The procedures outlined in **Table 1** attempt to summarize the considerable amount of work involved in toxicity tests.

Table 1 Consensus of basic procedure comprising acute, subchronic and chronic oral toxicity tests

	Acute oral	Subchronic oral	Chronic oral
Animals	Rats preferred	Rodent and non-rodent species	Rodent and non-rodent species
Sex		Males and females equally distributed per dose level	
Age and weight	Young adult weight variation within 20% of mean	Rodents 6 weeks; dogs 4–6 months old	
No. per dose level	At least 10 animals (5 per sex)	At least 20 for rodents (10 per sex)	50 per sex group for rodents
Minimum no. of treatment groups	3 spaced appropriately to produce test groups with mortality rates between 10% and 90%	3 but not more than 10% mortality in high-dose group	3: low-dose should reflect expected human exposure. High-dose must produce an effect but not more than 10% mortality
Untreated control	Not necessary	Yes	Yes
Vehicle control	Yes, if suspending agent of unknown toxicity is used	Yes	Yes
Fasting	Rat overnight	Not appropriate	Not appropriate
Dosing	By gavage; single dose, same dose of vehicle. If necessary use divided doses over 24 h	Diet, gavage, drinking-water	Diet, gavage, drinking-water
Duration of study	At least 14 days	90 days	24 months in rats
Body weight determination	To be recorded before dosing, weekly thereafter and at death	Weekly and at termination	Weekly for first 13 weeks. Every 2 weeks thereafter and at termination
Food consumption	Weekly	Weekly	Weekly for first 13 weeks. Every 2 weeks thereafter and at termination
Necropsy	All animals	All test animals. Organ weights of liver, kidney, heart, lungs, brain, gonads, adrenals and spleen	
Histopathology	Examination of organs showing evidence of gross pathological change	All tissues high-dose and control groups. Liver, kidney, heart, lungs, target organs and any gross lesion in mid- and low-dose groups	All tissues all animals
Frequency of observation	Frequently during day of dosing. Once each morning and late afternoon thereafter	Daily	Daily
Observations to be made	Nature, onset, severity and duration of any effect observed	Ophthalmoscopy pretest and at termination on control and high-dose	
		Haematology/clinical chemistry: pretest monthly or dosing mid-point termination	Pretest 3, 6, 12, 18, 24 months
		Urinalysis: dosing mid-point termination	Pretest 3, 6, 12, 18, 24 months

TESTING FOR ACUTE TOXICITY

The objectives of an acute study are to define the intrinsic toxicity of a chemical, to assess the susceptible species, to identify the target organs of toxicity, to provide information for risk assessment after acute exposure to the chemical and to provide information for the design and selection of dose levels for more prolonged studies. In the absence of data on the toxicity of a chemical, acute studies also help in formulating safety measures/monitoring procedures for all workers involved in the development and testing of a chemical. Accordingly, a battery of tests under different conditions and exposure routes should be conducted. In general, these tests should include determination of a chemical's oral (Chapter 28) cutaneous (Chapter 30) and inhalation (Chapter 31) toxicities, as well as skin and eye irritation studies (Chapter 43 and 40).

From a regulatory viewpoint, acute toxicity data are essential in the classification, labelling and transportation of a chemical (van den Heuvel *et al.*, 1987). From an academic standpoint, a carefully designed acute toxicity study can often produce information on the mechanism of toxicity and the structure–activity relationships within a particular class of chemicals. Therefore, acute toxicity tests should aim to record all lethal and non-lethal parameters.

Choice of Animal Species

In part, the choice of species depends on the intended use of the chemical, but as humans will be intimately involved in its manufacture, distribution and use, acute toxicity tests, like all toxicity tests, should be conducted on an animal which will elicit compound-related responses similar to those which can be expected to occur in man. However, it should be appreciated that responses caused by a compound can vary greatly among species, owing to differences in metabolism and pharma-

cokinetics (Tee *et al.*, 1987) and sometimes other factors such as receptor differences or differences in structure of animal organs or systems. Therefore, a sensible approach is to conduct acute oral toxicity studies in a variety of species of experimental animal under the assumption that if the toxicity of a compound is consistent in all the species tested, then there is a greater chance that such a similar response will occur in man. Although the response in different species is often consistent, it is better to err on the safe side, with risk assessment being based on the most sensitive species. There may be good reasons for concluding that results in a particular species are not likely to be relevant for man. However, the information to draw such a conclusion often arises later in the course of development, for example during phase 1 studies of pharmaceuticals or, with other chemicals, when occupational exposure data become available. This means that the information arrives too late to inform the choice of animal model, although such information is, of course, invaluable in data interpretation. Therefore, there is no absolute criterion for selecting a particular species, and most commonly rats, mice, rabbits and guinea-pigs are chosen for acute toxicity studies. However, toxicity within a particular species can vary with age, sex and health conditions, as well as genetic makeup (**Figure 2**). For example, immature animals may lack an effective xenobiotic metabolizing system. This may result in greater toxicity of the compound in an immature animal if an enzyme is responsible for detoxification or decrease toxicity if the enzyme system is responsible for activation (**Table 2**). Therefore, it is important to document all data on the animals' source, strain, sex, age, body weight and general health conditions.

Selection of Dose Levels

The purpose of an acute toxicity study is to establish the degree of toxicity of a new chemical entity, and the

Table 2 Consequences of metabolism

Process	Effect		Example	
	Pharmacological	Toxicological		
Inactive compound activated by metabolism	Activation	—	Prontosil	
	—	Intoxication	Fluoroacetate	
Active compound changed into another active compound	Change in activity	—	Imipramine to desmethylimipramine	
		Detoxication or intoxication	Isoniazid	Peripheral neuropathy greater in slow acetylators Hepatic damage greater in rapid acetylators
Active compound inactivated by metabolism	Inactivation	Detoxification	Barbiturates	

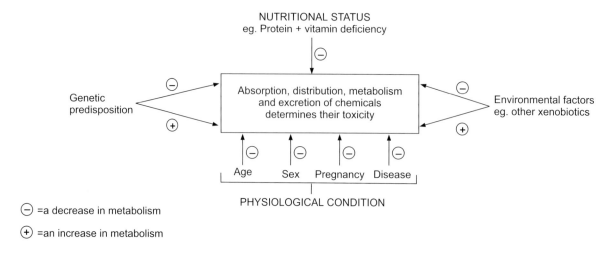

Figure 2 Factors affecting metabolism and toxicity.

reader is reminded that formal determination of the LD_{50} value is not considered necessary nowadays and is more often measured in a semiquantitative limit test. Additionally, the LD_{50} test has been criticized on scientific and humane grounds (British Toxicology Society, 1984; Society of Toxicology, 1989; van den Heuvel, 1990). The Society of Toxicology document makes the point that much of the information supplied by the LD_{50} test can be supplied by other forms of acute toxicity test. Moreover, the Society of Toxicology noted that the reproducibility of the test was poor. In general, dose levels should be sufficient in number, at least three, to allow a clear demonstration of the dose–response relationship. In practice, a pilot study will be needed to determine the order of toxicity. The British Toxicology Society's approach (van den Heuvel *et al.*, 1987) is to perform a preliminary 'sighting' study, using just three or four animals. Following administration, observations for effects are made. When toxicity is not evident at the chosen dose level or where a severe toxic reaction requires, for animals welfare reasons, the removal of the animals from the study, the substance should be re-tested at the next higher or lower dose level. Three alternative guidelines to LD_{50}-type studies have been adopted by the OECD. They are the fixed dose procedure (OECD, 1992), the acute toxic class method (OECD, 1996) and the up-and-down method (OECD, 1998). The fixed dose procedure is based on the administration of one of the following fixed doses, 5, 50, 500 or 2000 mg kg^{-1} body weight, the object being to produce clear signs of toxocity, but not death. The acute toxic class method uses as a starting dose 25, 200 or 2000 mg kg^{-1} body weight. What happens next depends on the number of animals that die at the chosen starting dose, and is described in an annex to OECD (1996), in which there are flow charts which describe how to proceed. The up-and-down method does not use fixed

doses: one animal is given the test material at a dose believed to be the best estimate of the LD_{50}: if the animal dies the dose given to the next animal is reduced, whereas if the first animal survives, the dose is increased. The procedure is repeated until the point is reached where increasing or decreasing the dose reverses the mortality; four additional animals are then dosed. Essentially, therefore the up-and-down procedure is an iterative strategy designed to bracket the median lethal dose. All three alternative methods use considerably fewer animals than conventional LD_{50} studies, but the fixed dose procedure specifically does not use death as an endpoint.

Principles of Acute Oral Tests

The test substance is dissolved in water, or corn oil/appropriate solvents if it is insoluble in aqueous media. If all attempts to dissolve the material fail, then appropriate suspending agents such as 0.5% methyl cellulose or gum tragacanth in water can be used, provided that a homogeneous dosing preparation be produced. The dosing solution is administered by gastric intubation, and animals in the control groups should receive the same volume of vehicle, it being borne in mind that there are two methods of dosing the test material: (1) by varying the dosing volume, which means that animals are given different volumes of the same dosing solution; (2) by varying the concentration of the dosing solutions so that animals are given the same volume of vehicle.

The different methods of dosing can result in different toxicities for the same compound being obtained. For instance, when a large volume of corn oil is given orally, it will increase gastrointestinal mobility and have a laxative effect which may decrease the time the test substance is in the gut and available for absorption. Conversely, irritation of the gut will be decreased when the test substance is given in a diluted form. As the objective of an acute oral toxicity study is to determine systemic toxicity, which may include gastrointestinal irritation, many toxicologists may choose constant concentration versus constant dose volume. However, most regulatory guidelines wish for constant dose volume. But, the choice should be based on sound scientific judgement. If the dose is too large to be administered at a single time, it can be divided into equal doses with 3–4 h between them. Food should be withheld until the last dose, which should be given within 24 h of the first.

Principles of Acute Skin Tests

Skin exposure probably represents the most important route of exposure in the workplace, and, accordingly, knowledge of a chemical's dermal toxicity is prerequisite to its classification by regulatory authorities. The tests are commonly performed on rabbits and three types of dosing procedure are employed—namely unocclusive, semiocclusive and occlusive. The back or a band around the trunk of the animal is clipped free of hair, care being taken not to abrade the skin. The test substance should be applied uniformly to approximately 10% of the body surface of the animal. Liquid test substances are generally applied undiluted. If the test substances is a solid, it is pulverized and moistened to a paste with physiological saline or appropriate solvent and spread evenly on the closely shaved skin. For the study to be meaningful, the effect of the vehicle on the dermal penetration of the test substance should be fully evaluated prior to the toxicity study. For occlusive or semiocclusive application, the application site is covered with an impervious material such as plastic sheet or with a porous gauze dressing, respectively. For unocclusive exposure, the test substance is applied to the skin as near to the head as possible, to prevent ingestion by preening of the application site. Alternatively, the correct amount of a liquid test substance may be applied underneath a plastic cuff with a long feeding needle, followed by gently rubbing the cuff to distribute evenly the test material.

The length of exposure ranges from 4 to 24 h, depending on the guidelines followed, which, in general, agree that if no test-substance-related mortality is observed at 2 g kg^{-1}, testing at higher doses is not necessary. After 4–24 h of exposure the site of application is inspected after gently removing the compound with cotton wool soaked in the appropriate solvent, and skin irritation can be assessed according to the scoring system described by Draize et al. (1944). However, the primary purpose of an acute dermal toxicity study is to provide information on the adverse, systemic effects of the test substance following percutaneous absorption.

Acute Inhalation Tests

Acute inhalation tests—technically difficult and specialized studies—may not be needed if inhalation exposure is not expected to occur. This might be because the physicochemical properties of the test substance are such that respirable particles cannot be generated even under the most favourable laboratory conditions. It is generally recognized that particles greater than 100 μm in diameter are unlikely to be inhaled, as they settle too rapidly. Those with diameters of 10–50 μm are likely to be retained in the nose and upper parts of the respiratory tract. Particles with diameters of less than 7 μm can reach the alveoli and are regarded as respirable. When inhalation studies are required, the exposure duration is usually 4–6 h and comprises either whole-body or head-only exposure. For details of the design of the different types of chambers as well as a discussion of the advantages/limitations of different methods of exposure, see Chapter 31 and Kennedy and Trochimowicz (1982). In brief, gases, followed by volatile liquids, are the simplest atmospheres to generate and quantify. The quantity of a solid test substance in aerosols needs to be expressed in terms of both concentration and particle size.

Accordingly, the actual conduct of an inhalation experiment will differ for each type of material under study but the primary objective of an inhalation study is to derive a median lethal concentration (LC$_{50}$) following a single exposure, in much the same way as an LD$_{50}$ is derived from acute oral or dermal toxicity tests. The LC$_{50}$, which must be qualified by the duration of exposure, can then be used to derive short-term occupational exposure limits. Sometimes the median lethal dose for an inhaled toxicant is expressed as the LCt$_{50}$, that is, the product of LC$_{50}$ and time, often expressed as mg min m^{-3}. Were gases and vapours to obey Haber's law ($Ct = K$), this expression of dose would be constant regardless of duration of exposure. Gases and vapours rarely obey this law, hence the LCt$_{50}$ usually has to be qualified by the conditions of exposure. Although the LCt$_{50}$ thus offers no great advantage, the concept is much favoured by military establishments.

Interpretation of Data

It is accepted that all chemicals can produce toxicity under some experimental conditions, if a sufficiently large dose is given. However, it would be misleading to conduct toxicity studies at unreasonably high dose levels just for the sake of demonstrating lethality/toxicity which may be irrelevant to human experience of the compound. Effects may non-specific: for example, extremely high oral doses of a practically non-toxic compound can cause blockage of the gastrointestinal tract and death (Chapter 1). However, such toxicity should not be related to the intrinsic characteristics of the test substance but rather to the fact that toxicity is a direct result of the physical blockage that was produced essentially by an inert substance. Accordingly, there must be a point where the toxicologist is confident in concluding that the test substance is practically non-toxic after acute exposure. For this reason an oral test limit of 5 g kg^{-1}, a cutaneous test limit of 2 g kg^{-1}, and an inhalation test limit of 50 mg m^{-3} are generally accepted. At these levels the investigator should conclude that administration of higher doses is not necessary.

REPEATED-DOSE (SUBACUTE AND SUBCHRONIC) TOXICITY STUDIES

Repeated-dose (subacute or subchronic) toxicity studies are designed to examine the adverse effects resulting from repeated exposure to a chemical at lower doses than used in acute studies. Primarily such studies demonstrate whether the accumulation of a compound, which may be virtually non-toxic in an acute study, disrupts vital body functions, rendering it toxic. Also, as repeated dose studies are conducted over longer periods of time, up to 10% of the animal's life-span, than acute studies, they also demonstrate whether there is a latent period for the development of toxicity. Thus, although an animal may survive the acutely toxic action of a chemical, some irreversible change that overcomes normal mechanisms may have occurred. A classical example of such an effect is the delayed neuropathy caused by many organophosphorus insecticides, which can manifest itself some weeks after the chemical has been eliminated from the body.

Such non-lethal adverse effects are obviously undesirable, and so repeated-dose studies are considered to be essential for all new chemicals before their specific hazard can be assessed. Thus, unlike acute studies, the major end-point in a repeated-dose study is not mortality but some non-lethal parameter which can be defined by functional, biochemical, physiological or pathological effects **(Table 3)**. Furthermore, the toxicological responses observed in a low-dose repeated-dose study may be quite different from those observed in a high-dose acute study. Repeated administration of a test material can have very profound differences from administration of the same material in a single dose. Cumulation may occur after multiple dosing, increasing toxic effects. On the other hand enzyme induction may occur, decreasing toxicity when the test material is itself toxic, or increasing toxicity when the test material is metabolized to a more toxic metabolite. The complexity of the situation is exemplified by cyanides, which are highly toxic when administered as a single dose (Ballantyne, 1987). Cyanides are the subject of a low capacity but otherwise highly effective endogenous detoxication system, so that presented as small doses

Table 3 Types of toxicity

(1) Functional: based on clinical observations – e.g. behavioural toxicology, immunotoxicity
(2) Biochemical: e.g. mechanism underlying dysfunction; absorption, distribution, metabolism and excretion of toxins
(3) Structural: e.g. pathology based at the level of organs/ tissues, including carcinogenesis
(4) Environmental: e.g. Fear what? Monitor what? Ban what?
(5) Newer aspects: e.g. irritancy, endocrine toxicology, genetic toxicology, reproductive toxicology, including fertility, teratology, postnatal development

cyanides can be tolerated almost indefinitely (McNamara, 1976). On the other hand, very long exposure to cyanides in humans can result in a variety of neurological diseases, that appear to result, at least in part, from depletion of substances that act as cofactors in detoxication (Wilson, 1987). Other effects can occur on repeated dosing, such as tolerance, which has been frequently observed with anticholinesterases (see Lotti, 1992). Conversely, induction of the chemical's metabolism may lead to detoxification, depending on whether the parent compound or a metabolite is the toxic species (see **Table 2**). In view of the complicated changes in the disposition and metabolism of a chemical that can occur during prolonged exposure, a properly designed subchronic study will monitor a variety of clinical, haematological, biochemical and histopathological parameters (see **Table 1**) in order to detect a wide variety of effects. Such nonlethal adverse effects may be reversible, and therefore a reversibility phase is usually included in most subchronic studies. Clearly, irreversible changes will be weighted more heavily in reaching conclusions on the hazard a chemical may pose for humans.

Finally, the results of repeated-dose studies are generally extremely important in defining the no observable effect level and in selecting dose levels for chronic (Chapter 3), reproductive (Chapter 52), developmental (Chapter 53) and carcinogenicity (Chapters 50 and 51) studies.

Choice of Animal Species

Any common laboratory animal may be selected, but it is recommended that repeated-dose studies be conducted on at least two species, one being a rodent and the other a non-rodent. As with acute studies, the animal of choice should have a similar response to the test substance to that of humans. If this information is lacking, as is often the case, it is good practice to select the most sensitive species to evaluate the safety of a substance. Similarly, repeated-dose studies should always attempt to expose the animal by the route by which man is most likely to come into contact with the substance. In practice, dogs are the most commonly used non-rodent species, as, owing to their size, they have the advantage that blood samples can be collected during the study without it being necessary to kill the animal. There are also pharmacodynamic, pharmacokinetic and metabolic factors for the use of the dog (Parkinson and Grasso, 1993), while the use of monkeys, the main practicable alternative to dogs, presents particular problems not encountered with other species, which militate against the use of these animals except when absolutely necessary (Dayan, 1987; Lansdown and Conning, 1990). There is, of course the presumption that metabolically these animals are more likely to resemble man than other mammals, but this has to be weighed against the cost and there is the added consideration that monkeys may carry infections transmissible to humans. Rabbits are often used in irritancy and teratology studies while guinea-pigs are used in immunological work and, occasionally, in inhalation toxicology. Hens are used to screen for the potential of organophosphate anticholinesterases to cause delayed polyneuropathy as they are more sensitive to the delayed neuropathic effects of such chemicals than rodents (Johnson, 1992). Dogs, cats and farm animals may be used in safety evaluation of veterinary medicines, when such substances are intended for those animals. The use of exotic and unusual animals in toxicology is rare in regulatory work; the most serious difficulty is frequently the lack of background information on such animals. The most common routes of administration employed in repeated-dose toxicity studies are oral, skin and respiratory. Thus, as repeated-dose studies, they are usually carried out over 10% of the animal's life-span, oral and inhalation studies are usually carried out over 3 months in rodents and 1 year in dogs or monkeys, while repeated-dose skin studies are performed in 1 month or less.

Young and still-growing animals are preferred at the start of a subchronic study. Commonly rats and mice of 6–8 weeks of age are used, and, when dogs are chosen, these are 4–6 months old. Variation in responses due to sex differences may be important, and so each dose group should consist of equal numbers of male and female animals—usually 10–20 animals per sex per dose group for rodents, and 6–8 per sex per dose group for dogs. The number of animals will need to be increased if interim kills are to be made and if the reversibility of effects is to be examined. In reversibility studies the animals are removed from the test compound at the end of the study and 2–4 weeks later are subjected to the same analyses as the animals comprising the main study.

Selection and Maintenance of Dose Levels

The purpose of a repeated-dose study is to define a no observable effect level as well as to determine which organs have the greatest susceptibility to the toxic effects of the chemical. The reason for the first of these objectives is the already discussed desire of regulators to set acceptable exposure levels on the basis of NOELs. Accordingly, ideal dose levels will be those that do not result in toxicity at the low dose, although this should be higher than the expected level of human exposure, only slight toxicity at the intermediate level and toxicity at the high dose, but not high enough to result in the death of more than 10% of the group. In practice, this can only usually be achieved with a range-finding study of about 2 weeks duration prior to initiating the study. Toxicity in the pilot study is defined and based on the same measurements that will be employed in the main study.

In both repeated-dose and chronic toxicity studies the test substance is often incorporated into the diet or added to the drinking-water. The doses are commonly expressed in terms of concentration (parts per million; ppm) of the test substance in the diet or drinking-water or more usefully in terms of the test substance received by the animal [mg (kg body weight)$^{-1}$ day^{-1}]. In order to determine this, the exact amount of food or fluid consumed needs to be known. The approximate relationship of parts per million in the diet to mg (kg body weight)$^{-1}$ day^{-1} is shown in **Table 4**; however, the use of these relationships is a less satisfactory procedure than measured test material intake, in determining daily dose. Moreover, food consumption varies from weaning to maturity, with younger animals consuming more food on a body weight basis. Therefore, in order to ensure constant dosing throughout the study, it will be necessary for the investigator to predict on a weekly basis changes in body weight and food consumption, until they both stabilize, and adjust the concentration of the test substance in the diet according to the formulae shown in **Table 5**.

To avoid differences in food consumption due to changes in the calorific value of different batches of animal feed, the same batch of diet and, for that matter, the test substance should be used throughout the experiment. If different lots of test substance are used, purity and chemical, composition should not alter and should certainly be assayed. Also, adequate mixing of the test substance with the diet should be ensured by monitoring its concentration at the top, middle and bottom of a batch of diet. In addition, samples of diet that have been kept at room temperature for the same duration as that for which the animals have been exposed to it should also be analysed to ensure the stability of the test material.

Finally, whenever food consumption appears excessive, account should be taken of the spillage of food. This can be very easily estimated if the animals are housed in cages with wire-grid bottoms and spilt food is collected on a sheet of absorbent paper. Obviously, faecal contributions to spilt food and food in the hopper are taken into account. In contrast, when a chemical is dosed via the drinking-water, spillage is more disastrous, because it cannot be recovered as easily as spilled feed. All oral dosing regimens are on a 7 days per week basis. A 5

Table 4 Approximate relation of parts per million in the diet to mg per kg body weight per day

Animal	Weight (kg)	Food consumed per day (g) (liquids omitted)	Type of diet	Conversion factors	
				1 ppm in diet to mg (kg body weight)$^{-1}$ day^{-1}	1 mg (kg body weight)$^{-1}$ day^{-1} to 1 ppm in diet
Mouse	0.02	3	Dry laboratory chow diets	0.150	7
Chick	0.40	50		0.125	8
Rat (young)	0.10	10		0.100	10
Rat (old)	0.40	20		0.050	20
Guinea-pig	0.75	30		0.040	25
Rabbit	2.0	60		0.030	33
Dog	10.0	250		0.025	40
Cat	2	100	Moist, semi-solid diets	0.050	20
Monkey	5	250		0.050	20
Dog	10	750		0.075	13
Man	60	1500		0.025	40
Pig or sheep	60	2400	Relatively dry grain forage mixtures	0.040	25
Cow (maintenance)	500	7500		0.015	65
Cow (fattening)	500	15000		0.030	33
Horse	500	10000		0.020	50

Source: WHO (1987).

Table 5 Formulae for dietary studies

(1) Amount of test compound to be added to the diet to give a specified achieved intake in terms of body weight:

$$\frac{\text{projected mid} - \text{week average body weight (g rat}^{-1}) \times \text{average food eaten body week)}}{\text{average mid-week body weight (g rat}^{-1}) \text{ week}^{-1}} = \text{Amount of test compound to add to diet (ppm)}$$

(2) Achieved intake of test compound:

$$\frac{\text{inclusion level of test compound in the diet (ppm)} \times \text{average food eaten (g rat}^{-1} \text{ week}^{-1})}{\text{average mid-week body weight (g rat}^{-1}) \times 7} = \text{Average achieved intake of test compound (mg kg}^{-1} \text{ rat}^{-1} \text{ day}^{-1})$$

Source: Dr C. J. Powell, personal communication.

days a week basis is usually sufficient for repeated-dose skin and inhalation studies.

Other methods of administration of the test substance include parenteral dosing (Chapter 26), which is frequently used for pharmaceutical preparations, and subcutaneous or intramuscular implantation, which is commonly used for evaluating the toxicity of materials used in medical devices.

TESTING FOR CHRONIC TOXICITY

Nowadays the term 'chronic toxicity' encompasses investigations that include multigeneration reproduction studies and carcinogenicity tests. However, only classical chronic toxicity studies which are undertaken to define a safety factor between proposed use/exposure levels and

toxicity will be described here. Chronic toxicity studies usually consist of three treatment groups plus a control group, and the xenobiotic is administered 7 days a week for 2 years to rats or for 18 months to mice.

Carcinogenicity studies are generally done on rats and mice. One important consideration in the choice of strain with both the rat and the mouse is overall survival in the control group. A study may have to be terminated prematurely when the survival is less than 25–30%. Indeed, regulatory bodies often specify a minimum proportion of surviving animals at termination (OECD, 1981; Ministry of Health and Welfare, Japan, 1990).

Dose levels are usually selected after a 3 month range-finding study with enough doses to find a level which suppresses body weight gain slightly, i.e. by 10%. This dose, defined as the maximum tolerated dose (MTD), is selected as the highest dose. Alternatively, with a relatively non-toxic compound the dose may be chosen as not exceeding 100–200 times the anticipated human dose. Dose setting also requires careful consideration of the end-use of the chemical under study. For example, if the chemical is intended as a pharmaceutical which will only be used under medical supervision, then the dose levels may never be set at the MTD but rather will be related to the maximum therapeutic dose. Similarly, if the compound is expected to contaminate foodstuffs, the highest dose is likely to be 100 times the maximum detectable level in food. The intermediate dose is often half of the top dose, less frequently one third or one quarter, while the low dose may be one quarter of the top dose or one eighth or one tenth (Bucher *et al.*, 1996). It is not infrequent that the doses have to be changed in the course of the study, because of unacceptable mortality; almost always it is only the top dose that is reduced, with the result that some studies end up with unusual factors between the doses. An example is a long-term rat study on the insecticide mevinphos (FAO/WHO, 1997).

Pharmacokinetic data (see Chapters 4 and 5) are also particularly pertinent in selecting the dose levels to be employed. For example, in its simplest form comparison of the day 1 and day 90 LD_{50} values, the so-called 'chronicity factor', will indicate something about the *in vivo* handling of the chemical. Thus, if the 90 day LD_{50} is much lower than the LD_{50} value derived from the acute study, it is probable that the compound is slowly metabolized and will accumulate within the animal during a chronic toxicity study. In such cases where the metabolism and/or excretion of a chemical becomes saturated, relatively minor pathways of metabolism may become of major significance to the toxic effects observed. Whatever dose levels are chosen, they are maintained in the same way as that described for repeated-dose studies.

INTERPRETATION OF THE RESULTS OF REPEATED-DOSE AND CHRONIC TOXICITY STUDIES

In Life Observations

Because all subacute, subchronic and chronic toxicity studies are expensive to perform, observations should be made frequently, and the onset, severity and duration of any observed effect recorded in plain English. Similarly, loss of valuable tissues due to autolysis must be avoided, and severely moribund animals should be killed and necropsied. An important observation is, of course, survival and an adverse effect upon survival will be treated as an adverse effect in the study. Moreover survival, especially of control and low dose groups, may effect study duration (see above). Animals found dead should be refrigerated, not frozen, if necropsy cannot be performed immediately. Finally, food and fluid consump-

tion and growth rates should be determined on a fixed schedule and double-checked to avoid dosing errors which may invalidate the study. Also, expression of the food consumed per unit weight gain is a useful way of assessing the effect of a treatment on eating habits and food utilization. Fluid consumption is a useful way of identifying an agent with a diuretic action.

Organ Weights

In terms of the total cost of a subchronic or chronic study, weighing the organs at necropsy is both cheap and may reveal a specific target organ response which could be confirmed by histopathological examination (see Chapter 16). The most easily dissected organs are the liver, lung, kidney, spleen and testes. However, considerable variation in the weight of other organs can occur, e.g. of heart due to entrapped blood, of adrenals due to adhering fat, of brain due to where the spinal cord is cut, but these variations can be avoided by careful dissection technique to a standardized protocol. Organ weights are best expressed as a percentage of the animal's body weight, in most cases.

Histopathology

See Chapter 16 for details of appropriate techniques. Much emphasis is placed on histopathological changes which are supported by clinical chemistry (Chapter 17).

Ophthalmoscopy

Ophthalmoscopy will reveal damage to the retina but examination may be difficult in rodents if they are bled, for haematology and clinical chemistry, from the retro-orbital sinus.

Haematology

Blood can easily be collected by venepuncture from large species and from the retro-orbital sinus in rodents under anaesthesia, it being borne in mind that this will interfere with subsequent ophthalmoscopy. Bleeding from the tail-tip of rodents avoids this complication but the tendency of investigators to 'milk' blood from the animal often results in anomalous results due to extrusion of extracellular fluids. At termination, rodents may be bled from the abdominal aorta or inferior vena cava. Bleeding should be performed at the same time of day and the treatment groups should be randomized to avoid spurious changes in blood constituents due to circadian rhythms, which can occur as a result of the time involved if the dose groups are bled in sequence.

The clinical characteristics of blood are determined after treatment with an anticoagulant, the choice of which depends on the analyses to be performed, e.g. chelating agents such as EDTA may interfere with clinical chemistry assays and, therefore, the anticoagulant chosen should be checked out. Blood used for clinical chemistry must not be haemolysed, as not only will this result in a lower haematocrit and erythrocyte count, but also red cell constituents such as LDH, aminotransferases, potassium and creatinine will be released into the plasma and may lead to falsely high values.

The classic haematological measurements are erythrocyte, leukocyte and differential leukocyte counts, haemoglobin concentration, haematocrit, platelet and reticulocyte counts. From these data the mean corpuscular haemoglobin (MCH), mean corpuscular haemoglobin concentration (MCHC) and mean corpuscular volume (MCV) can be calculated and blood dyscrasias identified which may necessitate evaluation of the bone marrow (see Chapter 18).

CLINICAL CHEMISTRY

Standardized techniques need to be applied within any one laboratory, and intra-and inter-laboratory variance needs to be established before the values have any real meaning (see Chapter 17). Also, the introduction of automated equipment permits effortless analysis of nearly every biochemical parameter that can be measured, but before requesting a multitude of analyses the toxicologist should carefully think about selecting a battery of tests to identify specific target organ effects in the acute and subchronic studies and then focus on the area of concern in more depth in the chronic study.

URINALYSIS

Urinalysis is easy to perform but interpretation is fraught with difficulty due to the crude procedures often used in collection. Hair, room dust, bacteria, food and even the contents of the drinking-water bottle have been known to settle in urine collected in trays placed below cages. If there is a real concern and reason to consider urinalysis important, then the urine should be collected from sufficient animals in a manner that makes the analyses meaningful (e.g. use of metabolism cages), as the clinical chemistry of urine can provide useful toxicological information:

(1) If carefully collected over a specified period of time, the volume of urine may be useful for fluid balance assessments; e.g. diuresis, dehydration, etc.
(2) *Osmolality*   Indicates the ability of the kidney to concentrate urine.
(3) *pH*   Urine has a pH of 4.6–8.0 with a mean around 6.0, but its pH is meaningless unless urine is collected directly from the bladder, as dissolved CO_2 quickly dissipates after urination. Starvation and ketosis increase the acidity of urine.
(4) *Glucose*   High levels of reducing sugars, which can be measured by simple dipstick methods, occur in diabetes.
(5) Coloration/turbidity increases when urine becomes supersaturated, and microscopy may show crystals indicating formation of kidney or bladder stones. Red coloration is indicative of haemoglobinuria, haematuria or hepatic porphyria.

CONCLUSION

The life of modern man has been greatly improved by the development of chemicals employed in all spheres of human activity. However, in doing so we must ensure that our own existence is not endangered by their uncontrolled use, about which we know so little but are beginning to learn more. What we do know is obtained from animal studies conducted under controlled conditions on a short-, intermediate-or long-term basis. All of these studies are looking for dose-response relationships so that we may extrapolate them to the human situation, which is often uncontrollable. Animal studies can tell us about no observable effect levels, which are used to derive acceptable daily intakes for environmental contaminants and other chemicals.

The toxicological studies described in this chapter are applicable to most xenobiotics and, when coupled with tests for reproductive toxicity, mutagenicity/genotoxicity, and carcinogenicity, will usually satisfy the regulatory requirements of most countries. Because of this overriding ambition, many toxicological experiments have become rather stereotyped. However, a toxicological experiment should not be different from an experiment in any other scientific discipline. Thus, its experimental design should be logical and, hence, there is no valid reason to adhere to a standard protocol if this is inappropriate for the specific test material. Regulatory guidelines are only a useful index of what is required and should not be used as a rigid checklist, because there are virtually no findings in experimental toxicology that can be simply extrapolated to man and his ecosystem without careful thought. When it is considered appropriate to modify an approach recommended by a particular regulatory agency, it is wise to discuss this with, and get agreement from, the agency in order to avoid subsequent administrative complications.

Furthermore, by performing experiments to a standardized protocol, toxicologists are missing real opportunities to unravel some of the most fascinating problems of biology by identifying chemical tools to probe life processes. There may often be too much emphasis on the generation of data with very little time available for scientific interpretation. It is this aspect of toxicological research that must be encouraged to survive or else the science will become as stereotyped as the studies conventionally performed for economic/regulatory purposes. Therefore, consider abandoning a standard protocol if it is inappropriate, and feel free to increase the number of animals employed, particularly with regard to reversibility studies, because the best way of reducing the number of experiments performed on living animals is to conduct them properly. However, as noted above, studies carried out for regulatory agencies should be discussed with the agency before proceeding with extensive modifications.

It is essential to randomize the animals at the beginning of the study as well as during intermediate and terminal investigations. Always look for dose–response relationships and compare the data obtained with the controls as well as appropriate historical values for animals of the same age, sex and physiological condition. Above all, ensure that all observations are recorded in plain English. Remember that the primary purpose of a toxicological experiment is the same as that of any other scientific study—that is, that it can be repeated, blemishes and all!

REFERENCES

Draize, J. H., Woodward, G. and Calvery, H. O. (1944). Methods for the study of irritations and toxicity of substances applied topically to the skin and mucous membranes. *J. Pharmacol. Expt. Ther.* **82**, 377–390.

Ballantyne, B. (1987). Toxicology of cyanides. In Ballantyne, B. and Marrs, T. C. (Eds), *Clinical and Experimental Toxicology of Cyanides*. John Wright, Bristol, pp. 41–126.

British Toxicology Society (1984). Working party on toxicity. A new approach to the classification of substances and preparations on the basis of their acute toxicity. *Hum. Toxicol.*, **3**, 85–92.

Bucher, J. R., Portier, C. J., Goodman, J. I., Faustman, E. M. and Lucier, G. W. (1996). National toxicology program studies: principles of dose selection and applications to mechanistic based risk assessment. *Fundam. Appl. Toxicol*, **31**, 1–8.

Calabrese, E. J. (1983). *Principles of Animal Extrapolation*. Wiley-Interscience, New York, pp. 538–539.

Dayan AD (1987). Editorial. A framework for the use of primates? *Hum. Toxicol.* **6**, 449–450.

Dixit, R. and Kacew, S. (1997). Use of moderate dietary restriction in safety assessment. *Fundam. Appl. Toxicol.* **36**, Suppl., 106.

FAO/WHO (1997). *Pesticide Residues in Food. Joint FAO/WHO Meeting on Pesticide Residues. Evaluations 1996, Part II: Toxicology*. WHO, Geneva, pp. 179–194.

Haseman, J. K., Barbone, J. and Eustis, S. L. (1994). Effect of individual housing and other experimental design factors on tumor incidence in B6C3F1 mice. *Fundam. Appl. Toxicol.*, **23**, 44–52.

Hayes, A. W. (Ed.) (1982). *Principles and Methods of Toxicology*. Raven Press, New York.

Johnson, M. K. (1992). Molecular events in delayed neuropathy: experimental aspects of neuropathy target esterase. In Ballantyne, B. and Marrs, T. C. (Eds), *Clinical and Experimental Toxicology of Organophosphates and Carbamates*. Butterworth-Heinemann, Oxford, pp. 90–113.

Kennedy, G. L. and Trochimowicz, H. J. (1982). Inhalation toxicology. In Hayes, A. W. (Ed.), *Principles and Methods of Toxicology*. Raven Press, New York, pp. 185–208.

Lansdown, A. B. G. and Conning, D. M. (1990). Animal husbandry. In Anderson, D. and Conning, D. M. (Eds), *Experimental Toxicology the Basic Issues*. pp. 83–106. The Royal Society of Chemistry, Cambridge.

Lotti, M. (1992). Central neurotoxicity and behavioural effects of anticholinesterases. In Ballantyne, B. and Marrs, T. C. (Eds), *Clinical and Experimental Toxicology of Organophosphates and Carbamates*. Butterworth-Heinemann, Oxford, pp. 75–83.

Lumley, C. E., Parkinson, C. and Walker, S. R. (1992). An international comparison of the maximum duration of chronic animal toxicity studies. *Hum. Exp. Toxicol.*, **11**, 155–162.

McNamara, B. P. (1976). *Estimates of the Toxicity of Hydrocyanic Acid Vapors in Man*. Edgewood Arsenal Technical Report EG-TR-76023. Edgewood Arsenal, Maryland.

Ministry of Health and Welfare, Japan (1990). *Guidelines for Toxicity Studies of Drugs Manual, New Drugs Division*. Pharmaceutical Affairs Bureau, Tokyo.

OECD (1981). *OECD Guidelines for the Testing of Chemicals, Carcinogenicity Studies*. OECD Guideline 451. Organization for Economic Cooperation and Development, Paris.

OECD (1992). *OECD Guideline for the Testing of Chemicals, Acute Oral Toxicity—Fixed Dose Method*. OECD Guideline 420. Organization for Economic Cooperation and Development, Paris.

OECD (1996). *OECD Guideline for the Testing of Chemicals, Acute Oral Toxicity–Acute Toxic Class Method*. OECD Guideline 423. Organization for Economic Cooperation and Development, Paris.

OECD (1998). *OECD Guideline for the Testing of Chemicals, Acute Oral Toxicity–up-and-down Procedure*. OECD Guideline 425. Organization for Economic Cooperation and Development, Paris.

Parkinson, C. and Grasso, P. (1993). The use of the dog in toxicity tests on pharmaceutical compounds. *Hum. Exp. Toxicol.*, **12**, 99–109.

Society of Toxicology (1989). SOT position paper comments on the LD_{50} and acute eye and skin irritation test. *Fundam. Appl. Toxicol.* **13**, 621–623.

Tee, L. B. G., Davies, D. S., Seddon, C. E. and Boobis, A. R. (1987). Species differences in the hepatotoxicity of paracetamol are due to differences in the rate of conversion to its cytotoxic metabolite. *Biochem. Pharmacol.*, **36**, 1041–1052.

Tucker, M. J. (1979). The effect of long-term food restriction on tumours in rodents. *Int. J. Cancer*, **23**, 803–808.

Tucker, M. J. (1987) Editorial. Factors influencing carcinogenicity testing in rodents. *Hum. Toxicol.*, **6**, 107–109

van den Heuvel (1990). Editorial. An alternative to the LD_{50}? *Hum. Exp. Toxicol.*, **9**, 369–370.

van den Heuvel, M. J., Dayan, A. D. and Shillaker, R. O. (1987). Evaluation of the BTS approach to testing of substances and preparations for their acute toxicity. *Hum. Toxicol.*, **6**, 279–291.

WHO (1987). *Principles for the Safety Assessment of Food Additives and Contaminants in Food.* Environmental Health Criteria No. 70. World Health Organization, Geneva.

Wilson, J. (1987). Cyanide in human disease. In Ballantyne, B. and Marrs, T. C. *Clinical and Experimental Toxicology of Cyanide.* John Wright, Bristol, pp. 292–311.

ADDITIONAL READING

Anderson, D. and Conning, D. M. (Eds.) (1993). *Experimental Toxicology. The Basic Issues, 2ⁿᵈ Edn.* Royal Society of Chemistry, Cambridge.

Ecobichon, D. J. (1992). *The Basis of Toxicity Testing.* CRC Press, Boca Raton, Fl.

Galli, C. L., Murphy, S. D. and Paoletti, R. (Eds.) (1980). *The Principles and Methods in Modern Toxicology.* Elsevier/North Holland Biomedical Press, Amsterdam.

Gorrod, J. W. (Ed) (1981). *Testing for Toxicity.* Taylor and Francis, Ltd., London.

Hayes, A. W. (Ed) (1994). *Principles and Methods of Toxicology, 3ʳᵈ Edn.* Raven Press, New York.

Svendson, P. and Hau, J. (Eds.) (1994). *Handbook of Laboratory Animal Science, Vols. 1 and 2.* CRC Press, Boca Raton, Fl.

Symposium (1998). Nutrition and toxicity modulation. *Int. J. Toxicol.*, **17**, 1–134.

WHO (1978). Principles and Methods for the Evaluation of the Toxicity of Chemicals. *Environmental Health Criteria, Vol. 6.* World Health Organization, Geneva.

Chapter 16
Pathological Techniques in Toxicology

Peter Greaves

CONTENTS

- General Approaches
- Methods Applicable to Specific Organ Systems
- References

GENERAL APPROACHES

For over 100 years microscopic evaluation of pathological alternations in human tissues has made major contributions to our understanding of diseases and remains a significant diagnostic tool in human medicine. Rather than diminish in importance in the face of novel imaging techniques, recent advances in immunology and biotechnology have served to reaffirm the central role of histopathology in the diagnoses of human diseases. This has occurred because the transfer of new technologies into the pathology laboratory has led to the development of new histological visualization procedures. These new methods represent a logical extension to the use of special stains on tissue sections and have provided the pathologist with powerful new objective techniques which allow more precise morphological and functional correlation of changes in tissues.

A similar spectrum of both classical histological and new technologies has also made important contributions in both experimental pathology and toxicology. Histopathological evaluation of tissue sections represents a major technique in experimental studies of human diseases. It also has a central role in conventional toxicology studies which are performed to assess the toxicity of xenobiotics, including novel therapeutic agents and industrial chemicals. The particular contribution of histopathology is its unique ability to assess a broad range of effects of xenobiotics on body and organ systems and processes.

The important place of histological assessment of tissues in regulatory toxicology has given rise to the development of the discipline of the toxicological pathologist. The work of the toxicological pathologist requires training in comparative pathology and clinical pathology in addition to an understanding of the principles of toxicology and experimental method. It is also important to understand the kinetics and metabolism of administered xenobiotics, particularly therapeutic agents. In this way, pathological alterations can be related to the degree of exposure of organs and tissues to administered agents and their metabolites (Zbinden, 1988).

A thorough knowledge of pathological techniques applicable to experimental pathology and problem solving in toxicology is an important and integral component of the skills needed by the toxicological pathologist. This needs to be linked to a good understanding of the latest methods in molecular biology and their application to histopathology. The aim of this chapter is to describe pathological techniques and technologies applicable to the morphological evaluation of alterations produced in laboratory animals during the toxicity testing of chemicals and place them in the context of specific organs and organ systems.

Basic techniques in autopsy and histology practice

Fundamental to good histopathological evaluation of tissue sections is a detailed autopsy which implies careful observation of the organs for any abnormalities and appropriate selection of tissues. The autopsy is the responsibility of the pathologist. It is conducted or supervized by an experienced pathologist, usually with the help of trained prosectors.

Whereas in human autopsy practice and in experimental pathology studies tissue sampling is usually directed towards particular lesions or organs of direct relevance to the problem under study, a more systematic approach is usually adopted in conventional toxicity studies. Most international regulatory guidelines require 30–40 tissues to be taken from all animals in most conventional toxicity studies. These are usually defined by the standard protocols of laboratories performing regulatory work. However, it is important to remain acutely aware that even the most complete tissue list remains a selective process and a careful inspection of the tissues for abnormalities at autopsy remains mandatory.

However, the precise selection of blocks and number of slides among different laboratories to achieve complete tissue lists can be very different. For instance, some laboratories will take two blocks of tissue from the rat liver in carcinogenicity bioassays, others as many as four (Maronpot et al., 1989). Thorough histological examination of the heart of the beagle dog requires at least five or six blocks to provide reasonable sampling of the four chambers, coronary arteries and areas sensitive to ischaemic damage such as the papillary muscles of the left ventricle. However, this number of sections appears unreasonably large to many laboratories examining large numbers of dogs for toxicity studies. This underlines the need for careful inspection of tissues at autopsy and adjustment of the tissue sampling procedure to take account of the particular chemical under study.

For routine purposes, tissues are fixed in formalin or formol–saline by most laboratories for practically all organs. Exceptions are eyes and testes, where formalin is a poor fixative. Here, Bouin's, Zenker's or Davidson's fixatives are used. Occasionally, Bouin's fluid is employed routinely for all tissues (Taradach and Greaves, 1984). Although fixation in Bouin's fluid produces excellent cytology, its cost effectiveness leaves much to be desired when used routinely and the simplicity of formalin is usually preferred. Moreover, formalin when used under stringent conditions can be employed as a fixative for many immunocytochemical and molecular biological techniques on tissue sections. Microwave fixation has potential for the pathology laboratory engaged in toxicology (Boon and Kok, 1987), but it has not been exploited to any great extent in this context and initial results have not been entirely satisfactory.

Haematoxylin and eosin remains the most widely used stain in most laboratories, supplemented where appropriate by a Romanovsky stain for haemopoietic cells, PAS for hepatic glycogen, glomerular basement membrane and the acrosome on testicular germ cells, trichrome and elastic stains for the myocardium and blood vessels and oil red O for neutral lipids.

Immunocytochemical techniques have now superseded traditional tinctorial stains for the demonstration of polypeptide hormones.

Organ weights

Some regulatory guidelines indicate that certain organs should be weighed during the course of the autopsy in conventional repeat dose toxicity studies (Alder and Zbinden, 1988). The extent to which organs are weighed varies between laboratory but organ weighing is a useful adjunct to macroscopic assessment. Therefore, the selection of organs for weighing is the primary responsibility of the study pathologist. Weighing helps to focus the histopathological examination on key target organs such as the liver and kidney, the weights of which are frequently altered be administration of xenobiotics. Heart weight is a guide to potential cardiac alterations and especially important in the assessment of cardiovascular drugs. Likewise, the lungs are weighed in inhalation studies as this can provide a useful indication of the extent of oedema or accumulation of exudate. Brain weight is employed as a stable reference point in adult animals as it is fairly independent of body weight changes. The weights of endocrine organs are useful guides to alterations in the endocrine status of laboratory animals. However, weighing a small and firmly attached organ such as the thyroid can severely disrupt its quality and orientation in the sections to offset any apparent advantage.

Testicular weights correlate with testicular toxicity and weights can be compared with in-life measurement of testicular size (Heywood and James, 1978; Creasy, 1998). Weighing the testis is a useful precaution at the early phase of development of a novel drug prior to any assessment of male fertility. By contrast, ovarian weight is highly variable as a consequence of cyclical ovarian development and is therefore a less sensitive indicator of treatment induced-changes in the female reproductive system(Long et al., 1998).

Histopathological evaluation of conventional toxicological studies

Much has been written on methods in histopathological assessment. However, it requires, above all, a systematic and meticulous approach to the assessment of tissue sections, correlating in-life observations, autopsy findings, organ weight and clinical pathology changes with histopathological alterations. Careful selection of diagnostic terminology is essential because many of the terms utilized in experimental pathology have been borrowed from human pathology where they may be applied to specific clinical conditions not relevant to laboratory animal species. Lucid summary reports are essential.

In conventional subacute and chronic toxicity studies and in carcinogenicity bioassays, a complete set of tissues from the top dose and control animals is routinely examined. In addition, any target organs or tissues showing tumours or other macroscopic alterations at autopsy in animals from intermediate dose groups are also assessed. This baseline approach is outlined in some of the regulatory guidelines. However, some pathologists avoid this selective approach and examine all tissues sampled from all animals. This approach is perhaps more costly from a histological processing point of view but has the merit of completeness and forms a more satisfactory basis for the rapid reporting of all the salient histopathological findings in every dose group. Cause of death assignment is another component of the assessment of carcinogenicity studies in rodents which is widely practised to aid statistical evaluation (Kodell et al., 1995).

The error which develops from the increased awareness of a lesion by the pathologist only after examining a considerable number of animals has been aptly termed by Roe (1977) 'diagnostic drift'. It is important to have a good understanding of the nature of any lesion before grading is undertaken and particular care given to selection of the 'cut-off' point for each grade (Greaves and Faccini, 1984). The appropriateness of blind slide reading as a means to avoid bias is another point of debate. However, blind slide reading as a routine process conflicts with the need to have relevant clinical, clinical pathology and macroscopic data to make an appropriate tissue diagnosis. For this reason, only doubtful lesions which persist after a careful and integrated non-blind review of tissue sections are those which should be evaluated in a properly designed blind review (Newberne and de la Iglesia, 1985).

Peer review of pathological findings and quality assurance audit of the processes in histopathological assessment have also become more important components of regulatory toxicology studies in recent years. Peer review is a relatively recent process so it remains a topic of debate and correspondence in the relevant journals. However, peer review serves to ensure integrity of the pathological diagnoses, encourages consistency and facilitates learning (Ward *et al.*, 1995). Moreover, it is generally accepted that a peer review or check of a percentage of the diagnoses in a particular study by a second pathologist provides a level of security for regulatory authorities. Some regulatory authorities have taken a clear stance on the audit of the processes which take place in the office of the toxicological pathologist. For instance, the UK regulatory authorities require a critical phase audit of this part of the study which includes evaluation of the completeness, quality and labelling of glass slides given to the pathologist, review of the remarks made by the pathologist on missing or poor quality slides and verification that the pathologist has sufficient time to carry out the work required in the study protocol (Department of Health, 1988).

Another point that relates to the practice of toxicological pathology under the regulations of Good Laboratory Practice (GLP) is the definition of raw data. However, as slides, tissue blocks and wet tissues are retained as specimens under GLP, the pathologist's *final* signed and dated report is usually accepted as the raw data and not the various notes and memoranda that may be necessary in the construction of the definitive report (Lepore, 1996).

For over a decade the pathologist has been assisted in the evaluation of toxicity and carcinogenicity studies by computer recording, storage and collation of macroscopic findings and their corresponding histopathological diagnoses (Faccini and Naylor, 1979; Herrick *et al.*, 1983; Clapp and McNamee, 1985). This has been a particularly important contribution to the timely and accurate reporting of carcinogenicity studies where the number of observations in older animals renders hand recording and tabulation a time-consuming process, prone to transcription error. This has had a significant impact in the development of novel drugs as the carcinogenicity studies are usually performed towards the end of the development programme where the results from these studies may be needed before the drug can be extensively employed for therapeutic purposes.

Finally, it is worth noting that as new strategies are developed for the use of new models such as mouse transgenics to shorten the time taken and increase the accuracy of carcinogen identification, the same basic principles of evaluation of tumours in tissues are needed (Mahler *et al.*, 1998).

Histochemistry and cytochemistry

Histochemistry is a tool which is a system of chemical morphology that adds another dimension to the characterization of alterations in tissues. Changes to structures, cells or organelles can be assessed by the changes in their chemical structure or enzymatic activity. For instance, the well studied methods for alkaline phosphatase demonstrate activity at the cell membrane where active transport occurs. This can be used to localize and detect changes in structures such as the surface of the intestinal epithelium and the brush border of proximal renal tubules (Faccini, 1982). The histochemical method for 5'-nucleotidase is also an excellent marker for plasma membrane. Measures of peroxidase activity can be used to localize peroxisomes. Succinate dehydrogenase is used as an indicator for the Kreb's cycle and mitochondrial enzyme activity (Chayen *et al.*, 1973). The enzyme, γ-glutamyl transpeptidase is regarded as the classical marker for neoplastic foci in the rodent liver. Glucose-6-phosphate dehydrogenase, the regulatory enzyme of the pentose phosphate shunt, which provides ribose for the synthesis of nucleic acids, is elevated in a number of malignant conditions in man (Ibrahim *et al.*, 1983) and can also be used as a marker for foci of hepatocellular alteration in rats (Greaves *et al.*, 1986).

It is important to note that the use of histochemical methods for the simple localization of tissue constituents or pathological alterations is conceptually different to *quantitative cytochemistry*. This form of cytochemistry combines procedures for the production of insoluble chromophores by rigorous, controlled biochemical reactions with optical methods for their measurement (Chayen, 1984). To achieve enzyme measurement in this way it is imperative to avoid techniques such as fixation and the use of clearing agents and embedding media, all of which produce loss of enzymatic activity. Supercooling of tissues and the use of colloid stabilizers are essential in order to facilitate chemical reactions and the precipitation of insoluble reaction products close to the sites of active groups where they are generated

(Chayen, 1984). Coloured reaction products can then be visualized and measured by a spectrophotometer built around a microscope. This is coupled to a system to assess optically heterogeneous areas using methods such scanning and integrating microdensitometry.

Quantitative cytochemistry has advantages over biochemical measurements. It is non-disruptive, retains spatial relationships, relates activity measurement to histology and requires only small pieces of tissue. However, these advantages are offset by the fact that it is a labour-intensive technology. Quantitative cytochemical analysis has been undertaken to measure the effects of hormones in target tissues (Chayen, 1984) and in the characterization of the distribution of glycogen, glutathione and enzymatic activity within the liver lobule of rodents treated with xenobiotics (Irisarri and Mompon, 1983; Mompon et al., 1987).

Immunocytochemistry

Immunocytochemistry of routinely fixed and processed tissues has been one of the major technological advances in the histopathological evaluation and diagnosis of human diseases because it represents an independent, objective method of cell identification against which traditional subjective morphological criteria can be compared (Taylor and Kledzig, 1981). Immunocytochemistry has been particularly useful in the characterization of human neoplasms. However, unlike enzyme cytochemistry, it can usually only demonstrate the presence of antigenic determinants and is less able to demonstrate activity of cellular systems. Nevertheless, it represents a powerful tool for solving certain problems in toxicology. Many of the commercially available monoclonal and polyclonal antisera cross-react well with the tissues of laboratory animals and can be used in the histopathological evaluation of toxicity studies, provided that appropriate controls are applied. Examples include polypeptide and protein hormones, metabolizing enzymes, structural proteins and cell markers such as S100 protein and intermediate filaments (Schlage et al., 1998). An increasingly important measure in risk or safety assessment is cell proliferation (reviewed by Jones et al., 1996). The use of peroxidase-labelled or biotinated antibodies against bromodeoxyuridine (BrdUrd) represents an alternative to autoradiographic detection of cell proliferation using tritiated thymidine. Both of these methods require the administration of tritiated thymidine or BrdUrd prior to sacrifice. Another method which requires no prior administration of marker is the immunocytochemical staining of an auxiliary protein required in cell proliferation, the so-called proliferating cell nuclear antigen or PCNA (Jones et al., 1993; 1996).

Although haemopoietic cells retain species-specific surface markers, monoclonal antibodies to lymphocytic and monocytic surface membrane markers are available for rodents and dogs and can be used in the characterization of xenobiotic-induced alterations in the haemopoietic and lymphoid systems.

Lectin histochemistry

A technique closely allied to immunocytochemistry is that of lectin histochemistry. The term 'lectin' is applied to proteins and glycoproteins extracted from invertebrates and lower vertebrates that have the capacity to bind sugar groups and glycoproteins in specific ways. For many years studies on red blood cells have been performed with the lectin concanavalin A, which possesses haemagglutination properties. More recently, lectins labelled with peroxidase or fluorocene have been used to demonstrate specific sugar groups and glycoproteins histochemically in tissue sections (Nicholson, 1974; Spicer and Schulte, 1982). Lectin histochemistry has been used for the characterization of mucins, the demonstration of cell structures in normal tissues and changes in cell surface expression in malignant cells (Walker, 1985). In toxicology, the primary use is in the characterization of changes induced by xenobiotics in structures which are well delineated by labelled lectins such as the biliary canaliculus, testicular germ cell acrosome, renal tubule and bronchial and gastrointestinal epithelium (Geleff et al., 1986; Masson et al., 1986). The lectin Griffonia simplicifolia isolectin B$_4$ has also been used to stain microglia in the study of the toxic effects of xenobiotics on the rat cerebral cortex (Fix et al., 1996). Conventional formalin fixation and paraffin wax embedding are frequently adequate for the application of labelled lectin histochemistry, although alcoholic fixation or unfixed frozen sections may provide superior results in some cases.

Electron microscopy

Although electron microscopy is widely used as a basic research tool, transmission electron microscopy also has a well established role in the characterization of subcellular structural alterations in tissues which have been modified by the effects of xenobiotics. Despite the fact that electron microscopy only provides a static morphological assessment of cells, its ability to characterize changes in subcellular organelles can provide valuable information about any functional deficit. A common, almost routine, application of electron microscopy in regulatory toxicology studies is the characterization of cytoplasmic alterations associated with liver weight changes and hepatocellular hypertrophy. Electron microscopy allows the characterization of changes such as proliferation of the smooth endoplasmic reticulum, peroxisomal or mitochondrial proliferation, apoptosis and phospholipidosis. It is also important in the exclusion of subcellular degeneration in vital organs such as the heart when unexplained macroscopic or weight changes are seen without a light microscopic correlate.

A variety of methods for the selection, perfusion and immersion fixation of tissues have been proposed for the application of electron microscopy in toxicity studies. Optimum fixation is obtained by whole body perfusion with an aldehyde fixative, but this may conflict with procedures necessary for other components of a toxicity study such as routine histopathological examination, biochemical, metabolism and kinetic studies. One good compromise is perfusion fixation of freshly isolated samples of organs such as lung or liver. This provides superior tissue preparation to that obtained by immersion fixation (Roberts et al., 1990).

Despite the technological advances in transmission electron microscopy, especially semi-automated tissue processing and staining, it remains a demanding and labour-intensive process. Furthermore, it is highly selective and only small samples of tissues can be examined. Therefore, any electron microscopic work performed within the context of a toxicity study should have precisely defined objectives so that appropriate samples are selected and examined. Electron microscopy is not a method for speculative study of tissues in toxicity studies and defining no-effect dose levels.

The use of larger, semithin (1–3 μm thick) plastic- or resin-embedded sections is a cost-effective compromise between electron microscopy and conventional light microscopy. Sometimes termed 'high-resolution light microscopy', light microscopic evaluation of semi-thin sections provides a means of avoiding extensive use of the electron microscope because it can locate cytoplasmic organelles in a way sometimes not possible in paraffin-embedded material.

Scanning electron microscopy has some applications in the study of early chemical-induced changes on epithelial surfaces such as the gastrointestinal mucosa and the bladder epithelium. It also forms the basis for a robust technique for the examination of the middle ear in laboratory animals treated with ototoxic agents (Astbury and Read, 1982).

Immunocytochemistry can also be applied to electron microscopic study in order to define the subcellular distribution of antigenic sites. Ultrastructural autoradiography using tritium-labelled xenobiotics, especially when performed using quantitative methods such as the so-called hypothetical grain analysis, is valuable for the identification of sites of accumulation of drugs and chemicals within cells and may provide information on mode of cellular action (Read et al., 1985).

Confocal microscopy

Recent advances in microscopy have led to the application of confocal microscopy to the study of biological systems and this has found uses in toxicological pathology. Confocal imaging systems are based on the principle that both the illumination and detection systems are focused on the same single volume element of the specimen. This permits the examination of optical sections through intact tissue without the need for fixation, embedding, sectioning and staining. This has been applied to the study of a number of tissues but notably to the translucent tissues of the eye in ocular toxicity studies (Jester et al., 1996).

Morphometric methods

Morphometry represents a powerful tool applicable to the light and electron microscopic evaluation of xenobiotic-induced cellular and tissue changes. Morphometric study supports subjective histopathological descriptions or diagnoses by sharpening the distinction between normal and altered structures on a quantitative basis. It also allows different variables to be compared and correlated (Pesce, 1987). Morphometry has been applied to the study of a variety of organ toxicity, notably in the liver, pulmonary tract and brain (Weibel, 1979; de la Iglesia and McGuire, 1981; de la Iglesia et al., 1982; Barry and Crapo, 1985). Morphometric analysis requires good statistical methods in the choice of numbers of animals, number of samples per animal, the quantity of data points per sample and in the mode of data analysis. In the measurement of basic parameters such as volume density, surface density and numerical density, account should be taken of potential artefacts due to shrinkage of tissues following fixation and processing as well as the problems posed by magnification factors (Barry and Crapo, 1985). Semiautomated digital image analysis is also useful in the quantitation of immunocytochemical staining in the toxicology laboratory (Levine et al., 1987).

Application of molecular biology technology

Recombinant DNA technology represents the most recent transfer of basic research technology into the pathology laboratory. Molecular probes have been used to examine the structure and expression of specific genes in both normal and neoplastic human tissues. Current applications in clinical and anatomic pathology include rapid microbiological diagnosis, study of oncogene expression, gene amplification and drug resistance of tumours and molecular characterization of inherited diseases and their parental diagnosis (Fenoglio-Preiser and Willman, 1987).

These techniques have been widely applied in experimental pathology where they provide the pathologist with new opportunities for the study of mechanisms in pathological processes (DeLellis and Wolfe, 1987). They have been used in the study of experimental tumorigenesis, notably activated oncogenes in hepatic neoplasms in mice (Reynolds *et al.*, 1987). Other applications have been the examination of cell proliferation and gene rearrangements in various rodent organs (Malarkey and Maronpot, 1996; Hong *et al.*, 1998) and the study of mRNA expression such as in renin-excreting cells of the kidney (Doughty *et al.*, 1995). Some of the most important methods for the assessment of apoptosis in tissue sections are based on DNA polymerase-mediated or terminal deoxynucleotidyl transferase-mediated incorporation of biotinylated nucleotides to DNA strand breaks, so-called *in situ* end-labelling methods (Wheeldon *et al.*, 1995; Goldsworthy *et al.*, 1996; Pritchard and Watson, 1996).

METHODS APPLICABLE TO SPECIFIC ORGAN SYSTEMS

Skin and subcutaneous tissue

Careful visual inspection remains the principle component of the assessment of skin alterations or changes in the pelage of laboratory animals in conventional toxicity studies. In studies in which compounds are administered systematically, any skin abnormalities detected during life or at autopsy should be examined histologically. In addition, sections taken from carefully selected standard sites should also be sampled for routine histopathological examination. Haematoxylin and eosin staining is sufficient for most purposes. Drugs and chemicals given systematically may affect the skin in a number of ways. Pigmented skin or hair may lose its normal colour and albino skin may become coloured by administration of pigmented compounds or chemicals with pigmented metabolites. Agents with effects on sebaceous glands may alter the normal glossy pelage of laboratory animals. Compounds such as bleomycin which adversely effect mitotic activity in squamous epithelium lead to ulceration and inflammation in zones subjected to minor spontaneous trauma of everyday life such as the feet and tail (Thompson *et al.*, 1972; Szczech and Tucker, 1985).

Studies conducted to study topical irritancy, contact sensitization, or phototoxic activity usually employ rabbits or guinea pigs. Here, reliance is commonly placed on visual inspection and a semiquantitative assessment of the degree of erythema, swelling, erosion and ulceration of the treated skin without histopathological examination. A mouse ear model has been proposed for study of skin irritancy because it can be quantified more accurately by the measurement of ear thickness (Patrick *et al.*, 1985). Although histopathological techniques are not routinely practised in the assessment of skin irritation

and sensitization, histological examination can serve to define the nature of any induced changes. Moreover, semiquantitative histological examination has also been shown to be a useful adjunct to naked eye assessment of the epidermis in experimental irritancy studies (Ingram and Grasso, 1975).

Immunohistochemical study of Ia antigen expression in antigen presenting cells of the epidermis has been used in studying delayed hypersensitivity reactions in the guinea pig skin (Sobel and Colvin, 1986). The ultrastructural appearances of Langerhan's cells have also been shown to be modulated by topical application of sensitising or irritating substances. Irritating agents cause their degeneration and vacuolation, whereas sensitization increases numbers of cytoplasmic Birkbeck granules and coated vesicles (Kolde and Knop, 1987).

Histological examination of injection site injury and the local damage around subcutaneously implanted biomaterials is an essential part of the assessment of their irritancy potential. It is important to evaluate not only the character and severity of the surrounding cellular reaction to these materials but also the time course of the inflammatory and healing process in comparison with known negative and positive control substances (Autian 1972; Darby 1987; Henderson *et al.*, 1987).

In carcinogenicity studies performed in rodents, tumours of the skin and subcutaneous tissues are usually adequately diagnosed by conventional microscopic techniques. In certain instances, immunocytochemistry and electron microscopy are helpful in the characterization of soft tissue tumours. Mesenchymal cells can be more accurately defined by the presence of immune-reactive myoglobin, lysozyme, alpha-1 antichymotrypsin, intermediate filaments and other cytoplasmic antigens and also by electron microscopic evaluation of subcellular structures such as myofilaments, cross-striations, basal lamina and lysosomes (Greaves and Barsoum, 1990).

Mammary gland

In laboratory animals, the mammary gland represents a sensitive indicator of the pituatary–gonadal axis. It is liable to develop neoplasms either spontaneously with advancing age or following prolonged hormonal derangement induced by administration of xenobiotics. For these reasons mammary glands are examined carefully in conventional toxicity studies both during life and at autopsy and this is followed by histological examination.

The basic structure of the mammary gland is similar in all laboratory animal species. It is composed of a system of alveolar buds or acini connected by a system of branching ducts which eventually converge on the nipple. Ducts and alveolar tissues are not static structures but respond to changes of the oestrous or menstrual cycles, pregnancy and lactation and to those xenobiotics which induce analogous hormonal alterations. Therefore, histological assessment of treatment-induced changes in these structures provides useful information about the nature of hormonal derangements.

As laboratory rodents and beagle dogs possess several pairs of mammary glands, routine histological examination is usually conducted on a selected number of sites, frequently on one gland from each side plus any other showing macroscopic abnormality. Orientation remains a difficulty in small inactive glands but an attempt is made to take a section which includes the nipple, adjacent skin and underlying mammary ducts and acini.

Conventional haematoxylin and eosin stained sections are sufficient for mammary gland assessment. Myoepithelial cells which surround the ducts and acini may be difficult to visualize without special techniques, but immunocytochemical staining for cytokeratins and myosin is helpful in making this distinction (Warburton et al., 1982; Dulbecco et al., 1986). Myoepithelial and epithelial cells in the rat mammary gland have also been delineated on the basis of their activity in the histochemical reaction for ATPase. Myoepithelial cells show a reaction with Na^+, K^+-ATPase but epithelial cells only with Mg^{2+}-ATPase (Russo et al., 1982)

Haemopoietic and Lymphatic Systems

In conventional toxicity studies, blood smears, haemopoietic organs and lymphoid tissues are routinely examined by light microscopy in conjunction with automated analysis of peripheral red and white blood cells. Weighing and careful histological examination of thymus, spleen and lymph nodes are widely considered to be an important component in the examination of effects of xenobiotics on the immune system and forms part of the first tier of procedures adopted in immunotoxicity testing batteries in the National Toxicology Program and at the Chemical Industry Institute of Toxicology (Dean et al., 1986; Dean and Thurmond, 1987; Luster et al., 1988).

Blood smears are commonly examined using classical Romanowsky stains and conventional histological sections are taken from spleen, selected lymph nodes, thymus and decalcified bone marrow sections. The cellularity of bone marrow varies between different sites in laboratory animals. In rodents, bone marrow from the femur, sternum and vertebral bodies is considered to be the most representative (Cline and Maronpot, 1985; Wright, 1989). The cytology of bone marrow cells in decalcified, paraffin-embedded sections is not ideal and Romanowsky-stained bone marrow smears provide better cytological detail. The technical problems posed by the need to decalcify bone have been surmounted in some toxicology laboratories by the use of 3 μm thick methyl methacrylate-embedded sections stained with modified Giemsa or gallamine blue–Giemsa supplemented by Gomori's stain for reticulin, a technique originally developed by Burkhardt et al. (1982) for human bone marrow biopsies.

Critical histological examination of lymph nodes requires good orientation of the tissue to provide the basis for a clear assessment of the relative sizes of cortex, paracortex and medulla and their three-dimensional orientation. A semiquantitative assessment based on a standard approach defined by the World Health Organization (WHO) represents a good method for the characterization of functional alterations in the B and T cell zones of the lymphoid system (Cottier et al., 1972; van der Valk and Maijer, 1987).

Whereas the spleen functions as a blood storage organ and a site of extramedullary haemopoiesis, its discrete nature and small size in rodents makes it a useful organ to weigh and undertake morphometric analysis of the periarteriolar lymphoid sheaths (T cell zones) and germinal follicles (B cell areas). Spleen weight does not appear to be a reliable indicator of haemopoietic cellularity in the dog.

Conventional histological stains are readily supplemented by a variety of antibodies for the immunohistochemical localization of monocytic cells and lyphoid subsets. Whilst most reagents are monoclonal antibodies which require the use of frozen tissue sections or smear preparations, many are commercially available for specific cells in the common laboratory animal species. For the mouse, these include antibodies to Thy-1 for T lymphocytes and thymocytes, Lyt-1 for helper T cells and Lyt-2 for cytotoxic/suppressor T cells (Ahmed and Smith, 1983). An antibody to asialo GM1 (ganglio-n-tetrosylceramide) has been employed as a marker for murine natural killer cells in the study of the toxicity of human recombinant interleukin-2 in the mouse (Anderson et al., 1988). Mouse monoclonal antibodies W3/13, W3/25 and MRC OX8 have been employed immunocytochemically as pan-T, helper-T and suppressor/cytotoxic-T lymphocytes respectively, in the study of the effects of immune modulators in the laboratory rat using both tissue sections and immunogold staining of peripheral blood smears (Evans et al., 1988a). A mouse monoclonal antibody to Thy-1 can also be used to label canine T-lymphocytes (Evans et al., 1988b).

Antibodies to immunoglobulins or immunoglobulin light chains can be used in the characterization of B-lymphocytes in paraffin wax-embedded sections.

Musculoskeletal System

An assessment of long bone growth is conveniently made by measurement of long bone length. The femur is frequently used for this purpose in laboratory animals. Measurement can also be conducted by radiographic means, which is an effective in vivo measure of bone growth in immature animals when treated by agents affecting bone (Robinson et al., 1982).

Appropriate laboratory processing of bone is a prerequisite for good histological assessment. Formalin is adequate for most purposes, followed by decalcification using acidic fluids and embedding in paraffin wax. The use of polarized light microscopy is helpful in the identification of bone types in decalcified sections for such use can demonstrate the patterns of collagen orientation. Undecalcified sections using methacrylate or similar hard embedding media, supplemented by stains such as von Kossa, Goldner trichrome or solochrome cyanine, are essential for the assessment of bone mineralization.

The choice of sampling site is particularly important in toxicity studies in laboratory animals. It should be an identical site in all animals within a particular study, as it has been shown that even modest differences in sampling site can influence histomorphological variables of bone (Anderson and Danylchuk, 1978). In long bones, histological examination is usually directed to the metaphysis. Chondrocytes dividing in the metaphysis as columns of proliferating cells and maturing into hypertrophic cells are responsible for bone growth. Therefore, examination of this zone, particularly if morphometric analysis is also carried out, is an ideal place to evaluate bone formation and resorption in studies designed to evaluate xenobiotics which affect this process (Schenk et al., 1986).

The use of vital fluorescent labels such as tetracycline, alizarin red S, calcein, procion or haematoporphyrin can be used to visualize sites of bone mineralization in tissue sections of bone from laboratory animals (Solheim, 1974).

Articular cartilage reacts to chemical insult only in a limited way (Mankin, 1974). Like bone, cartilage represents a stratified structure growing from the chondrosseous junction of the epiphysis which can be assessed histologically using conventional processing and staining procedures. Special stains such as toluidine blue and safranine O, lectin histochemistry and immunocytochemistry or electron microscopy represent further tools for the study of chondrocytes, glycosaminoglycans and collagen in the matrix (Mankin, 1974; Brighton et al., 1984; Gough et al., 1985; Kirivanta et al., 1987; Farnum and Wilsman, 1988).

Conventionally processed and stained sections are employed for routine purposes for the appraisal of intramuscular irritancy of locally injected drugs and embedded biomaterials. As at other sites of local damage, is important to assess the extent and nature of local damage and the time course of the repair process. The rabbit sacrospinalis muscle is the model of choice in the assessment of intramuscular preparations (Gray, 1981), but muscles in rat and dog are also used. Histological evaluation of muscle damage can be supplemented by histochemical methods for enzymes such as succinate dehydrogenase and acid phosphatase which correlate with damage and repair activity (Salthouse and Willigan, 1972). Immunohistochemical stains for structural components such as myosin isoforms, collagen, fibronectin, myoglobin, laminin and desmin have also be used as adjuncts to assess alterations induced by xenobiotics in skeletal muscle (Helliwell, 1988).

It should be remembered that skeletal muscle fibres are heterogeneous in type and different types may respond differently to adverse stimuli. Although an over-simplification, two main types of fibres exist, the slow twitch or type I fibres and the fast twitch or type II fibres. These fibres are usually distinguished histochemically in frozen sections using their differences in myosin ATPase activity (Brooke and Kaiser, 1970; Pierobon-Bormioli et al., 1980, 1981; Billeter et al., 1981).

Pulmonary System

Nasal chambers are the structures which are first subjected to the effects of inhaled substances. Although they are not studied in great detail in conventional toxicity studies, it is vital that they are examined histologically when drugs and other chemicals are administered by inhalation. In rodents, the small size of the bones of the nose and nasal sinuses make a simple transverse blocking procedure following decalcification a cost-effective way to provide standardized histological sections (Young, 1981). A series of standard diagrams for the examination and recording of lesions in the nasal passages of rats and mice have been devised (Mery et al., 1994). For large animals, a complex dissection is required for histological assessment of the nasal mucosa.

Careful inspection of the lungs in a good light after opening the thoracic cavity at autopsy provides important information about pathological alterations. Changes may be manifest by uneven collapse, enlargement or overinflation, patchy discoloration or stiffness of the lung parenchyma as well as the presence of oedema or pleural effusions. Total weight or dry/wet weight ratios can be sensitive indicators of lung damage and oedema, although vascular congestion may be a confounding factor (Nemery et al., 1987).

Various methods of lung fixation are available. Immersion fixation in neutral buffered formalin is widely employed for most routine purposes and has the advantage of retaining exudates and fluids within the air spaces and airways. Instillation of fixative via the trachea under constant pressure (25–30 cm water) shows structural alterations well, although it has a tendency to dislodge exudates. Use of formalin vapour, perfusion fixation via the vasculature and freezing in liquid nitrogen are other methods which are employed (Tyler et al., 1985; Nemery et al., 1987).

Ultrastructural study has a place in the elucidation of selective structural damage to the pulmonary parenchyma, but the size of the lungs and the diversity of its cellular components create problems of fixation and sampling. The technical considerations for fixation for ultrastructural study of the lung in toxicological studies have been reviewed by Tyler *et al.*, (1985). Extensive use of semi-thin sections is helpful for the selection of samples and a rigorous, tiered approach to random sampling is necessary for morphometric study (Barry and Crapo, 1985).

As in other tissues, immunocytochemical, cytochemical and autoradiologic techniques are important in the study of the effects of xenobiotics on lung tissue. For instance, the pulmonary vascular leak syndrome of human recombinant interleukin-2 in mice has been studied by the use of an immunocytochemical method to demonstrate T lymphocytes, macrophages and natural killer and lymphokine-activated killer cells (Anderson *et al.*, 1988). Monoxygenase enzymes and important structural components such as collagen, cytokeratins and laminin can also be studied in this way (Gil and Martinez-Hernandez, 1984; Linnoila and Petrusz, 1984; Schlage *et al.*, 1998). Mucin histochemistry is helpful in the study of changes in the lining epithelium of the bronchi (Sturgess and Reid, 1973; Sturgess, 1985).

Cardiovascular System

Of key importance to the pathological evaluation of the heart in toxicity studies is the careful visual inspection of the pericardium, myocardium, endocardium and valve cusps of each cardiac chamber. Cardiac weight in laboratory animals varies with body weight, body length, age, sex and circulatory demand. For this reason, weighing the heart is not only a useful guide to the toxic effects of xenobiotics on the myocardium but is also a measure of functional adaptation to cardiac work load. This is particularly true if individual ventricles are also weighed or ventricular wall thickness is measured as this may provide information about any changes affecting either the pulmonary or the systemic circulation.

Careful sampling of representative sections of each cardiac chamber is also important for adequate histological assessment (Piper, 1981). These should include segments of the coronary arteries, valves and zones sensitive to ischaemia such as the endocardium and papillary muscles of the left ventricle (Greaves, 1998). Histological examination of the cardiac conducting tissue is not conducted routinely in regulatory toxicity studies as it requires a large number of tissue sections for thorough study. However, a simplified method for the examination of the sinuatrial and atrioventricular nodes in the dog has been proposed which can be more routinely applied (Palate *et al.*, 1995).

Conventional fixation, paraffin wax embedding, haematoxylin and eosin with connective tissue, fibrin and elastic stains are the cornerstones for the detection of myocardial and vascular alterations. Polarized light microscopy using formalin-fixed sections stained with picrosirius red is a powerful technique for the assessment of the distribution, size and orientation of collagen fibres

within myocardial scar tissue (Pick *et al.*, 1989; Whittaker *et al.*, 1989).

Other histological techniques include the detection of early myocardial damage in formalin-fixed tissue using demonstration of the loss of myosin, tropomyosin ATPase, creatine kinase or lactate dehydrogenase from muscle fibres (Block *et al.*, 1983; Hayakawa *et al.*, 1984; Spinale *et al.*, 1989). Damaged muscle fibres stain red with the basic fuchsin–picric acid method or develop fluorescence in haematoxylin-stained sections (Al-Rufaie *et al.*, 1983).

Digestive System

The mouth is subjected to visual inspection in conventional toxicity studies and the tongue is commonly sectioned for histopathological examination of the oral mucosa. Major salivary glands are examined using conventional processing and staining techniques although mucin histochemical stains are useful in the study of alterations in mucin secretion in these glands. The mature dentition is not usually affected by xenobiotics but some drugs such as anticancer agents have been shown to affect the immature dentition (Stene and Koppang, 1976; Robinson and Harvey, 1989). For this reason, it may be necessary to examine the dentition histologically in animals treated with xenobiotics. This is performed using the techniques employed for bone. Standardized sections for examination of rat incisors have been proposed (Kuijpers *et al.*, 1996).

Histological examination of the gastrointestinal tract itself is complicated by its great length and the fragility of the mucosa before fixation. Careful inspection without vigorous washing is essential both to locate lesions and to avoid artefacts in histological sections which mimic inflammation and ulceration. Although selective blocking is usually appropriate if preceded by careful macroscopic inspection, the so-called 'Swiss roll' techniques are valuable for a detailed histological survey of the gastrointestinal epithelium. These methods can be adjusted for use in laboratory rodents, larger animal species and man. They may be performed on fresh tissue or after fixation (Filipe and Branfoot, 1974; Greaves *et al.*, 1980; Moolenbeck and Ruitenberg, 1981).

Mucin stains are useful tools in the study of xenobiotic-induced changes in the gastrointestinal mucosa. This can be approached by both conventional mucin histochemistry or lectin histochemistry on formalin-fixed and paraffin wax-embedded material. The techniques are applicable to the study of the gastrointestinal mucosa from laboratory animals and man although there are considerable interspecies difference in the distribution of glycoconjugates demonstrated by these methods (Sheahan and Jarvis, 1978; Tsiftis *et al.*, 1980; Greaves and Boiziau, 1984; Ishihara *et al.*, 1984). Argyrophil staining is useful in the characterization of enterochromaffin cells of the stomach and intestine because of their endogenous reducing activity. Argyrophil staining has been widely employed in the study of the effects of hist-amine H2 receptor blockers on enterochromaffin cells in the rodent gastrointestinal tract (Hirth *et al.*, 1988; Betton *et al.*, 1988; Streett *et al.*, 1988). Immunohisto-chemistry is also used for the characterization of these enterochromaffin cells in the mucosa, notably using anti-sera to histamine, histidine decarboxylase, neurone-specific enolase and chromogranin A (Hirth *et al.*, 1988; Betton *et al.*, 1988). The use of immunocytochem-istry for the study of cell proliferation using PCNA or BrdUrd is also important in the study of the effects of xenobiotics on the gastrointestinal tract. The various techniques used for the characterization of apoptosis complete the repertoire in the study of the effects of drugs on cell turnover in the gastrointestinal tract (reviewed by Pritchard and Watson, 1996).

Monoclonal antibodies against lymphoid surface markers are used for the study of the mucosa-associated lymphoid system or MALT in laboratory animals (Bland and Warren, 1985; Ermak and Owen, 1986; Martin *et al.*, 1986). The so-called M cells overlying Peyer's patches can only be adequately demonstrated at the ultrastruc-tural level or by the paucity of alkaline phosphatase activity (Owen and Bhalla, 1983). Mucosal mast cells in rats have been shown to be demonstrable in convention-ally processed tissues by prolonged toluidine blue stain-ing (Widgren and Enerbäck, 1983).

As the principle site of metabolism and detoxification of drugs and other xenobiotics, the liver is a frequent site of alterations in toxicity studies and is therefore the focus of careful histopathological assessment. In conven-tional studies, the liver is weighed prior to fixation and selection of blocks for processing for light and electron microscopy as well as other techniques. The relatively large size of the liver presents problems of selection of tissue blocks and considerable interlaboratory variation exists in the hepatic blocking schedule exists. For instance, blocks processed from the rat liver for routine histological examination in conventional toxicity studies may vary from between one to over five (personal obser-vations). In the National Toxicology Program (NTP) rat carcinogenicity studies, the procedure involves the selec-tion of two blocks taken from the widest parts of the left lobe and the right median lobe (Maronpot *et al.*, 1989). Selection of two blocks appears to be the generally accepted practice for routine rodent liver histopatholog-ical examination in many laboratories. Fine needle aspiration of hepatic tissue from rodents, fixation in ethanol and staining with the Papanicolaou stain, in a manner similar to that used in human medicine, repre-sents a method of sampling which can be used *in vivo* (Giampaolo *et al.*, 1989).

Electron microscopy, enzyme cytochemistry, immun-ocytochemistry and molecular biological methods have well accepted roles in the characterization of changes in induced by xenobiotics in the liver of laboratory animals. It is frequently necessary to characterize the proliferation of smooth endoplasmic reticulum, peroxi-somes or mitochondria and lysosomal alternations such as phospholipidosis when treatment-induced changes in liver weight are recorded or there is light microscopic evidence of hepatocyte hypertrophy. Quantification of both hepatic cell proliferation using PCNA or BrdUrd and apoptosis with methods such as *in situ* end-labelling are becoming increasingly important in toxicology (Goldsworthy *et al.*, 1996; Wheeldon *et al.*, 1995).

As the liver possesses considerable functional hetero-geneity within the lobule (Jungerman and Katz, 1982), cytochemical methods for reactions such as catalase, uri-case, various dehydrogenases, alkaline phosphatase, 5′-nucleotidase and NADH$_2$ diaphorases as well as glu-tathione form a bridge between morphology and activity measured by classical biochemical techniques (Chayen, 1984; Mompon *et al.*, 1987). Although cytochrome P450 activity is difficult to measure directly by cytochemical techniques, immunocytochemistry localizes immune-reactive metabolizing enzymes in tissue sections (Moody *et al.*, 1985; Foster *et al.*, 1986).

A number of histochemical methods have been applied to the study of foci of cellular alteration in the rodent liver. These include the classical marker γ-glutamyl transpeptidase, glucose-6-phosphate dehydrogenase and immunohistochemical demonstration of placental glutathione *S*-transferase (Farber, 1984; Greaves *et al.*, 1986; Tatematsu *et al.*, 1987). Immunocytochemical detection of oncogene proteins has also been used in the study of oncogene expression in the liver of carcinogen-treated rodents (Richmond *et al.*, 1988).

Another histochemical technique of potential import-ance is the direct Schiff reaction, which can detect the presence of cellular aldehydes or free radicals produced *in vivo* when it is performed on cryostat sections (Rushmore *et al.*, 1987; Taper *et al.*, 1988).

Urinary Tract

The kidney is particularly important in toxicology because many xenobiotics or their metabolites are eliminated primarily through the urinary tract. In addition, the kidney is liable to be exposed quickly to peak concentrations of circulating xenobiotics by virtue of its high blood flow. Its ability to concentrate toxic solutes in renal tubular cells or in the tubular lumen is an additional risk factor.

Renal weight changes are a useful guide to renal tox-icity, although renal weight may also alter as a physiolog-ical response to changes in renal demand. Hence it is essential that the assessment of renal toxicity includes careful visual inspection of the renal parenchyma at autopsy for appearances of toxicity such as swelling, pallor, congestion and haemorrhage, and this should be followed by histopathological examination. Inspection of the contents of the renal pelvis for crystals, mineral and cellular debris is also important at autopsy as these substances may be lost in subsequent tissue handling and processing.

Conventional fixation and processing followed by haematoxylin and eosin staining supplemented by PAS are usually appropriate for most conventional toxicity studies. It is important that all parts of the nephron are examined microscopically, so histological sections should comprise both cortex and medulla and include the tip of the papilla.

A variety of techniques are available for more detailed study of xenobiotic-induced alterations in the nephron. Electron microscopy has a time-honoured place in the study of pathological alterations in both the glomerulus and renal tubule, although perfusion fixation may be needed for good preservation of tubular cells for ultra-structural study (Verlander, 1998). Light microscopy of plastic embedded sections 1–3 μ m thick is a useful compromise which provides excellent resolution of renal structures (Gregg et al., 1990).

Various parts of the renal tubule show different enzyme activities which relate to the function of different segments (Guder and Ross, 1984; Lock and Reed, 1998). Histochemical demonstration of enzyme activities can therefore be used as markers for components of the nephron and for structural–functional studies. For instance, lysosomal enzyme activity is highest in the proximal tubule, reflecting the role of this segment in the degradation of reabsorbed macromolecules. Therefore, enzyme cytochemical demonstration of acid phosphatase or other lysosomal enzymes outlines the proximal tubule. Demonstration of acid phosphatase at the electron microscopic level using the cerium technique has been employed in the characterization of drug-induced alterations in proximal tubular lysosomes (Read et al., 1988). Of special interest to the pathologist as cytochemical markers are brush border enzymes, alkaline phosphatase, $5'$-nucleotidase and γ-glutamyl transpeptidase, which are useful in the study of tubular damage (Faccini, 1982). Measurement of enzyme activity in the urine is also a useful complementary, non-invasive technique for the assessment of tubular toxicity in man and laboratory animals because cellular enzymes from damaged tubular cells spill into the urine in increased amounts (Kluwe, 1981; Zbinden et al., 1988; Clemo, 1998).

Immunocytochemistry can also be used to demonstrate the presence of brush border enzymes such as γ-glutamyl transpeptidase (Yasuda and Yamashita, 1985). Immunocytochemical demonstration of Tamm–Horsfall proteins, localized at the surface membrane of the thick ascending loop of Henle, has also been used for the study of renal tubular changes induced by xenobiotics (Howie et al., 1990).

In the study of drug-induced alterations to the juxtaglomerular apparatus, immunocytochemical staining using antisera to renin is superior to the classical, non-specific techniques for renin-containing granules such as the Bowie and Hartroft stains (Faraggiana et al., 1982; Zaki et al., 1982). More recently, drug-induced modification in renin mRNA expression in rat juxtaglomerular cells has been demonstrated in tissue sections by in situ hybridization (Doughty et al., 1995).

It is worth recording that labelled lectins can be used to localize different segments of the nephron histochemically and this can often be performed on formalin-fixed, paraffin wax-embedded material (Schulte and Spicer, 1983; Holthofer, 1983; Murata et al., 1983). For instance, peanut lectin (Phaseolus vulgaris, PNA) and Ricinus comminis (RCA) stain the S1 and S2 segments of the rat proximal tubule whereas the S2 segment remains poorly stained. The mouse proximal tubule brush border stains with Lotus tetragonolobus (LTA) (Schulte and Spicer, 1983).

Histological study of the bladder mucosa requires special care. The best orientation of the epithelium is obtained following inflation of the bladder with fixative at autopsy, as this removes folds which can give a misleading impression of the thickness of the epithelium. However, this procedure may dislodge exudates and other material from the bladder lumen, so care should be exercised in its application. Assessment of cell proliferation can be important in the assessment of hyperplasia and neoplasia of the bladder epithelium. Scanning electron microscopy is a useful special technique for the examination of chemically induced alterations to the superficial transitional epithelium.

Reproductive System

The effects of xenobiotics on reproduction are usually examined in special reproductive studies in which histopathological examination plays relatively little part. However, histopathological examination of the male and female reproductive tract is an important component of conventional toxicity studies. At an early stage of the development of a new medicine this histopathological examination may represent the only assessment of treatment-related effects on the reproductive organs and germ cells and therefore needs to be performed with care. Special fixatives are routinely employed for light microscopic examination of the testes because formalin is a poor method of preservation of the germinal epithelium prior to embedding in paraffin wax. Immersion in Bouin's, Zenker's or Helly's fluids is commonly used, followed by paraffin wax embedding and staining with haematoxylin and eosin. PAS is used for the demonstration of the germ cell acrosome as this permits the most precise staging of the germ cell cycle in laboratory animals and in humans (Clermont, 1972). More recently, the cycle of the seminiferous epithelium has been defined in formalin-fixed plastic-embedded testis stained with toluidine blue (Russell and Frank, 1978; Ulvik *et al.*, 1982). This method provides excellent cytology of the germinal epithelium.

A number of quantitative and semiquantitative methods have been devised for the assessment of the effects of xenobiotics on testicular germ cells. These involve measurement of the cross-sectional area of seminiferous tubules and of germ cell–Sertoli cell ratios and counting the number of spermatids per tubule (Creasy, 1997).

The female reproductive system is examined histologically using conventional histological techniques, paying close attention to the cyclical alteration in the endometrium, vaginal mucosa and ovarian tissue. The ovary requires careful orientation if sections are to include cortex, medulla and hilar tissue. As ovarian function is closely linked to the endocrine system, it is important that in any assessment of the reproductive tract, account is taken of endocrine organs. In the National Toxicology Program (NTP), alterations in reproductive organs induced by a variety of different chemicals, were frequently associated with changes in the pituitary gland and adrenal cortex (Maronpot, 1987).

Endocrine System

The capacity of the mammalian organism to function as an integral and independent unit depends on the endocrine system operating in concert with the nervous system. Interrelationships between endocrine organs are complex. There are close links between the hypothalamus, the pituitary gland and the rest of the endocrine and nervous systems. The nervous system releases substances which act as circulating hormones and hormones released by endocrine cells also have local effects. As a consequence, endocrine organs are extremely sensitive to stimulation and inhibition by trophic or antitrophic substances, end organ feedback and systemic perturbations induced by administration of high doses of active chemicals. Furthermore, the close link between secretory function of endocrine tissue and proliferative activity (Pawlikowski, 1982) concords with the frequent observation in toxicity studies that a common response to excessive stimulation is endocrine hyperplasia and neoplasia. By contrast, endocrine cells often appear resistant to the direct cellular toxic effects of xenobiotics.

For these reasons histological examination of endocrine tissues is important in toxicity studies. Such studies should carefully designed to avoid the effects of environmental and other experimental variables on the endocrine system and hormone measurements (Davies, 1993). Where technically possible, histological examination is preceded by weighing of the organs. However, this may not be advisable for firmly bound organs such as the thyroid gland owing to the risk of disruption of histological sections. Moreover, total adrenal weight is not a good indicator of adrenal medullary size as it represents only 10–20% of adrenal size (Neville, 1969).

Important for the examination of peptide-containing endocrine organs is immunocytochemistry. Antisera to many peptide hormones are widely available and provided that appropriate dilution and absorption controls are employed, they can be used in the examination of the endocrine tissues of most conventional laboratory animal species. They have superseded the tinctoral stains in the examination of the pituitary gland altered by drugs and hormones (El Etreby and Fath el Bab, 1977; El Etreby *et al.*, 1977; Zak *et al.*, 1985; Lloyd and Landefeld, 1986; Lloyd and Mailloux, 1987). Islet cell pathology can be demonstrated in rats, primates and dogs by immunocytochemical staining for insulin, somatostatin, glucagon and pancreatic polypeptide (Spencer *et al.*, 1986; Wieczorek *et al.*, 1998). C-cells in the thyroid gland are clearly delineated in the thyroid by immunocytochemistry for calcitonin (DeLellis *et al.*, 1987). Immunohistochemical demonstration of the acidic protein chromogranin A is also a good marker in different species for many endocrine cells containing secretory granules (Hawkins *et al.*, 1989). Techniques of *in situ* hybridization for the detection of mRNA are also applicable to the identification of peptide-producing cells in the endocrine system (Bloch, 1985).

Immunostaining for non-polypeptide hormones such as steroids and catecholamines is less well developed and conventional methods for histopathological assessment are still widely employed. Standard special stains for lipids using frozen sections and electron microscopy are applicable to the characterization of changes in the adrenal cortex. Immunocytochemical approaches have been used in the study of cytochromes P450 in the adrenal cortex (Le Goascogne *et al.*, 1987).

The chromaffin reaction, with darkening on exposure to aqueous solutions of potassium dichromate as a result of oxidation and polymerization of catecholamines, remains a useful stain in the study of catecholamine activity in the medulla (Tischler *et al.*, 1985). More reliable may be formaldehyde vapour or glycoxylic acid treatment and fluorescence microscopy (Tischler and DeLellis, 1988). Neurone-specific enolase is consistently present in the rat and mouse adrenal medulla and can be used as a histochemical marker for proliferative and neoplastic alteration in this tissue (Wright *et al.*, 1990). The examination of electron-dense granules in the medulla is also useful for the detailed characterization of medullary cells (Rhodin, 1974).

Nervous System and Special Sense Organs

Careful histological examination of the nervous system frequently reveals subtle structural alterations which precede evidence of functional abnormality. However, this sensitivity is dependent on the identification of vulnerable zones and determination of the nature of the tissue alterations under study (Spencer *et al.*, 1980). This requires careful selection of nervous tissues and their appropriate fixation, processing and staining, often in ways that are different from the techniques employed for other tissues.

Perfusion fixation of the brain is ideal for the avoidance of fixation artefact, although immersion fixation followed by conventional processing is adequate for most routine purposes. It is essential to be aware of the artefacts which can develop in the immersion fixation of brain so that they are not confounded with treatment-induced alterations (reviewed by Garman, 1990).

It is important that blocks for histological examination are carefully selected to ensure that appropriate cerebral nuclei and fibre tracts are examined. In toxicity studies performed with pharmaceutical agents possessing central nervous system activity, appropriate cerebral nuclei and fibre tracts should be examined histologically. Guidelines for testing under the Toxic Substances Control Act (TOSCA) suggest that cross-sections of forebrain, centre of the cerebrum, midbrain, pons, medulla oblongata, cervical and lumbar spinal cord, Gasserian and dorsal root ganglia, dorsal and ventral root fibres, proximal sciatic, sural and tibial nerves should be examined in a full neurotoxicological assessment (Environmental Protection Agency, 1985).

Standard sections can be obtained by the use of a metal mould with cross channels for accurate slicing of the fixed brain and appropriate zones assessed by use of a stereotaxic atlas of neuroanatomy such as that of Paxinos and Watson (1986) for the laboratory rat.

In addition to haematoxylin and eosin, special stains for myelin, neuronal bodies, axons and glial cells are of additional help. Changes in peripheral nerve fibres are particularly well characterized in semi-thin plastic- or epoxy resin-embedded, toluidine blue-stained sections (Spencer *et al.*, 1980). Teased nerve fibre preparations are helpful in the demonstration of Wallerian degeneration, demyelination and regeneration (Griffin, 1990). Morphometric analysis of brain pathology, particularly neuronal loss, is also helpful in the characterization of neuronal toxicity (Robertson *et al.*, 1987).

Immunocytochemistry is important for the localization of neuropeptides, particularly in the hypothalamus. For instance, specific depletion of growth hormone-releasing factor has been demonstrated using immunocytochemistry in the median eminence of rats treated with monosodium glutamate (Bloch *et al.*, 1984). Immunocytochemical localization of neurotransmitters can be combined with anterograde tracing with peanut lectin for the study of target fibre systems or neurons (Luiten *et al.*, 1988). Immunocytochemistry using antisera to glial fibrillary acid protein (GFA), S100 protein, neurone specific enolase and cytoskeletal components

may also provide valuable information in the identification of cell types and characterization of changes within them (Koestner, 1990). The topographical distribution of S100 and GFA proteins appears similar in most species but has been well studied in the rat (Ludwin *et al.*, 1976). Immunocytochemical localization of GFA protein is now becoming a useful addition to the assessment of the effects of toxins on the central nervous system, particularly when used together with more conventional stains (Fix *et al.*, 1996).

It is possible to localize cytochrome P450 enzymes in neurones and glial cells of experimental animals by immunocytochemistry (Köhler *et al.*, 1988). Conventional quantitative enzyme cytochemistry is also applicable to neural tissues (Kuger, 1988). Electron microscopy also remains a valuable tool for problem solving in neuropathology, although it is technically demanding and labour intensive (Jones, 1988).

Eyes are examined by use of conventional histological techniques after use of special fixatives such as Davidson's fluid to avoid as much artefact as possible to the cornea, lens and retina (Taradach and Greaves, 1984). The lens poses particular problems in histological processing but excellent results can be achieved using plastic embedding procedures (Heywood and Gopinath, 1988). Recently, confocal microscopy has been shown to be a potentially powerful technique in the histological study of corneal irritation because it can be applied in a non-invasive manner (Jester *et al.*, 1996).

The middle and inner are can be examined histologically after decalcification of the petrous bone and preparation of conventional sections. However, sectioning the cochlea to achieve the correct orientation requires considerable skill and this method can only demonstrate small numbers of sensory cells in the organ. Engström *et al.* (1966) developed the surface preparation technique which involves dissection of the cochlea and subdivision of the organ of Corti into short segments for examination by phase contrast microscopy. A modification of this technique using scanning electron microscopy is relatively simple to perform and can be used in the rat and other experimental animals (Astbury and Read, 1982; Liberman, 1990).

REFERENCES

Ahmed, A. and Smith, A. H. (1983). Surface markers, antigens and receptors on murine T and B cells. Part 2. *CRC Crit. Rev. Toxicol.*, **4**, 19–94.

Alder, S. and Zbinden, G. (1988). *National and International Drug Safety Guidelines*. MTC Verlag, Zollikon, pp. 20–182.

Al-Rufaie, H. K., Florio, R. A. and Olsen, E. G. J. (1983). Comparison of the haematoxylin basic fuchsin picric acid method and the fluorescence of haematoxylin and eosin stained sections for the identification of early myocardial infarction. *J. Clin. Pathol.*, **36**, 646–649.

Anderson, C. and Danylchuck, K. D. (1978). Bone remodeling rates of the beagle: a comparison between different sites on the same rib. *Am. J. Vet. Res.*, **39**, 1763–1765.

Anderson, T. D., Hayes, T. J., Gately, M. K., Bontempo J. M., Stern, L. L. and Truitt, G. A. (1988). Toxicity of human recombinant interleukin-2 in the mouse is mediated by interleukin-activated lymphocytes. Separation of efficacy and toxicity by selective lymphocyte subset depletion. *Lab. Invest.*, **59**, 598–612.

Astbury, P. J. and Read, N. G. (1982). Improved morphological technique for screening potentially ototoxic compounds in laboratory animals. *Br. J. Audiol.*, **16**, 131–137.

Autian, J. (1987) The new field of plastics toxicology—methods and results. *CRC Crit. Rev. Toxicol.*, **2**, 1–40.

Barnes J. L. (1998). *In situ* hybridization in the study of remodeling in proliferative glomerulonephritis. *Toxicol. Pathol.*, **26**, 43–51.

Barry, B. E. and Crapo, J. D. (1985). Application of morphometric methods to study diffuse and focal injury in the lung caused by toxic agents. *CRC Crit. Rev. Toxicol.*, **14**, 1–32.

Betton, G. R., Dormer, C. S., Wells, T., Pert, P., Price, C. A. and Buckley, P. (1988). Gastric ECL-cell hyperplasia and carcinoids in rodents following chronic administration of H2-antagonists SK&F 93479 and oxmetidine and omeprazole. *Toxicol. Pathol.*, **16**, 288–298.

Billeter, R., Heizmann, C. W., Howald, H. and Jenny, E. (1981). Analysis of myosin light and heavy chain types in single human skeletal muscle fibres. *Eur. J. Biochem.*, **116**, 389–395.

Bland, P. W. and Warren, L. G. (1985). Immunohistologic analysis of the T-cell macrophage infiltrate in 1,2-dimethylhydrazine-induced colon tumors in the rat. *J. Natl. Cancer Inst.*, **75**, 757–764.

Bloch, B. (1985). L'hybridation *in situ*: méthodologie et applications à l'analyse des phénomènes d'expression génique dans les glands endocrines et le système nerveux. *Ann. Endocrinol.*, **46**, 253–261.

Bloch, B., Ling, N., Benoit, R., Wehrenberg, W. B. and Guillemin, R. (1984). Specific depletion of immunoreactive growth hormone-releasing factor by monosodium glutamate in rat median eminence. *Nature*, **307**, 272–273.

Block, M. I., Said, J. W., Siegel, R. J. and Fishbein, M. C. (1983). Myocardial myoglobin following coronary artery occlusion. An immunohistochemical study. *Am. J. Pathol.*, **111**, 374–379.

Boon, M. E. and Kok, L. P. (1987). Microwave stabilization of unfixed tissue by microwave fixation. In *Microwave Cookbook of Pathology*. Coulomb Press Leyden, Leiden, Chap. 9, pp. 71–77.

Brighton, C. T., Kitajima, T. and Hunt, R. M. (1984). Zonal analysis of cytoplasmic components of articular cartilage chondrocytes. *Arth. Rheum.*, **27**, 1290–1299.

Brooke, M. H. and Kaiser, K. K. (1970). Muscle fiber types: How many and what kind? *Arch. Neurol.*, **23**, 369–379.

Burkhardt, R., Firsch, B. and Bartl, R. (1982). Bone biopsies in haematological disorders. *J. Clin. Pathol.*, **25**, 257–284.

Chayen, J. (1984). Quantitative cytochemistry: a precise form of cellular biochemistry. *Biochem. Soc. Trans.*, **12**, 884–898.

Chayen, J., Bitensky, L. and Butcher R. G. (1973). *Practical Histochemistry*. Wiley, Chichester.

Clapp, M. J. L. and McNamee, J. A. (1985). The integration of modern computer technologies for effective toxicological data handling. *Med. Inform.*, **10**, 115–121.

Clemo, F. A. S. (1998). Urinary enzyme evaluation of nephrotoxicity in the rat. *Toxicol. Pathol.*, **26**, 29–32.

Clermont, Y. (1972). Kinetics of spermatogenesis in mammals: seminiferous epithelium cycle and spermatogonial renewal. *Am. J. Anat.*, **112**, 35–45.

Cline, J. M. and Maronpot, R. R. (1985). Variations in the histologic distribution of rat bone marrow cells with respect to age and anatomic site. *Toxicol. Pathol.*, **13**, 349–355.

Cottier, H., Turk, J. A. and Sobin, L. (1972). A proposal for a standardardized system of reporting human lymph node morphology in relation to immunological function. *Bull. WHO*, **47**, 375–408.

Creasy, D. M. (1997). Evaluation of testicular toxicity in safety evaluation studies. *Toxicol. Pathol.*, **25**, 119–131.

Darby, T. D. (1987). Safety evaluation of polymer materials. *Annu. Rev. Pharmacol. Toxicol.*, **27**, 157–167.

Davies, D. T. (1993). Assessment of rodent thyroid endocrinology: advantages and pit-falls. *Comp. Haematol. Int.*, **3**, 142–152.

Dean, J. H. and Thurmond L. M. (1987). Immunotoxicology: an overview. *Toxicol. Pathol.*, **15**, 265–271.

Dean, J. H., Lauer, L. D., House, R. V. and Thurmond, L. M. (1986). Immunomodulation: assessing the immunoenhancing and immunosuppressive properties of xenobiotics. In *Toxicology in the Nineties, 1985 Ciba-Geigy International Workshop*. Mary Ann Liebert, New York, pp. 245–285.

de la Iglesia, F. A. and McGuire, E. J. (1981). Quantitative stereology: toxicologic pathology applications. *Toxicol. Pathol.*, **9**, 21–28.

de la Iglesia, F. A., Sturgess, J. M. and Feuer, G. (1982). New approaches for the assessment of hepatotoxicity by means of quantitative functional-morphological interrelationships. In Plaa, G. L. and Hewitt W. R. (Eds), *Toxicology of the Liver*. Raven Press, New York, pp. 47–102.

DeLellis, R. A. and Wolfe, H. J. (1987). New techniques in gene product analysis *Arch. Pathol. Lab. Med.*, **111**, 620–627.

DeLellis, R. A., Wolfe, H. J. and Mohr, U. (1987). Medullary thyroid carcinoma in the Syrian golden hamster: an immunocytochemical study. *Exp. Pathol.*, **31**, 11–16.

Department of Health. (1988). *The Quality Assurance Unit's Role in the Monitoring of Specialist Toxicology Disciplines. The Department of Health GLP Monitoring Unit Response to Clarification Sought by Quality Assurance Group, England.*

Doughty, SE., Ferrier, R. K., Hillan, K. J. and Jackson, D. G. (1995). The effects of ZENECA ZD8731, an angiotensin II antagonist, on renin expression by juxtaglomerular cells in the rat: comparison of protein and mRNA expression as detected by immunohistochemistry and *in situ* hybridization. *Toxicol. Pathol.*, **23**, 256–261.

Dulbecco, R., Allen, W. R., Bologna, M. and Bowman, M. (1986). Marker evolution during the development of the rat mammary gland: stem cells identified by markers and the role of myoepithelial cells. *Cancer Res.*, **46**, 2449–2456.

El Etreby, M. F. and Fath el Bab, M. R. (1977). Effect of cyproterone acetate on cells of the pars distalis of the adenohypophysis in the beagle bitch. *Cell Tissue Res.*, **183**, 177–189.

El Etreby, M. F., Schilk, B., Soulioti, G., Tüshaus, U., Wieman, H. And Günzel, P. (1977). Effect of 17β-estradiol on cells of the pars distalis of the adenohypophysis in the beagle bitch: an immunocytochemical and morphometric study. *Endokrinologie*, **69**, 202–216.

Engström, H., Ades, H. W. and Andersson, A. (1966). *Structure Patterns of the Organ of Corti*. Almqvist and Wiksell, Stockholm.

Environmental Protection Agency, (1985). Toxic Substances Control Act Guidelines, 40 DFR, Part 798, Subpart G, Section 798.6400, Neuropathology. *Fed. Regist.* **50**, No. 188, 39461–39463.

Ermark, T. H. and Owen, R. L. (1986). Differential distribution of lymphocytes and accessory cells in mouse Peyer's patches. *Anat. Rec.*, **215**, 144–152.

Evans, G. O., Flynn, R. M. and Lupton, J. D. (1988a). An immunogold labelling method for rat T lymphocytes. *Lab. Anim.*, **2**, 332–334.

Evans, G. O., Flynn, R. M. and Lupton, J. D. (1988b). An immunogold labelling method for the enumeration of canine T-lymphocytes. *Vet. Q.*, **10**, 273–276.

Faccini, J. M. (1982). A perspective on the pathology and cytochemistry of renal lesions. In Bach, P. H., Bonner, F. W., Bridges J. W. and Lock E. D. (Eds), *Nephrotoxicity Assessment and Pathogenesis*. Wiley, Chichester, pp. 82–97.

Faccini, J. M. and Naylor, D. (1979). Computer analysis and integration of animal pathology data. *Arch. Toxicol.*, Suppl. 2, 517–520.

Faraggiana, T., Gresik, E., Tanaka, T., Inagami, T. and Lupo, A. (1982). Immunohistochemical localization of renin in the human kidney. *J. Histochem. Cytochem.*, **30**, 459–465.

Farber, E. (1984). Chemical carcinogenesis: a current biological perspective. *Carcinogenesis*, **5**, 1–5.

Farnum, C. E. and Wilsman, N. J. (1988). Lectin-binding histochemistry of intracellular glycoconjugates of the reserve cell zone of growth plate cartilage. *J. Orthop. Res.*, **6**, 166–179.

Fenoglio-Preiser, C. and Willman, C. L. (1987). Molecular biology and the pathologist. General principles and applications. *Arch. Pathol. Lab. Med.*, **111**, 601–619.

Filipe, M. I. and Branfoot, A. C. (1974). Abnormal patterns of mucous secretion in apparently normal mucosa of the large intestine with carcinoma. *Cancer*, **34**, 282–290.

Fix, A. S., Ross, J. F., Stitzel, S. R. and Switzer, R. C. (1996). Integrated evaluation of central nervous system lesions: stains for neurones, astrocytes, and microglia reveal the spatial and temporal features of MK-801-induced neuronal necrosis in the rat cerebral cortex. *Toxicol. Pathol.*, **24**, 291–304.

Foster, J. R., Elcombe, C. R., Boobis, A. R., Davies, D. S., Sesardic, D., McQuade, J., Robson, R. T. Hayward C. and Lock, E. A. (1986). Immunocytochemical localization of cytochrome P-450 in hepatic and extra-hepatic tissues of the rat with a monoclonal antibody against cytochrome P-450c. *Biochem. Pharmacol.*, **35**, 4543–4554.

Garman, R. H. (1990). Artefacts in routinely immersion fixed nervous tissue. *Toxicol. Pathol.*, **18**, 149–153.

Geleff, S., Böck, P. and Stockinger, L. (1986). Lectin binding affinities of the epithelium in the respiratory tract. A light microscopical study of ciliated epithelium in rat, guinea pig, and hamster. *Acta Histochem.*, **78**, 83–95.

Giampaolo, C., Bray, K., Kowalski, B. and Rogers, A. E. (1989). Cytologic characteristics of neoplastic and regener-

ating hepatocytes in fine needle aspirates of rat liver. *Toxicol. Pathol.*, **17**, 743–753.

Gil, J. and Martinez-Hernandez, A. (1984). The connective tissue of the rat lung: electron immunocytochemical studies. *J. Histochem. Cytochem.*, **32**, 230–238.

Goldsworthy, T. L., Fransson-Steen, R. and Maronpot, R. R. (1996). Importance of and approaches to quantification of hepatocyte apoptosis. *Toxicol. Pathol.*, **24**, 24–35.

Gough, A. W., Barsoum, N. J., Renlund, R. C., Sturgess, J. M. and de la Iglesia, F. A. (1985). Fine structural changes during reparative phase of canine drug-induced arthropathy. *Vet. Pathol.*, **22**, 82–84.

Gray, J. E. (1981). Appraisal of the intramuscular irritation test in the rabbit. *Fundam. Appl. Toxicol.*, **1**, 290–292.

Greaves, P. (1998). Patterns of drug-induced cardiovascular pathology in the beagle dog: relevance for humans. *Exp. Toxicol. Pathol.*, **50**, 283–293.

Greaves, P. and Boiziau, J.-L. (1984). Altered patterns of mucin secretion in gastric hyperplasia in mice. *Vet. Pathol.*, **21**, 224–228.

Greaves, P. and Barsoum, N. J. (1990). Tumours of soft tissues. In V. S. Turusov (Ed.), *Pathology of Laboratory Animals, Vol. 1, Tumours of the Rat*, 2nd edn. IARC, Lyon, pp. 597–623.

Greaves, P. and Faccini J. M. (1984). The pathological evaluation of toxicological studies. In *Rat Histopathology. A Glossary For Use In Toxicity and Carcinogenicity Studies*. Elsevier, Amsterdam, pp. 240–245.

Greaves, P., Filipe, M. I. and Branfoot, A. C. (1980). Transitional mucosa and survival in human colorectal cancer. *Cancer*, **46**, 764–770.

Greaves, P., Irisarri, E. and Monro, A. M. (1986). Hepatic foci of cellular and enzymatic alteration and nodules in rats treated with clofibrate or diethylnitrosamine followed by phenobarbital: their rate of onset and their reversibility. *J. Natl. Cancer Inst.*, **76**, 475–484.

Gregg, N. J., Courtauld, E. A. and Bach, P. H. (1990). High resolution light microscopic morphological and microvascular changes in an acutely induced renal papillary necrosis. *Toxicol. Pathol.*, **18**, 47–55.

Griffin, J. W. (1990). Basic pathology in the nervous system. *Toxicol. Pathol.*, **18**, 83–88.

Guder, W. G. and Ross, B. D. (1984). Enzyme distribution along the nephron. *Kidney Int.*, **26**, 101–111.

Hawkins, K. L., Lloyd, R. V. and Toy, K. A. (1989). Immunohistochemical localization of chromogranin A in normal tissues from laboratory animals. *Vet. Pathol.*, **26**, 488–498.

Hayakawa, B. N., Jorgensen, A. O., Gotlieb, A. I., Zhao, M.-S. and Liew, C.-C. (1984). Immunofluorescent microscopy for the identification of human necrotic myocardium. *Arch. Pathol. Lab. Med.*, **198**, 284–286.

Helliwell, T. R. (1988). Lectin binding and desmin staining during bupicicaine-induced necrosis and regeneration in rat skeletal muscle. *J. Pathol.*, **155**, 317–326.

Henderson,. J. D., Jr, Mullarky, R. H. and Ryan D. E. (1987). Tissue biocompatability and kevlar aramid fibres and polymethyl methacrylate composites in rabbits. *J. Biomed. Mater. Res.*, **21**, 59–64.

Herrick, S. S., Davis, C., Donnelly, D. V., Lockhart, T., Marek, L. and Russell, H. (1983). Histopathology automated system. *Drug Inf. J.*, **17**, 287–295.

Heywood, R. and Gopinath, C. (1988). Morphological assessment of visual dysfunction. *Toxicol. Pathol.*, **18**, 204–217.

Heywood, J. and James, R. W. (1978). Assessment of testicular toxicity in laboratory animals. *Environ. Health Perspect.*, **24**, 73–80.

Hirth, R. S., Evans, L. D., Buroker, R. A. and Oleson, F. B. (1988). Gastric enterochromaffin-like cell hyperplasia and neoplasia in the rat: an indirect effect of the histamine H2-receptor antagonist, BL-6341. *Toxicol. Pathol.*, **16**, 273–287.

Holthofer, H. (1983). Lectin binding sites in kidney. A comparative study of 14 animal species. *J. Histochem. Cytochem.*, **31**, 531–537.

Hong, H-H. L., Devereux, T. R., Roycroft, J. H., Boorman, G. A. and Sills, R. C. (1998). Frequency of *ras* mutations in liver neoplasms from B6C3F$_1$ mice exposed to tetrafluoroethylene for two years. *Toxicol. Pathol.*, **26**, 646–650.

Howie, A. J., Gunson, B. K. and Sparke, J. (1990). Morphometric correlates of renal excretory function. *J. Pathol.*, **160**, 245–253.

Ibrahim, K. S., Husain, O. A., Bitensky, L. and Chayen, J. (1983). A modified tetrazolium reaction for identifying malignant cells from gastric and colonic cancer. *J. Clin. Pathol.*, **36**, 133–136.

Ingram, A. J. and Grasso, P. (1975). Patch testing in the rabbit using a modified patch test method. *Br. J. Dermatol.*, **92**, 131–142.

Irisarri, E. and Mompon, P. (1983). Hepatic effects of fasting on 6 and 12 week old mice: a quantitative histochemical study. *J. Pathol.*, **140**, 176.

Ishihara, K., Ohar, S., Azuumi, Y., Goso, K. and Hotto, K. (1984). Changes of gastric mucus glycoproteins with aspirin administration in rats. *Digestion*, **29**, 98–102.

Jester, J. V., Maurer, J. K., Petroll, W. M., Wilkie, D. A., Parker, R. D. and Cavanagh, H. W. (1996). Application of *in vivo* confocal microscopy to the understanding of surfactant-induced ocular irritation. *Toxicol. Pathol.*, **24**, 412–428.

Jones, H. B. (1988). The role of ultrastructural investigations in neurotoxicology. *Toxicology*, **49**, 3–15.

Jones, H. B., Clarke N. A. B. and Barrass N. C. (1993). Phenobarbital-induced hepatocellular proliferation: anti-bromodeoxyuridine and anti-proliferating cell nuclear antigen immunocytochemistry. *J. Histochem. Cytochem.*, **41**, 21–27.

Jones, H. B., Eldridge, S. H., Butterworth, B. E. and Foster, J. R. (1996). Measures of cell replication in risk/safety assessment of xenobiotic-induced, nongenotoxic carcinogenesis. *Reg. Toxicol. Pharmacol.*, **23**, 117–127.

Jungerman, K. and Katz, N. (1982). Functional hepatocellular heterogeneity. *Hepatology*, **2**, 385–395.

Kirivanta, I., Jurvelin, J. Tammi, M., Säämänen, A.-M. and Helminen, H. H. (1987). Weight bearing controls glycosaminoglycan concentration and articular cartilage thickness in the knee joints of young beagle dogs. *Arth. Rheum.*, **30**, 801–809.

Kluwe, W. (1981). Renal function tests as indicators of kidney injury in subacute toxicity studies. *Toxicol. Appl. Pharmacol.*, **57**, 414–424.

Kodell, R. L., Blackwell, B.-N., Bucci, T. J. and Greenman, D. L. (1995). Cause-of-death assignment at the National Center for Toxicological Research. *Toxicol. Pathol.*, **23**, 241–247.

Koestner, A. (1990). Characterization of *N*-nitrosourea-induced tumors of the nervous system; their prospective value of studies of neurocarcinogenesis and brain tumor therapy. *Toxicol. Pathol.*, **18**, 186–192.

Köhler, C., Eriksson, L. G., Hansson, T., Warner, M. and Ake-Gustafsson, J. (1988). Immunohistochemical localization of cytochrome P-450 in the rat brain. *Neurosci. Lett.*, **84**, 109–114.

Kolde, G. and Knop, J. (1987). Different cellular reaction patterns if epidermal Langerhans cells after application of contact sensitizing, toxic and tolerogenic compounds. A comparative ultrastructural and morphometric time course analysis. *J. Invest. Dermatol.*, **89**, 19–23.

Kuger, P. (1988). Quantitative enzyme histochemistry in the brain. *Histochemistry*, **90**, 99–107.

Kuijpers, M. H. M., Van de Kooij, A. J. and Slootweg, P. J. (1996). The rat incisor in toxicologic pathology. *Toxicol. Pathol.*, **24**, 346–360.

Le Goascogne, C., Robel, P., Gouézou, M., Sananès, N., Baulieu, E.-E. and Waterman, M. (1987). Neurosteroids: cytochrome P-450scc in rat brain. *Science*, **237**, 1212–1215.

Lepore, P. D. (1996). Pathology raw data. *Toxicol. Pathol.*, **24**, 147.

Levine, G. M., Brousseau, P. and O'Shaughnessy, D. J. and Losos G. J. (1987). Quantitative immunocytochemistry by digital image analysis. Application to toxicologic pathology. *Toxicol. Pathol.*, **15**, 303–307.

Liberman, M. C. (1990). Quantitative assessment of inner ear pathology following ototoxic drugs or acoustic trauma. *Toxicol. Pathol.*, **18**, 138–148.

Linnoila, I. and Petrusz, P. (1984). Immunohistochemical techniques and their application in the histology of the respiratory system. *Environ. Health Perspect.*, **56**, 131–148.

Lloyd, R. V. and Landefeld, T. D. (1986). Detection of prolactin messenger RNA in rat anterior pituitary *in situ* hybridization. *Am. J. Pathol.*, **125**, 35–44.

Lloyd, R. V. and Mailloux, J. (1987). Effect of diethylstibestrol and propylthiouracil on the rat pituitary. An immunohistochemical study. *J. Natl. Cancer Inst.*, **79**, 865–873.

Lock, E. A. and Reed, C. J. (1998). Xenobiotic metabolizing enzymes of the kidney. *Toxicol. Pathol.*, **26**, 18–25.

Long, G. G., Symanowski, J. T. and Roback, K. (1998). Precision in data acquisition and reporting of organ weights in rats and mice. *Toxicol. Pathol.*, **26**, 316–318.

Ludwin, S. K., Kosek, J. C. and Eng, L. F. (1976). The topographical distribution of S-100 and GFA proteins in adult rat brain: an immunohistochemical study using horseradish peroxidase-labelled antibodies. *J. Comp. Neurol.*, **165**, 197–208.

Luiten, P. G. M., Wouterlood, F. G., Matsuyama, T., Strosberg, A. D., Buwalder, B. and Gaykema, R. P. A. (1988). Immunocytochemical applications in neuroanatomy. Demonstration of connections, transmitters and receptors. *Histochemistry*, **90**, 85–97.

Luster, M. I., Munson, A. E., Thomas, P. T., Holsapple, M. P., Fenters, J. D., White, K. L., Jr, Lauer, L. D., Germolec, D. R., Rosenthal, G. J. and Dean, J. H. (1988). Development of a testing battery to assess chemical induced immunotoxicity: National Toxicology Program's guidelines for immunotoxicity evaluation in mice. *Fundam. Appl. Toxicol.*, **10**, 2–19.

Mahler, J. F., Flagler, N. D., Malarkey, D. E., Mann, P. C., Haseman, J. K. and Eastin, W. (1998). Spontaneous and chemically induced proliferative lesions in Tg.AC transgenic and p53-heterozygous mice. *Toxicol. Pathol.*, **26**, 501–511.

Malarkey, D. E. and Maronpot, R. R. (1996). Polymerase chain reaction and *in situ* hybridization: applications in toxicological pathology. *Toxicol. Pathol.*, **24**, 13–23.

Mankin, H. J. (1974). The reaction of articular cartilage to injury and osteoarthritis. *N. Engl. J. Med.*, **291**, 1285–1292.

Maronpot, R. R. (1987). Ovarian toxicity and carcinogenicity in eight recent National Toxicology Program studies. *Environ. Health Perspect.*, **73**, 125–130.

Maronpot, R. R., Harada, T., Murthy, A. S. K. and Boorman, G. A. (1989). Documenting foci of hepatocellular alteration in two-year carcinogenicity studies: current practices of the National Toxicology Program. *Toxicol. Pathol.*, **17**, 675–683.

Martin, M. S., Hammann, A. and Martin, F. (1986). Gut-associated lymphoid tissue and 1,2-dimethylhydrazine intestinal tumours in the rat: a histological and immunocytochemical study. *Int. J. Cancer*, **38**, 75–80.

Masson, M. T., Villanove, F. and Greaves, P. (1986). Histological demonstration of wheat germ lectin binding sites in the liver of normal and ANIT treated rats. *Arch. Toxicol.*, **59**, 121–123.

Mery, S., Gross, E. A., Joyner, D. R., Godo, M. and Morgan, K. T. (1994). Nasal diagrams: a tool for recording the distribution of nasal lesions in rats and mice. *Toxicol. Pathol.*, **22**, 353–372.

Mompon, P., Greaves P., Irisarri E., Monro, A. M. and Bridges, J. W. (1987). A cytochemical study of the livers of rats treated with diethylnitrosamine/phenobarbital, with benzidine/phenobarbital, with phenobarbital, or with clofibrate. *Toxicology*, **46**, 217–236.

Moody, D. E., Taylor, L. A. and Smuckler, E. A. (1985). Immunofluorescent determination of the lobular distribution of a constitutive form of hepatic microsomal cytochrome P-450. *Hepatology*, **5**, 440–451.

Moolenbeck, C. and Ruitenberg, E. J. (1981). The 'Swiss roll': a simple technique for histological studies of rodent intestine. *Lab. Anim.*, **15**, 57–59.

Murata, F., Tsuyama, S., Suzuki, S., Hamada, H., Ozawa, M. and Muramatsu, T. (1983). Distribution of glycoconjugates in the kidney studied by use of labelled lectins. *J. Histochem. Cytochem.*, **31**, 139–144.

Nemery, B., Dinsdale, D. and Verschoyle, R. D. (1987). Detecting and evaluating chemical-induced lung damage in experimental animals. *Bull. Eur. Physiopathol. Respir.*, **23**, 501–528.

Neville, A. M. (1969). The adrenal medulla. In T. Symington (Ed.), *Functional Pathology of the Human Adrenal Gland, Part II*. Livingstone, Edinburgh, pp. 219–234.

Newberne, P. M. and de la Iglesia, F. A. (1985). Philosophy of blind slide reading in toxicological pathology. *Toxicol. Pathol.*, **13**, 255.

Nicholson, G. L. (1974). The interactions of lectins with animal cell surfaces. *Int. Rev. Cytol.*, **39**, 89–190.

Owen, R. L. and Bhalla, D. K. (1983). Cytochemical analysis of alkaline phosphatase and esterase activities and of lectin binding and anionic sites in rat and mouse Peyer's patch M cells. *Am J. Anat.*, **168**, 199–212.

Palate, B. M., Denoel, S. R. and Roba, J. L. (1995). A simple method for performing routine histopathological examina-

tion of the cardiac conduction tissue in the dog. *Toxicol. Pathol.*, **23**, 56–62.

Patrick, E., Maibach, H. I. and Burkalter, A. (1985). Mechanisms of chemically induced skin irritation. 1. Studies of time course, dose response and components of inflammation in the laboratory mouse. *Toxicol. Appl. Pharmacol.*, **81**, 476–490.

Pawlikowski, M. (1982). The link between secretion and mitosis in the endocrine glands. *Life Sci.*, **30**, 315–320.

Paxinos, G. and Watson, C. (1986). *The Rat Brain in Stereotaxic Coordinates*, 2nd edn. Academic Press, Sydney.

Pesce, C. M. (1987). Biology of disease. Defining and interpreting diseases through morphometry. *Lab. Invest.*, **56**, 568–575.

Pick, R., Jalil, J. E. Janicki, J. S. and Weber K. T. (1989). The fibrillar nature and structure of isoproterenol-induced myocardial fibrosis in the rat. *Am. J. Pathol.*, **134**, 365–371.

Pierobon-Bormioli, S., Sartore, S., Vitadello, M. and Schiaffino, S. (1980). 'Slow' myosins in vertebrate skeletal muscle. An immunofluoresence study. *J. Cell Biol.*, **85**, 672–681.

Pierobon-Bormioli, S., Sartore, S., Vitadello, M. and Schiaffino, S. (1981). 'Fast' isomyosins and fibre types in mammalian skeletal muscle. *J. Histochem. Cytochem.*, **29**, 1179–1188.

Piper, R. C. (1981). Morphologic evaluation of the heart in toxicology studies. In Balazs, T. (Ed.), *Cardiac Toxicology*. CRC Press, Boca Raton, FL, pp. 111–136.

Pritchard, D. M. and Watson, A. J. M. (1996). Apoptosis and gastrointestinal pharmacology. *Pharmacol. Ther.*, **72**, 149–169.

Read, N. G., Beesley, J. E., Blackett, N. M. and Trist, D. G. (1985). The accumulation of an aryloxyalkylamidine (501C) and polymorphonuclear leucocytes: a quantitative electron microscopic study. *J. Pharm. Pharmacol.*, **37**, 96–99.

Read, N. G., Astbury, P. J., Morgan, R. J. I., Parsons, D. N. and Port, C. J. (1988). Induction and exacerbation of hyaline droplet formation in the proximal tubular cells of the kidneys from male rats receiving a variety of pharmacological agents. *Toxicology*, **52**, 81–101.

Reynolds, S. H., Stowers, S. J., Patterson, R. M., Maronpot, R. R., Aaronson, S. A. and Anderson M. W. (1987). Activated oncogenes in B6C3F1 mouse liver tumours: implications for risk assessment. *Science*, **237**, 1309–1316.

Rhodin, J. A. G. (1974). Adrenal (suprarenal) glands. In *Histology. A Text and Atlas*. Oxford University Press, New York, pp. 456–466.

Richmond, R. S., Pereira, M. A., Carter, J. H., Carter, H. W. and Long, R. E. (1988). Quantitative and qualitative immunohistochemical detection of myc and src oncogene proteins in normal, nodule, and neoplastic rat liver. *J. Histochem. Cytochem.*, **36**, 179–184.

Roberts, J. C., McCrossan, M. V. and Jones, H. B. (1990). The case for perfusion fixation of large tissue samples for ultrastructural pathology. *Ultrastruct. Pathol.*, **14**, 177–191.

Robertson, D. G., Gray, R. H. and de la Iglesia. F. A. (1987). Quantitative assessment of trimethyltin induced pathology of the hippocampus. *Toxicol. Pathol.*, **15**, 7–17.

Robinson, P. B. and Harvey, W. (1989). Tooth root resorption induced in rats by diphenylhydantoin and parathyroidectomy. *Br. J. Exp. Pathol.*, **70**, 65–72.

Robinson, P. B., Harris, M., Harvey, W. and Papadogeargakis, N. (1982). Reduced bone growth on rats treated with anticonvulsant drugs: a type II pseudohypoparathyroidism? *Metab. Bone Dis. Rel. Res.*, **4**, 269–275.

Roe, F. J. C. (1977). Quantitation and computerisation of histopathological data. Paper presented at a Ciba Symposium (unpublished).

Rushmore, T. H., Ghazarian, D. M., Subrahmanyan, V., Farber, E. and Ghoshal, A. K. (1987). Probable free radical effects on rat liver nuclei during early hepatocarcinogenesis with a choline-devoid low methionine diet. *Cancer Res.*, **47**, 6731–6740.

Russell, L. D. and Frank, B. (1978). Characterization of rat spermiogenesis after plastic embedding. *Arch. Androl.*, **1**, 5–18.

Russo, J., Tay, L. K. and Russo, I. H. (1982). Differentiation of the mammary gland and susceptibility to carcinogenesis. *Breast Cancer Res. Treat.*, **2**, 5–73.

Salthouse, T. N. and Willigan, D. A. (1972). An enzyme histochemical approach to the evaluation of polymers for tissue compatibility. *J. Biomed. Res.*, **6**, 105–113.

Schenk, R., Eggli, P. and Rosini, S. (1986). Quantitative morphometric evaluation of the inhibitory activity of new aminobisphosphonates on bone resorption in the rat. *Calcif. Tissue Int.*, **38**, 342–349.

Schlage, W. K., Bülles, H., Friedrichs, D., Kuhn, M. and Teredesai, A. (1998). Cytokeratin expression patterns in the rat respiratory tract as markers of epithelial differentiation in inhalation toxicology. I. Determination of normal cytokeratin expression patterns in nose, larynx, trachea and lung. *Toxicol. Pathol.*, **26**, 324–343.

Schulte, B. A. and Spicer, S. S. (1983). Histochemical evaluation of mouse and rat kidneys with lectin-horseradish peroxidase conjugates. *Am. J. Anat.*, **168**, 345–362.

Sheahan, D. G. and Jarvis, H. R. (1978). Comparative histochemistry of gastrointestinal mucosubstances. *Am. J. Anat.*, **146**, 103–132.

Sobel, R. A. and Colvin, R. B. (1986). Responder strain-specific enhancement of endothelial and mononuclear cell Ia in delayed hypersensitivity reactions in (strain 2 × strain 13) F1 guinea pigs. *J. Immunol.*, **137**, 2132–2138.

Solheim, T. (1974). Pluricolor fluorescent labeling of mineralizing tissue. *Scand. J. Dent. Res.*, **82**, 19–27.

Spencer, A. J., Andreu, M. and Greaves, P. (1986). Neoplasia and hyperplasia of pancreatic endocrine tissue in the rat: an immunocytochemical study. *Vet. Pathol.*, **23**, 11–15.

Spencer, P. S., Bischoff, M. C. and Schaumburg, H. H. (1980). Neuropathological methods for the detection of neurotoxic disease. In Spencer, P. S. and Schaumburg. H. H. (Eds), *Experimental and Clinical Neurotoxicology*. Williams and Wilkins, Baltimore, pp. 743–757.

Spicer, S. S. and Schulte, B. A. (1982). Identification of cell surface constituents. *Lab. Invest.*, **47**, 2–4.

Spinale, F. G., Schulte, B. A. and Crawford, F. A. (1989). Demonstration of early ischemic injury in porcine right ventricular myocardium. *Am. J. Pathol.*, **134**, 693–704.

Stene, T. and Koppang, H. S. (1976). The effect of vincristine on dentinogenesis in the rat incisor. *Scand. J. Dent. Res.*, **84**, 342–344.

Streett, C. S., Robertson, J. L. and Crissman, J. W. (1988). Morphologic stomach findings in rats and mice treated with the H2 receptor antagonists, ICI 125, 211 and ICI 162, 846. *Toxicol. Pathol.*, **16**, 299–304.

Sturgess, J. M. (1985). Mucociliary clearance and mucus secretion in the lung. In Witschi, H. P. and Brain, J. D. (Eds), *Toxicology of Inhaled Materials. General Principles of Inhalation Toxicology*. Springer, Berlin, pp. 319–367.

Sturgess, J. and Reid, L. (1973). The effect of isoprenaline and pilocarpine on (a) bronchial mucus-secreting tissue and (b) pancreas, salivary glands, heart, thymus, live and spleen. *Br. J. Exp. Pathol.*, **54**, 388–403.

Szczech, G. M. and Tucker, W. E. (1985). Nail loss and footpad erosions in beagle dogs given BW 134U, a nucleoside analog. *Toxicol. Pathol.*, **13**, 181–184.

Taper, H. S., Somer, M. P., Lans, M., de Gerlache, J. and Roberfroid, M. (1988). Histochemical detection of the *in vivo* produced cellular aldehydes by means of direct Schiff's reaction in CC14 intoxicated liver. *Arch. Toxicol.*, **61**, 406–410.

Taradach, C. and Greaves, P. (1984). Spontaneous eye lesions in laboratory animals: incidence in relation to age. *CRC Crit. Rev. Toxicol.*, **12**, 121–147.

Tatematsu, M., Tsuda, H., Shirai, T., Masui, T. and Ito, N. (1987). Placental glutathione *S*-transferase (GST-P) as a new marker for hepatocarcinogenesis: in vivo short-term screening for hepatocarcinogenesis. *Toxicol. Pathol.*, **15**, 60–68.

Taylor, C. R. and Kledzig, G. (1981). Immunohistochemical techniques in surgical pathology—a spectrum of 'new' special stains. *Hum. Pathol.*, **12**, 590–596.

Thompson, G. R., Baker J. R., Fleischman, R. W., Rosenkranz, H., Schaeppi, U. H., Cooney, D. A. and Davis, R. D. (1972). Preclinical toxicologic evaluation of bleomycin (NSC 125 006), a new anti-tumor antibiotic. *Toxicol. Appl. Pharmacol.*, **22**, 544–555.

Tischler, A. S. and DeLellis, R. A. (1988). The rat adrenal medulla. 1. The normal adrenal. *J. Am. Coll. Toxicol.*, **7**, 1–19.

Tischler, A. S., DeLellis, R. A., Perlman, R. L., Allen, J. M., Costopoulos, D., Lee, Y. C., Nunnemacher, G., Wolfe, H. J. and Bloom, S. R. (1985). Spontaneous proliferative lesions of the adrenal medulla in ageing Long–Evans rats. Comparison to PC12 cells, small granule-containing cells, and human adrenal medullary hyperplasia. *Lab. Invest.*, **53**, 486–498.

Tsiftis, D., Jass, J. R., Filipe, M. I. and Wastell, C. (1980). Altered patterns of mucin secretion in precancerous lesions induced in the glandular part of the rat stomach by the carcinogen *N*-methyl-*N*-nitro-*N'*-nitrosoguanidine. *Invest. Cell. Pathol.*, **3**, 339–408.

Tyler, W. S., Dungworth, D. L., Plopper, C. G., Hyde, D. M. and Tyler, N. K. (1985). Structural evaluation of the respiratory system. *Fundam. Appl. Toxicol.*, **5**, 405–422.

Ulvik, N. M., Dahl, E. and Hars, R. (1982). Classification of plastic-embedded rat seminiferous epithelium prior to electron microscopy. *Int. J. Androl.*, **5**, 27–36.

van der Valk, P. and Maijer, C. J. L. M. (1987). Histology of reactive lymph nodes. *Am. J. Surg. Pathol.*, **11**, 866–882.

Verlander, J. W. (1998). Normal ultrastructure of the kidney and lower urinary tract. *Toxicol. Pathol.*, **26**, 1–17.

Walker, R. (1985). The use of lectins in histopathology. *Histopathology*, **9**, 1121–1124.

Warburton, M. J., Mitchell, D., Ormerod, E. J. and Rudland, P. (1982). Distribution of myoepithelial cells and basement membrane proteins in the resting, pregnant, lactating and involuting rat mammary gland. *J. Histochem. Cytochem.*, **30**, 667–676.

Ward, J. M., Hardisty J. F., Hailey, J. R. and Streett, C. S. (1995). Peer review in toxicologic pathology. *Toxicol. Pathol.*, **23**, 226–234.

Weibel, E. R. (1979). The lung and its gas exchange apparatus: an example of the use of stereology in studies of structure–function correlation. In Weibel, E. R. (Ed.), *Stereological Methods, Vol. 1, Practical Methods for Biological Morphometry*. Academic Press, New York, pp. 322–331.

Wheeldon, E. B., Williams, S. M., Soames, A. R., James, N. H. and Roberts, R. A. (1995). Quantitation of apoptotic bodies in rat liver by *in situ* end labelling (ISEL): correlation with morphology. *Toxicol. Pathol.*, **23**, 410–415.

Whittaker, P., Boughner, D. R. and Kloner, R. A. (1989). Analysis of healing after myocardial infarction using polarized light microscopy. *Am. J. Pathol.*, **134**, 879–893.

Widgren, U. and Enerbäck, L. (1983). Mucosal mast cells of the rat intestine: a re-evaluation of fixation and staining properties, with special reference to protein blocking and solubility of the granular glycosaminoglycans. *Histochem. J.*, **15**, 571–582.

Wieczorek, G., Pospischil, A. and Parentes, E. (1998). A comparative immunohistochemical study of pancreatic islets in laboratory animals (rats, dogs, minipigs, nonhuman primates). *Exp. Toxicol. Pathol.*, **50**, 151–172.

Wright, J. A. (1989). A comparison of rat femoral, sternebral and lumbar vertebral bone marrow fat content by subjective and image analysis of histological assessment. *J. Comp. Pathol.*, **100**, 419–426.

Wright, J. A., Wadsworth, P. F. and Stewart, M. G. (1990). Neurone-specific enolase in rat and mouse phaeochromocytomas. *J. Comp. Pathol.*, **102**, 475–478.

Yasuda, K. and Yamashita, S. (1985). Immunohistochemical study on gamma glutamyl transpeptidase in the rat kidney with monoclonal antibodies. *J. Histochem. Cytochem.*, **34**, 111.

Young, J. T. (1981). Histopathologic examination of the rat nasal cavity. *Fundam. Appl. Toxicol.*, **1**, 309–312.

Zak, M., Kovaks, K., McComb, D. J. and Heitz, P. U. (1985). Aminoglutethimide stimulated corticotrophs. An immunocytologic, ultrastructural and immunoelectron microscopic study of the rat adenohypophysis. *Virchows Arch. Cell. Pathol.*, **49**, 93–106.

Zaki, F. G., Keim, G. R., Takii, Y, and Inagami, T. (1982). Hyperplasia of the juxtaglomerular cells and renin localization in kidneys of normotensive animals given captopril. *Ann. Clin. Lab. Sci.*, **12**, 200–215.

Zbinden, G. (1988). Biopharmaceutical studies, a key to better toxicology. *Xenobiotica*, **18**, Suppl. 1, 9–14.

Zbinden, G., Fent, K. and Thouin, M. H. (1988). Nephrotoxicity screening in rats; general approach and establishment of test criteria. *Arch. Toxicol.*, **61**, 344–348.

Chapter 17
Clinical Chemistry

M. D. Stonard and G. O. Evans

C O N T E N T S

INTRODUCTION

In the early stages of the safety evaluation of development compounds, a variety of tests should be chosen to evaluate the broadest possible range of physiological and metabolic functions, and to provide evidence of target organ toxicity (**Table 1**). At later stages, a tiered approach using more specialized and targeted measurements may be required to characterize treatment-induced changes—e.g. urinary enzymes for monitoring nephrotoxicity (Kallner and Tryding, 1989). Few of the common biochemical parameters are independent of each other, and several measurements may be used to determine damage in a single organ—for example, plasma enzymes in the assessment of hepatotoxicity. As the liver and kidneys are frequently the target organs in toxicity studies, several of the traditional clinical chemistry measurements applied in human clinical practice can be applied to detect damage to these organs. For the smaller laboratory animals, the number of analytes which can be measured is governed partially by the restricted volume of plasma available for analysis.

The use of plasma enzymes as markers of organ damage continues to be a significant part of the safety evaluation process (**Table 2**). The plasma activity of an enzyme depends on several factors, including the enzyme concentrations in different tissues, the intracellular location of the enzyme, the severity of tissue and cellular damage, the molecular site of the enzyme, and the rate of clearance of the enzyme from plasma.

The distribution of enzymes in different tissues varies between species, and therefore influences their diagnostic effectiveness in particular species (Clampitt and Hart, 1978; Keller, 1981; Lindena et al., 1986; Evans, 1996a). For example, plasma alkaline phosphatase (ALP) and lactate dehydrogenase (LDH) activities show greater variability in rats and monkeys when compared with humans, and therefore have a poorer predictive value in these species. In young animals the osseous ALP iso-enzyme is the dominant form in plasma, but in the adult

Table 1 Blood, plasma or serum tests suggested by regulatory authorities for toxicology studies

Acid/base balance	Creatinine
Alanine aminotransferase	Glucose
Albumin	γ-Glutamyl transferase
Alkaline phosphatase	Hormones (miscellaneous)
Aspartate aminotransferase	Inorganic phosphate
Bile acids	Lactate dehydrogenase
Bilirubin (total)	Lipids (triglycerides, non-esterified fatty acids)
Calcium	Potassium
Chloride	Sodium
Cholesterol	Total protein
Creatine kinase	Urea (or urea nitrogen)

Table 2 Enzymes, their abbreviations and enzyme commission (EC) numbers

Abbreviation	Recommended name	EC number
ALT (GPT)	Alanine aminotransferase	2.6.1.2
AAP	Alanine aminopeptidase	3.4.1.2
ALP	Alkaline phosphatase	3.1.3.1
AMY	Amylase	3.2.1.1
AST (GOT)	Aspartate aminotransferase	2.6.1.1
CHE	Cholinesterase	3.1.1.8
CK (CPK)	Creatine kinase	2.7.3.2
GGT	γ-Glutamyl transferase	2.3.2.2
GLDH	Glutamate dehydrogenase	1.4.1.3
ICDH	Isocitrate dehydrogenase	1.1.1.42
LDH	Lactate dehydrogenase	1.1.1.27
LAAP	Leucine arylamidase	3.4.11.2
LAP	Leucine aminopeptidase	3.4.11.1
LIP	Lipase	3.1.1.3
NAG	N-Acetyl-β-glucosaminidase	3.2.1.30
5'NT	5'-Nucleotidase	3.1.3.5
OCT	Ornithine carbamoyltransferase	2.1.3.3
SDH	Sorbitol dehydrogenase	1.1.1.14

rat the proportion of intestinal ALP in plasma is greater than in other species. Plasma γ-glutamyl transferase (GGT) activities are lower in most rodent species compared with the activity found in human, but the enzyme is a good marker of chemically induced cholestasis (Leonard *et al.*, 1984).

This general consideration of the diagnostic effectiveness of plasma enzyme measurements in different species also extends to other measurements, particularly hormones. For example, corticosterone is the primary glucocorticosteroid of rat adrenal tissue, and is therefore the plasma marker of choice in the rat. In canine plasma there are substantial quantities of both cortisol and corticosterone in comparison with human and guinea-pig plasma, where cortisol is the dominant glucocorticosteroid.

Pre-analytical Variables

It is necessary to distinguish between treatment-induced responses to a test material and normal biological variation, particularly where statistical differences are found for data in the absence of any other findings. When biological variation is considered, several pre-analytical variables must be considered; these include species, genetic influences, sex, age, environmental conditions, chronobiochemical changes or cyclic biorhythms, diet and water intake, stress, exercise and the route chosen for the administration of the test material (Robinson and Evans, 1996).

Clearly, there are major differences between species for reference clinical chemistry values in healthy laboratory animals (Mitruka and Rawnsley, 1977; Caisey and King, 1980; Loeb and Quimby, 1989; Matsuzawa *et al.*,

1993), and these differences are not necessarily related to size or relative organ weight (Garattini, 1981). Genetic differences may occur in healthy animals—e.g. glomerular filtration rates vary between inbred strains of rats (Hackbarth *et al.*, 1981)—or the responses to a particular compound may vary between strains (Berdanier and Baltzell, 1986). Differences related to sex and age of laboratory animals are often observed (Nachbaur *et al.*, 1977; Nakamura *et al.*, 1983; Uchiyama *et al.*, 1985).

Several environmental factors which affect biological systems have been recognized including caging density, lighting, room temperature, relative humidity, cage bedding and cleaning procedures (Fouts, 1976). To some extent rodent accommodation is now designed to minimize the effects of such factors, but dogs may undergo periodic changes of housing, which may affect biochemical values (Kuhn and Hardegg, 1988). Parasitic or viral infections present in the animal stock may also affect some measurements—e.g. plasma proteins.

Cyclic variation of some analytes, particularly hormones, occurs in several laboratory animals (Jordan *et al.*, 1980; Orth *et al.*, 1988). Circadian rhythms may be altered by changing the light–dark cycles of the animal's accommodation, or they may be adapted by other experimental procedures—e.g. intravenous infusion effects of nutrients on blood glucose levels (Sitren and Stevenson, 1980). Other cyclic variations may be related to reproductive cycles or seasonal changes.

While in recent years attention has been drawn to the effects of differing diets in long-term carcinogenicity studies, diet or feeding regimens may also cause a marked effect on biochemical values, particularly in small rodents. Food restriction for 16–24 h in rats may produce changes in the composition of plasma enzymes, urea, creatinine and glucose (Jenkins and Robinson, 1975;

Kast and Nishikawa, 1981; Matsuzawa and Sakazume, 1994). Fasting may also lead to haemoconcentration effects.

The practice of fasting small laboratory animals overnight prior to blood collection may produce changes which differ from the findings for animals that have been fed. These differences may be due to (1) an alteration of the absorption or uptake of the test material, (2) changes in the competitive binding of proteins with the test material, (3) changes in metabolism rates or detoxification mechanisms or (4) modification of renal clearance. Treatment prior to sequential blood sampling in toxicology studies should be similar in respect to food and water intake. Fasting prior to blood collection also produces a transient reduction in body weight which affects the growth curve.

Mineral imbalances in the diets may predispose some species to particular conditions—e.g. nephrocalcinosis with associated changes in plasma and urine biochemistry (Stonard et al., 1984; Bertani et al., 1989; Meyer et al., 1989). Reduction of dietary protein may cause changes of plasma analytes (Schwartz et al., 1973), and changes in the composition of dietary fat or the use of corn oil as a vehicle for test materials may also produce effects on plasma chemistry measurements (Meijer et al., 1987).

Biochemical changes occur in stress situations, and include changes of plasma corticosterone/cortisol, catecholamines and other analytes, although toxic effects may be variable in these situations (Vogel, 1987). Transport between breeding colonies and user laboratories or different environments (Bean-Knudsen and Wagner, 1987; Garnier et al., 1990), caging arrangements (Riley, 1981) and restraint during experimental procedures (Pearl et al., 1966; Gartner et al., 1980) appear to be stressful, with the potential to affect the levels of several analytes.

There are several general points to consider when collecting blood from laboratory animals, including the use of anticoagulants and the changes in blood composition which occur with time. When collecting blood, it is important to separate the plasma or serum as soon as possible; this reduces the effects of glycolysis which result in reduced glucose levels and increased lactate, inorganic phosphate and potassium levels. Sodium fluoride or fluoride/oxalate anticoagulants may be used to minimize the effects of glycolysis, but these anticoagulants interfere with other measurements, including enzymes and electrolytes.

Heparin and lithium heparinate are suitable anticoagulants for most plasma measurements. Inappropriate use of anticoagulants and incorrect proportions of anticoagulant to blood volumes may also cause errors. Samples collected with sequestrene (EDTA) or sodium citrate for haematological investigations are not suitable for several electrolyte and enzyme measurements.

For several enzyme measurements, it is preferable to use plasma rather than serum, owing to the relatively high erythrocytic concentrations of those enzymes, or other enzymes which may interfere with their measurements (Korsrud and Trick, 1973; Friedel and Mattenheimer, 1976).

Several other factors to be considered when collecting blood, particularly from smaller laboratory animals, include the sampling site, the choice of anaesthetic agent and the method for drawing the blood from the site of collection. In general, the collection of blood from dogs and most primates does not cause particular problems in terms of the sample volume required for clinical chemistry (Mitruka and Rawnsley, 1977; Fowler, 1982). The use of restraining procedures and sedatives for either large or small primates may affect biochemical values (Davy et al., 1987).

For rodents, various sites and anaesthetic agents have been used, and the choice of blood collection procedure may markedly affect some biochemical measurements (Neptun et al., 1985). For interim blood collections the retro-orbital plexus, tail or jugular veins may be used, whereas the major blood vessels (e.g. abdominal aorta) or cardiac puncture may be used at necropsy (McGuill and Rowan, 1989).

Anaesthetic agents used for rodents include halothane, ether, barbiturate, methoxyfluorane, and carbon dioxide. Repeated anaesthesia may affect the analyte values, and blood collections repeated too frequently may cause anaemia. The collection of 0.5 ml of blood from a 20 g mouse represents more than a 20% loss of blood volume for that animal. Combinations of different methods of blood collection within the same study for interim and terminal sampling points may confound interpretation of data and should be avoided if at all possible.

When collecting the blood with either a syringe or vacuum-container device, the choice of needle in relation to the proposed blood vessel site for collection is important (Conybeare et al., 1988). Additionally, forcing blood from a syringe into the collection tube through a fine needle frequently increases the degree of haemolysis observed in the plasma samples.

Haemolysis and lipaemia may interfere with analyte determinations (Young, 1990), although the degree of interference may vary with a particular method (Powers et al., 1986). Haemolysis may be compound-induced, but more frequently is due to problems in sample collection (Fowler, 1982); additional haematological data may be generated to elucidate this situation. Interference due to haemolysis may affect the analytical results in several different ways.

A change in plasma analyte concentration may occur because of a higher analyte concentration in erythrocytes—e.g. potassium. Some enzymes occurring at relatively high concentrations in erythrocytes compared with plasma may interfere with the measurement of other enzymes—e.g. adenylate kinase interferes with creatine kinase (CK) measurements. The presence of haemoglobin may affect absorbance measurements for a selected analyte, or haemoglobin may interfere with a chemical reaction—e.g. diazotisation reactions for bilirubin (Chin *et al.*, 1979; Leard *et al.*, 1990). Some coloured compounds such as naphthoquinones may impart a pink or red colour to plasma which may be misinterpreted as haemolysis.

Turbidity caused by hyperlipaemic plasma may also interfere with the measurement of some analytes; this hyperlipaemia may be induced by the test material (Steinberg *et al.*, 1986) or may be caused by conditions such as severe ketosis. The turbidity due to lipaemia may be reduced by ultracentrifugation or precipitation techniques (Thompson and Kunze, 1984), but these procedures may disguise significant changes of analyte concentrations.

Analytical Procedures

The introduction of Good Laboratory Practice (GLP) requiring proven equipment maintenance, calibration and documentation, and, more importantly, the use of analytical equipment such as centrifugal analysers, has led to an overall improvement in analytical procedures when small volumes of plasma (3–50 μl per test) are used. Most laboratories use automated analytical methods for the common biochemical measurements, and adhere to quality control procedures within the laboratory; these laboratories may also participate in external quality assessment schemes. The level of precision or imprecision intra-assay is usually less than 5% (expressed as a coefficient of variation) for most assays, but may be slightly higher for specialized assays—e.g. hormones or manual analytical methods.

Despite improvements in analytical procedures, large differences for reference (or control) ranges are observed between laboratories. Some of these differences are due to the use of methods and reagents formulated for the analysis of human samples, and these methods may not be suitable for all laboratory animal species. Dooley (1979) reported that substrate concentrations required for measurements of aspartate aminotransferase (AST) differed substantially between rat, dog, monkey and human sera. Other examples include the measurement of plasma creatinine using alkaline picrate reagent, in which the contribution of non-creatinine chromogens is greater in some laboratory species compared with humans (Evans, 1986b), and the differing affinities of various dyes for plasma albumin in different species (Evans and Parsons, 1988).

Xenobiotics may interfere with the analytical methods in several different ways. Direct interference with an assay may be chemical or physical, and the interference may be either negative or positive. Various guidelines have been proposed for testing for drug interference in clinical chemistry measurements (Kallner and Tryding,

1989), but seldom are the metabolites studied individually for possible interference with analytes. Additionally, the interference of a particular compound may vary with the analytical method (Evans, 1985). Comprehensive databases have been established for pharmaceuticals known to cause analytical interference with clinical chemistry methods (Young, 1990). Early recognition during *in vivo* studies of potential interference in plasma or urine measurements can be further investigated by alternative analytical methods or *in vitro* studies.

In general, the analytical variation is less than the biological variation, and the intra-animal variability differs for each analyte—e.g. Leissing *et al.* (1985) found in healthy dogs that intra-animal variability for sodium was less than 1%, whereas it was more than 40% for ALP. This intra-animal variation differs between species—e.g. the analytical variation for glucose is small (with a coefficient of variation of $< 2\%$ for the method) but the biological variation observed in the marmoset was greater than in the dog, probably owing to stress during blood collection procedures (Fowler, 1982).

Although several analytes exhibit a normal (or Gaussian) distribution, other analytes show a skewed distribution to the right or are not continuous in nature. The distribution of analyte values may vary between and within long-term studies (Weil, 1982).

In rodent toxicology studies conducted for regulatory purposes, it is usual to compare differences between the treatment groups and a concurrent control group, whereas in studies using larger animals (primates, dogs, etc.), where group sizes of 4–6 animals per sex are common, the emphasis is both on differences, as already stated, and comparison with pretreatment values in the same animals. Where the number of animals within a study is small, it is advisable to take at least one baseline measurement and preferably more as a guide to intra-animal variations. It is sometimes necessary to compare the values obtained for a concurrent control group with the historical database, to ensure that differences between the concurrent control and treatment groups are not the consequence of an aberrant control group. Although historical reference ranges may be useful, there may be slight differences in the treatments (e.g. test vehicle, route of dosing) or animal populations studied. With samples taken from moribund animals in the absence of a concurrent control group, it is often difficult to distinguish between results expected due to toxicity and those results which would occur in moribund but untreated animals.

LIVER

Hepatic damage is not uncommon as a toxicological problem, but the fact that the damage is not a single entity is reflected by the choice of tests that may be used to detect hepatotoxicity. Xenobiotics may or may not produce functional impairment as a consequence of hepatic damage. The liver undertakes a diverse range of functions, and it is therefore unrealistic to expect a single test to determine the functional status of this organ.

Diagnostic tests for the evaluation of hepatic damage or dysfunction may be arbitrarily grouped as (1) plasma enzymes, (2) functional or clearance tests which measure hepatic transport, uptake, conjugation and excretion and (3) tests to assess hepatic metabolism of proteins, lipids and carbohydrates. A major deficiency of most of these tests is that they do not provide a current assessment of liver integrity, but rather a retrospective view of hepatic status over the preceding days and weeks. However, their value lies in serial measurements in blood samples taken periodically, which can be used to monitor the progression of the damage. The assessment of hepatic function and damage in animal species has been reviewed in the light of current practice in the UK (Woodman, 1988a, 1996).

Plasma Enzymes

Various factors affecting plasma enzyme measurements were discussed earlier in this chapter. In the early stages of tissue damage, cytoplasmic enzymes may leak from cells where membrane permeability has altered. As the severity of tissue damage progresses, enzymes normally present in subcellular organelles may be released into the circulation. Increased plasma enzyme activities may indicate loss of hepatocyte integrity with changes of parenchymal enzymes, or 'biliary' enzymes may indicate obstruction, proliferation, inflammation or neoplasia of the biliary system. Reduced plasma enzyme activities are also observed in some forms of liver injury—e.g. cholinesterase (see later discussion). In addition, some enzyme changes are the result of enzyme induction—e.g. the increase of ALP that occurs with glucocorticosteroids (Dorner et al., 1974; Wellman et al., 1982; Eckersall, 1986).

Many of the enzymes listed in **Table 2** have been used or tested as markers of hepatotoxicity. The value of standard 'liver function tests', which includes the listed enzymes, in the diagnosis of liver disease in humans has been comprehensively covered (Johnson, 1989). It should not be assumed, however, that enzymes applied in human clinical practice show the same diagnostic value in various animal species (Woodman, 1981). The majority of plasma enzyme measurements for detecting hepatotoxicity are not specific to the liver and show a wide tissue distribution.

Alanine aminotransferase (ALT, previously called GPT) is widely used as a sensitive marker of hepatotoxicity but does lack some specificity. In the dog the concentration of ALT found in the hepatic tissue is approximately five times that found in any other tissues, but tissue enzyme distribution studies show that this difference is much less in the guinea-pig, rat and rabbit (Clampitt and Hart, 1978; Lindena et al., 1986). In some species plasma ALT activity is low and is less useful as a marker of hepatotoxicity (Davy et al., 1984; Cowie and Evans, 1985). Plasma AST may also be elevated in hepatotoxicity where cellular and subcellular injury has occurred; the proportional activity of the two isoforms of the enzyme (mitochondrial and cytosolic) may indicate the extent of liver injury.

Several dehydrogenases have been used as screening tests for liver injury. The diagnostic value of LDH is limited, because it is widely distributed in the tissues and the tissue isoenzyme patterns vary between species. Glutamate dehydrogenase and sorbitol dehydrogenase are two of the more specific tests for hepatotoxicity, since both show high activities in the liver, relative to other tissues.

ALP is widely used as a marker of liver injury, particularly for cholestasis. However, the variable composition of plasma ALP alters its diagnostic value in different species. The dominant ALP isoenzyme in dog plasma is the hepatic form, but the osseous and intestinal isoenzymes are the dominant forms in rat plasma. The concentration of ALP in rat liver is very low, which limits its usefulness as an index of hepatic injury in this species. In the rat, the food intake affects the proportion of intestinal ALP in plasma (Pickering and Pickering, 1978a, b). In the majority of species, age-related changes are found owing to the presence of osseous ALP. Methods for the separation of ALP isoenzymes have been reviewed (Moss, 1982).

GGT is a useful marker of cholestasis, but its use as a marker of enzyme induction in animals is less predictive compared with data from human studies. The relative enzyme activity of GGT is highest in the kidney, of all the major organs. In the rat kidney the level of GGT is approximately 200 times higher than the level found in the liver. Although plasma GGT activity is lower in rodents than in other species, including human, it remains a good marker of cholestasis (Braun et al., 1987).

Of the other plasma enzymes, ornithine carbamoyl transferase (OCT) is a sensitive liver-specific enzyme (Baumann and Berauer, 1985), and 5'-nucleotidase has been used for the diagnosis of hepatobiliary disease. Whether through lack of technical simplicity, suitability for use with automated laboratory analysers or readily available reagents, some of the enzyme determinations mentioned are rarely used in regulatory toxicology studies—e.g. OCT.

The family of enzymes collectively known as glutathione S-transferases, which catalyse reactions between reduced glutathione and various electrophiles, have been proposed as markers of liver disease. Glutathione S-transferase α is a specific and sensitive marker of damage to hepatocytes. It comprises approximately 5% of the soluble protein of hepatocytes, and is readily released into the plasma in response to hepatic damage.

Its rapid release into and removal from the circulation provide an early marker of hepatic damage (Campbell *et al.*, 1991). An enzyme immunoassay for the alpha form has been validated (Rees *et al.*, 1995). In contrast to the alpha form, the pi form of glutathione *S*-transferase is localized in the biliary epithelium (Beckett and Hayes, 1993) and can be measured by an ELISA method in both bile and plasma.

Plasma Bilirubin

Increased plasma concentrations of total bilirubin (icterus) may follow excessive haem turnover by the reticulo-endothelial system, alterations of hepatic clearance by microsomal conjugation, intrahepatic obstruction of the bile canaliculi, or extrahepatic obstruction of the bile duct. Where one of these conditions is truly severe, the measurement of conjugated (direct) and unconjugated (indirect) bilirubin may be helpful.

Plasma total bilirubin is lower (less than 8μ mol l^{-1}) in many laboratory animal species compared with the levels found in human plasma. Species such as the rat and dog have a low renal threshold for bilirubin. The very low values found in rats are close to the limit of detection for many photometric methods commonly used for total bilirubin assays (Rosenthal *et al.*, 1981); this methodological problem is exacerbated when measurements of conjugated bilirubin are required.

When haemolytic jaundice occurs, the presence of plasma haemoglobin and other pigments may cause analytical interference at these low concentrations of plasma bilirubin. This has led to the suggestion that measurement of plasma total bilirubin is inappropriate in species such as the rat (Waner, 1990), although plasma bilirubin measurements still can be useful where cholestasis occurs. In addition to the unconjugated and conjugated forms of bilirubin, there exists a third form, known as Δ-bilirubin, which is irreversibly bound to plasma albumin (Lauff *et al.*, 1981). This Δ-bilirubin is present in human serum in liver disorders associated with increased serum conjugated bilirubin, but has a significantly longer half-life (Weiss *et al.*, 1983). It is unclear whether this third form offers any significant diagnostic advantage over the measurement of total and conjugated bilirubin. The binding of bilirubin by plasma proteins is complex in the presence of xenobiotics (Gautam *et al.*, 1984; Blanckaert *et al.*, 1986), and in the rat there are marked sex differences in hepatic conjugation of bilirubin (Muraca *et al.*, 1983).

Plasma Bile Acids

Total bile acids may be subdivided into primary (cholic and chenodeoxycholic) and secondary (deoxycholic and lithocholic) bile acids, with their taurine and glycine conjugates. The relative proportions of individual bile acids differ with species (Parraga and Kaneko, 1985). For example, the secondary bile acid β-muricholate is a prominent component of cholestasis in the rat (Greim *et al.*, 1972), but the reaction leading to its formation in man is absent (Hofmann, 1988). Secretion of bile acids alters after food intake, and the timing of blood sampling in relation to food intake can be critical for the detection of changes. When measured 2 h after a meal, plasma bile acids have shown a high specificity for detecting hepatic dysfunction; however, their measurement may offer little advantage over plasma aminotransferases for detecting mild liver disease in humans (Fromm and Albert, 1987). Hepatic uptake and the carrier-mediated transport system for bile acids differ from the mechanisms responsible for the transport of bilirubin and exogenous dyes (Alpert *et al.*, 1969; Schardsmidt *et al.*, 1975; Erlanger *et al.*, 1976).

The development of sensitive and inexpensive test kits has encouraged several investigators to recommend the plasma measurement of 3α-hydroxy bile acids as an indicator of cholestasis (Gopinath *et al.*, 1980; Woodman and Maile, 1981; Woodman, 1988a). This measurement can be applied to most species and is an alternative to the measurement of individual bile acids (Thompson, 1996; Azer *et al.*, 1997); however, more evidence is required to support bile acid measurements in rodent toxicology before they become a core test in regulatory studies (Evans, 1993).

Urine Bilirubin, Urobilinogen and Urobilin

Bilirubinuria can be a useful marker of hepatic necrosis or bile duct obstruction, but the low renal threshold in some animals reduces the usefulness of this test in borderline cases—e.g. increases of bilirubin may occur in the urine in the dog before changes of plasma total bilirubin (de Schepper and van der Stock, 1972).

Urobilinogen and stercobilinogen are formed from bile by the bacterial action of the intestinal flora, and enter the extrahepatic circulation to be excreted as urobilinogen. Urobilinogen may be increased following excessive breakdown of haemoglobin or hepatic dysfunction, including situations where there is a bypass via the enterohepatic circulation; urobilinogen is not elevated in cases of extrahepatic obstruction.

If exposed to strong light, urobilinogen is rapidly converted to urobilin. Both urobilinogen and urine bilirubin may be detected qualitatively by the use of test strips.

Exogenous Dyes

Of several major quantitative liver function tests applied in a broad range of circumstances in human clinical practice (Tredger and Sherwood, 1997), only dye clearance has occasionally been used in animal species. Several dye clearance and excretion tests have been used as indices of hepatic function. Bromosulphthalein (BSP or sulphbromophthalein) and indocyanine green (ICG) are the two commonly used cholephilic dyes (Jablonski and Owen, 1969; Ott, 1998). When administered intravenously, BSP binds principally to albumin and to a lesser extent to lipoprotein. In the hepatocytes the bound dye is removed from the circulation by conjugation with glutathione in the presence of glutathione transferase; the conjugated dye and a proportion of the free dye are excreted in the bile. These clearance measurements require numerous blood collection procedures and accurately timed blood samples.

Approximately 50% of liver functional mass has to be lost before the BSP clearance changes. Delayed dye clearance may be due to hepatic necrosis, cholestasis, reduced hepatic blood flow or renal dysfunction; obstruction of biliary excretion causes BSP retention.

Marked differences are observed for BSP clearance determinations in various species. Both the rat and rabbit show greater ability to clear the dye than the dog—i.e. approximately 1 mg min^{-1} kg^{-1} in the first two species compared with 0.2 mg min^{-1} kg^{-1} in the dog. Therefore, it is essential to optimize BSP dosage and the timing of blood collections for each species studied (Klaassen and Plaa, 1967). The relationships of dosages and clearances for ICG between species is not identical with those determined with BSP (Klaassen and Plaa, 1969). The quantitation of hepatic blood flow poses a technical challenge, but the clearance of ICG, with constant intravenous infusion, may provide an indirect measure of hepatic blood flow (Caesar et al., 1961).

Plasma Coagulation Factors

Most coagulation factors are synthesized in the liver. The measurement in plasma of prothrombin time and activated partial thromboplastin time provides indications of the status of the extrinsic and intrinsic coagulation pathways, respectively (Theus and Zbinden, 1984). As several of the coagulation factors have short half-lives, their measurement provide an indication of current functional status in hepatic damage (Pritchard et al., 1987).

Plasma Lipids

Lipid accumulation in the liver often reflects changes in the rate of lipoprotein synthesis or a reduced ability to catabolize the non-esterified fatty acids which are formed when triglycerides are mobilized and degraded. Several compounds of diverse structure have the ability in some rodent species to produce a hypolipidaemic response characterized by reductions in the circulating concentrations of triglycerides and/or cholesterol. These reductions in circulating lipids appear to reflect both structural and functional changes in the liver leading to differences in the metabolic handling of saturated fatty acids (Lock et al., 1989). Fat accumulation in hepatocytes does not necessarily lead to necrosis of the cells, but some conditions involving fat accumulation may lead to the disruption of cellular integrity. Plasma lipid changes associated with hepatotoxicity may be detected by measuring plasma total cholesterol, triglycerides, ratio of esterified to free cholesterol, non-esterified fatty acids (Degen and van der Vies, 1985) and individual lipoprotein fractions. Techniques for the measurement of plasma lipids and lipoproteins can be found elsewhere (Evans, 1996c).

Urinary Taurine

Exposure of rats to several toxic agents which cause hepatic necrosis (and steatosis in some cases) caused an elevation of urinary taurine (a β-amino acid) output (Waterfield et al., 1993a). The excretion of urinary taurine was shown to be increased by compounds which inhibit glutathione and protein synthesis and, conversely, decreased by compounds which deplete glutathione and stimulate protein synthesis (Waterfield et al., 1993b). No significant increases in urinary taurine were found after treatment of rats with agents known to damage kidneys, heart or testes; thus damage to extra-hepatic organs is unlikely to be a confounding factor in the use of urinary taurine as a marker of hepatic damage (Waterfield et al., 1993b).

KIDNEY

The primary functions of the kidneys are in volume regulation, excretion of waste products, regulation of acid–base balance, regulation of electrolyte balance and endocrine functions, including the renin–aldosterone axis, erythropoietin synthesis, 1,25-dihydroxycholecalciferol and synthesis of prostaglandins and kinins. Nephrotoxic substances may impair some or all of these functions by a variety of toxic mechanisms (Commandeur and Vermeulen, 1990). It is important to recognize that renal function tests do not ensure identification of nephrotoxicity in all cases where structural alterations of the kidneys can be demonstrated by histopathology (Sharratt and Frazer, 1963). However, a combination of screening tests based on qualitative and quantitative measurements can be used to detect nephrotoxicity (Bovee, 1986; Fent et al., 1988). The timing of the measurements is often critical in detecting transient changes of diagnostic significance. Many xenobiotics are known to affect renal function, and these effects may vary between species because of the relative morphological differences of the kidneys (Mudge, 1982). The assessment of renal function and damage in animal species has been reviewed in the light of current practices in the UK (Stonard, 1990, 1996).

Glomerular Function

Glomerular function is commonly measured using creatinine and/or urea as both of these endogenous substances are normally filtered from the plasma and reabsorbed or secreted by the kidneys to a minor extent, dependent upon the species used. The plasma concentrations of both compounds are affected by diet (Evans, 1987). Although plasma creatinine is generally thought to be a better marker than urea of glomerular function, plasma creatinine measurements may be subject to analytical interference by endogenous non-creatinine chromogens or some xenobiotics—e.g. some cephalosporins (Evans, 1986b; Grotsch and Hajdu, 1987). The term 'BUN' should be used strictly for the determination of blood urea nitrogen (not plasma or serum urea).

The glomerular filtration rate (GFR) may be determined by endogenous creatinine clearance or following administration of exogenous inulin (with or without radiolabel) or iodothalamate. These determinations require infusion and accurately timed blood and/or urine collection procedures. These measurements may be affected by the use of particular anaesthetic agents for blood collection from small laboratory animals.

As glomerular filtration reduces, plasma creatinine and/or urea will increase. The relationship between the loss of glomerular filtration capacity and plasma creatinine/urea is not linear. Approximately 50% or more of renal capacity can be lost before plasma creatinine levels become abnormal and renal disease is detectable clinically (Berndt, 1981). Glomerular function, plasma creatinine and urea, to a lesser extent, all show variations with age (Corman et al., 1985; Goldstein, 1990).

Urinalysis

Urinalysis can be a valuable non-invasive technique for monitoring nephrotoxicity, but it is important to give particular attention to the conditions for urine collection. Contamination of urine samples by diet and/or faeces may cause erroneous results for many parameters. Some assays may require the use of a preservative and/or cooling of the samples during collection. Simple observations of the urine appearance and colour may be useful, as the colour may be altered by the presence of exogenous and endogenous substances—e.g. blood, bilirubin, porphyrin and some drugs.

Several of the urinary measurements—e.g. glucose, pH, blood, ketones, urobilinogen, can be made using one of several commercial test strips (or dipsticks). Cer-

tain pitfalls may be encountered as the test strips are designed for use in human clinical rather than laboratory animal practice; these pitfalls are primarily related to sensitivity and/or specificity—e.g. protein, osmolality (Allchin and Evans, 1986c; Evans and Parsons, 1986; Allchin et al., 1987).

Urine volume and concentration may act as markers of nephrotoxicity. Many nephrotoxins will produce oliguria, whereas persistent polyuria may indicate an alteration of renal concentrating ability. Polyuria may also be a desired pharmacological diuretic response. Osmolality, specific gravity, or refractometric measurements can be used to measure urine concentration, and additional information on tubular concentrating ability may be obtained by using water deprivation or water loading techniques. The maximum osmolality that can be achieved varies with species, with both rat and dog giving values approximately twofold greater than in humans (Schmidt-Nielsen and O'Dell, 1961).

Glycosuria may be detected conveniently by the use of a test strip. Urinary glucose may reflect enhanced excretion because of elevated blood levels or more likely is due to damage to the proximal tubules, where glucose is reabsorbed.

Changes of hydrogen ion concentration (pH) may reflect changes in tubular function or they may simply reflect dietary protein composition. Delays in analysing urine samples may cause hydrogen ion concentration values to be altered by ammonia produced by microorganisms. Low pH values may reflect catabolic states associated with severe toxicity.

Urine Cytology

Microscopic examination of urine sediment for the presence of erythrocytes, leucocytes, renal epithelial cells, bladder cells, spermatozoa, etc., may be used to detect urinary tract damage, particularly to the kidneys. The sediment may be examined unstained, although the use of stains helps to distinguish between renal epithelial cells and leucocytes (Prescott and Brodie, 1964; Hardy, 1970). Methodology needs to be standardized to minimize any variations within and between studies.

As the normal background of celluria differs from one species to another, and on the basis of the few published data on urine sediments in species other than man (Davies and Kennedy, 1967; Prescott, 1982), celluria appears to be of little benefit for monitoring renal injury, except for acute proximal tubular damage. When acute injury occurs to this region, cells in urine may be a sensitive but unreliable indicator (Prescott and Ansari, 1969). Hyaline or granular casts associated with Tamm–Horsfall glycoprotein may be found in the tubular lumen and urine sediment.

The presence of blood in the urine may reflect non-specific bleeding or renal or post-renal injury. Contamination of urine samples by blood from superficial injuries (e.g. skin abrasions) must always be considered as a possible explanation for blood in the urine. The presence of leucocytes in the urine may indicate bacterial infection.

Crystalluria may be due to the pH-dependent precipitation of urates or phosphates. Occasionally crystalluria may be due to the high urinary concentration of a xenobiotic or its metabolite(s).

Urine Protein

Increased urinary protein levels are often the first sign of renal injury. Commercial test strips offer a simple method for the assessment of proteinuria, but they react mainly with albumin and are therefore not particularly useful in detecting the presence of proteins other than albumin. This is well recognized in laboratory rodents which show several qualitative and quantitative differences in protein excretion in comparison with dogs and humans. The major protein in male rat urine is not albumin as in most species, but a low molecular weight protein, α_2-globulin (Roy and Neuhaus, 1967). Moreover, the amount of protein excreted increases, and changes in the composition of protein excreted occur, with age (Neuhaus and Flory, 1978; Alt et al., 1980). Several methods are available for the quantitative measurement of urinary total protein (McElderry et al., 1982; Dilena et al., 1983).

Proteins such as albumin and transferrin, which originate from the plasma, are normally filtered to a slight extent through the glomeruli, and subsequently reabsorbed by the tubules. When tubular reabsorption of proteins is normal, as reflected by a normal excretion of low molecular weight proteins, then increases in the excretion of albumin and transferrin indicate alterations in glomerular permeability. There are several immunoassay techniques available for the measurement of specific proteins, especially albumin, although the range of proteins which can be measured in animal species is restricted by the lack of suitable purified proteins and specific antisera.

Primary tubular disorders may be distinguished from glomerular damage by the ratio of high and low molecular weight proteins in the urine. Techniques using various electrophoretic support media and buffers can provide additional information on the composition of urinary proteins (Boesken et al., 1973; Allchin and Evans, 1986a; Stonard et al., 1987).

Urine Enzymes

Urinary enzyme measurements provide useful information on the site of renal injury, whereas plasma enzymes are poor markers of nephrotoxicity (Wright and Plummer, 1974; Stroo and Hook, 1977; Price, 1982;

Guder and Ross, 1984; Stonard, 1987). However, of the many urinary enzyme measurements investigated, relatively few have proved to be of diagnostic value. In several acute studies with nephrotoxic substances, reasonable correlations between renal pathology and urinary enzyme excretion have been demonstrated (Cottrell et al., 1976; Bhargava et al., 1978). However, there are a few examples where urinary enzymes do not appear to be as sensitive as other renal function indices (Stroo and Hook, 1977; Kluwe, 1981).

The enzymes which have received most attention are those localized in the proximal tubules. Those enzymes located on the brush border of the renal proximal tubules—e.g. ALP, GGT and alanine aminopeptidase (AAP)—appear generally to act as earlier indicators of renal damage compared with other tests of renal toxicity (Wright et al., 1972; Jung and Scholz, 1980; Salgo and Szabo, 1982). N-Acetyl-β-glucosaminidase (NAG) appears to be a useful enzyme marker of damage to the papilla of the kidney (Price, 1982). Several studies with papillotoxic agents have shown that the excretion of a voluminous, dilute urine is accompanied by an increased urinary excretion of NAG (Bach and Hardy, 1985; Stonard et al., 1987).

The presence of endogenous low molecular weight inhibitors in the urine may cause problems when urinary enzymes are being analysed, and these inhibitors require removal by dialysis, gel filtration or ultrafiltration (Werner et al., 1969; Werner and Gabrielson, 1977). Several urinary enzymes are unstable and rapid analysis following collection is advisable. A possible effect on the enzymes by the presence in urine of the test material and/or its metabolite(s) should also be considered. There is evidence of the effects of age, sex, urinary flow and biorhythms on urinary enzyme excretion (Grotsch et al., 1985; Pariat et al., 1990).

For some urinary enzymes which exist in isoenzymic forms—e.g. NAG—the measurements of the isoenzymes can be more informative than the measurement of the total enzyme activity (Halman et al., 1984). Similarly, glutathione S-transferase isoenzymic forms show regional specificity within the renal tubules, with the α form found primarily in the proximal convoluted tubule, and the π form found in the distal convoluted tubule, thin loop of Henle and collecting ducts (Campbell et al., 1991; Sundberg et al., 1994a). This difference in distribution can be exploited to distinguish between certain pathological processes in the kidney (Sundberg et al., 1994b).

A comprehensive text on urinary enzymology has detailed accomplishments in this field of interest (Jung et al., 1992).

Electrolyte Balance

Urinary electrolyte values are highly dependent not only on water and dietary intake but also water loss arising from vomitus or diarrhoea. Measurement of the cations potassium and sodium, which can be secreted or re-absorbed at various sites along the nephron, does not usually provide any additional diagnostic information of value. Urinary magnesium and calcium determinations may be important for some nephrotoxic substances—e.g. cisplatin (Magil et al., 1986).

Perturbations of acid–base balance will often accompany severe electrolyte changes, but these measurements require controlled conditions, particularly for small laboratory animals. Measurements of renin, aldosterone and atrial natriuretic hormone are generally reserved for xenobiotics where the mode of action suggests that these assays will be useful for the understanding of the pathogenesis of renal changes.

The kidneys receive 20–25% of the cardiac output, and it is sometimes important to measure the effective renal plasma flow (ERPF). This can be demonstrated by the active uptake and tubular secretion of the organic anion p-aminohippurate (PAH): the PAH transport is so efficient in many species that the PAH clearance indicates ERPF. A reduction of PAH clearance may be due to an alteration of renal blood flow, by an effect on vasculature, or a disruption of the active secretory process for organic anions.

NMR Spectroscopy

NMR is a non-invasive and non-destructive technique which can be used to monitor potential changes in the spectra of endogenous intermediary metabolites in biological fluids, e.g. urine. Characteristic changes in the normal urinary profile can be detected in the urine from animals treated with nephrotoxic agents which have a common site of injury (Gartland et al., 1989). The mild nephrotoxic effects in rabbits of several cephalosporin antibiotics can be clearly distinguished by NMR urinalysis, but not by conventional urinalysis (Halligan et al., 1995). This rapid multi-component analysis technique offers a sensitive approach for the early detection of nephrotoxicity, and the opportunity to characterize profiles indicative of damage to selective areas of the kidney.

The search for new biomarkers of renal damage includes cytokines, growth factors, extracellular matrix components (collagen, glycoproteins and proteoglycans), lipid mediators, transcription factors, cell adhesion molecules and protooncogenes (Finn et al., 1997; Mueller et al., 1997). Epidermal growth factor (EGF), the origin of which appears to be the kidney (Olsen et al., 1984), may provide an indication of distal tubular damage, which may be more closely related to changes in GFR than some other markers (Finn et al., 1997). In rats, renal excretion of EGF has been shown to fall immediately in response to the release of ischaemia (Safirstein et al., 1990).

GASTROINTESTINAL TRACT

Nutritional status may influence the bioavailability and, hence, toxic effects on the gastrointestinal tract in several ways (George, 1984; Aungst and Shen, 1986; Omaye, 1986). Disturbances of gastrointestinal function are often accompanied by electrolyte imbalance due to fluid losses either by emesis (vomiting), volvulus (dilatation) or diarrhoea. Excessive salivation may also cause electrolyte perturbations. Prolonged or excessive losses of fluid via the gastrointestinal tract will affect packed cell volume (haematocrit) and plasma total protein, albumin, electrolytes, acid–base balance and osmolality values (Smith, 1986).

Electrolyte Balance

Hypo- or hypernatraemia may occur, depending on the proportional losses of electrolyte to water; these electrolyte changes are also reflected by plasma osmolality. In the presence of osmotically active solutes (e.g. mannitol) there may be significant differences between measured and calculated osmolality; similar differences may occur in the presence of hyperlipidaemia and hyperproteinaemia. These electrolyte measurements emphasize the need to separate plasma from erythrocytes as rapidly as possible in order to avoid changes in plasma potassium concentrations, although these changes are less in the dog than with other species.

Excessive losses of chloride-rich fluids (e.g. pancreatic secretion) may be monitored by plasma chloride measurements; changes in plasma chloride concentration which are not accompanied by a change in plasma sodium are usually associated with disturbances of acid–base balance where chloride concentration varies inversely to plasma bicarbonate.

Occult Blood

For compounds suspected of causing gastrointestinal bleeding or having ulcerogenic properties (e.g. non-steroidal anti-inflammatory compounds), the detection of faecal occult or frank blood may be of value. There are a number of available procedures for the detection of occult blood, and the majority of colorimetric qualitative tests are based on the pseudoperoxidase activity of haemoglobin. The sensitivity of these tests varies with the reagents used, and is subject to interferences from peroxidases and pseudoperoxidases present in food (Aldercreutz et al., 1984; Johnson, 1989). Additionally, in animal studies it may be necessary to alter the sensitivity of a particular method in order to avoid false positive reactions associated with animal diets, particularly for carniverous species (Dent, 1973). False positive reactions may also be caused by some cleaning fluids used in animal housing—e.g. hypochlorite solutions. Alternative methods for the detection of faecal occult blood include the use of radiolabelled erythrocytes (Walsh, 1982) or the detection of porphyrins by fluorescence (Boulay *et al.*, 1986), but these methods are not used widely.

Enzymes

Several enzyme measurements are available for assessing gastrointestinal function and toxicity, but these assays are not usually included in the majority of toxicology studies. Relatively simple assays are used for assessing pancreatic exocrine function (Boyd *et al.*, 1988), whereas the measurement of intestinal disaccharidases is more complex. Some of these enzyme measurements require the collection of gastric, pancreatic and other intestinal fluids, faeces or tissues.

The two enzymes amylase and lipase have been widely used to detect pancreatitis, although there are wide variations in plasma amylase levels and the tissue distribution of amylase and its isoenzymes in different species (Rajasingham *et al.*, 1971; McGeachin and Akin, 1982). Pancreatic chymotrypsin activity can be measured in plasma following oral administration of *N*-benzoyl-1-tyrosyl-*p*-aminobenzoic acid.

Of the proteolytic enzymes, pepsin and trypsin can be measured by relatively simple techniques. Pepsinogen is the precursor of the proteolytic enzyme pepsin (EC 3.4.23.1) and is secreted by gastric parietal cells; it may be measured in plasma or gastric fluid by colorimetric, fluorimetric or radioimmunometric methods (Will *et al.*, 1984; Ford *et al.*, 1985; Tani *et al.*, 1987). Pepsinogen activities may be increased following peptic ulceration and by parasitic infections. Trypsin (EC 3.4.21.4) can be measured in faeces by gelatin digestion, chromogenic assays or immunoenzymometric methods (Fletcher *et al.*, 1986; Simpson and Doxey, 1988).

Measurement of intestinal disaccharidases may be useful, but these enzymes are subject to various factors, including age, nutritional status, hormonal influences due to glucocorticoids and thyroid hormones, diurnal variations etc. (Henning, 1984). Duodenal or intestinal ALP is markedly reduced with some ulcerogens—e.g. cysteamine (Japundzic and Levi, 1987). Other enzyme changes occur in miscellaneous gastrointestinal conditions such as intestinal infarction or obstruction (Kazmlerczak *et al.*, 1988) and parasitic infections.

Endocrine, Pancreatic Function and Carbohydrate Metabolism

For plasma glucose measurements, the use of an inhibitor (i.e. sodium fluoride) or rapid separation of the plasma is recommended to prevent glycolysis. Plasma glucose levels below 1.7 mmol l^{-1}, which would give rise to clinical signs of hypoglycaemia in man, do not appear to produce similar adverse effects in some other primates. With some rodent species it appears that the animals have to be fasted for much longer periods than other species to achieve similar reductions in plasma glucose. The ability of certain primates to store food in their buccal pouches often prevents the true measurement of 'fasting' glucose. Blood collection procedures may cause a marked elevation of plasma glucose where the animal is subject to stress, including restraint (Gartner *et al.*, 1980).

The measurement of plasma and urinary glucose, and additional measurements of ketosis (i.e. urinary ketones), plasma 3-hydroxybutyrate, lipids and osmolality will all act as indicators of the severity of the disturbance to carbohydrate metabolism. The additional measurement of glycosylated haemoglobin may be useful when monitoring the effects of hypoglycaemic agents (Higgins *et al.*, 1982; Neuman *et al.*, 1994).

The molecular structures of the pancreatic hormones insulin and glucagon vary with animal species, and this prevents the universal application of immunoassays across different species, although there are degrees of cross-reactivity between some species (Berthet, 1963; Young, 1963).

Other Tests

Drug-induced pancreatitis may be accompanied by gross plasma lipid changes, and hypocalcaemia due to excessive loss of pancreatic secretion. Gross examination of faeces may show evidence of undigested fat in animals with severe pancreatic deficiency.

Other more specialized investigations for detecting gastrointestinal toxicity include measurement of intestinal permeability with polyethylene glycol polymers (Walsh, 1982), xylose absorption tests, and hydrogen or carbon isotopic pulmonary or 'breath' tests. Plasma gastrin measurements may be a useful adjunct to studies where antiulceration drugs are being investigated, but gastrin has a relatively short half-life (Koop *et al.*, 1982; Larsson *et al.*, 1986). Where gastrointestinal toxic effects are prolonged, marked reductions in the intake of essential nutrients such as vitamins (folate), amino acids, etc., may occur.

HEART

Enzymes

Enzymes are used as primary markers of cardiotoxicity, but timing and the methods of sample collection are particularly critical for the detection of cardiac damage;

the importance of sample times has been shown in several studies where myocardial lesions have been induced by the administration of isoprenaline (Balazs and Bloom, 1982; Barrett et al., 1988). Following cardiac damage, a large number of tissue enzymes are released into the plasma, but only a few of these enzymes are used commonly for the diagnosis of myocardial damage and congestive cardiac failure. These enzymes are CK, LDH, AST and, to a lesser extent, ALT. None of these enzyme measurements is specific for cardiac tissue, and this has led to the use of isoenzymes, particularly for CK and LDH, to obtain additional information.

CK is a dimeric molecule with subunits B and M; there are three cytosolic enzymes—the muscle dimer MM, the brain dimer BB and the myocardial dimer MB (Lang, 1981). There are also mitochondrial isoenzymes and isoforms of CK. The tissue distribution of CK is not confined to the heart and the distribution pattern varies between species.

Plasma CK activities may be markedly affected by skeletal muscle damage by either simple intramuscular injections or toxic myopathies. Various compounds such as pethidine, lidocaine, diazepam, digoxin, chlorpromazine and tetracycline have been reported to increase CK activity in rats and dogs (Meltzer et al., 1970; Gloor et al., 1977; Steiness et al., 1978; Swain et al., 1994). Occasionally, increased plasma CK activity and muscle necrosis may be caused by the osmolality, hydrogen ion concentration, volume of administered formulation or an excipient (Surber and Dubach, 1989).

LDH is a cytosolic tetrameric enzyme with five major isoenzymes in plasma consisting of H (heart) and M (muscle) subunits. The five isoenzymes are numbered according to decreasing anodic mobility during electrophoretic separation: LDH1 has four H subunits, LDH5 has four M subunits and LDH2, LDH3 and LDH4 are hybrid combinations, containing HHHM, HHMM and HMMM, respectively (Markert and Whitt, 1975). The tissue distribution of LDH is widespread, and differences occur between the various species (Karlsson and Larsson, 1971). The broad normal ranges for plasma total LDH activity encountered in laboratory animals makes interpretation difficult; in the rat LDH5 is a major isoenzyme in plasma, and therefore a considerable increase of LDH1 is required before total plasma LDH values change significantly. Additional isoenzymes of LDH have been described, and some LDH isoenzymes may complex with some drugs—e.g. streptokinase (Poldlasek and McPherson, 1989).

The isoenzymes of CK and LDH may be separated by a variety of electrophoretic techniques or immuno-inhibition methods, but the latter are limited by the specificity of the monoclonal antibodies currently available (Lang, 1981; Landt et al., 1989). The plasma activities of the aminotransferases AST and ALT may also change following cardiac damage, although these enzymes are used more commonly as markers of hepatotoxicity.

Troponins

The troponins form the protein filament components of the contractile and skeletal muscles. There are three genetically and biochemically distinct troponins: troponin I (TnI), which inhibits ATPase, troponin T(TnT), which binds to tropomyosin, and troponin C (TnC), which binds to calcium (Katus et al., 1992; Adams et al., 1993). Troponin I and T measurements have been described in the rat and dog, and further evaluations of the troponins in cardiotoxicity models are required (Saggin et al., 1990; Malouf et al., 1992; Dameron et al., 1997).

Other plasma measurements which may be altered by cardiotoxic compounds include electrolytes, proteins other than enzymes and lipids (Evans, 1991, 1996b). Some of the preanalytical factors discussed previously may contribute to cardiotoxicity—e.g. obesity, nutritional status, genetic variations, anaemia and thyroid function.

Electrolyte Balance

Disturbances of the intra-and extracellular equilibria of the cations sodium, potassium, calcium and magnesium may result in increased irritability of cardiac tissue and be associated with arrhythmias. As the balance of these cations is interrelated, an extreme change in the ionic balance of one cation may influence the concentrations of the other cations. The divalent cations—calcium and magnesium—are partially bound to plasma proteins, particularly albumin, and it is necessary to consider the ionized and metabolically more important plasma fractions in relation to plasma proteins.

Cationic changes are accompanied invariably by disturbances of plasma anionic concentrations and acid–base balance. Where there are alterations of fluid balance such as occur with congestive cardiac failure, these may be reflected by changes in plasma osmolality and protein concentrations, particularly albumin. Following cardiotoxic changes, there may be alterations of the plasma protein pattern with increases in acute phase proteins—e.g. myoglobin, C-reactive protein and fibrinogen; these changes may be detected by electrophoretic techniques or selective methods for quantifying individual protein fractions.

The interpretation of changing values for plasma electrolytes may be complex where cardiac output is a consequence of the failure of other organ functions (e.g. the kidneys) and, conversely, where impaired cardiac damage affects renal function. This interrelationship of organ functions is seen with several anthracycline antitumour agents, which may cause cardiotoxic and nephrotoxic effects (Sinha, 1982). The procedures used for blood collection may affect the measurements of enzymes, cations and proteins used for the detection of cardiotoxicity.

Although haemoglobinuria, proteinuria and enzymuria may occur following myocardial infarction or damage to pulmonary arteries, urine tests are generally not helpful in the detection of cardiotoxicity.

Lipoproteins and Lipids

Various lipoproteins transport lipids in the plasma, and these lipoproteins are classified according to their physico-chemical properties. The lipoproteins may be separated into chylomicra, very low density lipoproteins (VLDL), low-density lipoproteins (LDL) and high-density lipoproteins (HDL). The lipid and protein contents (apolipoproteins) also vary with the individual lipoprotein fractions. Adverse toxic and/or pharmacological effects on lipid metabolism can be monitored by measuring plasma cholesterol (total and free), triglycerides, non-esterified fatty acids, total lipids, phospholipids, lipoproteins (high- and low-density) and apolipoproteins. These measurements may be made using a variety of techniques, including chromogenic enzymatic assays, solvent extraction, electrophoresis, immunoassay, gas–liquid chromatography and ultracentrifugation. Initial information concerning alterations of plasma lipids may be obtained by measuring total cholesterol and triglycerides and by qualitative lipoprotein electrophoresis.

Plasma lipoproteins vary with age, sex, diet and the period of food withdrawal prior to sample collection. The proportion of chylomicra present in plasma is reduced after a period of fasting, but this selective food withdrawal may enhance the absorption of the test material and, hence, its toxic or pharmacological effect.

Quantitative and qualitative differences of lipoproteins and lipids occur between species. These differences are observed for the rates of absorption, synthesis and metabolism (Beynon, 1988). Some of these differences are reflected by the plasma lipoprotein patterns; for example, the major plasma lipoprotein fraction in rats, dogs, mice, rabbits and guinea-pigs are the HDL fractions, whereas in old-world monkeys, the LDL fraction is the dominant fraction (Alexander and Day, 1973; Terpstra et al., 1981; Lehmann et al., 1993). These species differences lead to some additional methodological considerations when samples are analyzed (Evans, 1986a). The testing of pharmaceutical agents such as hypolipidaemics in animal models, where atherosclerosis has been deliberately induced, may yield different responses from those obtained in healthy animals.

The effect of lipids on other plasma measurements has been briefly mentioned, and it is particularly relevant to the measurement of electrolytes. Sodium and potassium may be measured by the use of flame photometry or specific ion electrodes, and the differences observed between these two methods is accentuated in plasma samples with increased lipid content (Weisberg, 1989).

PLASMA PROTEINS

Perturbations of Plasma Proteins

Hypoproteinaemias are characterized by reductions in albumin and/or globulin fractions. In addition to reduced hepatic synthesis or increased renal excretion (discussed in previous sections on hepatotoxicity and nephrotoxicity), hypoproteinaemia may result from impaired nutritional status, some parasitic infections, haemorrhage and impaired intestinal or pancreatic function. Severe hypoproteinaemia may be associated with oedema and ascites due to the osmotic influence of albumin, whereas hyperproteinaemia may be observed with dehydration. In some situations a compensatory increase in globulin fractions may occur where there are reductions in plasma albumin and total protein concentrations—e.g. plasma protein changes in rats treated with warfarin (Colvin and Lee Wang, 1974). Few protein changes are pathognomonic.

Albumin has an important colloidal osmotic effect and this protein fraction is also associated with binding of xenobiotics perhaps more frequently than other protein fractions; marked changes of drug-binding plasma proteins may clearly affect the apparent blood concentrations of test materials, and hence toxicity. Other plasma proteins are involved in chelation of cations (e.g. caeruloplasmin, transferrin and metallothionein), binding of calcium and magnesium, antibody functions, clotting mechanisms, hormone metabolism, etc.

Protein measurements may be used to monitor inflammatory responses, although the timing of sample collection is again critical for the measurement of acute phase proteins (Betts et al., 1964; Nakagawa et al., 1984). Following inflammatory stimuli, several changes in the pattern of proteins synthesized by the liver occur, with elevations of the acute phase proteins and some reductions of other proteins. There are considerable variations of the acute phase response patterns found in different species, particularly for C-reactive protein, amyloid protein and α_2-macroglobulin (Kushner and Mackiewicz, 1987). Plasma amyloid protein is the major acute phase protein in the mouse, whereas α_2-macroglobulin is the major acute phase protein in the rat.

For rats and other small rodents, the site used for blood collection has a marked effect on the plasma protein values (Neptun et al., 1985). Age and sex differences occur in the plasma protein values obtained for laboratory animals (House et al., 1961; Reuter et al., 1968; Coe and Ross, 1983; Wolford et al., 1987).

Analytical Methods

Methods for assessing changes of plasma protein concentrations usually include measurement of total protein and albumin and qualitative or quantitative separation of proteins by various electrophoretic techniques. Plasma protein values are slightly higher than corresponding serum values, owing to the presence of fibrinogen, although this protein fraction may precipitate during cold storage. Globulin values are usually determined as the difference between total protein and albumin concentrations, although the plasma globulin value will also include a contribution due to fibrinogen.

The bromocresol green dye-binding method for plasma albumin appears to be suitable for a majority of laboratory animal species, unlike some other albumin-binding dyes (Witiak and Whitehouse, 1969; Evans and Parsons, 1988). Simple electrophoretic techniques using cellulose acetate or agarose support media can be used to assess changes of albumin and globulin fractions, although the support media may affect the electrophoretic pattern (Allchin and Evans, 1986b).

Although albumin is usually the dominant electrophoretic band, there are marked species differences in the electrophoretic patterns. Using techniques such as two-dimensional immunoelectrophoresis, it is possible to demonstrate changes of plasma proteins which are not apparent using one-dimensional electrophoresis—e.g. in rats given hypolipidaemic agents (Hinton et al., 1985).

Using electrophoretic methods, it is possible to observe increases in plasma α-and β-globulins following the injection of known irritants into rats (e.g. carrageenan). With quantitative immunoelectrophoretic techniques applied in the same model of irritancy, it is possible to demonstrate changes which occur for over 20 individual proteins in acute phase response (Scherer et al., 1977).

For compounds which act as immunomodulators, immunoglobulins may be measured by various immunological techniques. Immunoassay of individual proteins is dependent on obtaining specific antisera, although some antisera cross-react with several species (Hau et al., 1990), and allow the use of such techniques as immunoturbidimetry and single radial immunodiffusion.

CHOLINESTERASES

Cholinesterase enzymes are known targets for organophosphate and carbamate esters, which are used as insecticides. Two principal types of cholinesterase enzyme have been identified in blood:

(1) Erythrocyte acetylcholinesterase (AChE) (EC 3.1.1.7). This enzyme is bound to the stroma of erythrocytes and is characterized by preferential affinity for acetylcholine as substrate. It is also referred to as 'true' cholinesterase.

(2) Plasma or serum cholinesterase (ChE) (EC 3.1.1.8). This enzyme exhibits heterogeneity (Ecobichon and Comeau, 1972; Unakami et al., 1987) and shows less substrate specificity than AChE. It is also referred to as 'butyryl', 'pseudo-' or 'non-specific' cholinesterase.

AChE in erythrocytes is identical in function with AChE found in the central nervous system, sympathetic ganglia and motor end plates, where it serves to inactivate the neurotransmitter, acetylcholine. Its functional role in erythrocytes is unclear, but it may have a protective role by acting as a 'sink' for part of the absorbed dose of anticholinesterase compounds (Wills, 1972). Even more conjectural is the physiological role of plasma ChE, which is also found in the liver (the major site of synthesis), intestinal mucosa and several other tissues. Most of the cholinesterase activity in brain can be accounted for by AChE; however, it has been estimated that some 15% of the total activity may be attributable to pseudo/non-specific ChE in certain areas of white matter (Ecobichon and Joy, 1982). It is known that the distribution and activities of AChE vary in different regions of the central nervous system.

Several methods have evolved for the measurement of cholinesterase activity (cf. review by Whittaker, 1986). The electrometric pH method (Michel, 1949) was for many years the method of choice in many laboratories, but has been superseded by a superior colorimetric method (Ellman et al., 1961) and its modifications for human and animal species (Voss and Sachsse, 1970; Pickering and Pickering, 1971). This latter method and its modifications offer significant advantages in speed, sensitivity and reliability. There are, however, some difficulties with the measurement of erythrocyte AChE using this method, where the Soret band of haemoglobin at 415–420 nm may interfere with colour development. For this and other reasons, the US EPA has encouraged the development of a more robust method, in consultation with interested parties. A standard operating procedure has now been proposed by the US EPA as part of its overall approach to risk assessment of anti-ChE compounds (Padilla and Hooper, 1992).

There are significant pitfalls associated with the measurement of cholinesterases, especially when spontaneous reactivation of the inhibited enzyme occurs relatively rapidly. If the incubation time for the assay is significant in relation to the rate of reactivation, then the degree of inhibition may be underestimated. Also, further inhibition of cholinesterase may occur after blood sampling and is usually indicative of the presence of free inhibitor. Thus, if the rate of inhibition by free inhibitor exceeds the rate of reactivation, then the degree of inhibition may be overestimated. It is essential, therefore, that the time which elapses between blood sampling and assay (including the pre-incubation and incubation periods) should be reduced to a minimum. The length of pre-incubation period in automated spectrophotometric analyses may be a major factor in the reactivation of ChE activity in tissues from carbamate-treated animals (Hunter *et al.*, 1997).

In toxicological studies where organophosphates or carbamates are to be evaluated, it is usual (and essential) to measure cholinesterase activities in blood at various intervals, and brain AChE activity at termination, during acute, subchronic and chronic studies in more than one species: the dog and the rat are the preferred species. The more toxic the compound, the more frequent should be the sampling. While concurrent control groups are used routinely in these studies, the study design for dog studies where the group sizes are smaller than for rodents, should incorporate two or more baseline measurements prior to treatment. This is important since the variation in erythrocyte AChE and plasma ChE between individuals exceeds the variation between successive determinations in the same individual (Callaway *et al.*, 1951; Gage, 1967). The percentage difference from the mean baseline value which achieves statistical significance is, of course, dependent upon which enzyme is being assayed and upon the number of baseline measurements (Hayes, 1982). The interpretation of cholinesterase inhibition data is confounded by the various sources of variability. Historically, at least 20% inhibition of either enzyme activity has been used as the determinant of biological significance. The basis of this is a combination of analytical inter-and intra-person variability seen in the human population (Callaway *et al.*, 1951; Gage, 1967; Hackathorn *et al.*, 1983). Plasma ChE may be reduced for reasons other than inhibition by organophosphates and carbamates. These reasons have been tabulated (Whittaker, 1986), and include inherited, physiological, acquired and iatrogenic conditions.

The comparative sensitivity to man has been examined for a variety of organophosphates and carbamates in the preferred species—dog and rat. In all examples where cholinesterase inhibition was the critical effect, the dog was equally sensitive as or more sensitive than the rat (Appelman and Feron, 1986). These findings add substance to an earlier recommendation that cholinesterases should be measured in two species, one of which is the dog, because 'when plasma ChE or erythrocyte AChE provide the most sensitive index of cumulative effect, the response in the dog has approached very closely that in the human' (Lehman, 1959). However, it must be recognized that the mode of administration and differences in eating habits between the various species, including man, may influence the data regarding species sensitivity.

ENDOCRINE FUNCTION

Major toxic effects on the endocrine system appear to be relatively uncommon, on the basis of published literature. The extent to which this reflects the lack of relevant measurements or dismissal of any changes as non-specific or secondary to other effects is unclear. The susceptibility of the endocrine tissues to compound-induced lesions has been shown to be ranked in the following decreasing order of frequency: adrenal, testis, thyroid, ovary, pancreas, pituitary and parathyroid (Ribelin, 1984). Similar findings have been revealed by the Centre for Medicines Research **(Table 3)**. Compounds affecting the adrenal and testis total approximately 70% of all reports reviewed.

Table 3 Frequency of toxicity to endocrine glands

Organ	Number of compounds with an effect	Weight change only	Species
Adrenal glands	44	27	Rat, dog, primate
Testes	24	10	Rat, dog
Thyroid gland	17	9	Rat, dog
Ovaries	14	7	Rat, dog
Pituitary gland	11	6	Rat, dog, primate
Pancreas	4	0	Rat, dog, primate

The release of peripheral hormones is controlled by the secretion of trophic hormones from the pituitary, which in turn are regulated by releasing hormones secreted by the hypothalamus **(Table 4)**. The endocrine feedback axis

Table 4 Hypothalamic–pituitary endocrine target axis, with examples of releasing and trophic hormones

Hypothalamus	Releasing hormones—e.g. corticotrophic releasing hormone (CRH), thyrotrophic releasing hormone (TRH), follicle stimulating releasing hormone (FRH), luteinizing releasing hormone (LRH)
Pituitary	Trophic hormones—e.g. adrenocorticotrophic hormone (ACTH), thyroid stimulating hormone (TSH), follicle stimulating hormone (FSH), luteinizing hormone (LH)
Endocrine target organ	Peripheral hormones—e.g. cortisol, corticosterone, aldosterone, thyroxine (T4), triiodothyronine (T3)
Peripheral circulation	Transport proteins, peripheral metabolism and excretion
End organ target	Receptor binding

is completed by circulating hormones modulating the output of releasing/trophic hormones from the hypothalamic–pituitary axis. Clearly, the measurements of circulating levels of one or more hormones together with other specific endocrine organ indicators of function are powerful tools in defining the level at which functional impairment occurs (Woodman, 1997).

The majority of non-polypeptide hormones do not show species differences, and therefore several commercial test kits for human clinical use can be applied, although the circulating levels in some animal species present difficulties in analytical sensitivity. In contrast, the trophic hormones are polypeptides and require the use of species-specific reagents, which are often only available from relatively few sources. The majority of hormone assays utilize radioisotopes; however, several alternative approaches are now available—e.g. enzyme immunoassay, bioluminescence.

Adrenal Gland

The hormones of the adrenal cortex fall into three classes: (1) glucocorticoids, which influence the metabolism of carbohydrates, lipids and proteins, with the liver, muscles and adipose tissue as the major sites of action; (2) mineralocorticoids, which influence electrolyte transport by regulating renal sodium and potassium reabsorption and excretion, thereby affecting blood pressure homeostasis; and (3) androgens and oestrogens.

The biosynthesis and secretion of these adrenal cortical hormones is under the direct control of a trophic hormone, adrenocorticotrophic hormone (ACTH), released by the pituitary. The secretion of ACTH is under a negative feedback control mechanism exercised by the circulating cortical hormones, of which cortisol is the most important in humans and dogs, and corticosterone in rats.

The circulating level of adrenal cortical hormone in rats depends on several factors, including age, season and strain (Kuhn et al., 1983; Wong et al., 1983a) sex and light (Critchlow et al., 1963). It is also readily apparent that experimental (and pre-experimental) disturbance of animals has a pronounced effect upon the measurement of plasma cortisol (or corticosterone). It has been demonstrated that relatively innocuous stimuli, such as handling and change in environment, may induce significant increases in plasma corticosterone levels in rats (Barrett and Stockham, 1963; Jurcovicova et al., 1984). Plasma corticosterone levels are high in young rats and decrease dramatically during sexual development, reflecting a highly active adrenal gland during puberty.

The need for standardization in plasma corticosterone (and cortisol) measurements is illustrated by the circadian rhythm (D'Agostino et al., 1982). In the dog a circadian rhythm is not apparent (Johnston and Mather, 1978); however, episodic secretion of cortisol and ACTH has been seen (Kemppainen and Sartin, 1984).

The need for standardization extends also to the methods of blood collection, although the differences in corticosterone levels were less apparent than for some other hormones (Dohler et al., 1978). Sequential termination and caging density may also affect plasma corticosterone measurements in laboratory animals (Dunn and Scheving, 1971).

The determination of plasma cortisol during periods of rest and following stimulation with ACTH can be used to diagnose whether adrenocortical function is perturbed (Garnier et al., 1990). To evaluate further the functional status, direct assay of ACTH can be combined with administration of metyrapone, which is known to inhibit adrenal 11β-hydroxylase activity and cause a transient reduction in cortisol synthesis; this is normally sufficient to stimulate ACTH secretion from the pituitary, followed by a resultant increase in the secretion of 11-deoxycortisol (Orth et al., 1988).

Toxic agents appear to interfere with the adrenal cortex by one of three direct mechanisms: (1) altering cholesterol synthesis; (2) altering conversion of cholesterol to 5-pregnenolone; and (3) altering 11β-hydroxylation. The plasma levels of unbound and metabolically active corticosteroids may also be measured indirectly by the effects on hepatic steroid metabolism or upon the plasma transport proteins (Harvey, 1996).

Plasma volume and circulating electrolytes are the key regulators of mineralocorticoid secretion. The secretion of aldosterone is governed largely by the renin-angiotensin system and by plasma potassium and sodium concentrations. A circadian rhythm has been demonstrated for plasma aldosterone in the rat (Gomez-Sanchez et al., 1976).

Thyroid Gland

The hormones of the thyroid gland arise from the iodination of tyrosine residues at positions 3 and 5 of the aromatic moiety to yield mono-and diiodotyrosines, which in combination give rise to triiodotyrosine (triiodothyronine, T3) and tetraiodotyrosine (thyroxine, T4). The requirement for iodine by the thyroid gland is met by dietary intake of iodide and uptake into the gland against a concentration gradient. Within the thyroid gland, the iodide is 'activated' by a peroxidase, and the receptors for this 'activated' iodine are the tyrosine residues in the protein, thyroglobulin (TBG). Most of the iodine within the gland is in a bound form as mono-and diiodotyrosines, with much smaller amounts as T3 and T4. Secretion and release of T3 and T4, the active hormones of the thyroid gland, are effected by proteolytic degradation of thyroglobulin (Davies, 1996).

The biosynthesis and secretion of these thyroid hormones is under the direct control of a trophic hormone, thyroid stimulating hormone (thyrotrophin, TSH), released by the pituitary. A reciprocal relationship exists between T3 and T4 production and TSH secretion, in which low circulating levels of thyroid hormones stimulate TSH release from the pituitary.

The problems of interspecies differences and relevance of findings to human are reflected well in the pituitary–thyroid axis—in particular, the binding and transport of these hormones by plasma proteins. Over 99.95% of T4 and more than 99.5% of T3 in blood are bound to carrier proteins (Robbins and Johnson, 1982). It is the unbound form of each hormone which is metabolically active, and for all species this generally amounts to less than 1%. Several species are known to have plasma proteins which bind with either high affinity and low capacity or low affinity and high capacity. The low-affinity, high-capacity binding is provided mainly by albumin and/or a prealbumin in all species. However, differences exist between T3 and T4 binding to plasma proteins in different species (Woodman, 1988b). The low-affinity, high-capacity binding in the rat leads to a more rapid removal of thyroid hormones from the blood and conjugation by the liver such that metabolic half-lives in rat and human are widely different.

The two thyroid hormones differ in their physiological activity. Not only is T3 almost twice as active as T4, but also its onset of action is more rapid. Removal from the body involves hepatic uptake, conjugation with glucuronic acid and elimination of the conjugate in the bile.

Diurnal variations of plasma TSH, T4 and T3 have been observed in rats. Peak TSH levels occurred in the light period prior to peaks of T3 and T4 later (Jordan et al., 1980; Ottenweiler and Hedge, 1982). The circulating levels of both TSH and thyroid hormones in rats show a 24 h periodicity which is influenced by strain of rat and season of year but not age (Wong et al., 1983b); however, significant changes in 24 h mean serum levels of TSH and T3 occur during pubertal development. Starvation of rats leads to reduced thyroid gland function, with thyroid concentrations of T3 and T4 increased, circulating levels of T3 and T4 decreased, and TSH secretion markedly depressed (Donati et al., 1966; Harris et al, 1978). Peripheral metabolism of T4 is also decreased, which reflects both reduced deiodination and faecal excretion (Ingbar and Galton, 1975).

Sex-related differences in plasma concentrations of canine TSH, T3 and T4 have been found, with TSH and T4 levels higher in males and T3 higher in females (Fukuda et al., 1975). Species differences in the levels of total and free T3 and T4 have been found in the serum of vertebrates—cattle, goats, guinea-pigs, horses, pigs, rats and sheep (Refetoff et al., 1970; Anderson et al., 1988).

Several commercial immunoassay kits are available for the measurement of T3 and T4. Few require any modifications for the measurement of these hormones in laboratory animal species. In contrast, the measurement of TSH requires species-specific reagents because of the polypeptide nature of the hormone; methods for this assay have been developed using a double-antibody RIA.

Testis

The weights of accessory glands, testes and epididymides are the primary indicators of a possible alteration in androgen status. Reductions in weight are indicative that androgen secretion is suboptimal or that testicular function has been compromised. The measurement of circulating hormones can often assist in the diagnosis of suspected reproductive toxicity. The testis can be functionally separated into the interstitial or Leydig cells, and the seminiferous tubular compartments, which produce a complex fluid containing spermatozoa and a number of largely uncharacterized proteins. The morphological, physiological and biochemical aspects of male reproduction have been described elsewhere (Desjardins, 1985; Foster, 1989).

The major function of the Leydig cells is the maintenance of spermatogenesis, which is partially mediated by the production of testosterone and dihydrotestosterone. Several radioimmunoassays have been described for testosterone and dihydrotestosterone, and the development of these sensitive assays has led to an assessment of Leydig cell function.

The endocrine control of testicular function is mainly exercised by the gonadotrophic hormones, luteinizing hormone (LH), and follicle-stimulating hormone (FSH), which are dimeric glycoproteins of similar molecular mass synthesized and released by the anterior pituitary gland. The principal targets of the gonadotrophic hormones are the Leydig and Sertoli cells for LH and FSH, respectively. The homeostatic control of the hypothalamo–pituitary–testicular (HPT) axis is complex, involving feedback modulation at several sites. Elevations of gonadotrophins are usually evidence of testicular injury. Leydig cell dysfunction usually leads to an increase in LH production, whereas increases in plasma FSH are usually indicative of damage to seminiferous tubules.

Apart from the technical aspects of performing these assays, there remain the questions of how and when to sample. LH is secreted in a pulsatile manner, and these pulses may cause plasma levels to vary by a factor of 2.5 or more from baseline values (Santen and Bardin, 1973). Collection procedures and storage procedures should be standardized to minimize any losses due to instability. Radioimmunoassay techniques for these gonadotrophins, when performed competently, are sufficiently accurate to detect changes of 20% in mean blood hormone levels, with group sizes of 20 or more (Thorell and Larson, 1978).

Seminiferous tubular function cannot be studied as easily, since many of its products are released into the tubular lumen which is contained within the 'blood–testis barrier'. This barrier has been shown to be capable of excluding from the tubular lumen many substances normally present in blood (Steinberger, 1981). It is clear that blood-borne components such as hormones and nutrients which can successfully permeate the blood–testis barrier can gain direct access to germ cells. Conversely, damage to this barrier caused by toxic substances or in disease would be expected to lead to release of extracellular and possible intracellular contents into blood, offering a possible screening mechanism of testicular dysfunction.

An androgen binding protein (ABP) has been detected in the testis of rat, and appears to be identical with that in the epididymis. It is a heat-stable glycoprotein which is synthesized and released by Sertoli cells with a high affinity for testosterone and dihydrotestosterone (Gunsalus et al., 1981). The role of ABP is ill-defined at present. In the rat this protein has been isolated by affinity chromatography and a radioimmunoassay has been developed for its detection in tissues and body fluids, especially blood (Gunsalus et al., 1978). The ability to measure an androgen binding protein of testicular origin in blood provides a novel method for the investigation of seminiferous tubular function (Gunsalus et al., 1978; Spitz et al., 1985).

The study of androgen-binding proteins in some species, including humans, has been confounded by the existence of a closely related protein in serum. Testosterone–oestradiol binding globulin (TEBG) or sex hormone binding globulin (SHBG) is a glycoprotein of hepatic origin which has a greater affinity for androgens than for oestrogens. Further studies are needed to clarify the relationship between ABP and TEBG (Bardin et al., 1981; Cheng et al., 1985). Inhibin, a glycoprotein of Sertoli cell origin, is known to be present in blood and seminiferous tubular fluid. It is believed to inhibit FSH secretion from the pituitary, and thereby provides a role in the feedback regulation of the pituitary–ovarian hormonal axis.

Several mammalian enzymes exist in testis-specific forms. The most widely studied of these is the testis-specific isoenzyme of LDH, referred to as LDH-C4 or LDH-X. This isoenzyme possesses several properties which are distinct from the other isoenzymes of LDH. The synthesis of this unique gene product has been shown to occur during the mid-pachytene stage of spermatocyte development, and continues throughout spermatid differentiation (Meistrich et al., 1977; Wheat et al., 1977). LDH-C4 is not normally detected in circulating blood; however, several studies of acute testicular toxicity in the rat have shown that elevations of plasma LDH-C4 can be detected (Haqqi and Adhami, 1982; Itoh and Ozasa, 1985; Reader et al., 1991).

The measurement of enzymes in seminal fluid and a variety of other fluids in animals as possible indicators of testicular damage is dependent upon a knowledge of the origin of these enzymes, since several accessory glands can contribute to the composition of semen. Enzymes may in future be useful markers of testicular damage, e.g. phosphoglycerate kinase (Kramer, 1981; Vandeberg et al., 1981) and branched-chain amino acid transferase (Mantamat et al., 1978).

Ovary

The ovaries have two main functions, namely the production of ova and the biosynthesis of steroid hormones. Several hormones of the hypothalamic–pituitary–ovarian axis are involved in the hormonal control of the female reproductive system. Both FSH and LH act on specific ovarian receptors to stimulate production of steroid hormones. FSH stimulates the growth and secretion of follicles, and stimulates steroid hormone production by the granulosa cells. LH stimulates hormone production by the theca cells and corpus luteum and promotes ovulation (Erickson et al., 1985; Wilson and Leigh, 1992; Gangolli and Phillips, 1993). The steroid hormone 17β-oestradiol is the most potent oestrogenic hormone released from the ovaries.

The absolute length of the reproductive cycle varies greatly between species. The mouse and dog regulate the normal reproductive cycle at comparatively low 17β-oestradiol levels, in contrast to the monkey, rat and human, which require much higher levels at particular phases of the cycle (Gunzel et al., 1989). Both specific high affinity binding proteins and non-specific low affinity binding proteins exist for oestrogens. The morphological, physiological and biochemical aspects of female reproduction can be found elsewhere (Korach and Quarmby, 1985; Cooper et al., 1989).

The duration of pregnancy is also known to vary greatly across species. Progesterone, a steroid hormone, which is produced in the corpus luteum and placenta, plays a key role in the maintenance of pregnancy. The relative affinity of progesterone for receptors varies from species to species, and probably also from organ to organ. Monkeys regulate pregnancy at a significantly lower progesterone level than all other experimental animal species (Gunzel et al., 1989).

Prolactin is a single-chain polypeptide produced by the adenohypophysis. It stimulates the secretion of milk and promotes the functional activity of the corpus luteum. Substances that possess oestrogenic activity can stimulate prolactin secretion, which can suppress gonadotrophin secretion.

The hormonal regulation of the female reproductive system can be perturbed in a variety of ways by exogenous agents. Toxicity may result from a direct action in which the toxicant has a structural similarity with an endogenous hormone, e.g. oral contraceptives, and anti-oestrogens which alter the normal feedback regulation of oestrogen production. In contrast, toxicity may be as a consequence of an indirect action such as an alteration in the microsomal mixed function oxidase activities of the ovaries (Haney, 1985; Wilson and Leigh, 1992; Ratcliffe *et al.*, 1993).

SUMMARY

Clinical chemistry has a key role in toxicology studies, since it can provide advance warning of adverse effects that may be anticipated, e.g. by histopathology. By employing a combination of tests, it is possible to identify potential target organs and also to evaluate the functional status of major organs. As a general approach to the investigation of toxicity, a phased approach is recommended in which the first phase should include the traditional clinical chemistry tests, many of which have evolved from clinical practice. However, the timing of these tests is often governed by rigid protocols designed for regulatory submissions which therefore may not be appropriate to determine the period of maximal damage. The majority of these tests can be performed on automated equipment with a good throughput of samples per unit time, with high precision and with the use of relatively small volumes of body fluids. If confirmation is required of the first phase results which may be indicative of toxicity in a single target organ, further studies should be targeted at this organ in order to characterize, where possible, the anatomical and subcellular localization of the lesion, the severity of the damage and functional impairment and whether the changes observed are reversible or not. These further tests may be chosen on the basis of the known or suspected mechanism of action, using a more flexible study design with the sampling times geared to the evaluation of peak damage and/or dysfunction and recovery phase. The diagnostic effectiveness of the various analytes, enzymes and hormones, etc., has to be evaluated on a case-by-case basis for the relevant species. Some measurements (e.g. polypeptide hormones) require species-specific reagents, which may limit their application.

Several factors can contribute to biological variation, including husbandry practice, environmental control, genetic difference, diurnal rhythm and diet. Thus, values generated in any given laboratory are unique to that laboratory. It cannot be emphasized too strongly that a concurrent control group must be a feature of the design of toxicologicol studies and therefore allows reference ranges from clinical chemistry parameters to be established. Equally important to the generation of meaningful data is the application of sound laboratory practices when collecting body fluids and the use of the same

sampling site when making repeated measurements of the same analytes at intervals throughout a study. There are many examples of problems which can be overcome by reliance on the expertise and experience of the clinical chemist. These include a knowledge of the potential interferences (both endogenous and exogenous) which may lead to erroneous values, the lability of several analytes that require immediate analysis, and the need to adopt and optimize assays to improve sensitivity in a particular species.

Finally, adherence to Good Laboratory Practice in the form of proven equipment maintenance, calibration and documentation is an absolute requirement in the clinical chemistry laboratory. A combination of internal quality control procedures with participation in an external quality assessment scheme permits the management and output of the laboratory to be monitored routinely and for unwanted trends and practices to be eliminated at the earliest opportunity.

REFERENCES

Adams, J. E., Bodor, G. S., Davila-Roman, V. G., Delmez, J. A., Apple, F. S., Ladenson, J. H. and Jaffe, A. S. (1993). Cardiac troponin 1: a marker with a high specificity for cardiac injury. *Circulation*, **88**, 101–106.

Aldercreutz, H., Partanen, P., Virkola, P., Liewendahl, K. and Turunen, M. J. (1984). Five guaiac-based tests for occult blood in faeces compared *in vitro* and *in vivo*. *Scand. J. Clin. Lab. Invest.*, **44**, 519–528.

Alexander, C. and Day, C. E. (1973). Distribution of serum lipoproteins of selected vertebrates. *Comp. Biochem. Physiol.*, **46B**, 295–312.

Allchin, J. P. and Evans, G. O. (1986a). A simple rapid method for the detection of rat urinary proteins by agarose electrophoresis and nigrosine staining. *Lab. Anim.*, **20**, 202–205.

Allchin, J. P. and Evans, G. O. (1986b). Serum protein electrophoresis patterns of the marmoset, *Callithrix jacchus*. *J. Comp. Pathol.*, **96**, 349–352.

Allchin, J. P. and Evans, G. O. (1986c). A comparison of three methods for determining the concentration of rat urine. *Comp. Biochem. Physiol.*, **85A**, 771–773.

Allchin, J. P., Evans, G. O. and Parsons, C. E. (1987). Pitfalls in the measurement of canine urine concentration. *Vet. Rec.*, **120**, 256–257.

Alpert, E., Mosher, M., Shankse, A. and Arias, I. M. (1969). Multiplicity of hepatic excretory mechanisms for organic anions. *J. Gen. Physiol.*, **53**, 238–247.

Alt, J. M., Hackbarth, F., Deerberg, F., and Stolte, H. (1980). Proteinuria in rats in relation to age-dependent renal changes. *Lab. Anim.*, **14**, 95–101.

Anderson, R. R., Nixon, D. A. and Akasha, M. A. (1988). Total and free thyroxine and triiodothyronine in blood serum of mammals. *Comp. Biochem. Physiol.*, **89A**, 401–404.

Appelman, L. M. and Feron, V. J. (1986). Significance of the dog as 'second animal species' in toxicity testing for establishing the lowest 'no-toxic effect level'. *J. Appl. Toxicol.*, **6**, 271–279.

Aungst, B. and Shen, D. D. (1986). Gastrointestinal absorption of toxic agents. In Rozman, K. and Hanninen, O. (Eds), *Gastrointestinal Toxicology*. Elsevier, Amsterdam, pp. 29–52.

Azer, S.A., Klaassen, C.D. and Stacey, N.H. (1997). Biochemical assay of serum bile acids: methods and applications. *Brit. J. Biomed. Sci.*, **54**, 118–132.

Bach, P. H. and Hardy, T. L. (1985). Relevance of animal models to analgesic-associated papillary necrosis in humans. *Kidney Int.*, **28**, 605–613.

Balazs, T. and Bloom, S. (1982). Cardiotoxicity of adrenergic bronchodilator and vasodilating antihypertensive drugs. In Van Stee, E. W. (Ed.), *Cardiovascular Toxicology*, Raven Press, New York, pp. 199–200.

Bardin, C. W., Musto, N., Gunsalus, G., Kotiten, N., Cheng, S. L., Larrea, F. and Becker, R. (1981). Extracellular androgen binding proteins. *Annu. Rev. Physiol.*, **43**, 189–198.

Barrett, A. M. and Stockham, M. A. (1963). The effect of housing conditions and simple experimental procedures upon the corticosterone level in the plasma of rats. *J. Endocrinol.*, **26**, 97–105.

Barrett, R. J., Harleman, H. and Joseph, E. C. (1988). The evaluation of HBDH and LDH isoenzymes in cardiac cell necrosis. *J. Appl. Toxicol.*, **8**, 233–238.

Baumann, M. and Berauer, M. (1985). Comparative study on the sensitivity of several serum enzymes in detecting hepatic damage in rats. *Arch. Toxicol., Suppl.* **8**, 370–372.

Bean-Knudsen, D. E. and Wagner, J. E. (1987). Effect of shipping stress on clinicopathologic indicators in F344/N rats. *Am. J. Vet. Res.*, **48**, 306–308.

Beckett, G. J. and Hayes, J. D. (1993). Glutathione *S*-transferases: biomedical applications. *Adv. Clin. Chem.*, **30**, 281–380.

Berdanier, C. D. and Baltzell, J. K. (1986). Comparative studies of the responses of two strains of rats to an essential fatty acid deficient diet. *Comp. Biochem. Physiol.*, **85A**, 725–727.

Berndt, W. O. (1981). Use of renal function tests in the evaluation of nephrotoxic effects. In: Hook, J. B. (ed.), *Toxicology of the Kidney*, (Raven Press, New York), 14.

Bertani, T., Zoja, C., Abbate, M., Rossini, M. and Remuzzi, G. (1989). Age-related nephropathy and proteinuria in rats with intact kidneys exposed to diets with different protein content. *Lab. Invest.*, **60**, 196–204.

Berthet, J. (1963). Pancreatic hormones: glucagon. In von Euler, U. S. and Heller, H. (Eds), *Comparative Endocrinology*. Academic Press, London, pp. 410–423.

Betts, A., Tanguay, R. and Freidell, G. H. (1964). Effect of necrosis on hemoglobin, serum protein profile and erythroagglutination reaction in golden hamsters. *Proc. Soc. Exp. Biol. Med.*, **116**, 66–69.

Beynon, A. C. (1988). Animal models for cholesterol metabolism. In Beynon, A. C. and Solleveld, H. A. (Eds), *Biosciences*. Martinus Nijhoff, Dordrecht, pp. 279–288.

Bhargava, A. S., Khater, A. R. and Gunzel, P. (1978). The correlation between lactate dehydrogenase activity in urine and serum and experimental renal damage in the rat. *Toxicol. Lett.*, **1**, 319–323.

Blanckaert, N., Servaes, R. and Leroy, P. (1986). Measurement of bilirubin–protein conjugates in serum and application to human and rat sera. *J. Lab. Clin. Med.*, **108**, 77–87.

Boesken, W. H., Kopf, K. and Schollmeyer, P. (1973). Differentiation of proteinuric diseases by disc electrophoretic molecular weight analysis of urinary proteins. *Clin. Nephrol.*, **1**, 311–318.

Boulay, J. P., Lipowitz, A. J., Klausner, J. S., Ellefson, M. L. and Schwartz, S. (1986). Evaluation of a fluorimetric method for the quantitative assay of fecal hemoglobin in the dog. *Am. J. Vet. Res.*, **47**, 1293–1295.

Bovee, K. C. (1986). Renal function and laboratory evaluation. *Toxicol. Pathol.*, **14**, 26–36.

Boyd, E. J. S., Rinderknecht, H. and Wormsley, K. G. (1988). Laboratory tests in the diagnosis of the chronic pancreatic diseases. Part 4. Tests involving the measurement of pancreatic enzymes in body fluid. *Int. J. Pancreatol.*, **3**, 1–16.

Braun, J. P., Siest, G. and Rico, A. G. (1987). Uses of gammaglutamyl transferase in experimental toxicology. *Adv. Vet. Sci. Comp. Med.*, **31**, 151–172.

Caesar, J., Shaldon, S., Chiandussi, L., Guevara, L. and Sherlock, S. (1961). The use of indocyanine green in measurement of hepatic blood flow and as a test of hepatic function. *Clin. Sci.*, **21**, 43–57.

Caisey, J. D. and King, D. J. (1980). Clinical chemistry values for some common laboratory animals. *Clin. Chem.*, **26**, 1877–1879.

Callaway, S., Davies, D. R. and Rutland, J. P. (1951). Blood cholinesterase levels and a range of personal variation in a healthy adult population. *Br. Med. J.*, **2**, 812.

Campbell, J. A., Corrigall, A. V., Guy, A. and Kirsch, R. E. (1991). Immunohistologic localization of alpha, mu, and pi class glutathione *S*-transferases in human tissues. *Cancer*, **67**, 1608–1613.

Cheng, C. Y., Musto, N. A., Gunsalus, G. L., Frick, J. and Bardin, C. W. (1985). There are two forms of androgen binding protein in human testes. *J. Biol. Chem.*, **260**, 5631–5640.

Chin, B. H., Tyler, T. R. and Kozbelt, S. J. (1979). The interfering effects of hemolyzed blood on rat serum chemistry. *Toxicol. Pathol.*, **7**, 19–22.

Clampitt, R. J. and Hart, R. J. (1978). The tissue activities of some diagnostic enzymes in ten mammalian species. *J. Comp. Pathol.*, **88**, 607–621.

Coe, J. E. and Ross, M. J. (1983). Hamster female protein. A divergent acute phase protein in male and female Syrian hamsters. *J. Exp. Med.*, **157**, 1421–1433.

Colvin, H. W. and Lee Wang, W. (1974). Toxic effects of warfarin in rats fed different diets. *Toxicol. Appl. Pharmacol.*, **28**, 337–348.

Commandeur, J. N. M. and Vermeulen, N. P. E. (1990). Molecular and biochemical mechanisms of chemically induced nephrotoxicity: a review. *Chem. Res. Toxicol.*, **3**, 171–194.

Conybeare, G., Leslie, G. B., Angles, K. and Barrett, R. J. (1988). An improved technique for the collection of blood samples from rats and mice. *Lab. Anim.*, **22**, 177–182.

Cooper, R. L., Goldman, J. M. and Rehnberg, G. L. (1989). Regulation of ovarian function. In Working, P. K. (Ed.), *Toxicology of the Male and Female Reproductive Systems*. Hemisphere Publishing, New York, pp. 15–29.

Corman, B., Pratz, J. and Poujeol, P. (1985). Changes in the anatomy, glomerular filtration rate and solute excretion in aging rat kidney. *Am. J. Physiol.*, **248**, r282–r287.

Cottrell, R. C., Agrelo, C. E., Gangolli, S. D. and Grasso, P. (1976). Histochemical and biochemical studies of chemically induced acute kidney damage in the rat. *Food Cosmet. Toxicol.*, **14**, 593–598.

Cowie, J. R. and Evans, G. O. (1985). Plasma aminotransferase measurements in the marmoset (*Callithrix jacchus*). *Lab. Anim.*, **19**, 48–50.

Critchlow, V., Liebelt, R. A., Bar-Sela, M., Mountcastle, W. and Lipscomb, H. S. (1963). Sex difference in resting pituitary–adrenal function in the rat. *Am. J. Physiol.*, **205**, 807–815.

D'Agostino, J. B., Vaeth, G. F. and Henning, S. J. (1982). Diurnal rhythm of total and free concentration of serum corticosterone in the rat. *Acta Endocrinol.*, **100**, 85–90.

Dameron, G. W., Beck, M. L, Brandt, M. A. and O'Brien, P. J. (1997). Tissue and species specificity of two generations of cardiac troponin-T immunoassays. *Clin. Chem.*, **43**, S192.

Davies, D. J. and Kennedy, A. (1967). The excretion of renal cells following necrosis of the proximal convoluted tubule. *Br. J. Exp. Pathol.*, **48**, 45–50.

Davies, D. T. (1996) Thryoid endocrinology. In Evans, G. O. (Ed.), *Animal Clinical Chemistry: A Primer for Toxicologists.* Taylor and Francis, London, pp. 105–122.

Davy, C. W., Jackson, M. R. and Walker, J. M. (1984). Reference intervals for some clinical chemical parameters in the marmoset (*Callithrix jacchus*): effect of age and sex. *Lab. Anim.*, **18**, 135–142.

Davy, C. W., Trennery, P. N., Edmunds, J. G., Altman, J. F. B. and Eichler, D. A. (1987). Local myotoxicity of ketamine hydrochloride in the marmoset. *Lab. Anim.*, **21**, 60–67.

Degen, A. J. M. and van der Vies, J. (1985). Enzymatic microdetermination of free fatty acids in plasma of animals using paraoxon to prevent lipolysis. *Scand. J. Clin. Lab. Invest.*, **45**, 283–285.

Dent, N. J. (1973). Occult blood detection in faeces of various animal species. *Lab. Pract.*, **22**, 674–676.

de Schepper, J. and van der Stock, J. (1972). Increased urinary bilirubin excretion after elevated free plasma haemoglobin levels. 1. Variations in the calculated renal clearance of bilirubin in whole dogs. *Arch. Int. Physiol. Biochim.*, **80**, 279–281.

Desjardins, C. (1985). Morphological, physiological, and biochemical aspects of male reproduction. In Dixon, R. L. (Ed.), *Reproductive Toxicology.* Raven Press, New York, pp. 131–146

Dilena, B. A., Penberthy, L. A. and Fraser, C. G. (1983). Six methods for determining urinary protein compared. *Clin. Chem.*, **29**, 553–557.

Dohler, K. D., Wong, C. C., Gaudssuhn, D., von zur Muhlen, A., Gartner, K. and Dohler, U. (1978). Site of blood sampling in rats as a possible source of error in hormone determinations. *J. Endocrinol.*, **79**, 141–142.

Donati, R. M., Warnecke, M. A. and Gallagher, N. I. (1966). The effect of acute starvation on thyroid function in rodents. *Experientia*, **22**, 270–272.

Dooley, J. F. (1979). The role of clinical chemistry in chemical and drug safety evaluation by use of laboratory animals. *Clin. Chem.*, **25**, 345–347.

Dorner, J. L., Hoffman, W. E. and Long, G. B. (1974). Corticosteroid induction of an isoenzyme of alkaline phosphatase in the dog. *Am. J. Vet. Res.*, **35**, 1457–1458.

Dunn, J. and Scheving, L. (1971). Plasma corticosterone levels in rats killed sequentially at the 'trough' or 'peak' of the adrenocortical cycle. *J. Endocrinol.*, **49**, 347–348.

Eckersall, P. D. (1986). Steroid induced alkaline phosphatase in the dog. *Isr. J. Vet. Med.*, **42**, 253–259.

Ecobichon, D. J. and Comeau, M. (1972). Pseudocholinesterases of mammalian plasma: physiochemical properties and organophosphate inhibition in eleven species. *Toxicol. Appl. Pharmacol.*, **24**, 92–100.

Ecobichon, D. J. and Joy, R. M. (1982). *Pesticides and Neurological Disease.* CRC Press, Boca Raton, FL.

Ellman, G. L., Courtney, K. D., Andres, V. and Featherstone, R. M. (1961). A new and rapid colorimetric determination of acetylcholinesterase activity. *Biochem. Pharmacol.*, **7**, 88–95.

Erickson, G. F., Magoffin, D. A., Dyer, C. A. and Hofeditz, C. (1985). The ovarian androgen producing cells: a review of structure/function relationships. *Endocrinol. Rev.*, **6**, 371–399.

Erlanger, S., Glasinovic, J. C., Poupon, R. and Dumont, M. (1976). In Taylor, W. (Ed.), *The Hepatobiliary System.* Plenum Press, New York, pp. 433–452.

Evans, G. O. (1985). Changes of methodology and their potential effects on data banks for drug effects on clinical laboratory tests. *Ann. Clin. Biochem.*, **22**, 397–401.

Evans, G. O. (1986a). The use of three esterase kits to measure plasma cholesterol concentration in the rat and three other species. *J. Comp. Pathol.*, **96**, 551–556.

Evans, G. O. (1986b). The use of an enzymatic kit to measure plasma creatinine in the mouse and three other species. *Comp. Biochem. Physiol.*, **85B**, 193–195.

Evans, G. O. (1987). Post-prandial changes in canine plasma creatinine. *J. Small Anim. Pract.*, **28**, 311–315.

Evans, G. O. (1991). Biochemical assessment of cardiac function and damage in animal species. *J. Appl. Toxicol.*, **11**, 15–21.

Evans, G. O. (1993). Clinical pathology testing recommendations for nonclinical toxicity and safety studies. *Toxicol. Pathol.*, **21**, 513–514.

Evans, G. O. (1996a). General enzymology. In Evans, G. O. (Ed.), *Animal Clinical Chemistry: a Primer for Toxicologists.* Taylor and Francis, London, pp. 59–70.

Evans, G. O. (1996b). Assessment of cardiotoxicity and myotoxicity. In Evans, G. O. (Ed.), *Animal Clinical Chemistry: a Primer for Toxicologists.* Taylor and Francis, London, pp. 147–154.

Evans, G. O. (1996c). Lipids. In Evans, G.O. (Ed.), *Animal Clinical Chemistry: a Primer for Toxicologists.* Taylor and Francis, London, pp. 177–185.

Evans, G. O. and Parsons, C. E. (1986). Potential errors in the measurement of total protein in male rat urine using test strips. *Lab. Anim.*, **20**, 27–31.

Evans, G. O. and Parsons, C. E. (1988). A comparison of two dye binding methods for the determination of dog, rat and human plasma albumins. *J. Comp. Pathol.*, **98**, 453–460.

Fent, K., Mayer, E. and Zbinden, G. (1988). Nephrotoxicity screening in rats: a validation study. *Arch. Toxicol.*, **61**, 349–358.

Finn, W. F., Nolan, C., Lash, L. H., Lorenzon, G., Manley, S. E. and Safirstein, R. (1997). Urinary biomarkers to detect significant effects of environmental and occupational exposure to nephrotoxins; VI. Future research needs. *Renal Failure*, **19**, 575–594.

Fletcher, T. S., Tsukamoto, H. and Largman, C. (1986). Immunoenzymometric determination of trypsin/alpha 1 protease inhibitor complex in plasma of rats with experimental pancreatitis. *Clin. Chem.*, **32**, 1738–1741.

Ford, T. F., Grant, D. A. W., Austen, B. M. and Hermon-Taylor, J. (1985). Intramucosal activation of pepsinogens in the pathogenesis of acute gastric erosions and their prevention by the potent semi-synthetic amphipathic inhibitor pepstatinyl-glycyl-lysyl-lysine. *Clin. Chim. Acta.*, **145**, 37–47.

Foster, P. M. D. (1989). Testicular structure and physiology: a toxicologist's view. In Working P. K. (Ed.), *Toxicology of the Male and Female Reproductive Systems*. Hemisphere Publishing, New York, pp. 1–14.

Fouts, J. R. (1976). Overview of the field: environmental factors affecting chemical or drug effects in animals. *Fed. Proc.*, **35**, 1162–1165.

Fowler, J. S. L. (1982). Animal clinical chemistry and haematology for the toxicologist. *Arch. Toxicol., Suppl.*, **5**, 152–159.

Friedel, R. and Mattenheimer, H. (1976). Release of metabolic enzymes from platelets during blood clotting of man, dog, rabbit and rat. *Clin. Chim. Acta*, **30**, 37–46.

Fromm, H. and Albert, M. B. (1987). Serum bile acid assays for liver disease; when and how to use them. *Gastroenterology*, **92**, 829–830.

Fukuda, H., Greer, M. A., Roberts, L., Allen, C. F., Critchlow, V. and Wilson, M. (1975). Nyctohemeral and sex-related variations in plasma thyrotropin, thyroxine and triiodothyronine. *Endocrinology*, **97**, 1424–1431.

Gage, J. C. (1967). The significance of blood cholinesterase activity measurements. *Residue Rev.*, **18**, 159–173.

Gangolli, S. D. and Phillips, J. C. (1993). Assessing chemical injury to the reproductive system. In Anderson, D. and Conning, D. M. (Eds), *Experimental Toxicology*, 2nd edn. Royal Society of Chemistry, Cambridge, pp. 376–404.

Garattini, S. (1981). Toxic effects of chemicals: difficulties in extrapolating data from animals to man. *CRC Crit. Rev. Toxicol.*, **16**, 1–29.

Garnier, F., Benoit, E., Virat, M., Ochoa, R. and Delatour, P. (1990). Adrenal cortical response in clinically normal dogs before and after adaptation to a housing environment. *Lab. Anim.*, **24**, 40–43.

Gartland, K. P. R., Bonner, F. W. and Nicholson, J. K. (1989). Investigations into the biochemical effects of region-specific nephrotoxins. *Mol. Pharmacol.*, **35**, 242–250.

Gartner, K., Buttner, D., Dohler, K., Friedel, R., Lindena, J. and Trautshold, I. (1980). Stress response of rats to handling and experimental procedures. *Lab. Anim.*, **14**, 267–274.

Gautam, A., Seligson, H., Gordon, E. R., Seligson, D. and Boyer, J. L. (1984). Irreversible binding of conjugated bilirubin to albumin in cholestatic rats. *J. Clin. Invest.*, **73**, 873–877.

George, C. F. (1984). Food, drugs and bioavailability. *Br. Med. J.*, **289**, 1093–1094.

Gloor, H. O., Vorburger, C. and Schadelin, J. (1977). Intramuskulare injektionen und serumkreatinphosphokinaseaktivität. *Schweiz. Med. Wochenschr.*, **107**, 948–952.

Goldstein, R. S. (1990). In Volans, G. N., Sims, J., Sullivan, F. M. and Turner, P. (Eds), *Basic Science in Toxicology*. Taylor and Francis, London, pp. 412–421.

Gomez-Sanchez, C., Holland, O. B., Higgins, J. R., Kem, D. C. and Kaplan, N. M. (1976). Circadian rhythms of serum renin activity and serum corticosterone, prolactin and aldosterone concentrations in the male rat on normal and low-sodium diets. *Endocrinology*, **99**, 567–572.

Gopinath, C., Prentice, D. C., Street, A. E. and Crook, D. (1980). Serum bile acid concentration in some experimental lesions of rat. *Toxicology*, **15**, 113–127.

Greim, H., Truzsch, D., Roboz, J., Dressler, K., Czygan, P., Hutterer, F., Schaffner, F. and Popper, H. (1972). Mechanism of cholestasis. 5. Bile acids in normal rat liver and in those after bile ligation. *Gastroenterology*, **63**, 837–845.

Grotsch, H. and Hajdu, P. (1987). Interference by the new antibiotic Cefipirome and other cephalosporins in clinical laboratory test, with specific regard to the Jaffe reaction. *J. Clin. Chem. Clin. Biochem.*, **25**, 49–52.

Grotsch, H., Hropot, M., Klaus, E., Malerczyk, V. and Mattenheimer, H. (1985). Enzymuria of the rat: biorhythms and sex differences. *J. Clin. Chem. Clin. Biochem.*, **23**, 343–347.

Guder, W. G. and Ross, B. D. (1984). Enzyme distribution along the nephron. *Kidney Int.*, **26**, 101–111.

Gunsalus, G. L., Musto, N. A. and Bardin, C. W. (1978). Immunoassay of androgen binding protein in blood: a new approach for study of the seminiferous tubule. *Science* **200**, 65–66.

Gunsalus, G. L., Larrea, F., Musto, N. A., Becker, R. R., Mather, J. P. and Bardin, C. W. (1981). Androgen binding protein as a marker for Sertoli cell function. *J. Steroid Biochem.*, **15**, 99–106.

Gunzel, P., Putz, B., Lehman, M., Hasan, S. H., Humpel, M. and El Etreby, M. F. (1989). Steroid toxicology and the 'pill': comparative aspects of experimental test systems and the human. In Dayan, A. D. and Paine A. J. (Eds), *Advances in Applied Toxicology*. Taylor and Francis, London, pp. 19–49.

Hackathorn, D. R., Brinkman, W. J., Hathaway, T. R., Talbot, T. D. and Thompson, L. R. (1983). Validation of whole blood method for cholinesterase monitoring. *Am. Ind. Hyg. Assoc. J.*, **44**, 547–551.

Hackbarth, H., Baunack, E. and Winn, M. (1981). Strain differences in kidney function of inbred rats. 1. Glomerular filtration rate and renal plasma flow. *Lab. Anim.*, **15**, 125–128.

Halligan, S., Byard, S. J., Spencer, A. J., Gray, T. J. B., Harpur, E. S. and Bonner, F. W. (1995). A study of the nephrotoxicity of three cephalosporins in rabbits using ^{1}H NMR spectroscopy. *Toxicol. Lett.*, **81**, 15–21.

Halman, J., Price, R. G. and Fowler, J. S. L. (1984). Urinary enzymes and isoenzymes of N-acetyl-β-glucosaminidase in the assessment of nephrotoxicity. In Goldberg, D. M. and Werner, M. (Eds), *Selected Topics in Clinical Enzymology*. Walter de Gruyter, Berlin, pp. 435–444.

Haney, A. F. (1985). Effect of toxic agents on ovarian function. In *Endocrine Toxicology*, Target Organ Toxicology series. Raven Press, New York, pp. 181–210.

Haqqi, T. M. and Adhami, U. M. (1982). Testicular damage and change in serum LDH isoenzyme patterns induced by multiple sub-lethal doses of apholate in albino rats. *Toxicol. Lett.*, **12**, 199–205.

Hardy, T. L. (1970). Identification of cells exfoliated from the rat kidney in experimental nephrotoxicity. *Ann. Rheum. Dis.*, **29**, 64–66.

Harris, A. R. G., Fang, S. L., Azizi, F., Lipworth, L., Vagenakis, A. G. and Braverman, L. E. (1978). Effect of starvation on hypothalamic – pituitary – thyroid function in the rat. *Metabolism* **27**, 1074–1083.

Harvey, P. W. (1996). *The Adrenal in Toxicology*. Taylor and Francis, London.

Hau, J., Nilsson, M., Skovgaard-Jensen, H. J., de Souza, A., Eriksen, E. and Wandall, L. T. (1990). Analysis of animal serum proteins against human analogous proteins. *Scand. J. Lab. Anim. Sci.*, **17**, 3–7.

Hayes, W. J. (1982). *Pesticides Studied in Man*. Williams and Wilkins, Baltimore.

Henning, S. J. (1984). Hormonal and dietary regulation of intestinal enzyme development. In Schiller, C. M. (Ed.), *Intestinal Toxicology*. Raven Press, New York, pp. 17–32.

Higgins, P. J., Garlick, R. L. and Bunn, H. F. (1982). Glycosylated hemoglobin in human and animal red cells. *Diabetes* **26**, 743–748.

Hinton, R. H., Price, S. C., Mitchell, F. E., Mann, A., Hall, D. E. and Bridges, J. W. (1985). Plasma protein changes in rats treated with hypolipidaemic drugs and with phthalate esters. *Hum. Toxicol.*, **4**, 261–271.

Hofmann, A. F. (1988): Bile acids. In Arias, I. M., Jakoby, W. B., Popper, M., Schacter, D. and Shafritz, D. A. (Eds), *The Liver, Biology and Pathobiology*. Raven Press, New York, pp. 553–572.

House, E. L., Pansky, B. and Jacobs, M. S. (1961). Age changes in blood of the golden hamster. *Am. J. Physiol.*, **200**, 1018–1022.

Hunter, D. L., Marshall, R. S. and Padilla, S. (1997). Automated instrument analysis of cholinesterase activity in tissues from carbamate-treated animals: a cautionary note. *Toxicol. Methods*, **7**, 43–53.

Ingbar, D. H. and Galton, V. A. (1975). The effect of food deprivation on the peripheral metabolism of thyroxine in rats. *Endocrinology*, **96**, 1525–1532.

Itoh, R. and Ozasa, H. (1985). Changes in serum lactate dehydrogenase isozyme X activity observed after cadmium administration. *Toxicol. Lett.*, **28**, 151–154.

Jablonski, P. and Owen, J. A. (1969). The clinical chemistry of bromsulfophthalein and other cholephilic dyes. *Adv. Clin. Chem.*, **12**, 309–386.

Japundzic, I. and Levi, E. (1987). Mechanism of action of cysteamine on duodenal alkaline phosphatase. *Biochem. Pharmacol.*, **36**, 2489–2495.

Jenkins, F. P. and Robinson, J. A. (1975). Serum biochemical changes in rats deprived of food or water for 24 h. *Proc. Nutr. Soc.*, **34**, 37A.

Johnson, D. A. (1989). Fecal occult blood testing. Problems, pitfalls and diagnostic concerns. *Postgrad. Med.*, **85**, 287–299.

Johnston, S. D. and Mather, E. C. (1978). Canine plasma cortisol (hydroxycortisone) measured by radioimmunoassay: clinical absence of diurnal variation and results of ACTH stimulation and dexamethasone suppression tests. *Am. J. Vet. Res.*, **39**, 1766–1770.

Jordan, D., Rousset, B., Perrin, F., Fournier, M. and Orgiazzi, J. (1980). Evidence for circadian variations in serum thyrotropin, 3,5,3'-triiodothyronine, and thyroxine in the rat. *Endocrinology*, **107**, 1245–1248.

Jung, K. and Scholz, D. (1980). An optimised assay of alanine aminopeptidase activity in urine. *Clin. Chem.*, **26**, 1251–1254.

Jung, K., Mattenheimer, H. and Burchardt, U. (1992). *Urinary Enzymes in Clinical and Experimental Medicine*. Springer, Berlin.

Jurcovicova, J., Vigas, M., Klir, P. and Jezova, D. (1984). Response of prolactin, growth hormone and corticosterone secretion to morphine administration or stress exposure in Wistar–AVN and Long–Evans rats. *Endocrinol. Exp.*, **18**, 209–214.

Kallner, A. and Tryding, N. (1989). I.F.C.C. guidelines to the evaluation of drug effects in clinical chemistry. *Scand. J. Clin. Lab. Invest.*, **49**, Suppl. 195, 1–29.

Karlsson, B. W. and Larsson, G. B. (1971). Lactic and malic dehydrogenases and their multiple molecular forms in the mongolian gerbil as compared with the rat, mouse and rabbit. *Comp. Biochem. Physiol.*, **40B**, 93–108.

Kast, A. and Nishikawa, J. (1981). The effect of fasting on oral acute toxicity of drugs in rats and mice. *Lab. Anim.*, **15**, 359–364.

Katus, H. A., Scheffold, T., Remppis, A. and Zehlein, J. (1992). Proteins of the troponin complex. *Lab. Med.*, **23**, 311–317.

Kazmlerczak, S. C., Lott, J. A. and Caldwell, J. H. (1988). Acute intestinal infarction or obstruction: search for better laboratory tests in an animal model. *Clin. Chem.*, **34**, 281–288.

Keller, P. (1981). Enzyme activities in the dog: tissue analyses, plasma values, and intracellular distribution. *Am. J. Vet. Res.*, **42**, 575–582.

Kempainnen, R. J. and Sartin, J. L. (1984). Evidence for episodic but not circadian activity in plasma concentrations of adrenocorticotrophin, cortisol and thyroxine in dogs. *J. Endocrinol.*, **103**, 219–226.

Klaassen, C. D. and Plaa, G. L. (1967). Species variation in metabolism, storage and excretion of sulfobromophthalein. *Am. J. Physiol.*, **213**, 1322–1326.

Klaassen, C. D. and Plaa, G. L. (1969). Plasma disappearance and biliary excretion of indocyanine green in rats, rabbits and dogs. *Toxicol. Appl. Pharmacol.*, **15**, 374–384.

Kluwe, W. M. (1981). Renal function tests as indicators of kidney injury in subacute toxicity studies. *Toxicol. Appl. Pharmacol.*, **57**, 414–424.

Koop, H., Schwab, E., Arnold, R. and Creutzfeldt, W. (1982). Effect of food deprivation on gastric somatostatin and gastrin release. *Gastroenterology*, **82**, 871–876.

Korach, K. S. and Quarmby, V. E. (1985). Morphological, physiological, and biochemical aspects of female reproduction. In Dixon, R. L. (Ed.), *Reproductive Toxicology*. Raven Press, New York, pp. 47–68.

Korsrud, G. O. and Trick, K. D. (1973). Activities of several enzymes in serum and heparinised plasma from rats. *Clin. Chim. Acta*, **48**, 311–315.

Kramer, J. M. (1981). Immunofluorescent localization of PGK-1 and PGK-2 isozymes within specific cells of the mouse testis. *Dev. Biol.*, **87**, 30–36.

Kuhn, E. R., Bellon, K., Huybrechts, L. and Heyns, W. (1983). Endocrine differences between the Wistar and Sprague–Dawley laboratory rat: influence of cold adaptation. *Horm. Metab. Res.*, **15**, 491–498.

Kuhn, G. and Hardegg, W. (1988). Effects of indoor and outdoor maintenance of dogs upon food intake, body weight and different blood parameters. *Z. Versuchstierkd.*, **31**, 205–214.

Kushner, I. and Mackiewicz, A. (1987). Acute phase proteins as disease markers. *Dis. Markers*, **5**, 1–11.

Landt, Y., Vaidya, H. C., Porter, S. E., Dietzler, D. N. and Ladenson, J. H. (1989). Immunoaffinity purification of creatine kinase-MB from human, dog, and rabbit heart with use of a monoclonal antibody specific for CK-MB. *Clin. Chem.*, **35**, 985–989.

Lang, H. (1981). *Creatine Kinase Isoenzymes*. Springer, Berlin.

Larsson, H., Carlsson, E., Mattsson, H., Lundell, L., Sundler, F., Sundler, G., Wallmark, B., Wanatabe, T. and Hakanson, R. (1986). Plasma gastrin and gastric enterochromaffin like cell activation and proliferation. *Gastroenterology*, **90**, 391–399.

Lauff, J. J., Kasper, H. E. and Ambrose, R. T. (1981). Separation of bilirubin species in serum and bile by high performance liquid chromatography. *J. Chromatogr.*, **226**, 629–639.

Leard, B. L., Alsaker, R. D., Porter, W. P. and Sobel, L. P. (1990). The effect of haemolysis on certain canine serum chemistry parameters. *Lab. Anim.*, **24**, 32–35.

Lehman, A. J. (1959). *Appraisal of the Safety of Chemicals in Foods, Drugs and Cosmetics*. Association of FDA Officials, Topeka.

Lehmann, R., Bhargava, A. S. and Gunzel, P. (1993). Serum lipoprotein patterns in rats, dogs and monkeys including method comparison and influence of menstrual cycle in monkeys. *Eur. J. Clin. Chem. Clin. Biochem.*, **31**, 633–637.

Leissing, N., Izzo, R. and Sargent, H. (1985). Variance estimates and individuality ratios of 25 serum constituents in beagles. *Clin. Chem.*, **31**, 83–86.

Leonard, T. B., Neptun, D. A. and Popp, J. A. (1984). Serum gamma glutamyl transferase as a specific indicator of bile duct lesions in the rat liver. *Am. J. Pathol.*, **166**, 262–269.

Lindena, J., Sommerfeld, U., Hopfel, C. and Trautschold, I. (1986). Catalytic enzyme activity concentration in tissues of man, dog, rabbit, guinea pig, rat and mouse. *J. Clin. Chem. Clin. Biochem.*, **24**, 35–47.

Lock, E. A., Mitchell, A. M. and Elcombe, C. R. (1989). Biochemical mechanisms of induction of hepatic peroxisome proliferation. *Annu. Rev. Pharmacol.* Toxicol., **29**, 145–163.

Loeb, W. F. and Quimby, F. W. (1989). *The Clinical Chemistry of Laboratory Animals*. Pergamon Press, New York.

McElderry, L., Tarbit, I. F. and Cassells-Smith, A. J. (1982). Six methods for urinary protein compared. *Clin. Chem.*, **28**, 356–360.

McGeachin, R. L. and Akin, J. R. (1982). Amylase levels in the tissues and body fluids of several primate species. *Comp. Biochem. Physiol.*, **72A**, 267–269.

McGuill, M. W. and Rowan, A. N. (1989). Biologic effects of blood loss: implications for sampling volumes and techniques. *ILAR News*, **31**, 5–18.

Magil, A. B., Mavichak, V., Wong, N. L. M., Quamme, G. A., Dirks, J. H. and Sutton, R. A. L. (1986). Long-term morphological and biochemical observations in cisplatin induced hypomagnesaemia in rats. *Nephron*, **43**, 223–230.

Malouf, N. M., McMahon, D., Oakeley, A. E. and Anderson, P. A. W. (1992). A cardiac troponin T epitope conserved across phyla. *J. Biol. Chem.*, **267**, 9269–9274.

Mantamat, E. E., Moreno, J. and Blanco, A. (1978). Branched-chain amino acid transferase in mouse testicular tissue. *J. Reprod. Fertil.*, **53**, 117–123.

Markert, C. L. and Whitt, G. S. (1975). Evolution of a gene. *Science*, **189**, 102–114.

Matsuzawa, T. and Sakazume (1994). Effect of fasting on haematology and clinical chemistry values in the rat and dog. *Comp. Haematol. Int.*, **4**, 152–156.

Matsuzawa, T., Nomura, M. and Unno, T. (1993). Clinical pathology reference ranges of laboratory animals. *J. Vet. Med. Sci.*, **55**, 351–362.

Meijer, G. W., de Bruijne, J. J. and Beynen, A. C. (1987). Dietary cholesterol–fat type combinations and carbohydrate and lipid metabolism in rats and mice. *Int. J. Vit. Nutr. Res.*, **57**, 319–326.

Meistrich, M. L., Trostle, P. K., Frapart, M. and Erickson, R. P. (1977). Biosynthesis and localization of lactate dehydrogenase X in pachytene spermatocytes and spermatids of mouse testes. *Dev. Biol.*, **60**, 428–441.

Meltzer, H. Y., Mrozak, S. and Boyer, M. (1970). Effect of intramuscular injections on serum creatine phosphokinase activity. *Am. J. Med. Sci.*, **259**, 42–48.

Meyer, O. A., Kristiansen, E. and Wurtzen, G. (1989). Effects of dietary protein and butylated hydroxytoluene on the kidneys of rats. *Lab. Anim.*, **23**, 175–179.

Michel, H. O. (1949). An electrometric method for the determination of red blood cell and plasma cholinesterase activity. *J. Lab. Clin. Med.*, **34**, 1564–1568.

Mitruka, B. M. and Rawnsley, H. M. (1977). *Clinical Biochemical and Hematological Reference Values in Normal Experimental Animals*. Masson, New York.

Moss, D. W. (1982). Alkaline phosphatase isoenzymes. *Clin. Chem.*, **28**, 2007–2016.

Mudge, G. H. (1982). Comparative pharmacology of the kidney; implications for drug-induced renal failure. In Bach, P. H., Bonner, F. W., Bridges, J. W. and Lock, E. A. (Eds), *Nephrotoxicity: Assessment and Pathogenesis*. Wiley, Chichester, pp. 504–518.

Mueller, P. W., Lash, L., Price, R. G., Stolte, H., Gelpi, E., Maack, T. and Berndt, W. O. (1997). Urinary biomarkers to detect significant effects of environmental and occupational exposure to nephrotoxins; 1. Categories of tests for detecting effects of nephrotoxins. *Renal Failure*, **19**, 505–521.

Muraca, M., de Groote, J. and Fevery, J. (1983). Sex differences of hepatic conjugation of bilirubin determine its maximal biliary excretion in non-anaesthetised male and female rats. *Clin. Sci.*, **64**, 85–90.

Nachbaur, J., Clarke, M. R., Provost, J. P. and Dancia, J. L. (1977). Variations of sodium, potassium and chloride plasma levels in the rat with age and sex. *Lab. Anim. Sci.*, **27**, 972–975.

Nakagawa, H., Watanabe, K. and Tsurufuji, S. (1984). Changes in serum and exudate levels of functional macroglobulins and anti-inflammatory effect of alpha-2-acute-phase-macroglobulin on carrageenin-induced inflammation in rats. *Biochem. Pharmacol.*, **33**, 1181–1186.

Nakamura, M., Itoh, T., Miyata, K., Higashiyama, N., Takesue, H. and Nishiyama, S. (1983). Difference in urinary *N*-acetyl-β-D-glucosaminidase activity between male and female beagle dogs. *Renal Physiol. (Basel)*, **6**, 130–133.

Neptun, D. A., Smith, C. N. and Irons, R. (1985). Effect of sampling site and collection method on variations in baseline clinical pathology parameters in Fischer 344 rats. *Fundam. Appl. Toxicol.*, **5**, 1180–1185.

Neuhaus, O. W. and Flory, W. (1978). Age dependent changes in the excretion of urinary proteins by the rat. *Nephron*, **22**, 570–576.

Neuman, R. G., Hud, E. and Cohen, M. P. (1994). Glycated albumin: a marker of glycaemic status in rats with experimental diabetes. *Lab. Anim.*, **28**, 63–69.

Olsen, P. S., Nexo, E., Poulsen, S. S., Hansen, H. F. and Kirkegaard, P. (1984). Renal origin of rat urinary epidermal growth factor. *Regul. Pept.*, **10**, 37–45.

Omaye, S. T. (1986). Effects of diet on toxicity testing. *Fed. Proc.*, **45**, 133–135.

Orth, D. N., Peterson, M. E. and Drucker, W. D. (1988). Plasma immunoreactive propiomelanocortin peptides and cortisol in normal dogs and dogs with Cushing's syndrome: diurnal rhythm and responses to various stimuli. *Endocrinology*, **122**, 1250–1262.

Ott, P. (1998). Hepatic elimination of indocyanine green with special reference to distribution kinetics and the influence of plasma protein binding. *Pharmacol. and Toxicol.*, **83**, Suppl. 2, 1–48.

Ottenweller, J. E. and Hedge, G. A. (1982). Diurnal variations of plasma thyrotropin, thyroxine and triiodothyronine in female rats are phase shifted after invasion of the photoperiod. *Endocrinology*, **111**, 509–514.

Padilla, S. and Hooper, M. J. (1992). Cholinesterase measurements in tissues from carbamate-treated animals: cautions and recommendations. In *Proceedings of the U.S. EPA Workshop on Cholinesterase Methodologies, Washington, D. C: Office of Pesticide Programs*. Environmental Protection Agency, Washington, DC, pp. 63–81.

Pariat, C. I., Ingrand, P., Cambar, J., de Lemos, E., Piriou, A. and Courtois, P. (1990). Seasonal effects on the daily variations of gentamicin-induced nephrotoxicity. *Arch. Toxicol.*, **64**, 205–209.

Parraga, M. E. and Kaneko, J. J. (1985). Total serum bile acids and the bile acid profile as tests of liver function. *Vet. Res. Commun.*, **9**, 79–88.

Pearl, W., Balazs, T. and Buyske, D. A. (1966). The effect of stress on serum transaminase activity in the rat. *Life Sci.*, **5**, 67–74.

Pickering, C. E. and Pickering, R. G. (1971). Methods for the estimation of acetylcholinesterase activity in the plasma and brain of laboratory animals given carbamates or organophosphorus compounds. *Arch. Toxicol.*, **27**, 292–310.

Pickering, C. E. and Pickering, R. G. (1978a). Studies of rat alkaline phosphatase. 1. Development of methods for detecting isoenzymes. *Arch. Toxicol.*, **39**, 249–266.

Pickering, C. E. and Pickering, R. G. (1978b). Studies of rat alkaline phosphatase. 2. Some applications of the methods for detecting the isoenzymes of plasma alkaline phosphatase in rats. *Arch. Toxicol.*, **39**, 267–287.

Poldlasek, S. J. and McPherson, R. A. (1989). Streptokinase binds to lactate dehydrogenase subunit-M, which shares an epitope with plasminogen. *Clin. Chem.*, **35**, 69–73.

Powers, D. M., Boyd, J. C., Glick, M. R., Kotschi, M. L., Letellier, G., Miller, W. G., Nealon, D. A. and Hartmann, A. E. (1986). *Interference Testing in Clinical Chemistry: Proposed Guidelines*. NCCLS Document 6.13.EP7/P, Villanova, PA.

Prescott, L. F. (1982). Assessment of nephrotoxicity. *Br. J. Clin. Pharmacol.*, **13**, 303–311.

Prescott, L. F. and Ansari, S. (1969). The effects of repeated administration of mercuric chloride on exfoliation of renal tubular cells and urinary glutamic–oxaloacetic transaminase activity in the rat. *Toxicol. Appl. Pharmacol.*, **14**, 97–107.

Prescott, L. F. and Brodie, D. E. (1964). A simple differential stain for urinary sediment. *Lancet*, **ii**, 940.

Price, R. G. (1982). Urinary enzymes, nephrotoxicity and renal disease. *Toxicology.*, **23**, 99–134.

Pritchard, D. H., Wright, M. G., Sulsh, S. and Butler, W. H. (1987). The assessment of chemically-induced liver injury in rats. *J. Appl. Toxicol.*, **7**, 229–236.

Rajasingham, R., Bell, J. L. and Baron, D. N. (1971). A comparative study of the isoenzymes of mammalian alpha amylase. *Enzyme*, **12**, 180–186.

Ratcliffe, J. M., McElhatton, P. R. and Sullivan, F. M. (1993). Reproductive toxicity. In Ballantyne, B., Marrs, T. and Turner, P. (Eds), *General and Applied Toxicology*. Stockton Press, New York, pp. 989–1021.

Reader, S. C. J., Shingles, C. and Stonard, M. D. (1991). Acute phase testicular damage in the rat following 1,3-dinitrobenzene or ethylene glycol monomethyl ether. The use of biochemical markers of testicular function/dysfunction. *Fundam. Appl. Toxicol.*, **16**, 61–70.

Rees, G. W., Trull, A. K. and Doyle, S. (1995). Evaluation of an enzyme-immunometric assay for serum α-glutathione S-transferase. *Ann. Clin. Biochem.*, **32**, 575–583.

Refetoff, S., Robin, N. I. and Fang, U. S. (1970). Parameters of thyroid function in serum of 16 selected vertebrate species: a study of PBI, serum T4, free T4 and the pattern of T4 and T3 binding to serum protein. *Endocrinology*, **86**, 793–805.

Reuter, A. M., Kennes, F., Leonard, A. and Sassen, A. (1968). Variations of the prealbumin in serum and urine of mice, according to strain and sex. *Comp. Biochem. Physiol.*, **25**, 921–928.

Ribelin, W. E. (1984). The effects of drugs and chemicals upon the structure of the adrenal gland. *Fundam. Appl. Toxicol.*, **4**, 105–119.

Riley, V. (1981). Psychoneuroendocrine influences on immuno-competence and neoplasia. *Science*, **212**, 1100–1102.

Robbins, J. and Johnson, M. L. (1982). Possible significance of multiple transport proteins for the thyroid hormones. In Albertini, A. and Ekins, R. P. (Eds), *Free Hormones in Blood*. Elsevier Biomedical, New York, pp. 53–64.

Robinson, J. and Evans, G. O. (1996). Preanalytical and analytical variables. In Evans, G. O. (Ed.), *Animal Clinical Chemistry: a Primer for Toxicologists*. Taylor and Francis, London, pp. 21–43.

Rosenthal, P., Blanckaert, N., Kabra, P. M. and Thaler, M. M. (1981). Liquid chromatographic determination of bilirubin and its conjugates in rat serum and human amniotic fluid. *Clin. Chem.*, **27**, 1704–1707.

Roy, A. K. and Neuhaus, O. W. (1967). Androgenic control of a sex-dependent protein in the rat. *Nature*, **214**, 618–620.

Safirstein, R., Price, P. M., Saggi, S. J. and Harris, R. C. (1990). Changes in gene expression after temporary renal ischaemia. *Kidney Int.*, **37**, 1515–1521.

Saggin, L., Gorza, L., Ausoni, S. and Schiaffino, S. (1990). Cardiac troponin T in developing regenerating and denervated rat skeletal muscle. *Development*, **110**, 547–554.

Salgo, L. and Szabo, A. (1982). Gamma-glutamyl transpeptidase activity in human urine. *Clin. Chim. Acta*, **126**, 9–16.

Santen, R. J. and Bardin, C. W. (1973). Episodic LH secretion in man: pulse analysis, clinical interpretation, physiologic mechanisms. *J. Clin. Invest.*, **52**, 2617–2628.

Schardsmidt, B. F., Waggoner, J. G. and Berk, P. D. (1975). Hepatic organic anion uptake in the rat. *J. Clin. Invest.*, **56**, 1280–1292.

Scherer, R., Abd-el-Fattah, M. and Ruhenstroth-Bauer, G. (1977). In Willoughby, D. A., Giroud, J. P. and Velo, G. P. (Eds), *Perspectives in Inflammation, Future Trends and Development*. MTP, Lancaster, pp. 437–444.

Schmidt-Neilsen, B. and O'Dell, R. (1961). Structure and concentrating mechanism in the mammalian kidney. *Am. J. Physiol.*, **200**, 1119–1124.

Schwartz, E., Tornaben, J. A. and Boxill, G. C. (1973). The effects of food restriction on hematology, clinical chemistry and pathology in the albino rat. *Toxicol. Appl. Pharmacol.*, **25**, 515–524.

Sharratt, M. and Frazer, A. C. (1963). The sensitivity of function tests in detecting renal damage in the rat. *Toxicol. Appl. Pharmacol.*, **39**, 423–434.

Simpson, J. W. and Doxey, D. L. (1988). Evaluation of faecal analysis as an aid to the detection of exocrine pancreatic insufficiency. *Br. Vet. J.*, **144**, 174–178.

Sinha, B. K. (1982). Myocardial toxicity of anthracyclines and other antitumour agents. In van Stee, E. W. (Ed.), *Cardiovascular Toxicology*. Raven Press, New York, pp. 181–198.

Sitren, H. S. and Stevenson, N. R. (1980). Circadian fluctuations in liver and blood parameters in rats adapted to a nutrient solution by oral, intravenous and discontinuous intravenous feeding. *J. Nutr.*, **110**, 558–566.

Smith, P. L. (1986). In Rozman, K. and Hanninen, O. (Eds), *Gastrointestinal Toxicology*. Elsevier, Amsterdam, pp. 1–23.

Spitz, I. M., Gunsalus, G. L., Mather, J. P., Thau, R. and Bardin, C. W. (1985). The effects of the imidazole carboxylic acid derivative, tolmidamine, on testicular function. 1. Early changes in androgen binding protein secretion in the rat. *J. Androl.*, **6**, 171–178.

Steinberg, K. K., Freni-Titulaer, L. W. J., Rogers, T. N., Burse, V. W., Mueller, P. W., Stehr, P. A. and Miller, D. T. (1986). Effects of polychlorinated biphenyls and lipemia on serum analytes. *J. Toxicol. Environ. Health*, **19**, 369–381.

Steinberger, E. (1981). Current status of studies concerned with evaluation of toxic effects of chemicals on the testes. *Environ. Health Perspect.*, **38**, 29–33.

Steiness, E., Rasmussen, F., Svendsen, O. and Nielsen, P. (1978). A comparative study of serum creatine phosphokinase (CPK) activity in rabbits, pigs and humans after intramuscular injection of local damaging drugs. *Acta Pharmacol. Toxicol.*, **42**, 357–364.

Stonard, M. D. (1987). In Bach, P. H. and Lock, E. A. (Eds), *Nephrotoxicity in the Experimental and Clinical Situation*. Martinus Nijhoff, Dordrecht, pp. 563–592.

Stonard, M. D. (1990). Assessment of renal function and damage in animal species. *J. Appl. Toxicol.*, **10**, 267–274.

Stonard, M. D. (1996). Assessment of nephrotoxicity. In Evans, G. O. (Ed.), *Animal Clinical Chemistry: a Primer for Toxicologists*. Taylor and Francis, London, pp. 87–98.

Stonard, M. D., Samuels, D. M. and Lock, E. A. (1984). The pathogenesis of nephrocalcinosis induced by different diets in female rats, and the effect on renal function. *Food Cosmet. Toxicol.*, **22**, 139–146.

Stonard, M. D., Gore, C. W., Oliver, G. J. A. and Smith, I. K. (1987). Urinary enzymes and protein patterns as indicators of injury to different regions of the kidney. *Fundam. Appl. Toxicol.*, **9**, 339–351.

Stroo, W. E. and Hook, J. B. (1977). Enzymes of renal origin in urine as indicators of nephrotoxicity. *Toxicol. Appl. Pharmacol.*, **39**, 423–434.

Sundberg, A., Appelkvist, E. L., Dallner, G. and Nilsson, R. (1994a). Glutathione transferases in the urine: sensitive methods for detection of kidney damage induced by nephrotoxic agents in humans. *Environ. Health Perspect.*, **102**, Suppl. 3, 293–296.

Sundberg, A., Appelkvist, E. L., Backman, L. and Dallner, G. (1994b). Urinary π-class glutathione transferase as an indicator of tubular damage in the human kidney. *Nephron*, **67**, 308–316.

Surber, C. and Dubach, U. C. (1989). Tests for local toxicity of intramuscular drug preparations. Comparison of *in vivo* and *in vitro* findings. *Arzneim. Forsch.*, **39**, 1586–1589.

Swain, R., Williams, G. and Cochran, J. (1994). Elevation and clearance of serum creatine kinase in Fischer rats. *Clin. Chem.*, **40**, 990.

Tani, S., Ishikawa, A., Yamazaki, H. and Kudo, Y. (1987). Serum pepsinogen levels in normal and experimental peptic ulcer rats measured by radioimmunoassay. *Chem. Pharm. Bull.*, **35**, 1515–1522.

Terpstra, A. H. M., Woodward, C. J. H. and Sanchez-Muniz, F. J. (1981). Improved techniques for the separation of serum lipoproteins by density gradient ultracentrifugation: visualization by prestaining and rapid separation of serum lipoproteins from small volumes of serum. *Anal. Biochem.*, **11**, 149–157.

Theus, R. and Zbinden, G. (1984). Toxicological assessment of the hemostatic system, regulatory requirements, and industry practice. *Regul. Toxicol. Pharmacol.*, **4**, 74–95.

Thompson, M.B. (1996). Bile acids in the assessment of hepatocellular function. *Toxicologic Pathol.*, **24**, 62–71.

Thompson, M. B. and Kunze, D. J. (1984). Polyethylene glycol-6000 as a clearing agent for lipemic serum samples from dogs and the effect on 13 serum assays. *Am. J. Vet. Res.*, **45**, 2154–2157.

Thorell, J. I. and Larson, S. M. (1978). *Radioimmunoassay and Related Techniques*. C. V. Mosby, St. Louis, MO.

Tredger, J. M. and Sherwood, R. A. (1997). The liver; new functional, prognostic and diagnostic tests. *Ann. Clin. Biochem.*, **34**, 121–141.

Uchiyama, T., Tokoi, K. and Deki, T. (1985). Successive changes in the blood composition of the experimental normal beagle dogs accompanied with age. *Exp. Anim.*, **34**, 367–377.

Unakami, S., Suzuki, S., Nakarishi, E., Ichonohe, K., Hirata, M. and Taninoto, Y. (1987). Comparative studies on multiple forms of serum cholinesterase in various species. *Exp. Anim.*, **36**, 199–204.

Vandeberg, J. L., Yu Lee, C. and Goldberg, E, (1981). Immunohistochemical localization of phosphoglycerate kinase isozymes in mouse testes. *J. Exp. Zool.*, **217**, 435–441.

Vogel, W. H. (1987). Stress—the neglected variable in experimental pharmacology and toxicology. *Trends Pharmacol. Sci.*, **8**, 35–38.

Voss, G. and Sachsse, K. (1970). Red cell and plasma cholinesterase activities in microsamples of human and animal blood determined simultaneously by a modified acetylcholine/DTNB procedure. *Toxicol. Appl. Pharmacol.*, **16**, 764–772.

Walsh, C. T. (1982). Methods in gastrointestinal toxicology. In Hayes, A. W. (Ed.), *Principles and Methods of Toxicology*. Raven Press, New York, pp. 475–486.

Waner, T. (1990). Clinical chemistry in regulatory toxicology: the state of the art. In Kaneko, J. J. (Ed.), *Proceedings, IVth Congress, International Society for Animal Clinical Biochemistry, University of California*, pp. 61–68.

Waterfield, C. J., Turton, J. A., Scales, M. D. C. and Timbrell, J. A. (1993a). Investigations into the effects of various hepatotoxic compounds on urinary and liver taurine levels in rats. *Arch. Toxicol.*, **67**, 244–254.

Waterfield, C. J., Turton, J. A., Scales, M. D. C. and Timbrell, J. A. (1993b). Effect of various non-hepatotoxic compounds on urinary and liver taurine levels in rats. *Arch. Toxicol.*, **67**, 538–546.

Weil, C. S. (1982). Statistical analysis and normality of selected hematologic and clinical chemistry measurements used in toxicological studies. *Arch. Toxicol., Suppl.* **5**, 237–253.

Weisberg, L. S. (1989). Pseudohyponatremia: a reappraisal. *Am. J. Med.*, **86**, 315–318.

Weiss, J. S., Gautam, A., Lauff, J. J., Sundberg, M. W., Jatlow, P., Boyer, J. L., *et al.* (1983). The clinical importance of a protein-bound fraction of serum bilirubin in patients with hyperbilirubinemia. *N. Engl. J. Med.*, **309**, 147–150.

Wellman, M.L., Hoffmann, W. E., Dorner, J. L. and Mock, R. E. (1982). Comparison of the steroid-induced, intestinal, and hepatic isoenzymes of alkaline phosphatase in the dog. *Am. J. Vet. Res.*, **43**, 1204–1207.

Werner, M. and Gabrielson, D. (1977). Ultrafiltration for improved assay of urinary enzymes. *Clin. Chem.*, **23**, 700–704.

Werner, M., Maruhn, D. and Atoba, M. (1969). Use of gel filtration in the assay of urinary enzymes. *J. Chromatogr.*, **40**, 254–263.

Wheat, T. E., Hintz, M., Goldberg, E. and Margoliash, E. (1977). Analysis of stage specific multiple forms of lactate dehydrogenase and of cytochrome *c* during spermatogenesis in the mouse. *Differentiation*, **9**, 37–41.

Whittaker, M. (1986). *Cholinesterase*, Monographs in Human Genetics, Vol. II. Karger, Basle.

Will, P. C., Allbee, W. E., Witt, C. G., Bertko, R. J. and Gaginella, T. S. (1984). Quantification of pepsin A activity in canine and rat gastric juice with the chromogenic substrate Azocoll. *Clin. Chem.*, **30**, 707–711.

Wills, J. H. (1972). The measurement and significance of changes in the cholinesterase activities of erythrocytes and plasma in man and animals. *CRC Crit. Rev. Toxicol.*, **1**, 153–201.

Wilson, C. A. and Leigh, A. J. (1992). Endocrine toxicology of the female reproductive system. In Atterwill, C. K. and Flack, J. (Eds) *Endocrine Toxicology*. Cambridge University Press, Cambridge, pp. 313–399.

Witiak, D. T. and Whitehouse, M. W. (1969). Species differences in the albumin binding of 2,4,6-trinitrobenzaldehyde, chlorophenoxyacetic acids, 2-(4′-hydroxybenzeneazo)benzoic acid and some other acidic drugs—the unique behaviour of plasma. *Biochem. Pharmacol.*, **18**, 971–977.

Wolford, S. T., Schroer, R. A., Gallo, P. P., Gohs, F. X., Brodeck, M., Falk, H. B. and Ruhren, R. (1987). Age-related changes in serum chemistry and hematology values in normal Sprague–Dawley rats. *Fundam. Appl. Toxicol.*, **8**, 80–88.

Wong, C. C., Dohler, K. D., Atkinson, M. J., Geerlings, H., Hesch, R. D. and von zur Mehlen, A. (1983a). Influence of age, strain and season on diurnal periodicity of thyroid stimulating hormone, thyroxine, tri-iodothyronine and parathyroid hormone in the serum of male laboratory rats. *Acta Endocrinol.*, **101**, 377–385.

Wong, C. C., Dohler, K. D., Geerlings, H. and von zur Mehlen, A. (1983b). Influence of age, strain and season on circadian periodicity of pituitary, gonadal and adrenal hormones in the serum of male laboratory rats. *Horm. Res.*, **17**, 202–215.

Woodman, D. D. (1981). In Gorrod, J. W. (Ed.). *Aspects of Drug Toxicity Testing Methods*. Taylor and Francis, London, pp. 145–156.

Woodman, D. D. (1988a). Assessment of hepatic function and damage in animal species. *J. Appl. Toxicol.*, **8**, 249–254.

Woodman, D. D. (1988b). In Keller, P. and Bogin, E. (Eds), *The Use of Clinical Biochemistry in Toxicologically Relevant Animal Models and Standardization and Quality Control in Animals Biochemistry*. Hexagon-Roche, Basle, pp. 63–77.

Woodman, D. D. (1996). Assessment of hepatotoxicity. In Evans, G. O. (Ed.), *Animal Clinical Chemistry: a Primer for Toxicologists*. Taylor and Francis, London, pp. 71–86.

Woodman, D. D. (1997). Laboratory animal endocrinology: hormonal action, control mechanisms, and interactions with drugs. John Wiley & Sons Ltd., Chichester, England.

Woodman, D. D. and Maile, P. A. (1981). Bile acids as an index of cholestasis. *Clin. Chem.*, **27**, 846–848.

Wright, P. J. and Plummer, D. T. (1974). The use of urinary enzyme measurements to detect renal damage caused by nephrotoxic compounds. *Biochem. Pharmacol.*, **23**, 65–73.

Wright, P. J., Leathwood, P. D. and Plummer, D. T. (1972). Enzymes in rat urine: alkaline phosphatase. *Enzymologia*, **42**, 317–327.

Young, D. S. (1990). *Effects of Drugs on Clinical Laboratory Tests*. AACC Press, Washington, DC.

Young, F. G. (1963). Pancreatic hormones: insulin. In von Euler, U. S. and Heller, H. (Eds). *Comparative Endocrinology*. Academic Press, London, pp. 371–402.

Chapter 18
Haematology and Toxicology

Timothy C. Marrs and Simon Warren

C O N T E N T S

INTRODUCTION

Haematological investigations are of importance in toxicology in two different sets of circumstances. First, toxicological effects on the blood and blood-forming organs may occur in humans; these effects will often show charactistic changes in haematological studies. Second, toxicological parameters are routinely measured during toxicological studies, regardless of whether the test compound is thought to be specifically haematotoxic, and guidelines are available about how these investigations should be carried out (e.g. Weingand *et al.*, 1996). Both in humans and in experimental animals, abnormalities observed may be due to toxicity to the haematopoietic organs such as the bone marrow, or be produced indirectly through effects on animal nutrition, or on organs such as the kidney, which affect haematopoiesis. Moreover, some xenobiotics can affect the peripheral blood directly, an example being the production of haemolysis by certain drugs. One of the most interesting aspects of haematology in humans is the frequent interaction of inherited traits, for example porphyria, glucose-6-phosphate dehydrogenase deficiency, with xenobiotics.

STRUCTURE AND FUNCTIONS OF THE BLOOD AND ASSOCIATED ORGANS

Blood is a fluid containing a number of cellular elements, including the red cells, which contain the oxygen-transporting pigment, the white cells and the platelets. The white cells can be subdivided into neutrophils, eosinophils, basophils, monocytes and lymphocytes.

Haematopoiesis

Haematopoiesis occurs from stem cells. In studies with irradiated mice it was noted that certain bone marrow cells had the ability to form haematopoietic colonies in irradiated mice (Till and McCulloch, 1961). It appears that the stem cells in the marrow can give rise to all types of blood cells and these stem cells are thus known as pluripotent stem cells (Barton *et al.*, 1980). The pluripotent stem cells are also known as colony-forming units spleen (CFU-S) from their properties in *in vitro* studies and they have a marked ability for self-renewal. The colony-forming unit spleen (CFU-S) assay can be used to quantitate pluripotent stem cells.

The pluripotent stem cell can differentiate into stem cells that are capable of giving rise to myeloid cell types, the colony-forming unit granulocyte/erythroid/monocyte/megakaryocyte (CFU-GEMM), which in turn to give rise to progenitor cells, whose potential is more restricted, such as the colony-forming unit granulocyte macrophage (CFU-GM) and the colony-forming unit erythroid (CFU-E) (Chanarin, 1985; Irons, 1991; Means, 1997; Young and Weiss, 1997).

In most mammals, including man, haematopoiesis is first seen in the yolk sac and later in foetal life, in the liver and spleen. After birth, the bone marrow is, in humans, the major site of haematopoiesis. In rats and mice, virtually all the bone medullary space is occupied by haematopoietic tissue, whereas in adult humans, dogs and rabbits such tissue becomes limited to the proximal epiphyses of the long bones and skull, the remainder of the marrow being occupied by fat. Increased haematopoietic activity is, in man, usually confined to the medullary space, except under conditions of extreme demand. In the mouse and the rat, this is not the case and splenic (and hepatic) haematopoiesis is much more common in conditions of very high demand. The bone marrow contains a network of thin-walled branching vessels called the venous sinuses. The wall of the sinuses consists of the endothelium, basement membrane and the adventitia, the last of which is associated with adventitial reticular cells. The endothelium is complete, i.e. not fenestrated, but the basement membrane is discontinuous. Mature blood cells cross the wall of the sinuses to enter the circulation (Chanarin, 1985). In normal circumstances, the cellular component of the marrow remains fairly constant, unless disturbed by factors such as loss of blood; in such conditions, the marrow can respond rapidly to bring the number of cells in the peripheral circulation back to normal; this is controlled by a number of factors that stimulate haematopoiesis, such as erythropoietin (see below).

The Red Cell and Haemoglobin— Erythropoiesis

The main role of the red blood cell is to bind reversibly to oxygen. The erythroid series of cells is derived from the stem cell and thence the CFU-GEMM. The earliest progenitor restricted to the red cell lineage is the burst-forming unit erythroid (BFU-E), from which is derived the CFU-E. This gives rise to the precursor cells, the various normoblasts (Irons, 1991; Means, 1997). The last stage in maturation to the non-nucleated biconcave erythrocyte is the reticulocyte, so-called because of its fine basophil reticular network (see Sieff and Nathan, 1996). In situations in which erythrocyte production has been stimulated, reticulocytes may be seen in the peripheral blood. The regulation of production of red cells is dependent upon the oxygen requirement of the tissues, being controlled by humoral factors, including erythropoietin, whose main source is the kidney (Spivak and Graber, 1980; Koury *et al.*, 1988), with a contribution from the liver (Chanarin, 1985).

Haemoglobin is one of a number of oxygen-binding proteins that have evolved in the animal and plant kingdoms, and contains a tetrapyrrole ring system, with ferrous iron at the centre.

Chlorophyll, in the plant kingdom, resembles haemoglobin in so far as it has a similar ring, although magnesium takes the place of the iron of haemoglobin. Copper, found in haemocyanin, replaces the iron atom in many invertebrates and, in some sea squirts, vanadium is present. The structure of haemoglobin can be summarized: each molecule of haemoglobin consists of four amino acid chains: a pair of alpha chains and a pair of beta chains (Perutz, 1967–68). The chains are folded and each carries a haem group, attached to a histidine residue at position 87 in the alpha chains and 92 in the beta chains. The haem group comprises a tetrapyrrole ring with a central ferrous iron atom. The iron remains in the ferrous state during binding to both oxygen and carbon monoxide. If oxidized to the ferric state, methaemoglobin is produced; this is discussed below.

The iron atoms of haemoglobin can each accept electrons from a maximum of six oppositely charged ions or neutral substances, ligands (Strang, 1977). Each iron atom forms six bonds: four with the nitrogen atoms of the tetrapyrrole ring, one with the histidine residue of the amino acid chain and one with oxygen or, in cases of poisoning, with carbon monoxide. As the haemoglobin molecule takes up oxygen, its quaternary structure changes owing to changes in the extent of loose bonding, or attraction, of the iron atom to other amino acid residues in the amino acid chains. These conformational changes lead to the haemoglobin molecule passing from a 'tense' configuration when in the deoxygenated state to a 'relaxed' state as oxygen atoms are taken up. In the relaxed state the affinity for oxygen is high: saturation occurs when the haemoglobin molecule has bound four molecules of oxygen. This sequential change in affinity for oxygen defines the sigmoid shape of the oxyhaemoglobin dissociation curve. It is interesting to note that if haemoglobin bound only one oxygen atom, i.e. consisted of only one amino acid chain with a single haem group, the dissociation curve could be represented by a hyperbola: this is the case with myoglobin, a one-chain molecule. The structure of haemoglobin differs in different species and that in the foetus is different from that in the adult human. Abnormal haemoglobins in humans can produce diseases such as sickle cell anaemia and some types of hereditary methaemoglobinaemia.

In addition to haemoglobin, the red cell contains enzymes, such as glucose-6-phosphate dehydrogenase (G6PD). G6PD is of great importance in maintaining NADPH levels. NADPH is essential for reducing oxidized glutathione, reduced glutathione being required for the protection of intraerythrocytic sulphydryl groups and the structural integrity of the cell. Maintenance of the reducing potential of the red cells is also necessary to prevent methaemoglobinaemia. Oxidant stress of the red cells will produce haemolytic anaemia, methaemoglobinaemia and/or Heinz bodies (see below).

White Cells

Granulocytes

The granulocytic series are derived from the CFU-GEMM, which gives rise to the colony-forming unit granulocyte/macrophage (CFU-GM). Three lineages give rise to mature granulocytes, which are known as polymorphonuclear leucocytes or polymorphs. They have segmented nuclei and cytoplasmic granules and are divided into neutrophils, eosinophils and basophils according to the staining characteristics of their cytoplasmic granules (Irons, 1991; Liesveld and Lichtman, 1997). The granules contain a variety of enzymes and other substances characteristic of the inflammatory response and phagocytosis, and the cells have a turnover rate of a few hours (Marsh, 1985). The primary role of polymorphs is phagocytosis, and they perform the major part of this role in the tissues, into which they pass between the capillary endothelial cells. The granules of neutrophils are notable for their high alkaline phosphatase activity and polymorph leucocytosis is characteristic of bacterial infection, but may also occur in other conditions, e.g. myeloid leukaemias. Eosinophils have a distinct progenitor cell, the colony-forming unit eosinophil (CFU-EO) (Young and Weiss, 1997), and are frequently present during allergic phenomena and in parasite infestations. The granules of eosinophils have high peroxidase activity and contain a variety of hydrolytic enzymes. Basophils are the circulating equivalent of mast cells and the granules contain heparin and histamine. Granulocytopoiesis is under the control of factors such as granulocyte colony-stimulating factor.

Monocytes

Monocytes are derived from the CFU-GM, in common with neutrophils. Once they reach the tissues they transform to tissue macrophages or more specialized forms such as the Kupffer cells of the liver. Monocytes are large cells, whose function is phagocytosis.

Lymphocytes

Lymphocytes can be divided into T-lymphocytes and B-lymphocytes. These are so-called because of the involvement of the thymus in T-lymphocyte production, whereas in birds the site of B-lymphocyte development is the Bursa of Fabricius (see Chapter 47). In mammals the primary lymphoid organs are the thymus and bone marrow.

Platelets and Coagulation

Platelets are formed in the bone marrow by fragmentation of megakaryocytes, large cells (diameter 50–200 μm), which are derived from megakaryoblasts (Tarallo, 1985; Irons, 1991). The function of platelets is to stop bleeding: thus platelet aggregation can produce primary haemostasis, while platelets are also concerned in the initiation of coagulation, by liberating various molecules. In addition, thrombocytopenia results in increased capillary fragility. If the platelet count falls below about 50 000 μl^{-3}, spontaneous haemorrhage and haemorrhage after minor trauma are likely to occur (Chanarin, 1985). The process of coagulation involves both plasma factors and platelets to produce the so-called cascade. There is an opposing system, fibrinolysis, which removes unwanted fibrin.

Interspecies Differences

There are notable differences in the ratios of the various cell types of the blood in different laboratory animals. Thus in the rat, guinea pig and certain types of primate (e.g. lemurs), lymphocytes predominate over polymorphs in the blood, whereas in other animals, including man, polymorphs predominate. Thus haematological data should be compared with control data from the same species. Historical control data, where used, should be from the same species and, as strain differences can occur, also from the same strain. In addition to quantitative differences between blood cell numbers, there are some notable morphological differences between species. There are major differences in red cell morphology between some species not commonly used in the laboratory, but the red cell of nearly all laboratory species resembles that in humans in being a biconcave disc; however, central pallor is not seen in cat red cells. Reticulocytosis is frequently observed in rats, whereas in other species it is an indicator of increased red cell production. The size of erythrocytes varies considerably between species, being about 8 μm in humans and as small as 3 μm in the goat (Irons, 1991). The life span of the human red cell is approximately 120 days (Ashby, 1919), whereas in many other species it is considerably shorter, e.g. 30 days in the mouse (Irons, 1991). Amongst the white cells, amphophils, pseudoeosinophils or heterophils are the rabbit equivalent of the neutrophils of other species, as are the pseudoeosinophils of guinea pigs (Loeb et al., 1978); although these cells carry out approximately the same functions as do neutrophils in other species, the specific granules stain orange–red with Romanowsky stains. The size of the granules in basophils varies considerably depending upon the species. The bone marrow of mice and rats is notable for the paucity of fat by comparison with human marrow, while rat haematopoietic tissue is remarkable for its large number of mast cells.

PRACTICAL ASPECTS OF HAEMATOLOGY IN TOXICOLOGICAL STUDIES

Among the advantages conferred by modern automation, and possibly not yet adequately recognized in guidelines or in standard study designs, is that data can potentially be processed extremely rapidly. It is therefore possible, even with shorter term studies, to use basic parameters to screen for an effect at a pre-terminal investigation and then to design a further examination to characterize better the nature of the effect using the larger blood samples available at termination. This option should be considered (on both welfare and economic grounds) if it might usefully spare additional animals being included in a new study.

Blood Sampling

Modern haematology is heavily automated, to such an extent that the procedure for obtaining blood samples probably represents one of the major sources of variability. This variability can be markedly reduced if sampling is conducted by well trained and experienced personnel, with adequate preparation and time to perform the procedure to a constant standard. Coupled with the obvious possible consequences of the sampling procedure for the well-being of the animals, it is essential that any sampling procedure strikes the best compromise between welfare of the animal, minimization of stress to animals and to staff and fulfilment of the aims of the experiment or study. For small species such as rats and mice it is usually necessary that the volume of each blood sample is kept to a minimum, and therefore it follows that blood sampling equipment and analytical instrumentation should be designed to ensure that 'dead volume', or other sources of sample loss, are minimized.

Rules, guidelines and regulations relating to animal experimentation may also have a strong influence in different parts of the world on the methodology available for blood sampling and anaesthesia. The following few paragraphs should therefore not be taken as a recommendation to apply any particular technique, merely as guidance for consideration.

A useful discussion of blood sampling procedures for various species, and of appropriate volumes of blood which might be taken, was given by the BVA/FRAME/RSPCA/UFAW Joint Working Group on Refinement (Morton and Abbot, 1993). This publication has the aim of reducing pain, distress or discomfort for the animals to the minimum necessary, provides good practice guidelines, and should be regarded as important reading for the toxicologist responsible for planning blood sampling procedures in study designs. Further discussion by Evans (1994) and Morton and Jennings (1994) illuminates situations where flexibility in these guidelines may be appropriate.

Small volumes of blood (0.1 ml or less) may be drawn by simple venepuncture, without anaesthetic being necessary. For repeated sampling (intervals of 3–4 weeks), Morton and Abbot (1993) suggest up to 10% of the circulating volume can be drawn on each occasion. The circulating blood volume is cited as 55–70 ml (kg body weight)$^{-1}$, suggesting that for a 250 g rat 1.5 ml or for a 30 g mouse 0.2 ml might be an appropriate maximum sample size. The available sample size from rabbits or dogs is unlikely to be a limiting factor for haematological investigations.

The recommended blood sampling sites for various of the common species used in toxicology studies are given in **Table 1**.

Morton and Abbot (1993) discuss the use of the rodent orbital venous sinus but recommend this as not appropriate particularly for the rat, and also recommend against sampling from the sublingual vein of small rodents. This conclusion differs from the opinion of many practitioners, since a large sample (of 1 ml or more in the rat) can be drawn relatively easily. A Study

Table 1 Recommended sampling sites for blood

Species	Site
Mouse	Amputation of the tail tip or venepuncture of the tail vein
Rat	Venepuncture of the tail vein or of the jugular vein
Rabbit	Venepuncture of the ear vein
Dog	Venepuncture of the cephalic vein (forelimb) or jugular vein

Director should always consider if an alternative site may be more appropriate. Some authors have in the past suggested that anaesthesia or analgesia might not be necessary for orbital sinus bleeding; however, it should be noted that such a practice would be unacceptable in some countries and the authors of this chapter cannot condone it. If sampling a large volume from the rodent tail vein (with practice as much as 1 ml might be obtained from a rat), it is helpful if the animal be warmed in a thermostatically controlled hot box for some minutes. This promotes dilatation of, and good blood flow through, the vein. Insufficient warming, or dipping the tail in warm water to dilate the vein, is usually insufficient to allow, for example, a sample of as much as 0.5 ml to be taken from a rat.

If larger samples are required, blood sampling can be performed as a terminal procedure. Techniques such as decapitation or exsanguination under deep anaesthesia from the jugular vein may result in wastage and excessive contamination by hair or skin scales. A useful alternative for both rats and mice, particularly if necropsy is performed, is venepuncture of the abdominal vena cava, which can be performed as long as 10 min after death, although the procedure is best conducted as soon as possible.

Blood drawn from different sampling sites may give slightly different values and therefore confound results, a point that should be kept in mind on occasions when, for example, a large terminal blood sample is drawn from a different location to those samples drawn during the in-life part of the study.

Anaesthesia

Use of general anaesthesia, other than to reduce pain to the animal, will aid restraint of the animal during the sampling procedure and may well reduce the incidence of injury associated with sampling. Dogs are usually sufficiently docile and compliant that blood samples can be drawn without anaesthesia, whereas for rats and mice subject to more invasive methods such as orbital sinus bleeding and cardiac puncture, use of anaesthesia should be mandatory. There are several inhalation anaesthetic agents which are used with smaller animals. All have the advantage of being convenient, with rapid recovery, but it should be recognized that all may affect the quality of blood samples to a slight extent. Use of ether should no longer be considered acceptable except in the most unusual circumstances; not only is the vapour potentially flammable and explosive, but also, if not used in a closed system, ether may affect the well-being of the operator (as is a general property of the volatile anaesthetics), and it appears irritant to the nasal mucosa of the rat. More modern volatile anaesthetics (e.g. methoxyfluorane) in a closed system are a preferred alternative. A gas mixture of 70% carbon dioxide and 30% oxygen may be permitted, but it is questionable whether such a procedure is truly anaesthetic (i.e. whether it really prevents pain). Moreover, the risk of death of the animal through anaesthetic accident, remote if anaesthesia is performed by an experienced operator, is probably greater than by use of a well metered volatile anaesthetic. The risk is somewhat greater if 100% CO_2 is used. Use of CO_2 will not be appropriate if simultaneous samples are drawn for blood gas or electrolyte analysis, since this agent causes alkalosis. Injectable agents may also be used, particularly for large species, but do not have the popularity of inhalation agents.

Anticoagulants

Anticoagulants are necessary for haematological investigations. Those generally recommended are EDTA for blood cellular investigations and citrate for tests of clotting function. It is good practice to ensure that tubes containing samples are gently agitated for the period between collection and analysis.

Commercially available containers pre-treated with these anticoagulants are readily available. However, it should be noted that these commercially available tubes are generally of a size appropriate to samples drawn for humans, where sample volume is not usually a major restraint. The toxicologist performing a standard haematology and blood chemistry screen in smaller species will usually find the available sample volume restrictive and wish to make best use of every microlitre. The volume devoted to haematology can often be the smaller portion of a 1 ml sample. It may be a useful technique to mark containers at a level less than full, to give a volume which is more appropriate to the array of assays intended. For example, if the haematology assay requires only 0.3 ml of blood then it will be helpful to mark tubes at this volume rather than to collect to a commercially available 0.5 ml mark. It should be recognized that using pre-prepared tubes with any volume of sample other than that for which the tube is intended will lead to a concentration of anticoagulant which is different, but (hopefully) greater, than is optimum. This may lead, for instance, to slight cell shrinkage, but must not permit coagulation. If all samples in the study are subject to the same conditions, this should not affect the ability to detect a treatment-related change. The consideration is particularly important if the test groups, particularly at high dose levels, are adversely affected by their treatment

such that it may be difficult to obtain a full-size blood sample. There would then be a possibility that the mean sample size of affected groups would be smaller than that of controls, with correspondingly greater concentrations of anticoagulant, potentially leading to an artefactual dose-related effect.

Useful Parameters

Parameters recommended in standard study guidelines, e.g. those of the OECD, provide a screen to identify if the blood be a principal target organ. These parameters are red blood cell count, haematocrit (packed cell volume, PCV), haemoglobin, white cell count and platelet (thrombocyte) count, and can all be determined by automated equipment easily and quickly from a relatively small blood sample easily obtained from most laboratory mammalian species. This section will not deal with the large variety of other tests which might be used to explore further any abnormalities detected. Haematology samples do not require separation, e.g. into cells and supernatant, and thus all of the sample may be used. This is in contrast to clinical chemistry investigations, where discarding the cellular portion of blood is a comparatively inefficient process.

Erythrocytes and Platelets

The red cell parameters are usually determined by measuring cell size and number, by light scattering or changes in resistivity as cells are passaged through a pore, hence the primary values obtained are mean cell volumes and counts. Modern automated laboratories should therefore easily be able to report mean cell volume (MCV), and often indices such as mean cell haemoglobin (MCH) and mean corpuscular haemoglobin concentration (MCHC), in addition to the guideline expectations. There is generally little variation in the values obtained for these parameters between equipment and laboratories, which should in any case be periodically subject to quality-control analysis of standard samples. There is no major species difference in these parameters between the principal laboratory mammalian species, although it should be noted that cell sizes vary slightly between species and that different automated analysers may therefore flag abnormal samples with varying degrees of success, dependent on the ability of the equipment software to deal with samples from non-human species.

Should the results indicate an anaemia, examination of a blood film is useful for information on the mechanism. A blood smear requires a very small quantity of blood, and it is probably good practice to ensure that a smear is made and fixed (even if not routinely examined) each time a haematology sample is drawn. Smears are examined for features such as variation in degree of staining, shape and appearance of cells and detection of cellular inclusions. As an example, polychromasia usually indicates uptake of dye by the residual nucleic acids in young erythrocytes, so a treatment-related increase may be suggestive of reticulocytosis. Confirmation of reticulocytosis, however, requires the use of a vital stain on a fresh blood sample. The observation of spherocytes may indicate a problem with the osmolarity, while Heinz bodies are indicative of abnormality in the oxidative status of the red cell.

White Blood Cell (WBC, Leucocyte) Parameters

WBC counts are usually measured from the same sample as used for RBC counts. Techniques to differentiate between WBCs and RBCs rely on the fact that WBCs contain a nucleus and are larger. A typical WBC differential count would score lymphocytes, neutrophils (banded and segmented), monocytes, basophils and eosinophils. Differential WBC counts can be determined from the EDTA sample by some autoanalysers, by a variety of methods dependent on the equipment. Techniques which might be used include cell size differentials, oxidative ability or, at the most sophisticated (and expensive), image analysis of cell morphology. The expression and terminology of white cell sub-populations will therefore differ according to the type of instrumentation. Other than image analysis, none of the automated techniques are ideal for the differentiation of cell types into the types generally recognized for use by toxicologists. These techniques might, however, be used automatically to detect if differences are present between groups. It is usually appropriate to verify the nature of any abnormalities visually. Alternatively, blood smears may be prepared easily by trained staff from a single drop of blood; however, these smears are generally suitable primarily for manual microscopic examination, which is time consuming and more expensive. Testing guidelines such as those of the OECD therefore permit such smears to be examined only from control and high-dose animals, with other groups being subsequently investigated (e.g. to determine a no-effect level) only if high-dose animals show different results to controls.

Differential WBC counts are usually expressed as '%WBC', i.e. each cell type as a proportion of the total WBC population. Since WBC and differential counts show greater interindividual variation than do RBC parameters, it is often more helpful to see differential counts expressed in units of cells/volume since it may be easier to determine if a particular WBC subtype is affected.

Standard guidelines for carcinogenicity studies usually require blood smears to be taken at 52 and 104 weeks for differential cell counts, without requiring examination of other haematology parameters. The use of these slides is primarily for the detection and diagnosis of haemato-

logical neoplasia, of which the differential count is only indicative. Routine determination of differential blood counts in these slides is otherwise a questionable use of resources, although it may be useful owing to the potentially large number of samples taken if differential count changes are seen in other investigations (which will typically involve a minority percentage of the population of animals under test).

Bone Marrow Sampling

In cases where anaemia may be due to abnormalities of cell production, it is desirable to carry out examination of the bone marrow. Histopathology of bone marrow sections is not usually useful for differential counts and smears of bone marrow should be considered. This is generally done as a terminal procedure, in which case it should be carried out as soon as possible after the death of the animal. In the case of large animals, it is possible to draw a known volume of marrow into a syringe for further dilution and cell quantitation. With small laboratory animals this is more technically challenging, but it is possible to snip off the ends of long bones, such as the femur, and flush out the marrow with saline solution. Cell suspensions may subsequently be diluted to an appropriate density for differential counts. An alternative procedure is to crack the bones, take marrow on to a fine saline-moistened paintbrush and smear the cell suspension on to a slide. A long smear (e.g. several times up and down the slide) is recommended, to increase the probability of an appropriate cell density for differential counts at some area of the slide.

Tests of Clotting Function

Toxicity testing guidelines require some measure of clotting function and, although platelet counts are routinely part of a standard haematology screen, these are probably not in isolation an adequate measure. Although it logically follows that a decrease in platelet numbers may result in impairment of coagulation, it is also possible that impairment of coagulation can occur without an obvious change in platelet numbers. However, it need also be recognized that tests of clotting function require in general a larger blood sample than do the standard haematology parameters described previously. Clotting is often measured in automated equipment by the clot mechanically impairing the movement of a sensor. This may rule out the possibility of getting sufficient blood from a young rat to allow a clotting function test in addition to the standard haematology screen described above, particularly if blood samples for clinical chemistry are also required. It may not be possible to obtain sufficient sample from a mouse to allow a clotting test, even if this be the only assay required. Hence it is understandable that clotting function tests are conducted perhaps less often than regulators might wish. The analytical determination of coagulation proteins as part of a clinical chemistry screen may be an alternative. However, there should be less difficulty in obtaining sufficient blood sample for the conduct of clotting tests from larger laboratory species, or from animals at termination.

Selection of the most relevant clotting function test is a further problem. The most comprehensive would be the bleeding time, but this is technically challenging and time consuming in the animal room and is relatively seldom conducted. Preferred tests, owing to their relative simplicity, are prothrombin time (the quick, or one-stage test, a measure of the effectiveness of the extrinsic system), followed in popularity by the activated partial thromboplastin time, a measure of the effectiveness of the intrinsic system. In screening studies in dogs, it is not unusual for both of these tests to be performed.

Should abnormalities in either of these tests be detected, it may be prudent to investigate further where in the coagulation cascade the impairment has occurred. It should be noted that an additional specialized study with additional animals may be more appropriate for this investigation than to add to the burden of investigations in a standard screening study, particularly with small laboratory animals.

ABNORMALITIES IN HAEMATOLOGICAL TESTS

As has been discussed at the beginning of this chapter, xenobiotics can affect the blood in numerous different ways. Experimental animals are, of course, generally used as models for human toxicological disease, but it must be remembered that experimental animals are not perfect models. As a generalization, laboratory animals are better predictors of dose-related haematological phenomena than of idiosyncratic human responses.

In both experimental animals and humans, increases and decreases in the numbers of particular blood cell types may be observed: a decrease in the number of red cells is characteristic of anaemia, while a diminution in the number of white cells is called leucopenia. A low platelet count is called thrombocytopenia. Leucopenia can affect all white cell types, or be more specific (e.g. granulocytopenia or lymphopenia). Cytopenias can be due to decreased production of the affected cell type or to increased destruction. Increases in circulating cell types can also be seen: an increase in circulating red cells is called polycythaemia, and that of white cells, leucocytosis and platelets is called thrombocytosis. Again, specific white cell types may be affected, giving rise, for example, to lymphocytosis. An increase in circulating eosinophils is often called eosinophilia. A feature of haematotoxicity is that changes in cell types rarely occur alone. Thus aplastic anaemia brings about a reduction in all formed elements of the blood and polycythaemia rubra vera is often characterized by increased circulating granulocytes and platelets, in addition to red cells.

Anaemia

Anaemia is a decrease in the number of red cells in the circulation, in the mean corpuscular volume (MCV) or the haemoglobin content (MCH) or any combination of these three (Irons, 1991). There are a number of mechanisms whereby xenobiotics may cause anaemia **(Table 2)**. In some instances this may be a result of an interaction between an inherited predisposition: this is clearly the case in the haemolytic anaemia associated with glucose-6-phosphate dehydrogenase deficiency and certain compounds foreign to the body, where anaemia will only occur in the minority of the population carrying the enzyme deficiency. Toxic anaemias can be normocytic (e.g. aplastic anaemia), megaloblastic or microcytic (toxic microcytic anaemias are often sideroblastic).

Aplastic Anaemia

Aplastic anaemia is but one example of a group of conditions, the cytopenias, which result from bone marrow failure. Bone marrow failure may have various effects, granulocytopenia, thrombocytopenia, etc., depending on the species, individual, xenobiotic involved or precise experimental conditions. These differences may be related to factors such as the rate of production and turnover of the various cell populations; a good example is sulphur mustard, where in experimental animals studies, all types of bone marrow failure can be produced depending on the type of study and the period that has elapsed after dosing (see Chapter 98). Conditions where leukopenia or thrombocytopenia predominate are discussed below; those including anaemia are discussed in this section.

Aplastic anaemia consists of pancytopenia. A number of xenobiotics, both drugs and other chemicals, give rise to bone marrow depression and, ultimately, aplastic anaemia **(Table 2)**. There is a marked decrease in the cellularity of the bone marrow associated with a decrease in the number of circulating red cells, white cells and platelets. Immunosuppression may occur. In some cases, e.g. with cytotoxic drugs, the condition is inevitable if the dose is sufficient, and the effect is dose-related, whereas in other cases the reaction is an idiosyncratic one, and is not dose-related. A large number of drugs have been reported to give rise to idiosyncratic aplastic anaemia on occasion. There is often difficulty in demonstrating a cause and effect relationship and this has also been a difficulty with some non-drug xenobiotics, e.g. lindane (IPCS, 1991; Irons, 1992).

Table 2 Xenobiotic-induced anaemia

Type of anaemia	Mechanism	Example

Aplastic		Benzene
		Trichothecene toxins
		Drugs:
		    Chloramphenicol
		    Phenylbutazone
		    Gold salts

Megaloblastic	Interference with vitamin B_{12} absorption or action	Nitrous oxide Drugs: PAS

	Dihydrofolate reductase inhibitors	Drugs:
		    Methotrexate
		    Trimethoprim

	Interference with other aspects of folate utilization	Drugs:
		    Phenitoin
		    Primidone
		    Barbiturates

	Antimetabolites	Drugs: 6-Mercaptopurine
Microcytic, including sideroblastic		Alcohol Drugs: Isoniazid Lead

Haemolytic	Oxidant materials	Aminophenols
		Anilines
		Nitrites
		Drugs:
		    Dapsone
		    Salazopyrin
		    Phenacetin
		Pesticides
		    Propanil
		    Sodium chlorate

	Immune mechanisms	Various drugs including:
		    α-Methyldopa
		    PAS
		    Sulphonamides
		    Sulphonylureas
		    Penicillin
		    Cephalosporins

	Glucose-6-phosphate dehydrogenase deficiency Others	Various drugs and other xenobiotics Copper Arsine

Sources: Ueno (1983); Fisher (1992); Amess (1993); Hoffbrand (1996); Weatherall (1996).

In the case of benzene, excessive exposure results in pancytopenia, and in severe cases aplastic anaemia (USDHHS, 1997), while low-dose exposure may cause falls in specific cell counts (i.e. anaemia, leucopenia or thrombocytopenia may occur separately). Lymphocytopenia seems to be a particularly reliable indicator of repeated benzene exposure (Irons, 1991). In animal studies, abnormalities of cellular and humoral immunity have been noted, while benzene and its metabolites may interfere with uptake of iron into bone marrow precursors, and reactive metabolites may play a part in benzene toxicity (USDHHS, 1997). Exposure to benzene is associated with leukaemia (see below).

Chloramphenicol has been known for many years to be haematotoxic. The precise mechanism whereby the toxcity arises is still unknown but has been ascribed to single-stranded DNA breaks produced by the chloramphenicol metabolite nitrosochloramphenicol, to the production of reactive oxygen species and to actions on mitochondria (Holt *et al.*, 1993, 1997).

A number of other compounds can cause anaemia as part of pancytopenia, but the leukopenia is usually more prominent than the anaemia, for example trichothecene mycotoxins (see below).

Pure selective red cell aplasia is unusual as a toxic effect, but can occur as an immune reaction to phenytoin and 6-sulphathiazides (Krantz, 1983).

Megaloblastic Anaemia

Megaloblastic anaemia is characterized by large erythrocytes (macrocytosis), so that the haemoglobin is reduced and the MCV increased; additionally, there is anisocytosis and poikilocytosis. The morphology of red cell precursors in the bone marrow is abnormal: changes are seen in the erythroid, granulocytic and megakaryocytic precursor cells, including large nuclei and Howell–Jolly bodies. The underlying abnormality is often disturbance of DNA synthesis, most commonly in human medicine as a result of an effect on vitamin B_{12} or folate. Megaloblastic anaemia as a toxic end-point may result from interference with the absorption or metabolism of vitamin B_{12} or folate or by a direct action on DNA metabolism. In fact, interference with the absorption of vitamin B_{12} by xenobiotics rarely causes severe deficiency, although a number of substances, such as ethanol, PAS and colchicine, are known to cause malabsorption of vitamin B_{12} (Hoffbrand, 1996). A number of drugs can interfere with folate metabolism: dihydrofolate reductase inhibitors interfere with the conversion of dihydrofolates to terahydrofolates and include methotrexate and trimethoprim. Anticonvulsants such as phenytoin, primidone and barbiturates can cause a deficiency of folate, possible due to poor absorption, enzyme induction, excess utilization or a combination of these three.

Sideroblastic and Other Microcytic Anaemias

In microcytic anaemia, the haemoglobin is reduced as is the MCV. Sideroblastic anaemia is one type of microcytic anaemia, in which there is excess iron in the bone marrow. The erythroblasts in the haematopoietic organs contain granules of iron arranged in a ring around the nucleus ('ring sideroblasts'), these granules staining very easily with Prussian Blue (Weatherall, 1996). Alcohol intoxication is said to be the most common cause cause of toxic sideroblastic anaemia (Hines, 1969). Sideroblastic anaemia is characteristic of toxicants which interfere with the biosynthesis of haem and thus occurs in lead poisoning, and after exposure to antituberculous drugs and chloramphenicol. The microcytic anaemia of lead poisoning is only sometimes characterized by sideroblastic change in the bone marrow, but this anaemia is characterized in the periphery by prominant basophil stippling of the erythrocyte (Fried, 1997). Increased δ-aminolaevulinic acid appears in the urine. Lead interferes with haem biosynthesis (see below) and also increases the fragility of the erythrocyte by binding to its membrane (Irons, 1992).

Haemolytic Anaemia

Haemolytic anaemias are characterized by reduced red cell survival, often accompanied by a raised bilirubin, reticulocytosis and, if severe, the presence of nucleated red cells in the peripheral circulation. Hyperplasia of erythropoietic tissue occurs and extramedullary haematopoiesis can cause splenomegaly, which may be particularly prominent in rodents (Irons, 1991). There are two main mechanisms for xenobiotic-induced haemolytic anaemia: (1) oxidative stress and (2) immune mechanisms. A combination of inherited G6PD deficiency and certain foreign compounds can give rise to a severe type of oxidative haemolysis, sometimes accompanied by intravascular haemolysis. With some drugs, e.g. primaquine, the dose required to produce haemolysis of normal human erythrocytes is very much greater than that required in cells that are enzyme-deficient (Dern et al., 1955), but this is not the case with all drugs. At least three mechanisms have been identified for immune haemolytic anaemia. Methyldopa is associated with an autoimmune reaction, while immune complexes can be responsible for PAS-, sulphonamide- and sulphonylurea-induced haemolytic anaemia. Penicillin and cephalosporins can act as membrane-associated haptenes. The Coombs test is usually positive in drug-induced immune haemolytic anaemia (Hoffbrand and Pettit, 1984; Jacobs et al., 1990). Haemolytic anaemia due to oxidative stress may be accompanied by methaemoglobinaemia, sulphaemoglobinaemia and/or the appearance of Heinz bodies (see below). There are some compounds, which can cause haemolytic anaemia, where the cause remains unclear, e.g. copper (Fisher, 1992).

Polycythaemia

Polycythaemia is the opposite of anaemia and is characterized by an increase in the haemoglobin and red blood cell count. An apparent polycythaemia will be observed in dehydration. Polycythaemia is seen in both experimental animals and humans as a compensatory phenomenon, where potential for tissue hypoxia exists. In human populations, polycythaemia is seen in those who dwell at high altitudes and in smokers, because of their intake of carbon monoxide. Cobalt is another cause of polycythaemia, apparently due to stimulation of renal erythropoietin release (Templeton, 1992). Polycythaemia rubra vera is an uncommon myeloproliferative disease seen in humans in which the polycythaemia is often accompanied by an increase in granulocytes and/or platelets. In most cases the aetiology is not known, but cases have been described in personnel who took part in a test of nuclear weapons (Caldwell *et al.*, 1984).

Toxicants Affecting Haemoglobin

The physiology of haemoglobin is considered at the beginning of this chapter. Toxicants can affect haemoglobin by (1) influencing the synthetic pathway for haem (e.g. lead), (2) altering the final haemoglobin (e.g. various oxidant materials to produce methaemoglobin) or (3) reacting with haemoglobin (e.g. carbon monoxide). The first process may cause anaemia, whereas methaemoglobinaemia and carbon monoxide poisoning both effectively decrease the oxygen-carrying power of the blood, without causing anaemia.

Porphyria

The synthesis of haem involves the synthesis of porphyrins. This process involves the condensation of glycine and succinyl-coenzyme A to form δ-aminolaevulinic acid (ALA), and this is followed by a number of steps to protoporphyrin into which iron is inserted to form haem. Porphyrias are mostly hereditary diseases, but their importance to the toxicologist is twofold: (1) certain toxicants, e.g. lead, can cause acquired porphyria in normal human subjects and in experimental animals and (2) the acute porphyrias are often precipitated by various drugs in those predisposed to these diseases. These diseases are characterized by increased excretion of porphyrin precursors. Acute intermittent porphyria is the most severe and most common of these conditions and it is characterized by gastro-intestinal, neurological and psychiatric abnormalities. In variegate porphyria there is notable photosensitivity (McColl *et al.*, 1996). Lead acts by inhibiting the haem biosynthetic enzyme ALA dehydratase, while the activity of ferrochelatase is also reduced. By contrast, the activity of ALA synthetase is increased. As a result, levels of ALA in the blood and urine are increased, as are coproporphyrin III and zinc protoporphyrin (Feldman, 1999). A number of other chemicals are porphyrogenic, e.g. the organochlorine pesticides lindane and heptachlor (Simon and Siklósi, 1974; Mylchreest and Charbonneau, 1997; Taira and San Martin de Viale, 1998) and certain herbicides (Jinno *et al.*, 1999).

Oxidant and Other Changes in Haemoglobin

Methaemoglobinaemia and carboxyhaemoglobinaemia, the latter resulting from the binding of carbon dioxide to haemoglobin, cause changes in the colour of the blood; carboxyhaemoglobin is cherry red and methaemoglobin is brown. In addition, a number of other derivatives of haemoglobin have been described **(Table 3)**.

Methaemoglobin

Methaemoglobin is the pigment that results when the iron of haemoglobin, normally in the ferrous (Fe^{2+}) state, is oxidized to the ferric (Fe^{3+}) state. The toxicological importance of methaemoglobin is twofold:

(1) Methaemoglobin is incapable of carrying oxygen reversibly in the way that haemoglobin does, with the result that methaemoglobinaemia represents a loss of oxygen-carrying power of the blood and very high levels of methaemoglobin ($> 50\%$) are thus potentially lethal.
(2) Methaemoglobin can combine with cyanide, sulphide and azides and thereby ameliorate their toxic effects (see Chapter 20).

A large number of compounds that produce other oxidant changes in the erythrocytes **(Table 3)** can also produce methaemoglobinaemia. However, there are also other causes of methaemoglobinaemia, some of which are non-toxicological. Two methaemoglobin reductase enzymes serve to keep methaemoglobin levels in the red cells low; deficiency, which may be inherited, causes raised level of methaemoglobin. In human populations, certain unusual haemoglobins are more susceptible than normal haemoglobin to oxidation. This can result in high levels of methaemoglobin. Methaemoglobin levels after exposure to methaemoglobin-generating xenobiotics are determined by levels of the xenobiotic or its active metabolite, the intrinsic sensitivity of the haemoglobin to oxidation and the activity of methaemoglobin reductase (Bright and Marrs, 1986; Marrs and Bright, 1986; Marino *et al.*, 1997), but the marked interspecies differences that have been observed appear mainly to result from differences in the ability of the erythrocyte to reduce red cell methaemoglobin levels, laboratory rodents having a high capacity and dogs, cats and

Table 3 Oxidant and other derivatives of haemoglobin

Pigment	How formed
Methaemogobin	Oxidation of Fe^{2+} to Fe^{3+} in haemoglobin
Sulphaemoglobin	Ill-characterized pigment associated with oxidant changes in the erythrocyte
Cyanmethaemoglobin	Reaction of cyanide with methaemoglobin
Sulphmethaemoglobin	Reaction of sulphide with methaemoglobin
Carboxyhaemoglobin	Reaction of carbon monoxide with haemoglobin

humans and (probably) non-human primates having a much lower capacity (Kiese and Weis, 1943; Malz, 1962; Robin and Harley, 1966; Smith and Beutler, 1966; Stolk and Smith, 1966; Smith *et al.*, 1967; Agar and Harley, 1972; Bolyai *et al.*, 1972; Hawkins *et al.*, 1981; Marrs *et al.*, 1987). In toxicological studies, where only rodents are used, the low propensity of rodents for demonstrating methaemoglobinaemia may cause the potential of a xenobiotic to cause toxic methaemoglobinaemia to be missed. In practice, dogs are probably the best models for humans.

Chemically induced methaemoglobinaemia can result from exposure to a very large number of toxicants, many of which are aniline derivatives, aminophenols or nitrites **(Table 4)**.

Aminophenols and their derivatives, including 4-dimethylaminophenol, appear to form methaemoglobin by establishing an intraerythrocytic cycle in which a quinoneimine is formed by oxidation of the aminophenol by the oxygen from oxyhaemoglobin. On the reduction of the quinoneimine to the aminophenol, the Fe^{2+} iron of haemoglobin is oxidized to its trivalent state. With the aniline derivatives, including 4-aminopropiophenone (*p*-hydroxypropiophenone, PAPP), a nitroso intermediate is involved in the formation of methaemoglobin. The methaemoblobin formation observed with the antileptic drug dapsone appears to be mediated by hydroxylamine metabolites (Vage *et al.*, 1994). Methaemoglobin formation is strongly influenced by PO_2 (Kiese, 1974; Mansouri, 1985; Marrs *et al.*, 1987).

Methaemoglobin levels may be measured by spectrophotometric means either directly or before and after the addition of cyanide (the latter is the principle of the method of Evelyn and Malloy, 1938).

Table 4 Some compounds producing methaemoglobinaemia

Chemical or drug group	Examples
Aminophenols and derivatives	2-Aminophenol 4-Aminophenol 4-Dimethylaminophenol Propanil
Anilines	Aniline 4-Aminopropiophenone
Antimalarials	Chloroquine Primaquine
Antileprotics	Dapsone
Chlorates	Sodium chlorate
Nitrites	Amyl nitrite Sodium nitrite
Hydroxylamines	Hydroxylamine Phenylhydroxylamine
Sulphonamides	Sulphamethoxazole

Sources: Kiese *et al.* (1950); Beutler (1985); Hall *et al.* (1986).

Methaemoglobinaemia may be treated with methylene blue or toluidine blue (Kiese *et al.*, 1972; IPCS/CEC, 1993).

Heinz Bodies

Heinz bodies are inclusions in red blood cells that consist of denatured globin (White *et al.*, 1951). Heinz bodies can be seen in wet preparations of blood, using phase contrast microscopy, and they can also be stained with methyl violet (Bushby, 1970). Their appearance may be an accompaniment to haemolytic anaemia, produced by oxidant xenobiotics ('Heinz body anaemia'), including those substances that produce methaemoglobin. However, there does not appear to be a close correlation between ability to produce methaemoglobin and Heinz bodies or of the latter with erythrocytic depletion of reduced glutathione (Miller and Smith, 1970). Moreover, in toxicological studies, there can be marked species differences in the production of Heinz bodies with the same substance (Marrs *et al.*, 1984).

Sulphaemoglobin

Sulphaemoglobin is an ill-characterized pigment that differs from methaemoglobin by resistance to reducing agents. It should be distinguished from sulphmethaemoglobin **(Table 3)**.

Carboxyhaemoglobin

Carbon monoxide binds to haemoglobin in precisely the same way as does oxygen, although the affinity of carbon monoxide for haemoglobin is about 245 times that of oxygen. This means that if the carbon monoxide saturation of haemoglobin is plotted against the partial pressure of carbon monoxide, a curve of precisely the same shape as the standard oxyhaemoglobin dissociation curve would be obtained. Indeed, if one adjusted the scales on the partial pressure axes, the curves could be superimposed. It is also worth recalling that, at saturation, 1.34 ml of either oxygen or carbon monoxide is carried per gram of haemoglobin. If haemoglobin is exposed to a mixture of oxygen and carbon monoxide, the gases will compete for the binding sites. At equilibrium the relative concentrations of oxyhaemoglobin and carboxyhaemoglobin are given by the Haldane equation:

$$[COHb]/[O_2Hb] = M PCO/PO_2$$

where M is referred to as the Haldane coefficient.

The effect of the great affinity of carbon monoxide on the uptake of the gas relative to that of oxygen is discussed in Chapter 57.

In addition to reducing the capacity of haemoglobin to carry oxygen, carbon monoxide inhibits the release of oxygen by haemoglobin. Under normal circumstances, as oxygen atoms dissociate from haemoglobin the affinity of the molecule for oxygen drops rapidly. This produces the sudden change in gradient at the shoulder of the oxyhaemoglobin dissociation curve. To move from the relaxed, high oxygen affinity state to the tense, low affinity state, oxyhaemoglobin must lose oxygen atoms. In carbon monoxide poisoning haemoglobin molecules do not carry either oxygen alone or carbon monoxide alone; on the contrary, haemoglobin molecules will probably carry a mixture of oxygen and carbon monoxide molecules. As the partial pressure of oxygen falls, at the tissues, for example, oxygen molecules would normally be released and haemoglobin would move from the relaxed to the tense state. However, if the haemoglobin molecule is carrying carbon monoxide molecules in addition to oxygen, the carbon monoxide molecules will not be released and the relaxed, high oxygen affinity state will be maintained. This effect can be summed up as follows: the binding of carbon monoxide molecules to haemoglobin inhibits the release of oxygen, which is seen in carbon monoxide poisoning as a shift of the oxyhaemoglobin dissociation curve to the left. This shift is sometimes referred to as the Haldane shift, although the term is confusing as it is also used to describe the shift in affinity of haemoglobin for carbon dioxide that occurs when haemoglobin loses oxygen molecules. The above details were worked out by J. S. Haldane and his son J. B. S. Haldane in the early years of the century (Douglas et al., 1912; Haldane, 1912).

The shift in the dissociation curve causes a major problem for the release of oxygen at the tissues. An often quoted example is the difference between the effects of anaemia, with the haemoglobin concentration reduced to 50% of normal, and carbon monoxide poisoning, with a carboxyhaemoglobin concentration of 50%. In the case of the anaemia the venous PO_2 would be about 3.6 kPa (27 mmHg); in the case of carbon monoxide poisoning the venous PO_2 would be about 1.9 kPa (14 mmHg), very significantly lower (Nunn 1993).

Exposure to carbon monoxide results in equilibration of the gas across the alveolar/capillary barrier. As has been already stated, the equilibrium conditions are given by the Haldane equation. The rate of increase of carboxyhaemoglobin conforms to a 'wash in' exponential function. More detailed modelling of the kinetics of carbon monoxide uptake has been undertaken (Coburn et al., 1965; Coburn, 1979) and complex equations have been produced.

Carbon monoxide poisoning is relatively common because the gas, which is odourless, can be formed by partial combustion of natural gas, a fuel commonly used for heating in many countries. At high concentrations (> 50%), carbon monoxide causes death, while concentrations as low as 3–4% may cause angina, presumably through impaired oxygen transport (DOE, 1994). Additionally, delayed effects can occur in the central nervous system after apparent recovery.

The affinity of foetal haemoglobin for oxygen is greater than that of adult haemoglobin (Power and Longo, 1975; Longo, 1976; Garvey and Longo, 1978). In addition, the foetal oxyhaemoglobin dissociation curve is displaced to the left of the equivalent adult curve. Foetal haemoglobin also has a greater affinity for carbon monoxide than adult haemoglobin, although the foetal/adult difference in affinity is not as great as that for oxygen. Engel et al., 1969 gave the CO/O_2 affinity ratio as 175 for foetal haemoglobin compared with 245 for adult haemoglobin.

As in the adult, carbon monoxide shifts the foetal oxyhaemoglobin dissociation curve to the left. This is particularly dangerous as the foetus is always at a significantly lower partial pressure of oxygen than the adult. A 10% level of carboxyhaemoglobin will move the maternal venous PO_2 to 26 mmHg but the foetal venous PO_2 to 11 mmHg. Uptake into, and release of, carbon monoxide from the foetus are delayed compared with the mother. This is a reason for considering treatment with hyperbaric oxygen whenever carbon monoxide poisoning occurs during pregnancy.

It should be noted that carboxyhaemoglobinaemia can occur due to metabolism of methylene chloride, commonly used as a paint remover (Hughes and Tracy, 1993).

Changes in White Cells

Reductions in the number of white cells (neutropenia) may affect all, a few or just one type of white cell. It may be part of a pancytopenia or, even if all blood cell types are affected, the leucopenia may predominate; this is common with T-2 mycotoxin, poisoning with which is often characterized by some degree of anaemia, but a marked leukopenia and thrombocytopenia are usually the most prominant feature (Smalley, 1973; Hayes et al., 1980; Ueno, 1984). Tricothecene toxins produced by fungal species such as *Fusarium* are responsible for a number of syndromes, including alimentary toxic aleukia (ATA) in Russia and red mould disease in Japan. ATA occurs after the consumption of overwintered mouldy grain and includes leucopenia, haemorrhages, sepsis and bone marrow failure (Lutsky, 1981; Ueno, 1983, 1984; Lautraite et al., 1995; Wang et al., 1998).

Neutropenia/granulocytopenia/ agranulocytosis

Severe neutropenia or granulocytopenia is often called agranulocytosis. Neutropenia may result from inadequate production or increased destruction, while an apparent neutropenia can result from a shift into the blood marginal pool (Marsh, 1985). The former may occur as part of aplastic anaemia, but many compounds capable of producing aplastic anaemia sometimes affect granulocytes and their precursors more severely than cells of the erythrocyte series, perhaps because of the erythrocyte's longer life span.

Granulocytopenia can be a dose-related predictable effect as with radiation (Cronkite, 1949), various anticancer drugs, chloramphenicol and the mustards [including the chemical warfare agent sulphur mustard (Marrs et al., 1996; see also Chapter 98)] or an idiosyncratic response. Idiosyncratic neutropenias fall into two groups. The slowly developing dose-dependent type has been reported with chloramphenicol, phenothiazines, sulphonamides and numerous other substances. The rapidly developing type of idiosyncratic neutropenia is rare, often accompanied by eosinophilia and sometimes catastrophic. There is often a history of prior exposure (Marsh, 1985) and the effect is notoriously difficult to predict from animal studies. Amongst compounds producing this effect are chloramphenicol, gold salts and non-steroidal anti-inflammatory drugs. It will have been noted that chloramphenicol can produce several types of neutropenia.

Neutropenia, analogous to haemolytic anaemia, can occur because of increased cell destruction which may result from immunological mechanisms, e.g. with antipyrine.

Increases in the polymorph count are found in acute infections, in leukaemias of the myeloid series and also with lithium carbonate. A notable toxicological cause of eosinophilia was the eosinophilia–myalgia syndrome seen in the early 1990s, after contamination of certain preparations of the food supplement and essential amino acid L-tryptophan with a contaminant (Harati, 1994).

Leukaemias

Leukaemias are a heterogeneous group of malignant diseases involving the precursors of peripheral blood cells. Most arise in the bone marrow and exhibit high levels of circulating white cells. They are classified by the cell type involved and also into acute and chronic (Tsongas, 1985). Leukaemias are seen in many species, including man and experimental animals such as mice and rats (for a review of appearances and diagnostic criteria in experimental animals, see Della Porta et al., 1979 and Ward et al., 1990). There are notable strain differences in the susceptibility of mice to leukaemia.

Exposure to a number of drugs and other chemicals can be associated with leukemias, as can radiation. A notable example is benzene (see also above), where exposure of human populations seems causally related to acute non-lymphocytic leukaemia (Paxton et al., 1994; Jex and Wyman, 1996). Benzene causes chromosomal abnormalities in a number of cell types, including blood. The precise mechanisms of benzene leukaemogenesis have not been elucidated: benzene is metabolized to benzene oxide and thence to phenol in the liver (Tunek et al., 1978;

Sawahata et al., 1985) and chronic exposure to benzene results in the presence of metabolites in the bone marrow, including hydroquinone and, additionally, benzene itself. These compounds produce a reduction in circulating lymphocytes and are immunotoxic (Pyatt et al., 1998) and they also bring about an increase in cells of the granulocyte series. Further, benzene and its metabolities have been shown to induce DNA damage, which may contribute to leukaemogenesis, plausibly perhaps in combination with the increased replication of primitive progenitor cells, as has been observed in laboratory animals (Farris et al., 1997). Another possibility is that activation of protein kinase C may alter the activation and expression of cellular protooncogenes (see review by Snyder and Kalb, 1994). There is some evidence that benzene may be associated with other malignant conditions, including Hodgkin's disease (Jex and Wyman, 1996).

Drugs where there is an association with leukaemias in laboratory rodents include anticancer drugs (Schmahl and Habs, 1978). Hydrocarbons such as methylcholanthrene, benzopyrene and dimethylbenzanthracene can also produce leukaemias in rodents (Rappaport and Baroni, 1962). Exposure to a number of chemicals in humans is associated with an increased prevalence of leukaemia; furthermore, there is an association of increased risk of leukaemia and certain occupations where, however, the precise causative agent is not known (Irons, 1992).

Thrombocytopenia

Thrombocytopenia is amongst the commonest blood dyscrasias reported as due to xenobiotics, especially drugs (Irons, 1991). The results are purpura and spontaneous haemorrhage or bleeding in response to minor trauma. As with red cells and granulocytes, a reduction in circulating platelets can result from decreased production or increased destruction. Decreased production of platelets may be seen with thiazide diuretics, which are toxic to megakaryocyte precursors (Levin, 1974). Other drugs which may cause thrombocytopenia by toxicity to the bone marrow include chloramphenicol (Yunis, 1973), sulphonamides (Pena et al., 1985) and phenytoin (Brown and Chun, 1986); however, many drugs that cause thrombocytopenia by an effect on the bone marrow can also produce other signs of bone marrow failure depending on the circumstances and isolated thrombocytopenia with some drugs, e.g. chloramphenicol, may proceed to aplastic anaemia. Increased destruction of platelets is generally of immunological origin, although not in the case of ristocetin, an antibiotic which has a dose-related effect on platelets, by a non-immunological mechanism. Drugs that produce thombocytopenia by immune mechanisms include quinine and quinidine (Christie et al., 1985) and gold salts (Stavem et al., 1988).

Drugs Affecting the Coagulation System

Anticoagulants of the coumarin group, some of which are used as rodenticides, interfere with vitamin K-dependent blood-clotting factors (Proudfoot, 1996; see also Chapter 97). Coumarol, in mouldy sweet clover, is an important cause of haemorrhagic disease in cattle (Blood *et al.*, 1983).

CONCLUSIONS

The components of the blood can be affected by many xenobiotics, most particularly therapeutic drugs. Many of the techniques used in human and veterinary medicine have not been widely applied to laboratory animal toxicology studies. This limits the use to which information from routine laboratory animal toxicology studies may be put. Part of the reason for this is that haematology is often the Cinderella of disciplines in the toxicology laboratory in comparison with clinical chemistry and particularly histopathology; there is also the tendency for guidelines rapidly to become a recipe, which has to be followed but whose scope should not be exceeded unless specifically required by regulators. This is a great pity, because the haematological data in toxicology studies represent a great deal of effort and investment and, in so far as satellite groups of animals are employed, a cause of usage of additional experimental animals. It is therefore only right that such data should be exploited to the hilt and used to their best possible advantage.

REFERENCES

Agar, N. S. and Harley, J. D. (1972). Erythrocytic methaemoglobin reductases of various mammalian species. *Experientia*, **28**, 1248–1249.

Amess, J. (1993). Haematotoxicology. In Ballantyne, B., Marrs, T.C. and Turner, P. (Eds), *General and Applied Toxicology*, 1st edn. Macmillan, Basingstoke, and Stockton Press, New York, pp. 839–867.

Ashby, M. (1919). Determination of length of life of transfused blood corpuscles in man. *J. Exp. Med.*, **29**, 267–271.

Barton, J. C., Conrad, M. E. and Parmley, R. T. (1980). Acute lymphoblastic leukemia in idiopathic sideroblastic anemia: evidence for a common lymphoid and myeloid progenitor cell. *Am. J. Hematol.*, **9**, 109–115.

Beutler, E. (1985). Chemical toxicity of the erythrocyte. In Irons, R. D. (Ed.), *Toxicology of the Blood and Bone Marrow*. Raven Press, New York, pp. 39–49.

Blood, D. C., Rastotits, O. M. and Henderson, J. A. (1983). *Veterinary Medicine*. Ballière-Tindall, London, p. 306.

Bolyai, J. Z., Smith, R. P. and Gray, C. T. (1972). Ascorbic acid and chemically-induced methemoglobinemias. *Toxicol. Appl. Pharmacol.*, **21**, 176–185.

Bright, J. E. and Marrs, T. C. (1986). Kinetics of methaemoglobin production (2). Kinetics of the cyanide antidote p-aminopropiophenone during oral administration. *Hum. Toxicol.*, **5**, 303–307.

Brown, J. J. and Chun, R. W. (1986). Phenytoin-induced thrombocytopenia. *Pediatr. Neurol.*, **2**, 99–101.

Bushby, S. R. M. (1970). Haematological studies during toxicity tests. In Paget, G. E. (Ed.), *Methods in Toxicology*. Blackwell, Oxford, pp. 238–371.

Caldwell, G. G., Kelley, D. B., Heath, C. W. and Zack, M. (1984). Polycythemia vera among participants of a nuclear weapons test. *J. Am. Med. Assoc.*, **252**, 662–664.

Chanarin, I. (1985). Function of the bone marrow. In Irons, R. D. (Ed.), *Toxicology of the Blood and Bone Marrow*. Raven Press, New York, pp. 1–16.

Christie, D. J., Mullen, P. C. and Aster, R. H. (1985). Fab-mediated binding of drug-dependent antibodies to platelets in quinidine-and quinine-induced thrombocytopenia. *J. Clin. Invest.*, **75**, 310–314.

Coburn, R. F. (1979). Mechanisms of carbon monoxide toxicity. *Prev. Med.*, **8**, 310–322.

Coburn, R. F., Forster, R. E. and Kane, P. B. (1965). Considerations of the physiological variables that determine the blood carboxyhemoglobin concentration in man. *J. Clin. Invest.*, **44**, 1899–1910.

Cronkite, E. P. (1949). Ionizing radiation injury: its diagnosis by physical examination and clinical laboratory procedures. *J. Am. Med. Assoc*, **139**, 366–369.

Della Porta, G., Chieco-Bianchi, L. and Pennelli, N. (1979). Tumours of the haematopoietic system. In Turosev, V. S. (Ed.), *Pathology of Tumours in Laboratory Animals. Vol. 2, The Mouse* International Agency for Research on Cancer, Lyon, pp. 527–576.

Dern, R. J., Beutler, E. and Alving, A. S. (1955). The hemolytic effect of primaquine. V. Primaquine sensitivity as a manifestation of a multiple drug sensitivity. *J. Lab. Clin. Med.*, **45**, 40–50.

DOE (1994). Department of the Environment, Expert Panel on Air Quality Standards. *Carbon Monoxide*. HMSO, London.

Douglas, C. G., Haldane, J. S. and Haldane, J. B. S. (1912). The laws of combination of haemoglobin with carbon monoxide and oxygen. *J. Physiol.*, **44**, 275–304.

Engel, R. F., Rodkey, F. L., O'Neal, J. D. and Collison, H. A. (1969). Relative affinity of human foetal haemoglobin for carbon monoxide and oxygen. *Blood*, **33**, 37–45.

Evans, G. O. (1994). Letter to the Editor. Removal of blood from laboratory mammals and birds. *Lab. Anim.*, **28**, 178–179.

Evelyn, K. A. and Malloy, H. T. (1938). Microdetermination of oxyhemoglobin, methemoglobin, and sulfhemoglobin in a single sample of blood. *J. Biol. Chem.*, **126**, 655–660.

Farris, G. M., Robinson, S. N., Gaido, K. W., Wong, B. A., Wong, V. A., Hahn, W. P. and Shah, R. S. (1997). Benzene-induced hematotoxicity and bone marrow compensation in B6C3F1 mice. *Fundam. Appl. Toxicol.*, **36**, 119–129.

Feldman, R. G. (1999). *Occupational and Environmental Neurotoxicology*. Lippincott-Raven, Philadelphia.

Fisher, D. (1992). Copper. In Sullivan, J. B. and Krieger, G. R. (Eds), *Hazardous Materials Toxicology*. Williams and Wilkins, Baltimore, pp. 860–864.

Fried, W. (1997). Evaluation of red cells and erythropoiesis. In Bloom, J. C., Sipes, I. G., McQueen, C. A. and Gandolfi, A.

J. (Eds), *Comprehensive Toxicology*, Vol. 4. Pergamon Press, Oxford, pp. 35–54.

Garvey, D. J. and Longo, L. D. (1978). Chronic low level maternal carbon monoxide exposure and fetal growth and development. *Biol. Reprod.*, **19**, 8–14.

Haldane, J. B. S. (1912). The dissociation of oxyhemoglobin in humans during partial CO poisoning. *J. Physiol.*, **45**, pp. B434–B436.

Hall, A. H., Kulig, K. W. and Rumack, B. H. (1986). Drug- and chemical-induced methaemoglobinaemia clinical features and management. *Med. Toxicol.*, **1**, 253–260.

Harati, Y. (1994). Eosinophilia–myalgia syndrome and its relation to toxic oil syndrome. In de Wolff, F. A. (Ed.), *Handbook of Clinical Neurology, Vol. 20, Intoxications of the Nervous System, Part 1*. Elsevier, Amsterdam, pp. 249–271.

Hawkins, S. F., Groff, W. A., Johnson, R. P., Froehlich, H. L., Kaminskis, A. and Stemler, P. M. (1981). Comparison of the *in vivo* formation of methemoglobin by 4-dimethylaminophenol and sodium nitrite by the cynomolgus monkey. *Fed. Am. Soc. Exp. Biol. Proc.*, **40**, 718.

Hayes, M. A., Bellamy, J. E. C. and Schiefer, H. B. (1980). Subacute toxicity of dietary T-2 toxin in mice: morphological and hematological effects. *Can. J. Comp. Med.*, **44**, 203–218.

Hines, J. D. (1969). Reversible megaloblastic and sideroblastic marrow abnormalities in alcoholic patients. *Br. J. Haematol.*, **16**, 87–101.

Hoffbrand, A. V. (1996). Megaloblastic anaemia and miscellaneous deficiency anaemias. In Weatherall, D. J., Ledingham, J. G. G. and Warrell, D. A. (Eds), *Oxford Textbook of Medicine*. Oxford University Press, Oxford, pp. 3484–3500.

Hoffbrand, A. V. and Pettit, J. E. (1984). *Essential Haematology*. Blackwell, Oxford, pp. 243–244.

Holt, D. E., Hurley, R. and Harvey, D. (1993). Chloramphenicol toxicity. *Adv. Drug. React. Acute Pois. Rev.*, **12**, 83–95.

Holt, D. E., Ryder, T. A., Fairbairn, A., Hurley, R. and Harvey, D. (1997). The myelotoxicity of chloramphenicol: *in vitro* and *in vivo* studies: *in vitro* effects on cells in culture. *Hum. Exp. Toxicol.*, **16**, 570–576.

Hughes, N. J. and Tracy, J. A. (1993). A case of methylene chloride (Nitromors) poisoning, effects on carboxyhaemoglobin levels. *Hum. Exp. Toxicol.*, **12**, 159–160.

IPCS (1991). International Program on Chemical Safety. *Environmental Health Criteria 124, Lindane*. Geneva, World Health Organization p. 125.

IPCS/CEC (1993). International Program on Chemical Safety/ Commission of the European Communities. *Evaluation of Antidotes Series, Vol. 2. Antidotes for Cyanide Poisoning*. Cambridge University Press, Cambridge, pp. 145–158.

Irons, R. D. (1991). Blood and bone marrow. In Haschek, W. M. and Rousseaux, C. G. (Eds), *Handbook of Toxicologic Pathology*. Academic Press, San Diego, pp. 389–419.

Irons, R. D. (1992). Benzene and other hemotoxins. In Sullivan, J. B. and Krieger, G. R. (Eds), *Hazardous Materials Toxicology*. Williams and Wilkins, Baltimore, pp. 718–731.

Jacobs, D. S., Kasten, B. L., Demott, W. R. and Wolfson, W. L. (1990). *Laboratory Test Handbook*. Williams and Wilkins, Baltimore, pp. 847–851.

Jex, T. T. and Wyman, D. O. (1996). A minireview of benzene. *Toxic Subst. Mech.*, **15**, 135–p144.

Jinno, H., Hatakayema, N., Hanioka, N., Yoda, R., Nishimura, T. and Ando, M. (1999). Cytotoxic and porphyrino-

genic effects of diphenyl ethers in cultured rat hepatocytes: chlornitrofen (CNP), CNP-amino, chlormethoxyfen and bifenox. *Food Chem. Toxicol.*, **37**, 69–74.

Kiese, M. (1974). *Methemoglobinemia: a Comprehensive Treatise*. CRC Press, Cleveland, OH.

Kiese, M. and Weis, B. (1943). Die Reduktion des Hämiglobins in den Erythrozyten verschiedener Tiere. *Naunyn-Schmiedebergs Arch. Exp. Pathol. Pharmakol.*, **202**, 493–501.

Kiese, M., Reinwein, D. and Waller, H. D. (1950). Kinetik der Hämiglobinbildung. IV Mitteilung. Die Hämiglobinbildung durch Phenylhydroxylamin und Nitrosobenzol in roten Zellen *in Vitro*. *Naunyn-Schmiedebergs Arch. Exp. Pathol. Pharmakol.*, **210**, 393–398.

Kiese, M., Lörcher, W., Weger, N. and Zierer, A. (1972). Comparative studies on the effects of toluidine blue and methylene blue on the reduction of ferrihaemoglobin in man and dog. *Eur. J. Clin. Pharmacol.*, **4**, 115–118.

Koury, S. T., Bondurant, M. L. and Koury, M. J. (1988). Localization of erythropoietin synthesizing cells in murine kidneys by *in situ* hybridization. *Blood*, **71**, 524–527.

Krantz, S. B. (1983). In Aram, M. C. and McCulloch, P. B. (Eds), *Current Therapy in Hematology–Oncology 1983–1984*. Mosby, St Louis.

Lautraite, S., Parent-Massin, D., Rio, B. and Hoellinger, H. (1995). Comparison of toxicity induced by T-2 toxin on human and rat granulo-monocytic progenitors with an *in vitro* model. *Hum. Exp. Toxicol.*, **14**, 672–678.

Levin, J. (1974). Effects of oral antidiabetic and diuretic agents on platelets. In Dimitrov, N. V. and Nodine, J. H. (Eds), *Drugs and Hematological Reactions*. Grune and Stratton, New York, pp. 263–270.

Liesveld, J. L. and Lichtman, M. L. (1997). Evaluation of granulocytes and mononuclear phagocytes. In Bloom, J. C., Sipes, G., McQueen, C. A. and Gandolfi, A. J. (Eds.) *Comprehensive Toxicology*, 4, pp. 123–144. Pergamon, Oxford.

Loeb, W. F., Bannerman, R. M., Rininger, B. F. and Johnson, A. J. (1978). Hematological disorders. In Bernischke, K., Garner, F. M. and Jones, T. C. (Eds), *Pathology of Laboratory Animals*. pp. 331–336. Springer, New York.

Longo, L. D. (1970). Carbon monoxide in the pregnant mother and fetus and its exchange across the placenta. *Ann. N. Y. Acad. Sci.*, **174**, 313–341.

Longo, L. D. (1976). Carbon monoxide: effects on oxygenation of the fetus *in utero*. *Science*, **194**, 523–525.

Lutsky, I. I. (1981). Alimentary toxic aleukia (septic angina, endemic panmyelotoxicosis, alimentary hemorrhagic aleukia). T-2 toxin-induced intoxication of cats. *Am. J. Pathol.*, **104**, 189–191.

Malz, E. (1962). Vergleichende Untersuchungen über die Methämoglobinreduktion in kernhaltigen und kernlosen Erythrozyten. *Folia Haematol. (Leipzig)*, **78**, 510–515.

Mansouri, A. (1985). Review: methemoglobinemia. *Am. J. Med. Sci.*, **289**, 200–209.

Marino, M. T., Urquhart, M. R., Sperry, M. L., Bredow, J. V., Brown, L. D., Lin, E. and Brewer, T. G. (1997). Pharmacokinetics and kinetic dynamic modelling of aminophenones as methaemoglobin formers. *J. Pharm. Pharmacol.*, **49**, 282–287.

Marrs, T. C. and Bright, J. E. (1986). Kinetics of methaemoglobin production (1). Kinetics of methaemoglobinaemia induced by the cyanide antidotes, *p*-aminopropiophenone, *p*-hydroxyaminopropiophenone or *p*-dimethylaminophenol after intravenous administration. *Hum. Toxicol.*, **5**, 295–301.

Marrs, T. C., Scawin, J. and Swanston, D. W. (1984). The acute intravenous and oral toxicity in mice, rats and guinea-pigs of 4-dimethylaminophenol (DMAP) and its effects on haematological variables. *Toxicology*, **31**, 165–173.

Marrs, T. C., Bright, J. E. and Woodman, A. C. (1987). Species differences in methaemoglobin production after addition of 4-dimethylaminophenol, a cyanide antidote, to blood *in vitro*: a comparative study. *Comp. Biochem. Physiol. B*, **86**, 141–148.

Marrs, T. C., Maynard, R. L. and Sidell, F. (1996). *Chemical Warfare Agents, Toxicology and Treatment*. Wiley, Chichester.

Marsh, J. C. (1985). Chemical toxicity of the granulocyte. In Irons, R. D. (Ed.), *Toxicology of the Blood and Bone Marrow*. Raven Press, New York, pp. 51–63.

McColl, K. E. L., Dover, S., Fitzsimons, E. and Moore, M. R. (1996). Porphyrin metabolism and the porphyrias. In Weatherall, D. J., Ledingham, J. G. G. and Warrell, D. A. (Eds.), *Oxford Textbook of Medicine*. Oxford University Press, Oxford, pp. 1388–1399.

Means, R. T. (1997). Toxic effects on erythrogenesis. In Bloom, J. C., Sipes, I. G., McQueen, C. A. and Gandolfi, A. J. (Eds), *Comprehensive Toxicology, Vol 4*. Pergamon Press, Oxford, pp. 87–106.

Miller, A. and Smith, H. C. (1970). The intracellular and membrane effects of oxidant agents on normal red cells. *Br. J. Haematol.*, **19**, 417–419.

Morton, D. B. and Abbot, D. (1993). Removal of blood from laboratory mammals and birds. First report of the BVA/FRAME/RSPCA/UFAW Working Group on Refinement. *Lab. Anim.*, **27**, 1–22.

Morton, D. B. and Jennings, M. (1994). Letter to the Editor. Removal of blood from laboratory mammals and birds: reply. Lab. Anim., **28**, 179.

Mylchreest, E. and Charbonneau, M. (1997). Studies on the mechanism of uroporphyrinogen decarboxylase inhibition in hexachlorobenzene-induced porphyria in the female rat. *Toxicol. Appl. Pharmacol.*, **145**, 23–33.

Nunn, J. F. (1993). *Nunn's Applied Respiratory Physiology*, 4th edn. Butterworth-Heinemann, London.

OECD (1997). *OECD Guidelines for the Testing of Chemicals. Section 4—Health Effects*. Organization for Economic Cooperation and Development, Paris.

Paxton, M. B., Chinchilli, V. M., Brett, S. M. and Rodricks, J. V. (1994). Leukemia risk associated with benzene exposure in the plioform cohort II. Risk estimates. *Risk Anal.*, **14**, 155–157.

Pena, J. M., Gonzalez-Garcia, J. J., Garcia-Alegria, J., Barbado, F. J. and Vazquez, J. J. (1985). Thrombocytopenia and sulfasalazine. *Ann. Int. Med.*, **102**, 277–278.

Perutz, M. F. (1967–68). The structure and function of haemoglobin. *Harvey Lectures, Series 63*. pp. 213–261.

Power, G. G. and Longo, L. D. (1975). Fetal circulation times and their implications for tissue oxygenation. *Gynecol. Invest.*, **6**, 342–355.

Proudfoot, A. (1996). *Pesticide Poisoning Notes for the Guidance of Medical Practitioners*. HMSO, London.

Pyatt, D. W., Stillman, W. S. and Irons, R. D. (1998). Hydroquinone, a reactive metabolite of benzene, inhibits NF-κB in primary human CD4$^+$ T lymphocytes. *Toxicol. Appl. Pharmacol.*, **149**, 178–184.

Rappaport, H. and Baroni, C. (1962). A study of the pathogenesis of malignant lymphoma induced in the Swiss mouse by 7, 12-dibenz[*a*]anthracene injected at birth. *Cancer Res.*, **22**, 1067–1074.

Robin, H. and Harley, J. D. (1966). Factors influencing response of mammalian cells to the methaemoblobin reduction test. *Aust. J. Exp. Biol. Med. Sci.*, **44**, 519–526.

Sawahata, T., Rickert, D. E. and Greenlee, W. F. (1985). Metabolism of benzene and its metabolites in bone marrow. In Irons, R. D. (Ed.), *Toxicology of the Blood and Bone Marrow*. Raven Press, New York, pp. 141–148.

Schmahl, D. and Habs, M. (1978). Experimental carcinogenesis by antitumor drugs. *Cancer Treat. Rev.*, **5**, 175–184.

Sieff, C. A. and Nathan, D. G. (1996). Haemopoietic stem cells. In Weatherall, D. J., Ledingham, J. G. G. and Warrell, D. A. (Eds), *Oxford Textbook of Medicine*. Oxford University Press, Oxford, pp. 3381–3390.

Simon, N. and Siklósi, C. S. (1974). Experimentellen Porphyrie-Modell mit Hexachlorocyclohexan. *Z. Hautkr.*, **49**, 497–504.

Smalley, E. B. (1973). T-2 toxin. *J. Am. Vet. Med. Assoc.*, **163**, 1278–1281.

Smith, J. E. and Beutler, E. (1966). Methemoglobin formation and reduction in man and various animal species. *Am. J. Physiol.*, **210**, 347–350.

Smith, R. P., Alkaitis, A. A. and Schafer, P. R. (1967). Chemically-induced methemoglobinemias in the mouse. *Biochem. Pharmacol.*, **16**, 317–328.

Snyder, R. and Kalb, G. F. (1994). A perspective on benzene leukemogenesis. *Crit. Rev. Toxicol.*, **24**, 177–209.

Spivak, J. L. and Graber, S. E. (1980). Erythropoietin and the regulation of erythropoiesis. *Johns Hopkins Med. J.*, **146**, 311–320.

Stavem, P., Stromme, J. and Bull, O. (1988). Immunological studies in a case of gold salt-induced thrombocytopenia. *Scand. J. Haematol.*, **5**, 271–277.

Stolk, J. M. and Smith, R. P. (1966). Species differences in methemoglobin reductase activity. *Biochem. Pharmacol.*, **15**, 343–351.

Strang, L. B. (1977). *Neonatal Respiration: Physiological and Clinical Studies*. Blackwell, Oxford.

Taira, M. C. and San Martin de Viale, L. C. (1998). Effect of lindane and heptachlor on δ-aminolaevulinic acid synthetase. *Arch. Toxicol.*, **72**, 722–730.

Tarallo, P. (1985). Platelets. In Siest, G., Schiele, F., Henny, J. and Young, D. S. (Eds), *Interpretation of Clinical Laboratory Tests*. Biomedical Publications, Foster City, CA, pp. 379–391.

Templeton, D. M. (1992). Cobalt. In Sullivan, J. B. and Krieger, G. R. (Eds), *Hazardous Materials Toxicology*. Williams and Wilkins, Baltimore, pp. 853–859.

Till, J. E. and McCulloch, E. A. (1961). A direct measurement of the radiation sensitivity of normal mouse bone marrow cells. *Radiation Res.*, **14**, 213–222.

Tsongas, T. A. (1985). Occupational factors in the epidemiology of chemically-induced lymphoid and hemopoietic cancers. In Irons, R. D. (Ed.), *Toxicology of the Blood and Bone Marrow*. Raven Press, New York, pp. 149–177.

Tunek, A., Platt, K. L., Bentley, P. and Oesch, F. (1978). Microsomal metabolism of benzene to species irreversibly binding to microsomal protein and effects of modifications of this metabolism. *Mol. Pharmacol.*, **14**, 920–929.

Ueno, Y. (1983). Trichothecenes. In *Chemical, Biological and Toxicological Aspects. Developments in Food Science.* Elsevier, New York, pp. 1–6.

Ueno, Y. (1984). Toxicological features of T-2 toxin. *Fund. Appl. Toxicol.*, **4**, S124–S132.

USDHHS (1997). *Toxicological Profile for Benzene.* US Department of Health and Human Services, Public Health Service, Agency for Toxic Substances and Disease Registry, Atlanta GA.

Vage, C., Saab, N., Woster, P. M. and Svensson, G. K. (1994). Dapsone-induced hematologic toxicity: comparison of the methemoglobin-forming ability of hydroxylamine metabolites of dapsone in rat and human blood. *Toxicol. Appl. Pharmacol.*, **129**, 309–316.

Wang, J.-S., Kensler, T. W. and Groopman, J. D. (1998). Toxicants in food: fungal contaminants. In Ioannides, C. (Ed.), *Nutrition and Chemical Toxicology.* Wiley, Chichester, pp. 29–57.

Ward, J. M., Rehm, S. and Reynolds, C. W. (1990). Tumours of the haematopoietic system. In Turosev, V. and Mohr, U. (Eds.), *Pathology of Tumours in Laboratory Animals, Vol. I, Tumours of the rat,* 2nd edn. International Agency for Research on Cancer, Lyon. pp. 625–645.

Weatherall, D. J. (1996). Other anaemias resulting from defective red cell metabolism. In Weatherall, D. J., Ledingham, J. G. G. and Warrell, D. A. (Eds), *Oxford Textbook of Medicine.* Oxford University Press, Oxford, pp. 3521–3524.

Weingand, K., Brown, G., Hall, R., Davies, D., Gossett, K., Neptun, D., Waner, T., *et al.* (1996). Harmonization of animal clinical pathology testing in toxicity and safety studies. *Fundam. Appl. Toxicol.*, **29**, 198–201.

White, J. C., Dacie, J. V., Holliday, E. R., Beavan, G. R. and Johnson, E. A. (1951). Heinz body abnormality. *Br. Med. J.*, **2**, 357–358.

Young, K. M. and Weiss, L. (1997). Hematopoiesis: structure–function relationships in bone marrow and spleen. In Bloom, J. C., Sipes, I. G., McQueen, C. A. and Gandolfi, A. J. (Eds), *Comprehensive Toxicology,* Vol. 4. Pergamon Press, Oxford, pp. 11–34.

Yunis, A. A. (1973). Chloramphenicol-induced bone-marrow suppression. *Semin. Hematol.*, **10**, 225–234.

Chapter 19
Alternatives to *In Vivo* Studies in Toxicology

Shayne C. Gad

CONTENTS

INTRODUCTION

The key assumptions underlying modern toxicology are (1) that other organisms can serve as accurate predictive models of toxicity in man, (2) that the selection of an appropriate model to use is the key to accurate prediction in man, and (3) that understanding the strengths and weaknesses of any particular model is essential to understanding the relevance of specific findings to man. The nature of models and their selection in toxicological research and testing has only recently become the subject of critical scientific review. Usually in toxicology, when we refer to 'models', we really have meant test organisms, although, in fact, the manner in which parameters are measured (and which parameters are measured to characterize an end-point of interest) are also critical parts of the model (or, indeed, may actually constitute the 'model').

Although there have been accepted principles for test organism selection, these have not generally been the final basis for such selection. It is a fundamental hypothesis of both historical and modern toxicology that adverse effects caused by chemical entities in higher animals are generally the same as those induced by those entities in man. There are many who point to individual exceptions to this and conclude that the general principle is false. Yet, as our understanding of molecular biology advances and we learn more about the similarities of structure and function of higher organisms at the molecular level, the more it becomes clear that the mechanisms of chemical toxicity are largely identical in humans and animals. This increased understanding has caused some of the same people who question the general principle of predictive value to suggest in turn that our state of knowledge is such that mathematical models or simple cell culture systems could be used just as well as intact animals to predict toxicities in man. This last suggestion also missed the point that the final expressions of toxicity in man or animals are frequently the summations of extensive and complex interactions on cellular and bio-chemical levels. Zbinden (1987a) and Gad (1996) have published extensively in this area, including a very advanced defence of the value of animal models. Lijinsky (1988) has reviewed the specific issues about the predictive value and importance of animals in carcinogenicity testing and research. Although it was once widely believed, and still is believed by many animal rights activists, that *in vitro* mutagenicity tests would entirely replace animal bioassays for carcinogenicity, this is clearly not the case on either scientific or regulatory grounds. Although there are differences in the responses of various species (including man) to carcinogens, the overall predictive value of such results, when tempered by judgment, is clear. At the same time, a well reasoned use of *in vitro* or other alternative test model systems is essential to the development of a product safety assessment program is both effective and efficient (Gad, 1990a, 1996).

The subject of intact animal models and their proper selection and use has been addressed elsewhere (Gad and Chengelis, 1992) and will not be further addressed here. However, alternative models which use other than intact higher organisms are seeing increasing use in toxicology for a number of reasons.

The first and most significant factor behind the interest in so-called *in vitro* systems has clearly been political—an unremitting campaign by a wide spectrum of individuals concerned with the welfare and humane treatment of laboratory animals (Singer, 1975). In 1959, Russell and Burch first proposed what have come to be called the 3 Rs of humane animal use in research—replacement, reduction and refinement. These have served as the conceptual basis for reconsideration of animal use in research.

Replacement means utilizing methods that do not use intact animals in place of those that do. As examples: veterinary students may use a canine cardiopulmonary – resuscitation simulator, Resusci-Dog, instead of living dogs; and cell cultures may replace mice and rats that are fed new products to discover substances poisonous to humans. In addition, using the preceding definition of animal, an invertebrate (e.g. a horseshoe crab) could replace a vertebrate (e.g. a rabbit) in a testing protocol.

Reduction refers to the use of fewer animals. For instance, changing practices allow toxicologists to estimate the lethal dose of a chemical with as few as one-tenth the number of animals used in traditional tests. In biomedical research, long-lived animals, such as primates, may be used in multiple sequential protocols, assuming that they are not deemed inhumane or scientifically conflicting. Designing experimental protocols with appropriate attention to statistical inference can lead to decreases or to increases in the numbers of animals used. Through coordination of efforts among investigators, several tissues may be taken simultaneously from a single animal. Reduction can also refer to the minimization of any unintentionally duplicative experiments, perhaps through improvements in information resources.

Refinement entails the modification of existing procedures so that animals are subjected to less pain and distress. Refinements may include administration of anaesthetics to animals undergoing otherwise painful procedures; administration of tranquillizers for distress; humane destruction prior to recovery from surgical anaesthesia; and careful scrutiny of behavioural indices of pain or distress, followed by cessation of the procedure or the use of appropriate analgesics. Refinements also include the enhanced use of non-invasive imaging technologies that allow earlier detection of tumours, organ deterioration or metabolic changes and the subsequent early euthanasia of test animals.

Progress towards these first three Rs has been reviewed previously (Gad, 1990b, 1994; Salem, 1995). However, there is a fourth R—responsibility, which was not in Russell and Burch's initial proposal. To toxicologists this is the cardinal R. They may be personally committed to minimizing animal use and suffering, and to doing the best possible science of which they are capable, but at the end of it all toxicologists must stand by their responsibility to be conservative in ensuring the safety of the people using or exposed to the drugs and chemicals produced by our society.

Since 1980, issues of animal use and care in toxicological research and testing have become one of the fundamental concerns of both science and the public. Are our results predictive of what may or may not be seen in man? Are we using too many animals, and are we using them in a manner that gets the answer we need with as little

discomfort to the animals as possible? How do we balance the needs of man against the welfare of animals?

In 1984, the Society of Toxicology (SOT) held its first symposium and addressed scientific approaches to these issues. The last such symposium for SOT was in 1988. Each year that passes has brought new regulations, attempts at federal and state legislation in the USA and legislation in other countries, and demonstrations that directly affect the practice of toxicology. Increasing amounts of both money and scientific talent have been dedicated to progress in this area. At the same time, the public clearly supports animal use in research when they see a need and benefit. This is shown in **Table 1**.

During the same time-frame, interest and progress in the development of *in vitro* test systems for toxicity evaluations have also progressed. Early reviews by Hooisma (1982), Neubert (1982) and Williams *et al.* (1983) record the proceedings of conferences on the subject, but Rofe's 1971 review was the first found by this author. Although it is hoped that in the long term some of these (or other) *in vitro* methods will serve as definitive tests in place of those that use intact animals, at present it appears more likely that their use in most cases will be as screens. Frazier (1992), Gad (1994) and Gad and Chengelis (1997) have given recent overviews of the general concepts and status of *in vitro* alternatives.

The entire product safety assessment process, in the broadest sense, is a multistage process in which none of the individual steps is overwhelmingly complex, but the integration of the whole process involved fitting together a large complex pattern of pieces. The single most important part of this product safety evaluation programme is, in fact, the initial overall process of defining and developing an adequate data package on the potential hazards associated with the product life-cycle (the manufacture, sale, use and disposal of a product and associated process materials). To do this, one must ask a series of questions in a highly interactive process, with many of the questions designed to identify and/or modify their successors. The first is—what information is needed?

Required here is an understanding of the way in which a product is to be made and used, and the potential health and safety risks associated with exposure of humans

Table 1 Public opinion on animal use in research

A 1989 survey conducted for the American Medical Association (1989) sampled almost 1500 households and found that:

- 64% opposed organizations attempting to stop the use of animals in research testing.
- 77% thought that animal research was necessary for progress in medicine.
- Other polls have give the same results in terms of medical research or general issues of animal research and testing, but a majority has been found to oppose animal testing of cosmetics as unwarranted (Cowley *et al.*, 1988).

who will be associated with these processes. Such an understanding is the basis of a hazard and toxicity profile. Once such a profile has been established (as illustrated in **Figure 1**), the available literature is searched to determine what is already known.

Taking into consideration this literature information and the previously defined exposure profile, a tier approach **(Table 2)** has traditionally been used to generate a list of tests or studies to be performed. There is also the special case of pharmaceutical and pesticide products, where there are regulatory mandated minimum test batteries). What goes into a tier system is determined by regulatory requirements imposed by government agencies and also the philosophy of the parent organization, economics and available technology. How such tests are actually performed is determined on one of two bases. The first (and most common) is the menu approach: selecting a series of standard design tests as 'modules' of data. The second is an interactive literative approach, where strategies are developed and studies are designed, based on both needs and what has been learned to date about the product. This process has been previously examined in some detail. Our interest here, however, is in the specific portion of the process involved in generating data—the test systems.

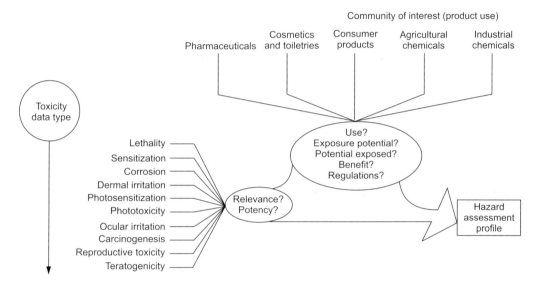

Figure 1 The hazards associated with a new product are a multi-dimensional problem depending on the product's intended use, its innate toxicity, its physiochemical properties and the potential human and environmental exposure. This matrix diagrammatically illustrates the key questions involved in developing the final hazard assessment profile.

Table 2 Tier testing

Testing tier	Mammalian toxicology	Genetic toxicology	Remarks
0	Literature review	Literature review	Upon initial identification of a problem, database of existing information and particulars of use of materials are established
1	Cytotoxicity screens Dermal sensitization Acute systemic toxicity Lethality screens	Ames test *In vitro* SCE *In vitro* cytogenetics Forward mutation/CHO	R&D material and low-volume chemicals with severely limited exposure
2	Subacute studies Metabolism Primary dermal irritation Eye irritation	*In vivo* SCE *In vivo* cytogenetics	Medium-volume materials and/or those with a significant chance of human exposure
3	Subchronic studies Reproduction Developmental toxicity Chronic studies Mechanistic studies		Any materials with a high volume or a potential for widespread or long-term human exposure or one that gives indications of specific long-term effects

The usual way of characterizing the toxicity of a compound or product is to develop information in a tier approach manner. More information is required (a higher tier level is attained) as the volume of production and potential for exposure increase. A common scheme is shown.

TEST SYSTEMS: CHARACTERISTICS, DEVELOPMENT AND SELECTION

Any useful test system must be sufficiently sensitive to ensure that the incidence of false negatives is low. Clearly, a high incidence of false negatives is intolerable. In such a situation, large numbers of dangerous chemical agents would be carried through extensive additional testing only for it to be found that they possess undesirable toxicological properties after the expenditure of significant time and money. One the other hand, a test system that is overly sensitive will give rise to a high incidence of false positives, which will have the deleterious consequence of rejecting potentially beneficial chemicals. The 'ideal' test will fall somewhere between these two extremes and thus provide adequate protection without unnecessarily stifling development.

The 'ideal' test should have an end-point measurement that provides data such that dose–response relationships can be obtained. Furthermore, any criterion of effect must be sufficiently accurate in the sense that it can be used reliably to resolve the relative toxicity of two test chemicals that produce distinct (in terms of hazard to humans) yet similar responses. In general, it may not be sufficient to classify test chemicals into generic toxicity categories. For instance, if a test chemical falls into an 'intermediate' toxicity category, yet is borderline to the next more severe toxicity category, it should be treated with more concern than a second test chemical that falls at the less toxic extreme of the same category. Therefore, it is essential for a test system to be able both to place test chemicals in an established toxicity category and to rank materials relative to others in the category.

The end-point measurement of the 'ideal' test system must be objective. This is important, to ensure that a given test chemical will give similar results when tested using the standard test protocol in different laboratories. If it is not possible to obtain reproducible results in a given laboratory over time or between various laboratories, then the historical database against which new test chemicals are evaluated will be time and laboratory dependent. If this condition is the case, then there will be significant limitations on the application of the test system since it could potentially produce conflicting results. From a regulatory point of view this possibility would be highly undesirable. Along these lines, it is important for the test protocol to incorporate internal standards to serve as quality controls. Hence test data could be represented utilizing a reference scale based on

Table 3 Rationale for using *in vivo* test systems

(1) Provides evaluation of action/effects on intact animal on organ–tissue interactions
(2) Either neat chemicals or complete formulated products (complex mixtures) can be evaluated
(3) Either concentrated or diluted products can be tested
(4) Yields data on the recovery and healing processes
(5) Required statutory tests for agencies under such laws as the Federal Hazardous Substances Act (unless data are already available), Toxic Substances Control Act, Federal Insecticides, Fungicides and Rodenticides Act (FIFRA), Organization for Economic Cooperation (OECD) and Food and Drug Administration Laws
(6) Quantitative and qualitative tests with scoring system generally capable of ranking materials as to relative hazards
(7) Amenable to modifications to meet the requirements of special situations (much as multiple dosing or exposure schedules)
(8) Extensive available database and cross-reference capability for evaluation of relevance to human situation
(9) The ease of performance and relative low capital costs in many cases
(10) Tests are generally both conservative and broad in scope, providing for maximum protection by erring on the side of overprediction of hazard to man
(11) Tests can be either single end-point (such as lethality, corrosion, etc.) or shot-gun (also called multiple end-point, including such test systems as a 13 week oral toxicity study).

Table 4 Limitations of *in vivo* testing systems which serve as a basis for seeking *in vivo* alternatives for toxicity tests

(1) Complications and potential confounding or masking findings of *in vivo* systems
(2) *In vivo* systems may only assess short-term site of application or immediate structural alterations produced by agents. Specific *in vivo* tests may only be intended to evaluate acute local effects (i.e. this may be a purposeful test system limitation)
(3) Technician training and monitoring are critical (particularly in view of the subjective nature of evaluation)
(4) *In vivo* tests in animals do not perfectly predict results in humans if the objective is to exclude or identify severe-acting agents
(5) Structural and biochemical differences between test animals and humans make extrapolation from one to the other difficult
(6) Lack of standardization of *in vivo* systems
(7) Variable correlation with human results
(8) Large biological variability between experimental units (i.e. individual animals)
(9) Large, diverse and fragmented databases which are not readily comparable

the test system response to the internal controls. Such normalization, if properly documented, could reduce interest variability.

From a practical point of view, there are several additional features of the 'ideal' test which should be satisfied. Alternatives to current *in vivo* test systems basically should be designed to evaluate the observed toxic response in a manner as closely predictive of the outcome of interest in man as possible. In addition, the test should be fast enough to ensure that the turnaround time for a given test chemical is reasonable for the intended purpose, very rapid for a screen and timely for a definitive test. Obviously, the speed of the test and the ability to conduct tests on several chemicals simultaneously will determine the overall productivity. The test should be inexpensive, so that it is economically competitive with current testing practices. Finally, the technology should be easily transferred from one laboratory to another without excessive capital investment (relative to the value of the test performed) for test implementation.

It should be kept in mind that although some of these practical considerations may appear to present formidable limitations for any given test system at the present time, the possibility of future developments in testing technology could overcome these obstacles. In reality, these practical considerations are grounds for consideration of multiple new candidate tests on the basis of competitive performance. The most predictive test system in the universe of possibilities will never gain wide acceptance if it takes years to produce an answer or costs substantially more than other test systems that are only marginally less predictive. The point is that these characteristics of the 'ideal' test system provide a general framework for evaluation of alternative test systems in general. No test system is likely to be 'ideal'. Therefore, it will be necessary to weigh the strengths and weaknesses of each proposed test system in order to reach a conclusion on how 'good' a particular test is.

In both theory and practice, *in vivo* and *in vitro* tests have potential advantages. **Tables 3** and **4** summarize their advantages. How, then, might the proper tests be selected, especially in the case of the choice of staying with an existing test system or adopting a new one? The next section will present the basis for selection of specific tests.

CONSIDERATIONS IN ADOPTING NEW TEST SYSTEMS

Conducting toxicological investigations in two or more species of laboratory animals is generally accepted as being a prudent and responsible practice in developing a new chemical entity, especially one that is expected to receive widespread use and to have exposure potential over human lifetimes. Adding a second or third species to

the testing regimen offers an extra measure of confidence to the toxicologist and the other professionals who will be responsible for evaluating the associated risks, benefits and exposure limitations or protective measures. Although undoubtedly broadening and deepening a compound's profile of toxicity, the practice of enlarging on the number of test species is an indiscriminate scientific generalization, as has been demonstrated in multiple points in the literature (Gad and Chengelis, 1997). Moreover, such a tactic is certain to generate the problem of species-specific toxicosis. This is defined as a toxic response or an inordinately low biological threshold for toxicity that is evident in one species or strain, while all other species examined are either unresponsive or strikingly less sensitive. Species-specific toxicosis usually implies that either different metabolic pathways for converting or excreting xenobiotics or anatomical differences are involved. The investigator confronting such findings must be prepared to address the all-important question, 'are humans likely to react positively or negatively to the test agent under similar circumstances?' Assuming that numerical odds prevail and that humans automatically fit into the predominant category would be scientifically irresponsible, whether on the side of being safe or at risk. Such a confounded situation can be an opportunity to advance more quickly into the heart of the search for predictive information. A species-specific toxicosis can frequently contribute towards a better understanding of the general case if the underlying biological mechanism either causing or enhancing toxicity is defined, and especially if it is discovered to uniquely reside in the sensitive species.

The design of our current tests appears to serve society reasonably well (i.e. significantly more times than not) in identifying hazards that would be unacceptable. However, the process can just as clearly be improved from the standpoint of both improving our protection of society and doing necessary testing in a manner that uses fewer animals in a more humane manner.

IN VITRO MODELS

In vitro models, at least as screening tests, have been with us in toxicology for some 25 years now. The last 10–15 years have brought a great upsurge in interest in such models. This increased interest is due to economic and animal welfare pressures and technological improvements.

Criteria against which an *in vitro* model should be evaluated for its suitability in replacing (partially or entirely) an accepted *in vivo* model are incorporated in the process detailed in **Table 5**, which presents the proposed steps for taking a new *in vitro* testing technology from being a research construct to a validated and accepted test system.

Table 5 Multistage scheme for the development, validation and transfer of *in vitro* test system technology in toxicology

STAGE I: STATEMENT OF TEST OBJECTIVE
(A) Identify existing test system and its strengths and weaknesses
(B) Clearly state objectives for alternative test system
(C) Identify potential alternative test system

STAGE II: DEFINE DEVELOPMENTAL TEST DESIGN
(A) Identify relevant variables
(B) Evaluate effects of variables on test system
(C) Optimize test performance
(D) Understand what the test does in a functional sense
    (1) Is it a simulation of an *in vivo* event?
    (2) Is this simply a response to the presence of the agent?
    (3) Is the measured response a functional step or link in the *in vivo* event of interest?
    (4) Is the measured response a functional step or link in the *in vivo* event of interest or some intermediate stage?
    (5) Is this an effect on some structure or function analogous to the *in vivo* structure or function?

STAGE III: EVALUATE PERFORMANCE OF OPTIMUM TEST
(A) Develop library of known positive-and negative-response materials of diverse structure and a range of response potencies (i.e. if the end-point is irritation, then materials should range from non-irritating to severely irritating)
(B) Use optimum test design to evaluate the library of 'knowns' under 'blind' conditions
(C) Compare correlation of test results with those of other test systems and with real case of interest—results in humans

STAGE IV: TECHNOLOGY TRANSFER
(A) Present and publish results through professional media (at Society meetings, in peer-reviewed journals).
(B) Provide hands-on training to personnel from other facilities and facilitate internal evaluations of test methods.

STAGE V: VALIDATION
(A) Arrange for test of coded samples in multiple laboratories (i.e. interlaboratory validation)
(B) Compare, present and publish results
(C) Gain regulatory acceptance

STAGE VI: CONTINUE TO REFINE AND EVALUATE TEST SYSTEM PERFORMANCE AND UTILIZATION
(A) Continually strive for an understanding of why the test 'works' and its relevance to effects in man
(B) Remain sceptical. Why should any one of us be the one to make the big breakthrough? Clearly, there is some basic flaw in the design or conduct of the study which has given rise to these promising results. Doubt, check and question; let your most severe critic review the data; go to a national meeting and give a presentation; then go back home and doubt, check and question some more!

Table 6 Possible interpretations when *in vitro* data do not predict results of *in vivo* studies

(1) Chemical is not absorbed at all or is poorly absorbed in *in vivo* studies
(2) Chemical is well absorbed but is subject to 'first-pass effect' in the liver
(3) Chemical is distributed so that less (or more) reaches the receptors than would be predicted on the basis to its absorption
(4) Chemical is rapidly metabolized to an active or inactive metabolite that has a different profile of activity and/or different duration of action from that of the parent drug
(5) Chemical is rapidly eliminated (e.g. through secretory mechanisms)
(6) Species of the two test systems used are different
(7) Experimental conditions of the *in vitro* and *in vivo* experiments differed and may have led to different effects from those expected. These conditions include factors such as temperature or age, sex and strain of animal
(8) Effects elicited *in vitro* and *in vivo* by the particular test substance in question differ in their characteristics
(9) Tests used to measure responses may differ greatly for *in vitro* and *in vivo* studies, and the types of data obtained may not be comparable
(10) The *in vitro* study did not use adequate controls (e.g. pH, vehicle used, volume of test agent given, samples taken from sham-operated animals), resulting in 'artifacts' of method rather than results
(11) *In vitro* data cannot predict the volume of distribution in central or in peripheral compartments
(12) *In vitro* data cannot predict the rate constants for chemical movement between compartments
(13) *In vitro* data cannot predict the rate constants of chemical elimination
(14) *In vitro* data cannot predict whether linear or non-linear kinetics will occur with specific dose of a chemical *in vivo*
(15) Pharmacokinetic parameters (e.g. bioavailability, peak plasma concentration, half-life) cannot be predicted solely on the basis of *in vitro* studies
(16) *In vivo* effects of chemical are due to an alteration in the higher order integration of an intact animal system, which cannot be reflected in a less complex system.

There are substantial potential advantages in using an *in vitro* system in toxicological testing which include isolation of test cells or organ fragments from homeostatic and hormonal control, accurate dosing and quantification of results. It should be noted that, in addition to the potential advantages, *in vitro* systems *per se* also have a number of limitations which can contribute to their not being acceptable models. Findings from an *in vitro* system that either limit their use in predicting *in vivo* events or make them totally unsuitable for the task include wide differences in the doses needed to produce effects or differences in the effects elicited. Some reasons for such findings are detailed in **Table 6**.

Tissue culture has the immediate potential to be used in two very different ways by industry. First, it has been used to examine a particular aspect of the toxicity of a compound in relation to its toxicity *in vivo* (i.e. mechanistic or explanatory studies). Second, it has been used as a form of rapid screening to compare the toxicity of a group of compounds for a particular form of response. Indeed, the pharmaceutical industry has used *in vitro* test systems in these two ways for years in the search for new potential drug entities.

The theory and use of screens in toxicology have previously been reviewed (Gad, 1988a, 1989a, b, 1999). Mechanistic and explanatory studies are generally called for when a traditional test system gives a result that is either unclear or is one for which the relevance to the real-life human exposure is doubted. *In vitro* systems are particularly attractive for such cases because they can focus on very defined single aspects of a problem or pathogenic response, free of the confounding influence of the multiple responses of an intact higher level organism. Note, however, that first one must know the nature (indeed the existence) of the questions to be addressed. It is then important to devise a suitable model system which is related to the mode of toxicity of the compound.

There is currently much controversy over the use of *in vitro* test systems—will they find acceptance as 'definitive tests systems' or only be used as preliminary screens for such final tests?—or, in the end, not be used at all? Almost certainly, all three of these cases will be true to some extent. Depending on how the data generated are to be used, the division between the first two is ill-defined at best.

Before trying to definitely answer these questions in a global sense, each of the end-points for which *in vitro* systems are being considered should be overviewed and considered against the factors outlined up to this point.

LETHALITY

Many of the end-points of interest in toxicology present a fundamental limitation to the development and use of an *in vitro* or non-mammalian system in place of established *in vivo* methods. While cytotoxicity is a component mechanism in many of these toxic responses, disruption or diminution of the integrated function of multiple cells and systems is just as important.

The evaluation of lethality (symbolized in the public mind by the LD_{50} test) would seem to offer a unique opportunity for the development and use of alternatives. Approaches to alternatives for lethality testing include no living materials at all (the SAR or computer model approaches), those that use no intact higher organisms (but rather cultured cells or bacteria), and those that use lower forms of animal life (invertebrates and fish, for example). Each of these approaches presents a different approach to the objective of predicting acute lethality in humans or, rarely, economic animals, and will be examined in turn.

There are systems that do not directly use any living organisms but, rather, seek to predict the lethality (in particular, the LD_{50}) of a chemical on the basis of what is known about structurally related chemicals. Such structure–activity relationship (SAR) systems have improved markedly over the last 10 years (Enslein *et al.*, 1983a; Lander *et al.*, 1984), but are still limited. Accurate predictions are usually possible only for those classes of structures where data have previously been generated on several members of the classes. For new structural classes, the value of such predictions in minimal. Accordingly, this approach is valuable when working with analogues in a series but not for novel structures. It is also a strong argument for getting as many data as possible into the published literature.

A more extensive and seemingly fruitful approach has been the use of various cultured cell systems. Kurack *et al.* (1986), for example, have developed and suggested a system based on cultured mammalian hepatocytes. The system does metabolize materials in a manner like mammalian target species, and has shown promise in a limited battery of chemicals. Such mammalian cell culture and bacterial screening systems have significant weaknesses for assessing the lethality of many classes of chemicals, since they lack any of the integrative functions of a larger organism. Thus, they would miss all agents that act by disrupting functions such as the organophosphate pesticides, most other neurologically mediated lethal agents and agents that act by modifying hormonal or immune systems.

Clive *et al.* (1979) have reported on the correlation of the LC_{50}s of a variety of chemicals in mouse lymphoma cell cultures with their oral LD_{50}s in mice, as shown in **Figure 2**. No linear correlation is present, but highly cytotoxic substances (in this group) are significantly more toxic orally. Given the impression of some LD_{50} values, due to such factors as steepness of slope of the lethality curve, the lack of linear correlation should be no surprise. Most recently, Ekwall *et al.* (1989) have reported on the MEIC program system, which utilizes a

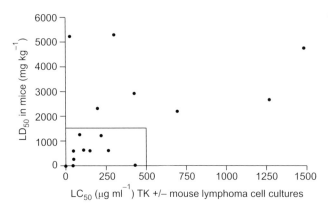

Figure 2 Graph showing a comparison of the lethalities of a group of 18 drugs of diverse structure in *in vivo* (mouse) and *in vitro* (cultured mouse lymphoma cells) test systems. Correlation of these LD_{50}/LC_{50} values is very poor, though extreme high- and low-scale values seem to be more closely associated in the two systems.

battery of five cellular systems. For a group of ten chemicals, the system provided good correlation with, or predictive power of, rat LD_{50}s.

Parce *et al.* (1989) reported on a biosensor technique in which cultured cells are confined to a flow chamber through which a sensor measures the rate of production of acidic metabolites. It is proposed to use this as a functional measure of cytotoxicity and as a screening technique for a number of uses, including *in vivo* lethality.

Three lower species of intact animals have been proposed for use in screening or testing of the lethal effects of chemicals. First, some researchers have shown a good correlation between the lethality of chemicals to *Daphnia magnus* (the LC_{50} of the material dissolved in water) and the oral LD_{50} of the same chemicals in rats. This correlation is non-linear, but still suggests that more toxic materials could be at least initially identified and classified in some form of screening system based on *Daphnia*. A broader range of chemical structures will need to be evaluated, however, and some additional laboratories will need to confirm the finding. It must also be kept in mind that the metabolic systems and many of the other factors involved in species differences (as presented by Gad and Chengelis, 1988, 1992) contribute to a non-linear correlation and may also make the confidence in the prediction of human effects in cases somewhat limited.

Earthworms have been one of the more common species used to test chemicals for potential hazardous impact on the environment. The 48 h contrast test has proved to be a fast and resource-effective way of assessing acute toxicity of chemicals in earthworms and is outlined in **Table 7**. The standardized method, approved by the EEC, was discussed by Neuhauser *et al.* (1986). This test is for environmental impact assessment where

cross-laboratory comparisons are important. If, however, one wishes to adopt this technology for the purpose of screening new chemicals or releasing batches of antibiotics, then variants of this method may be acceptable, as internal consistency is more important than inter-laboratory comparisons. There are two important considerations. First, because of seasonal variation in the quality of earthworms obtained from suppliers, positive controls or comparator chemicals should be included on every assay run. Second, distilled water must be used, as worms are sensitive to contaminants that may occur in chlorinated water. The filter-paper should completely cover the sides of the vessel, otherwise the worms will simply crawl up the sides to escape the adverse stimulus the chemical contact may provide.

Using these techniques, Roberts and Dorough (1984, 1985) and Neuhauser *et al.* (1986) compared acute toxicity in a variety of organic chemicals in several earthworm species. While there are some obvious differences between worm species, in general the rank order of toxicity is about the same. *Lumbricus rubellus* tends to be the most sensitive species. All earthworms are very sensitive to carbofuran under the conditions of this test. Neuhauser *et al.* (1985a, b) proposed a toxicity rating scheme based on acute lethality in the earth worms which is similar to the more familiar scheme based on acute toxicity in rodents **(Table 8)**. Roberts and Dorough (1985) and Neuhauser *et al.* (1986) published extensive compilations of acute lethality in worms and compared these with acute lethality in rats and mice. A selection of these is shown in **Table 9**. Applying the rating scheme of Neuhauser *et al.*, most chemicals receive about the same toxicity rating based on results in *Eisenia foetida* and mice. This may suggest that replacing the LD_{50} with the LC_{50} for rating toxicity (for transportation permits, for example) deserves serious consideration.

Table 7 Earthworm 48 h contact test—acute lethality

(1) Place filter-paper of known size (9 cm or 12×6.7 cm) in a Petri dish or standard scintillation vial
(2) Dilute test article in acetone or some other volatile solvent
(3) Slowly and evenly deposit known amounts of test article solution on filter-paper
(4) Dry thoroughly with gentle stream of air or nitrogen
(5) Add 1.0 ml of distilled water to filter-paper
(6) Add worm (*L. rubellus*). Use 400–500 mg body weight range
(7) Ten replicate vials per concentration
(8) Store/incubate in the absence of light at 15–20 °C for 48 h
(9) Examine for lethality (swollen, lack of movement upon warming up to room temperature, lack of response to tactile stimulation)
(10) Express dose as μg cm^{-2} and mortality as usual. Calculate LD_{50} using standard techniques
(11) Always include negative and positive (benchmark) controls

Table 8 Earthworm toxicity—toxicity rating

Rating	Designation	Rat LD_{50} (mg kg^{-1})	*Eisenia foetida* LC_{50} (μg cm^{-2})
1	Supertoxic	< 5	< 1.0
2	Extremely toxic	5–50	1.0–10
3	Very toxic	50–500	10–100
4	Moderately toxic	500–5000	100–1000
5	Relatively non-toxic	> 5000	> 1000

From Neuhauser *et al.* (1985a, b).

Table 9 Earthworm acute lethality—comparative values

Chemical	*Eisenia foetida* (LC_{50})	*Mouse* (LD_{50})
2,4-Dinitrophenol	0.6(1)[a]	45(2)[a]
Carbaryl	14(3)	438(3)
Benzene	75(3)	4700(4)
1,1,1-Trichloroethane	83(3)	11240(5)
Dimethyl phthalate	550(4)	7200(5)

[a] Values in parentheses are toxicity ratings as described in **Table 8**.

The main advantages of the 40 h contact test are the savings of time and money. The cost savings fall into three categories. First, earthworms are cheap. One hundred *L. rubellus* will cost about US $2. The 100 mice they could replace in screens and quality control (QC) testing, for example, would cost $125–175. Second, earthworms require no vivarium space, and their use could reduce the number of rodents used, resulting in a net decrease in vivarium use. Third, adapting the 48 h contact test would require little capital investment, other than a dedicated under-the-counter refrigerator set at 15–20 °C. Otherwise, the assay can be easily performed in a standard biochemistry laboratory. With regard to time savings, the standard lethality test with rodents requires 7–14 days of post-dosing observations. The 48 h contact test is completed in 48 h. Not only is the turnaround time faster, but also the amount of time that technical personnel will have to spend observing animals and recording observations will be reduced. An incidental advantage of earthworms is that they are cold-blooded vertebrates, and thus as exempt from current animal welfare laws.

There are two main disadvantages to the use of earthworms in acute toxicity testing. First, there are a limited number of end-points. Other than death and a few behavioural abnormalities (Stenersen, 1979; Drewes *et al.*, 1984), the test does not yield much qualitative information. Second, there is probably some institutional bias. Because the test is basically low technology (no tissue culture) and uses a non-mammalian model, it may be easy to dismiss the utility of the test.

Finally, the use of smaller species of fish as a surrogate for man has gained some supporters. Although, to date, the Medaka and rainbow trout have been proposed

primarily as models for aquatic toxicity and carcinogenicity, there is no reason why they could not be used for screening water-soluble compounds for extreme acute toxicity.

Although the intact organisms would seem to be the most utilitarian on the face of it, they still will not totally replace mammalian systems, owing to the need to be concerned about those systems that are significantly different in the higher organisms. Still, it would appear that for those compounds for which human exposure is not intentional, testing in an intact lower organism systems (or perhaps even in a cell culture system) should be sufficient to identify agents of significant concern. In these cases, lethality testing in intact mammals is probably unwarranted.

SPECIFIC AREAS

Ocular Irritation

Testing for potential to cause irritation or damage to the eyes remains the most active area for the development (and validation) of alternatives and the most sensitive area of animal testing in biomedical research. This has been true since the beginning of the 1980s. **Table 10** presents an overview of the reasons for pursuing such alternatives. The major reason, of course, has been the pressure from public opinion.

Indeed, many of the *in vitro* tests now being evaluated for other end-points (such as skin irritation and lethality) are adaptations of test systems first developed for eye irritation uses. A detailed review of the underlying theory of each test system is beyond the scope of this chapter. Frazier *et al.* (1987) and Gad (1994) performed such reviews, and **Table 11** presents an updated version of the list of test systems overviewed in those volumes.

There are six major categories of approach to *in vitro* eye irritation tests. Because of the complex nature of the eye, the different cell types involved and interactions between them, it is likely that a successful replacement for existing *in vivo* systems (such as the rabbit) would require some form of battery of such test systems. Many individual systems, however, might constitute effective screens in defined situations. The first five of these aim at assessing portions of the irritation response, including alterations in tissue morphology, toxicity to individual component cells or tissue physiology, inflammation or immune modulation and alterations in repair and/or recovery processes. These methods have the limitation that they assume that one of the component parts can or will predict effects in the complete organ system. While each component may serve well to predict the effects of a set of chemical structures which determine part of the ocular irritation response, a valid assessment across a broad range of structures will require the use of a collection or battery of such tests.

Table 10 Rationales for seeking *in vitro* alternatives for eye irritancy tests

(1) Avoid whole-animal and organ *in vivo* evaluation
(2) Strict Draize scale testing in the rabbit assesses only three eye structures (conjuctiva, cornea, iris) and traditional rabbit eye irritancy tests do not assess cataracts, pain, discomfort or clouding of the lens
(3) *In vivo* tests assess only inflammation and immediate structural alterations produced by irritants (not sensitizers, photoirritants or photoallergens). Note, however, that the test was (and generally is) intended to evaluate any pain or discomfort
(4) Technician training and monitoring are critical (particularly in view of the subjective nature of evaluation)
(5) Rabbit eye tests do not perfectly predict results in humans, if the objective is either the total exclusion of irritants or the identification of truly severe irritants on an absolute basis (that is, without false positives or negatives). Some (such as Reinhardt *et al.*, 1985) have claimed that these tests are too sensitive for such uses
(6) There are structural and biochemical differences between rabbit and human eyes which make extrapolation from one to the other difficult. For example, Bowman's membrane is present and well developed in man (8–12 μm thick) but not in the rabbit, possibly giving the cornea greater protection
(7) Lack of standardization
(8) Variable correlation with human results
(9) Large biological variability between experimental units
(10) Large, diverse and fragmented databases which are not readily comparable

Table 11 *In vitro* alternatives for eye irritation tests

(I) MORPHOLOGY
(1) Enucleated superfused rabbit eye system (Burton *et al.*, 1981)
(2) Balb/c 3T3 cells/morphological assays (HTD) (Borenfreund and Puemer, 1984)

(II) CELL TOXICITY
(1) Adhesion/cell proliferation
  (a) BHK cells/growth inhibition (Reinhardt *et al.*, 1985)
  (b) BHK cells/colony formation efficiency (Reinhardt *et al.*, 1985)
  (c) BHK cells/cell detachment (Reinhardt *et al.*, 1985)
  (d) SIRC cells/colony forming assay (North-Root *et al.*, 1982)
  (e) Balb/c 3T3 cells/total protein (Shopsis and Eng, 1985)
  (f) BCL/D1 cells/total protein (Balls and Horner, 1985)
  (g) Primary rabbit corneal cells/colony forming assay (Watanabe *et al.*, 1988)
(2) Membrane integrity
  (a) LS cells/dual dye staining (Scaife, 1982)
  (b) Thymocytes/dual fluorescent dye staining (Aeschbacher *et al.*, 1986)
  (c) LS cells/dual dye staining (Kemp *et al.*, 1983)
  (d) RCE-SIRC-P815-YAC-1/Cr release (Shadduck *et al.*, 1985)
  (e) L929 cells/cell viability (Simons, 1981)
  (f) Bovine red blood cell/haemolysis (Shadduck *et al.*, 1987)
  (g) Mouse L929 fibroblasts–erythrocin C staining (Frazier, 1988)
  (h) Rabbit corneal epithelial and endothelial cells/membrane leakage (Meyer and McCulley, 1988)
  (i) Agarose diffusion (Barnard, 1989)
  (j) Corneal protein profiles (Eurell and Meachum, 1994)
(3) Cell metabolism
  (a) Rabbit corneal cell cultures/plasminogen activator (Chan, 1985)
  (b) LS cells/ATP assay (Kemp *et al.*, 1985)
  (c) Balb/c 3T3 cells/neutral red uptake (Borenfreund and Puerner, 1984)
  (d) Balb/c 3T3 cells/uridine uptake inhibition assay (Shopsis and Sathe, 1984)
  (e) HeLa cells/metabolic inhibition test (MIT-24) (Selling and Ekwall, 1985)
  (f) MDCK cells/dye diffusion (Tchao, 1988)

(III) CELL AND TISSUE PHYSIOLOGY
(1) Epidermal slice/electrical conductivity (Oliver and Pemberton, 1985)
(2) Rabbit ileum/contraction inhibition (Muir *et al.*, 1983)
(3) Bovine cornea/corneal opacity (Muir, 1984)
(4) Proposed mouse eye/permeability test (Maurice and Singh, 1986)

(Continued)

Table 11 *(Contd)*

(IV) INFLAMMATION/IMMUNITY
(1) Chlorioallantoic membrane (CAM)
    (a) CAM (Leighton *et al.*, 1983)
    (b) HET-CAM (Luepke, 1985)
(2) Bovine corneal cup model/leucocyte chemotactic factors (Elgebaly *et al.*, 1985)
(3) Rat peritoneal cells/histamine release (Jacaruso *et al.*, 1985)
(4) Rat peritoneal mast cells/serotonin release (Dublin *et al.*, 1984)
(5) Rat vaginal explant/prostaglandin release (Dublin *et al.*, 1984)
(6) Bovine eye cup/histamine (Hm) and leukotriene C4 (Lt/C4) release (Benassi *et al.*, 1986)

(V) RECOVERY/REPAIR
(1) Rabbit corneal epithelial cells–wound healing (Jumblatt and Neufeld, 1985).

(VI) OTHER
(1) EYTEX assay (Gordon and Bergman, 1986; Soto *et al.*, 1988)
(2) Computer-based structure–activity relationship (SAR) (Enslein, 1984; Enslein *et al.*, 1988)
(3) *Tetrahymena*/motility (Silverman, 1983)

The sixth category contains tests that have little or no empirical basis, such as computer-assisted structure–activity relationship models. These approaches can only be assessed in terms of how well or poorly they perform. **Table 11** presents an overview of all six categories and some of the component tests within them, updated from the assessment by Frazier *et al.* (1987) along with references for each test.

Given that there are now some 80 or more potential *in vitro* alternatives, the key points along the route to the eventual objective of replacing the *in vivo* test systems are thus: (1) how do we select the best candidates from this pool? (2) how do we want to use the resulting system (as a screen or test?)? (3) how do we gain regulatory and user acceptance of the appropriate test systems?

There have been some large-scale validations of some of these tests (IRAG, 1993). Most of the individual investigators have performed smaller 'validations' as part of their development of the test system, and in a number of cases trade associations have sponsored comparative and/or multilaboratory validations. At least for screening, several systems should be appropriate for use and, in fact, are used now by several commercial organizations. However, the Intraagency Regulatory Alternatives Group (IRAG, 1993) and the Interagency Coordinating Committee on the Validation of Alternative Methods (ICCVAM, 1997) have coordinated and reported on large-scale evaluations. In terms of use within defined chemical structural classes, use of *in vitro* systems for testing of chemicals for non-human exposure should supplant traditional *in vivo* systems once validated on a broad scale by multiple laboratories. Broad use of single tests based on single end-points (such as cytotoxicity) is not likely to be successful, as demonstrated by such efforts as those of Kennah *et al.* (1989).

Skin Irritation

Extensive progress has been made in devising alternative (*in vitro*) systems for evaluating the dermal irritation potential of chemicals since this author first reviewed the field (Gad and Chengelis, 1988). **Table 12** overviews 20 proposed systems which now constitute five very different approaches.

The first approach (I) uses patches of excised human or animal skin maintained in some modification of a glass diffusion cell which maintains the moisture, temperature, oxygenation and electrolyte balance of the skin section. In this approach, after the skin section has been allowed to equilibrate for some time, the material of concern is placed on the exterior surface and wetted (if not a liquid). Irritation is evaluated either by swelling of the skin (a crude and relatively insensitive method for mild and moderate irritants), by evaluation of inhibition of uptake of radiolabeled nutrients, or by measurement of leakage of enzymes through damaged membranes.

The second set of approaches (II) utilizes a form of surrogate skin culture comprising a mix of skin cells which closely mirror key aspects of the architecture and function of the intact organ. These systems seemingly offer a real potential advantage but, to date, the 'damage markers' employed (or proposed) as predictors of dermal irritation have been limited to cytotoxicity.

The third set of approaches (III) is to use some form of cultured cell (either primary or transformed), with primary human epidermal keratinocytes (HEKs) preferred. The cell cultures are exposed to the material of interest, then either cytotoxicity, release of inflammation markers or decrease of some indicator of functionality (lipid metabolism, membrane permeability or cell detachment) is measured.

Table 12 *In vitro* dermal irritation test systems

System	End-point	Validation data?[a]	Reference
I.			
Excised patch of perfused skin	Swelling	No	Dannenberg (1987)
Mouse skin organ culture	Inhibition of incorporation of [^{3}H]thymidine and [^{14}C]leucine labels	No	Kao *et al.* (1982)
Mouse skin organ culture	Leakage of LDH and GOT	Yes	Bartnik *et al.* (1989)
II.			
TESTSKIN—cultured surrogate skin patch	Morphological evaluation (?)	No	Bell *et al.* (1988)
Cultured surrogate skin patch	Cytotoxicity	No	Naughton *et al.* (1989)
III.			
Human epidermal keratinocytes (HEKs)	Release of labeled arachidonic acid	Yes	DeLeo *et al.* (1988)
Human polymorphonuclear cells	Migration and histamine release	Yes (surfactants)	Frosch and Czarnetzki (1987)
Fibroblasts	Acid		Lamont *et al.* (1989)
HEKs	Cytotoxicity	Yes	Gales *et al.* (1989)
HEKs	Cytotoxicity (MTT)	Yes	Swisher *et al.* (1988)
HEKs, dermal fibroblasts	Cytotoxicity	Yes	Babich *et al.* (1989)
HEKs	Inflammation mediator release	No	Boyce *et al.* (1988)
Cultured Chinese hamster ovary (CHO) cells	Increases in β-hexosaminidase levels in media	No	Lei *et al.* (1986)
Cultured C$_3$H10T$_{1/2}$ and HEK cells	Lipid metabolism inhibition	No	DeLeo *et al.* (1987)
Cultured cells—BHK21/C13	Cell detachment	Yes	Reinhardt *et al.* (1987)
BHK21/C13	Growth inhibition		
Primary rat thymocytes	Increased membrane permeability		
Rat peritoneal mast cells	Inflammation mediator release	Yes (surfactants)	Prottey and Ferguson (1976)
IV.			
Hen's egg	Morphological evaluation		Reinhardt *et al.* (1987)
SKINTEX—protein mixture	Protein coagulation	Yes	Gordon *et al.* (1989)
V.			
Structure—activity relationship (SAR) model	NA[b]	Yes	Enslein *et al.* (1987)
SAR model	NA	No	Firestone and Guy (1986)

[a] Evaluated by comparison of predictive accuracy for a range of compounds compared with animal test results. Not validated in the sense used in this chapter.
[b] NA = not available.

The fourth group (IV) contains two miscellaneous approaches—the use of a membrane from the hen's egg with a morphological evaluation of damage being the predictor end-point (Reinhardt *et al.*, 1987) and the SKINTEX system, which utilizes the coagulation of a mixture of soluble proteins to predict dermal response.

Finally, in group V there are two structure–activity relationship models which use mathematical extensions of past animal results correlated with structure to predict the effects of new structures.

Many of these test systems are in the process of evaluation of their performance against various small groups of compounds for which the dermal irritation potential is known. Evaluation by multiple laboratories of a wider range of structures will be essential before any of these systems can be generally utilized.

Irritation of Parenterally Administered Pharmaceuticals

Intramuscular (im) and intravenous (iv) injection of parenteral formulations of pharmaceuticals can produce a range of discomfort resulting in pain, irritation and/or damage to the muscular or vascular tissue. These are normally evaluated for prospective formulations before use in humans by evaluation in intact animal models— usually the rabbit (Gad and Chengelis, 1988).

Currently, a protocol utilizing a cultured rat skeletal muscle cell line (the L6) as a model is in an interlaboratory validation programme among more than 10 pharmaceutical company laboratories. This methodology (Young *et al.*, 1986) measures creatine kinase levels in media after exposure of the cells to the formulation of interest, and predicts *in vivo* intramuscular damage based on this end-point. It is reported to give excellent rank-correlated results across a range of antibiotics (Williams *et al.*, 1987), and in a recent multilaboratory evaluation a broader structural range of compounds (PMA Drusafe *In Vitro* Task Force, 1994).

Another proposed *in vitro* assay for muscle irritancy for injectable formulations is the red blood cell haemolysis assay (Brown *et al.*, 1989). Water-soluble formulations are gently mixed at a 1:2 ratio with freshly collected human blood for 5 s, then mixed with a 5% w/v dextrose solution and centrifuged for 5 min. The percentage red blood cell survival is then determined by measuring differential absorbance at 540 nm, and this is compared with values for known irritants and non-irritants. Against a very small group of compounds (four), this is reported to be an accurate predictor of muscle irritation.

There is no current candidate alternative for the venous irritation test, but the *in vitro* alternative for pyrogenicity testing, the *Limulus* test, is one of the success stories for the alternatives movement. It has totally replaced the classical intact rabbit test in both research and product release testing. The test is based on the jelling or colour development of a pyrogenic preparation in the presence of the lysate of the amoebocytes of the horseshoe crab (*Limulus polyphemus*). It is simpler, more rapid and of greater sensitivity than the rabbit test that it replaced (Cooper, 1975).

Sensitization

There are actually several approaches available for the *in vitro* evaluation of materials for sensitizing potential. These use cultured cells from various sources and, as end-points, look at either biochemical factors (such as production of MIF—migration inhibition factor) or cellular events (such as cell migration or cell 'transformation').

Milner (1970) reported that lymphocytes from guinea pigs sensitized to dinitrofluorobenzene (DNFB) would transform in culture, as measured by the incorporation of tritiated thymidine, when exposed to epidermal proteins conjugated with DNFB. This work was later extended to guinea pigs sensitized to *p*-phenylenediamine. Milner (1971) also reported that his method was capable of detecting allergic contact hypersensitivity to DNFB in humans, using human lymphocytes from sensitized donors and human epidermal extracts conjugated with DNFB.

Miller and Levis (1973) reported the *in vitro* detection of allergic contact hypersensitivity to DNCB conjugated to leucocyte and erythrocyte cellular membranes. This indicated that the reaction was not specifically directed towards epidermal cell conjugates. Thulin and Zacharian (1972) extended others' earlier work on MIF-induced

Table 13 Requested reference compounds for skin sensitization studies (US Consumer Product Safety Commission)

Hydroxylamine sulphate	Penicillin G
Ethyl aminobenzoate	*p*-Phenylenediamine
Iodochlorohydroxyquinoline (clioquinol, chinoform)	Epoxy systems (ethylenediamine, diethylenetriamine, diglycidyl ethers)
Nickel sulphate	Toluene-2,4-diisocyanate
Monomethyl methacrylate	Oil of bergamot
Mercaptobenzothiazole	

migration of human peripheral blood lymphocytes to a test for delayed contact hypersensitivity. Burka *et al.* (1981) reported on an assay system based on isolated guinea pig trachea. No further mention of this has been found in the literature. None of these approaches has yet been developed as an *in vitro* predictive test, but work is progressing. Milner published a review of the history and state of this field in 1983 which still provides an accurate and timely overview.

Any alternative (*in vitro* or *in vivo*) test for sensitization will need to be evaluated against a battery of 'known' sensitizing compounds. The Consumer Product Safety Commission in 1977 proposed such a battery, which is shown in **Table 13**. This has not yet been done for any of the proposed systems. Owing to the complexity of the system involved, it is unlikely that a suitable *in vitro* replacement system will be available soon.

Gad *et al.* (1986) have published comparative data on multiple animal and human test system data for 72 materials. Such a database should be considered for the development and evaluation of new test systems.

Phototoxicity and Photosensitization

The Daniel test for phototoxicity (also called photoirritant contact dermatitis) utilizes the yeast *Candida albicans* as a test species and has been in use for more that 20 years (Daniel, 1965). The measured end-point is simply cell death. The test is simple to perform and cheap, but does not reliably predict the phototoxicity of all classes of compounds (e.g. sulphanilamide). Test systems utilizing bacteria have been suggested as alternatives over the last 20 years (Harter *et al.*, 1976; Ashwood-Smith *et al.*, 1980) for use in predicting the same end-point.

Most recently, ICI has conducted studies on an *in vitro* phototoxicity assay which involves using three cultured cell lines: the A431 human epidermal cell line (a derived epidermal carcinoma), normal human epidermal keratinocytes (a primary cell line derived from cosmetic surgery) and the 3T3 Swiss mouse fibroblast cell line. The protocol for this assay involves subculturing the particular cell type into microtitre tissue culture grade plates and incubating them over a period of 24 h. Following

Table 14 Alternative developmental toxicity test systems

Category	Test system	Model	Reference
(I) Lower organisms	Sea urchins	Organism	Kotzin and Baker (1972)
	Drosophila	Intact and embryonic cells	Abrahamson and Lewis (1971)
	Trout	(Fish species)	MacCrimmon and Kwain (1969)
	Planaria	Regeneration	Best *et al.* (1981)
	Brine shrimp	Disruption of elongation; DNA and protein levels in *Artemia nauplii*	Kerster and Schaeffer (1983); Sleet and Brendel (1985)
	Animal virus	Growth of poxvirons in culture	Keller and Smith (1982)
	Slime mould	Dictyostelium discoidem	Durston *et al.* (1985)
	Medaka	(Fish species)	Cameron *et al.* (1985)
	'Artificial embryo'	*Hydra attenuata*	Johnson *et al.* (1982)
(II) Cell culture	Protein synthesis of cultured cells	Pregnant mouse and chick lens epithelial cells	Clayton (1979)
	Avian neural crest	Differentiation of cells	Sieber-Blum (1985)
	Neuroblastoma	Differentiation of cells	Mummery *et al.* (1984)
	Lectin-mediated attachment	Tumour cells	Braun and Horowicz (1983)
(III) Organ culture	Frog limb	Regeneration	Bazzoli *et al.* (1977)
	Mouse embryo limb bud	Inhibition of incorporation of precursor and of DNA synthesis	Kochhar and Aydelotte (1974)
	Metanephric kidney organ cultures	From 11 day mouse embryos	Saxen and Saksela (1971)
(IV) Submammalian embryo	Chick embryo		Gebhardt (1972)
	Frog embryo	*Xenopus laevis*	Davis *et al.* (1981)
(V) Mammalian embryo	Rat embryo culture	Whole postimplantation embryos	Brown and Fabro (1981); Cockroft and Steele (1989)
	Chernoff	Mouse embryo short test	Chernoff and Kaviock (1980)
	'Micromass cultures'	Rat embryo midbrain and limb	Flint and Orton (1984)
(VI) Other	Structure–activity relationships (SAR)	Mathematical correlations of activity with structural features	Enslein *et al.* (1983b); Gombar *et al.* (1990)

Table 15 Developmental toxicity test system considerations

Possibility	*In vivo*	Organ culture	Cell culture	Lower organisms	Mammalian embryo culture	Submammalian embryos	Other[a]
To study maternal and organ factors	Yes	No	No	No	No/Yes	No/Yes	NA
To study embryogenesis as a whole	Yes	No	No	No	Yes	Somewhat	NA
To eliminate maternal confounding factors (nutrition, etc.)	No	Yes	Yes	No	Yes	Yes	NA
To eliminate placental factors (barrier differences)	No	Yes	Yes	No	Yes	No	NA
To study single morphogenetic events	Difficult	Yes	No	Maybe	Yes	Yes	NA
To create controllable, reproducible conditions	Difficult	Yes	Yes	Yes	Yes	Yes	NA
For exact exposure and timing	Difficult	Yes	Yes	Yes	Yes	Yes	NA
For microsurgical manipulations	Difficult	Yes	No	Maybe	Yes	Yes	NA
For continuous registration of the effects	Difficult	Yes	Yes	No	Yes	Yes	NA
To collect large amounts of tissue for analysis	Yes	Difficult	Yes	No	Yes	No	NA
To use human embryonic tissue for testing	No	Yes	Yes	No	No	No	NA
Screening	Expensive	Yes	Yes	Yes	Yes	Yes	Yes

[a] NA = not available.

incubation, the cultures are exposed to the test compound at a concentration predetermined as non-toxic. After a 4 h exposure to the compound, the cell cultures are exposed to either UV A (320–400 nm) or UV A/B (280–400 nm) radiation for various lengths of time. The degree of enhanced toxicity effected by either UV A or UV A/B radiation in the presence of the test compound relative to the control is assessed, using the MTT assay. MTT, abbreviated from 3-(4,5-dimethylthiazol-2-yl)-2,5-diphenyltetrazolium bromide, undergoes a reduction reaction which is specific to mitochondrial dehydrogenases in viable cells. Work on validation of this test using 30 compounds of know phototoxic potential has shown a high degree of correlation between *in vitro* and *in vivo* results. Jackson and Goldner (1989) have described several other *in vitro* assay systems for this end-point.

The area of development of *in vitro* photosensitization assays has been a very active one, as the review of McAuliffe *et al.* (1986) illustrates. Such tests have focused on being able to predict the photosensitizing potential of a compound and variously employed cultured mammalian cell lines, red blood cells, microorganisms and biochemical reactions. McAuliffe's group has developed and proposed a test that measures the incorporation of tritiated thymidine into human peripheral blood mononuclear cells as a predictive test (Morison *et al.*, 1982). They claim to have internally validated the test, using a battery of known photosensitizers.

Bockstahler *et al.* (1982) have developed and proposed another *in vitro* test system which uses the responses of two *in vitro* mammalian virus – host cell systems to the photosensitizing chemicals proflavine sulphate and 8-methoxypsoralen (8-MOP) in the presence of light as a predictive system. They found that infectious simian virus 40 (SV40) could be induced from SV40-transformed hamster cells by treatment with proflavine plus visible light or 8-MOP plus near-UV radiation. The same photosensitizing treatments inactivated the capacity of monkey cells to support the growth of herpes simplex virus. SV40 induction and inactivation of host cell capacity for herpes virus growth might be useful as screening systems for testing the photosensitizing potential of chemicals. Advantages (ease and speed of conduct) and disadvantages (use of potentially infective agent and the limited range of compounds evaluated to date) were found to be associated with both of these test systems.

Development Toxicity

The area of developmental toxicology is one of the earliest to have alternative models suggested for it, and has one of the most extensive and oldest literatures. This is, of course, partly due to such models originally being used to elucidate the essential mechanisms and process of embryogenesis.

Because of the complicated and multiphasic nature of the developmental process, it has not been proposed that any of these systems be definitive tests, but rather that they serve as one form or another of a screen. As such, these test systems would either preclude or facilitate more effective full-scale evaluation in one or more of the traditional whole-animal test protocols.

The literature and field are much too extensive to review comprehensively here. There are a number of extensive review articles and books on the subject (Wilson, 1978; Clayton, 1981; Kochhar, 1981; Saxen, 1984; Homburger and Goldberg, 1985; Faustman, 1988; Daston and D'Amato, 1989), which should be consulted by those with an in-depth interest.

The existing alternative test systems fall into six broad classes: (1) lower organisms; (2) cell culture systems; (3) organ culture systems; (4) submammalian embryos; (5) mammalian embryos; and (6) others.

Table 14 provides an overview of the major representatives of these six groups, along with at least one basic reference to the actual techniques involved and the system components for each.

The comparative characteristics of these different classes of test systems are presented in **Table 15**. The key point is that these systems can be used for a wide range of purposes, only one of which is to screen compounds to determine the degree of concern for developmental toxicity.

The utility of these systems for screening is limited by the degree of dependability in predicting effects primarily in people and secondarily in the traditional whole-animal test systems. Determining the predictive performance of alternative test systems requires the evaluation of a number of compounds for which the 'true' (human) effect is known. In 1983, a consensus workshop generated a so-called 'gold standard' set of compounds of known activity (Smith *et al.*, 1983). The composition of this list has been open to a fair degree of controversy over the years (Flint, 1989; Johnson, 1989; Johnson *et al.*, 1989). However, an agreed-upon 'gold standard' set of compounds of known activity is an essential starting point for the validation of any single test system or battery of test systems because of the multitude of mechanisms for developmental toxicity. It is unlikely that any one system will be able to stand in place of segment II studies in two species, much less to predict activity in humans accurately. Their use as general screens or as test systems for compounds with little potential for extensive or intended human exposure will, however, probably be appropriate.

Target Organ Toxicity Models

This last model review section addresses perhaps the most exciting potential area for the use of *in vitro* models—as specific tools to evaluate and understand discrete target organ toxicities. Here the presumption is that there is reason to believe (or at least suspect) that some specific target organ (nervous system, lungs, kidney, liver, heart, etc.) is or may be the most sensitive site of adverse action of a systemically absorbed agent. From this starting point, a system that is representative of the target organ's *in vivo* response would be useful in at least two contexts.

First, as with all the other end-points addressed in this chapter, a target organ predictive system could serve as a predictive system (in general, a screen) for effects in intact organisms, particularly man. As such, the ability to identify those agents with a high potential to cause damage in a specific target organ at physiological concentrations would be extremely valuable.

The second use is largely specific to this set of *in vitro* models. This is to serve as tools to investigate, identify and/or verify the mechanisms of action for selective target organ toxicities. Such mechanistic understandings then allow for one to know whether such toxicities are relevant to man (or to condition of exposure to man), to develop means either to predict such responses while they are still reversible or to develop the means to intervene in such toxicosis (i.e. first aid or therapy) and finally potentially to modify molecules of interest to avoid unwanted effects while maintaining desired properties (particularly important in drug design).

In the context of these two uses, the concept of a library of *in vitro* models (Gad, 1989c, 1996) becomes particularly attractive. If one could accumulate a collection of 'validated', operative methodologies that could be brought into use as needed (and put away, as it were, when not being used), this would represent an extremely valuable competitive tool. The question becomes one of selecting which systems/tools to put into the library, and how to develop them to the point of common utility.

Additionally, one must consider what forms of markers are to be used to evaluate the effect of interest. Initially, such markers have been exclusively either morphological (in that there is a change in microscopic structure), observational (is the cell/preparation dead or alive or has some gross characteristic changed?) or functional (does the model still operate as it did before?). Recently, it has become clear that more sensitive models do not just generate a single-end-point type of data, but rather a multiple set of measures which in aggregate provide a much more powerful set of answers.

There are several approaches to *in vitro* target organ models.

The first and oldest is that of the isolated organ preparation. Perfused and superfused tissues and organs have been used in physiology and pharmacology since the late nineteenth century. There is a vast range of these available, and a number of them have been widely used in toxicology (Mehendale, 1989, presented an excellent overview). Almost any end-point can be evaluated in most target organs (the CNS being a notable exception), and these are closest to the *in vivo* situation and therefore generally the easiest to extrapolate or conceptualize

from. Those things that can be measured or evaluated in the intact organism can largely also be evaluated in an isolated tissue or organ preparation. However, the drawbacks or limitations of this approach are also compelling.

An intact animal generally produces one tissue preparation. Such a preparation is viable generally for a day or less before it degrades to the point of losing utility. As a result, such preparations are useful as screens only for agents that have rapidly reversible (generally pharmacological or biomechanical) mechanisms of action. They are superb for evaluating mechanisms of action at the organ level for agents that act rapidly, but not generally for cellular effects of for agents that act over a course of more than a day.

The second approach is to use tissue or organ culture. Such cultures are attractive, owing to maintaining the ability for multiple cell types to interact in at least a near-physiological manner. They are generally not as complex as perfused organs, but are stable over a longer period of time, increasing their utility as screens. They are truly a middle ground between perfused organs and cultured cells. Only for relatively simple organs (such as the skin and bone marrow) are good models which perform in a manner representative of the *in vitro* organ available.

The third and most common approach is that of cultured cell models. These can be either primary or transformed (immortalized) cells, but the former have significant advantages in use as predictive target organ models. Such cell culture systems can be utilized to identify and evaluate interactions at the cellular, subcellular and molecular level on an organ-and species-specific basis (Acosta *et al.*, 1985). The advantages of cell culture are that single organisms can generate multiple cultures for use, that these cultures are stable and useful for protracted periods of time and that effects can be studied very precisely at the cellular and molecular levels. The disadvantages are that isolated cells cannot mimic the interactive architecture of the intact organ, and will respond over time in a manner that becomes decreasingly representative of what happens *in vivo*. An additional concern is that, with the exception of hepatocyte cultures, the influence of systemic metabolism is not factored in unless extra steps are taken. Stammati *et al.* (1981) and Tyson and Stacey (1989) presented excellent reviews of the use of cell culture in toxicology. Any such cellular systems would be more likely to be accurate and sensitive predictors of adverse effects if their function and integrity were evaluated while they were operational. For example, cultured nerve cells should be excited while being exposed and evaluated.

A wide range of target organ-specific models have already been developed and used. Their incorporation into a library-type approach requires that they be evaluated for reproducibility of response, ease of use and predictive characteristics under the intended conditions of use. These evaluations are probably at least somewhat specific to any individual situation. **Tables 16–21** present

Table 16 Representative *in vitro* test systems for respiratory system toxicity

System[a]	End-point	Evaluation	Reference
Isolated perfused rat and rabbit lungs (S)	Damage markers: exuadate of hormones	Correlation with results *in vivo*	Anderson and Eling (1976); Roth (1980); Mehendale (1989)
Alveolar macrophages (S)	Cytotoxicity: as a predictor of fibrogenicity	Correlation with *in vivo* fibrogenicity across a broad range of compounds	Reiser and Last (1979)
Lung organ culture (M, S)	Morphological: structure and macromolecular composition	Proposed from prior experience in pharmacology	Placke and Fisher (1987)
Hamster lung culture (M)	Morphological: structure and cell death	Correlation of *in vivo* effects of cigarette smoke	Stammati *et al.* (1981)

[a] Letters in parentheses indicate primary employment of system: S = screening system; M = mechanistic tool.

Table 17 Representative *in vitro* test systems for neurotoxicity

System[a]	End-point	Evaluation	Reference
Perfused rat phrenic nerve—hemidiaphragm (M)	Functional: release of ACh, conduction velocities, muscle response	Correlates with *in vivo* effects of trialkyltins	Bierkamper (1982)
Primary rat cerebral cells (S)	Observational: cell growth and differentiation	Cell diameter and outgrowth	Hooisma (1982)
Primary rat tissue culture (S)	Functional: receptor–ligand binding	Binding rates	Bondy (1982); Volpe *et al.* (1985)
Organotypic neural cultures (S)	Functional: electrophysiological and pharmacological properties	Correlation with *in vivo* results for a range of known active agents	Spencer *et al.* (1986); Kontur *et al.* (1987)
Isolated perfused brain (M)	Functional: biochemical and electrophysiological	Unknown	Mehendale (1989)
Cultured mouse otocyst (M)	Morphological	Unknown—a tool for potentially evaluating ototoxins	Harpur (1988)

[a] Letters in parentheses indicate primary employment of system: S = screening system; M = mechanistic tool.

Table 18 Representative *in vitro* test systems for renal toxicity

System[a]	End-point	Evaluation	Reference
Rat proximal tubular cells (S)	Functional: α-methylglucose uptake or organic ion transport	Correlation with effects of known nephrotoxin	Boogaard *et al.* (1989)
Rat cortical epithelial cells (S)	Functional: biochemical	Good correlation with *in vivo* for nephrotoxic metals and acetaminophen	Smith *et al.* (1986, 1987); Rylander *et al.* (1987)
Isolated perfused kidney (M)	Functional: biochemical and metabolic. Morphological	Correlation with *in vivo* findings for some nephrotoxins	Mehendale (1989)
Renal slices (S, M)	Full range of functional (biochemical and metabolic)	Correlation with *in vivo* findings for a range of nephrotoxins. Still allows evaluation of a degree of cell-to-cell and nephron-to-nephron interactions	Smith *et al.* (1988)

[a] Letters in parentheses indicate primary employment of system: S = screening system; M = mechanistic tool.

Table 19 Representative *in vitro* test systems for cardiovascular toxicity

System[a]	End-point	Evaluation	Reference
Coronary artery smooth muscle cells (S)	Morphological evaluation—vacuole formation	Correlates with *in vivo* results	Ruben *et al.* (1984)
Isolated perfused rabbit or rat heart (M, S)	Functional: operational, electrophysiological, biochemical and metabolism	Long history of use in physiology and pharmacology	Mehendale (1989)
Isolated superfused atrial and heart preparations (S, M)	Functional: operational and biochemical	Correlation with *in vivo* findings for antioxidants	Gad *et al.* (1977, 1979)

[a] Letters in parentheses indicate primary employment of system: S = screening system; M = mechanistic tool.

Table 20 Representative *in vitro* test systems for hepatic toxicity

System[a]	End-point	Evaluation	Reference
Primary hepatocytes (S, M)	Multiple: Biotransformation Genotoxicity Peroxisome proliferation Biliary dysfunction Membrane damage Ion regulation Energy regulation Protein synthesis	NA[b]	Tyson and Stacey (1989)[c]; Stammati *et al.* (1981)
Hamster hepatocytes (S)	Functional: biochemical	Correlates with *in vivo* effects of acetaminophen	Harman and Fischer (1983)
Rat liver slices (S)	Functional: alterations in ion content, leakage of damage markers, changes in biosynthetic capability. Morphological: histopathological evaluation	Rank correlation with *in vivo* findings for a wide range of chemicals	Gandolfi *et al.* (1989); Adams (1995); Fisher *et al.* (1995)
Isolated perfused liver (M)	Functional: biochemical and metabolic	Correlation with *in vivo* findings for a wide range of chemicals	Mehendale (1989); Wyman *et al.* (1995)

[a] Letters in parentheses indicate primary employment of system: S = screening system; M = mechanistic tool.
[b] NA = not available.
[c] Tyson and Stacey estimated in 1989 that there were 800 unpublished studies of a toxicological nature on cultured hepatocytes.

Table 21 Representative *in vitro* test systems for other target organ studies

Organ	System[a]	End-point	Evaluation	Reference
Pancreas	Isolated perfused intestines (M)	Functional: biochemical and metabolic	Correlation with *in vivo* findings for methylprednisolone	Mehendale (1989)
GI tract	Isolated perfused intestines (M)	Functional: biochemical and metabolic	Limited	Mehendale (1989)
Reticuloendothelial	Erythrocytes (S)	Observational: cytotoxicity Functional: inhibition of colony formation	Correlation with haemolytic effects	Stammati *et al.* (1981)
Testicular	Sertoli and germ cell cultures (S)	Observational: cytotoxicity Functional: steroid and hormone production	Correlation with *in vivo* effects for phytholate esters and glycol ethers	Garside (1988)
Adrenal gland	Primary adrenocortical ADC cell cultures (S, M)	Functional: cortisol production	Correlation with *in vivo* effects for three known ADC toxicants	Wolfgang *et al.* (1994)
Thyroid	Cultured thyroid cells (S, M)	Functional: biochemical and metabolic	Correlation with *in vivo* findings for a wide range of agents with thyroid-specific toxicity; evaluation against 'negative' compounds not significant	Brown (1988)

[a] Letters in parentheses indicate primary employment of system: S = screening system; M = mechanistic tool.

overviews of representative systems for a range of target organs: respiratory, nervous system, renal, cardiovascular, hepatic, pancreatic, gastro-intestinal and reticuloendothelial. These tables do not mention any of the new co-culture systems in which hepatocytes are 'joined up' in culture with a target cell type to produce a metabolically competent cellular system.

CONCLUSION

The tools are currently at hand (or soon will be) to provide the practising toxicologist with unique oppor-tunities both for identifying potentially toxic compounds in a much more rapid and efficient manner than before and for teasing apart the mechanisms underlying such toxicities on an integrated basis (from the level of the molecule to that of the intact organism). The *in vitro* systems overviewed here, once understood (by investig-ators and regulators) in how they function and fail (just as *in vivo* systems have come to be understood), will allow this to happen while reducing the need to have recourse to intact mammalian test systems. However, the intact animal models—and, indeed, man for pharmaceuti-cals—will still be an essential element in the safety assess-ment armamentarium for the foreseeable future.

REFERENCES

Abrahamson, S. and Lewis, E. B. (1971). The detection of mutations in *Drosophila melanogaster*. In Hollaender, A. (Ed.), *Chemical Mutagens. Principles and Methods of Their Detection*, Vol. 2. Plenum Press, New York, pp. 461–488.

Acosta, D., Sorensen, E. M. B., Anuforo, D. C., Mitchell, D. B., Ramos, K., Santone, K. S. and Smith, M. A. (1985). An *in vitro* approach to the study of target organ toxicity of drugs and chemicals. *In Vitro Cell. Devel. Biol.*, **21**, 495–504.

Adams, P. E. (1995). *In vitro* methods to study hepatic drug metabolism. In *Emphasis*. Corning Hazleton, Madison, WI, p. 6(2).

Aeschbacher, M., Reinhardt, C. A. and Zbinden, G. (1986). A rapid cell membrane permeability test using fluorescent dyes and flow cytometry. *Cell Biol. Toxicol.*, **2**, 247.

American Medical Association (1989). Public support for animals in research. *Am. Med. News*, 9 June.

Anderson, M. W. and Eling, T. E. (1976). Studies on the uptake, metabolism, and release of endogenous and exogenous chemicals by the use of the isolated perfused lung. *Environ. Health Perspect.*, **16**, 77–81.

Ashwood-Smith, M. J., Poulton, G. A., Barker, M. and Midenberger, M. (1980). 5-Methoxypsoralen, an ingredient in several suntan preparations, has lethal mutagenic and clastogenic properties. *Nature*, **285**, 407–409.

Babich, H., Martin-Alguacil, N. and Borenfreund, E. (1989). Comparisons of the cytotoxicities of dermatotoxicants to human keratinocytes and fibroblasts *in vitro*. In Goldberg, A. M. (Ed.), *In Vitro Toxicology: New Directions*. Mary Ann Liebert, New York, pp. 153–167.

Balls, M. and Horner, S. A. (1985). The FRAME interlaboratory program on *in vitro* cytotoxicology. *Food Chem. Toxicol.*, **23**, 205–213.

Barnard, N. D. (1989). A Draize alternative. *Anim. Agenda*, **6**, 45.

Bartnik, F. G., Pittermann, W. F., Mendorf, N., Tillmann, U. and Kunstler, K. (1989). Skin organ culture for the study of skin irritancy. Presented at the Third International Congress of Toxicology, Brighton, UK.

Bazzoli, A. S., Manson, J., Scott, W. J. and Wilson, J. G. (1977). The effects of thalidomide and two analogues on the regenerating forelimb of the newt. *J. Embryol. Exp. Morphol.*, **41**, 125–135.

Bell, E., Parenteau, N. L., Haimes, H. B., Gay, R. J., Kemp, P. D., Fofonoff, T. W., Mason, V. S., Kagan, D. T. and Swiderek, M. (1988). Testskin: A hybrid organism covered by a living human skin equivalent designed for toxicity and other testing. In Goldberg, A. M. (Ed.), *Progress in In Vitro Toxicology*. Mary Ann Liebert, New York, pp. 15–25.

Benassi, C. A., Angi, M. R., Salvalaoi, L. and Bettero, A. (1986). Histamine and leukotriene C4 release from isolated bovine sclerachoroid complex: a new *in vitro* ocular irritation test. *Chim. Agg.*, **16**, 631–634.

Best, J. B., Morita, M., Ragin, J., and Best, J., Jr. (1981). Acute toxic responses of the freshwater planarian, *Dugesia dorothocephala*, to methylmercury. *Bull. Environ. Contam. Toxicol.*, **27**, 49–54.

Bierkamper, G. G. (1982). *In vitro* assessment of neuromuscular toxicity. *Neurobehav. Toxicol. Teratol.*, **4**, 597–604.

Bockstahler, L. E., Coohill, T. P., Lytle, C. D., Moore, S. P., Cantwell, J. M. and Schmidt, B. J. (1982). Tumor virus induction and host cell capacity inactivation: possible *in vitro* test for photosensitizing chemicals. *J. Nat. Cancer Inst.*, **69**, 183–187.

Bondy, S. C. (1982). Neurotransmitter binding interactions as a screen for neurotoxicity. In Prasad, K. N. and Vernadakis, A. (Eds), *Mechanisms of Actions of Neurotoxic Substances*. Raven Press, New York, pp. 25–50.

Boogaard, P. J., Mulder, G. J. and Nagelkerke, J. F. (1989). Isolated proximal tubular cells from rat kidney as an *in vitro* model for studies on nephrotoxicity. *Toxicol. Appl. Pharmacol.*, **101**, 135–157.

Borenfreund, E. and Puerner, J. A. (1984). A simple quantitative procedure using monolayer cultures for cytotoxicity assays (HTD/NR-NE). *J. Tissue Cult. Methods*, **9**, 7–10.

Boyce, S. T., Hansbrough, J. F. and Norris, D. A. (1988). Cellular responses of cultured human epidermal keratinocytes as models of toxicity to human skin. In Goldberg, A. M. (Ed.), *Progress in In Vitro Toxicology*. Mary Ann Liebert, New York, pp. 27–37.

Braun, A. G. and Horowicz, P. B. (1983). Lectin-mediated attachment assays for teratogens. Results with 32 pesticides. *J. Toxicol. Environ. Health*, **11**, 275–286.

Brown, C. G. (1988). Application of thyroid cell culture to the study of thyrotoxicity. In Atterwill, C. K. and Steele, C. E. (Eds), *In Vitro Methods in Toxicology*. Cambridge University Press, New York, pp. 165–188.

Brown, N. A. and Fabro, S. (1981). Quantitation of rat embryonic development *in vitro*: a morphological scoring system. *Teratology*, **24**, 65–78.

Brown, S., Templeton, L., Prater, D. A. and Potter, C. J. (1989). Use of an *in vitro* haemolysis test to predict tissue irritancy in an intramuscular formulation. *J. Parent. Sci. Technol.*, **43**, 117–120.

Burka, J. F., Ali, M., McDonald, J. W. D. and Paterson, N. A. M. (1981). Immunological and non-immunological synthesis and release of prostaglandins and thromboxanes from isolated guinea pig trachea. *Prostaglandins*, **2**, 683–690.

Burton, A. B. G., York, M. and Lawrence, R. S. (1981). The *in vitro* assessment of severe eye irritants, *Food Cosmet. Toxicol.*, **19**, 471–480.

Cameron, I. L., Lawrence, W. C. and Lum, J. R. (1985). Medaka eggs as a model system for screening potential teratogens. In Prevention of Physical and Mental Congenital Defects, Part C, *Prog. Clin. Biol. Res.*, **198**, 163C, pp. 239–243.

Chan, K. Y. (1985). An *in vitro* alternative to the Draize test. In Goldberg, A. M. (Ed.), *In Vitro Toxicology. Alternative Methods in Toxicology*, Vol. 3. Mary Ann Liebert, New York, pp. 405–422.

Chasin, M., Scott, C., Shaw, C. and Persico, F. (1979). A new assay for the measurement of mediator release from rat peritoneal in most cells. *Int. Arch. Allergy Appl. Immunol.*, **58**, 1–10.

Chernoff, N. and Kavlock, R. J. (1980). A potential *in vivo* screen for the determination of teratogenic effects in mammals. *Teratology*, **21**, 33A–34A.

Clayton, R. M. (1979). In Rowan, A. N. and Stratmann, C. J. (Eds), *Alternatives in Drug Research*. Macmillan, London, p. 153.

Clayton, R. M. (1981) An *in vitro* system for teratogenicity testing. In Rowan, A. N. and Stratmann, C. J. (Eds), *The*

Use of Alternatives in Drug Research. University Park Press, Baltimore, pp. 153–173.

Clive, D., Johnson, K., Spector, J., Batson, A. and Brown, M. (1979). Validation and characterization of the L5178Y/TK mouse lymphoma mutagen assay system. *Mutat. Res.*, **59**, 61–108.

Cockroft, D. L. and Steele, C. E. (1989). Postimplantation embryo culture and its application to problems in teratology. In Atterwill, C. K. and Steele, C. E. (Eds), *In Vitro Methods in Toxicology*. Cambridge University Press, New York, pp. 365–389.

Cooper, J. F. (1975). Principles and applications of the Limulus test for pyrogen in parenteral drugs. *Bull. Parent. Drug Assoc.*, **3**, 122–130.

Cowley, G., Hager, M., Drew, L., Namuth, T., Wright, L., Murr, A., Abbot, N. and Robins, K. (1988). The battle over animal rights. *Newsweek*, 26 December.

Daniel, F. (1965). A simple microbiological method for demonstrating phototoxic compounds. *J. Invest. Dermatol.*, **44**, 259–263.

Dannenberg, A. M., Moore, K. G., Schofield, B. H., Higuchi, K., Kajjki, A., Au, K., Pula, P. J. and Bassett, D. P. (1987). Two new *in vitro* methods for evaluating toxicity in skin (employing short-term organ culture). In Goldberg, A. M. (Ed.), *Alternative Methods in Toxicology*, Vol. 5. Mary Ann Liebert, New York, pp. 115–128.

Daston, G. P. and D'Amato, R. A. (1989). *In vitro* techniques in teratology. In Mehlman, M. (Ed.), *Benchmarks: Alternative Methods in Toxicology*. Princeton Scientific, Princeton, NJ, pp. 79–109.

Davis, K. R., Schultz, T. W. and Dumont, J. N. (1981). Toxic and teratogenic effects of selected aromatic amines on embryos of the amphibian *Xenopus laevis*. *Arch. Environ. Contam. Toxicol.*, **10**, 371–391.

DeLeo, V., Midlarsky, L., Harber, L. C., Kong, B. M. and Salva, S. D. (1987). Surfactant-induced cutaneous primary irritancy: an *in vitro* model. In Goldberg, A. M. (Ed.), *Alternative Methods in Toxicology*, Vol. 5. Mary Ann Liebert, New York, pp. 129–138.

DeLeo, V., Hong, J., Scheide, S., Kong, B., DeSalva, S. and Bagley, D. (1988). Surfactant-induced cutaneous primary irritancy: an *in vitro* model-assay system development. In Goldberg, A. M. (Ed.), *Progress in In Vitro Toxicology*. Mary Ann Liebert, New York, pp. 39–43.

Drewes, C., Vining, E. and Callahan, C. (1984). Non-invasive electrophysiological monitoring: a sensitive method for detecting sublethal neurotoxicity in earthworms. *Environ. Toxicol. Chem.*, **3**, 559–607.

Dubin, N. H., De Blasi, M. C., *et al.* (1984). Development of an *in vitro* test for cytotoxicity in vaginal tissue: effect of ethanol on prostanoid release. In Goldberg, A. M. (Ed.), *Acute Toxicity Testing: Alternative Approaches. Alternative Methods in Toxicology*, Vol. 2. Mary Ann Liebert, New York, pp. 127–138.

Durston, A., Van de Wiel, F., Mummery, C. and de Loat, S. (1985). *Dictyostelium discoideum* as a test system for screening for teratogens. *Teratology*, **32**, 21A.

Ekwall, B., Bondesson, I., Castell, J. V., Gomez-Lechon, M. J., Hellberg, S., Hagberg, J., Jover, R., Ponsoda, X., Romert, L., Stenberg, K. and Watum, E. (1989). Cytotoxicity evaluation of the first ten MEIC chemicals: acute lethal toxicity in man predicted by cytotoxicity in five cellular assays and by oral LD50 tests in rodents. *J. Anim. Tech. Lab. Assoc.*, **17**, 83–100.

Elgebaly, S. A., Nabawi, K., Herkbert, N., O'Rourke, J. and Kruetzer, D. L. (1985). Characterization of neutrophil and monocyte specific chemotactic factors derived from the cornea in response to injury. *Invest. Ophthalmol. Vis. Sci.*, **26**, 320.

Enslein, K. (1984). Estimation of toxicology end points by structure–activity relationships, *Pharmacol. Rev.*, **36**, 131–134.

Enslein, K., Lander, T. R., Tomb, M. E. and Craig, P. N. (1983a). *A Predictive Model for Estimating Rat Oral LD50 Values*. Princeton Scientific, Princeton, NJ.

Enslein, K., Lander, T. R. and Strange, J. L. (1983b). Teratogenesis: a statistical structure–activity model. *Teratog Carcinog Mutagen.*, **3**, 289–309.

Enslein, K., Borgstedt, H. H., Blake, B. W. and Hart, J. B. (1987). Prediction of rabbit skin irritation severity by structure–activity relationships. *In Vitro Toxicol.*, **1**, 129–147.

Enslein, K., Blake, V. W., Tuzzeo, T. M., Borgstedt, H. H., Hart, J. B. and Salem, H. (1988). Estimation of rabbit eye irritation scores by structure–activity equations. *In Vitro Toxicol.*, **2**, 1–14.

Eurell, T. E. and Meachum, S. H. (1994). *In vitro* evaluation of ocular irritants using tissue isoelectric focusing protein profiles from human, rabbit, and bovine corneal specimens. *Toxicol. Methods*, **4**, 66–75.

Faustman, E. M. (1988). Short-term tests for teratogens. *Mutat. Res.*, **205**, 355–384.

Firestone, B. A. and Guy, R. H. (1986). Approaches to the prediction of dermal absorption and potential cutaneous toxicity. In Goldberg, A. M. (Ed.), *In Vitro Toxicology. Alternative Methods in Toxicology*, Vol. 3. Mary Ann Liebert, New York, pp. 526–536.

Fisher, R. L., Hasal, S. J., Sanuik, J. T., Gandolfi, A. J. and Brendel, K. (1995). Determination of optimal incubation media and suitable slice diameters in precision-cut tissue slice culture, Part 2. *Toxicol. Methods*, **5**, 115–130.

Flint, O. P. (1989). Reply to Letter to the Editor. *Toxicol. Appl. Pharmacol.*, **99**, 176–180.

Flint, O. P. and Orton, T. C. (1984). An *in vitro* assay for taratogens with cultures of rat embryo midbrain and limb bud cells. *Toxicol. Appl. Pharmacol.*, **76**, 383–395.

Frazier, J. M. (1988). Update: a critical evaluation of alternatives to acute ocular irritancy testing. In Goldberg, A. M. (Ed.), *Progress in In Vitro Toxicology*. Mary Ann Liebert, New York, pp. 67–75.

Frazier, J. M. (1992). *In Vitro Toxicity Testing*. Marcel Dekker, New York.

Frazier, J. M., Gad, S. C., Goldberg, A. M. and McCulley, J. P. (1987) *A Critical Evaluation of Alternatives to Acute Ocular Irritation Testing*. Mary Ann Liebert, New York.

Frosch, P. J. and Czarnetzki, B. M. (1987). Surfactants cause *in vitro* chemotaxis and chemokinesis of human neutrophils. *J. Invest. Dermatol.*, **88**(3), Suppl., 52s.

Gad, S. C. (1999). Defining product safety information and testing requirements. In Gad, S. C. (Ed.), *Handbook of Product Safety Evaluation*, 2nd Edn. Marcel Dekker, New York, pp. 1–24.

Gad, S. C. (1988a). An approach to the design and analysis of screening data in toxicology. *J. Am. Coll. Toxicol.*, **7**, 127–138.

Gad, S. C. (1989a). Principles of screening in toxicology: with special emphasis on applications to neurotoxicology. *J. Am. Coll. Toxicol.*, **8**, 21–27.

Gad, S. C. (1989b). Statistical analysis of screening studies in toxicology: with special emphasis on neurotoxicology. *J. Am. Coll. Toxicol.*, **8**, 171–183.

Gad, S. C. (1989c). A tier testing strategy incorporating *in vitro* testing methods for pharmaceutical safety assessment. *Humane Innov. Alt. Ani. Exp.*, **3**, 75–79.

Gad, S. C. (1990a). Industrial applications for *in vitro* toxicity testing methods: a tier testing strategy for product safety assessment. In Frazier, J. (Ed.), *In Vitro Toxicity Testing*, pp. 253–280 Marcel Dekker, New York.

Gad, S. C. (1990b). Recent developments in replacing, reducing and refining animal use in toxicologic research and testing. *Fundam. Appl. Toxicol.*, **15**, 8–16.

Gad, S. C. (1994). *In Vitro Toxicology*. Raven Press, New York.

Gad, S. C. (1996). Preclinical toxicity testing in the development of new therapeutic agents. *Scand. J. Lab. Anim. Sci.*, **23**, 299–314.

Gad, S. C. and Chengelis, C. P. (1992). *Animal Models in Toxicology*. Marcel Dekker, New York.

Gad, S. C. and Chengelis, C. P. (1997). *Acute Toxicology*, 2nd edn. Academic Press, San Diego, CA.

Gad, S. C., Leslie, S. W., Brown, R. G. and Smith, R. V. (1977). Inhibitory effects of dithiothreitol and sodium bisulfate on isolated rat ileum and atrium. *Life Sci.*, **20**, 657–664.

Gad, S. C., Leslie, S. W. and Acosta, D. (1979). Inhibitory actions of butylated hydroxytoluene (BHT) on isolated rat ileal, atrial and perfused heart preparations. *Toxicol. Appl. Pharmacol.*, **48**, 45–52.

Gad, S. C., Dunn, B. J., Dobbs, D. W. and Walsh, R. D. (1986). Development and validation of an alternative dermal sensitization test: the mouse ear swelling test (MEST). *Toxicol. Appl. Pharmacol.*, **84**, 93–114.

Gales, Y. A., Gross, C. L., Karebs, R. C. and Smith, W. J. (1989). Flow cytometric analysis of toxicity by alkylating agents in human epidermal keratinocytes. In Goldberg, A. M. (Ed.), *In Vitro Toxicology: New Directions*. Mary Ann Liebert, New York, pp. 169–174.

Gandolfi, A. J., Brendel, K., Tisher, R., Azri, S., Hanan, G., Waters, S. J., Hanzlick, R. P. and Thomas, C. M. (1989). Utilization of precision-cut liver slices to profile and rank-order potential hepatotoxins. Presented at the PMA-Drusafe East Spring Meeting, 2 May.

Garside, D. A. (1988). Use of *in vitro* techniques to investigate the action of testicular toxicants. In Atterwill, C. K. and Steele, C. E. (Eds), *In Vitro Methods in Toxicology*. Cambridge University Press, New York, pp. 411–423.

Gebhart, D. O. E. (1972). The use of the chick embryo in applied teratology. In Woolam, D. H. M. (Ed.), *Advances in Teratology*, Vol. 5. Academic Press, London, pp. 97–111.

Gombar, V. K., Borgstedt, H. H., Enslein, K., Hart, J. B. and Blake, B. W. (1990). A QSAR model of teratogenesis. *Quant. Struct.–Activity Relat.*, **10**, 306–332.

Gordon, V. C. and Bergman, H. C. (1986). *Eytex, an In Vitro Method for Evaluation of Optical Irritancy*. National Testing Corporation Report, 26.

Gordon, V. C., Kelly, C. P. and Bergman, H. C. (1989). SKIN-TEX, an *in vitro* method for determining dermal irritation. Presented at the International Congress of Toxicology, Brighton, UK.

Harman, A. W. and Fischer, L. J. (1983). Hamster hepatocytes in culture as a model for acetaminophen toxicity: studies with inhibitors of drug metabolism. *Toxicol. Appl. Pharmacol.*, **71**, 330–341.

Harpur, E. S. (1988). Ototoxicity. In Atterwill, C. K. and Steele, C. E. (Eds), *In Vitro Methods In Toxicology*. Cambridge University Press, New York, pp. 37–58.

Harter, M. L., Felkner, I. C. and Song, P. S. (1976). Near-UV effects of 5,7-dimethoxycoumarin in *Bacillus subtilis*. *Photochem. Photobiol.*, **24**, 491–493.

Homburger, F. and Goldberg, A. M. (1985). *In Vitro Embryotoxicity and Teratogenicity Tests*. Mary Ann Liebert, New York.

Hooisma, J. (1982). Tissue Culture and Neurotoxicology. *Neurobehav. Toxicol. Teratol.*, **4**, 617–622.

ICCVAM (1997). *Validation and Regulatory Acceptance of Toxicological Test Methods*. NIEHS, Research Triangle Park, NC.

IRAG (1993). *Washington Group Reports*. IRAG, Washington, DC.

Jacaruso, R. B., Barlett, M. A., Carson, S. and Trombetta, L. D. (1985). Release of histamine from rat peritoneal cells *in vitro* as an index of irritational potential. *J. Toxicol. Cut. Ocular Toxicol.*, **4**, 39–48.

Jackson, E. M. and Goldner, R. (1989). *Irritant Contact Dermatitis*. Marcel Dekker, New York.

Johnson, E. M. (1989). Problems in validation of *in vitro* developmental toxicity assays. *Fundam. Appl. Toxicol.*, **13**, 863–867.

Johnson, E. M., Gorman, R. M., Gabel, B. E. C. and George, M. E. (1982). The *Hydra attenuata* system for detection of teratogenic hazards. *Teratog. Carcinog. Mutagen.*, **2**, 263–276.

Johnson, E. M., Newman, L. M. and Fu, L. (1989). Letter to the Editor. *Toxicol. Appl. Pharmacol.*, **99**, 173–176.

Jumblatt, M. M. and Neufeld, A. H. (1985). A tissue culture model of the human corneal epthelium. In Goldberg, A. M. (Ed.), *In Vitro Toxicology, Alternative Methods in Toxicology*, Vol. 3. Mary Ann Liebert, New York, pp. 391–404.

Kao, J., Hall, J. and Holland, J. M. (1982). Quantitation of cutaneous toxicity: an *in vitro* approach using skin organ culture. *Toxicol. Appl. Pharmacol.*, **68**, 206–217.

Keller, S. J. and Smith, M. (1982). Animal virus screens for potential teratogens: poxvirus morphogenesis. *Teratog. Carcinog. Mutagen.*, **2**, 361–374.

Kemp, R. V., Meredith, R. W. J., Gamble, S. and Frost, M. (1983). A rapid cell culture technique for assaying to toxicity of deteragent based products *in vitro* as a possible screen for high irritants *in vivo*. *Cytobios*, **36**, 153–159.

Kemp, R. V., Meredith, R. W. J. and Gamble, S. (1985). Toxicity of commercial products on cells in suspension: a possible screen for the Draize eye irritation test. *Food Chem. Toxicol.*, **23**, 267–270.

Kennah, H. E., Albulescu, D., Hignet, S. and Barrow, C. S. (1989). A critical evaluation of predicting ocular irritancy potential from an *in vitro* cytotoxicity assay. *Fundam Appl. Toxicol.*, **12**, 281–290.

Kerster, H. W. and Schaeffer, D. J. (1983). Brine shrimp (*Artemia salina*) Nauplia as a teratogen test system. *Ecotoxicol. Environ. Saf.*, **7**, 342–349.

Kochhar, D. M. (1981). Embryo explants and organ cultures in screening of chemicals for teratogenic effects. In Kimmel, C.

A. and Buelbe-Saw, J. (Eds), *Developmental Toxicology*. Raven Press, New York, pp. 303–319.

Kochhar, D. M. and Aydelotte, M. B. (1974). Susceptible stages and abnormal morphogenesis in the developing mouse limb, analyzed in organ culture after transplacental exposure to vitamin A (retinoic acid) *J. Embryol. Exp. Morphol.*, **31**, 721–734.

Kontur, P. J., Hoffman, P. C. and Heller, A. (1987). Neurotoxic effects of methamphetamine assessed in three-dimensional reaggregate tissue cultures. *Dev. Brain Res.*, **31**, 7–14.

Kotzin, B. L. and Baker, R. F. (1972). Selective inhibition of genetic transcription in sea urchin embryos. *J. Cell. Biol.*, **55**, 74–81.

Kurack, G., Vossen, P., Deboyser, D., Goethals, F. and Roberfubid, M. (1986). An *in vitro* model for acute toxicity screening using hepatocytes freshly isolated from adult mammals. In Goldberg, A. M. (Ed.) *In Vitro Toxicology*, pp. 235–242. Mary Ann Liebert, New York.

Lamont, G. S., Bagley, D. M., Kong, B. M. and DeSalva, S. J. (1989). Developing an alternative to the Draize skin test: comparison of human skin cell responses to irritants *in vitro*. In Goldberg, A. M. (Ed.), *In Vitro Toxicology: New Directions*. Mary Ann Liebert, New York, pp. 175–181.

Lander, T., Enslein, K., Craig, P. and Tomb, N. (1984). Validation of a structure–activity model of rat oral LD50. In Goldberg, A. M. (Ed.), *Acute Toxicity Testing: Alternative Approaches*. Mary Ann Liebert, New York, pp. 183–184.

Lei, H., Carroll, K., Au, L. and Krag, S. S. (1986). An *in vitro* screen for potential inflammatory agents using cultured fibroblasts. In Goldberg, A. M. (Ed.), *In Vitro Toxicology. Alternative Methods in Toxicology*, Vol. 3. Mary Ann Liebert, New York, pp. 74–85.

Leighton, J., Nassauer, J., Tchao, R. and Verdon, J. (1983). Development of a procedure using the chick egg as an alternative to the Draize test. In Goldberg, A. M. (Ed.), *Product Safety Evaluation. Alternative Methods in Toxicology*, Vol. 1. Mary Ann Liebert, New York, pp. 165–177.

Lijinksy, W. (1988). Importance of animal experiments in carcinogenesis research. *Environ. Mol. Mutagen.*, **11**, 307–314.

Luepke, N. P. (1985) Hen's egg chorioallantoic membrane test for irritation potential. *Food Chem. Toxicol.*, **23**, 287–291.

McAuliffe, D. J., Hasan, T., Parrish, J. A. and Kochevar, I. E. (1986). Determination of photosensitivity by an *in vitro* assay as an alternative to animal testing. In Goldberg, A. M. (Ed.), *In Vitro Toxicology*. Mary Ann Liebert, New York, pp. 30–41.

MacCrimmon, H. R. and Kwain, W. H. (1969). Influences of light on early development and meristic characters in the rainbow trout (*Salmo gairdneri* Richardson). *Can. J. Zool.*, **47**, 631–637.

Maurice, D. and Singh, T. (1986). A permeability test for acute corneal toxicity. *Toxicol. Lett.*, **31**, 125–130.

Mehendale, H. M. (1989). Application of isolated organ techniques in toxicology. In Hayes, A. W. (Ed.), *Principles and Methods of Toxicology*. Raven Press, New York, pp. 699–740.

Meyer, D. R. and McCulley, J. P. (1988). Acute and protracted injury to cornea epithelium as an indication of the biocompatibility of various pharmaceutical vehicles. In Goldberg, A. M. (Ed.), *Progress in In Vitro Toxicology*. Mary Ann Liebert, New York, pp. 215–235.

Miller, A. E., Jr, and Levis, W. R. (1973). Studies on the contact sensitization of man with simple chemicals. I. Specific lymphocyte transformation in response to dinitrochlorobenzene sensitization. *J. Invest. Dermatol.*, **61**, 261–269.

Milner, J. E. (1970). *In vitro* lymphocyte responses in contact hypersensitivity. *J. Invest. Dermatol.*, **55**, 34–38.

Milner, J. E. (1971). *In vitro* lymphocyte responses in contact hypersensitivity II. *J. Invest. Dermatol.*, **56**, 349–352.

Milner, J. E. (1983). *In vitro* tests for delayed skin hypersensitivity: lymphokine production in allergic contact dermatitis. In Marzulli, F. N. and Maibach, H. D. (Eds), *Dermatotoxicology*. Hemisphere, New York, pp. 185–192.

Morison, W. L., McAuliffe, D. J., Parrish, J. A. and Bloch, K. J. (1982). *In vitro* assay for phototoxic chemicals, *J. Invest. Dermatol.*, **78**, 460–463.

Muir, C. K. (1984). A simple method to assess surfactant-induced bovine corneal opacity *in vitro*: preliminary findings. *Toxicol. Lett.*, **23**, 199–203.

Muir, C. K., Flower, C. and Van Abbe, N. J. (1983). A novel approach to the search for *in vitro* alternatives to *in vivo* eye irritancy testing. *Toxicol. Lett.*, **18**, 1–5.

Mummery, C. L., van den Brink, C. E., van der Saag, P. T. and de Loat, S. W. (1984). A short-term screening test for teratogens using differentiating neuroblastoma cells *in vitro*. *Teratology*, **29**, 271–279.

Naughton, G. K., Jacob, L. and Naughton, B. A. (1989). A physiological skin model for *in vitro* toxicity studies. In Goldberg, A. M. (Ed.), *Progress in In Vitro Toxicology*. Mary Ann Liebert, New York, pp. 183–189.

Neubert, D. (1982). The use of culture techniques in studies on prenatal toxicity. *Pharmacol. Ther.*, **18**, 397–434.

Neuhauser, E., Durkin, P., Malecki, M. and Antara, M. (1985a). Comparative toxicity of ten organic chemicals to four earthworm species. *Comp. Biochem. Physiol.*, **83C**, 197–200.

Neuhauser, E., Loehr, C., Malecki, M., Milligan, D. and Durkin, P. (1985b). The toxicity of selected organic chemicals to the earthworm *Eisenia fetida*. *J. Environ. Qual.*, **14**, 383–388.

Neuhauser, E., Loehr, C. and Malecki, M. (1986). Contact and artificial soil tests using earthworms to evaluate the impact of wastes in soil. In Petros, J., Lacy, W. and Conway, R. C. (Eds), *Hazardous and Industrial Solid Waste Testing: Fourth Symposium*. ASTM STP 886. American Society for Testing and Materials, Philadelphia, PA, pp. 192–202.

North-Root, H., Yackovich, K., Demetrulias, F. J., Gucula, N. and Heinze, J. E. (1982). Evaluation of an *in vitro* cell toxicity test using rabbit corneal cells to predict the eye irritation potential of surfactants. *Toxicol. Lett.*, **14**, 207–212.

Oliver, G. J. A. and Pemberton, N. A. (1985). An *in vitro* epidermal slice technique for identifying chemicals with potential for severe cutaneous effects. *Food Chem. Toxicol.*, **23**, 229–232.

Parce, J. W., Owicki, J. C., Kercso, D. M., Sigal, G. B., Wada, H. G., Muir, V. C., Bousse, L. J., Ross, K. L., Sikic, B. I. and McConnell, H. M. (1989). Detection of cell-affecting agents with a silicon biosensor. *Science*, **246**, 243–247.

Placke, M. E. and Fisher, G. L. (1987). Adult peripheral lung organ culture—a model for respiratory tract toxicology. *Toxicol. Appl. Pharmacol.*, **90**, 284–298.

PMA/Drusafe *In Vitro* Task Force (1994). A collaborative evaluation of an *in vitro* muscle irritation assay. *Toxicol. Methods*, **4**, 215–223.

Prottey, C. and Ferguson, T. F. M. (1976). The effect of surfactants upon rat peritoneal mast cells *in vitro*. *Food Chem. Toxicol.*, **14**, 425.

Reinhardt, C. A., Pelli, D. A. and Zbinden, G. (1985). Interpretation of cell toxicity data for the estimation of potential irritation. *Food Chem. Toxicol.*, **23**, 247–252.

Reinhardt, C. A., Aeschbacher, M., Bracker, M. and Spengler, J. (1987). Validation of three cell toxicity tests and the hen's egg test with guinea pig eye and human skin irritation data. In Goldberg, A. M. (Ed.), *In Vitro Toxicology—Approaches to Validation. Alternative Methods in Toxicology*, Vol. 5. Mary Ann Liebert, New York, pp. 463–470.

Reiser, K. M. and Last, J. A. (1979). Silicosis and fibrogenesis: fact and artifact. *Toxicology*, **13**, 51–72.

Roberts, R. and Dorough, H. (1984). Relative toxicities of chemicals to the earthworm *Eisenia foetida*. *Environ. Toxicol.*, **3**, 67–78.

Roberts, R. and Dorough, H. (1985). Hazards of chemicals to earthworms. *Environ. Toxicol. Chem.*, **4**, 307–323.

Rofe, P. C. (1971). Tissue culture and toxicology. *Food Cosmet. Toxicol.*, **9**, 685–696.

Roth, J. A. (1980). Use of perfused lung in biochemical toxicology. *Rev. Biochem. Toxicol.*, **1**, 287–309.

Ruben, Z., Fuller, G. C. and Knodle, S. G. (1984). Disobutamide-induced cytoplasmic vacuoles in cultured dog coronary artery muscle cells, *Arch. Toxicol.*, **55**, 206–212.

Russell, W. M. S. and Burch, R. L. (1959). *The Principles of Humane Experimental Technique*. Methuen, London.

Rylander, L. A., Phelps, J. S., Gandolfi, A. J. and Brendel, K. (1987). *In vitro* nephrotoxicity: response of isolated renal tubules to cadmium chloride and dichlorovinyl cysteine. *In Vitro Toxicol.*, **1**, 111–127.

Salem, H. (1995) *Animal Test Alternatives*. Marcel Dekker, New York.

Saxen, L. (1984). Test *in vitro* for teratogenicity. In Gorrod, J. W. (Ed.), *Testing for Toxicity*. Taylor and Francis, London, pp. 185–197.

Saxen, L. and Saksela, E. (1971). Transmission and spread of embrymic induction. Exclusion of an assimilatory transmission mechanism in kidney tubule induction. *Exp. Cell Res.*, **66**, 369–377.

Scaife, M. C. (1982). An investigation of detergent action on *in vitro* and possible correlations with *in vivo* data. *Int. J. Cosmet. Sci.*, **4**, 179–193.

Selling, J. and Ekwall, B. (1985). Screening for eye irritancy using cultured Hela cells. *Xenobiotica*, **15**, 713–717.

Shadduck, J. A., Everitt, J. and Bay, P. (1985). Use of *in vitro* cytotoxicity to rank ocular irritation of six surfactants. In Goldberg, A. M. (Ed.), *In Vitro Toxicology: Alternative Methods in Toxicology*, Vol. 3. Mary Ann Liebert, New York, pp. 641–649.

Shadduck, J. A., Render, J., Everitt, J., Meccoli, R. A. and Essexsorlie, D. (1987). An approach to validation: comparison of six materials in three tests. In Goldberg, A. M. (Ed.), *In Vitro Toxicology—Approaches to Validation. Alternative Methods in Toxicology*, Vol. 5. Mary Ann Liebert, New York.

Shopsis, C. and Eng, B. (1985). Uridine uptake and cell growth cytotoxicity tests: comparison, applications and mechanistic studies. *J. Cell. Biol.*, **101**, 87a.

Shopsis, C. and Sathe, S. (1984). Uridine uptake inhibition as a cytotoxicity test: correlation with the Draize test. *Toxicology*, **29**, 195–206.

Sieber-Blum, M. F. (1985). Differentiation of avian neural crest cells *in vitro* (quail, chick, rodent). *Crisp Data Base*, HD15311–04.

Silverman, J. (1983). Preliminary findings on the use of protozoa (*Tetrahymena thermophila*) as models of ocular irritation testing in rabbits. *Lab. Anim. Sci.*, **33**, 56–59.

Simons, P. J. (1981). An alternative to the Draize test. In Rowan, A. N. and Stratmann, C. J. (Eds), *The Use of Alternatives in Drug Research.*, pp. 147–152. Macmillan, London.

Singer, P. (1975). *Animal Liberation: A New Ethic for Our Treatment of Animals*. Random House, New York.

Sleet, R. B. and Brendel, K. (1985). Homogenous populations of *Artemia nauplii* and their potential use for *in vitro* testing in developmental toxicology. *Teraog. Carcinog. Mutagen.*, **5**, 41–54.

Smith, M. A., Acosta, D. and Bruckner, J. V. (1986). Development of a primary culture system of rat kidney cortical cells to evaluate the nephrotoxicity of xenobiotics. *Food Chem. Toxicol.*, **24**, 551–556.

Smith, M. A., Acosta, D. and Bruckner, J. V. (1987). Cephaloridine toxicity in primary cultures of rat renal epithelial cells. *In Vitro Toxicol.*, **1**, 23–29.

Smith, M. A., Hewitt, W. R. and Hook, J. (1988). *In Vitro* methods in renal toxicology. In Atterwill, C. K. and Steele, C. E. (Eds), *In Vitro Methods in Toxicology*. Cambridge University Press, New York, pp. 13–36.

Smith, M. K., Kimmel, G. L., Korchhar, D. M., Shepard, T. H., Spielberg, S. P. and Wilson, J. C. (1983). A selection of candidate compounds for *in vitro* teratogenesis test validation. *Teratog. Carcinog. Mutagen.*, **3**, 461–480.

Soto, R. J., Servi, M. J. and Gordon, V. C. (1988). Evaluation of an alternative method of ocular irritation. In Goldberg, A. M. (Ed.), *Progress in In Vitro Toxicology*. Mary Ann Liebert, New York, pp. 289–296.

Spencer, P. S., Crain, S. M., Bornstein, M. B., Peterson, E. R. and van de Water, T. (1986). Chemical neurotoxicity: detection and analysis in organotypic cultures of sensory and motor systems. *Food Chem. Toxicol.*, **24**, 539–544.

Stammati, A. P., Silano, V. and Zucco, F. (1981). Toxicology investigations with cell culture systems. *Toxicology*, **20**, 91–153.

Stenersen, J. (1979). Action of pesticides on earthworms. Part I: toxicity of cholinesterase-inhibiting insecticides to earthworms as evaluated by laboratory tests. *Pestic. Sci.*, **10**, 66–74.

Swisher, D. A., Prevo, M. E. and Ledger, P. W. (1988). The MTT *in vitro* cytotoxicity test: correlation with cutaneous irritancy in two animal models. In Goldberg, A. M. (Ed.), *Progress in In Vitro Toxicology*. Mary Ann Liebert, New York, pp. 265–269.

Tchao, R. (1988). Trans-epithelial permeability of fluorescein *in vitro* as an assay to determine eye irritants. In Goldberg, A. M. (Ed.), *Progress in In Vitro Toxicology*. Mary Ann Liebert, New York, pp. 271–284.

Thulin, H. and Zacharian, H. (1972). The leukocyte migration test in chromium hypersensitivity. *J. Invest. Dermatol.*, **58**, 55–58.

Tyson, C. A. and Stacey, N. H. (1989). *In vitro* screens from CNS, liver and kidney for systemic toxicity. In Mehlman, M. (Ed.), *Benchmarks: Alternative Methods in Toxicology*. Princeton Scientific, Princeton, NJ, pp. 111–136.

Uyeki, E. M., Ashkar, A. E., Shoeman, D. W. and Bisel, J. U. (1977). Acute toxicity of benzene inhalation of hemopoietic precursor cells. *Toxicol. Appl. Pharmacol.*, **40**, 49–57.

Volpe, L. S., Biagioni, T. M. and Marquis, J. K. (1985). *In vitro* modulation of bovine caudata muscarinic receptor number by organophosphates and carbamates. *Toxicol. Appl. Pharmacol.*, **78**, 226–234.

Watanabe, M., Watanabe, K., Suzuki, K., Nikaido, O., Sugahara, T., Ishii, I. and Konishi, H. (1988). *In vitro* cytotoxicity test using primary cells derived from rabbit eye is useful as an alternative for Draize testing. In Goldberg, A. M. (Ed.), *Progress in In Vitro Toxicology*. Mary Ann Liebert, New York, pp. 285–290.

Williams, G. M., Dunkel, V. C. and Ray, V. A. (Eds) (1983). *Cellular Systems for Toxicity Testing. Ann. N.Y. Acad. Sci.*, **407**.

Williams, P. D., Masters, B. G., Evans, L. D., Laska, D. A. and Hattendorf, G. H. (1987). An *in vitro* model for assessing muscle irritation due to parenteral antibiotics. *Fundam. Appl. Toxicol.*, **9**, 10–17.

Wilson, J. G. (1978). Survey of *in vitro* systems; their potential for use in teratogenicity screening. In Wilson, J. G. and Frazer, F. C. (Eds.), *Handbook of Teratology*, pp 135–154. Plenum Press, New York.

Wolfgang, G. H. I., Vernetti, L. A. and MacDonald, J. R. (1994). Isolation and use of primary adrenocortical cells from guinea pigs, dogs and monkeys for *in vitro* toxicity studies. *Toxicol. Methods*, **4**, 149–160.

Wyman, J., Stokes, J. S., Goehring, M., Buring, M. and Moore, T. (1995). Data collection interface for isolated perfused rat liver: Recording oxygen consumption, perfusion pressure and pH. *Toxicol. Methods*, **5**, 1–14.

Young, M. F., Trombetta, L. D. and Sophia, J. V. (1986). Correlative *in vitro* and *in vivo* study of skeletal muscle irritancy. *Toxicologist*, **6**, 1225.

Zbinden, G. (1987). *Predictive Value of Animal Studies in Toxicology*. Centre for Medicines Research, Carshalton.

Chapter 20
Antidotal Studies

Nicholas Bateman and Timothy C. Marrs

C O N T E N T S

INTRODUCTION

An antidote is defined in *Webster's Ninth New Collegiate Dictionary* (Webster, 1986) as a remedy to counteract the effects of a poison. Remedies in this sense are usually visualized to be specific chemical entities, but sometimes the definition is broadened to include non-specific measures such as charcoal, haemoperfusion, dialysis and so on (Bateman and Chaplin, 1989). This chapter deals solely with chemical antidotes.

Experimental studies on antidotes are carried out for the same reasons as on other drugs, to demonstrate efficacy and to assess safety in use. However, antidotes differ from many other drugs both in the way they are used and in the manner in which their effectiveness and toxicity need to be assessed. Antidotes are usually only used in life-threatening situations and are often administered as a single dose or, at most, as a short treatment course. They are sometimes used, principally under conditions of war, in a prospective manner, but more often after exposure to the toxin. This means that many of the toxicological data required for drugs used over longer periods in less serious diseases may well be considered unnecessary by many people. Indeed, many antidotes, particularly older ones, have been introduced only after minimal animal toxicity studies and in many cases the impetus to the introduction of antidotes has been military. A further difference from many other drugs is that randomized clinical trials, including placebo groups, are rarely possible because of ethical considerations. Although trials in humans can be designed, these often use a retrospective control group or a parallel group treated with an established antidote and may be less than totally satisfactory from a scientific point of view. This often means that one is more than usually reliant on animal studies for the evaluation of efficacy.

THE POISON

A programme of antidote development requires some knowledge of the toxicology of the poison. There are two purposes for this: first, to identify an antidotal approach that is likely to be successful, and second, to permit the design and interpretation of an antidote efficacy study.

The acute toxicity of a poison compound has traditionally been quantified by the LD_{50}. The use of the LD_{50} test has been criticized on both humane and scientific grounds (e.g. British Toxicology Society, 1984; Society of Toxicology, 1989), but most antidotal efficacy studies use experimental designs that require the use of this test. When the LD_{50} is carried out, the slope of the log dose–probit mortality line should be recorded because the slope is often changed by antidotal treatment (Natoff and Reiff, 1970); furthermore, the slope will be useful in calculating the dosing schedules of the poison in studies in which any antidote is to be administered. Ideally, acute toxicity studies should be carried out in several species of animal. Animals may show marked differences between one another and from humans in the quantitative or qualitative toxicity of the poison; such species differences will clearly influence the choice of a suitable animal model for experimental work.

Where the objective of the treatment is the amelioration of a non-lethal but crippling effect, for example, blindness in methanol poisoning, measurement of the ED_{50} (lowest dose giving the effect of interest in 50% of the animals) for the effect will be needed. In such cases species sensitivity to the appropriate toxic effect will be an important consideration in the choice of species in efficacy studies.

The subacute or chronic toxicity of a poison is not usually of interest specifically in the design of experiments to measure the effects of antidotes. However, delayed effects from acute toxicity may be important, for example the delayed exposure toxicity of carbon monoxide (Garland and Pearce, 1967: Werner *et al.*, 1985) and the 'intermediate syndrome' associated with acute organophosphorus toxicity (Senanayake and Karalleide, 1992). The ED_{50} may be a suitable measure of toxicity where the delayed effects are non-lethal.

It is reassuring for the toxicologist to know that the target organ is the same in an animal species as in man. Sometimes an indication of this may be gleaned from acute lethality studies, but on most occasions the effect of sublethal doses of the poison will have to be studied. This is usually necessary since death of some of the animals during acute lethal toxicity studies makes interpretation of the histology, a useful indicator of organs specific effects, difficult. Mechanistic studies on particular cell types within the target organ, while desirable and possibly helpful in the initial design of an antidotal approach, are in practice rarely necessary in the assessment of antidote efficacy.

Elucidation of the metabolic pathways of a poison is most useful where conversion to a toxic metabolite is a prerequisite for toxicity. In such instances it is essential that the species used in experimental studies handle the poison in a similar manner to man. In the situation where the antidote and poison directly react together, for example chelating agents and metals, differences in metabolic handling of the toxin or antidote are likely to be less important. Knowledge of the pharmacokinetics of the poison in animals and man, while less useful in identifying an antidotal mechanism, may be useful in designing animal efficacy studies, particularly with respect to the choice of an animal model and the choice of appropriate dosing regimes.

INTRODUCTION OF NEW ANTIDOTES

The introduction of new antidotes has only rarely occurred by the chance finding of antidotal action, for example, as part of a screening programme. It has usually been based on an extensive substructure of the knowledge of the mechanism of action of the poison. With application of pharmacological, biochemical or chemical expertise it has then been possible to find out a way in which the poison could be detoxified or its toxic effects reversed. If one considers the introduction of antidotes at present available, it is clear that most antidotes evolved from the study of an antidote which was less than optimal, a 'lead' compound (Burger, 1982). Analogous compounds were then studied and usually the one with the best therapeutic index was eventually adopted as the standard treatment. Examples of this approach include the introduction of sodium nitrite, a component of the classic therapy for cyanide which arose from the discovery by Pedigo (1888) of the usefulness of amyl nitrite in cyanide poisoning. Another example is the use of acetylcysteine for the treatment of paracetamol poisoning,

which followed the earlier introduction of cysteamine (Prescott, 1983). The discovery of the oxime organophosphorus antidotes 2-PAM, obidoxime and H16 followed from the discovery of the antidotal effect of hydroxylamine (Bismuth *et al.*, 1992). The introduction of dicobalt acetate as a cyanide antidote by Paulet (1960) was an attempt to improve upon the experimentally effective, but toxic, inorganic cobalt salts. Thus probably the single most challenging part of the process of bringing new antidotes into clinical practice is the discovery of 'lead' antidotes, and this is usually dependent on an hypothesis for the mechanism of toxicity of a particular poison.

MECHANISM OF ANTIDOTAL ACTION

It is difficult to produce a classification of antidotes that is satisfactory in all respects, although a number of workers have attempted to do so (Marrs, 1987, 1992; Bismuth, 1987; Bateman and Chaplin, 1989). To some extent this is because the mode of action of certain well known antidotes is controversial, while others appears to act in more than one way.

Table 1 Mechanism of action of antidotes (with examples of toxins in brackets)

Antidotes that act chemically

1. Direct chemical detoxicants:
    a. Chelating agents (metals)
    b. Cobalt compounds (cyanide)
    c. Antibodies and derivatives:
        i. Monoclonal antibodies (soman)
        ii. Fab fragments (digoxin)
2. Enzymatic detoxicants:
    a. Co-substrates:
        Sodium thiosulphate (cyanide)
    b. Enzymes:
        i. Rhodanese (cyanide)
        ii. Acetylcholinesterase (OPs)
    c. Prevention of formation of toxic metabolite:
        Ethanol (methanol, ethylene glycol)
3. Antidote gives rise to a detoxifying substance:
    Methaemoglobin formers (cyanide and sulphide)
4. Antidote reacts with enzyme–poison complex:
    Oximes (OPs)
5. Antidote reacts with toxic metabolite:
    N-Acetylcysteine and methionine (paracetamol)

Antidotes that act pharmacologically

1. Antagonism at characterized pharmacological receptors:
    a. Naloxone (opiates)
    b. Flumazanil (benzodiazepines)
    c. Prenalterol (β-blockers)
2. Antagonism at other macromolecules:
    Oxygen (carbon monoxide)

Functional

1. Diazepam as an anticonvulsant (OPs)
2. IV fluids (hypotensive agents)

It is possible to envisage a number of ways in the toxic of poisons might be opposed **(Table 1)**. Broadly they can be divided into three main classes: (1) antidotes that remove the active poison from its site of action, usually by bringing about chemical detoxification of the poison; (2) antidotes that act specifically at pharmacological receptors or other macromolecules; and (3) antidotes that act in a functional manner.

Antidotes that Act Chemically

Antidotes that Act Directly on the Poison

The simplest and most easily visualized mode of antidotal action is direct chemical reaction between an antidote and a poison to form a product which is less toxic or which is more rapidly excreted, or both. There are numerous examples of such antidotes, including the chelating agents used in poisoning with a variety of toxic metals and the cobalt-containing cyanide antidotes and Fab fragments used in digoxin poisoning. Studies *in vitro*, often unhelpful in antibody assessment, have been used in some of these examples to elucidate the chemistry of the reactions.

Chelating Agents

The term 'chelation' is often used with a lack of precision. The word comes from the Greek for a claw and it has been argued that monothiol compounds should not be described as chelating agents since they only have one reactive group. Nevertheless, the term is often used as a general term to describe those drugs whose action is to complex metals. The beneficial effect is the result of a number of processes: the complex may be less toxic than the free metal, mobilization from critical sites of toxic actions may occur or else elimination from the body takes place. In many instances all three processes contribute to antidotal efficacy.

One of the earliest chelating agents was dimercaprol (British anti-lewisite; BAL). Like many advances in toxicology, the introduction of this substance was stimulated by military considerations. Dimercaprol was intended for use in treatment of poisoning by the chemical warfare agent lewisite, an extremely toxic organic arsenical compound. The use of dimercaprol had its origin in the suspicion, subsequently confirmed, that the toxicity of arsenic was due to the ability to combine with sulphydryl groups in biological molecules, in particular in lipoic acid, part of the pyruvate decarboxylase complex. Dimercaprol and some similar compounds were extensively studied by Stocken and Thompson (1946), and dimercaprol was the first of the dithiol chelating agents to be used clinically. More recently, two more related drugs have been introduced, dimercaptosuccinic acid (DMSA) and dimercaptopropanesulphonic acid (DMPS). These possess the same dithiol

chelating grouping as dimercaprol but the molecules as a whole are more hydrophilic. Unlike dimercaprol, which has to be injected, DMSA and DMPS can be used orally and both have better therapeutic indices than the older drug (Aposhian *et al.*, 1984; Shum *et al.*, 1995; Mückter *et al.*, 1997).

The toxicity of many metals other than arsenic is due, at least in part, to reaction with sulphydryl groups. It is therefore not surprising that the active part of some other chelators also contain sulphydryl groups. Penicillamine, which is a monothiol chelator, has been used for some years for the treatment of Wilson's disease, a condition in which copper overload is responsible for hepatic and central nervous system damage. Therapy with penicillamine will chelate a variety of other metals, including lead. Other chelating agents contain active groups other than sulphydryl groups. Calcium disodium ethylenediaminetetraacetate (edetate) and its analogues chelate lead and zinc and can be used in acute cadmium poisoning. Desferrioxamine is a compound of natural origin that binds iron and aluminium. A considerable amount of work has been carried out on reactions of the chelating agents (ligands) with metals, and it is possible to predict the efficacy of particular chelating agents in individual metal poisonings on the basis of the affinity constant of the metal and chelator (Ringbom, 1963; Pearson, 1968). However, despite their logical derivation, net affinity (conditional stability) constants of metal complexes can be misleading. As discussed above, the beneficial action of chelating agents is probably the result of a combination of effects, including detoxication by complexation, mobilization and elimination. In order to detoxify effectively, chelating agents must gain access to the tissue where the metal is exerting its action. In the case of mobilization, the process must occur in a toxicologically desirable direction, that is, away from the critical site of toxic action of the metal. Unfortunately, net affinity constants cannot predict the extent to which chelation occurs *in vivo*, nor whether mobilization of the metal occurs in a beneficial direction. Thus, Catsch and Harmuth-Hoehne (1975) found that penicillamine was a more effective mobilizing agent in mercury poisoning than diethylenetriaminepentacetate, whereas the corresponding affinity constants would suggest otherwise. In an attempt to refine studies *in vitro*, Yokel and Kostenbauder (1987) hypothesized that hydrophobicity of the chelated complex was important in successful chelation therapy. They therefore studied chelating agents for use in aluminium poisoning *in vitro* in an octanol–aqueous system and *in vivo* in rabbits poisoned with this metal. They concluded that the ideal chelator should have sufficient affinity for the metal of interest, be sufficiently water soluble to take by mouth and be sufficiently lipid soluble to distribute to sites of accumulation of the metal. If this theoretical model were to be directly applicable to experimental investigations of antidotal efficacy *in vivo*, it would be a great advantage. Unfortunately, the *in vivo* situation cannot be adequately approximated *in vivo* even for chelating agents, a group of antidotes where *in vitro* studies would seem the most promising.

Cobalt-containing Cyanide Activities

It has been known for many years that transition metals can form stable and often relatively non-toxic complexes with cyanide. Clinically, this property of the transition metals has only been exploited in the case of iron (see methaemoglobin below) and cobalt. Cobalt is a metal whose toxicity is well recognized and it has therefore generally been considered that the toxicity of inorganic cobalt salts precludes their clinical use. Muschett *et al.* (1952) showed that hydroxocobalamin (vitamin B12$_a$) was an effective antidote in experimental cyanide poisoning in mice. In clinical practice, hydroxocobalamin presents a number of problems. The molecular weight is high and the compound binds cyanide in a ratio of 1 mol of hydroxocobalamin to 1 mol of cyanide. This means that very large quantities of hydroxocobalamin are necessary for meaningful cyanide antidotal action. Paulet (1960) studied a number of cobalt derivatives in order to find a compound of lower molecular weight which had the antidotal effectiveness of hydroxocobalamin, but which lacked the toxicity of inorganic cobalt salts. The cobalt compounds studied were the chloride, acetate, gluconate and glutamate salts and cobalt histidine and dicobalt edetate. The last two were effective and less toxic than the other compounds. On the basis of efficacy studies in dogs and acute lethality studies in mice, dicobalt edetate, in the formulation known as Kelocyanor, was widely adopted in Europe. Kelocyanor has given rise to adverse reactions, especially when given in the absence of substantial cyanide poisoning. More recently studies have been undertaken into other organic derivatives of cobalt, notably porphyrins (McGuinn *et al.*, 1994).

Fab Fragments and Monoclonal Antibodies

Antisera have long been used to treat poisoning with toxins of biological origin, such as botulinus toxin and toxins in snake venom: this approach can theoretically be adopted for other poisons. It is an attractive option for many poisons where no chemically detoxifying antidote of sufficient efficacy and an adequate lack of toxicity is available. Thus, monoclonal antibodies have reportedly been successful in experimental poisoning by the organophosphorus nerve agent soman (Lenz *et al.*, 1984), while monoclonal antibodies against paraquat have been produced (Johnston *et al.*, 1988). In the best known example of immunotherapy for poisoning with a drug, poisoning with digoxin, whole antibodies are not used. Instead, poisoning with this cardiac glycoside is treated with Fab antibody fragments (Stolshek *et al.*, 1988). Fab fragments have the advantages that they can be eliminated by glomerular filtration through the kidney (Cole and Smith, 1986) and they are less immunogenic than whole antibodies. Immunotherapy can in theory be used to treat any poisoning where detoxicating antibodies can be made against a toxicant. However, in practice, the size of the dose of poison makes the approach of limited practical value for many clinical poisonings. Biotechnology, making as it does large-scale manufacture of monoclonal antibodies easier, adds to the attractiveness of immunotherapy, making wider use more likely in the future.

Antidotes that Act on the Poison via an Enzyme-catalysed Reaction

The existence of enzymatic pathways of detoxication can be exploited in two main ways. Detoxifying co-substrates can be used, but will usually only be effective if the rate of reaction of that particular metabolic pathway is co-substrate limited. Alternatively, the amount of enzyme present can be increased by injecting enzyme derived from an exogenous source. A further way of influencing an enzymatic process is the exogenous supply of an alternative substrate, or the use of an enzyme inhibitor. This may be helpful where poisoning results from metabolism of an indirectly acting poison to a toxic metabolite.

Co-substrates

Sodium thiosulphate is probably not the physiological sulphur donor of the enzyme rhodanese. Nevertheless, this cyanide antidote appears to act by increasing the supply of sulphur for the enzyme, which is normally rate-limited by sulphane sulphur availability. The rhodanese reaction accelerates the rate of cyanide transulphuration to thiocyanate, an ion which is considerably less toxic than cyanide. Sodium thiosulphate, when used alone, is not particularly effective because, although it can increase the rate of cyanide transulfuration very considerably (Cristel *et al.*, 1977), the blood level of cyanide does not fall fast enough, in the context of acute cyanide poisoning, to counteract the poisoning effectively. The possible reason for this is that rhodanese is a mitochondrial enzyme, whereas sodium thiosulphate administered intravenously remains largely extracellular. Because of the slow nature of the fall in cyanide blood levels that are observed after the use of sodium thiosulphate, the main use of this cyanide antidote has been as a second-line antidote to one of the methaemoglobin formers (see below) such as sodium nitrate or 4-dimethylaminophenol.

Other sulphur compounds, including sodium ethane thiosulphonate and propane thiosulphonate, have been studied in the expectation that they would enter the mitochondria. In some animal studies these sulphonic acid derivatives were superior to sodium thiosulphate but they have not been used clinically. Cyanide detoxication by transulphuration has also been carried out using another endogenous enzyme, β-mecaptopyruvate sulphur transferase. In this case sodium β-mecaptopyruvate was the experimental antidote (Way *et al.*, 1985).

Exogenous Enzymes

Exogenous enzymes suffer from the disadvantage of being potentially foreign proteins, but have nevertheless been used experimentally as antidotes. Thus, in an attempt to place the rhodanese in the extra-cellular space, the use of intravenous bovine heart rhodanese accompanied by sulphur-containing cyanide antidotes has been studied in animals (Frankenberg, 1980). Another antidote that has been studied is acetylcholinesterase in the treatment of anticholinesterase poisoning. Thus Wolfe *et al.* (1992) found that foetal bovine serum acetylcholinesterase and horse serum butyrylcholinesterase were effective pretreatments in experimental soman toxicity in rhesus monkeys.

Alterations of Toxic Metabolite Formation

An enzymatic method of detoxication which is only applicable to indirectly acting poisons is the inhibition of the formation of a toxic metabolite. Clinically, such an approach is adopted when ethanol is used to compete at the active site of the enzyme alcohol dehydrogenase and thus to inhibit the formation of formic acid and formaldehyde in methanol poisoning (Cooper and Kini, 1962). Ethylene glycol poisoning can be treated in the same way. Additionally, in experimental studies, pyrazole or 4-methylpyrazole has been used to inhibit alcohol dehydrogenase in these poisons (Clay *et al.*, 1975).

Antidote Giving Rise to a Detoxifying Substance

Methaemoglobin-forming Antidotes

A group of antidotes that do not themselves act by chemically binding a poison but produce a substance that does are the cyanide antidotes that induce a therapeutic methaemoglobinaemia. Methaemoglobin is a form of haemoglobin in which the iron has been oxidized from Fe^{2+} to Fe^{3+}. Methaemoglobin is unable to carry oxygen reversibly in the way that haemoglobin does but it has a high affinity for cyanide and sulphide. The first of this group of antidotes introduced for the use of cyanide poisoning was amyl nitrite. Although this is still sometimes used, the most widely available methaemoglobin producer is sodium nitrite, and this is still used in the USA and elsewhere as a primary cyanide antidote. The more recently introduced 4-dimethylaminophenol (DMAP) is used in Germany, while 4-aminopropiophenone (PAPP) is primarily of military interest (Bright, 1987). Sodium nitrite and DMAP produce methaemoglobin, but in different ways, the former somewhat more slowly. The aim in both instances is to produce methaemoglobinaemia of sufficient degree to bind substantial quantities of cyanide, without producing such a high level of methaemoglobin as to produce an appreciable danger of tissue anoxia. In fact, there appear to be a number of instances where dangerously high levels of methaemoglobin have in fact been produced, perhaps

because of individual susceptibility, or over-enthusiastic use of the antidotes. It is unfortunate that the therapeutic monitoring of methaemoglobin during the treatment of cyanide poisoning is usually not possible, since common methods for measuring methaemoglobin do not separately measure haemoglobin, cyanmethaemoglobin and methaemoglobin. Cyanmethaemoglobin is the pigment produced by the reaction of cyanide with methaemoglobin. Adverse outcomes seem to be more common with DMAP than sodium nitrite, a fact which is surprising in view of the much longer time during which the latter has been used (Van Heijst *et al.*, 1987; Marrs, 1989). It is also worth noting that some authorities doubt whether the main action of sodium nitrite is for it to form methaemoglobin, and suggest a vasoactive action (Way *et al.*, 1987).

Antidotes that React with an Enzyme–Poison Complex

Oximes

Hydroxylamine was studied as an antidote to poisoning with organophosphate anticholinesterase because it was, in certain respects similar to the substrate of the enzyme, namely acetylcholine. It was superseded by the pyridinium oximes and organophosphate poisoning is now often treated with an oxime together with atropine, an anticholinergic drug. The oxime that is used in many countries is the monopyridinium oxime pralidoxime chloride (2-PAM). Additionally, one or two countries use other salts of pralidoxime; the methanesulfonate is used in the UK and the methylsulphate in France and some other countries. Furthermore, the methiodide is also available in certain pharmacopoeias. The bis-pyridinium oxime obidoxime has certain advantages in the therapy of organophosphate chemical warfare agents, particularly in that it is active in the treatment of tabun poisoning. However, there appears to be no major difference between 2-PAM and obidoxime in organophosphorus pesticide poisoning. The principle action of oximes is the dephosphorylation and consequent reactivation of acetylcholinesterase and, in this respect, the main weakness in their activity is against acetylcholinesterase which has undergone ageing. The ageing process, which involves monodealkylation of the dialkyl phosphorylated enzyme, renders the enzyme refractory to both oxime-induced and spontaneous reactivation (Bismuth *et al.*, 1992). It is probable that ageing occurs to some extent with all organophosphate anticholinesterases and it is possible that it may cause clinical problems in organophosphate pesticide poisoning where treatment is initiated very late. It is, however, a very serious problem with the nerve agent soman, whose complex with acetylcholinesterases ages with a half-life of a few minutes. Of the numerous oximes that have been studied, the only ones where much activity is exerted on aged enzyme complexes are the Hagedorn oximes such as

430 General and Applied Toxicology

HI-6. However, there is controversy whether the activity of this oxime in the situation where appreciable ageing has occurred is attributable to acetylcholinesterase reactivation or to other direct effects of the oxime (see Marrs *et al.*, 1996a).

Antidotes that Act on a Toxic Metabolite of the Poison

In the case of poisons requiring metabolism before they become toxic, any of the above antidotal methods could in principle be applied. In practice, however, poisoning with such materials is often treated by bringing about a direct reaction with a toxic metabolite. An example is in paracetamol poisoning. Paracetamol (acetaminophen) is toxic by virtue of its metabolic transformation to be a reactive metabolic *N*-acetyl-*p*-benzoquinoneimine (NABQI). Under normal conditions of use, paracetamol is harmless but in an overdosage causes cell damage which leads to, among other things, hepatic necrosis. The lead antidote cysteamine, although effective in animal models, caused adverse reactions in man, especially nausea. Acetylcysteine probably acts by conjugating with NABQI; methionine, an alternative antidote, may also do so, but only after conversion in the liver to homocysteine (Prescott, 1983; Seddon *et al.*, 1987).

Antidotes that Act Pharmacologically

It is convenient to divide antidotes that act pharmacologically into those antidotes where antagonism occurs at characterized pharmacological receptors and those where antagonism occurs at other macromolecules; this division, although somewhat artificial, is nevertheless useful.

Antidotes that Act at Characterized Pharmacological Receptors

Such antidotes include naloxone, an antidote for opiates (Evans *et al.*, 1973; Dollery, 1991) and flumazanil, which is effective in reversing the effects of benzodiazepines (Scollo-Lavgizzari, 1983) although not licensed for the management of poisoning in the UK. In severe poisoning with β-blockers, adrenergic agonists such as isoprenaline or the more specific and cardioselective prenalterol provide examples of receptor antagonism (Wallin and Hulting, 1983). Development of compounds within the class requires a knowledge of the pharmacological profile of a drug and the particular pharmacological property responsible for toxicity.

Antidotes that Antagonise at Other Macromolecules

Carbon monoxide is poisonous by virtue of its tight binding to haemoglobin and other cellular components. Carbon monoxide can be displaced competitively from such sites by oxygen.

Related Antidotal Mechanisms

Antagonism of clinical poisoning does not necessarily take place at the same receptor as that at which the poison acts. Atropine is an anticholinergic drug and acts upon muscarinic cholinergic receptors. However, this drug is used as an antidote in poisoning with organophosphate and carbamate anticholinesterases, substances whose major action is not directly on the cholinergic receptor. The macromolecule to which the anticholinesterases bind is the enzyme acetylcholinesterase, and the poisoning is a consequence of accumulation of acetylcholine, the normal substrate of that enzyme. It is this effect which is antagonized by atropine. Analogous to this is the use of physostigmine in atropine poisoning: this anticholinesterase promotes acetylcholine accumulation, which overcomes the effect of atropine.

Functional Antagonism

There are a number of antidotes which are used symptomatically in poisoning and as such are difficult to classify. In some cases, further study may show these to have antagonistic actions that belong to one of the above groups. An example is the use of diazepam to combat the convulsions and fasciculations produced by organophosphate poisoning (Sellström, 1992).

ASSESSMENT OF ANTIDOTAL EFFICACY

Antidotal efficacy can be assessed *in vitro*, in experimental animals and, to some extent, in human poisonings. All these approaches have limitations: studies *in vitro* cannot adequately simulate the situation *in vivo*, even in the case of the most straightforward antidotes which react with and detoxify the poison. Studies *in vitro*, however, are useful preliminaries to animal studies, particularly in narrowing down the choice amongst a series of related antidotes (Marrs, 1992). Moreover, in mechanistic studies of the action of antidotes, an *in vitro* approach is often extremely useful. Studies in experimental animals, possibly the most useful of the three approaches, are limited by the problems of extrapolation for two different substances, the toxin and the antidote, from animals to man, and by the need for very careful attention to experimental design. The limitations inherent in data on human poisonings are quite different: for example, Poison Centre data normally relate to suicidal and accidental exposure and so the dose of poison is uncontrolled and often unknown, so that while large multicentre trials are often very useful, they do not provide information which can properly replace animal studies.

Assessment of Antidotes in Experimental Animals

There are many ways in which studies of antidotal efficiency can be performed and some of the factors to be considered in experimental design are listed in **Table 2**.

Table 2 Variables

Animal model	a. Species, strain and sex
	b. Numbers and controls
Poison	a. Dose
	b. Route of administration
	c. Solvent and excipients
Antidote	a. Dose
	b. Route of administration
	c. Solvent and excipients
	d. Time between administration of poison and antidote
End-point	a. Lethality
	b. Other:
	i. Clinical
	ii. Biochemical
	iii. Haematological
	iv. Electrophysiological
	v. Histopathological
	vi. Behaviour

Animal Model

One of the main features requiring attention is the choice of species of experimental animal. However well constructed the study is in other respects, unless the behaviour of the poison and antidote are similar in the chosen species and in humans, the results will be valueless (see Calabrese, 1982; Marrs, 1987). Species suitability will be determined by similarity between the chosen species and humans in absorption, distribution, metabolism, excretion and response to the poison. The relative importance of these considerations depends on the mode of action of the poison: if it is a directly active poison, for example cyanide, similarity in rate of endogeneous detoxication would appear to be most important consideration, whereas for those substances which are toxic in humans only after a metabolic activation step, the occurrence of this conversion at a similar rate in the chosen species to that in man is probably the most important factor.

Major quantitative differences in lethality of chemicals between a given species and humans indicate that the species is probably a poor choice. Such differences exist with respect to methanol (Clay *et al.*, 1975), ethylene glycol (Gessner *et al.*, 1961) and certain organophosphates (Crawford *et al.*, 1976). It must be further borne in mind that the choice of scarce, large or exotic animals will increase the cost of the experiment and may thereby tend to reduce the numbers that can be used. This will clearly decrease the power of the study. Moreover, normative data on such animals is usually scanty or non-existent. All the forgoing considerations apply, of course, to the evaluation of any xenobiotic in animals; however, with antidotal studies the same considerations also apply with respect to the antidote, so that the species chosen must be similar to the human in its handling of both the poison and the antidote. This fact may greatly complicate the choice of animal model and indeed there may be no perfect solution.

The species having been decided upon, the numbers of animals and controls must be determined. Two main types of experimental design have been adopted for the evaluation of antidotes. In the first, 'LD$_{50}$ ratio', the LD$_{50}$ of the poison is measured with and without the administration of the antidote. This procedure has the advantage that the result produced is a single figure, the protection ratio, but is has the disadvantage that it is necessary to use a relatively large number of animals. Moreover, the slope of the treated and untreated log dose–probit mortality curves may not be the same (Natoff and Reiff, 1970), and this will impair the value of the single figure. The protection ratio design is usually employed when small laboratory animals are used, although there are instances of the use of this type of design with larger animals, such as sheep by Burrows and Way (1979), studying cyanide antidotes, and monkeys by Dirnhuber *et al.* (1979), studying pyridostigmine prophylaxis in soman poisoning. Although the performance of LD$_{50}$ ratio type studies sounds easy, multiple pilot experiments are often needed to bracket the median lethal dose.

The other principle design is the comparison of survival in groups of animals given the same supralethal dose of poison, one group being treated with the antidote and the other being left untreated. The number of animals used is much less than with protection ratio design, but the information supplied is also less. This approach has been criticized on the grounds that antidotes capable of increasing the LD$_{50}$ of the poison by comparatively small amounts can produce dramatic increases in the proportion of animals surviving (Way *et al.*, 1987); nevertheless, such experimental designs are frequently being used with large laboratory animals such as dogs. If this approach is adopted, it is essential to have an untreated but poisoned control group within the study. The reliance on literature LD$_{50}$s, where the animals normally of the same strain may have been studied under different conditions and with different formulations of poisons, is reprehensible and renders the study valueless.

Whichever type of design is adopted, consideration should be given to the inclusion of a treatment-only group.

Poison

The dose of poison used depends on the overall design of the study. Where a design of protection ratio type is used, dosing is, as with any LD_{50} estimate, designed to bracket the lethal dose. Adjustment of the dose range upwards may be required in the antidote-treated group. Often siting shots will be necessary preliminaries to a substantive experiment in both antidote-treated and untreated groups. Where survival is compared in two groups of animals, one poisoned and untreated and the other poisoned and treated with the antidote, the dose of poison chosen is usually a dose which will be supralethal in animals not treated with antidote. It must also be a dose against which there is a reasonable chance of survival with antidote. To obtain a reasonable idea of the maximum dose of toxicant against which an antidote will protect, it may be necessary to use several different doses of poison.

The poison should normally be given by the route by which it commonly gains access to man. In the case of a large number of poisons, this will be by mouth, so that gavage is appropriate in animals studies. Percutaneous and inhalation poisoning present problems, the former because the reproducibility of lethality figures tends to be poor, the latter because of the relative scarcity of inhalation facilities in laboratories. Intratracheal installation has been used as a substitute for inhalation studies, but it does not appear to be satisfactory particularly with toxicants acting locally on the lungs (Richards et al., 1989).

Where poisoning by a pharmaceutical preparation is being studied, formulations are readily available for experimental purposes and are often used. The use of the formulation, rather than the active ingredient by itself, should be considered with other formulated materials, such as pesticides.

Antidote

In the case of an antidote already in use in man, it may be appropriate to adjust the dose to the size of the animal in experimental studies. In certain instances, however, the choice of dose is more complicated. For example, it would be unwise to ignore species differences in methaemoglobin generation when studying methaemoglobin-producing cyanide antidotes.

The antidote is usually assessed after administration by the route by which it will be used. Furthermore, whereas in the early stages of development the antidote will be frequently studied in its pure state, at some point it should be evaluated in the formulation in which it will be used clinically.

One of the most difficult points to resolve is the time relationship between administration of the poison and the antidote. This is a problem which is particularly important with rapidly acting poisons, and careful attention must be applied to this aspect of the design of the study if data are to be produced which can be extrapolated to clinical human poisonings. The use of prophylactic administration of antidotes is not valid, except where mechanistic studies are being carried out or where the antidote is intended for prophylactic use (Way et al., 1987). Even when the antidote is given after poisoning, there is still the problem of the precise time interval between the challenge and the administration of the antidote. Usually the antidote is given at a fixed time after poisoning or at the onset of a well defined clinical sign. Unfortunately, the time interval has often been chosen so as to be unrealistic compared with the time between clinical poisoning and when clinical therapy is likely to be available. On the other hand, the use of clinical signs as a cue for antidote administration invites the possibility of observer bias. A possible solution is to use a fixed time interval but one somewhat longer than those customarily employed. In addition, it is of value to consider a study design in which the antidote is administered at intervals after the toxin, a situation that more closely resembles clinical poisoning. Temporal considerations discussed above tend to be much less important with poisons whose clinical effects have slow onset, or in the treatment of chronic or delayed poisoning, than in acute poisonings.

End-point

Although most antidote efficacy studies employ death or survival as the end-point, a possible alternative is change in time of survival. Clinical end-points other than lethality may be used, but observer bias should be carefully avoided. The efficacy of the antidote against sublethal effects, often behavioural ones, has also been used; this approach is attractive in military contexts where knowledge of a poisoned individual's ability to keep fighting is desired. Biochemical end-points such as reactivation of cholinesterase in organophosphate poisoning or mobilization of a metal in heavy metal poisoning may be used (e.g. Kreppel et al., 1995; Tandon et al., 1996). There is, however, a potential problem here, in that biochemical improvement does not always correlate with clinical efficacy of the antidote.

More Complex Studies

Comparison of Antidotes

It is frequently necessary to evaluate a new antidote against an existing one or to survey a series of structurally related antidotes. The aim should be to study the antidotes under reasonably realistic conditions. In this case the animal model chosen must be suitable for the evaluation of the toxic effects of the poison and of more than one antidote, as well as to be able to show comparative efficacy clearly. It may be appropriate to use control groups, these animals receiving each antidote alone, another group receiving the poison alone and further groups receiving the poison together with each treatment. Alternatively, a full dose–response evaluation which will yield a protection ratio for each antidote can be carried out and in fact has frequently been done (see, for example, Schwartz *et al.*, 1979). Although most of the variables discussed earlier will also apply to an evaluation of two or more antidotes in the same study, it is usually more difficult to standardize experimental conditions in a study employing more than one antidote.

Use of More than One Antidote in the Same Animal

More than one antidote, used together, may be used to treat a poisoning. Thus organophosphates are usually treated with atropine and an oxime, and cyanides frequently with sodium nitrite and sodium thiosulphate (see above). The combined effect of such treatments may be additive, synergistic or less than additive. There is no particular problem with assessing treatment regimes of this type, the usual procedure being to appraise each antidote separately in experimental animals and then together; an example is the study of the efficacy of dimercaptosuccinic acid and calcium disodium edetate in lead-intoxicated rats by Flora *et al.* (1995). It will frequently be necessary to use multiple dosing combinations and it should not be forgotten that antidotes may interact chemically if mixed together before administration.

Assessment of Antidotes in Human Beings

Provided that certain ethical guidelines are followed (e.g. Royal Colleges of Physicians of London, 1986) and given appropriate ethical committee approval, studies of poisons or antidotes may be carried out on human volunteers. Such studies would be performed for a number of different purposes.

It may be necessary to establish the pharmacokinetics or pharmacodynamics of a poison or antidote in man; further, the observer may wish to study the distribution and metabolism of both in humans. Thus a number of pesticides have been studied in human volunteers (Wilks and Woolen, 1994) as have chemical warfare agents (Marrs *et al.*, 1996b). Human studies may be carried out during clinical use, either as part of a control clinical trial or by observation during routine clinical use; antidotes can also be studied in human healthy volunteers.

Some compounds that are used as antidotes have already passed through such studies, since they are already used therapeutic substances in other clinical situations. An example is the use of β-adrenergic antagonists in the management of theophylline poisoning.

The second area where it may be necessary to study effects of antidotes in volunteers is in the evaluation of adverse effects. Sometimes, this may occur after the antidote has undergone clinical use, as is the case of the studies that were carried out on acetylcysteine. In these experiments intradermal acetylcysteine was given to volunteers and to patients who had undergone treatment for paracetamol poisoning and had suffered adverse reactions (Bateman *et al.*, 1984).

For antidotes that act as agonists and antagonists at pharmacological receptors sites, studies of the pharmacodynamic reaction in volunteers may be carried out prior to the administration of the drugs to patients. Thus, the opiate antagonist naloxone and the benzodiazepine antagonist flumazanil were studied in volunteers prior to being given to patients.

Clinical studies in patients may involve the use of single doses in intoxicated patients and comparison with control groups to assess response. This technique was used when naloxone was introduced, and had been shown to be efficacious in opiate poisoning but without affecting benzodiazepine and barbiturate poisoning. In addition, clinical studies need to be done in patients to establish the appropriate dosing regime, and this is particularly the case for pharmacological antagonists such as naloxone, for which studies were carried out to clarify the most appropriate dosing format (Goldfrank *et al.*, 1986).

REFERENCES

Aposhian, H. V., Carter, D. E., Hoover, T. E., Hsu, C.-H., Maiorino, R. M. and Stine, E. (1984). DMSA, DMPS and DMPH as arsenic antidotes. *Fundam. Appl. Toxicol.*, **4**, S58–S70.

Bateman, D. N. and Chaplin, S. (1989). Antidotes to human toxins. In Turner, P. and Volans, G. N. (Eds), *Recent Advances in Clinical Pharmacology and Toxicology*. Churchill Livingstone, Edinburgh, pp. 173–195.

Bateman, D. N., Woodhouse, K. W. and Rawlins, M. D. (1984). Adverse reactions to *N*-acetylcysteine. *Hum. Toxicol*, **3**, 393–398.

Bismuth, C. (1987). Generalités. In Bismuth, C., Baud, F. J., Conso, F., Fréjaville, J. P. and Garnier, R. (Eds), *Toxicologie Clinique*. Flammarion, Paris, pp. 2–24.

Bismuth, C., Inns, R. H. and Marrs, T. C. (1992). The efficacy, toxicity and clinical use of oximes in anticholinesterase poisoning. In Ballantyne, B. and Marrs, T. C. (Eds), *Clinical and Experimental Toxicology of Organophosphates and Carbamates*. Butterworth-Heinemann, Oxford, pp. 555–577.

Bright, J. E. (1987). A prophylaxis for cyanide poisoning. In Ballantyne, B. and Marrs, T. C. (Eds), *Clinical and Experimental Toxicology of Cyanides*. Wright, Bristol, pp. 259–382.

British Toxicology Society, Working Party on Toxicity (1984). A new approach to the classification of substances and preparations on the basis of their acute toxicity. *Hum. Toxicol.*, **3**, 85–92.

Burger, A. (1982). Drug design. In Hamner, C. E. (Ed.), *Drug Development*. CRC Press, Boca Raton, FL, pp. 53–72.

Burrows, G. E. and Way, J. L. (1979). Cyanide intoxication in sheep: enhancement of the efficacy of sodium nitrite, sodium thiosulfate and cobaltous chloride. *Am. J. Vet. Res.*, **40**, 613–617.

Calabrese, B. J. (1982). *The Principles of Animal Extrapolation*. Wiley, New York.

Catsch, A. and Harmuth-Hoehne, A. E. (1975). New developments in metal antidotal properties of chelating agents. *Biochem. Pharmacol.*, **24**, 1557–1562.

Clay, K. L., Murphy, R. C. and Watkins, W. D. (1975). Experimental methanol toxicity in the primate: analysis of metabolic acidosis. *Toxicol. Appl. Pharmacol.*, **34**, 49–61.

Cole, P. L. and Smith, T. W. (1986). Use of digoxin-specific Fab fragments in the treatment of digitalis intoxication. *Drug. Intell. Clin. Pharmacol.*, **20**, 267–269.

Cooper, J. R. and Kini, M. M. (1962). Biochemical aspects of methanol poisoning. *Biochem. Pharmacol.*, **11**, 405–416.

Crawford, N. J., Hutchinson, D. H. and King, P. A. (1976). Metabolic demethylation of the insecticide dimethylvinphos in rats, in dogs and *in vitro*. *Xenobiotica*, **6**, 745–762.

Cristel, D., Eyer, P., Hegemann, M., Kiese, M., Lörcher, W. and Weger, N. (1977). Pharmacokinetics of cyanide poisoning in dogs and the effect of 4-dimethylaminophenol or thiosulfate. *Arch. Toxicol.*, **38**, 177–189.

Dirnhuber, P., French, N. C. and Green, D. (1979). The protection of primates against soman poisoning by pre-treatment with pyridostigmine. *J. Pharm. Pharmacol.*, **31**, 295–299.

Dollery, C. T. (Ed.) (1991). *Naloxone in Therapeutic Drugs*, vol. 2. Churchill Livingstone, Edinburgh, pp. N17–N20.

Evans, L. J., Roscoe, P., Swainson, C. P. and Prescott, L. F. C. (1973). Treatment of drug over-dose with naloxone, a specific narcotic antagonist. *Lancet*, **i**, 452.

Flora, C. J. S., Seth, P. K., Prakash, A. O. and Mathur, R. (1995). Therapeutic efficacy of combined *meso*-2, 3-dimercaptosuccinic acid and calcium disodium edetate treatment during acute lead intoxication in rats. *Hum. Exp. Toxicol.*, **14**, 410–413.

Frankenberg, L. (1980). Enzyme therapy in cyanide poisoning: effect of rhodanese and sulphur compounds. *Arch. Toxicol.*, **45**, 315–323.

Garland, H. and Pearce, J. (1967). Neurological complications of carbon monoxide poisoning. *Q. J. Med.*, **36**, 445–455.

Gessner, P. K., Parke, D. E. and Williams, R. T. (1961). Studies in detoxification. *Biochem. J.*, **76**, 482–489.

Goldfrank, L., Weisman, R. S., Errick, J. K. and Lo, M. W. (1986). A dosing nomogram for continuous infusion intravenous naloxone. *Ann. Emergency Med.*, **15**, 566–570.

Johnston, S. C., Bowles, M., Winzor, D. J. and Pond, S. M. (1988). Comparison of paraquat-specific murine monoclonal antibodies produced by *in vitro* and *in vivo* immunisation. *Fundam. Appl. Toxicol.*, **11**, 261–267.

Kreppel, H., Reichel, F. X., Kleine, A., Szinicz, L., Singh, P. K. and Jones, M. M. (1995). Antidotal efficacy of newly synthesized dimercaptosuccinic acid (DMSA) monoesters in experimental arsenic poisoning in mice. *Fundam. Appl. Toxicol.*, **26**, 239–245.

Lenz, D. E., Brimfield, A. A. and Hunter, K. W. (1984). Studies using a monoclonal antibody against soman. *Fundan. Appl. Toxicol.*, **4**, S156–S164.

Marrs, T. C. (1987). Experimental approaches to the design and assessment of antidotal procedures. In Ballantyne, B. (Ed.), *Perspectives in Basic and Applied Toxicology*. Wright, Bristol, pp. 285–308.

Marrs, T. C. (1989). The antidotal treatment of acute cyanide poisoning. *Adv. Drug React. Acute Pois. Rev.*, **4**, 279–200.

Marrs, T. C. (1992). Principles in the development of antidotes to toxic materials. In O'Sullivan, J. B. and Krieger, G. B. (Eds), *Toxicology of Hazardous Materials*. Williams and Wilkins, Baltimore, pp. 46–60.

Marrs, T. C., Maynard, R. L. and Sidell, F. R. (1996a). *Chemical Warfare Agents Toxicology and Treatment*. Wiley, Chichester, p. 104.

Marrs, T. C., Maynard, R. L. and Sidell, F. R. (1996b). *Chemical Warfare Agents Toxicology and Treatment*. Wiley, Chichester, pp. 115–137.

McGuinn, W. D., Baxter, L., Pei, I., Petrikovics, I., Cannon, E. P. and Way, J. L. (1994). Antagonism of the lethal effects of cyanide by a synthetic water-soluble cobalt(III) porphyrin compound. *Fundam. Appl. Toxicol.*, **23**, 76–80.

Mückter, H., Liebe, B., Reichl, F.-X., Hunder, G., Walther, U. and Fichtl, B. (1997). Are we ready to replace dimercaprol (BAL) as an arsenic antidote? *Human Exper. Toxicol.* **16**, 460–465.

Muschett, C. W., Kelley, K. L., Boxer, G. E. and Rickards, J. C. (1952). Antidotal efficacy of vitamin B12a (hydroxo-cobalamin) in experimental cyanide poisoning. *Proc. Soc. Exp. Biol. Med.*, **81**, 234–237.

Natoff, I. L. and Reiff, B. (1970). Quantitative studies of the effects of antagonists on the acute toxicity of organophosphates in rats. *Br. J. Pharmacol.*, **40**, 124–134.

Paulet, G. (1960). *L'Intoxication Cyanhydrique et son Traitement*. Masson, Paris.

Pearson, R. G. (1968). Hard and soft acids and bases, HSAB. Part II. Underlying theories. *J. Chem. Educ.*, **45**, 643–648.

Pedigo, L. G. (1988). Antagonism between amyl nitrite and prussic acid. *Trans. Med. Soc. Virginia*, **19**, 124–131.

Prescott, L. F. (1983). Paracetamol overdosage. Pharmacological considerations and clinical management. *Drugs*, **25**, 290–314.

Richards, R. J., Atkins, J., Marrs, T. C., Brown, R. F. R. and Masek, L. (1989). The biochemical and pathological changes produced by the intratracheal instillation of certain components of zinc-hexachloroethane smoke. *Toxicology*, **54**, 79–88.

Ringbom, A. (1963). *Complexation in Analytical Chemistry*. Wiley-Interscience, New York.

Royal College of Physicians of London (1986). Research on healthy volunteers. *J. R. Coll. Phys. London*, **20**, 243–257.

Schwartz, C., Morgan, R. L. and Way, J. L. (1979). Antagonism of cyanide intoxication with sodium pyruvate. *Toxicol. Appl. Pharmacol.*, **10**, 437–441.

Scollo-Lavgizzari, G. (1983). First clinical investigation of the benzodiazepine antagonist TO 15-788 in comatose patients. *Eur. Neurol.*, **22**, 7–11.

Seddon, C. E., Boobis, A. R. and Davies, D. S. (1987). Comparative activation of paracetamol in the rat, mouse and man. *Arch. Toxicol.*, Suppl. II, 305–309.

Sellström, Å. (1992). Anticonvulsants. In Ballantyne, B. and Marrs, T. C. (Eds), *Clinical and Experimental Toxicology of Organophosphates and Carbamates.* Butterworth-Heinemann, Oxford, pp. 578–586.

Senanayake, N. and Karalleide, L. (1992). Interimediate syndrome in anticholinsterase neurotoxicity. In Ballantyne, B. and Marrs, T. C. (Eds), *Clinical and Experimental Toxicology of Organophosphates and Carbamates.* Butterworth-Heinemann, Oxford, pp. 126–134.

Shum, S., Whitehead, J., Vaughn, L., Shum, S. and Hale, T. (1995). Chelation of organoarsenate with dimercaptosuccinic acid. *Vet. Hum. Toxicol.*, **37**, 239–242.

Society of Toxicology (1989). SOT Position Paper comments on the LD_{50} and acute eye and skin irritation test. *Fundam. Appl. Toxicol.*, **13**, 621–623.

Stocken, L. A. and Thompson, R. H. S. (1946). British anti-lewisite, arsenic and thiol excretion in animals after treatment of lewisite burns. *Biochem. J.*, **40**, 548–554.

Stolshek, B. S., Osterout, S. K. and Dunham, G. (1988). The role of digoxin-specific antibodies in the treatment of digitalis poisoning. *Med. Toxicol.*, **3**, 167–171.

Tandon, S. K., Singh, S., Jain, V. K. and Prasad, S. (1996). Chelation in metal intoxication. XXXVIII: effect of structurally different chelating agents in the treatment of nickel intoxication in rat. *Fundam. Appl. Toxicol.*, **31**, 141–148.

Van Heijst, A. M. P., Douze, J. M. C., van Kesteren, R. T., van Bergen, J. E. A. M. and van Dijk, A. (1987). Therapeutic problems in cyanide poisoning. *Clin. Pharmacol.*, **25**, 383–398.

Wallin, G. J. and Hulting, J. (1983). Massive mataprolol poisoning treated with prenalterol. *Acta Med. Scand.*, **324**, 253–255.

Way, J. L., Holmes, R. and Way, J. L. (1985). Cyanide antagonism with mercaptopyruvate. *Fed. Proc.*, **44**, 718.

Way, J. L., Leuing, P., Sylvester, D. M., Burrows, G., Way, J. and Tamulinas, C. (1987). Methaemoglobin formation in the treatment of acute cyanide intoxication. In Ballantyne, B. and Marrs, T. C. (Eds), *Clinical and Experimental Toxicology of Cyanides.* Wright, Bristol, pp. 402–412.

Webster (1986). *Webster's Ninth New Collegiate Dictionary.* Merriam-Webster, Springfield, MA.

Werner, B., Back, W., Akerblom, H. and Barr, P. O. (1985). Two cases of acute carbon monoxide poisoning with delayed neurological sequelae after a 'free' interval. *J. Toxicol. Clin. Toxicol.*, **23**, 249–266.

Wilks, M. F. and Woolen, B. H. (1994). Human volunteer studies with non-pharmaceutical chemicals: metabolism and pharmacokinetic studies. *Hum. Exp. Toxicol.*, **13**, 383–392.

Wolfe, A. D., Blick, D. W., Murphy, M. R., Miller, S. A., Gentry, M. K., Hartgraves, S. L. and Doctor, B. P. (1992). Use of cholinesterases as pretreatment drugs for the protection of rhesus monkeys. *Toxicol. Appl. Pharmacol.*, **117**, 189–193.

Yokel, R. A. and Kostenbauder, H. B. M. (1987). Assessment of aluminum chelators in an octanol/aqueous system and in the aluminum-loaded rabbit. *Toxicol. Appl. Pharmacol.*, **91**, 281–294.

Chapter 21
Quality Assurance in Toxicology Studies

T. R. Stiles

CONTENTS

- Background
- Current GLP Standards
- Scope of GLP
- GLP Principles
- Conduct of Study
- Study Report
- Archives
- Application of GLP to Computer Systems
- Conclusion
- References

BACKGROUND

As in any science, the integrity of a toxicology study has its foundations or value based upon the assumption that others are able to reproduce the results of that study. In the conduct of preclinical safety studies, certain laboratory principles and practices entitled Good Laboratory Practice (GLP) were first introduced by legislation in 1979 in an attempt to assure regulatory receiving authorities of the integrity and reproducibility of work submitted to them.

These first GLPs were promulgated by the United States Food and Drug Administration (FDA) following evidence that a number of toxicological studies being submitted to the Agency contained deficiencies, inaccuracies and fraudulent data. An investigation of pharmaceutical and agrochemical companies, government laboratories and contract research laboratories was undertaken by the FDA in an attempt to confirm and then quantify the severity of their suspicions. The observations made during these investigations were summarized in the preamble to the proposed draft Good Laboratory Practice Regulations as published in 1976 and these were as follows:

1. Experiments were poorly conceived, carelessly executed or inaccurately analysed or reported.
2. Technical personnel were unaware of the importance of protocol adherence, accurate observations, accurate administration of test substance, and accurate record keeping and record transcription.
3. Management did not assure critical review of data or proper supervision of personnel.

4. Studies were impaired by protocol designs that did not allow the evaluation of all available data.
5. Assurance could not be given for the scientific qualifications and adequate training of personnel involved in the research study.
6. There was a disregard for the need to observe proper laboratory, animal care and data management procedures.
7. Sponsors failed to monitor adequately the studies performed in whole or in part by contract testing laboratories.
8. Firms failed to verify the accuracy and completeness of scientific data in reports of non-clinical laboratory studies in a systematic manner before submission to the FDA.

These problems were so severe in two companies, Industrial Bio-Test (IBT) and Biometric Testing Inc., that both contract laboratories were forced to stop performing such work. IBT had been one of the largest contract testing laboratories in the United States, with thousands of toxicology studies serving to support the safety of drugs, pesticides, and food additives. The FDA and the United States Environmental Protection Agency (US EPA) began reviewing all the studies that relied on IBT and Biometric data for support of safety submissions. From the audits of the IBT studies, the US EPA found 594 of 801 key studies, or 75%, to be invalid. The FDA's Bureau of Foods found 24 of 66 IBT studies, or 36%, to be invalid. Criminal charges of fraud were brought against four IBT officials, three of whom were later convicted.

From this investigation, it was concluded that fraudulent data from such studies could affect decisions relating to the safety of a product and such invalid data were alarming to Congress, industry and the public. Faced with this overwhelming evidence, the US Congress voted a special appropriation of 16 million dollars to support a Bioresearch Monitoring Program. Following the introduction of this programme came the first Draft GLP Standards in 1976. The intention of these 'quality standards' was to ensure, as far as possible, the quality and integrity of laboratory data used to support the safety assessment of compounds and to minimize the risk of a repeat of the problems identified at IBT and Biometric Inc.

CURRENT GLP STANDARDS

From these initial FDA GLP regulations, more and more countries that had pharmaceutical or agrochemical industries recognized the need for such standards and introduced some form of GLP regulation or standard. Today most countries in which safety toxicology is performed have some form of GLP principle in operation.

The Standards or Regulations which currently exist in various countries are given below.

United States of America

Within the USA, three Acts exist which cover the GLP Regulations, one from the FDA and two from the US EPA. The regulations are (1) FDA (1978), which has been amended on a number of occasions; the most recent amendment was published in the *Federal Register* on 4 September 1987; (2) US EPA (1983); and (3) US EPA (1989).

Japan

Japan has at least four Ministries which have published GLP Regulations; those of the Ministry of Health and Welfare and the Ministry of Labour are combined within one document. The references for the GLP documents from the four main agencies are: (1) Japan: Ministry of Health and Welfare (1987); (2) Japan: Ministry of Agriculture, Forestry and Fisheries (1984); and (3) Japan Ministry of International Trade and Industry (1984).

European Union

As the European Union (EU) began to develop in the 1980s, it was not long before it considered how to harmonize its approach to GLP. Within the EU, numerous Directives have now been issued covering the definition, application and implementation of GLP and the requirements for national inspection programmes.

The EU Directives require that the GLP standards to be applied across the EU Member States are those standards published by the OECD. (It should be noted that the actual reference to the OECD Principles within the various EU Directives are those OECD Principles published in 1982. However, it is anticipated that with time the Directives will be amended to refer to the recently revised OECD Principles of GLP (1997). In practice, most Member States are adopting the revised principles.) Each member state is required to establish through its national legislative programme a law covering the establishment of GLP and a monitoring body to monitor the conduct and performance of pre-clinical safety studies. To date, all current EU Member States have introduced such laws and are monitoring the conduct and performance of such pre-clinical studies within their own countries.

The following is a list of current EC Directives applicable to GLP.

Directive 79/831/EEC

The first European Community Directive requiring testing to be done in accordance with GLP was 79/831/EEC (EEC, 1979), the so-called Sixth Amendment, on notification of new industrial chemicals. It did not specify the GLP Principles, although from the time the OECD published their Principles of Good Laboratory Practice in 1982, little confusion was possible. Many European laboratories implemented GLP, therefore, before the first, more explicit, European directive was adopted by the end of 1986: Directive 87/18/EEC (EEC, 1987).

Directive 87/18/EEC

This Directive, the first one dealing with GLP, states that the OECD Principles of Good Laboratory Practice will apply whenever, in EU regulations, the application of GLP is required for the safety testing of chemicals and preparations. The Directive also requires the Member States to take the necessary enforcement measures and appoint responsible authorities. Apart from creating obligations on Member States, the Directive also restricts their rights: it is no longer acceptable to refuse the results of safety testing on GLP grounds if the OECD GLP has been applied. This provision is not limited to a specific geographical area and applies therefore equally to data originating from EU Member States and non-Member States.

Directive 88/320/EEC

The second GLP directive, 88/320/EEC (EEC, 1988), was adopted on 30 June 1988 and should have been implemented nationally before 1 January 1989. It elaborates on the obligation of Directive 87/18/EEC for national authorities to monitor compliance with the

OECD Principles of Good Laboratory Practice. The national authorities should follow the OECD guidance for compliance monitoring and, in a recent update of this directive, the full texts of the relevant OECD guidance documents have been attached. New in this Directive is the requirement for national monitoring units to submit, once a year, a report on the inspection activities to the Commission, with a summary of the findings. These reports will be circulated to other Member States.

Member States are obliged to accept the results of GLP compliance monitoring activities in other countries. The Directive 88/320/EEC provides, however, a procedure for solving problems, e.g. when a GLP authority or regulatory body in one country has questions on the compliance monitoring procedures in another country or when there is a specific concern on the GLP compliance for a specific study.

Other Directives

For completeness, another EU Directive should be mentioned; this is Directive 89/569/EEC, mandating the Commission to agree to the adoption of the 1989 OECD decision on GLP [C(89)87 (Final)] on behalf of the EU Member States (EEC, 1989).

United Kingdom

Within the UK, significant changes to the implementation of GLP occurred on 1 April 1997. Prior to this date the UK programme had been a voluntary scheme, Good Laboratory Practice, The United Kingdom Compliance Programme, Department of Health 1989. Whilst the scheme had been operating since 1986 very successfully, the programme had no legal status.

On 1 April 1997, in line with EU Directives, the UK Government published regulations (UK, 1997) which introduced the legal requirement for pre-clinical safety studies performed within the UK to be conducted in compliance with GLP. Under this legislation, all pre-clinical studies which are performed in the UK to assess the safety of a substance and/or used in support of a safety submission to a receiving authority must be conducted in compliance with GLP and at premises which are registered as members, or prospective members, of the GLP compliance programme as defined in the legislation.

The UK GLP Monitoring Authority (MA) is an entity within the Inspection and Enforcement Division of the Medicines Control Agency.

Prior to the conduct of any pre-clinical safety studies, the facilities within which the work is to be performed should be accredited by the MA. This can be achieved by a formal notification to the MA of one's intention to perform such studies. They will then arrange an inspection of those facilities and the systems and procedures in operation. On successful completion of the inspection a compliance statement will be issued.

Within the UK, any testing facility making a claim that it is operating in compliance with the UK GLP Regulations should hold a current certificate issued by the MA. Certificates are only issued following a satisfactory inspection performed by that Authority, such inspections being undertaken approximately every 2 years.

UK Good Laboratory Practice Advisory Leaflets

To assist in the application and understanding of Good Laboratory Practice, the UK GLP Monitoring Authority have produced advisory leaflets which cover specific areas of GLP. They cover Computer Systems (MA, 1995), the Application of GLP Principles to Field Studies (MA, 1990), Good Laboratory Practice and the Role of Quality Assurance (MA, 1991) and the Role of the Study Director (MA, 1992). A fifth advisory leaflet cover GLP in the Analytical Laboratory is also planned.

Organisation for Economic Cooperation and Development (OECD)

Although not a regulatory authority, the OECD has established over the years a series of test guidelines in a attempt to harmonize testing protocols in certain common areas. In such a role of harmonization, the OECD established an expert group in the early 1980s to produce a single set of GLP principles which it was hoped all member countries could accept. The resulting GLP Principles were accepted by all member countries and first published in 1982 (OECD, 1982).

In 1996, as a result of a broadening in the scope and application of GLP from the time the first principles were published, the OECD established a new group of experts to review the 1982 GLP Principles. This latest revision, which was published in 1998, provides a clearer understanding of some of the more complex situations which now impact upon the conduct of pre-clinical studies. The introduction of the principle investigator, clarification of the role and responsibility of facility management and the concept of multi-site studies are just a few of the modifications and modernization of the earlier OECD Principles of GLP (OECD, 1997). It is these GLP principles which now form the foundation of the 'International' Principles of Good Laboratory Practice.

The OECD currently consists of the following member countries: Australia, Austria, Belgium, Canada, Denmark, Finland, France, Germany, Greece, Iceland, Ireland, Italy, Japan, Luxembourg, Mexico, The Netherlands, New Zealand, Norway, Portugal, Spain, Sweden, Switzerland, Turkey, UK, USA, i.e. a large proportion of those countries that have pharmaceutical or chemical industries are members. Many countries have published their own GLP Regulations or principles but without exception these have all been based upon or closely reflect those of the OECD.

In addition to these principles of GLP, the OECD has produced a number of monographs which provide more detail in specific areas of the application and introduction of GLP. The topics of these monographs range from the role of the Study Director to the conduct of field trials with the role of quality assurance and many other topics in between.

The significance of these principles of GLP and the way in which they have influenced the application of GLP world-wide can be seen when we examine the GLP directives within the European Union.

SCOPE OF GLP

As GLP principles are continuing to be developed in new countries, so does their scope and application grow. Rather than attempting to identify the requirements of each country and run the risk of being out of date by the time this book is published, it is more accurate to state that any study undertaken to assess the safety of a test substance should be undertaken in compliance with GLP. This may include all types of toxicity studies from *in vitro* mutagenicity studies to acute, sub-chronic and long-term toxicity/carcinogenicity studies and metabolism and safety pharmacology on pharmaceuticals, agrochemicals, food additives and medical devices.

Although not all studies in a GLP facility will be destined for submission to a receiving authority, the overall quality of the both regulatory and non-regulatory studies should be the same. Dual standards within a laboratory can be detrimental to the overall quality of work within that laboratory. It is therefore recommended, where possible, that all the work within a GLP facility is performed to the same standard.

GLP PRINCIPLES

It would be very easy to write a book on GLP principles and their application, as the interpretation and application to different possible situations are numerous. However, this chapter will simply identify the essential elements of GLP as they apply to toxicology studies.

These elements themselves provide the environment within which good quality scientific work can be undertaken. It is worth noting that a study conducted in compliance with GLP is no guarantee of good science; good science is achieved through the application of good procedures, experienced and trained staff and the support of facility management in providing appropriate support, adequate resources, equipment and facilities.

To introduce GLP requires the interpretation and application of the GLP Regulations. This will inevitably mean that although the essential elements will be the same in any GLP facility, the detail at the operational level will be different. Therefore, no GLP facility will operate exactly the same as another. The way in which an organization implements the regulations should reflect the needs of that facility.

Management

As with any quality system, and GLP is no different, facility management commitment and support are a critical element required for the successful implementation of GLP within a facility.

Management is responsible for providing the environment within which toxicology studies are conducted. In GLP terms, this means ensuring that adequate Standard Operating Procedures (SOPs) exist, a Quality Assurance (QA) programme is in place, an archive is operated for the long-term retention of records, sufficient numbers of trained staff are available for the work being performed and appropriate facilities and equipment are available. Ultimately, it is facility management who are responsible for ensuring that the work conducted in a GLP facility is conducted in compliance with the GLP Regulations.

The responsibilities of 'Facility Management' defined in the various GLP standards/regulations include, but are not limited to, the following: management of the testing facility have responsibility for ensuring that the work, performed within the testing facility is carried out in accordance with the principles of GLP. As a minimum, management should:

- Designate a Study Director for each day.
- Replace the Study Director promptly if it becomes necessary to do so during the study, and record the action.
- Ensure that personnel employed on the study have sufficient training and experience to perform their duties, and that each individual clearly understands the functions he/she is to perform.
- Ensure that there are sufficient personnel for the proper conduct of studies and that their health, insofar as it may affect the integrity of studies, is monitored.
- Maintain a record of the qualifications, training and experience, together with a job description, for each professional and technical person involved in the study.
- Ensure that the laboratory facilities, equipment and experimental data handling procedures are of an adequate standard.
- Authorize all written SOPs. These SOPs should be adequate to ensure the quality and accuracy of data generated during the course of the study.

- Ensure that test and control articles or mixtures have been appropriately tested for identity, strength, purity, stability and uniformity as applicable.
- Ensure that a study protocol has been prepared for each study which is then approved by the sponsor prior to the study start. This document should also be authorized by management.
- Ensure that a system for tracking all studies works and a master schedule within the GLP facility is maintained. Such a system should enable the current status of existing or on-going work to be mapped. It must also serve as a mechanism to ascertain a historical listing of the progress of reported or completed work.
- Establish arrangements for a quality assurance programme and ensure that any problems reported during the monitoring of the study are communicated to the Study Director, and that corrective actions are taken and documented.
- Ensure that a historical file of all SOPs is maintained.
- Ensure that an individual is identified as responsible for the management of the archives.

Study Director

For each study, management should appoint a Study Director. The Study Director is the individual responsible for ensuring that the study is conducted in compliance with GLP, as well as being responsible for the interpretation, analysis, documentation and reporting of results. The Study Director is the single point of control in a study and fulfils the function of a Project Manager in ensuring that all goes according to the agreed plan. As a minimum, the responsibilities of a Study Director on any given study are to ensure that all aspects of the study are conducted in compliance with GLP. This includes, but is not limited to:

Study Plan (Protocol):

- Ensuring that a study plan is prepared which will include all the information required by GLP.
- Agreeing the final plan with management and the sponsor.
- Approving the study plan.
- Documenting and approving all/any changes to the study plan prior to effecting such changes in the form of a plan amendment.
- Ensuring prompt distribution of the plan, prior to animal arrival/study start, to all relevant individuals.

It should be noted that a study starts when the Study Director approves the final study plan. No data in a study should be generated prior to this date.

Study Conduct:

- Ensuring that the study is conducted in compliance with the study plan and all relevant SOPs.
- Documenting and approving prior to the event any planned deviations from SOPs.
- Ensuring that all experimental data including observations of responses of the test system are accurately recorded and verified.
- Promptly notifying the study sponsor, QA department and management of any unscheduled event which could compromise the integrity/outcome of the study and ensure such events are fully and completely/documented.

The Study Director should play an active and involved part in the conduct of the studies he/she directs. Whilst this may not include practical involvement, such as administering the test material, the Study Director should frequently visit the animal room and/or laboratory to discuss the progress of the study with those involved. Such involvement in the study should be documented in the study file.

Report Preparation:

- Being responsible for the preparation of a final report, which accurately records all the results generated during the course of the study and contains all the various information required by GLP.
- Preparing a GLP compliance statement for inclusion in the final report indicating the compliance of the reported study and accepting the responsibility of the validity of the data generated during the course of the study.
- Approving the final study report.

Data retention:

- Ensuring all raw data, specimens, slides, study protocols and other documentation, including the final report, are retained and transferred to archives as soon as practicable on completion of the study.
- On submission of data, and specimens to archives, ensuring the preparation of an inventory which details the type and amount of specimens and documentation sent for retention. This inventory should accompany the data to the archive as it will be used to account for the data sent.

Once archived, the continued retention of this material becomes the responsibility of facility management.

The Study Director is not required to observe every data collection event, but should ensure that data are collected, as specified by the study plan and SOPs, and that data collection includes the accurate recording of any unanticipated responses of the test system or study events. The Study Director should also review data periodically, to promote the accurate recording of data and to ensure that data are technically correct as well as compliant with GLP. Systems must be in place to ensure that the Study Director is notified promptly of unforeseen circumstances that may have an effect on the integrity of the study. Furthermore, as the Study Director is responsible for the GLP compliance of the study, it is important that he or she is fully aware of the requirements of the GLP Regulations.

Principal Investigator

Where a Study Director cannot exercise on-site supervisory control over any given phase of the study, a principal investigator will be identified/nominated to act on the Study Director's behalf for the defined phase. The principal investigator will be named in the study plan or by protocol amendment, and also the phase(s) of the study covered by each principal investigator's responsibilities will be delineated. The principal investigator will be an appropriately qualified and experienced individual suitably positioned to be able to supervise immediately the applicable phase.

The principal investigator, acting on behalf of the Study Director, will ensure that the relevant phase(s) of the study are conducted in accordance with the study plan, relevant SOPs and GLP. These responsibilities will include, but are not necessarily limited to, the following:

- Collaborating as appropriate with the Study Director and other study scientists in the drafting of the study plan.
- Ensuring that the study personnel are properly briefed, that such briefings are documented and that copies of the study plan and relevant SOPs are freely accessible to personnel as necessary.
- Ensuring that all experimental data, including unanticipated responses of the test system, are accurately recorded.
- Ensuring that all deviations from SOPs and the study plan (unforeseen occurrences or inadvertent errors) are noted when they occur and that, where necessary, corrective action is immediately taken; these are recorded in the raw data. As soon as practicable, the Study Director should be informed of such deviations. Amendments to the study plan (permanent changes, modifications or revisions), however, must be authorized in writing by the Study Director.
- Ensuring that all relevant raw data and records are adequately maintained to ensure data integrity and that they are transferred in a timely way to the Study Director or as directed in the study plan.
- Ensuring that all samples and specimens taken during the relevant study phase(s) are adequately protected against confusion and deterioration during

handling and storage; ensuring that these samples and specimens are dispatched in an appropriate manner as required by the study plan.
- Signing and dating a report of the relevant phase(s), certifying that the report accurately presents all the work done, and all the results obtained, and that the work was conducted in compliance with GLP. Sufficient commentary should be included in this report to enable the Study Director to write a valid final report covering the whole study, and send the report to the Study Director. The principal investigator may present the original raw data as his report, where applicable, including a statement of compliance with GLP.

The role of the principal investigator at a test site is to direct the work at the site and to ensure that the phase of the study is conducted in compliance with GLP. The role is similar to that of the Study Director with the exception that the role is limited to a site and a defined part of the study. The elements of the Study Director's role which cannot be performed by the principal investigator include approving the study plan or any amendments and authorizing the final study report.

The principal investigator will ensure that the delegated phases of the study are conducted in accordance with the applicable principles of GLP.

The key to the responsibilities of the Study Director and the principal investigator are:

- The study plan should identify the principal investigators and the role and responsibilities they are to take in the study.
- Any number of principal investigators may be appointed in a study; however, a principal investigator should not be appointed at the same site as the Study Director.
- The principal investigator is responsible to the Study Director for the GLP compliance of the work for which he or she is responsible.
- The principal investigator may be responsible for reporting the results of the work performed to the Study Director for inclusion in the final study report.
- Whilst taking responsibility for most GLP aspects of the part of the study for which he or she is responsible, the principal investigator may not approve the study plan, authorize plan amendments or authorize the final study report.
- The principal investigator should sign a statement of GLP compliance for that part of the study for which he or she is responsible.

Quality Assurance (QA)

There shall exist, within a testing facility, an individual or organizational group known as QA, separate from and independent to the personnel directly engaged in the control and conduct of a study. This individual or group shall give assurance to the management of the facility and the Study Director on individual projects that such work is conducted and reported to a high standard of quality and in accordance with existing GLP regulatory requirements.

The major purpose of QA is to assure facility management and the Study Director that the work within the facility and on individual studies has been conducted in compliance with GLP, company policy, SOPs and the study plan or if not, then to notify them of the deficiencies.

QA Operating Principles

- The test facility should have a documented QA programme to ensure that studies performed are in compliance with the GLP. QA should also confirm that those test facilities within which studies are performed comply with GLP.
- A copy of all study plans (protocol) and any amendments should be maintained.
- Written records of inspections undertaken by QA and any action taken by the Study Director and management to correct adverse findings should be kept.
- Management should be told if the facilities, equipment, personnel, methods, practices, records and controls are not considered to be in conformity with current GLP Regulations.

QA is a mechanism used to monitor ongoing studies to determine that the study plans and written SOPs have been followed. Thus the QA within a testing facility is charged with the responsibility for assuring the regulatory agency, the facility management and the Study Director that the facilities, equipment, personnel, methods, practices, procedures, records and controls are designed and function in conformance with GLP and the study plans for individual non-clinical laboratory studies.

The responsibilities of the QA personnel should be inclusive of, but not be limited to, the following functions:

- Verifying that the study plan contains information required for compliance with the principles of GLP; this verification should be documented.
- Ascertaining that the study plan and SOPs are available to personnel conducting the safety study.
- Ensuring that the study plan and SOPs are followed by periodic inspections of the laboratory and/or by auditing the safety study in progress. Records of such procedures should be retained.
- Promptly reporting to management and the Study Director unauthorized deviations from the study plan and from SOPs.

- Reviewing the final reports to confirm that the methods, procedures and observations are accurately described, and that the reported results accurately reflect the raw data of the safety study.
- Preparing and signing a statement to be included with the final report, which specifies the dates when inspections were made and the dates any findings were reported to management and to the Study Director.

The overall purpose of the QA programme should be to confirm to management and the Study Director that the work for which they are responsible is being conducted in compliance with GLP or, if not, to identify areas of concern and non-compliance. To achieve this objective the design and implementation of the QA programme will be different in each facility.

Personnel

Personnel involved in a toxicology study should:

- Have sufficient education, training and experience to enable them to undertake their assigned functions. Such training should include the requirements of GLP.
- Have a record of training and experience and a job description. The training record should indicate procedures in which the individual has attained competence. Such records and job description should be prepared not only for those individuals directly involved in the study but should also include staff from support areas.
- Take the necessary personal and health precautions to avoid contamination of test system and test articles by the study staff.
- Wear, and change as often as necessary, clothing appropriate for the duties performed, to prevent microbiological, radiological or any other form of contamination of test systems and test articles by staff.

Personnel working on GLP studies must be trained in GLP practice, have access to the appropriate SOPs and study plans and record study results accurately and in compliance with the GLP requirements.

- All study personnel involved in the conduct of study must be knowledgeable in those parts of the GLP which are applicable to their involvement in the study.
- Study personnel will have access to the study plan and appropriate SOPs applicable to their involvement in the study. It is their responsibility to comply with the instructions given in these documents. Any deviation from these instructions should be

documented and communicated directly to the Study Director and/or, if appropriate, the principal investigator(s).

■ All study personnel are responsible for recording raw data promptly and accurately and in compliance with GLP and are responsible for the quality of their data.

Laboratory Areas

GLP requires that a separate area should be provided, as necessary, for the various operations and activities on a study to prevent possible contamination or mix-ups occurring. The testing facilities should be of a suitable size and construction for the purpose intended.

If a testing facility is too small to handle its planned volume of work, there may be an inclination to mix incompatible functions. Examples might include the simultaneous conduct of studies involving incompatible species in the same room, setting up a small office in the corner of an animal housing area or housing an excessive number of animals in a room.

The facility should be constructed of materials which facilitate cleaning as appropriate for the species or study type involved. Heating, ventilation and air conditioning systems should be of adequate capacity to produce environmental conditions which comply with animal health and safety standards and should be designed to preclude any cross-contamination.

In principle, toxicity studies should be conducted in an appropriate facility to ensure the status of the test system plus the quality and integrity of study data generated within that facility.

Animal Care Facilities

A testing facility should have a sufficient number of animal rooms or areas to assure the proper separation of species or test systems, isolation of individual projects, quarantine of animals and routine or specialized procedures to be performed in a study.

Separate areas should be provided, as appropriate, for the diagnosis, treatment and control of laboratory animal diseases. These areas must provide effective isolation for the housing of animals either known to be or suspected of being diseased, or of being carriers of disease, from other animals.

Where animals are housed, facilities must exist for the collection and disposal of all animal waste and refuse or for safe sanitary storage of waste before removal from the testing facility. Disposal facilities must be provided and operated in such a way as to minimize vermin infestation, odours, disease hazards and environmental contamination.

There should also be storage areas, as needed, for feed, bedding, supplies and equipment. Storage areas for feed and bedding must be separated from areas housing the test systems and should be protected against infestation or contamination. Perishable supplies must be preserved by appropriate means.

Equipment

Equipment used in the generation, measurement, or assessment of data and equipment used for facility environmental control must be appropriate in design and of adequate capacity to function according to the study plan and be suitably located for operation, inspection, cleaning and maintenance.

Written records should be maintained of all inspection, maintenance, testing, calibrating and/or standardizing operations. These records, containing the date of the operation and the type performed, such equipment used for the generation, measurement, or assessment of data should also be adequately tested, calibrated and/or standardized before use.

Standard Operating Procedures (SOPs)

A testing facility must have SOPs in writing, setting forth the methods and procedures that the management is satisfied are adequate to ensure the quality and integrity of the data generated in the course of a study.

Where the Study Director, pathologist or other principal scientist recognizes a need for a variation in the SOPs for a given study, this is acceptable provided that the modification is agreed by the Study Director and is documented in the study raw data. Significant changes in established SOPs should be properly authorized in writing by management; this may require the revision or re-issue of the SOP.

Within each laboratory area, staff should have immediately available to them, the SOPs relating to the procedures performed in that area. Published literature such as operating manuals and text books may be used as supplementary information to the SOP. A historical file of SOPs, and all revisions thereof, including the dates of such revisions, should be maintained. SOPs should be periodically reviewed to maintain their accuracy. SOPs should be available for most procedures including the following categories of laboratory activities. The details given under each heading are to be considered as illustrative examples.

Test Substances (Including Control and Reference Substances)

■ Receipt, identification, characterization, handling, formulation and storage of substances, including expiry date, where appropriate.

- Testing of homogeneity and stability of test substance mixtures with carriers.
- Administration of test substance.

Test System

- Procedures for receipt, transfer, proper placement, identification and care of animals or other test system.
- Test system observations and examinations.
- Laboratory tests and analyses.
- Handling of animals found moribund or dead during the study.
- Experimental work using microorganisms.
- Autopsy procedures.
- Collection and identification of specimens.
- Histopathology and other post-mortem studies.
- Field studies.

Equipment

- Use of equipment.
- Maintenance, cleaning, calibration and/or standardization.
- Identification and instructions for use of computer hardware and software.

Documentation

- Data collection, handling, storage and retrieval.
- Preparation of reports.

SOPs should be treated as controlled documents, i.e. their distribution should be monitored to enable, when appropriate, an SOP can be re-issued and the old or out-of-date SOPs to be withdrawn.

It should be recognized that SOPs provide a mechanism by which the management of a facility can establish the quality level or standards they wish to be applied within the organization. The defining of the procedures to be followed within a facility is the first step in establishing any quality system.

Study Plan (Protocol)

For each study, a written approved study plan should be produced which indicates the work to be undertaken and the methodologies involved in the conduct of that study. Such a plan should be distributed and available to all staff engaged in the conduct of that study. Any changes to the plan must be in the form of an authorized amendment by the Study Director issued prior to the implementation of the change and maintained with each copy of the plan. The study plan should be prepared and distributed prior to the arrival of test system. Staff engaged in

the conduct of the study must have easy access to the study plan and any amendments.

The following is a guide to the items to be included in a study plan.

General

Study number. It is usual for a study to have a unique number by which it is identified. This number should appear on all data, records or specimens as a means of study identifications.

Name and address of the testing facility. The postal address of the testing facility. The address of any company or individual to which certain tests or analyses may be sub-contracted should also be identified.

Descriptive title. This should include the type of study, i.e. toxicity, metabolism, etc., the compound name or code number, species or the animal and, if appropriate, route of administration and duration of study in weeks.

Name and address of sponsor.

Name of sponsor's monitoring scientist.

Background to Study

Statement of study purpose.

Justification for test system selection. A number of possible justifications could include:

- Because this species/strain metabolizes the test compound in the same way as man.
- Because previous studies with the particular test compound have been done in this species/strain/substrain and the present work is required for comparison to be done in the same species.
- To meet the requirements/recommendations of governmental regulatory agencies.
- Because the sponsor instructed you to use this species/strain/substrain without giving further reasons, i.e. the statement "at sponsor request".
- Because the sponsor has substantial amounts of background data or experience with this species/strain/substrain.
- To compare findings with those obtained with other species/strains.
- Because of intended use of test compound (this applies, for example, with veterinary compounds when the target animal might be species of choice).

Reference to a test guideline. This is a requirement of OECD GLPs. If no test guideline is applicable then a statement to that effect is preferred to omission.

Name of Study Director. This is self explanatory; however, it must be pointed out that it is not possible to have two Study Directors for the same study.

Proposed Study Dates

These dates must be included in the study plan.

Delivery of animals. If animals were ordered specifically for the study, then the date of arrival at the test facility should be entered into the plan. If, however, the animals are selected from stock, it is the date on which the animals were allocated to the study from stock that should be placed in the plan.

First day of dosing. This is fairly straightforward except when a staggered start is to be operated, in which case all dates for the first day of dosing for each group or sex should be given; the time relative to first dose group or day of pregnancy (in a teratology study) is acceptable.

Interim sacrifice(s). The dates on which all interim sacrifices are to be made should be given in the protocol; again, times relative to first dose are acceptable.

Final sacrifice/completion of laboratory work. The date on which the final sacrifice is due to commence or the date of anticipated completion of laboratory work should be indicated in the plan.

Test System

Species. Dog, mouse, rat, rabbit, etc. Scientifically, 'primates' is not a species but a natural order. Both common names and generic and specific names are best given, e.g. cynomolgus monkey (*Macaca fascicularis*).

Strain. Beagle would be the strain of dog, New Zealand White the strain of rabbits, Large White the strain of pig, etc. In the case of the rat, Wistar and Sprague–Dawley are technically the strains and CFHB and CFY the substrains.

Supplier. The name and address of the animal supplier. In the case of primates and avian species, whether home bred or wild caught should be stated.

Bodyweight range. The bodyweight range of animals used should be stated and also the time point to which this range applies, i.e. on receipt, at first dose.

Age. This should be at the time of commencement of pre-dose period; however, provided sufficient information is given to be able to calculate this figure, then that is sufficient.

Test and Control Substances

Name/code number. The test substance name and/or code numbers plus alternative names should be given.

Identity. Chemical name or structure.

Strength. Concentration of solution, if applicable.

Purity. For radiochemicals, reference should be made to radiochemical purity and to specific activity.

Stability. The period over which the test material can be used.

Batch number(s). Purity data and batch number of the test material.

Test Substance: Mixtures

Method and frequency of preparation. A brief description of methods to be used in dose preparation and the frequency of preparation should be given. Frequency of dispensing should be provided in addition if appropriate.

Tests to determine homogeneity, stability and concentration. The study plan should state that tests to identify these parameters are being made and identify the organization who is performing them, if not your own.

Description of dosing vehicle. Details of any suspending/dispersing agents should be given.

Test System: Treatment and Maintenance

Location of study. Inclusion of building by name or number.

Environmental conditions. Temperature and humidity ranges and light/dark cycles.

Number of groups. The number of treatment and control groups in the study.

Number of each sex per group. Self-explanatory.

Method of animal identification. Tattoo, earmark, etc. The numbers used should be recorded in the study plan.

Route of administration. For all administrations it should be stated whether by capsules, dietary, gastric intubation, etc. (oral is not sufficient).

Reason for choice of route. The reason for choice to some extent will be covered in the Statement of Purpose, but a justification should still be given, e.g. because that is the route by which the test compound will be administered to man.

Dosage levels. This should include appropriate units and any control substances used as well as test compound.

Method, frequency and duration of dosing. The method of dosing should include brief details of the procedure to be followed. The frequency should be interpreted as number to times per day, number of days per week, number of weeks of administration. Duration is interpreted as the number of days or weeks the test system is exposed to the test compound. Any periods of recovery/withdrawal from treatment should be specified.

Description of experimental design. The study plan as a whole should define the design of the study.

Methods for the control of bias. This section should be used to identify the method used to ensure a random or bias-free allocation of animals to treatment groups or location within the animal unit.

Description and identification of diet. This should include the name of suppliers, commercial name and form of diet, i.e. powder, pellet, granules, etc. Any supplementary items of diet should also be identified, i.e. fruit, bread, blackcurrant juice, etc. Further description or identification is not necessary.

Identification of the level of any contaminant expected to be present in the diet at levels capable of affecting the study. The Study Director should be aware of any possible contaminant that could be present in the diet (or bedding) being used that could have an effect upon the test material or test system. All such possible contaminants should be identified in the study plan.

Reference to determine absorption. If this is to be done by the testing facility, the methods used should be stated in the study plan.

Observations

Type, frequency and methods of specified tests, analyses, observations, examinations and measurements. Self-explanatory and including bodyweights, food and water consumption, clinical signs, ophthalmoscopy, clinical pathology, gross pathological examination, organ weights, histopathological examination, etc.

Records to be maintained. It should suffice that a statement in the study plan indicates that all records will be maintained of all test measurements and analyses as listed in the plan.

Proposed statistical method. An outline of the methods to be used should be included with a comment that further examination using different statistical methods may be performed depending on the results generated.

Archiving. Location of archiving of all raw data samples and specimens associated with the study should be given.

GLP statement. The study plan should give an indication as to whether the study is to be conducted in compliance with GLP. If so, then the precise regulation should be specified in the study plan.

Dates and signatures of protocol approval. The study plan approval page should be signed and dated by the Study Director, facility management and the sponsor. The signature page should be numbered as part of the study plan.

It should always be remembered that the study plan is the intended plan for the study. It is the instruction from the Study Director to the study staff on what should be undertaken and when. Changes to this plan can be made via formal documented amendment which the Study Director must approve prior to the change.

CONDUCT OF STUDY

The study should be conducted as defined in the study plan and appropriate SOPs.

All data generated during the conduct of a study should be captured or recorded directly, promptly and legibly in ink. All data entries should be dated on the date of entry and signed or initialled by the person entering/recording the data.

Any change or corrections to raw data should be made so as not to obscure the original entry, should indicate the reason for such change and should be dated and signed or initialled at the time of the change. In automated data collection systems, the individual responsible for direct data input should be identified at the time of data input. Any change in automated data entries should be made so as not to lose the original entry, should indicate the reason for change and should be dated with the individual making the change being identified (an audit trail).

Specific Areas

The following are some specific areas of study conduct which are influenced by GLP requirements.

Refrigerators and Freezers

These should be kept neat and tidy with all items clearly labelled and identified. Items should be stored in a way to prevent cross-contamination. Monitoring the temperature of refrigerators and freezers should be appropriate for the type of samples being retained. Materials stored in freezers should be logged and tracked to control the duration and location of storage.

Snopake

Snopake or other such 'white out' material should never be used on raw data.

Availability of SOPs

SOPs need to be available and accessible in the workplace for those individuals who are required to follow them. The SOPs available should be the current versions with all appropriate SOPs for the work being conducted available. Staff should also be aware of the content of the SOPs and be appropriately trained in the performance of the procedures.

Equipment Maintenance

Records of equipment maintenance including routine and non-routine servicing should be maintained. Details of the maintenance performed should be retained.

Equipment Calibration

If appropriate, each piece of equipment should be calibrated at a suitable frequency. If required, such calibration should be traceable to a national standard.

Computer Systems Acceptance Testing

Computer systems are no different to any other piece of equipment in that they should be suitably calibrated and tested before use. Such acceptance testing should be documented.

Controlled Computer System Access

Computer systems should be password protected to ensure that only authorized access is permitted.

Labelling of Chemicals, Reagents and Solutions

All such materials within the laboratory should be suitably labelled. Such labelling may include material identity, concentration, storage conditions and use-by date. Other information such as the date of receipt, date first opened or re-assay date may also be included if appropriate.

Appropriate Storage for Consumables and Equipment

Consumables and equipment should be suitably stored. Often items are observed stacked on the floor or 'hidden' in other unsuitable locations.

Unofficial Notices

These can take many different forms, often a copy of a page from an SOP, a temporary instruction to staff or an instruction which is long out of date. Any documented instruction should be appropriately authorized, dated and controlled.

Sample Log-in and Sample Tracking

All samples entering the laboratory should be appropriately logged and their movement tracked whilst in the facility.

A Clean and Tidy Laboratory.

A clean, tidy and well-organised laboratory says a lot about the way the laboratory operates. Unnecessary material should be removed and regular housekeeping should be undertaken.

Accountability of the Test Substance

It is important that accurate records of test substance usage are maintained. It should be possible to account for all the test substance from the time of receipt in the laboratory to return or destruction.

Properly Corrected Data

Any corrections or alterations to raw data should be crossed through with a single line so as not to obscure the original entry, the revised value recorded, a reason for the change given and the dated signature of the individual making the change recorded.

Access to the Current Study Plan Plus any Amendments

Staff working on a particular study should have easy access to the study plan and all amendments.

Awareness of the GLP Regulations

Staff working in compliance with GLP should be aware of and trained in the GLP regulations and have access to a copy of the Statutory Instrument and/or the set of GLP regulations to which the study is being conducted.

Training Records

All individuals who take part in the conduct of a GLP study should maintain a personnel training record.

The purpose of the training record from a GLP perspective is to provide evidence to third parties, such as regulatory authorities or Study Director, that an individual involved in the conduct of a study is suitably trained and experienced to undertake, in the correct manner, those procedures they have been requested to perform.

In many organizations a "personnel training" file is maintained. Such a file may contain, in addition to an individual's training record, 'personal details' such as a CV and job description. In taking such an approach, all information relating to the qualifications, training and experience for that individual may be retained in one place and 'follows' that individual during his or her service with the organization.

STUDY REPORT

For each study, the boundaries of which are defined by the study plan, a final report should be produced. As a minimum this report should contain the following information:

- Name and address of the facility performing the study and the dates on which the study was initiated and completed.
- Objectives and procedures stated in the approved study plan, including any changes in the original study plan.
- Statistical methods employed for analysing the data.

- The test and control articles identified by name, Chemical Abstracts number or code number, strength, purity and composition or other appropriate characteristics.
- Stability of the test and control articles under the conditions of administration.
- Description of the methods used.
- A description of the test system used. Where applicable, the final report should include the number of animals used, sex, bodyweight range, source of supply, species, strain and substrain, age and procedures used for identification.
- A description of the dosage, dosage regimen, route of administration and duration.
- A description of all circumstances that may have affected the quality or integrity of the data.
- The name of the Study Director, the names of other scientists or professionals and the names of all supervisory personnel involved in the study.
- A description of the transformations, calculations or operations performed on the data, a summary and analysis of the data and a statement of the conclusions drawn from the analysis.
- The signed and dated reports of each of the individual scientists or other professionals involved in the study.
- The locations where all specimens, raw data and the final report are to be stored.

The final report should also contain the following signed and dated statements:

Study Director: The Study Director should prepare a statement indicating that the study was conducted in compliance, or not, as the case may be, with GLP. The statement should also indicate with which GLP Regulations compliance of the study is claimed.

Quality Assurance (QA). The QA Unit should prepare a statement to indicate that the final report has been audited and found to be a true, complete and accurate reflection of the data generated in the study. The dates on which study inspections were conducted and the dates on which management and the Study Director were informed should also be reported.

Once the final report has been issued changes to that report may only be made by formal amendment. On completion of the study, the final report and all records data and samples should be placed in the archive for their secure, long-term retention. It is the Study Director's responsibility to ensure this is done.

ARCHIVES

It is one of management's responsibilities to provide suitable facilities for the long term retention of data. Such facilities should be adequate to protect the data and ensure its integrity is maintained. Management

should appoint an individual to take responsibility for these records, known as the archivist. Records held by the archivist in the archive are held on behalf of facility management.

The Archive

The archive is a secure facility used for the storage of data and materials. It could be a file cabinet or purpose-built facility with mobile racking. Whilst in the archive, data should be protected against loss and be held in an environment which prevents deterioration and damage. The archive should also be maintained in a fashion which permits easy retrieval of materials with access being restricted to authorized personnel only.

Personnel

Access to the archive should be limited to authorized archive personnel. If company staff need to enter the archive they must be accompanied by archive staff. A log should be kept of *all* visitors to the archive. Should it be necessary for other personnel to enter the archive, records of their entry should be maintained. These records should indicate the reason for the entry, the date of entry, the purpose and the name of the archive staff accompanying them. The system of physical access restriction, i.e. keys/cards/electromagnetic codes, should be operated effectively.

Index of Material

All raw data, samples and specimens in the archives should be properly indexed and stored in an orderly manner which permits rapid retrieval. Samples of test compounds should be correctly labelled for test compound, batch number, quantity, date and be stored in accordance with the label and protocol. The way in which samples are indexed, be this a simple index card or computerized system, is not of importance provided that access to the information is maintained. The physical location of material within the archive is only important to protect the data or sample integrity. All data for one study do not need to be located in the same place. It is frequently found that records such as electronic computer files are held in a separate area. This is acceptable provided that the archivist maintains control over these records in the same way for all other records.

Retrieval of Material from the Archive

A procedure for the retrieval of material deposited in the archive should be established. A formal retrieval authorization should be obtained in writing from the facility management. The reason for the retrieval should also be recorded. The request is presented to a member of the archive staff who retrieves the required material from the storage area. A register of retrievals should be maintained in order that the tracking of items removed can be kept. When the material is returned, the information is recorded in the retrieval log. Retrieval of material from the archive should be restricted insofar as possible. Photocopies of data may be provided as opposed to the removal of records. By so doing, the raw data are kept under the control of the archivist. If material is loaned from the archive then checks on its return must be made to confirm all material has been returned.

Delayed Return of Retrievals

If retrieved materials from the archive are not returned by the date shown on the authorization form, a request is sent to the individual who requested the loan, with a copy to the manager who authorized the loan, requesting its return or renewed authorization. If no action is taken, a further reminder will be sent with a copy to the QA who will take action if the material remains outstanding.

Facility Management

The archivist should produce regular reports to management which detail problems/difficulties encountered during the operation of the archive, with evidence that these problems were resolved.

APPLICATION OF GLP TO COMPUTER SYSTEMS

When GLP was first promulgated, few companies had on-line data capture systems. As time has passed more and more computer systems have been developed and introduced within organizations. With this increase in computerization has come a growing interest from GLP monitoring bodies in the way such systems have been designed, developed, introduced, operated and controlled in order that compliance with GLP is maintained throughout an organization. In the UK, the Department of Health GLP Monitoring Unit first published in December 1988, revised in 1995, a document entitled 'The application of GLP principles to computer systems'. As the title suggests, this document identifies and applies those elements of GLP which relate to computer systems.

The US Food and Drug Administration (FDA), in the absence of any official regulatory intent, organized a meeting to which were invited 66 individuals from industry, government and academia on October 11, 1987, at the Red Apple Conference Center in Arkansas. The purpose of the meeting was to prepare a reference book which would present current concepts and procedures for the computer automation of toxicology laboratories and describe effective means for ensuring the quality of computerized data systems. The book from this consensus meeting was published in September 1988 (FDA, 1988).

The FDA has published new regulations concerning the use of electronic records and electronic signatures. This final rule will impact upon the use of such systems in the conduct of toxicology studies (FDA, 1997). The direction of organizations such as the FDA and the MCA GLP Monitoring Unit is to ensure as far as possible that computers involved in the capture and or manipulation of data used in support of safety assessment are developed, tested, introduced and operated in such a way as to ensure data integrity.

CONCLUSION

The purpose of GLP Regulations is to ensure as far as possible the quality and integrity of the data submitted to a receiving authority in support of the safety assessment of a product. To this end, most of the requirements of GLP would be considered familiar and reasonable by any conscientious scientist performing quality research. Study Plan and SOPs, adequate facilities and equipment, full identification of test substance, proper animal care, equipment maintenance, accurate recording of observations and accurate reporting of results are basic necessities for the conduct of high-quality, valid toxicology studies.

REFERENCES

EEC (1979). Council Directive of 18th September 1979 amending for the sixth time Directive 67/548/EEC on the approximation of the laws, regulations and administrative provisions relating to the classification, packaging and labelling of dangerous substances. *Off. J. Eur. Commun.*, No. L259, 10–28.

EEC (1987). Council Directive of 18th December 1986 on the harmonisation of laws, regulations and administrative provisions relating to the application of the principles of good laboratory practice and the verification of their application for tests on chemical substances. *Off. J. Eur. Commun.*, No. LO15, 29–30.

EEC (1988). Council Directive of the 9th June 1988 on the inspection and verification of good laboratory practice (GLP). *Off. J. Eur. Commun.*, No. L145, 35–37.

EEC (1989). Council Decision of 28th July 1989 on the acceptance by the European Economic Community of an OECD decision/recommendation on compliance with principles of good laboratory practice. *Off. J. Eur. Commun.*, No. L315, 1–17.

EPA (1983). US Environmental Protection Agency. Federal Insecticide, Fungicide and Rodenticide Act (FIFRA) Title 40. Code of Federal Regulations Part 160. *Federal Register*, 29 November 1983. US Government Printing Office, Washington, DC.

EPA (1989). US Environmental Protection Agency. Toxic Substances Control Act (TOSCA) Title 40. Code of Federal Regulations Part 160. *Federal Register*, 17 August 1989. US Government Printing Office, Washington, DC.

FDA (1978). US Food and Drug Administration. Title 21. Code of Federal Regulations Part 58. *Federal Register*, 22 December 1978. US Government Printing Office, Washington, DC.

FDA (1988). US Food and Drug Administration. *Computerised data systems for non-clinical safety assessment. Current concepts and quality assurance.* US Food and Drug Administration, Washington DC.

FDA (1997). US Food and Drug Administration. Electronic Records: Electronic Signatures; Final Rule. FDA 21. Code of Federal Regulations Part 2. *Federal Register*, 20 March 1997. US Government Printing Office, Washington, DC.

Japan: Ministry of Agriculture, Forestry and Fisheries (1984). 59 Nohsan, Notification No. 3850, Agricultural Production Bureau, 10 August 1984.

Japan: Ministry of Health and Welfare (1987). Notification No. Yakahatsu 313. Pharmaceutical Affairs Bureau, 31 March 1982 and subsequent ammendment Notification No. Yakahatsu 870, Pharmaceutical Affairs Bureau, 5 October 1988 and subsequently revised (Ministry of Health and Welfare Ordinance No. 21, March 1997).

Japan: Ministry of International Trade and Industry (1984). Directive, (Kanpogyo No. 39 Environmental Agency, Kikyoku No. 85, Ministry of International Trade and Industry), 31 March 1984.

OECD (1982). *Good Laboratory Practice in the Testing of Chemicals.* Organization for Economic Cooperation and Development, Paris.

OECD (1997). *Principles of Good Laboratory Practice.* Organization for Economic Cooperation and Development, Paris.

UK (1990). *The Application of GLP Principles to Field Studies.* Advisory Leaflet. UK GLP Monitoring Authority, London.

UK (1991). *Good Laboratory Practice and the Role of Quality Assurance.* Advisory Leaflet. UK GLP Monitoring Authority, London.

UK (1992). *Good Laboratory Practice and the Role of the Study Director.* Advisory Leaflet. UK GLP Monitoring Authority, London.

UK (1995). *The Application of GLP Principles to Computer Systems.* Advisory Leaflet. UK GLP Monitoring Authority, London.

UK (1997) *The Good Laboratory Practice Regulations 1997.* Statutory Instrument No. 654. HM Stationery Office, London.

Chapter 22

Toxicity Data Obtained from Human Studies

Martin F. Wilks and Neil A. Minton

CONTENTS

INTRODUCTION

The rationale for choosing animal or *in vitro* models for toxicity testing is based on the assumption that they offer a reasonable prediction of what may happen in humans as, in most cases, the ultimate species of interest. The main tasks of experimental toxicology have been defined as related to the spectrum of toxicity (detection of adverse effect and description of dose–response relationship), extrapolation from one species to another, particularly to humans, and prediction of safe levels of exposure (Zbinden, 1991). In contrast, most toxicity data from humans are observational and subject to much larger uncertainties and variations than animal toxicology studies (**Table 1**). Where experimental data in humans are obtained, they have to conform with strict ethical guidance and are constrained by practical limitations. Nevertheless, the continuing drive for a reduction in animal experimentation has stimulated the search for alternative methods of toxicity testing, including human studies (Volans *et al.*, 1991). Furthermore, both regulators and the concerned public are increasingly looking for actual human data to confirm or refute perceived health risks from chemical exposure.

The purpose of this chapter is to explore the benefits and limitations of various types of human studies which are of use in toxicity evaluations. This will be made in the context of specific subsets of human exposure to xenobiotics, e.g. exposure to industrial chemicals, pharmaceuticals or agricultural chemicals, in which certain types of studies have a particular relevance.

ETHICAL ISSUES

All research involving human subjects should only be conducted once ethical issues have been formally considered and documented. The principle of an ethical 'Code of Conduct' for such research was first enshrined following the trial of Nazi physicians who had conducted atrocious experiments on prisoners and detainees during the Second World War (USA, 1949). This so-called 'Nuremberg Code' was designed to protect the integrity of the individual, setting out conditions for the ethical conduct of research involving human subjects, in particular the principle of 'voluntary consent' to research. In 1966, the General Assembly of the United Nations adopted the International Covenant on Civil

Table 1 Some characteristics of animal experiments and human studies in toxicology

	Animal experiment	Human study
Genetic variability	Homogeneous	Heterogeneous
Age distribution	Uniform	Variable
Pre-existing morbidity	None	Frequent
Diet	Controlled	Uncontrolled
Environment	Controlled	Uncontrolled
Exposure	Onset and duration known	Onset and duration usually not known or variable
	Single agent exposure	Multiple agent exposure
	Exposure route defined	Multiple exposure routes
	Multiple dose levels	Dose unknown
Effect	Prospectively defined by observation, laboratory analysis and histopathology	Frequently established by retrospective analysis of morbidity and mortality data

and Political Rights, of which Article 7 states, 'No one shall be subjected to torture or to cruel, inhuman or degrading treatment or punishment. In particular, no one shall be subjected without his free consent to medical or scientific experimentation'.

The Declaration of Helsinki, adopted in 1964 by the World Medical Association, has become the fundamental document in the area of biomedical research and has formed the basis for international and national legislation and codes of conduct. The Declaration has been revised and updated several times, most recently at the South Africa Meeting of the Association in 1996. The Declaration sets out ethical guidelines for physicians engaged in clinical (patient) and non-clinical (non-patient volunteer) biomedical research (WMA, 1997). In view of special circumstances prevailing in developing countries, the Council for International Organizations of Medical Sciences (CIOMS) and the World Health Organization (WHO) issued in 1982 the 'Proposed International Guidelines for Biomedical Research Involving Human Subjects'. The purpose was to indicate how the ethical principles enshrined in the Declaration of Helsinki could be effectively applied particularly in developing countries. The 'Proposed Guidelines' were revised and subsequently adopted by the XXVIth CIOMS Conference in 1992 (Bankowski and Levine, 1993).

In the revision of the 'Proposed Guidelines', it became clear that special attention needed to be paid to epidemiological studies because of their growing importance, particularly in the public health sector, and the relative paucity of guidance available. The result was the issuing by CIOMS in 1991 of the 'International Guidelines for the Ethical Review of Epidemiological Studies'. These focus particularly on the safeguarding of confidentiality in the absence of informed consent.

Numerous pieces of legislation and other guidelines are available at national and international level (for details, see Bankowski and Levine, 1993). For example, in the USA the Federal Policy on Protection of Human Subjects (Common Rule) applies to all government-supported research involving volunteers (USA, 1991). In the UK there is no statutory legislation concerning human studies with limited exceptions under the Medicines (Administration of Radioactive Substances) Regulations (UK, 1978; ARSAC, 1993) and the Human Fertilisation and Embryology Act (UK, 1990). Apart from the Medical Research Council's statement on 'Responsibility in Investigations on Human Subjects' issued in 1962–63 and some limited guidance by the Association of the British Pharmaceutical Industry and the Department of Health and Social Security, little public debate took place until 1984, when fierce criticism was voiced in a national newspaper over a repeat dose tolerability study with a retinoid, leading to the study being abandoned. There were questions in parliament and calls for the closure of independent contract research organizations. In the same year, two deaths were reported of volunteers

participating in drug trials, and these events prompted a report by the Royal College of Physicians of London (Royal College of Physicians, 1986) dealing with research on healthy volunteers. This report was followed by further guidelines on research involving patients (Royal College of Physicians, 1990a) and on the practice of ethics committees (Royal College of Physicians, 1990b).

In 1995, a conference was held on the subject of 'Volunteers in Research and Testing' and a book based on the conference proceedings discusses the ethical and practical aspects of human volunteer studies in more detail (Close et al., 1997). In the case of non-patient human volunteer studies there is no direct benefit to the individual participating in the investigation. It follows that, where there is no direct benefit, the risk to the volunteer of coming to harm as a result of participation in the study should be no greater than minimal. The Royal College of Physicians of London (Royal College of Physicians, 1990b) has used the term 'minimal risk' to cover two situations. The first is where there is a small chance of a reaction which in itself is trivial, e.g. a headache or a feeling of lethargy. The second is where there is a very remote chance of a serious disability or death. This second risk to the volunteer should be no greater than that of flying as a passenger in a scheduled aircraft.

Where there is no direct benefit to the individual, the knowledge gained is expected somehow to benefit the community. This carries the burden of demonstrating the societal value of the research, something which is very dependent on the position of the enquirer (Dayan, 1997). For example, improving the therapy of a rare but particularly aggressive form of cancer might be regarded as a worthier cause than demonstrating that a particular deodorant does or does not cause itching. Yet we are all likely to use the latter, whereas the majority of us fortunately do not suffer the former.

All research involving volunteers must be approved by an appropriately constituted, independent ethics committee (in the USA the term 'institutional review board' is frequently being used). This requires a balance of medical and non-medical, scientific and lay men and women who act independently of the study sponsor. It is the ethics committee's duty to ensure that there is adequate justification for the proposal, that the previously mentioned acceptability criteria are being followed and that every effort is being made to safeguard the health and welfare of the volunteers. The ethics committee must be prepared to co-opt experts to advise on specific scientific aspects of the study or the risks involved. The committee will have to pay particular attention to adequate volunteer information and informed consent, and it approves payment of the volunteers. Ethics committees should be informed without delay of any significant untoward event occurring during the course of the study and should be consulted about significant changes in a project. For some types of studies a class approval may be given to avoid repetitive submissions of projects differing only in detail. This is particularly appropriate for projects that pose no risk of distress or injury to subjects (Royal College of Physicians, 1990b).

Most of the available legislation and guidance have stemmed from the need to regulate the development of medicines with particular attention being paid to human volunteer studies. The basic principles, however, are equally applicable to other areas of human studies. Thus, a framework has been established in which research on humans is permissible and is to be encouraged subject to controls and safeguards. The most important criteria which any human study needs to fulfil can be summarized as follows (Wilks and Woollen, 1994):

1. There must be a detailed experimental protocol including provisions for appropriate ethical review.
2. The objectives of the research must be scientifically sound and directed to an advancement of biomedical knowledge. The desired information must not be obtainable otherwise, e.g. through animal or *in vitro* studies. The study should use as few subjects as possible, but as many as necessary to ensure scientific validity.
3. The procedures must be justifiable in terms of the objectives. This requires respect for the individual and the avoidance of unnecessary, trivial or degrading procedures.
4. A formal risk–benefit analysis must have been carried out. As a general rule, the smaller the direct benefit to the individual involved, the lower the risk must be.
5. The responsible investigators must be appropriately qualified to carry out the research. The welfare of the individual participating in the study must be paramount and all data generated must be confidential.
6. Informed consent has to be obtained from all subjects participating in a study, except in clearly defined circumstances. For example, a retrospective analysis of hospital records may not require informed consent, provided that anonymity is guaranteed. Informed consent requires a full explanation of the study and the risks involved in language which the subject can understand. Subjects must be free to withdraw from the study at any time without the need for explanation and without penalty. Special consideration needs to be given to informed consent when studying population groups which are not considered to be independent, self-controlling individuals such as children, those with defects of cognition and people who do not enjoy a free life (e.g. prisoners, members of the armed forces).
7. Study subjects should be compensated for the inconvenience of participating in a study, but the level of compensation should not act as an inducement to participate against their better judgement and should never be for undergoing risk.

EVALUATION OF DATA FROM HUMAN STUDIES

As mentioned above, all human studies should be designed and conducted according to accepted scientific principles. This is nowhere more important than in the evaluation of data derived from the study. It is therefore paramount to establish *a priori* what the purpose of the study is and whether the data generated are likely to fulfil the objective. Human studies fall broadly into two categories: those which are used to generate a hypothesis and those which test a hypothesis (Cohrssen and Covello, 1989).

Hypothesis-generating studies are usually of a descriptive nature. They include single or multiple case reports, reports of adverse reactions and studies which demonstrate a correlation between the occurrence of illness and the existence of occupational or environmental hazards.

In contrast, hypothesis-testing studies are observational, looking at individuals or small groups of people. These studies are analysed using established statistical methods to determine if an association exists between presence of an exposure hazard and the occurrence of illness. Often, the hypothesis examined has been previously generated by a descriptive study. Examples include two widely used types of epidemiological studies: case-control and cohort studies, and also most human volunteer studies.

Qualitative Evaluation of Human Data

The process of human data evaluation has traditionally been one of inductive reasoning, beginning with fragments of data from which to derive a hypothesis which aims to explain the development of illness by attributing its origin to one or more causes or risk factors (Hoel and Landrigan, 1987). The observational nature of many of the studies has led to the establishment of principles to examine cause–effect relationships (Hill, 1962). While the focus has largely been on the traditional epidemiology studies, the six criteria proposed by Hill (1965) can and should be applied to any human data generated in the process of establishing whether an observed association represents causality:

1. *The strength of the association*. In epidemiological studies this is usually expressed in terms of relative risk, i.e. the stronger the relative risk, the greater is the likelihood that the association is of a causal nature. However, confounding factors need to be carefully taken into account, e.g. smoking when studying the chemical origins of respiratory disease or lung cancer.
2. *The consistency of the association*. The reproducibility of a finding 'by different persons, in different places,

circumstances and times' (Hill, 1965) is one of the strongest arguments for the existence of causality.

3. *The temporal relationship between cause and effect.* For causality to exist, exposure must have preceded illness. In the case of latency periods it is important to conduct the study at a time when the exposure is likely to have produced an effect.

4. *The biological gradient of the association.* The establishment of a dose–response relationship is a powerful argument for causation. Likewise, any alteration in exposure leading to a change in disease frequency supports a causal relationship.

5. *The specificity of the association.* If exposure to a specific hazard is associated with one type of illness and vice versa, there is strong evidence for causality. Although this is not very common in xenobiotic-induced illness, there are examples such as asbestos and mesothelioma, aromatic amines and bladder cancer, or vinyl chloride and haemangiosarcoma of the liver. However, absence of specificity does not exclude causality.

6. *The biological plausibility of the association.* A proposed causal relationship should not seriously conflict with knowledge of biological and pathophysiological disease mechanisms. This is by no means an absolute criterion, but consistency between findings in human studies and other experimental data strengthens the argument for a causal relationship.

Quantitative Evaluation of Human Data

Analysis of human data is considered a critical component of quantitative risk assessment. This is a stepwise process in which the occurrence of disease in an exposed population is related quantitatively to the intensity and duration of exposure. The individual steps in the process are:

1. *Hazard identification.* This answers the question of whether a particular agent can cause a specific biological effect or illness. Although hazard assessment is the domain of experimental studies, human data sometimes provide the initial information.

2. *Dose–response relationship.* Is there a linear, non-linear or threshold pattern in the relationship between exposure and effect?

3. *Exposure assessment.* What is the intensity, frequency and duration of human exposure to the agent in question? This is often the most difficult part of the assessment, particularly when direct exposure measurements are not available, as is the case for most retrospective studies.

The last two steps combine to form the *risk characterization* part of the process. This relies heavily on the use of models for the calculation of risk. However, any such calculations must be treated with great caution because of the uncertainties, in particular when combining data from animal studies, usually carried out using high doses, and estimates of human exposure which themselves are rarely precise. It is customary to include uncertainty or assessment factors when trying to quantify risk to account for some of these variables. Details of the methodologies involved and their applications can be found elsewhere (Richmond *et al.*, 1981; Cohrssen and Covello, 1989; Hallenbeck, 1993).

SOURCES OF HUMAN DATA

There are various ways of looking at sources of human data, depending on the their ultimate use. One which has already been mentioned is the classification into hypothesis-generating and hypothesis-testing studies. Another way would be to focus on the study subjects or populations in terms of whether an intervention is carried out, such as withdrawing a subject from exposure, or whether observations are being made without interventions. If the study focuses on the individual, it is often referred to as a clinical study, whereas epidemiological studies look at population groups or subsets. Finally, the nature of the study can be either retrospective, i.e. taking an individual's or population group's health status or disease incidence and trying to correlate it with past exposure, or prospective, where the development of the disease is followed in exposed and non-exposed subjects over time, possibly over many years.

Some principles of epidemiology have already been referred to above and further details can be found elsewhere in this book (Chapter 70). For the purpose of this chapter, those sources of human data are selected which allow a direct, although not always easily quantifiable, assessment of individual chemical exposure and health effects. Thus, the principle sources of information are case reports and surveillance schemes, use of chemicals as therapeutic agents, worker exposure and health surveys and human volunteer studies.

Case Reports and Surveillance Schemes

Case reports identify one or more cases of disease which have been detected, usually by clinicians, as a result of the treatment of a patient, whereas case series often stem from active surveillance (e.g. in occupational medicine) or passive reporting (e.g. adverse drug reaction reporting). In many instances, case reports have served to alert physicians to the existence of occupational or environmental illness. The earliest recorded examples of case series of occupational or environmental illness are reports of lung disease among potters and weavers (Ramazzini, 1713) and observations of scrotal cancer among chimney sweeps (Pott, 1775). Many of the known human carcinogens were identified through case reports (Miller, 1978). For example, the first three cases of haemangiosarcoma of the liver in vinyl chloride-exposed workers were reported by a company physician, John Creech, in a PVC resin manufacturing plant in Louisville, Kentucky (Creech and Johnson, 1974). Frequently, such case reports are then followed by further epidemiological studies and/or animal studies to confirm or refute the validity of the original observation. Thus, in most instances, case reports serve to generate a hypothesis.

A distinct advantage of case reports over most other types of studies is their low cost. Most of the work necessary to allow reporting of a case or case series is performed by health care workers in the course of their normal duties, hence the cost is largely absorbed by the medical care system. In addition, the time interval between identification of cases and publication is often short, indeed, many medical journals allow for the rapid publication of case reports by speeding up editorial review. Case reports are often highly specific: in many instances they contain extensive descriptions of symptoms and clinical signs. Frequently coupled with good exposure information (e.g. analytical verification in the case of drug overdose), they are uniquely able to define a dose–response relationship of chemical exposure.

Limitations of case reports are that they usually deal with single incidents or relatively small numbers. Extrapolation or generalization may therefore be difficult, especially since there is no information on the size or definition of the population at risk. They also rely on the individual effort of usually very busy health care workers who need to find the time for writing and literature searches. The role of case reports as 'early warning systems' is less useful when cases are sporadic, the relative risk is low, the outcome is a common disease, the aetiology is multifactorial or there is a long latency period between exposure and effect (Cone et al., 1987).

Case reports which are generated through a formal reporting system are of enormous use in disease surveillance, either as part of drug monitoring or toxicovigilance.

Drug Surveillance Schemes

These are used extensively to evaluate toxicity resulting from the use of pharmaceuticals, and may include chemicals which form part of prescription pharmaceuticals. Serious, but rare, toxicity, occurring with a frequency of 0.1% or less, may not manifest until after widespread general usage and general patterns of toxicity may not be recognized unless systematic drug surveillance schemes are employed. The statistical background to adverse drug reactions is well defined (Stephens et al., 1998) and gives an indication of the size of the exposed patient population required to manifest adverse drug reactions which occur infrequently.

The most common methods of post-marketing drug surveillance are described below.

Clinical trials

Development trials may be regarded as potentially artificial situations because of limitations on the types of patients entered and concurrent medications, defined dosage, duration of treatment and the use of comparators, including placebos. Nevertheless, clinical trials may provide useful information. During the course of clinical trials (whether pre-or post-marketing), pharmaceutical companies generally have an obligation to report all serious adverse events (fatal, life-threatening, disabling/incapacitating and those causing or prolonging hospitalization) to regulatory authorities in an expedited fashion. In general marketed usage, a wider spectrum of patients may receive a drug, occasionally even for an unlicensed (i.e. unproven/untested) indication and at higher doses and for longer periods. Previously unrecognized or unpredictable drug toxicity may also occur from such usage.

In many countries, there are legal requirements for pharmaceutical companies to submit periodic safety update reports (PSUR) to regulatory authorities on any new safety information which comes to light after a drug is marketed. However, there are rarely any formal requests for large-scale pharmacovigilance studies. Countries such as the USA and UK may request Post-marketing Surveillance Studies (PMS), particularly for drugs of a new class and for those where potentially significant but relatively infrequent adverse events have been seen (e.g. hepatic disturbance) in the development phase. Such large-scale, company-sponsored studies, involving many thousands of patients, may report a multitude of adverse events which are often difficult to interpret even when the studies are well designed. Indeed, it has often been considered that PMS can only give bad news about a new drug. However, with careful interpretation, such studies can yield useful safety information which will assist the passage of the drug into more widespread clinical usage. New (quintapartite) guidelines were issued in the UK in 1994 to ensure that these studies are conducted in an appropriate manner (Medicines Control Agency et al., 1994) and these are paralleled by European guidelines (European Commission, 1994).

Phase 4 clinical trials which are well controlled may yield useful safety information in the same manner as development trials.

Spontaneous Reporting

Much valuable safety information may be gleaned by the reporting of 'spontaneous' adverse events from routine clinical usage of a drug. Reports may be either from the consumer direct to the pharmaceutical company (commonly in the USA) or from a health care professional. Pharmaceutical companies have an obligation to submit an initial report on life-threatening and unexpected serious adverse events, received in this manner, to regulatory authorities within a given time frame (usually within 15 days of receipt). Clarification, obtained from a request for further information regarding concomitant disease, medication and outcome, may be submitted later in order to complete the overall assessment.

In the UK, the additional mechanism of the 'Yellow Card' scheme (administered by the Medicines Control Agency, MCA) encourages voluntary reporting of all suspected reactions to newly marketed drugs (defined as the first year of a drug's licence, although this may be extended; 'black triangle' designation) and serious or unusual reactions to established drugs. Reports number approximately 20 000 per year (Rawlins, 1995); however, it is estimated that only 10% of serious reactions and 2–4% of non-serious reactions are reported in this way. In contrast, in France physicians have a legal obligation to report to pharmacovigilance centres. The WHO also administers a scheme encompassing 33 countries. Reporting from these schemes may be influenced by many factors, including drug promotion, time on the market and adverse publicity. A balanced picture of a drug's safety may not necessarily be obtained, but this method is particularly useful in detecting signals worthy of further study.

Safety Assessment of Marketed Medicines (SAMM)

This is distinct from phase 4 studies as it involves primarily non-interventional studies in which a drug is prescribed in the usual way by the patient's physician. Their aim is to collect safety data from routine clinical use. SAMM studies involving any form of intervention (e.g. randomization and non-routine investigations), are subject to normal clinical trials ethics and regulatory requirements. In the UK, these latter studies are also subject to the quintapartite guidelines (Medicines Control Agency et al., 1994). They should have a protocol, study plan including precise objectives, stating whether the study is hypothesis testing (investigating known or putative safety issues) or generating (identifying previously unrecognized safety issues). SAMM studies are conducted by pharmaceutical companies, are approved and are sometimes required by regulatory authorities (e.g. MCA) as a condition of granting a product licence. Such studies should not be conducted for promotional purposes. Different types of study may be conducted. They include observational cohort studies, case control studies and case surveillance. Results of these studies are presented to regulatory bodies and are usually published. Reported adverse events from these are included in the PSUR. The various different types of study are described below.

Observational cohort studies. Patients who are about to receive a prescribed drug are identified and followed prospectively, whereby certain conditions apply:

1. The study population should reflect the population expected to receive the drug in normal clinical practice and is subject to the stipulated contraindications in the prescribing information.
2. The decision to prescribe the drug should have been made on clinical grounds before the patient is entered into the study.
3. The product is supplied by the family physician and not by the pharmaceutical company.
4. A control group of patients with the same condition should generally be prescribed an alternative therapy.
5. The physician reports adverse events during routine, rather than specially arranged consultations.

A special type of cohort study, commonly used in the UK since 1982 by the Drug Safety Research Trust, is where the patient is identified by the prescription (Prescription Event Monitoring, PEM, Mann, 1998). General Practitioners are, after an interval of 6 months, sent a questionnaire requesting information on 'events', i.e. new diagnoses, deterioration or improvement in a condition, any suspected adverse drug reaction or any other significant finding, including cessation of treatment and subsequent follow-up details. The results for one drug can be compared with those for other drugs subjected to this scrutiny.

Many general practices in the UK have computerized databases and there are many computerized healthcare systems (e.g. Kaiser–Permanente and Medicaid in the USA). These databases can be used either to investigate in greater detail previously identified clinical conditions that are suspected of being drug related (e.g. human insulin is associated with hypoglycaemia without warning) or to identify all patients on a specific drug or with a condition and follow them up to determine what clinical events subsequently occur. The latter is effectively an 'electronic' cohort study.

Case control studies. These are hypothesis testing, retrospective studies comparing the history of drug exposure of cases experiencing a disease or event with control patients without the disease or event. These studies have been employed to study associations between thromboembolism and oral contraceptives, endometrial cancer and hormone replacement therapy, and upper gastrointestinal haemorrhage and non-steroidal anti-inflammatory drugs.

Case surveillance. These are again retrospective studies studying patients with diseases or events that are likely to be related and ascertaining drug exposure.

In conclusion, each method has advantages and disadvantages in terms of ease of use, reliability and cost. The principal benefit is that otherwise unidentified associations can be detected by virtue of the population approach that these techniques employ.

Toxicovigilance

While drug surveillance schemes provide useful information on pharmaceuticals in 'normal use', they cover by their very nature only a very limited number of chemicals. There is a need to collect and review data related to drugs in overdose situations and also to the vast range of non-pharmaceutical chemicals to which people are exposed at work or in their everyday lives. Such information can be collected from various sources, such as statistics on mortality and morbidity and accident surveillance schemes.

Official statistics can provide overall numbers for deaths and hospital admissions and are useful for trend analysis, but they do not provide detailed clinical and toxicological information. Furthermore, the nature and extent of data collection vary enormously between countries and international comparisons are therefore extremely difficult. Accident surveillance schemes have been developed to facilitate health education and to monitor product safety. In the UK, for example, the Home Accident Surveillance Scheme administered by the Department of Trade and Industry monitors home and leisure accidents. However, experience has shown that suspected poisoning accounts for only 3–4% of such accidents and that, although overtly dangerous products can be identified, little information is collected from which to assess toxic effects and dose response (Volans et al., 1991). A special situation exists in the case of pesticide exposure. The UK Health and Safety Executive runs a scheme which allows pesticide operators, and also members of the general public, to report incidents relating to pesticide use. The data thus collected are evaluated by a panel of experts who decide, on the basis of the available information, whether the alleged health effect is likely to have been caused by the exposure (Health and Safety Executive, 1997).

The most important source of data on toxicovigilance comes from poison control centres (PCCs). Such centres now exist in many countries and their primary role is the provision of advice on potential risks and management of cases of suspected poisoning and toxicological emergencies. This advice is usually given by telephone, in many cases on a 24 h basis, either to health care professionals or to members of the general public. In order to be able to give accurate information, the PCC must receive details of the incident, patient information, the time course of symptoms and any treatment already given. This information has enormous potential as a source of human toxicology information and, increasingly, PCCs see it as their role to collect and evaluate such data for the purpose of health surveillance and promotion. As with other surveillance schemes, there are limitations in the way the data are collected and analysed, principally because of the lack of standardization of systems used to obtain and record information from the caller.

However, efforts are being made at a national and supranational level to improve the systems of toxicovigilance. In the USA, all PCCs accredited by the American Association of Poison Control Centers provide annually an agreed set of data on their incident-related activities which is reported in the Toxic Exposure Surveillance System (Litovitz et al., 1998). This database can be searched according to product, circumstances of exposure, therapy, type and severity of effect and medical outcome. The data thus obtained can be used for further analysis. For example, between 1985 and 1989 there were approximately 3.8 million exposure cases in children younger than 6 years (Litovitz and Manoguerra, 1992). Of these, some 2000 patients experienced a major outcome and there were 111 fatalities. The most commonly implicated substance categories were cosmetics (including personal care products), cleaning substances and plants. All had low hazard factors (sum of major and fatal outcomes per number of exposures), indicating that frequent exposure does not necessarily imply toxicity. Pharmaceutical preparations accounted for over half of the fatalities, with iron supplements being the single most frequent cause.

Many European countries require their PCCs to provide annual reports. Under the auspices of the European Association of Poison Control Centres and Clinical Toxicologists, efforts are being made towards better harmonization of data collection. In conjunction with the European Commission and the International Programme on Chemical Safety (IPCS), a standardized scheme for grading the severity of poisoning has been developed, tested and revised (Persson et al., 1998), involving 14 PCCs from different parts of the world. Initial application of the scoring system has shown that it is helpful in assessing accurately the initial clinical severity and the likelihood of further deterioration. Furthermore, it helps in deciding which enquiries to refer to a clinical toxicologist (Casey et al., 1998).

One of the aims of the IPCS is to encourage countries to establish PCCs and it has published a policy overview and technical guidance on PCC organization and management (WHO, 1997). These guidelines recommend the establishment of internationally agreed mechanisms for the collection, validation and analysis of data relating to poisonings. The IPCS has for a number of years developed a poison centre information system (Meredith and Haines, 1996). This 'INTOX' system is particularly aimed at helping developing countries to establish their own poison information services and contains a large volume of product and treatment information. At the same time the comprehensive incident recording facilities of the system help to foster standardization and integration of data collection and reporting not only across centres but also across countries.

Finally, it is worth noting the contribution of the analytical toxicology laboratory to toxicovigilance. The role of such specialist facilities has developed continuously over the past 30 years (Dawling and Volans, 1994). The rapid progress in analytical techniques has led to an increase in sensitivity of assays by orders of magnitude. While this has helped clinicians enormously in the accurate diagnosis of poisoning cases, it has to be said that our ability to interpret the significance of the presence of xenobiotics in biological systems at the parts per trillion (10^{-12}) level has yet to catch up with the technical abilities of the analytical laboratory.

Use of Chemicals as Therapeutic Agents

Chemicals have been used as therapeutics throughout history. Arsenic in its naturally occurring disulphide form was recommended by Hippocrates and Galen for treating ulcers and cautery of tumours by arsenic salts was practised by Avicenna in the tenth century. Potassium arsenite solution (Fowler's solution) was used extensively for treating numerous ailments, including until fairly recently in some treatments of leukaemia (Sollmann, 1957). Similarly, mercury ointments were used by Arab physicians in the tenth century. From around 1500 onwards, the use of mercury salts or vapour was standard treatment for syphilis (though it is a matter of debate whether more patients died from the disease or the treatment). The diuretic potential of mercury has been known at least since the seventeenth century, and mercurial diuretics were used as late as the mid-1970s.

The reason why the therapeutic use of chemicals is of interest for toxicologists is because of the first-hand, often extensive, human information which becomes available when a chemical is taken through the various stages of pharmaceutical development. There are three principal reasons why a chemical may become of interest for such development, as follows.

Incidental Discovery of Therapeutic Potential

Nitroglycerin (glycerol trinitrate) was discovered in 1847 and incorporated by Alfred Nobel into a major component of dynamite in 1867. Effects from occupational exposure were first described by Darlington (1890) as throbbing headaches, breathing difficulties, drowsiness, weakness and vomiting. These effects are due to the pharmacological action of nitroglycerin on the smooth muscle, producing relaxation.

The ability of organic nitrates to relieve anginal pain was discovered in 1867 by Lauder Brunton, who noticed that amyl nitrite caused marked flushing, tachycardia and a fall in blood pressure when its vapour was inhaled (cited in Rang and Dale, 1987). It was soon realized that the symptoms caused by nitroglycerin were due to the same action as that of amyl nitrite, and it was found to be just as effective in angina. It is still widely used but, because of its short action, other organic nitrates have been developed, the most commonly available being isosorbide di- or mononitrate and pentaerythritol tetranitrate.

Therapeutic Use as a Direct Consequence of the Known Properties of the Chemical

Treatment of human parasitic disease relies heavily on the use of insecticides. DDT was the first major chemical to be used with spectacular success by American troops during the Second World War in malaria vector control and against other insect pests (Smith 1991). During the 1940s and 1950s, it became an important element of public health campaigns, until concerns over its persistence in the human body and the environment and the development of insect resistance led to restriction of usage and an eventual ban in many countries. However, because of its cost-effectiveness and relatively low acute toxicity, DDT remains an important vector control agent in many parts of the world (IPCS, 1979). The widespread use of DDT prompted many investigations into possible health effects, including oral, dermal, inhalation and bioaccumulation volunteer studies at doses up to 1500 mg (for a summary, see Smith, 1991). Apart from its insecticidal use, DDT was also studied for a possible bilirubin-reducing effect in selected patients with jaundice (Thompson et al., 1969) at doses up to 3 mg kg^{-1} day^{-1} for 6 months. There were no side effects in this study, nor were there any when DDT was used as an antidote in phenobarbital intoxication as a single dose of 5000 mg (Rappolt, 1970)

The products nowadays used in ectoparasite control fall into different chemical categories, mainly organochlorines, organophosphates and pyrethroids. Lindane, malathion and permethrin are effective against scabies and malathion and permethrin are recommended for head lice.

Use as a Therapeutic Adjuvant

Many chemicals are used as co-formulants in medicinal preparations. For example, propylene glycol is used as a solvent in parenteral preparations, either on its own or in combination with ethanol. The chemically related diethylene glycol, an industrial solvent and antifreeze, was used in 1937 to prepare a liquid formulation of the newly introduced sulphanilamide antibacterial agent. The resulting deaths of over 100 people had profound consequences for the licensing of drugs in the USA, leading to new legislation which stipulated requirements for data submission to the Food and Drug Administration (Wax, 1995). Unfortunately, there have been at least five other mass poisonings with analgesic elixirs containing diethylene glycol, namely those in South Africa, India, Nigeria, Bangladesh and Haiti, resulting in the deaths of several hundred patients, the majority of them children (Wax, 1996). In each case, the cheaper diethylene glycol appears to have been substituted for the more expensive propylene glycol or glycerin.

Chlorofluorocarbons (CFCs) are still widely used as refrigerants, propellants, degreasers, fire extinguishers and industrial cleaning agents. Human health effects such as cardiac arrythmias and even fatalities from asphyxiation have been described at high concentrations (McGee *et al.*, 1990). On the other hand, CFCs are used as propellants in metered-dose inhalers prescribed for the treatment of asthma. Doses dispensed from these devices contain typically between 50 and 100 mg of CFCs, the most common ones being trichlorofluoro-methane (FC-11), dichlorodifluoromethane (FC-12) and dichlorotetrafluoroethane (FC-14) (Pierce *et al.*, 1991).

Worker Exposure and Health Surveys

Human studies of chemical exposure are at their most powerful if they include adequate information on both exposure and health effects. Such an ideal is rarely achieved; most studies concerned with exposure mea-surement look at relatively low levels of exposure over short periods which are unlikely to result in short-term health effects. Conversely, most epidemiological studies looking at health effects from chemical exposure suffer from a lack of verifiable exposure information, especially where there is a long latency period between exposure and onset of illness.

Exposure and health surveys can in theory be carried out wherever there is a likelihood of exposure occurring, including environmental exposure of the general public. In practice, it is mainly the surveillance of occupationally exposed workers which is likely to yield substantive information on the link between chemical exposure and health effects. Exposure and health surveys are useful as components of either risk assessment or risk manage-ment. The former takes place ideally before people are exposed to the chemical in question and the latter is part of an on going process to safeguard the health of the individual who may be exposed.

Methods for Exposure Assessment

Exposure can be determined by means of ambient mon-itoring or personal monitoring, a subset of the latter being biological monitoring. The choice of a method depends principally on the purpose of the investigation, the chemical involved, the conditions at the workplace and the resources available.

Ambient monitoring is designed to assess the concen-tration of chemicals either as particulate, gas or vapour in the workplace air. It is achieved by installing collection devices containing filters or other absorptive material (e.g. activated charcoal, silica gel) which can sub-sequently be analysed. The high sampling volume means that very low levels of detection can be achieved (Schlatter, 1992). This method is particularly suitable for process checks and for monitoring engineering controls designed to minimize exposure.

Personal monitoring is usually carried out to assess inhalation exposure. The distribution of a non-gaseous chemical depends largely on the physico-chemical prop-erties of the particle or droplet. In terms of inhalation risk assessment, two categories of airborne particulates are usually considered: the inhalable fraction (the mass frac-tion which is inhaled through the nose and mouth) can for sampling purposes be considered to be of a size below 100 μm. The respirable fraction (the mass fraction which penetrates into the unciliated airways) is considered to be below 15 μm (International Organization for Standardi-zation, 1995). The collection devices are attached to work clothing in the vicinity of the breathing zone and are connected to personal sampling pumps.

The contamination of workers' skin and clothing can be measured using a variable number of multi-layered gauze patches attached to defined areas of the body. However, because of the non-uniformity of dermal expo-sure, whole body monitoring using clothing which acts as a sampling medium has been proposed as an alternative (Chester, 1993). This has the advantage that the capture and retention properties of normal work clothing are mimicked as closely as possible.

Biological monitoring can be defined as the measure-ment of a chemical or its metabolites in the body fluids of exposed persons, and conversion to an equivalent absorbed dose of the chemical based on a knowledge of its human metabolism and pharmacokinetics (Woollen, 1993). Biological monitoring has the advantage that it provides an integrated estimate of exposure by all routes, respiratory, dermal and oral. A variant of biological monitoring is biological effect monitoring. This involves the use of biological markers as indicators signalling events in biological systems or samples and as tools to clarify the relationship between exposure and health impairment (Mercier and Robinson, 1993). Three types of biological markers can be distinguished:

1. *Biological markers of susceptibility.* These include genetic predisposition, such as acetylator status, or pre-existing disease.
2. *Biological markers of exposure.* These indicate an action of the chemical at the cellular or molecular level leading to measurable alteration of biochemistry or molecular interaction which may ultimately result in cell death or cell repair.
3. *Biological markers of disease.* These are the con-sequences of functional change or structural change as a result of organ or system pathology occurring.

The usefulness of biological monitoring depends on the exposure, metabolic and pharmacokinetic character-istics of the chemical in question. It is not suitable for detecting short-lasting peak exposure periods, but it is ideal for determining the body burden of slowly accumu-lating compounds such as heavy metals or chlorinated hydrocarbons. For such compounds, detection may be possible days, months or even years after exposure. The interpretation of biological monitoring relies on the understanding of kinetic parameters (e.g. organ distribution, elimination pattern and biological half-life). This information should ideally be obtained from controlled human studies (see below).

Medical Surveillance

Medical examinations form an important part of occupational health programmes. The content and frequency must depend on the results of the risk assessment process. In particular, the content of medical examinations should be related to the identified health hazards and to the characteristics of chemical exposure, while the frequency of periodical examinations should be determined on the basis of the magnitude of risk to human health and the natural course of the relevant adverse health effects (Tordoir and Maroni, 1994). There are three essential parts of medical surveillance:

1. *Pre-employment medical examinations.* These are carried out to determine the physical ability of the candidate to carry out the required job. They should also be designed to identify any medical condition which may be worsened by chemical exposure, or which would make the person more susceptible to health effects arising from the exposure. In addition, they should set a baseline from which to judge the significance of possible effects from future exposure.
2. *Specific periodical examinations.* These should be designed to detect adverse health effects which may have been caused by specific exposures or work conditions. They may also detect any significant changes in health status unrelated to exposure, but with potential consequences of the kind described under pre-employment medical examinations.
3. *Consultation when returning to work after significant illness.* The objectives are the same as in the pre-placement evaluation, but the baseline established at this examination will now supersede the original one. The content of this evaluation will be determined by the nature of the medical condition and the state of recovery.

Exposure and Health Surveys as Part of Risk Assessment

Risk assessment has already been defined as a stepwise process involving hazard identification, examination of dose–response relationships and exposure assessment. Human studies form a crucial part of this process, but with hundreds of thousands of chemicals in production and use, it is clearly neither possible nor desirable to establish a human database for all of them since the vast majority pose no appreciable risk to humans. Human data should therefore be obtained in a systematic, prior-

ity-based way with emphasis on those chemicals which are most likely to lead to adverse health effects as a result of their intrinsic hazard *and* the likely human exposure.

The registration and regulation of pesticides probably involves the most sophisticated risk assessment process outside the pharmaceutical area. This is not surprising given that pesticides are designed to have an effect on biological systems leading to the control or destruction of rodents, weeds, insects or fungi. Most countries operate regulatory systems, with the best known existing in the USA (Krieger and Ross, 1993) and the European Union. Internationally, the WHO and the Food and Agriculture Organization carry out toxicological evaluations of pesticides (Joint Meeting on Pesticide Residues, JMPR) for the purpose of setting acceptable daily intakes (IPCS, 1993).

It has been proposed to take a tiered approach to the generation and use of human data for the purpose of pesticide operator risk assessment (Henderson *et al.*, 1993; OECD, 1997). This is shown schematically in **Figure 1**. Each tier involves the comparison of an exposure data set with the appropriate No Observed Adverse Effect Level (usually obtained from animal toxicology studies) and applying an assessment or safety factor to account for uncertainties when extrapolating from animal data to human exposure, and also for inter-individual differences in human response.

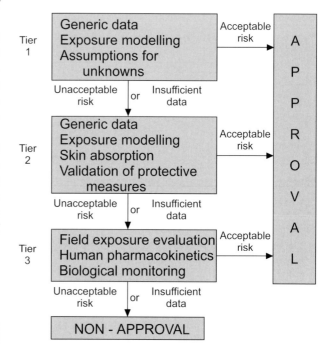

Figure 1 Three-tiered approach for the assessment of worker exposure in a risk assessment procedure for registration of a pesticide. Requirement of actual human data (field exposure evaluation, biological monitoring) depends on whether the calculated exposure shows an acceptable risk when considering the toxicology profile of the compound. Modified from OECD (1997) with permission.

The first tier in the risk assessment process would typically involve the use of generic databases which allow model calculations for the likely exposure level (Van Hemmen, 1993). The source and type of data used should be clearly identified and the database or model used must be validated and applied correctly. At this stage, very conservative assumptions are used (e.g. no protective equipment, 100% skin absorption). In the second tier the data set is refined, for example using actual skin absorption data (animal or human *in vitro*) and building in factors to account for personal protection. The third tier involves the generation of actual human data. These could be exposure measurements (Chester, 1993) or, ideally, biological monitoring backed by human pharmacokinetic information (Woollen, 1993). If the risk assessment still indicates excessive exposure, further risk mitigation factors may be considered to reduce the absorbed dose to an acceptable level.

Human health surveys can be of considerable benefit in the risk assessment process, particularly at the time of re-registration, when a considerable amount of human use experience data has accumulated. In addition, health surveys may help to refine assessment factors for the calculation of acceptable risk, particularly where there are questions about the applicability of animal data at high doses to the human use conditions which may involve exposure at doses several orders of magnitude lower than encountered in animal studies.

Exposure and Health Surveys as Part of Risk Management

Chemically induced occupational illnesses are prevented by the control of exposure to chemical hazards in the workplace. Sometimes this needs to be supplemented by surveillance of the people potentially exposed to chemicals at work. It is important that such surveillance is fully integrated in the risk management process (Tordoir and Maroni, 1994). If this is not the case, the surveillance will be out of focus and neither effective, nor efficient. Some of the basic principles which should be fulfilled are:

1. The surveillance should give information over and above that already available.
2. It should provide information which will assist in evaluating control measures.
3. If individual (biological) monitoring is involved, there must be an appropriate sampling strategy and analytical technique, preferably involving non-invasive sampling.
4. There must be clear criteria for interpreting the results.
5. There must be adequate consultation with employees, including feedback of the results.
6. Appropriate action is taken as a result of the surveillance and its effectiveness is evaluated.

In many countries, surveillance is a statutory requirement specified in health and safety regulations for workers exposed to well established health risks. **Table 2** lists the agents which require surveillance under various regulations in the UK, the most important being the Control of Substances Hazardous to Health Regulations 1988 (COSHH).

Any surveillance programme involving clinical care must contain appropriate safeguards for the participating individuals. Employees should be aware of the possible consequences of surveillance and individual medical records should be kept confidential. Before disclosing such information, the individual's consent needs to be obtained. However, as a result of surveillance employees may be transferred to a job that entails less exposure to a particular hazard, and this should be explained clearly to the participants in a programme at the outset. It is also important that surveillance programmes are not used to discriminate against specific employee groups (e.g. women or older workers).

Table 2 Health and safety regulations requiring statutory surveillance in the UK (Health and Safety Executive, 1990)

Agent	Regulation
Asbestos	Control of Asbestos at Work Regulations 1987
Carbon disulphide Disulphur dichloride Benzene, including benzol Carbon tetrachloride Trichloroethylene	COSHH
Compressed air (other than diving operations)	The Work in Compressed Air Special Regulations 1958
Diving operations	Diving Operations at Work Regulations 1981
Ionizing radiations	Ionising Radiations Regulations 1985
Lead	Control of Lead at Work Regulations 1980
Mine dusts	The Coal Mines (Respirable Dusts) Regulations 1975
1-Naphthylamine and its salts *o*-Tolidine and its salts Dianisidine and its salts Dichlorobenzidine and its salts Auramine Magenta Nitro or amino derivatives of phenol and of benzene or its homologues Pitch Potassium or sodium chromate or dichromate Vinyl chloride monomer	COSHH

Note: COSSH is the control of substances Hazardous to Health Regulations (1988)

Another crucial issue in occupational health surveillance is the possibility of epidemiological evaluations of the health status of the workforce (Tordoir and Maroni, 1994). Such evaluations, for example of the results of routine examinations of a group of workers, may reveal trends or abnormalities which are not evident from individual results. On the other hand, a group evaluation which shows no abnormalities may provide reassurance on the adequacy of measures taken to control exposure.

Record Keeping

Any occupational surveillance programme is critically dependent on the quality of data recording and retention. The records should document data relevant to individual workers, should be able to identify health trends and priority areas for action, fulfil legal requirements and enable future epidemiological studies to be carried out. It is important to keep records for sufficiently long periods; for example, in the case of exposure to ionizing radiation, 60 years are recommended. Ideally, records should contain information in the following areas:

1. Details which allow the identification of employees and facilitate their tracing and linkage in epidemiological research.
2. Job category and information on work circumstances (site, plant, process).
3. Information on chemicals and ambient exposure data.
4. Personal and biological monitoring data.
5. Medical (clinical) data.

It is recognized that ideal data records are rarely, if ever, available. Furthermore, data records may not follow the individual if they change their employer. Nevertheless, analysis of data records may be the only way to identify health effects from chemicals with long latency periods between exposure and the occurrence of illness.

Human Volunteer Studies

Human studies are commonplace in drug development. New chemical entities are taken through the stages of safety and efficacy testing, the former usually involving the administration of a single dose to volunteers (phase I testing). In contrast, there is very little information on human pharmacokinetics and toxicity for the majority of non-pharmaceutical chemicals. It is increasingly recognized that such information can be very useful, in some cases even essential, for the risk assessment process. Although the previously mentioned types of studies can all make a very valuable contribution to the understanding of the effects of chemicals in humans, they almost invariably suffer from a lack of control regarding expo-

sure. In contrast, human volunteer studies give information on health effects in relation to well defined exposures.

The Case for Human Volunteer Studies

The underlying principles and international guidelines on ethical aspects of research involving human subjects have already been extensively discussed (see above). Historically, safe exposure levels for chemicals were established through experience of safety in use. For less overtly toxic compounds it may have taken a long time to recognize the link between exposure and harmful effects. Even when this was achieved, certain effects may have been tolerated as an occupational hazard if the benefit from use was seen to be substantial. Increasing public awareness about the effects of chemical exposure has gradually led to the introduction of regulations covering the control of chemical exposure in the workplace. Biological monitoring has been established as a cornerstone of exposure surveillance (see above), but it requires an understanding of human metabolism and pharmacokinetics (Wilks *et al.*, 1993). It has also been argued that no new chemical entities should be introduced until carefully controlled human trials have been carried out (Hayes, 1983). To apply such a strategy rigorously would be both impractical and unnecessary, and it would also place undue emphasis on new chemicals rather than those already in existence. Human volunteer studies need, therefore, to be considered selectively for compounds where one or more of the following conditions apply (Wilks and Woollen, 1994):

1. There is a significant exposure potential in a large population.
2. There is a serious toxicological effect in animals with a reasonable likelihood that it might be relevant to man.
3. Structure–activity relationships suggest risk by analogy with other compounds.
4. The status of man in relation to a metabolic pathway relevant to toxicity (e.g. if it is known to differ in susceptible and non-susceptible species) needs to be established.
5. There is a need to use biological monitoring to demonstrate adequate safety in use.

A second line of argument concerns the use of human volunteer studies for the purpose of reduction, refinement or replacement of animal studies (Volans *et al.*, 1991). This is of particular importance in areas where public opinion is increasingly reluctant to accept animal testing for basic safety assessments. A typical example would be testing for topical effects of cosmetics and personal care and household products.

Public attitudes to human volunteer studies with non-pharmaceuticals vary widely from country to country. For example, in Germany such studies are difficult to carry out as a consequence of principles established post-1945. In the USA, they are uncommon mainly because of legal considerations in relation to the liability of investigators. However, the following factors have been instrumental in helping to change the balance in favour of carrying out studies in healthy volunteers:

1. Internationally accepted codes of practice have been established to safeguard the interests of the volunteer.
2. No-fault compensation is now commonplace in relation to such studies.
3. Progress in analytical techniques allows the administration of very low doses of chemicals which are relevant to human exposure.
4. Introduction of Good Laboratory Practice (GLP) (see Chapter 21) and Good Clinical Practice (GCP) have led to improved study design.
5. It is increasingly recognized that there is no single universally applicable animal model for human metabolism of chemicals.
6. The publication of human volunteer studies with non-pharmaceutical chemicals has demonstrated the safety and validity of this approach.

Preliminary Safety Data

An assessment of the risk to volunteers participating in any study involving the administration of drugs or chemicals can only be made on the basis of hazard information on the compound available at that time. There is a trend within the pharmaceutical industry to study new chemical entities in humans increasingly early in the development. This has led to a re-evaluation of the minimum toxicity information which must be available before administration to volunteers is acceptable. In contrast, a human dosing study with a non-pharmaceutical is almost invariably carried out comparatively late, e.g. in the case of pesticides, when data on operator exposure are required. This means that there will be substantially more toxicity information available than that which is required for a phase I single oral dosing study in drug development. The benefit of this situation in the case of the pesticide is that a risk assessment for humans will be improved as more toxicity information becomes available. On the other hand, there may be a tendency to overemphasize adverse effects occurring in chronic and lifetime studies in animals at high dose levels, which may have little or no relevance for possible effects expected from a single low dose administered to volunteers. A minimum toxicity data-set has therefore been suggested which should be available before considering a human volunteer study with non-pharmaceutical chemicals (Wilks and Woollen, 1994). This would, of course, need to be adjusted depending on the type of study and the chemical in question, but for a single oral dosing study it should contain at least the following, carried out according to OECD guidelines:

1. *In vitro* and *in vivo* tests of genotoxicity.
2. Acute oral toxicity tests in one rodent and one non-rodent species.
3. Sub-chronic (90 days) toxicity in one rodent and one non-rodent species.
4. Balance and biotransformation studies in one species.
5. Assessment of fertility in a single generation study.
6. Teratology in one species (in case of participation of female volunteers).

Particular attention should be given to the results of short-term tests which are most relevant to a single exposure of humans. For a single dose dermal study, additional information would be required on:

1. Acute dermal toxicity in one rodent species.
2. Percutaneous absorption, either using animal *in vivo* or human skin *in vitro* data.

In addition to any toxicological information, human experience in use should be considered whenever possible.

Types of Human Volunteer Studies

Two principal types of human volunteer studies with non-pharmaceutical chemicals need to be distinguished. There are studies which look at an adverse or toxic effect as the outcome measurement. The second type involves the administration of chemicals to study their metabolic fate and pharmacokinetic behaviour.

Effect Studies
The term 'minimal risk' in human volunteer studies has already been discussed, and this is of paramount importance when considering effect studies. It therefore follows that the study of adverse or toxic effects in volunteers can only be justified on the assumption that no lasting damage will occur. In practice, this restricts such studies to acute and inherently reversible changes at dose levels which people are likely to encounter at their workplace or in the general environment. For example, the acute neurobehavioural effects of solvents have been studied in volunteers at exposures around permitted occupational exposure limits (Iregren and Gamberale, 1990). Such studies include the effects of exercise and alcohol as modifiers of the CNS effects of solvents. Another example is the study of sensory effects of pyrethroid insecticides. Synthetic pyrethroids have the potential to induce transient, fully reversible paraesthesia (variously described as tingling, burning or numbness) in exposed skin of susceptible individuals (LeQuesne *et al.*, 1980). The underlying mechanisms of this effect and the potential for therapy have been studied using human volunteers (Flannigan and Tucker, 1985; Flannigan *et al.*, 1985).

Organophosphorus insecticides have been tested in volunteer studies for their potential to inhibit cholinesterase (ChE) activity as biochemical marker of exposure. Oral administration of malathion at doses up to 16 mg person^{-1} day^{-1} for up to 47 days had no significant effect on either plasma or red cell ChE activity and the volunteers remained asymptomatic (Moeller and Rider, 1962). Parathion-methyl has been studied in a whole series of volunteer studies, with oral doses between 1 and 22 mg person^{-1} day^{-1} producing no significant effect on plasma or red cell ChE (for a summary, see Rider et al., 1969). A dose of 30 mg person^{-1} day^{-1}, or approximately 0.4–0.5 mg kg^{-1} day^{-1}, showed a maximal mean red cell ChE depression of 37%, thus being defined as the level of minimal incipient toxicity for parathion-methyl (Rider et al., 1971). In studies designed to test the safety of dichlorvos as a disinfectant of aircraft, 15 volunteers were intermittently exposed to a concentration of 0.5 mg m^{-3} for 5 h per night, 4 nights per week over 2 weeks (Rasmussen et al., 1963). There was no effect on red cell ChE activity, but a gradual reduction of plasma ChE with the lowest single plasma value observed being 34% of normal. No clinical signs were seen and detailed studies of visual performance, complex reaction time, neurological function and airways resistance showed no abnormalities.

The largest number of effect studies is carried out in the testing of consumer products for topical irritancy and sensitization. It is now recognized that the standard animal tests, such as the Draize skin and eye irritation tests (Draize et al., 1944; Draize, 1959) frequently overpredict the severity of effects occurring in humans (Nixon et al., 1975; Freeberg et al., 1984). With regard to eye effects, volunteer studies have been employed to establish the threshold of effects seen with mild to moderate irritants (Freeberg et al., 1986). This has shown that a modification of the Draize test using a lower instillation volume is more representative of human effects. For the predictive testing of skin irritancy a human 4 h patch test has been developed (Basketter et al., 1994; Dykes et al., 1995; York et al., 1995). It has been proposed to use this test as an alternative to the Draize test for the classification and labelling of substances and preparations (York et al., 1996).

Metabolism and Pharmacokinetic Studies

These types of studies have two main purposes. The first is the identification of metabolic pathways and target metabolites which can subsequently be used in biological monitoring studies at the workplace or in the general population. Secondly, in order to interpret the results of biological monitoring studies and extrapolate back from the excretion of a metabolite to exposure to the parent compound, a detailed knowledge about the human pharmacokinetics of the compound is required. When a compound is administered to humans for the first time, it is prudent to carry out a pilot study with a single volunteer. This serves several purposes. It provides

assurance that adverse reactions are unlikely, confirms whether the dose is adequate in terms of analytical sensitivity, provides material for the improvement of analytical methods and allows the sample collection times to be optimized. For the main study, it may be desirable to study more than one dose level and, where dermal or inhalation uptake is important, more than one route of administration. In certain circumstances it may be appropriate to administer a radioactively labelled form of the compound. Special restrictions apply to the use of human volunteers in such studies which, in the UK for example, require prior authorization by the Administration of Radioactive Substances Advisory Committee (ARSAC, 1993).

For example, the pyrethroid insecticide cypermethrin was administered to volunteers as a single oral and dermal dose (Woollen et al., 1992). Urine was collected for 120 h after dosing and analysed for the metabolites cis- and trans 3-(2,2-dichlorovinyl)-2,2-dimethylcyclopropanecarboxylic acid (DCVA), 3-phenoxybenzoic acid (3PBA) and 3-(4-hydroxyphenoxy)benzoic acid (4OH3PBA). Following oral dosing, the ratio of trans- to cis-DCVA metabolites was approximately 2:1 and similar amounts of DCVA and PBA (3PBA + 4OH3PBA) metabolites were excreted. In contrast, the dermal study of the ratio of trans- to cis-DCVA metabolites excreted in urine was approximately 1:1 and the total amount of PBA metabolites recovered was four times higher than the total DCVA metabolites. In comparison, the metabolite excretion profiles in a field worker exposure study involving hand-held spraying were consistent with a predominance of absorption by the oral rather than the dermal route, since the ratios of trans- to cis-DCVA were usually close to 2:1 and similar amounts of DCVA and PBA metabolites were excreted in urine (Wilks et al., 1993). These data illustrate route-specific metabolism of cypermethrin which may not have been predicted from animal studies, and also the importance of both oral and dermal volunteer studies and the usefulness of measuring multiple metabolites. The results could be used to provide indicators of the main route of absorption during occupational exposure, thus allowing better targeting of safety advice and protective measures.

Di-2-ethylhexyl adipate (DEHA) is a plasticizer which is added to PVC to produce 'cling-film'-type food wrappings. DEHA can migrate into foods, particularly those with a high fat content, and the maximum likely daily intake has been estimated to be around 8 mg day^{-1} (MAFF, 1990). An oral human volunteer study was carried out using deuterium-labelled compound to distinguish between metabolites derived from the test substance and background levels (Loftus et al., 1993). The most abundant metabolite found was 2-ethylhexanoic acid (EHA), whereas mono-2-ethylhexyl adipate, the major metabolite found in a primate study at a 100-fold higher dose level, was not found. This example illustrates a potential problem in risk assessment. Certain metabolic pathways may become overloaded at higher doses and bring other pathways into operation. Consequently, there will be some uncertainty about comparisons between animal toxicology studies at high dose levels and human volunteer studies at much lower doses. Follow-up biological studies were carried out using EHA as a biological marker in 24 h urine samples from 112 individuals from five geographic locations in the UK. Estimates of daily intake of DEHA showed a skewed distribution with a median value of 2.7 mg (Loftus *et al.*, 1994).

CONCLUSION

The use of toxicity data from human studies is still very much the domain of the safety assessment for pharmaceuticals. This is likely to remain the case for some time to come but the benefits of the collection of human data are being increasingly recognized in other areas, most notably those involving exposure to industrial chemicals and pesticides, and also the safety assessment of consumer products. This chapter has looked at the main sources of human data in toxicity assessment, in particular for non-pharmaceutical chemicals. They all have their unique advantages and limitations, and no single type of human study is able to answer all questions.

Case reports often contain a high level of detailed and verified exposure and give a rare insight into dose–response relationships. In the case of adverse reaction reporting they also allow an estimate of the likelihood of adverse effects occurring. Their main limitation is that they are reactive, not controlled and rely on the individual effort of clinicians or relatively few data collection systems, e.g. those of poison control centres and the pharmaceutical industry.

In the case of human therapeutic use of chemicals, the much more systematic use of human data normally seen with pharmaceuticals applies through a combination of volunteer studies and adverse data reporting. However, this is only applicable to a small number of chemicals.

Worker exposure studies and health surveillance provide invaluable information on the presence or absence of effects from long-term exposure to chemicals in the workplace or environment. However, they can be time consuming and expensive, and the link between exposure and effect may be difficult to verify, particularly for retrospective studies.

Human volunteer studies with non-pharmaceutical chemicals have the advantage of well characterized exposure combined with information on the pharmacokinetic behaviour and/or effects of the compound. Nevertheless, outside the area of consumer products their usefulness has up until now been limited by ethical concerns and practical issues such as study design and small study populations. It is hoped that the establishment of clear ethical guidelines and international standards and the

demonstration of the usefulness of such studies through publications will overcome those difficulties. Much has been learnt here from the practices and standards used in drug development.

In the end, it is not so much the type of human study which will determine the ultimate usefulness of the data generated, but the rigorous application of established scientific principles. For the reasons discussed in this chapter, it is neither feasible nor desirable that human studies will replace experimental toxicology, but the two should be complementary. The danger is that toxicologists will continue to do experiments and epidemiologists will continue to collect data, but they fail to constructively interact with each other (Wilks *et al.*, 1996). As observed by Sir Richard Doll, most occupational hazards of cancer have been discovered as a result of clinical intuition or epidemiological observation. However, most could have been avoided if modern laboratory techniques had been employed to test the substances used before men and women were exposed to them in an industrial environment (Doll, 1984).

REFERENCES

ARSAC (1993). *Notes for Guidance on the Administration of Radioactive Substances to Persons for Purposes of Diagnosis, Treatment or Research*. Administration of Radioactive Substances Advisory Committee. HMSO, London.

Bankowski, Z. and Levine, R. J. (1993). *Ethics and Research on Human Subjects—International Guidelines*. CIOMS, Geneva.

Basketter, D. A., Whittle, E., Griffiths, H. A. and York, M. (1994). The identification and classification of skin irritation hazard by a human patch test. *Food Chem. Toxicol.*, **32**, 769–775.

Casey, P. B., Dexter, E. M., Michell, J. and Vale, J. A. (1998). The prospective value of the IPCS/EC/EAPCCT Poisoning Severity Score in cases of poisoning. *J. Toxicol. Clin. Toxicol.*, **36**, 215–217.

Chester, G. (1993). Evaluation of agricultural worker exposure to, and absorption of, pesticides. *Ann. Occup. Hyg.*, **37**, 509–523.

Close, B., Combes, R., Hubbard, A. and Illingworth, J. (Eds) (1997). *Volunteers in Research and Testing*. Taylor and Francis, London.

Cohrssen, J. J. and Covello, V. T. (1989). *Risk Analysis: a Guide to Principles and Methods for Analyzing Health and Environmental Risks*. United States Council on Environmental Quality, Executive Office of the President, Washington, DC.

Cone, J. E., Reeve, G. R. and Landrigan, P. J. (1987). Clinical and epidemiological studies. In Tardiff, R. G. and Rodricks, J. V. (Eds), *Toxic Substances and Human Risk—Principles of Data Interpretation*. Plenum Press, New York, pp. 95–120.

Creech, J. L. and Johnson, M. N. (1974). Angiosarcoma of liver in the manufacture of polyvinyl chloride. *J. Occup. Med.*, **16**, 150–151.

Darlington, T. (1890). The effects of the products of high explosives, dynamite and nitroglycerin on the human system. *Med. Rec.*, **38**, 661–662.

Dawling, S. and Volans, G. N. (1994). Poisons. In Noe, D. A. and Rock, R. C. (Eds), *Laboratory Medicine—The Selection and Interpretation of Clinical Laboratory Studies*. Williams and Wilkins, Baltimore, pp. 580–617.

Dayan, A. (1997). The volunteer subject, encouragement and protection. In Close, B., Combes, R., Hubbard, A. and Illingworth, J. (Eds), *Volunteers in Research and Testing*, Taylor and Francis, London, pp. 5–21.

Doll, R. (1984). Epidemiological discovery of occupational cancers. *Ann. Acad. Med. Singapore*, **13**, 2 Suppl., 331–339.

Draize, J.H. (1959). Dermal toxicity. In *Appraisal of the Safety of Chemicals in Foods, Drugs and Cosmetics*. Association of Food and Drug Officials of the United States, Littleton, CO, pp. 46–59.

Draize, J. H., Woodard, G. and Calvary, H. O. (1944). Methods for the study of irritation and toxicity of substances applied topically to the skin and mucous membranes. *J. Pharmacol. Exp. Ther.*, **82**, 377–390.

Dykes, P. J., Black, D. R., York, M., Dickens, A. D. and Marks, R. (1995). A stepwise procedure for evaluating irritant materials in normal volunteer subjects. *Hum. Exp. Toxicol.*, **14**, 204–211.

European Commission (1994). *Draft Notice to Applicants*. European Commission, Brussels, pp. 85–90.

Flannigan, S. A. and Tucker, S. B. (1985). Variation in cutaneous perfusion due to synthetic pyrethroid exposure. *Br. J. Ind. Med.*, **42**, 773–776.

Flannigan, S. A., Tucker, S. B., Key, M. M., Ross, C. E., Fairchild, E. J., II, Grimes, B. A. and Harrist, R. B. (1985). Synthetic pyrethroid insecticides: a dermatological evaluation. *Br. J. Ind. Med.*, **42**, 363–372.

Freeberg, F. E., Griffith, J. F., Bruce, R. D. and Bay, P. H. S. (1984). Correlation of animal test methods with human experience for household products. *J. Toxicol. Cutaneous Ocul. Toxicol.*, **1**, 53–64.

Freeberg, F. E., Nixon, R. A., Reer, P. J., Weaver, J. E., Bruce, R. E., Griffith, J. F. and Sanders, L. W., III (1986). Human and rabbit eye responses to chemical insult. *Fundam. Appl. Toxicol.*, **7**, 626–634.

Hallenbeck, W. H. (1993). *Quantitative Risk Assessment for Environmental and Occupational Health*, 2nd edn. Lewis Publishers, Boca Raton, FL.

Hayes, W. J. (1983). Ethical considerations involving studies of pesticides and other xenobiotics in man. In Miyamoto, J. and Kearney, P. C. (Eds), *IUPAC Pesticide Chemistry: Human Welfare and Environment. Volume 3: Mode of Action, Metabolism and Toxicology*. Pergamon Press, Oxford, pp. 387–394.

Health and Safety Executive (1990). *Surveillance of People Exposed to Health Risks at Work*. HS (G) 61. HMSO, London.

Health and Safety Executive (1997). *Pesticide Incidents Report 1996/97*. HSE Books, Sudbury.

Henderson, P. T., Brouwer, D. H., Opdam, J. J. G., Stevenson, H. and Stouten, J. T. J. (1993). Risk assessment for worker exposure to agricultural pesticides: review of a workshop. *Ann. Occup. Hyg.*, **37**, 499–507.

Hill, A. B. (1962). *Statistical Methods in Clinical and Preventive Medicine*. Oxford University Press, New York.

Hill, A. B. (1965). The environment and disease. Association or causation? *Proc. R. Soc. Med.*, **58**, 295–300.

Hoel, D. G. and Landrigan, P. J. (1987). Comprehensive evaluation of human data. In Tardiff, R. G. and Rodricks, J. V. (Eds), *Toxic Substances and Human Risk—Principles of Data Interpretation*. Plenum Press, New York, pp. 121–130.

International Organization for Standardization (1995). *Air Quality—Particle Size Fraction Definitions for Health-related Sampling*. ISO 7708: 1995 (E). International Organization for Standardization, Geneva.

IPCS (1979). International Programme on Chemical Safety. *Environmental Health Criteria 9: DDT and Its Derivatives*. World Health Organization, Geneva.

IPCS (1993). International Programme on Chemical Safety. *Summary of Toxicological Evaluations Performed by the Joint FAO/WHO Meeting on Pesticide Residues [JMPR]*. WHO/PCS/94.1. World Health Organization, Geneva.

Iregren, F. and Gamberale, F. (1990). Human behavioural toxicology. Central nervous effects of low-dose exposure to neurotoxic substances in the work environment. *Scand. J. Work Environ. Health*, **16**, Suppl. 1, 17–25.

Krieger, R. I. and Ross, J. H. (1993). Risk assessments in the pesticide regulatory process. *Ann. Occup. Hyg.*, **37**, 565–578.

LeQuesne, P. M., Maxwell, I. C. and Butterworth, T. G. (1980). Transient facial sensory symptoms following exposure to synthetic pyrethroids: a clinical and electrophysiological assessment. *Neurotoxicology*, **2**, 1–11.

Litovitz, T. and Manoguerra, A. (1992). Comparison of pediatric poisoning hazards: an analysis of 3.8 million exposure incidents. *Pediatrics*, **89**, 999–1006.

Litovitz, T. L., Klein-Schwartz, W., Dyer, K. S., Shannon, M., Lee, S. and Powers, M. (1998). 1997 Annual Report of the American Association of Poison Control Centers Toxic Exposure Surveillance System. *Am. J. Emerg. Med.*, **16**, 443–497.

Loftus, N. J., Laird, W. J. D., Wilks M. F., Steel, G. T. and Woollen, B. H. (1993). Metabolism and pharmacokinetics of deuterium-labelled di-2-(ethylhexyl) adipate (DEHA) in humans. *Food Chem. Toxicol.*, **31**, 609–614.

Loftus, N. J., Woollen, B. H., Steel, G. T., Wilks M. F. and Castle, L. (1994). An assessment of the dietary uptake of di-2-(ethylhexyl) adipate (DEHA) in a limited population study. *Food Chem. Toxicol.*, **32**, 1–5.

MAFF (1990). *Plasticisers: Continuing Surveillance*. Ministry of Agriculture, Fisheries and Food, Food Surveillance Paper No. 30. HMSO, London.

Mann, R. D. (1998). Prescription-event monitoring - recent progress and future horizons. *Br. J. Clin. Pharmacol.*, **46**, 195–201.

McGee, M. B., Meyer, R. F. and Jejurikai, S. G. (1990). A death resulting from trichlorotrifluoromethane poisoning. *J. Forensic Sci.*, **35**, 1453–1460.

Medicines Control Agency, Committee on Safety of Medicines, Royal College of Physicians, British Medical Association and Association of the British Pharmaceutical Industry (1994). Guidelines for company-sponsored safety assessment of marketed medicines. *Br. J. Clin. Pharmacol.*, **38**, 93–97.

Mercier M. J. and Robinson, A. E. (1993). Use of biologic markers for toxic end-points in assessment of risks from exposure to chemicals. *Int. Arch. Occup. Environ. Health*, **65**, S7–S10.

Meredith, T. and Haines, J. (1996). International data collection and evidence-based clinical toxicology. *J. Toxicol. Clin. Toxicol.*, **34**, 647–649.

Miller, R. W. (1978). The discovery of human teratogens, carcinogens and mutagens: lessons for the future. In Hollaender, R. and DeSerres, F. J. (Eds), *Chemical Mutagens—Priorities and Mechanisms for Their Detection*, Vol. 5. Plenum Press, New York, pp. 101–126.

Moeller, H. C. and Rider, J. A. (1962). Plasma and red blood cell cholinesterase activity as indications of the threshold of incipient toxicity of ethyl-*p*-nitrophenyl thionobenzenephosphonate (EPN) and malathion in human beings. *Toxicol. Appl. Pharmacol.*, **4**, 123–130.

Nixon, G. A., Tyson, G. A. and Warts, W. C. (1975). Interspecies comparisons of skin irritancy. *Toxicol. Appl. Pharmacol.*, **31**, 481–490.

OECD (1997). *Guidance Document for the Conduct of Studies of Occupational Exposure to Pesticides During Agricultural Application*. OECD Environmental Health and Safety Publications, Series on Testing and Assessment, No. 9. Environment Directorate, Organization for Economic Cooperation and Development, Paris.

Persson, H. E., Sjöberg, G. K., Haines, J. A. and Pronczuk de Garbino, J. (1998). Poisoning severity score. Grading of acute poisoning. *J. Toxicol. Clin. Toxicol.*, **36**, 205–213.

Pierce, R. J., Seale, J. P. and Ruffin, R. E. (1991). Inhaled medications and the use of chlorofluorocarbons (CFCs). *Med. J. Aust.*, **154**, 701–704.

Pott, P. (1775). *Chirurgical Observations Relative to the Cataract, the Polypus of the Nose, the Cancer of the Scrotum, the Different Kinds of Rupture, and the Mortification of the Toes and Feet*. Hawes, Clark and Collins, London.

Ramazzini, B. (1713). *Diseases of Workers*. Translated by Wilmer Cave Wright, Hafner, New York, 1964.

Rang, H. P. and Dale, M. M. (1987). *Pharmacology*. Churchill Livingstone, Edinburgh.

Rappolt, R. T. (1970). Use of oral DDT in three human barbiturate intoxications: CNS arousal and/or hepatic enzyme induction by reciprocal detoxicants. *Ind. Med. Surg.*, **39**, 319.

Rasmussen, W. A., Jensen, J. A., Stein, W. J. and Hayes, W. J., Jr (1963). Toxicological studies of DDVP for disinfection of aircraft. *Aerosp. Med.*, **34**, 594–600.

Rawlins, M. D. (1995). Pharmacovigilance: paradise lost, regained or postponed? *J. R. Coll. Physicians London*, **29**, 41–49.

Richmond, C. R., Walsh, P. J. and Copenhaver, E. D. (1981). *Health Risk Analysis*. Franklin Institute Press, Philadelphia.

Rider, J. A., Moeller, H. C., Puletti, E. J. and Swader, J. I. (1969). Toxicity of parathion, Systox, octamethyl pyrophosphoramide and methyl parathion in man. *Toxicol. Appl. Pharmacol.*, **14**, 603–611.

Rider, J. A., Swader, J. I. and Puletti, E. J., (1971). Anticholinesterase toxicity studies with methyl parathion, Guthion and phosdrin in human subjects. *Fed. Proc.*, **30**, 443.

Royal College of Physicians (1986). *Research on Healthy Volunteers. A Working Party Report*. Royal College of Physicians, London.

Royal College of Physicians (1990a). *Research Involving Patients. A Working Party Report*. Royal College of Physicians, London.

Royal College of Physicians (1990b). *Guidelines on the Practice of Ethics Committees in Medical Research Involving Human Subjects*, 2nd edn. Royal College of Physicians, London.

Schlatter, C. (1992). Personal sampling, biomonitoring or periodic medical examination: selecting the appropriate method for surveillance. In *Medichem—Occupational Health in the Chemical Industry*. World Health Organization Regional Office for Europe, Copenhagen, pp. 1–12.

Smith A. G. (1991). Chlorinated hydrocarbon insecticides. In Hayes, W. J. and Laws, E. R. (Eds), *Handbook of Pesticide Toxicology*, Vol. 2. Academic Press, San Diego, pp. 731–915.

Sollmann, T. (1957). *A Manual of Pharmacology and Its Applications to Toxicology and Therapeutics*, 8th edn. Saunders, Philadelphia.

Stephens, M. D. B., Routledge, P. A. and Talbot, J. C. C. (1998). *Detection of New Adverse Drug Reactions*, 4th edn. Macmillan, London.

Thompson, R. P. H., Pilcher, C. W. T., Robinson, J., Stathers, G. M., McLean, A. E. M. and Williams, R. (1969). Treatment of unconjugated jaundice with dicophane. *Lancet*, **2**, 4–6.

Tordoir, W. F. and Maroni, M. (1994). Basic concepts in the occupational health management of pesticide workers. *Toxicology*, **91**, 5–14.

UK (1978). *The Medicines (Administration of Radioactive Substances) Regulations. SI 1978 No. 1004*. HMSO, London.

UK (1990). *Human Fertilisation and Embryology Act*. HMSO, London.

USA (1949). *Nuremberg Code. Reprinted from Trials of War Criminals Before the Nuremberg Military Tribunals under Control Law*, No. 10, Vol. 2. US Government Printing Office, Washington, DC.

USA (1991). Federal Policy on Protection of Human Subjects (Common Rule) (40 CFR Part 26). 56FR 28012, 28022.

Van Hemmen, J. J. (1993). Predictive exposure modelling for pesticide registration purposes. *Ann. Occup. Hyg.*, **37**, 541–564.

Volans, G., Blain, P., Bennett, P., Berry, C., Sims, J. and Warrington, S. (1991). Toxicity data derived from man. In Balls, M., Bridges, J. and Southee, J. (Eds), *Animals and Alternatives in Toxicology*. Macmillan, London, pp. 201–221.

Wax, P. M. (1995). Elixirs, diluents and the passage of the 1938 Federal Food, Drug and Cosmetic Act. *Ann. Intern. Med.*, **122**, 456–461.

Wax, P. M. (1996). It's happening again—another diethylene glycol mass poisoning. *J. Toxicol. Clin. Toxicol.*, **34**, 517–520.

WHO (1997). *Guidelines for Poison Control*. World Health Organization, Geneva.

Wilks, M. F. and Woollen, B. H. (1994). Human volunteer studies with non-pharmaceutical chemicals: metabolism and pharmacokinetic studies. *Hum. Exp. Toxicol.*, **13**, 383–392.

Wilks M. F., Woollen, B. H., Marsh, J. R., Batten, P. L. and Chester, G. (1993). Biological monitoring for pesticide exposure—the role of human volunteer studies. *Int. Arch. Occup. Environ. Health*, **65**, S189–S192.

Wilks, M. F., Volans, G. N. and Smith, L. L. (1996). Environmental endocrine modulators—where toxicology meets epidemiology. *Hum. Exp. Toxicol.*, **15**, 692–693.

WMA (1997). World Medical Association: Declaration of Helsinki. Recommendations guiding physicians in biomedical research involving human subjects. *J. Am. Med. Assoc.*, **277**, 925–926.

Woollen, B. H. (1993). Biological monitoring for pesticide absorption. *Ann. Occup. Hyg.*, **37**, 525–540.

Woollen, B. H., Marsh, J. R., Laird, W. J. D. and Leeser, J. E. (1992). The metabolism of cypermethrin in man: differences in metabolite profile following oral and dermal administration. *Xenobiotica*, **22**, 983–993.

York, M., Basketter, D. A., Cuthbert, J. A. and Neilson, L. (1995). Skin irritation testing in man for hazard assessment—evaluation of four patch systems. *Hum. Exp. Toxicol.*, **14**, 729–734.

York, M., Griffiths, H. A., Whittle, E. and Basketter, D. A. (1996). Evaluation of a human patch test for the identification and classification of skin irritation potential. *Contact Dermatitis*, **34**, 204–212.

Zbinden, G. (1991). Predictive value of animal studies in toxicology. *Regul. Toxicol. Pharmacol.*, **14**, 167–177.

Chapter 23
Information Resources for Toxicology

Philip Thomas Copestake

C O N T E N T S

INTRODUCTION

We are told often that we live in an Information Age. The latter half of the twentieth century indeed saw a huge growth in the generation of information of all kinds, commensurate with monumental advances in our ability to store and manage that information effectively. Information handling and dissemination have developed their own science, from the dusty card files and classification schemes in the libraries of not so many years ago, through the advent of high-density storage media and the super-fast searching capabilities of computers, and on to the global information repository that is the Internet. Toxicology as a science has grown in parallel with these developments and toxicological information today is disseminated in a multitude of ways. It is essential that we have not only a knowledge of what information resources are available, but also an understanding of the process by which they have been produced.

Toxicological insights are sought by a diverse array of people and their reasons for looking will differ widely. They may be research scientists in industry or academia, seeking to understand the mechanisms by which materials are causing adverse effects, or consultants advising on the risks to employees of a particular set of exposure conditions. They may be regulators, trying to establish, on a wider level, guidance or legislation to protect public health. They even might be lawyers, entering the fray when something has gone seriously wrong. Librarians or information staff may assist with the identification of toxicological data and the maintenance of special collections as part of an alerting service. Poisons control centres will assist the medical profession with responding to acute emergencies. Even the general public may seek information to satisfy an interest in the chemicals that have become an everyday part of their modern lives. Whether it is a highly specific question that is being addressed, or a more general requirement for data, the ultimate aim usually is to understand the hazards that are inherent to a particular chemical or product and to determine the risks that may be associated with a certain level of exposure. Armed with such information, appropriate management of those risks, whether it be on a local, national or international scale, can be attempted. Alternatively, communication of those risks can be made to those who may have reason to be exposed to them. Such is the world in which we live that toxicological information and its application invariably become entwined with commercial and political influences. Wide and open access to existing knowledge in this area is the ideal if we are to ensure consumer safety, minimize environmental damage and, on animal welfare grounds, reduce the level of unnecessary toxicity testing.

It is not the aim of this chapter to provide a shopping list of resources that are currently available in the area of toxicology. Whole books have, in fact, been devoted to this topic itself, and it is certainly not within the scope of a single, short chapter to give a comprehensive overview of what is available. In any case, not only can such compilations leave their author(s) open to criticism from those whose favoured tomes or preferred databases have been omitted, but they can also quickly go out of date. Rather, an attempt is made to offer what is hoped will be more fruitful discussion about the various forms in which information is made available, their relative usefulness and some of the factors that need to be acknowledged in order that they may be used effectively. Practical advice will guide readers to where more comprehensive specific and current details can be found. The discussion should provide a useful basis on which the various available toxicological resources can be selected and used appropriately. Although examples may be given for illustrative purposes, these are by no means necessarily endorsements of these particular sources over others.

A particular problem with toxicology information is that it is found amongst the resources of a diverse array of disciplines. The reasons for this are related to the history of toxicology as a science and it is useful in this context first to look at how information resources in toxicology have evolved. Thus, following this section, the chapter briefly describes the history of information resources in toxicology. The chapter then discusses in more detail the various forms in which toxicological information is available, the importance of particular resource types and the mechanisms by which they are produced. An attempt is then made to consider the future, with the rapidly changing field of information technology, and some of the questions that it poses.

The chapter will try to focus on the specific subject of toxicological information rather than on the more general topic of health and safety, in which toxicology plays a part. Whilst there is an enormous overlap in some of the sources which may be useful here, there is a large proportion of health and safety information that is of little use to those seeking data of a toxicological bent.

HISTORY OF INFORMATION RESOURCES IN TOXICOLOGY

An independent scientific discipline is recognized by virtue of it having its own professional societies and specialist journals, textbooks and undergraduate courses. By these criteria, toxicology is regarded as being a relatively young science, its maturity being delayed until late on in the twentieth century. Its roots, of course, go back much further and are intertwined with those of pharmacology and general medicine. In many respects, toxicology may even pre-date these older sciences, as man first became aware of the toxic effects of animal venoms and poisonous plants and utilized this knowledge for hunting and warfare. An historical overview of information resources in toxicology reflects to a large degree the growth of the science of toxicology itself; the development of many systems for information dissemination, from early texts to computerized databases, has been marked by landmarks in its history.

Early resources demonstrate the intimate association with medicine. The Ebers Papyrus of around 1500 BC can probably be regarded as the birth of toxicological literature. This ancient Egyptian text includes descriptions of a number of 'poisons' and their effects, together with outlines for remedies for diseases. Later, around 900 BC, Indian medicine in the form of Ayurvedism provided

the Vedic texts. Early literature also includes many Greek and Latin documents which describe topics of a toxicological nature. Hippocrates, at around 400 BC, introduced rational medicine and described methods for controlling the absorption of toxic metals, whilst Theophrastus (370–286 BC) described numerous poisonous plants and Dioscorides (around AD 50) made an attempt to classify poisons. The physician Maimonides wrote a volume in 1198 entitled *Poisons and Their Antidotes*, which outlined treatments for poisonings.

In the sixteenth century, Paracelsus wrote his treatise *Bergsucht* (written in 1533–34) which included, for essentially the first time, descriptions of the health effects associated with exposure to chemicals found in mining, including arsenic and mercury poisonings, and the asthmatic and gastrointestinal symptoms common to miners' disease. Paracelsus had a profound influence at that time, presenting many ideas which remain important concepts of toxicology today. Developments in the Industrial Revolution gave rise to further information on occupational diseases. Percival Pott recognized the role of xenobiotics in human disease and linked the occupation of chimney sweep with cancer of the scrotum in a publication of 1775. The Spanish physician Orfelia, often cited as the founder of modern toxicology, produced his *A General System of Toxicology* in 1817, perhaps the first comprehensive textbook in the field.

Although many topics of a toxicological nature would have appeared in the medical journals of the nineteenth and early twentieth centuries, it was not until 1930 that the first scientific journal devoted to toxicology emerged. Published in Berlin, this was *Sammlung von Vergiftungsfällen*, the precursor of *Archives of Toxicology*, and this was followed in 1938 by *Farmakologiia i Toksikologiia*, which was published in Moscow, and by *Acta Pharmacologica et Toxicologica* (now *Pharmacology and Toxicology*) in Copenhagen, in 1945.

The growth of industry, particularly in the chemical and pharmaceutical sectors, following the Second World War was a major driving force for the increase in toxicological literature and many organizations devoted to the science of toxicology have their origins in this period. The journal *Toxicology and Applied Pharmacology* began publication in 1959 and became the official organ of the Society of Toxicology, founded in 1961. It was joined by the journal *Fundamental and Applied Toxicology*, first published in 1981. The 1960s and 1970s had seen the birth of the environmental movement, and the push for more detailed information was coupled to this growing public awareness of, and concern for, the effects of chemicals on health and the environment. The publication of Rachel Carson's book *Silent Spring* in 1962 highlighting the potential damage caused by the indiscriminate use of pesticides was a jolt to public consciousness and a major turning point in this aspect of the history of toxicology. Increased regulatory control in response to such demands frequently required companies to test their products and provide regulatory authorities with dossiers of data to assure safety. Such requirements were paralleled through the latter half of the twentieth century by a steep growth in the number of journal titles available. There was increased specialization in toxicology and this was reflected by the ever growing number of specialist journals, covering areas such as genetic toxicology and cancer, epidemiology, reproductive toxicology, contact dermatitis and ecotoxicology.

This enormous proliferation brought with it the problems of how to manage and track down important information and in its turn led to the increased importance of 'secondary' indexes to the literature. These secondary sources allowed the search, identification and retrieval of information by specific subject headings. Major publications included *Index Medicus* and *Excerpta Medica*, both of which cover the medical literature, *Biological Abstracts*, which took in the whole of the life sciences, and *Chemical Abstracts*, covering the entire field of chemistry. With the advent of computer technology, many of these resources became available in electronic form. Those required by law to provide information on the safety of chemicals had ready access to large volumes of information that was publicly available. Some regulations themselves involved the compilation of data sets in electronic form, establishing databanks of toxicological data made available in a standardized layout.

Towards the close of the twentieth century the move was toward increased standardization and harmonization of information requirements on an international scale, as it was recognized that differences acted as effective trade barriers.

THE SCIENTIFIC COMMUNITY: GENERATION AND DISSEMINATION OF TOXICOLOGICAL INFORMATION

Scientific knowledge is advanced principally through experimental research and observation. Data will first reside in the laboratories and offices of those who have been involved in its generation. Laboratory notebooks, correspondence and computer files may all be initial repositories for such raw information. Early dissemination is likely to take place on an informal level with immediate colleagues and peers. An extended group of outside contacts could also become included. Much research takes place on a collaborative basis, and scientists, perhaps widely separated geographically or spanning employment sectors, may all contribute. More formal presentation of results may occur at professional seminars and meetings, and such gatherings frequently represent the first outside disclosure of new data, albeit usually to a closed audience.

This 'invisible college' of scientists plays an essential part in the scientific process and the formation and possible rejection of ideas and hypotheses. These 'non-published' methods of dissemination can be major resources for toxicological information, particularly to those working in the research environment. Such communication reduces the time lag between completion of studies and dissemination of results, and allows for immediate analysis and discussion by the scientific community. The interdisciplinary nature of toxicology makes this human network and its organization critical to effective coordination and the spread of information. Often, toxicological topics find their way into meetings covering broader subject areas such as food technology or cosmetology.

The more tangible forms of information that result from such early processes may be the minutes or proceedings of meetings, news articles or company reports. Another early process is the circulation of preprints prior to publication. Direct contact with individuals or an organization may be the most effective means of acquiring such information.

Details on forthcoming major seminars and conferences are published in scientific magazines and journals, or may be sent directly to scientists who are a well established part of the invisible college in their particular specialist area. Other sources include online computer databases such as MediConf (Medical Conferences and Events) and, increasingly, the World Wide Web pages of scientific organizations.

PRIMARY LITERATURE

As is common with all science, the validity of toxicological findings presented at conferences is enhanced by formal publication. Most early data go through further organization before being made available to the public. The vehicle for the publication of results of scientific endeavour is generally the so-called primary journal (meaning first site of open publication). The primary journals form the backbone of what can be termed the 'scientific process'—that by which ideas or hypotheses are tested and results are reported, and are then scrutinized and re-evaluated by the wider scientific community through discussion, comment and further experimentation. The importance of these journals is such that the 'modus operandi' of their production warrants more detailed discussion.

Like most scientific journals, those in the toxicological arena are, of course, commercial ventures by publishers seeking to fill a niche in the market of scientific literature. Many, however, are also the official publications of distinguished associations, societies or other scientific organizations. Every journal will have its own particular aims and scope, and most issues publish a brief outline of these selection criteria. The reputation of a journal is a rather more nebulous concept and may have been built up over many years. The editorial policy and the list of those that sit on the editorial board may give some indication of its prestige. Citation statistics may also provide clues to how a journal is viewed by the scientific community at large, although these can often be misleading as a result of biases.

Whilst many items, such as short communications or letters, may take the form of a narrative, most journal editors expect papers to be submitted in a standard format, usually consisting of a Summary, Introduction, Methods, Results, Conclusion and References. The value of this format is straightforward: it should be clear what has been done, what was seen and noted, and what the results might mean. The Introduction should put the study into context and provide an indication of why the investigation was carried out. The Methods section should contain enough detail to allow the investigation to be repeated independently. The Results should indicate in quantitative and/or qualitative terms what was actually recorded and observed, and the Conclusion should present a discussion of how these results could be interpreted. Of particular interest in terms of information retrieval is the summary or abstract. Essentially used to judge in a short space of time whether a particular paper is likely to be of relevance, abstracts only rarely give sufficient detail to allow serious assessment of a study and often cannot be used as a replacement for the full text, only as a supplement to it. Although there have been recent moves by some journal editors to require abstracts in a standardized format, traditionally there has been no uniform structure and they may contain inadequate or even misleading information and analysis. These problems have been compounded by the frequent inclusion of abstracts in electronic bibliographic databases (see the section Databases), a feature which is fundamental to the way in which they are used for search and retrieval, and necessitated in reality by a lack of effective in depth indexing of the study by the database providers. Abstracts were developed in a pre-electronic era to provide a brief, readable and selective view of a full work. Neither their structure nor content is generally compatible with good indexing practice. Their inclusion effectively reduces the accuracy of retrieval of a well indexed paper, resulting frequently in large numbers of false hits. The abstract has then to be read as a method for refining the imprecise search results, in order to eliminate false drops and increase specificity, a costly strategy in scientist time and online costs. The ideal would be a database with a high quality of indexing which retrieves only information of relevance. The full text of these documents could then be scrutinized in the prior knowledge that it contains important information on the search topic.

Papers are generally submitted to the editor of the journal, who may make an initial decision as to the suitability for publication, whether, for example, the paper fits in with the aims and scope of the journal or whether it

is novel. An aspect of particular importance, however, and one on which the credibility of the journal is usually judged, is the so-called peer-review process. This mechanism involves the scrutiny of submitted papers by a number of independent referees (two is a generally accepted number) who are chosen as experts in the particular field of interest and who will use their judgement to accept the paper for publication or reject it. In most cases the referees will almost certainly make comments to which the authors must respond before it is deemed acceptable for publication. The peer-review process is often regarded as the basis of scientific credibility and ensures that much science of poor quality never appears in the good scientific literature. The mechanism has worked well over the years, although it is by no means infallible. It is a system which is dependent to a large degree on the goodwill and professionalism of the referees, who generally give their time and skill free of charge. It has been suggested that financial reward for such services would make for more efficient refereeing and reduce the delay between submission of a paper and publication, although such moves would inevitably lead to further increases in journal costs. Publications, including an increasing number of journals, that do not involve a recognizable peer-review process should certainly be treated as a potentially unreliable source of scientific information.

Once a paper has been accepted for publication, the process of copy editing and proof reading and the mechanisms of formal publication take over. This whole process, from first submission to final publication, can often take several months and perhaps as much as a year or longer, even using today's modern electronic mechanisms.

Many factors will influence investigators on whether to submit papers for publication in the scientific literature. Dissemination of information is perhaps the main motivation for publication, although improvement of prospects for further research funding and advancement of career can be other major driving forces. Approval for publication may need to be sought from the sponsor for work done under contract. Industry, for commercial reasons, may be less interested in information dissemination outside the parent organization, and this can be a major problem in toxicology.

Most science graduates will have some idea of the key journals in their particular specialist discipline and those moving into work in the toxicological arena are likely to have at their disposal an established library subscribing to a core list of journals which has evolved with the organization and clients that it serves. Those setting up an information service from scratch face a more difficult task, but assistance from established specialist libraries can generally be sought. The most appropriate method would be to draw up a core list of requirements through consultation with those they are to serve. Lists of journals can be obtained from the scientific publishers, who are also often most willing to supply sample copies for evaluation. International periodicals directories can also be consulted for a detailed compilation of the journals currently available. Scientists are likely to be alerted to the existence of important journals through their research, and discussion with colleagues.

The cost of subscribing to journals can be substantial. Journal costs have risen steeply in recent years and are likely to continue to do so, and libraries are frequently faced with stark choices and difficult deliberations with the scientists they serve over the merits or otherwise of subscribing to a particular journal. The costs of journal production can be offset by the introduction of page charges, whereby those submitting a paper are required to pay part of the cost, and this is common practice in the USA. It is less frequent in the UK and continental Europe, however, and any moves in that direction are likely to be resisted.

For specific published papers, many scientists will often rely on obtaining copies through national library systems, which are well established in most developed countries. This process is, however, affected by international copyright law, which can limit the quantity of material that can be copied from a particular document and generally requires a charge to be made. Some publishers may even prohibit any copying of material without their specific approval. A certain number of reprints are generally made available via the authors, so a direct approach may also prove fruitful.

There are currently well over 100 journals devoted primarily to toxicology. As the science has developed, emerging sub-disciplines have given rise to new titles. A very restricted core list for those interested primarily in hazard and risk assessment gives some indication of the range of titles available:

Archives of Environmental Contamination and Toxicology
Archives of Toxicology
Bulletin of Environmental Contamination and Toxicology
Carcinogenesis
CRC Critical Reviews in Toxicology
Drug and Chemical Toxicology
Ecotoxicology and Environmental Safety
Environmental Toxicology and Chemistry
Food and Chemical Toxicology
Fundamental and Applied Toxicology
Human and Experimental Toxicology
Journal of the American College of Toxicology
Journal of Applied Toxicology
Journal of Environmental Pathology, Toxicology and Oncology
Journal of Toxicology and Environmental Health
Mutagenesis
Mutation Research
Neurotoxicology and Teratology
Pharmacology and Toxicology

Regulatory Toxicology and Pharmacology
Reproductive Toxicology
Toxicology
Toxicology and Applied Pharmacology
Toxicology and Industrial Health
Toxicology In Vitro
Toxicology Letters
Veterinary and Human Toxicology

Other scientific journals also impinge vastly on the area of toxicology, most notably those dealing in medical, pharmacological or epidemiological research, and will, with varying degrees of frequency, publish useful data. More general, but highly prestigious, scientific periodicals such as *Nature* or *Science* also sometimes include reports which would be described as of toxicological significance. The increasing number of toxicological journal titles is testament to their position as the most important source of such information.

Keeping up-to-date with the primary literature can be a daunting task. Although abstracting and indexing services can play a valuable role, there is an inevitable time lag between publication of the journal article and its appearance in this type of secondary literature. Current awareness publications appear with greater frequency, often weekly, or even daily. *Current Contents* is perhaps one of the better known of these services in the biomedical field, but other, often more specialized, services are available, in both printed and electronic format, or as part of a service offered by an information unit. Such 'selective dissemination of information' (SDI) can provide a focused set of documents tailored to the specific requirements as outlined by the user.

Although it is unlikely that printed journals will be replaced completely, many full text journals are now available in electronic form on the Internet (see later). This allows material to be made available much more quickly, often months before the printed version, and also allows for additional information and comment to be included, along with multimedia applications such as sound and video. It permits full text searching and alerting services that serve individual interests and provide links to other relevant sites. Tables of contents can automatically be E-mailed to subscribers as they are published.

STANDARD TEXTS AND MONOGRAPHS

Standard reference works, or 'tertiary sources', compile and condense information into a form that can be seen to represent a culmination of the scientific process; they usually present a considered, and generally widely accepted, view in a particular area. They are often written, compiled or edited by distinguished experts in the field of interest. Many regularly used texts provide concise overviews or summary data on the toxicology of chemicals or chemical groups and can be useful for background material. As such, they are often the first port of call (and all too frequently the only port of call) by those seeking information. Most libraries or information units will have their favoured set of textbooks. General texts and books devoted to special areas within toxicology are abundant. They offer a comparatively cheap and easy way of gaining an often arbitary selection of the available information on a topic.

It is not within the scope of this chapter to commit to print a recommended reading list of particular books over others. New texts are constantly emerging and the usefulness of each will depend very much on the environment in which it is being used—the particular subject area of interest and the type and depth of information required. Some books have gained themselves enviable (sometimes perhaps misplaced) reputations as essential texts to grace the shelves of any self-respecting toxicologist. It is important, however, to acknowledge the limitations of some such material. One of the primary considerations is that of topicality. The gestation period and publication timetable of a large textbook are inevitably protracted. In a specialist area that is rapidly changing, the information may be somewhat out of date, perhaps by as much as 2–3 years, even as the text first appears on the bookshop shelves. Once published, well loved textbooks may remain on a library shelf for many years and that same book, consulted 10 years later, may present a very different view from that currently prevailing. Although generally making use of experts, the task of writing or contributing to a book is usually essentially unpaid and thus the authors may not have been able to afford the time and resources to conduct a comprehensive and in-depth evaluation of all the information that might be available on a particular topic. Typographical errors are, unfortunately, not uncommon within published works and the misplacement of a decimal point or the misprinting of a unit of measure, for instance, can have profound consequences to any dose–response analysis. Whilst such errors tend to be quickly picked up and corrected within the primary literature, no such process exists for published books, and errors are sometimes even repeated in citations by other works. It is always advisable if the reference is available, and resources permit, to check the original data. Unfortunately, referencing within textbooks tends to be poor, however, and sometimes even non-existent. It is certainly not usually as comprehensive as, say, that in a published journal article, often making it at best difficult to trace and verify data. Many texts are written with a very specific readership in mind and it is necessary to appreciate the context in which the book has been written, together with its aims. Frequently there is large overlap in the information provided by different texts so it is worth taking careful consideration of the merits of purchasing any particular book.

Current details of textbooks available are best sought from the catalogues and brochures of the major scientific publishers. Announcements of new books frequently appear in scientific journals and magazines and will inevitably be mailed directly to those whose contact details lie within the publisher's marketing department. Up-to-date details of books currently available can also be sought from published lists of scientific and technical books in print, which can generally be consulted in libraries and major book stores. It is also worth taking note of published book reviews which often appear in trade association journals, information bulletins and so on, along with the more mainstream primary biomedical journals. Advice on the suitability of various texts may also be sought from information units and experts working in the field. Clearly, it is important to evaluate the suitability of any particular text to personal requirements. Cost will certainly be a consideration and many large textbooks (or even those smaller ones with a more specialist, and thus limited, audience) are expensive.

A particular kind of tertiary source common to the toxicological information scene is the special monographic series. Well established publications of this type include, for instance, the *Monographs on the Evaluation of the Carcinogenic Risk (of Chemicals) to Humans*, published by the International Agency for Research on Cancer (IARC) of the World Health Organization (WHO), and the *Environmental Health Criteria*, published under the joint sponsorship of the United Nations Environment Programme, the International Labour Organization (ILO) and WHO. Other examples include the evaluations published by the Joint FAO (Food and Agriculture Organization)/WHO Expert Committee on Food Additives (JECFA) and those of the Joint FAO/WHO Meeting on Pesticide Residues (JMPR). A common feature of such reports is frequently the peer review and consensus process that is undertaken in their compilation by international working groups of experts in the particular field of interest and they are therefore held with high regard.

The aims of all such work are usually clearly defined and specific and, although such publications can be useful compilations of data, the context in which they have been written should be fully appreciated. Because of the part that toxicology plays in much of our lives, many similar *ad hoc* special reports are produced by both national and international committees of experts. These can be much more difficult to track down, and many would fall more squarely under the label of 'grey literature'.

GREY LITERATURE

One of the major difficulties in terms of information retrieval within the discipline of toxicology is the proliferation of so- called 'grey literature'. This term is a loose one, used to describe documents which do not fall easily within the primary, secondary and tertiary labels of mainstream science publication. Grey documents may include such material as conference or seminar proceedings, press releases, dissertations, internal reports and manufacturers' leaflets and brochures. The reports and pronouncements of expert groups convened to look at a particular toxicological issue may also fall within this category. Perhaps it is because toxicology impinges so much on our daily lives and thus is of interest, at some level, to virtually all of us that it suffers from problems posed by the grey literature more than any other of the scientific disciplines. For whatever reason, the prevalence of literature of this type presents particular difficulties to those whose job necessitates collating or seeking toxicology information. The problems stem largely from the fact that these documents do not arise as a result of the usual publication process and, as a consequence, do not pass to the cataloguers and indexers who would normally channel the details into the tools regularly used to search for information.

Although much can be highly valuable, by its very nature, there is no easy answer to the difficulties of tracking down or even being alerted to the existence of grey literature. If a known specific item is being sought, an approach to the responsible organization, particularly if it has an information unit or library, is the best route. Keeping track routinely of such publications is a more hit-and-miss affair. A place on a multitude of mailing lists is possibly one of the best strategies. Trade and research associations, societies and commercial information services that provide some form of alerting service are generally adept at tracking and receiving such information. Indeed, it is often part of their work to scan trade journals, notifications, reports and various publications lists in order to alert their clients. Such channels for obtaining grey literature may have been established and cultivated over many years and subscribing to these organizations can prove a worthwhile investment.

Perhaps one of the greatest improvements in the ability to track down documents of a grey complexion has been the emergence of the Internet (see later). Details and even the full texts of reports, news releases, agendas and minutes of specialist committees are now finding their way on to the Internet. Links to other sites can be an additional useful alert to other information that may be of value.

DEVELOPMENT AND USE OF ELECTRONIC SOURCES

Databases

The word database relates almost exclusively today to computer-held information. Traditionally it was a term which referred to any set of 'secondary' (or bibliographic) data compiled as an index to the primary literature. Secondary publications such as *Index Medicus, Chemical Abstracts* and *Biological Abstracts*, which were developed as search tools for the ever- expanding scientific literature, would therefore fall within this definition.

Computerized databases were developed in the mid-1960s as a spin-off from the computer phototypesetting process used in the production of these printed indexes; the bibliographic data were captured in machine-readable form so as to allow for reformatting and the creation of subject, author and cumulative indexes. Developments in computer and telecommunications technology during the 1960s and early 1970s made it possible for the machine-readable master tapes to be used directly for information retrieval. Although initially it was impossible to change the search strategy during the search, interactive online searching quickly became a reality; the results of any search could be viewed as the search progressed and the strategy employed to identify relevant information could be altered to provide a more focused or expanded set of data, as necessary. It was a revolution in the way information was held and disseminated and a huge advance in the mechanism by which searching was carried out.

Today, the reality of computer searching is taken very much for granted, but it is worth pondering on what a tremendous improvement such systems have made in locating relevant information. A search that would have taken many hours using traditional library sources can now be accomplished in a matter of minutes, and consequently at a fraction of the cost of a professional librarian's or information searcher's time. In addition, the computer databases are invariably more up-to-date than the printed equivalent, and they have greatly increased access points; it is possible to search an online database in many more ways than one can search its printed version.

Two large US corporations, Lockheed DIALOG and Systems Development Corporation (SDC), were the first to exploit these developments. They were followed, in the mid-1970s, by European services such as ESA-IRS, operated by the European Space Agency, and BLAISE, a system developed by the British Library. These were known as 'host' organizations and based their services on the large mainframe computers that they had at their disposal. The huge storage capacity of these computers enabled the hosts to mount numerous database files. The organizations that provide the database files are known as 'producer' organizations. They are generally separate, independent organizations, such as research associations or government agencies. They may make their particular files available to the host organizations free of charge or may require a certain percentage of the profits of the host to be passed over as royalties.

Medicine was one of the first sciences to benefit from this new information technology. The batch-processed MEDLARS (Medical Literature Analysis and Retrieval System) became operational at the US National Library of Medicine (NLM) in 1964, followed by MEDLINE, the interactive online version of *Index Medicus*, in 1971.

As has been discussed, this was a time when toxicology as a science was coming into its own, with a consequent huge expansion in its information base. Concern was expressed about the dispersion of toxicological information over a diverse array of published scientific literature. The Toxicology Information Program was established at the NLM in 1967 in an attempt to address this, and one of its early achievements was the development of TOXLINE in 1972. Now a family of computerized interactive bibliographic databases, TOXLINE was set up in the hope of providing a 'one-stop shop' for searching the toxicological literature. At the time, however, there was no available unified bibliography of toxicological information, as there was, for example, with medicine in the form of *Index Medicus*. The solution was to combine various subsets specifically relating to toxicology from a number of different secondary sources. Thus, relevant sections from *Index Medicus* and *Chemical Abstracts* were included, together with others such as from *Pesticides Abstracts* and *International Pharmaceutical Abstracts*. More specialist collections of bibliographic information were also included, such as the files of the Environmental Mutagen Information Center (EMIC) and the Environmental Teratology Information Center (ETIC). The precise group of subsets which goes to make up the TOXLINE databases has changed over the years, and presumably may do so in the future, but details of those currently included are available in documentation from the NLM or the hosts which make the databases available. Despite this heterogeneous array of subsets which go to make up the full files, the user of the TOXLINE databases is presented with a 'front end' interface which suggests a single, apparently homogeneous, system covering toxicology.

In terms of breadth of scope and size, the TOXLINE system remains the premier online bibliographic database in the field of toxicology. The number of records now runs into the millions. Thousands of journal titles are cited at least once, although a more limited core set of journals, running into the hundreds, provides the bulk of the records. As the system grew it was necessary to split the TOXLINE database, both in terms of time coverage and to separate the subsets whose producers required royalty charges from those that did not.

Toxicology and medicine are subjects where there are numerous general and more specialized online computer databases available, and TOXLINE cannot generally be relied upon alone for complete data retrieval; searches of other databases such as MEDLINE, BIOSIS Previews (the online equivalent of the indexing service *Biological Abstracts*), *Chemical Abstracts* and *Excerpta Medica* are certainly worth considering for a general and comprehensive trawl for toxicological information, whilst specialized and more selective databases may be more appropriate for a search in a particular subject category. With such a diverse selection of databases available it can be difficult to decide on the most appropriate one to search. Published directories of the online databases that are available, both generally and more specifically in the fields of biology and medicine, are produced not only as catalogues from the host organizations themselves, but frequently as independent compilations by scientific publishing houses or organizations in the business of library and information management. Such details can quickly go out of date as new databases regularly appear, so it is necessary to seek the most recent information available and, if necessary, supplement this with approaches to the host companies directly.

There can be a large overlap between databases in the information they select and index and it is certainly worth considering carefully whether a particular database will cover the area of interest comprehensively, but not be so broad as to generate masses of unwanted information. It should also be remembered that few computerized databases bother with the published literature prior to the mid-1960s and 1970s when they were first developed. Although some may have undergone a process of introducing older data, the date from which entries begin should be noted; toxicity hazard and risk assessment is unusual in that much of these missing older data may still be of critical importance. The scope of literature selection may also be an important factor in database choice. Whilst many bibliographic databases are fairly strong on conventionally published scientific information, they do not cope as well with the grey literature and, for reasons that have previously been discussed, this can represent a serious loss. Although most useful databases in the field of toxicology are updated frequently, it can still take several months, and perhaps up to as much as a year, between publication of a paper in a journal and its appearance on a database.

Many databases are available from a number of hosts, so the selection of which host organizations to register with can also require decision. The factors that should be considered are the particular databases available on the system, the need to learn the computer search command language and the cost of gaining access to databases of interest. The search languages used for interacting with the host computers tend to be unique to each system. To enable effective searching to be performed it is therefore necessary to have sufficient training and knowledge of the host system's own language. Generally, people can cope with learning and using several different languages, although the fewer command languages which need to be learnt and used, the more efficient searching is likely to be. Most database hosts produce weighty search guides or handbooks outlining the scope and coverage of the databases that they make available and the techniques for searching them. Training courses are frequently held for those needing to learn the basics of searching or wanting to improve their skills. Many databases also have free online 'training files', enabling new searchers to gain experience without running up large online costs. Details of these should be sought from the host organizations.

Demonstrations of databases can often be witnessed at seminars, workshops and conference exhibitions, and it may be worth visiting these prior to selection, or to keep abreast of what is available. Articles on searching for toxicological and medical information also often appear in the scientific journal literature, in both mainstream toxicology and biomedical journals, and also those in the area of library and information science. Journals such as *Toxicology, Journal of Chemical Information and Computer Science, Annual Review of Information Science and Technology, Chemosphere, American Journal of the Industrial Hygiene Association, Human and Experimental Toxicology* and *Toxicology and Environmental Chemistry* have all in the past published articles comparing the efficacy of different databases. Such papers can often provide useful discussion on searching techniques and on the value of particular databases in the search for toxicological information.

Although initial registration may be free, the hosts generally charge customers for using a database in the form of an online connect charge, plus a scale of charges for information viewed or printed, depending on the format required. There are also the telecommunication charges to take into account. Of more significance can be the initial costs of manuals and training courses. Overall, it should be appreciated, however, that charges for online searching are often trivial when compared with the cost of a professional information searcher's time saved.

Access to a particular host system is made traditionally via a computer terminal and keyboard linked to the telecommunications network. In this way, a user registered with a particular host organization can gain access to any of the databases available on the service. The great advantage of the computer-based systems over more conventional search methods is, of course, their interactive nature, by which a 'dialogue' can be established with the computer to modify or refine the search strategy in the light of initial results. Searches are essentially constructed and refined in most computer databases by combining search terms using the Boolean operators AND, OR and NOT. The inclusion of the operator AND will retrieve articles which are common to both sets, whilst OR will add the two sets together. For example, a search can be narrowed by indicating that documents that contain the search word CANCER must also contain the word MAN (viz. CANCER AND MAN), whilst it could be broadened by specifying that the document contains any of the words CANCER OR CARCINOGENICITY OR TUMOUR, as well as (AND), MAN OR HUMAN OR WORKER. The logi-

cal operator NOT will eliminate documents that contain the specified search term, for instance CANCER NOT STOMACH would retrieve any records that contain the search word CANCER, but not any that also contain the word STOMACH. It should be used with care, since documents that do contain useful information may be unintentionally eliminated. If the topic of interest is cancer of the colon, a paper which discusses both colon and stomach cancer would have been eliminated using the above strategy.

It is impossible here to describe in detail the established command languages and the tactics that can be employed to search the numerous databases available, as the online hosts have each developed their own set of search aids to enable refinement of strategies. In addition to the use of Boolean logic, common techniques involve the use of relational operators allowing a user to specify, for example, that two search words must appear adjacent to each other (STOMACH next to CANCER, for instance), or within a specified number of words from one another (say CANCER within four words of STOMACH, to retrieve both STOMACH CANCER and CANCER OF THE STOMACH). It may be possible also to require that words appear in a specified order, or within the same sentence or paragraph. The search may be limited to words appearing in the title only, or to just the keywords that have been added to the record by the databases indexers. Most systems allow the truncation of terms, such that MUTA-, for instance, could be used as a search term to include papers containing any of the words MUTATION, MUTANT, MUTAGEN, MUTAGENIC, MUTAGENICITY and so on. Again, the searcher needs to be aware that the truncated term might retrieve irrelevant information. In the above example, papers on the bacterium *Streptococcus MUTAns* would also be retrieved. Search statements can often be complex and need careful and expert construction. Once developed, many of the online hosts allow searches to be saved, so that they can be used at a later date, perhaps, for instance, with a different chemical. Thus a search which seeks to retrieve all documents relating to genotoxicity, or ecotoxicity, could be constructed by including all the various synonyms and permutations of words and phrases associated with these topics. On each occasion, such a saved search could be combined with terms for the new material(s) of interest. Some hosts include pre-constructed strategies covering common specialist topic areas and details of these are given in the search guides.

The use of these techniques will hopefully increase the probability of retrieving a set of documents that relates closely to that being sought.

The above examples allude to the main problems of searching: those of how the documents are indexed and the search strategies that need to be employed to obtain comprehensive but specific sets of results. Each record in a bibliographic database represents one scientific paper, journal article or document. The record generally has standard elements or fields which may include the Authors, Title, Publication Type and Reference, Language of the Paper, Year of Publication, Country of Publication, Organization(s) for which the authors work, Keywords or Descriptors and perhaps the Abstract. Each of these fields can be used as an entry point for searching or to limit the search using such methods as mentioned above. The Title, Keywords and Abstracts are most frequently used as the basis for searching.

The TOXLINE databases, as is common with many systems, are essentially 'free text', that is, there is no controlled vocabulary applied across all the subfiles for indexing and searching purposes. In order to search comprehensively on a particular subject, it is therefore necessary to include as many synonyms for each search term as possible. The computer will then look for any documents in the database where this word appears, in the title, abstract or keyword fields, for example, as specified. The keywords will be those terms highlighted from the text by the database indexers and will appear 'as is' in the keywords/descriptors field.

Other databases involve the use of a restricted and structured thesaurus of terms to index papers, for example, such that the word MAN would be used as a keyword to the exclusion of any others, even if these others, such as HUMAN, WORKER or CHILD, etc., were the only ones to appear in the text in relation to a paper that includes human data. In such an instance, a search restricted to the keywords field on MAN would retrieve all relevant papers and a list of synonyms is not needed. A controlled vocabulary like this is well developed, for instance, with the MEDLINE and BIOSIS Previews databases. The MEDLINE indexers have at their disposal a large hierarchical tree structure of terms, known as MeSH (Medical Subject Heading) terms. The indexers select the most appropriate of these descriptors to represent the subjects covered by a particular paper. The tree structure allows for broad and narrow concepts to be described. Whilst the most specific term available is applied in each case, explosion of a broader term on searching would retrieve this and related documents. The search word ASTHMA would miss any articles indexed under ASTHMA IN CHILDREN, unless the term ASTHMA was exploded in the search. The MeSH theasurus is continually evolving, with new terms added frequently, as the sciences that it describes grow and develop. Often the terms applied can be given added weight by the indexers as major or minor concepts in the article. This again allows refinement of searches if large sets are initially being retrieved.

The selection of keywords and, in particular, the use of structured vocabularies require particular knowledge and experience by both the database indexers themselves and by those wishing to search. Expert indexing is crucial to the effectiveness of a database and, unfortunately, on occasion is clearly lacking. Inappropriate or inadequate indexing of a particular paper will severely decrease the likelihood of it being retrieved during a specific search, or may lead to it appearing as a false drop. Similarly, errors during the entering of a paper's details, perhaps of a simple typographical nature, can result in an item failing to be retrieved.

Chemical names can present particular difficulties when searching for data, and thus are a major problem for those seeking information pertinent to toxicological hazard and risk assessment. Chemical nomenclature can be complex and all synonyms and permutations have to be included in a free text search, necessitating perhaps a high degree of chemical knowledge. Searching precisely on a parent compound without retrieving large numbers of papers on derivatives which include the parent name can also be a huge problem, as can searching for information on a generic class of substances, which would depend on a high degree of detailed chemical indexing, including generic details. Such comprehensive indexing is, unfortunately, lacking in many databases. The inclusion of Chemical Abstracts Service (CAS) Registry numbers in database records can eliminate many of the problems associated with chemical indexing. CAS Registry numbers are unique numbers for specific chemicals, assigned by the Chemical Abstracts Service. Unfortunately, few of the commonly used biomedical databases have comprehensive inclusion of CAS Registry numbers.

Another problem arises from the presence in the record of all chemicals mentioned in a paper, even those that are not central to the study being described. They may occur in the free text, or may specifically have been added by the indexers. Such indexing problems can be particularly acute, for instance, in relation to solvents, control substances or adjuvants. Eliminating large numbers of documents of no value can be difficult or impossible in many cases. The result frequently is that large numbers of 'hits' have to be scanned by title or abstract, a process that can be time consuming and expensive. Despite this, it is still a common misconception that the bigger the database, the better it is.

Although such considerations are often given little thought by those who use databases, the indexing policies and the expertise of the database indexing, together with the initial selection criteria for documents which should appear as records, clearly are vitally important aspects of database construction and the consequent use to which they can be put. The value of any bibliographic database must be judged by its ability to identify all relevant data sources. Two criteria are important in assessing performance. The first of these is the ability of any search to 'recall' information, which is defined as the number of relevant citations retrieved out of the total number of relevant citations in the database being searched, and can also be viewed as the 'sensitivity' of the search. The second criterion is 'specificity' (or 'precision'), which measures the ability of the search to discriminate between relevant and non-relevant citations and is the proportion of those records identified which prove, on final analysis, to be of relevance. Large, broad scope databases can perform very poorly on the basis of these criteria. The varied requirements of the different types of user—the basic research community, applied researchers, those charged with evaluating hazard and risk and so on—are accommodated at the expense of specificity, while the use of non-specialist selection and indexing reduces both specificity and recall. The ideal would be for a database to be subject specific, retrieving only information of relevance, which is easy to search, and comprehensive for that subject. In toxicological hazard and risk assessment, the loss of information may undermine an opinion on safety in use.

It may be no surprise that information searching, particularly in the biomedical field, has become a vocation in itself. The terms and command language used in searching have to be precise. Inexperienced searching of computer databases may not only miss relevant information or result in large numbers of irrelevant hits, but may also be costly. The complexity and vagaries of these systems have led to the emergence of specialist information searchers who, using their knowledge and experience of searching computer databases, act as an intermediary between those seeking the information and the information resource. Whilst such information specialists may have a scientific or biomedical background, they may not have knowledge of, or appreciate fully, the concepts of the highly specialized area being searched, and this again can introduce further potential for unfocused searching. The ideal would be for enquirers themselves to have detailed knowledge of the database construction and the initial selection and indexing policies, and to conduct the search and interact with the computer directly; the best database is one that is constructed with the close involvement of experts that need to use it.

Search techniques are continually evolving. Keeping up-to-date with database development can be a time-consuming process. Those with an account with a particular host will likely receive regular newsletters highlighting particular search aids and improvements that have been developed. Unless one is a regular searcher, remembering all this information is another matter altogether!

Databanks

Although the bibliographic databases retain their position as the most important resource for toxicological information, many people rely on compilations of hard facts in the form of databanks.

Under its precise definition, a databank provides factual information in the form of numeric data or textual statements. (In contrast, a database acts as an index, providing the bibliographic location of where that factual information can be found.) Whilst some of the issues discussed above in relation to the indexing and searching of databases would also apply to computer-based databanks, the factual nature of the latter presupposes some degree of value addition. The criteria for the selection and evaluation of the data become more crucial, and the nature and purpose of the databank should be considered carefully. An example of a commonly used databank is the Registry of Toxic Effects of Chemical Substances (RTECS), produced by the US National Institute for Occupational Safety and Health (NIOSH) in response to the US occupational safety and health regulations. It contains useful information on an enormous number of chemicals, although the data are limited in nature, and certainly are not intended to provide a complete assessment of hazard or risk. Nevertheless, it is surprising how many individuals rely on them for that purpose.

The Hazardous Substances Data Bank (HSDB) is another favoured and well resourced US databank, supported by the NLM. It contains extensive data including toxicity, safety and handling, emergency response, environmental fate and exposure potential information on a large number of potentially hazardous chemicals. Information is selected for inclusion by a scientific review panel, the initial aim of which was to establish a databank of 'evaluated' data. The result has been a predeliction for qualitative statements on hazard rather than quantitative insights on dose–response, essential to any evaluation of hazard and risk. Many of the records are also so large as to be almost unmanageable.

Efforts within Europe have given rise to the ECDIN (Environmental Chemicals Data and Information Network) database, which again is not comprehensive, and has failed to live up to the inital hopes. The IUCLID (International Uniform Chemicals Information Database) databank of accredited toxicity and ecotoxicity data on existing chemicals should prove valuable as it grows.

There is a seemingly desperate quest for good toxicological databanks that the layman can confidently use. The difficulty in producing them stems from the need to include large numbers of chemicals, if they are to be of any real general value, and the necessity to keep them up-to-date. The desire can only be realized, however, with substantial and ongoing investment.

Details of the wide range of databanks currently available in the area of toxicology can be sought from the catalogues and brochures of the online organizations which make them available. Many are also available on CD-ROM.

CD-ROM

The 1980s and 1990s saw huge advances in the accessibility and power of personal computers and the development of compact disc (CD-ROM) technology. This further revolutionized the information world, making available on a small disc at relatively low cost huge volumes of data, traditionally only accessible via the online services. Many of the database producers were quick to exploit the medium, making available large databases and databank collections, including such major resources as TOXLINE, MEDLINE and BIOSIS Previews. The major advantage of CD-ROM over online searching is that once the disc has been purchased there is unlimited access to the data, enabling an inexperienced searcher to explore their intricacies at relative leisure, without the fear of running up large online costs. Of course, the CD-ROM version of a database will inevitably not be as up-to-date as online versions, perhaps only a few updated discs being issued each year.

The relative ease with which compact discs can be produced and their low cost have also made the technology available directly to smaller organizations. Many more specialized products or sets of data in toxicology are now available. Details on CD-ROM products can be found, like the tertiary sources, in the brochures and catalogues of the scientific publishers or through fliers and advertisements of smaller producers. Specialist CD-ROM publishers are now in the market and, like the online hosts, may have a bewildering array of products available.

The Internet

The growth of the Internet, and particularly the World Wide Web, has seen substantial change in the traditional online market. The Internet has played a key role in restructuring the industry away from proprietary technologies and interfaces towards more open Internet standards. Although there have inevitably been teething problems, the developing technology is making it easier to find useful information, and the system is increasingly acting as an interface to the databases and databanks previously only available in equivalent form via the traditional online hosts. Access to a particular site is straightforward if the address, also referred to as the URL (Uniform Resource Locator), is known. Once at a site, pages can be browsed or printed. Of enormous use is the linking of sites to other pages of related or otherwise relevant information. More general searching can be achieved using the various search engines available, and the inclusion of terms or phrases, perhaps related by Boolean logic, as is common with the online host services. As has been mentioned, electronic versions of journals and books are now widely available. These may include the full text of the printed equivalent, but also allow for additional material to be made available, including multimedia applications such as sound or video. Once identified, a 'bookmark' can be inserted at the particular site, to allow rapid return at a future date.

Much 'grey literature' is available on the Internet and this has greatly improved the means of tracking and retrieving this type of information, much of it of great value. Many organizations are now using this as the sole method for dissemination of draft documents, minutes, agendas and reports. It is also possible for the system to alert users when new information has been added to a site of interest.

Whilst access to many valuable sites will be charged, a huge amount of information of a toxicological or biomedical nature is available free. This poses new considerations of information control and management to those seeking data, and greater thought needs to be given to the validation and verification of information. Anybody can make information available on the Internet and it is vital to establish the credentials of the authors of particular pages.

ORGANIZATIONAL RESOURCES

As has been touched on in some of the preceding sections, many sources of toxicological information emanate from national and international organizations. The nature of toxicology and its application are such that it has an extensive network of organizations that have some role in the generation, dissemination or use of toxicological information. Many of these will be governmental or quasi-governmental agencies, such as health, food or agriculture departments, or established research organizations. The industrial and consumer sectors will have their own interests represented by trade associations and consumer groups. On an international scale, organizations such as the WHO, ILO, Organization for Economic Cooperation and Development (OECD) and the European institutions will all have an input. Whilst many of these organizations publish using the traditional mechanisms, direct contact with an organization or individual may be an effective route to gaining current and relevant information or, at least, a pointer to where those details can be found. Academic, government and trade directories or yearbooks may help to target those organizations that are available.

CONCLUSION—QUALITY AND QUANTITY

With the huge growth in information and the diversification of media by which it is distributed, it is easy to lose sight of issues of quality. The proliferation of new sources not only brings tremendous advantages in terms of accessibility and speed, but also introduces new problems, in particular those of accuracy and verification. More is not necessarily better, and it is particularly important these days to consider how the information is being produced and compiled, and by whom. Unfortunately, the tremendous increase in toxicological data in recent times has not been matched by better quality control or analysis. Information is frequently misapplied or misunderstood. Expert selection and evaluation are something that comes at a price and the adage 'you get what you pay for' is an important one in the area of toxicological information. It is no easy task to assimilate a focused set of quality information from a diverse set of scientific disciplines, and particular expertise is required to add significant value to that information such that it becomes meaningful within the context in which it is being sought.

Another difficulty is presented by the nature of the science. Toxicology is often described as an 'art' as well as a science. The large subjective component in the interpretation of toxicological data can lead to conflicting views among experts in the field. Many of these areas are controversial and are thus open to political factors. Toxicology impinges so much of our daily lives that it perhaps suffers this more than many other sciences. The issue of independence can thus be an important factor.

It is difficult to predict what future moves will be made in information resources for toxicology. What is certain, however, is that the electronic revolution will continue to make a big impact. The trend is generally one of diversification of the media by which information can be accessed or disseminated. Predictions of the imminent demise of traditional methods such as the hard copy publication of primary journals have not been realized.

The printed textbook and journal article are still perhaps the most popular of media. The most important changes in information resources for toxicology are likely to be those prompted by the increasing specialization within the science and, of growing necessity, those of information quality control and analysis.

There has always been a move towards trying to provide data sources that can be readily accessible to the end (perhaps non-expert) user. The development of 'user-friendly' databanks, available at relatively low cost on CD-ROM, and the move of data collections to the Internet are progressions along this route. The danger is that the layman may not appreciate the issues of selectivity, validation and evaluation and the intricacies of chemical searching that are crucial to the effective and appropriate use of toxicological information. The hope is that the future will see a growing understanding of the benefit of quality, value-added over 'cheap and cheerful' quantity.

ACKNOWLEDGEMENTS

This chapter has been seen by colleagues of the Information and Advisory Service of BIBRA International, whose help and advice are gratefully acknowledged. The views expressed are the author's own and not necessarily those of the organization for which he works.

Chapter 24

Animal Welfare in the Toxicology Laboratory

Roy C. Myers

CONTENTS

INTRODUCTION

Animal welfare is not to be confused with 'animal rights', which is the concept that animals should have biological, social and legal status approaching that of humans. Those who adhere to this notion oppose the use of animals for research purposes and, indeed, for other human applications such as food, clothing or entertainment. The debate as to the legitimacy of this idea will be left to others, and the focus here will be the humane, considerate treatment of those animals used in the research laboratory.

Justification for proper care for and humane treatment of animal models should be obvious. From a moral standpoint, it contradicts our sense of decency purposely to cause pain and suffering in another species for no real benefit. Researchers should develop a measure of respect for laboratory animals and fully realize that they are living, breathing creatures that feel pain and have basic needs for sustaining good health. Most researchers have developed a strong interest in animals even before embarking upon a career involving animal research. Their concern for animal welfare naturally continues on throughout their scientific endeavours.

Beyond moral issues, it must be remembered that animal welfare is crucial for good science. Animals experiencing pain, stress or poor health do not make good test subjects. One of the basic precepts of science is that a test group must contain a minimal number of variables other than those purposely introduced (such as a chemical dose for assessing biological response). Subjects must be uniformly healthy and stress-free; otherwise, results are suspect and interpretations are difficult, if not impossible. Of course, some animal research by its nature may produce a certain level of pain or distress. This is especially true of acute toxicity testing and irritancy evaluations, where gross evidence of effect may be the desired endpoint. Still, the conscientious scientist will limit the degree of stress whenever possible while achieving the goals of the research project.

The pressures of society, including those from animal rights activists and the media, cannot be overlooked as another justification for animal welfare in the laboratory. All animal researchers feel the mounting public scrutiny of their work from the media, the government and various animal advocacy groups. Recently, a contract laboratory was the target of infiltration and public disclosure (via video footage) of apparent animal mistreatment. Of course, considerable negative publicity was generated against animal research in general. The specific laboratory involved may have lost several clients and, although the employment of those perpetrating the abuse was terminated, its reputation was possibly diminished as a result. The point is that all researchers must strive to avoid even a hint of animal abuse.

A final reason to be concerned about animal welfare is direct and critical—it is the law. Most nations and international governing bodies clearly prohibit animal misuse. As will be seen in subsequent sections, there are specific requirements regarding the care, treatment and disposition of laboratory animals. Failure to obey the laws can result in loss of licences, rejection of studies and even fines or imprisonment. These all are powerful inducements for the proper use of animals.

HISTORY OF ANIMAL WELFARE

For perspective, it might be helpful to take a brief look at how concern about animal use has evolved. A fairly concise account has been presented by King and Stephens (1991). These authors noted that animal welfare and antivivisection activities were relatively common by the end of the nineteenth century in the UK. By 1875, the British government was pressured to pass a bill regulating animal use, but opposition by scientists lead to a less restrictive law—the Animal Cruelty Act of 1876. Political and social pressure to prohibit animal research continued, however, and similar movements developed in the USA. In 1883, the American Antivivisection Society began a public outcry against experimental animal use. Other groups joined the cause and, through their protests, demonstrations and political actions, numerous bills prohibiting animal research were considered by various state legislatures. These bills, proposed between 1867 and 1906, were all defeated.

By 1908, the American Medical Association organized a Council for the Defense of Medical Research to consider the charges of antivivisectionists and to develop guidelines for animal experimentation in medicine. The advent of World War I and the growing enthusiasm for medical research tempered the opposition to animal use somewhat over the next several decades. However, a magazine story (*Life Magazine*, 1966) documented the poor living conditions for some dogs used in research and raised questions about possible theft of pets for research. The US Congress was flooded with mail demanding impositions of controls on animal research. Its response came in the form of new legislation (the Laboratory Animal Welfare Act, 1966) which prohibited the use of stolen dogs or cats for research, and required that research animals receive humane care and treatment. In 1970, this legislation became the Animal Welfare Act. Under this act, standards for care, treatment, and transportation of animals became the responsibility of the Secretary of Agriculture.

Possibly the most significant boost to the animal rights movement came from the publication of the book *Animal Liberation* (Singer, 1975). This work extended the philosophy of the civil rights movement of the 1960s to non-human animals. This philosophy, that animals have the same moral and legal rights as humans, has led to formation of modern animal activist groups and, in turn, to the pressures to control animal research that exist today. The result has been numerous legal actions and the establishment of a multitude of animal welfare agencies, as discussed below.

ANIMAL WELFARE LEGISLATION AND POLICY

Beginning with the Animal Welfare Act of 1966, several laws and regulations have been enacted in the USA to protect animals. Policies in other nations and international agreements are considered to be similar in content to the US policies. Some examples are the guidelines by the Canadian Council on Animal Care (Rowsell, 1991), the Australian Council for the Care of Animals in Research and Teaching (ACCART) (1990), the Netherlands Animal Welfare Society (1991), the International Council for Laboratory Animal Science (Cooper, 1990a, b) and so on. An effort to develop worldwide principles for laboratory animal use began in 1983, resulting in the 'International Guiding Principles for Biomedical Research Involving Animals', published in 1985 by the Council for International Organizations of Medical Sciences or CIOMS (Association for Assessment and Accreditation of Laboratory Animal Care (AAALAC) International, 1997a). CIOMS lists 11 'Basic Principles' which describe the circumstances and guidances for humane animal research. The system in the UK is defined by the Animals (Scientific Procedures) Act of 1986. This law requires researchers to obtain a personal licence, a project licence and a certificate for the research facility. Whenever new research techniques are proposed, amended licences must be obtained. Facility certificates designate a person responsible for enforcing the Animals Act (Association for Assessment and Accreditation of Laboratory Animal Care International, 1997b). Especially important in Europe is the European Directive 86/609 adopted by the Council of the European Communities (now the European Union) in 1986. This Directive is fairly comparable to the US Animal Welfare Act (Association for Assessment and Accreditation of Laboratory Animal Care International, 1997c).

Animal Welfare Act

The Animal Welfare Act (Public Law 89–544) has been amended in 1970 (P.L. 91–579), 1976 (P.L. 94–279), 1985 (P.L. 99–198) and 1990 (as part of the Food, Agriculture, Conservation and Trade Act). The US Department of Agriculture (USDA) has been empowered to implement the 'Act', which appears in Title 9, Code of Federal Regulations, Chapter 1 (USDA, 1995). Within the USDA, the Animal and Plant Inspection Service (APHIS) administers the 'Act' (USDA, 1996). APHIS is further divided into Regulatory Enforcement and Animal Care (REAC) units; the former unit (RE) was recently renamed the Investigative and Enforcement Services Unit.

The 'Act' provides standards for animal husbandry, veterinary care, exercise (dogs) and psychological health (primates). Specifically excluded are rats and mice, by far the most commonly used research models, and also farm animals not specifically used for research. To the extent possible, however, the conscientious investigator attempts to apply the principles of the 'Act' to rodents during toxicological research. Researchers are required, under specified circumstances, to administer anaesthesia or analgesics to minimize distress. Unnecessary research or duplication of animal testing is prohibited. A very important aspect of the 'Act' is the formation of an institutional animal care and use committee (IACUC) at each facility to oversee animal use. The IACUC must include three or more members, one being a veterinarian, another being an individual not affiliated with the facility and others being from a variety of backgrounds (USDA, 1995). It is often recommended that the 'outside' person be a non-scientist, possibly an ethicist or educator. The IACUC makes sure that the facility complies with the 'Act' through inspections (every 6 months), review of test protocols and formal reporting.

In considerable detail, the 'Act' specifies animal care conditions promoting a healthy and stress-free atmosphere. These cover housing, ventilation, lighting, temperature, interior surface composition, caging, sanitation, pest control, feed and water, record keeping, veterinary care and handling. Specially trained APHIS inspectors (veterinarians or animal health technicians) are given full access to all areas where regulated animals are kept. Any deficiencies discovered by the inspectors are made known to laboratory management along with deadlines for correction. Failure to address the deficiencies adequately could result in suspension of the facility's animal licence or in legal action.

Health Research Extension Act

Passed in 1985 (P.L. 99–158) and implemented 1986, the Health Research Extension Act has resulted in publication of the Public Health Service (PHS) Policy on Humane Care and Use of Laboratory Animals [Office for Protection from Research Risks (OPRR), 1996]. All facilities involved in PHS-sponsored projects must comply with this policy. Administration of the policy is the responsibility of the OPRR at the National Institutes of Health (NIH). Failure to comply results in a loss of NIH funding.

Like the Animal Welfare Act, the Health Research Extension Act details the requirements for facility maintenance, employee training, handling techniques, veterinary care and record keeping associated with animal research. Highlighted are the IACUC, certification of the facility, and compliance with the PHS 'Guide for the Care and Use of Laboratory Animals' (National Research Council, 1996). The 'Guide', considered by most researchers as the definitive source for animal welfare instruction, will be described more fully later. Also emphasized is the appropriate use of analgesia and anaesthesia, together with methods of euthanasia consistent with those recommended by the American Veterinary Medical Association (AVMA) Panel on Euthanasia (1993). The PHS Policy is summarized by nine US Government Principles (driven by the 'Guide') which must be agreed to through submission of an 'Assurance' of animal welfare prior to initiation of the study. The testing facility must be fully evaluated by an appropriate IACUC and/or accredited by the American Association for the Accreditation of Laboratory Animal Care (AALAC).

Good Laboratory Practice

With the adoption of the US Food and Drug Administration (FDA) Good Laboratory Practice (GLP) regulations (US Food and Drug Administration, 1978), animal care and use considerations have become part of an overall plan for the conduct of scientifically sound studies. Basically, research under FDA standards now must comply with the Animal Welfare Act and with animal treatment conditions recommended by the 'Guide'. GLP requirements for detailed standard operating procedures and a quality assurance unit review also help ensure appropriate attention to animal welfare. Other agencies in the USA followed suit, with the passing of GLP regulations under the US EPA Toxic Substance Control Act (US Environmental Protection Agency, 1989a) and the US EPA Federal Insecticide, Fungicide and Rodenticide Act (US Environmental Protection Agency, 1989b). Each of these provides some guidance on basic animal welfare, as does international GLP guidance from the Organization for Economic Cooperation and Development (OECD) (1981).

Specific Testing Guidance

Study guidance by the US EPA, FDA and OECD and many other agencies contains recommendations on the conduct of tests in a manner reflective of animal welfare. They especially promote the sacrifice of distressed or moribund animals, limits of numbers of animals used, non-animal screening and employment of available published data. As testing guidelines are updated, the emphasis on animal welfare issues typically increases.

ANIMAL WELFARE IN PRACTICE

It should be clear at this point that it is ethically and legally important to conduct animal research with as much attention to animal welfare as is practically possible. There are some very specific practices to achieve this, both from a standpoint of basic animal care and from the standpoint of humane research with animals. Responsibilities fall upon all personnel involved: institutional management, the investigator, technical staff and support staff (veterinary to maintenance). All must be committed to the proper treatment of animals and to maintaining a suitable environment.

Animal Care

It would be impossible to discuss all principles of animal care in detail within this chapter. Instead, some basic concepts as presented in the 'Guide' (National Research Council, 1996) and the Animal Welfare Act (USDA, 1995) are summarized below. An outline of the essential animal care considerations is given in **Figure 1**.

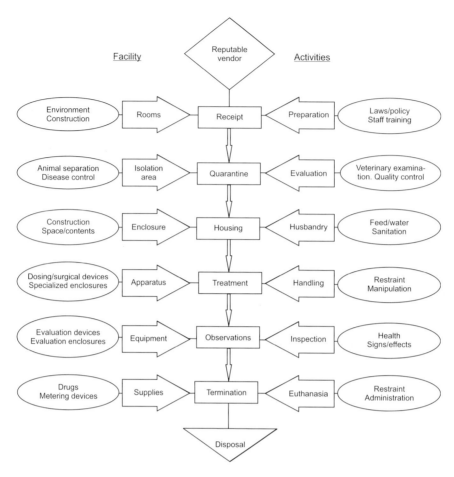

Figure 1 Essential considerations for animal care in the toxicology laboratory are shown diagrammatically. The central core includes the basic activities involving animals during their presence at the laboratory. Facility considerations and influencing factors are given on the left and animal care processes and influencing factors on the right.

Animal Environment

In general, facilities used for animal research should provide for the separation of animal rooms from those used for administrative purposes. Moreover, when possible, animals should be housed in areas isolated from laboratories where testing is conducted. Such areas permit minimal stress and confusion for the test animal. Surfaces within animal rooms should be resistant to moisture, vermin, cleansers and deterioration from frequent scrubbing. Porous surfaces and wooden surfaces, which allow the collection of dirt and microorganisms, must be avoided. Exposed plumbing, ductwork and lighting fixtures must be minimized. Animals must be obtained from only reputable vendors or bred under carefully controlled conditions within the facility. Newly received animals should be quarantined until their health status can be fully determined.

There should be space dedicated to sanitation of caging and supplies, storage of feed and bedding, performance of specialized animal treatment (dosing, surgery, necropsy, etc.) and storage of scientific apparatus and supplies. Humidity in animal rooms should be relatively consistent and controllable within the range 30–70%, and temperatures should be appropriate for the species housed and controllable within ±1°C. There must be adequate air filtration to control the spread of dust and pathogens, and provisions must be made for temporary ventilation in the event of a mechanical failure. Room lighting should be regulated by a timing device to provide a uniform diurnal cycle (typically 12 h of light and 12 h of darkness). To avoid excess noise, rooms should be constructed of sound-limiting materials. Moreover, sounds generated by personnel and equipment should be kept to a minimum.

If animal surgeries are to be performed, there should be adequate isolation from sources of contamination. It is suggested that separate areas be provided for support materials and equipment, prepping, surgery and recovery. The recovery area should permit adequate observation of treated animals.

Immediate Environment

Adequate control of the immediate surroundings is crucial to animal research projects. Primary enclosures (cages, boxes, pens) must provide for basic needs such as feeding, maintenance of body temperature, moving, urination/defaecation, access to adequate airflow and resting. They must be constructed of materials with a smooth, impervious surface that resist rust and damage from frequent handling. Their design must permit animal observation, efficient changing of feed and water and ease of cleaning and sanitation. Standard caging, especially for rodents and rabbits, typically is constructed of stainless steel with a mesh floor (although some researchers feel that a solid bottom with bedding is preferable). The wire mesh bottom permits animal waste to fall on to a collection tray underneath. A solid bottom (using plastics or vinyl-coated metal) may be more appropriate for larger animals. Some housing systems, for special types of research, involve closed boxes or cages with independent ventilation and air filtration systems. They also may have integral urine and faeces collection systems. Very large research models, such as sheep, goats or cattle, may require barns, corrals or pastures. The basic needs for these animals will be similar to those of smaller research

subjects, but with appropriate adjustments specific to each species.

Space recommendations are proportional to size, but are also based on expert judgment. These are detailed in the 'Guide' and summarized in **Table 1**. Attention must be given not only to floor area, but also to enclosure height. Volumes should be adjusted to account for special needs (pregnant animals, nursing animals, etc.) and for addition of feed/water containers or other objects. Moreover, required volumes for singly housed animals may differ from each animal housed in a group. It is essential that temperature be maintained within species-specific limits (**Table 1**). Extreme temperatures (above 29 C or below 4 C) may cause clinical effects including death. Relative humidity is not as critical, but for the sake of animal comfort and well being, should be controlled in the range 30–70%.

Animal enclosure ventilation provides a supply of breathing air, temperature control and removal of odours and contaminants. Under normal conditions, 10–15 air changes per hour are considered to be

Table 1 Recommended housing conditions for selected laboratory animal species[a]

Species	Housing type[b]	Size	Minimum cage/pen floor area	Minimum cage/pen height (cm)	Room temperature (°C)
Mouse	Group	10–15 g	39–52 cm^2	13	18–26
		15–25 g	52–77 cm^2	13	18–26
		25 g	97 cm^2	13	18–26
Rat	Group	100 g	110 cm^2	18	18–26
		100–200 g	110–148 cm^2	18	18–26
		200–400 g	148–258 cm^2	18	18–26
		400–500 g	258–387 cm^2	18	18–26
		500 g	452 cm^2	18	18–26
Hamster	Group	60–80 g	65–84 cm^2	15	18–26
		80–100 g	84–103 cm^2	15	18–26
		100 g	123 cm^2	15	18–26
Guinea pig	Group	350 g	387 cm^2	18	18–26
		350 g	651 cm^2	18	18–26
Rabbit	Single	2 kg	0.14 m^2	36	16–22
		2–4 kg	0.14–0.27 m^2	36	16–22
		4–5.4 kg	0.27–0.36 m^2	36	16–22
		5.4 kg	0.45 m^2	36	16–22
Rabbit (nursing)[c]	Single (plus litter)	2–4 kg	0.46 m^2	36	16–22
		4–5.4 kg	0.56 m^2	36	16–22
Cat	Single	4 kg	0.27 m^2	61	18–29
		4 kg	0.36 m^2	61	18–29
Dog	Single	15 kg	0.72 m^2	Species-specific[d]	18–29
		15–30 kg	1.1 m^2	Species-specific[d]	18–29
		30 kg	2.2 m^2	Species-specific[d]	18–29
Monkey	Single	1 kg	0.14 m^2	51	18–29
		1–10 kg	0.14–0.39 m^2	51–76	18–29
		10–25 kg	0.39–0.72 m^2	76–91	18–29
		25–30 kg	0.72–0.90 m^2	91–117	18–29
		30 kg	1.4 m^2	117	18–29
Ape	Single	20 kg	0.90 m^2	140	18–29
		20–35 kg	0.90–1.4 m^2	140–152	18–29
		35 kg	2.3 m^2	213	18–29

(Continued)

Table 1 *(Contd)*

Species	Housing type[b]	Size	Minimum cage/pen floor area	Minimum cage/pen height (cm)	Room temperature (°C)
Poultry[e]	Single	< 0.25 kg	0.02 m²	–[f]	16–27
		0.25–1.5 kg	0.02–0.09 m²	–	16–27
		1.5–3.0 kg	0.09–0.18 m²	–	16–27
		> 3.0 kg	> 0.27 m²	–	16–27
Sheep/goat	Single	< 25 kg	0.9 m²	–	16–27
		25–> 50 kg	0.9–1.8 m²	–	16–27
Swine	Single	< 15 kg	0.7 m²	–	16–27
		15–50 kg	0.7–1.4 m²	–	16–27
		50–200 kg	1.4–4.3 m²	–	16–27
		> 200 kg	> 5.4 m²	–	16–27
Cattle	Single	< 75 kg	2.2 m²	–	16–27
		75–350 kg	2.2–6.5 m²	–	16–27
		350–650 kg	6.5–11.2 m²	–	16–27
		> 650 kg	> 13.0 m²	–	16–27
Horse	Single	Adult	13.0 m²	–	16–27

[a] Recommendations for primary enclosure from the 'Guide' (National Research Council, 1996); larger animals may also require secondary enclosures for exercise, mating or other activities.
[b] Typical preference for housing; listed group-housed animals are frequently single-housed according to study protocol.
[c] Space recommendation from the Animal Welfare Act (USDA, 1995).
[d] Recommended cage height for dogs is 6 inches above the head during normal standing position.
[e] Based primarily on the chicken.
[f] Height recommendation not specified; allowance should be made for typical postures.

adequate. Special conditions, such as a large population density, presence of noxious gases, excessive heat generation by equipment or lighting or potential air contamination with toxic materials, would require upward adjustment of airflow. If the primary enclosure system contains its own ventilation and filtration system, the room airflow could be adjusted downward if so desired.

Lighting in an animal area must be carefully controlled, because factors such as intensity, duration, wavelength and schedule can affect the physical and behavioural well being of research subjects. Lighting should be diffuse throughout the housing area. The photoperiod should reflect each species' natural diurnal rhythm. For example, rodents are nocturnal and will feed mostly during darkness. They will maintain regular feeding patterns when lights are properly controlled. Moreover, rats are susceptible to phototoxic retinopathy; therefore, intensity should be maintained at 130–325 lux, according to the 'Guide'.

Many research animals are easily stressed by excess noise. They should be isolated from equipment, other animals (especially dogs, swine or non-humans primates) or human activity that produces intense, persistent, frequent or high-frequency sounds. Technical staff should be discouraged from loud talk, excessive banging of equipment and playing of radios. Animals that typically rest during daylight hours may be severely disturbed by such activities.

Some species may require special features in their primary enclosures. For example, cats prefer a raised resting area within their cage. Other species (notably higher species such as non-human primates) require perches, tunnels, swings, toys or foraging devices. These permit natural behaviours that, in turn, enhance the animal's physical and psychological health. Animals such as dogs should have frequent access to runs or large pens where they can exercise. Many species (dogs, cats, primates) may benefit from frequent contact with humans. Consideration should also be given to an animal's natural social environment. For many species, individuals may communicate with other individuals through tactile, visual, auditory and olfactory contact. Therefore, whenever not otherwise required by the testing protocol, such animals should be housed in groups or within a short distance of fellow members of the species. This may best be exemplified by the rat, which typically huddles with other rats during rest periods and tussles with its cage mates during active periods.

Husbandry

All research subjects must be provided nutritious, uncontaminated feed specific for the test species. Supplies of feed should be chosen carefully with special attention to feed content, methods of storage, vermin control and notations of manufacture date and shelf-life. Analytical reports should be available to the researcher who should review them for nutritional content and for the presence of contaminants that may cause unwanted physiological responses. Feed must be stored in a dry, cool, clean area.

It should be elevated from the floor using pallets, shelves or carts. Most feeds can be used for approximately 6 months after manufacture, although some special diets, such as those containing vitamin C supplements, may expire after just 3 months. Out-of-date feed should always be promptly discarded.

Feed containers should permit unimpeded access to their contents and should discourage contamination with animal waste. They must not be transferred between animals without being sanitized. In many instances feed should be restricted. This author has found, for example, that young rabbits received from a feed-restricted environment and placed into an *ad libitum* environment may initially overeat, then develop diarrhoea and then stop feed intake. These animals become severely anorexic if not treated and may have to be sacrificed. A useful practice is to restrict feed intake at first, gradually permitting *ad libitum* feeding. Sometimes intubation with fruit juice will stimulate normal feed patterns. There have been several studies (quoted in the 'Guide') indicating that unrestricted feed consumption will lead to obesity, shortened life spans and increased disease (including cancer). These are undesirable conditions in long-term research projects. Some species thrive on a variety of diets and on special additions such as fresh vegetables or grains.

Like feed, water supplied to animals must be palatable and uncontaminated. Water should be analysed by the facility or the supplier for contaminants, microbes and pH. Investigators should review reports from these analyses to ensure that the water is of sufficient quality. Water can be provided by individual bottles, pans or tubes, although automated systems may be preferable. For any system, the apparatus should be examined daily for operation and cleanliness. Automated systems should be flushed frequently, perhaps daily, and subjected to appropriate filtration and frequent sanitation. Some species may require training before they can learn to use the watering systems, usually by pressing the tips or levers to permit water flow and then holding the animal's mouth to the fluid. Care must be taken to avoid excess pressure in water systems for small animals such as mice. They may be unable to press the release devices and will quickly dehydrate as a result.

Choice of animal bedding can have considerable effect on animal well-being. It should not have strong odours (for example, cedar chips can induce enzymatic and cytotological changes) and should not produce excessive particulates. Bedding can consist of wood chips or other granular materials. Frequently, it is appropriate to place specially developed paperboard in trays under caging to collect waste. Such paperboard often minimizes odours and consists of materials that reduce microorganism growth. Like feed, bedding must be stored in a dry, clean area with elevation from the floor. The requirement for bedding change depends on the species, but typically varies from once a week to once a day. For rats and mice, at least three changes a week are recommended.

Cleaning and sanitation of cages, racks and feeders should occur at least every 2 weeks for typical research animals. Devices such as solid-bottom cages and water containers should be sanitized every week. Primary enclosures should be treated with hot water (typically 80°C) and/or chemical disinfectants. Water and feed containers must be treated with hot water and detergents so that microorganisms are killed. All room surfaces must be cleaned and disinfected to prevent disease. Special commercial solutions can be used to scrub floors and walls and they can be used in room foggers. The effectiveness of sanitation should be monitored through analysis of wipe samples for the presence of bacteria.

Other methods of controlling disease include incineration of animal carcasses and wastes. Pesticides may be used to control vermin outside the facility and in some areas inside. If chemical pest control is not practical or desirable, traps may be more appropriate for eliminating rodents.

Veterinary Care

A qualified veterinarian (certified and experienced in laboratory animal medicine) must be available to provide oversight of animal care and handling. This includes direct or indirect responsibility for administration of veterinary drugs, euthanasia and surgical procedures. The veterinarian should ensure that laboratory animals are healthy as received (free of injury or disease) and that proper care is provided while the animal remains in the research facility. Any health status reports provided by the vendor or generated by the facility should be reviewed by the designated veterinarian to ensure that only healthy animals are used and to prevent unhealthy new arrivals from infecting the rest of the colony. This means that each new animal shipment must be separated from other animals on site.

The facility should have a programme by which a schedule of animal examinations is followed and periodic quality control is conducted. Typically, several animals from large shipments or a few animals chosen periodically from smaller shipments are subjected to necropsy, evaluation for clinical pathology, haematology, serology, clinical chemistry, and possibly histopathology. These evaluations, to be completed under veterinary control, will help ensure that only disease-free animals are used in research projects. Otherwise, results could be confounded by the presence of disease or other anomalies. For example, certain rodent viruses can alter the toxicological response from test substances even though the animals may show no outward signs of disease. Any animals displaying infectious disease must be isolated from others, and preferably destroyed, before disease can spread. Any room contaminated by an infectious agent must be emptied and sanitized before reuse.

Technical Training

In typical research situations, substantial responsibility for the care of animals must fall on the animal technicians (**Figure 2**). As they tend to their feeding, watering, cleaning and observation duties, these persons will normally have daily contact with the animals. In a sense, they comprise the first line of defence against illness, injury or excess distress from treatment. No research facility can afford to leave such efforts to poorly trained or otherwise ill-equipped individuals.

Ideally, animal technicians will have received some training in biology or animal science prior to employment. A number of colleges or community colleges offer degrees in these fields. Whether such formal training is received or not, they must be given on the job training with experienced technical staff before being allowed to work alone. Research facilities should have a programme in place to provide theoretical and practical instruction in animal care. There should be standard operating procedures in place for reference and records of progress in the training programme should be maintained.

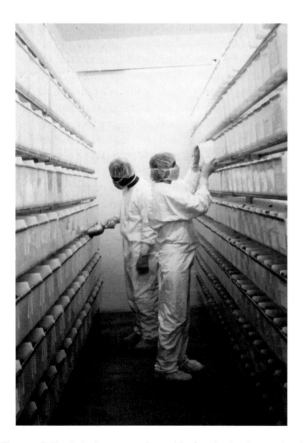

Figure 2 Technical personnel provide for the basic needs of research animals and serve as the 'front line' defence against animal distress. They must don appropriate attire and follow good hygienic procedures to prevent introduction of disease into the animal colony. Photograph courtesy of Harlan Sprague Dawley, Inc.

Probably the best insurance for adequate training of personnel is by formal certification. Through a programme offered by the American Association for Laboratory Animal Science (AALAS), technicians have the opportunity to become certified at three levels of achievement (American Association for Laboratory Animal Science, 1997). The beginning level of certification is for Assistant Laboratory Animal Technician (ALAT), followed by Laboratory Animal Technician (LAT) and Laboratory Animal Technologist (LATG). To determine qualification for certification at one of these levels, the candidate's education and experience are reviewed (up to 5 years of experience is required for a non-degreed LTAG certification, for example). AALAS provides a number of training materials for each level. In some instances, formal training programmes are conducted (by local AALAS chapters, facility management, etc.) to help candidates through a preparatory course. The candidate must submit a formal application and fee to take the required certification examination.

Difficulty and emphasis in the examination (and the training materials) reflect the level of certification involved. For the ALAT certification level, animal husbandry (anatomy, sanitation, nutrition, equipment) is emphasized. Less attention is given to animal health and welfare (disease, environment, anaesthesia, euthanasia) and the least emphasis is on facility management (regulations, records, safety, management). Course work and examination content for the LAT certification are slightly less concentrated on animal husbandry, with more emphasis on health and welfare and somewhat greater emphasis on facility management. For the highest level, the LATG certification, the relative order of emphasis is health and welfare, facility management and husbandry. The goal is to encourage technicians to become proficient in many phases of animal care, with achievement of appropriately higher certification levels as experience and education progress. AALAS members are also able to advance in their careers through attendance of local or national meetings, and through numerous educational resources that the association provides.

As a final note about technical certification, it is often desirable for non-technical staff, such as study coordinators or study directors, to complete one or more level of AALAS certification. It is a useful means of fully appreciating the needs of the animals and the function of technical staff. A bonus is that scientific decisions by researchers will more likely be reflective of humane animal use during study planning and conduct.

Laboratory Accreditation

Just as personnel should be certified for the proper use and care of animals, the research facility itself should be accredited. The organization that provides the standards of animal care excellence against which the facility can be measured is the Association for Assessment and Accreditation of Laboratory Animal Care International (AAALAC) (1997d). The core of this organization was formed in 1950 by a group of Chicago veterinarians who established the Animal Care Panel. Over time, one of the key functions of this panel, through a number of publications and specialized committees, became the establishment of professional standards for laboratory animal care. These standards were used to develop an accreditation programme. In 1965, AAALAC was incorporated as a voluntary accreditation body with 14 medical and veterinary charter member organizations.

Today, over 600 institutions have been accredited by AALAC International, including facilities in 10 countries. Over 100 consultants assist AAALAC International in evaluating animal care and use programmes, several of whom are international specialists. AAALAC International is administered by a Board of Trustees representing 43 member societies, several relating directly to toxicology research (Society of Toxicology, American College of Toxicology and others). Interaction with the member societies ensures that AAALAS International remains responsive to the research community. Actual accreditation is conducted by a Council of Accreditation consisting of 27 animal medical experts, research scientists and other specialists.

Any private or public organization using animals for research, teaching or testing may apply to AAALAC International for accreditation. AAALAC International assesses the institution's animal care and use programme by conducting a site visit. If the institution demonstrates excellence in animal welfare according to AAALAC International 'rules of accreditation' (including the principles presented in the 'Guide', EEC Directive 86/609 and individual national standards), full accreditation may be granted. Provisional accreditation may be awarded if correctable deficiencies are noted. Otherwise, accreditation is withheld. For accredited facilities, renewal visits are made every 3 years after which continued full accreditation, deferred continual accreditation (short-term deficiencies noted) or probationary accreditation (serious deficiencies seen) is awarded. Serious and uncorrected flaws will result in revoked accreditation.

Humane Animal Research

Certainly, the proper care of animals is a crucial aspect of animal welfare in the toxicology laboratory. However, the other major aspect, the humane use of research animals, is also crucial although somewhat more subject to interpretation. A number of organizations have published their policies on animal research, including the Society of Toxicology, the American College of Toxicology and many others. Basically, these policies state that there should not be repetitive animal procedures, unnecessary research, excessive numbers of animals in animal testing or excessive pain or discomfort in animal research. The conscientious researcher will make a serious commitment to these ends.

The basis for humane animal research is found in the 'three Rs' (Russell and Burch, 1959). These represent reduction, refinement and replacement, all important considerations while conducting animal testing. As the term suggests, reduction means limiting the numbers of animals to levels essential to meet the goals of the study. Refinement is improvement in test methods to reduce potential for pain and distress caused the test subjects. Replacement involves the use of alternative tests to substitute for whole-animal procedures. Recently, Salem and Katz (1998) have proposed a fourth R, responsibility. This introduces the commitment factor required for meeting the challenges of the first three Rs.

Reduction in Animal Numbers

Prior to recent concerns about animal use, many researchers paid little attention to the numbers of animals used in their research. The more animals were tested, the more statistically meaningful the results became. Moreover, results could often be obtained more quickly if larger numbers of animals were tested at the start rather than awaiting preliminary findings and then planning studies accordingly. Today, the approach has become very different. Through improved planning, more patient study conduct and better data analysis, fewer animals are needed for most research projects. Additionally (and very significantly), regulators around the world have decreased the numbers of animals required for testing protocols.

Possibly one of the fields most significantly changed over the last decade has been that of acute toxicity testing. Acute tests, by their nature, are more likely to result in distress and death as relatively high doses are administered by various routes (oral, cutaneous, intraperitoneal, intravenous, inhalation). In fact, for acute LD_{50} studies, the goal is determination of the dose that would be expected to kill half of the subject population. Animal rights activists find this test particularly objectionable. The classical method has been to dose several animals of each sex on each of several dose levels to give what was considered to be sufficient numbers for the LD_{50} calculation such as was required by the probit analysis method (Bliss, 1935; Finney, 1971). The end result was typically a total of 50–100 animals for a single LD_{50} test to fulfil the requirement of obtaining several treatment levels with fractional mortality. Numerous evaluations have now shown that acceptable LD_{50} values can be obtained with far fewer animals. For example, Weil et al. (1953) showed that for 24 compounds studied, the mean peroral LD_{50} in rats varied only from 4.64 and 4.76 g kg^{-1} when the number of animals per dose level was increased from 5 to 10. DePass et al. (1984) obtained similar results with 11 compounds, with a correlation coefficient of 0.98 for each sex. The same authors also concluded that additional dose levels did not affect the LD_{50} value, as a correlation coefficient of 0.99 was obtained from comparison of 2–3 levels with 3–7 levels per study.

The statistical method used to calculate the LD_{50} affects the number of animals required. The probit analysis, as noted above, typically requires many test animals. Other procedures, such as the moving average method (Thompson, 1947), approximate lethal dose method (Deichmann and LeBlanc, 1943) and up-and-down method (Bruce, 1985) require minimal numbers of test subjects. These methods have been summarized by DePass (1989), who reported that the conventional method (probit analysis) typically required roughly 50 animals (rats) per study, the moving average method required 10–20 animals, the approximate lethal dose method used about 5–10 animals and the up-and-down test required 6–8 rats. In the up-and-down method, a single rat is dosed at a time. If the animal dies, the next rat is administered a slightly lower dose. If the first animal lives, the second is given slightly higher doses. The process continues until multiple lethal and non-lethal levels are established. A series of calculations provides the LD_{50}. This method has recently been fully discussed and compared with other methodologies by Lipnick et al. (1995).

Another significant issue in the LD_{50} test is whether both sexes require investigation. In the work of DePass et al. (1984), it was found that mean LD_{50}s (from 91 rat oral tests) were 2.47 g kg^{-1} for males and 2.13 g kg^{-1} for females, with a correlation coefficient of 0.93. It has been the experience of several other researchers that females are somewhat more sensitive than males (although some have also disputed this), but that, overall, good correlation exists between the two sexes. Thus, several guidelines (US EPA, OECD) recommend using just one sex (the potentially more sensitive one) of animal for the LD_{50} determination and a few confirmatory animals of the opposite six at critical dose levels.

Whichever method is used for an LD_{50} determination, it is most useful to do a preliminary test with one or two animals at different dose levels suspected to be near the LD_{50} (based on chemical structure and/or literature data). After a day or two, additional animals may be treated to begin to fill in levels. It may take a few more days of 'wait-and-see' before all required animals are dosed. This approach has been detailed by Myers and DePass (1993).

In cutaneous irritation tests, the classic protocol (Draize et al., 1944) requires that at least six rabbits receive a small dose (0.5 ml or 0.5 g) of sample on the clipped skin. A number of investigators have indicated that fewer animals are sufficient. Derelanko et al. (1993) analysed data from 224 studies, which provided skin irritation classifications based on six rabbits. The data were randomly reduced to include three, four and five rabbits per study and skin irritation was reclassified for

each chemical tested. Agreements between classification with fewer animals and those with six animals ranged from 69 to 95% for negligible irritants, from 76 to 85% for mild irritants and from 90 to 100% for severe irritants. Absolute differences in dermal irritation indices between groups of three, four, five and six animals were small, with an average of no more than 0.3. The authors concluded that as few as three rabbits would normally be adequate. In fact, most guidelines (such as those of the OECD) have recommended three or four rabbits in the skin test in recent years (Organization for Economic Cooperation and Development, 1992). A practical approach to skin irritation evaluation is to start with a single rabbit and determine the degree of irritancy produced by a test substance. If the irritation is severe (necrosis or ulceration noted), additional testing is unnecessary. More moderate reaction should indicate the need for the full set of three animals. If results are equivocal, a few more rabbits may be dosed (up to six) to aid in the final interpretation.

Ocular irritation testing may be approached in a manner similar to that of the skin irritation procedures. The researcher should remember, however, that the 'Draize test' is probably one of the most controversial (to the public) of the short-term toxicity procedures. Every effort should be made to reduce animal use while not compromising the data required. Three eyes are probably sufficient, although some protocols may require more, especially if the benefit of washing out the eye is a desired end-point. A reasonable way to approach the eye test is first to review results of cutaneous testing if available. Severe skin irritants would be expected to cause substantial eye injury (of course, there are exceptions). This could be confirmed in a single eye test with a single animal if providing some ocular data is crucial. In any event, a single eye dose should be used, as a preliminary guide to the need for further testing. Just as in the skin irritation test, if one eye is severely affected, dosing should be terminated. Otherwise, a total of three eyes should be dosed, or up to six eyes for equivocal findings.

The above approaches or variations of these may also be applied to other types of toxicological evaluations. The USDA has recommended a few general methods for animal reduction (Bennett, 1994), including animal sharing, improved statistical design, phylogenetic reduction and better quality animals. In animal sharing, certain study animals may be reused for procedural development, training, alternative route testing (e.g. screening for oral toxicity following cutaneous irritancy testing), tissue harvesting or routine physiological or pathological measurements. This should only take place when animals are not stressed from the original study and there is little chance that the goals of the secondary procedure will be compromised. Another method for sharing animals involves the use of common controls. A negative control, vehicle control or positive group used for one study may sometimes be shared with other studies if test parameters are equivalent. An example would be a series of dermal sensitization studies conducted in tandem, using a single set of naive, vehicle and positive control groups.

Statistical design for a toxicological study may be improved by maintaining state of the art knowledge of applied statistics and by using the latest computer statistical packages. Inappropriate statistical design can result in failure to reach the study goals and, therefore, a necessary repetition of the project. Moreover, proper statistical analysis can permit the use of minimal numbers of animals. There must be sufficient numbers of animals to make a meaningful comparison among the treatment and control groups. No more subjects than statistically required should be used, as discussed by Erb (1990) and McCance (1989), among others. Phylogenetic reduction can be considered a type of reduction or replacement of animal use. It involves the use of the least advanced species that will permit the attainment of the study objectives. An example might be increased use of rodents and fewer dogs or non-human primates in a dietary inclusion project. The end result could be fewer animals used overall and/or fewer animals from a phylogenetic higher order used.

The use of better quality animals is easily overlooked as a means of reducing animal numbers. However, there is considerable logic in the practice of purchasing the most healthy and genetically consistent animals possible. The loss of animals to disease or abnormality can necessitate repetition of toxicity studies. Otherwise, study findings may become indecipherable from inherent flaws in inferior animal populations.

It is also important that animal quality be confirmed as soon as shipments arrive, preferably by veterinary personnel. In conjunction with the use of better animals should be the practice of ordering fewer animals. Typically, a few extra animals are ordered to compensate for losses prior to or during the study. The investigator should always make a habit of ordering only enough to meet study needs, and insist that the vendor only deliver the quantity ordered.

Refinement

Many, if not most, methodologies could be improved to provide for better science. Additionally, this process of *refinement* may frequently promote decreased pain and distress in the animal model. Several examples may apply to the acute toxicity procedures discussed previously.

In the LD_{50} test, there should be a practical dose limit beyond which further treatment is unnecessary. Most agencies recommended this 'limit test' years ago. As an example, acute peroral dosing with 2.0 or 5.0 g kg^{-1} of test substance (depending on the agency involved) will generally be sufficient if animals survive. The premise is that larger doses would be unlikely to be encountered by humans. There are exceptions, such as the need to evalu-

ate potential cumulative doses or clearance of very large doses, but reasonable limits should be established just the same. The 'limit test' effectively reduces total animal numbers and decreases the numbers of animals experiencing distress since sublethal doses are more frequently involved.

Many researchers have questioned the utility of using death as an end-point in acute toxicology. It may be sufficient to determine only levels producing observable clinical signs. This is the approach of the 'fixed dose procedure' (van den Heuvel *et al.*, 1990). Using a series of standardized dose levels, effect and no effect levels are established. Materials are assigned toxicity classifications according to a specified scheme. In an international validation study, these classifications were found to correlate well with those assigned on the basis of full LD_{50} studies. Like the limit test, the fixed dose procedure limits the degree of distress in animals since lethality is avoided as much as possible. A variation of this method, which does include death as an end-point, is the 'acute-toxic-class method' (Schlede *et al.*, 1994). It also uses a series of established dose levels to be given in a relatively complex pattern designed to determine efficiently lethal/non-lethal levels with few animals (usually three per group).

As fewer animals are employed in a toxicology study, it becomes more desirable to gather all the data reasonably possible from those animals studied. Rather than simply observe for lethality and gross signs on an acute study, one could consider evaluation for subtle behavioural effects, tissue changes, haematological alterations and so on. This type of approach was recommended by Gad *et al.* (1984). These authors proposed the inclusion of interval necropsies to help identify target organs before tissues have time to recover from treatment. A few animals euthanized at 3 or 4 days (instead of the typical 14 days) could have selected tissues (kidneys, liver, spleen, lungs, brain, reproductive organs, stomach, intestine) removed, weighed and processed. Comparisons are made with tissues of animals terminated at 14 days. Additionally, Gad *et al.* recommended the employment of a neurobehavioural screen designed to assess the peripheral and central nervous system. Benefits from such approaches, from an animal welfare standpoint, are decreased likelihood of additional testing to gather these data, better preparation for longer term studies and (perhaps) identification of subtle end-points for other tests on similar materials.

The author has found that a few relatively simple practices have substantially enhanced the value of acute tests. One is routinely to test animal urine for occult blood (with Ames HEMASTIX reagent strips), a potential early indication of kidney damage. Basic tests for righting reflex, grip strength, startle response and pupillary contraction give clues about neurological damage. Suspected target tissues can be saved from selected animals at death or sacrifice for possible subsequent evaluation. Whenever study results indicate a potential organ effect, appropriate tissues are available for histological assessment.

Skin and ocular irritancy tests can also be 'refined' to diminish stress in animals. Most regulatory agencies have already refined these procedures by eliminating the need for them when the pH is less than 2.0 or greater than 11.5, based on the assumption that strongly acidic or basic materials are severely irritating. However, this is not always a valid assumption, because irritation also depends on the characteristics (such as potential for buffering) of the chemical in question. In the skin test, lower dose amounts (0.05–0.1 ml instead of the usual 0.5 ml) might be administered for suspected severe irritants. Alternatively, diluted test substances may be applied. Of course, care must be taken to ensure the goals of the study and applicable regulations are fulfilled. Various transportation regulations, such as those of the US Department of Transportation (1991) or several international transportation agencies, require evaluation for several contact periods, typically 4 h (the standard contact time), 1 h and 1 min. Materials suspected to be severely irritating should first be applied for one of the shorter time periods (perhaps on only one or two animals) and results evaluated to determine whether longer contact periods are needed. Thus, a kind of range-finding study can be first conducted to establish irritant doses or contact times. If the specific test protocol permits, several doses may be applied simultaneously to a single animal set, with variations in dose amounts, contact times or even test substances. This process might be more appropriate for initial screens rather than definitive testing. A further refinement of the cutaneous irritation test could be the microscopic evaluation of dermal tissue. This will permit lesions not apparent grossly to be discovered, especially for low-dose or reduced contact period studies.

For ocular testing, one of the most effective methods to reduce distress is through low-volume doses. Instead of the typical dose of 0.1 ml, doses of 0.01 or 0.005 ml may be applied for potentially severe irritants (possibly in one or two animals). Additionally, treated eyes may be washed with lukewarm water at various times to limit the severity of response, as long as this does not interfere with the study goals (such as observation of healing time). Some of the most promising refinements in ocular testing have stemmed from improved techniques for assessing eye injury. These permit an increased likelihood of predicting ocular injury following doses that do not cause severe gross effects. Examples are measurements of intraocular pressure, examination by a slit-lamp biomicroscope and corneal thickness measurements (Ballantyne, 1986, 1993; Myers et al., 1998). These and other methods have been well correlated with traditional Draize scoring results and could become standard in the toxicology laboratory. A number of guidelines recommend use of a topical anaesthetic in eyes that exhibit severe injury, or even in conjunction with the initial treatment procedure. This may be acceptable wherever only the most basic ocular effects are to be evaluated (perhaps in comparative studies). However, topical analgesics or anaesthetics must be used with caution as they may substantially affect corneal permeability, with ocular injury underestimated (Myers et al., 1998) or possibly overestimated. Thus, the investigator will be compelled to find a balance between scientific objectives and animal welfare.

The preceding considerations, while specific for acute toxicology, should also be applicable to toxicology in general. The USDA (Bennett, 1994) has generalized some of these approaches, and others, into four categories: decreased invasiveness, improved instrumentation, improved control of pain and improved control of techniques. The first two (decreased invasiveness and improved instrumentation) are somewhat related. New technologies such as magnetic resonance imaging, improved clinical chemistry/haematology analysers, video systems, computer-driven activity detectors and modern monitoring devices (using microelectronics, fibre optics and laser instrumentation) may now be used to collect data that formerly required considerable animal surgery, manipulation or restraint. The end result is that more data may be obtained with fewer animals and less invasiveness. Even simple procedures, such as the use of HEMASTIX, may be considered a means of decreased invasiveness. As for the improved control of pain, the use of tranquillizers, analgesics and anaesthetics should be considered when test animals are experiencing discomfort. Certainly, these are imperative during surgery, invasive blood collection (for example, from the retro-orbital sinus) or invasive dose administration such as cannulation. Pain resulting after treatment, either the result of the procedure (such as surgery) or the result of a toxic response, should be relieved with the appropriate drug(s) if this does not conflict with the study objectives. An example might be application of an analgesic salve on sites of severe irritation following a repeated skin application study. In most instances, a qualified veterinarian should directly oversee administration of drugs controlling pain. The fourth USDA category for refinement, improved control of techniques, entails proficiency in the handling and restraint of animals. Animals need to be handled in a gentle, consistent fashion. Both the handler and the animal should be properly trained. The test animal can be preconditioned to accept conventional or unconventional handling methods required by the study protocol. In this way, there will be minimal stress during the study.

In any animal procedure, the ultimate relief from pain or distress is euthanasia. Two major elements must be considered here. The first is the recognition of distress that is sufficiently severe to warrant animal sacrifice. The second is the determination of the most appropriate method of euthanasia. Neither of these considerations is trivial for the investigator.

Nearly all toxicology protocols recommend euthanasia of animals experiencing pain or suffering. Difficulty arises, however, in defining when distress is sufficiently severe to justify early termination. Since the research animal cannot tell us how it feels, we must pay close attention to a number of visible signs. Recognition of pain and suffering has been discussed in the literature (Mroczek, 1992; National Research Council, 1992). Broadly, it can be manifested by any abnormal behaviour, unusual physical appearance or alteration of bodily function. More practically, only those signs indicative of prolonged, at least moderately severe, and possibly life-threatening abnormalities should trigger consideration of euthanasia. A number of these are listed in **Table 2**. By this reasoning, salivation or tremors may not indicate a need for euthanasia; laboured breathing or convulsions may indicate that euthanasia is advisable.

In acute studies, one must be very careful in determining the need for early sacrifice. By their nature, signs up to and including death are frequently observed. Premature euthanasia will skew LD_{50} calculations, eliminate the evaluation of reversal of signs and confound determination of survivability. This is where technical experience becomes crucial. Technical and veterinary personnel familiar with the various signs and probable outcomes should be consulted for advice. Again, a balance between science and animal welfare is needed. Clearly, moribund animals, those with lingering distress or severe local effects (such as ocular damage) should always be euthanized.

In longer term projects, the guidelines to euthanasia may be more flexible. Typically, the objectives are geared more toward subtle changes (such as altered tissue structure or function, weight effects, clinical chemistry or haematologic alterations, etc.) Animals showing substantial clinical signs, if suffering is clearly present, should be seriously considered for euthanasia, especially if the study is relatively long and sufficient numbers of animals remain available for evaluation. Of course, animals showing signs of disease (particularly contagious disease) should be euthanized quickly to avoid distortion of study data and possible infection of other animals.

The methodology for euthanasia, carried out either for the relief of distress or for scheduled study termination, should be considered thoughtfully. It is not automatically a matter of injecting the animal with a lethal dose of sodium pentobarbital (although it may often be). In fact, depending on the species and circumstances of the study, some methods may seem rather exotic (such as microwave irradiation or decapitation). One of the best known guidances for euthanasia is the Report of the American Veterinary Medical Association (AVMA) Panel on Euthanasia (1993). This document details the elements of humane euthanasia, common (and uncommon) agents, species-specific methods and Panel recommendations. According to the AVMA, euthanasia should be without pain or distress, preferably producing rapid unconsciousness followed by cardiac or respiratory arrest and loss of brain function. Moreover, it is helpful (more for the researcher than the animal, perhaps) if the

Table 2   Observable signs of severe pain or distress

Local effects [a]

Skin corrosion	Severe erosion or ulceration penetrating most or all of dermis, large areas of severe necrosis
Ocular injury	Severe corneal opacity, corneal ulceration, purulent or bloody discharge, severe periocular necrosis
Extremity injury	Severe swelling, ulcerative lesions, apparent fractures, severe cutaneous erosion/sloughing, gangrenous appearance

Systemic effects [a]

Nervous signs	Severe or persistent tremors, convulsions, narcosis, catalepsy
Locomotor/muscular signs	Ataxia, paralysis, prostration
Respiratory signs	Gasping or laboured breathing, very slow or rapid breathing, audible breathing (rales, wheezing)
Cardiovascular signs	Very slow or rapid heart rate, severe pallor, redness or cyanosis of extremities
Gastrointestinal signs	Persistent vomiting, severe diarrhoea, anorexia

Behavioural effects [b]

Excessive vocalization	Squealing, grunting, growling, whimpering, howling (especially during movement or handling)
Atypical actions	Self-mutilation, stereotypic activity, restlessness, head shaking, apparent apathy to stimulants
Direct response to pain	Licking, biting or scratching of affected area; unusual posture to relieve pressure on affected area (hunched or stretched appearance); excessive struggling or biting during handling; grimacing or baring teeth
Absence of actions	Failure to groom, decreased socialization, poor reflexes, marked decrease in feed/water intake

[a] Myers and DePass (1993).
[b] Mroczek, (1992); USDA (1995).

method produces little animal movement immediately following the procedure. Personnel performing euthanasia must be appropriately trained and experienced so that the process itself (handling, restraint, euthanasia technique) is relatively painless and stress-free. It is recommended that euthanasia should not take place in the presence of other animals, if possible, because they may become distressed by vocal or non-vocal (behaviour, odours) reactions of the euthanized animal.

Some common euthanasia procedures, and their advantages, are listed in **Table 3**. The AVMA has classified euthanization agents into those producing hypoxia (usually due to depression of vital organs or processes), depression of vital nerve function and physical disruption of brain or vital nerve function (such as by cervical dislocation). In some instances, inhalant anaesthetics (such as ether, halothane or methoxyflurane) are pre-ferred because of the rapid unconsciousness produced. These may be easily placed into a closed chamber to build up high vapour concentrations followed by introduction of the animal. Some species are more susceptible than others, and factors such as age or health status may affect reactions. A high concentration of carbon dioxide is useful for anaesthesia/euthanasia, especially for groups of small laboratory animals. Some inhalants may produce lung discoloration or other lesions and these agents should be avoided when pulmonary assessment is critical to a study.

Another major class of euthanasia agents consists of those typically injected intravenously (ear, tail, neck or limb veins) or, less commonly, intraperitoneally. Probably the most prevalent of these are the barbiturates such as sodium pentobarbital. The latter produces rapid anaesthesia with minimal apparent distress when

Table 3 Common methods of euthanasia in the toxicology laboratory[a]

Method	Species	Major advantages	Major limitations	AVMA recommendation
Barbiturate injection	Most	Rapid, safe, cheap	Requires training, restraint, drug control	Acceptable (preferred) method
Anaesthetic inhalation	Most	Rapid, multiple animals exposed	Initial irritation, hazardous to staff	Acceptable method for small species
Carbon dioxide inhalation	Several small laboratory animals	Rapid, safe, cheap, multiple animals	Some species stressed or very tolerant	Acceptable at high concentrations
Carbon monoxide inhalation	Most small	Rapid loss of consciousness	Hazardous to staff, difficult to detect	Acceptable method with appropriate generation
Microwave exposure	Mice, rats	Rapid, safe, brain enzymes fixed	Specialized training, equipment, costly	Acceptable method with appropriate equipment
Tricaine/benzocaine injection	Fish, amphibians	Rapid, safe	Costly	Acceptable method
Cervical dislocation	Birds, small rodents/rabbits	Rapid, safe, cheap, no drug residue	Requires training, unpleasant for staff	Conditionally acceptable method when justified
Decapitation	Most small	Rapid, no drug residue	Requires training, some hazard, unpleasant	Conditionally acceptable method when justified
Gunshot	Large farm or wildlife species	Rapid, ease for certain species	Requires training, dangerous, unpleasant	Conditionally acceptable method when necessary
Electrocution	Foxes, sheep, swine, mink	Rapid, cheap, no drug residue	Requires special equipment, hazardous, unpleasant, severe contractions	Conditionally acceptable method in specialized instances
Pithing	Small amphibians	Rapid, no drug residue	Requires training, unpleasant	Conditionally acceptable method in specialized instances
Nitrogen/argon inhalation	Most small	Rapid, safe, readily available	Stressful in some species, must limit O_2	Conditionally acceptable method in specialized instances
Exsanguination	Several	Safe, cheap	Very stressful	Unacceptable method without anasthesia
Rapid freezing	Several small	Safe, cheap	Very stressful	Unacceptable method without anaesthesia
Air embolism injection	Several	Safe, cheap	Causes convulsions, other sign of distress	Unacceptable method without anaesthesia
Drowning	Several	Safe, cheap	Very stressful, slow	Unacceptable method
Strychnine dosing	Several	Possibly convenient	Causes convulsions, painful contractions	Unacceptable method
Chloroform injection	Several	Possibly convenient	Very hazardous to staff	Unacceptable method
Cyanide dosing	Several	Possibly convenient	Unpleasant, hazardous	Unacceptable method
Stunning (blow to head)	Several	Rapid, no drug residue	Unpleasant, sufficient force required	Unacceptable method without other lethal procedure

[a] Summarized from the Report of the American Veterinary Medical Association (AVMA) Panel on Euthanasia (1993).

delivered in sufficient doses. For larger animals, chloral hydrate may be the preferred agent. Some available euthanasia solutions contain a barbiturate combined with local anaesthetics to make injection relatively painless.

The third method of euthanasia is by physical means such as cervical dislocation (by stretching and twisting the base of the skull from the first cervical vertebra), decapitation (by commercial guillotine), microwave irradiation (by equipment designed specifically for mice and rats) and exsanguination (by draining the blood from already unconscious animals). These procedures should be performed quickly and smoothly by experienced personnel. They typically are only used for specialized studies in which certain tissues or fluids must be preserved without drug contamination or degradation. Details of these and the other methods discussed are provided by the AVMA (1993).

Replacement

Much attention has been directed toward alternatives to animal research. While detailed discussion of them is beyond the scope of this chapter, they will be considered in general terms as means to reduce animal numbers and distress. Alternative test systems may be employed as screens and supplements to whole animal tests. They may permit rapid evaluation of multiple chemical substances for relative potential for toxicity or irritancy. They may also be used to predict reasonable starting doses for more definitive animal studies. Sometimes, alternative methods provide early indications of severe toxicity or irritancy so that methodologies can be appropriately adjusted to minimize animal discomfort. Additionally, the alternative techniques may provide insight into the most appropriate species, route, and other test conditions for a toxicity study.

Replacement methodologies may be divided into three general classifications: living systems, non-living systems, and computer simulations (Bennett, 1994). Living alternatives usually refer to *in vitro* models such as organ, tissue or cell cultures, invertebrate animals such as insects or simple marine species and microorganisms such as bacteria or yeasts. In non-living systems, chemicals or chemical matrices may be used to evaluate certain biological reactions, such as enzymatic or immunological action. For example, there are commercially available artificial skin systems, which may or may not contain human or animal cellular components. These are used to evaluate potential for cutaneous penetration and/or irritation. Recent advances in computer and mathematical modelling have resulted in some promising methods for predicting acute toxicity, chronic toxicity, carcinogenicity, genotoxicity, reproductive toxicity and primary irritancy of chemical substances. Essentially, the computer models are based on structure–activity relationships (SAR), the assumption being that similar chemical structures should produce similar biological effects. A few examples of the various types of alternatives are presented in **Table 4**. Extensive reviews of alternatives to animal testing can be found in the literature, such as the recent book by Salem and Katz (1998).

Before leaving the subject of animal alternatives, it may be useful to look at some specific examples of how they relate to animal welfare. A number of years ago, Kurt Enslein published his work on the predictability of oral LD_{50}s using a computer-assisted SAR approach (Enslein, 1988). He compared computer-estimated LD_{50}s and those derived from animal studies for over 2000 chemicals and found that 50% of the LD_{50}s were equivalent within a factor of two and 95% of the LD_{50}s were within a factor of eight. With improvements in his programs over the years, this procedure should be helpful in predicting relative toxicity for a number of actual or developmental molecules. At least in theory, numerous time-consuming and animal-intensive assays could be avoided and those chemicals with the best toxicity profiles would be pursued.

Ocular irritancy testing has been an area of intense alternative research, with considerable progress noted (Chu and Toft, 1993). A commercial alternative (EYE-TEX, National Testing Corp.) contains macromolecules of proteins, glycoproteins and mucopolysaccharides. In the presence of ocular irritants, resultant turbidity can be measured and is directly proportional to degree of irritancy and chemical concentration. Another system, using viable tissues, is the hen's egg chorioallantoic membrane (CAM) assay. This evaluates inflammation in fertilized eggs following the introduction of a test substance. Responses in the form of hyperaemia, haemorrhaging and/or coagulation are scored. Test systems such as EYETEX or CAM could give useful preliminary indications of the intensity of ocular response. The investigator could then adjust the conditions for *in vivo* testing (sample volume, number of animals, timing of washing) to provide the maximum benefit for the minimal animal distress.

One of the most animal-intensive studies is the chronic carcinogenesis assay. This costly, time-consuming work can be conducted only on selected test substances. An *in vitro* screen was developed by Ames *et al.* (1975) to assess the genotoxicity/carcinogenicity potential of chemicals. The Ames test utilizes mutated bacterial strains (*Salmonella typhimurium*) which are dependent on histidine for survival. These strains are sensitive to chemical carcinogens and react by reverting to histidine independence. Thus, colony growth in a histidine-free medium indicates genetic mutation and the potential for carcinogenicity. Frequently, this assay is included in a battery of acute tests as a relatively fast and inexpensive cancer screen. Such a battery may be the only testing done for many of the new materials being developed. No animals are used in the Ames test and subsequent long-term animal tests may or may not be indicated.

Table 4 Examples of alternative methods used for replacement of animals in toxicological research

Test system	Alternative classification	Potential toxicity end-point	Basis for procedure and measurement
Daphnia magnus[a]	Living system	Lethality	Correlation of LC_{50}s with LC_{50}s of other species
Cultured mammalian hepatocytes[a]	Living system	Metabolic changes	Prediction of and disturbance in metabolic pathways from chemical doses
Isolated perfused lung[b]	Living system	Lung injury	Evaluation of lung morphology and metabolic changes
Neutral red dye uptake[c]	Living system	Metabolism, ocular injury	Indication of cell injury by reduced dye uptake
Enucleated rabbit or bovine eye[d]	Living system	Corneal opacity	Evaluation of opacity, other morphological changes in isolated eyes
Computerized structure/ activity[e]	Computer simulation	Developmental toxicity, carcinogenicity	Prediction of effects based on computer input of chemical structure
Frog embryo teratogenesis assay[f]	Living system	Teratogenicity	Evaluation of microscopic morphological changes in frog embryos
SKIN[2] *in vitro* model[g]	Living/non-living system	Skin irritation, phototoxicity	Evaluation of metabolism, chemical change, structure change from chemical dose
Spermatozoa swimming analysis[h]	Living system/computer simulation	Cellular motion effects	Mathematical analysis of changes in cellular movement or structure
Mutatox bioluminescent bacterial test[i]	Living	Genotoxicity	Assessment of light produced in presence of genotoxic agents
Cultured human or mouse neurons[j]	Living	Neurotoxicity	Measurement of anticholinesterase activity
CORROSITEX *in vitro* system[k]	Non-living	Dermal corrosion	Assessment of lysis in biobarrier through determination of colour change

[a] Gad and Chengelis (1988a)
[b] Gad and Chengelis (1988b)
[c] Chu and Toft (1993); Zurlo *et al.* (1993)
[d] Chu and Toft (1993)
[e] Enslein (1988)
[f] Sklarew (1993)
[g] Rheins *et al.* (1998)
[h] Cohoon *et al.* (1998)
[i] Wang *et al.* (1998)
[j] Ehrich (1998)
[k] Gordon *et al.* (1998)

It must be remembered that most alternative toxicological methodologies are not fully validated and even those that are well accepted are not definitive replacements for animal use. Many are applicable to only certain chemical classes or under limited test conditions. Although they are continuously undergoing improvement, and their potential is endless, animal research will be required for the foreseeable future as a means of obtaining data from complete living systems.

Responsibility

The 'fourth R', responsibility, applies to all who have an influence on how animals are treated. Each person, organization and agency must make a commitment to conduct or promote the most stress-free animal research possible. The technical animal staff must be fully trained and observant in animal care and handling (**Figure 3**). SOPs must be understood and followed. Communica-

tions must be open between technical and supervisory personnel regarding animal health and well being. The facility management must be fully supportive of animal welfare and humane research. Even though pressures are high to keep costs low, finish projects rapidly and maintain a high volume of data output, these goals should not overshadow good science and animal welfare issues. Senior staff should make sure that the facility, personnel, policy and work environment are sufficiently directed toward this end. In the long term, this approach will project a respectable reputation for animal research. Along with this approach should be a commitment by those companies or organizations that sponsor animal research. They may have very special goals to reach from the research, but they must also be sensitive and supportive toward humane treatment of animals.

Since much research is guided by governmental or international agencies, it is most important that they keep current with validated animal research techniques.

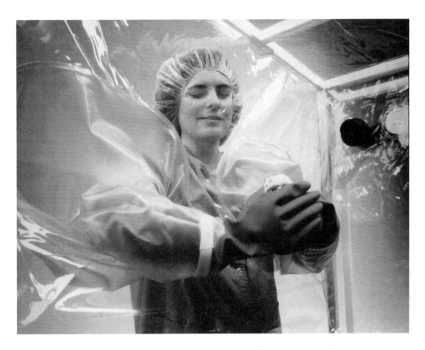

Figure 3 The tiniest of creatures play a crucial role in a research project. Thus, a respectful, gentle approach to animal handling is needed to ensure animal welfare and good science. Photograph courtesy of Harlan Sprague Dawley, Inc.

However, they should not cave in to political or social pressures to eliminate needed animal testing. Instead, refinements or replacements of animal testing should be carefully integrated into research guidelines. Importantly, agencies should formalize accepted improvements in animal testing quickly to avoid delays or confusion in procedural development in the toxicology laboratory. There must be continual efforts for harmonization among agencies of one nation and among the nations of the world. Unfortunately, tests must be frequently repeated because evaluation under the guidance of one agency may not fulfil the requirements of another agency or another country. International organizations such as the OECD and EEC are working hard to overcome such discrepancies.

The most significant and most direct responsibility for animal welfare falls on the investigators (study directors, primary researchers, project managers). They must be thoughtful and knowledgeable in their approach to animal research issues. It should become as much a part of study planning as the scientific aspects are. The investigator should first review the study goals and decide if sufficient work has been done previously. To do this, a review of available literature and historical data from the facility is helpful. If there is a precedence of similar testing, the new project should be aborted or at least altered to gain only the data still required. Throughout the process of protocol development, animal receipt, study conduct and study observations, animal welfare must be considered as in the approach shown in **Figure 4**.

If undue suffering or pain is anticipated or apparent during a research project, procedures must be revised and/or animals euthanized. Sometimes, this decision is made at the expense of study data and, therefore, it must be thought through carefully, with input from veterinary staff and the IACUC. Sponsoring organizations must be notified and the rationale provided. Moreover, animal welfare does not end with the termination of a toxicology project. Studies should be reviewed afterwards in the light of potential improvement of animal welfare. Whenever possible, serious consideration should be given to the publication of study findings so that other investigators will have access to them and avoid duplication of the work involved.

The Institutional Animal Care and Use Committee

As described briefly above, the Animal Welfare Act (USDA, 1995) requires the animal research facility to form an IACUC for oversight of animal-related issues, following the standards set forth by the 'Guide'. An active, well informed IACUC is one of the best guarantees that animal welfare policies are supported and adhered to. Although research facilities are sometimes criticized for self-policing (IACUC members are chosen by the management of the facility), there are numerous checks and outside (USDA, AAALAC) inspections that, along with practical considerations already noted, make most IACUCs effective. The required membership of an IACUC has been noted previously, and the total number of members depends on the size of the facility and the extent of its research. Beyond the mandated composition

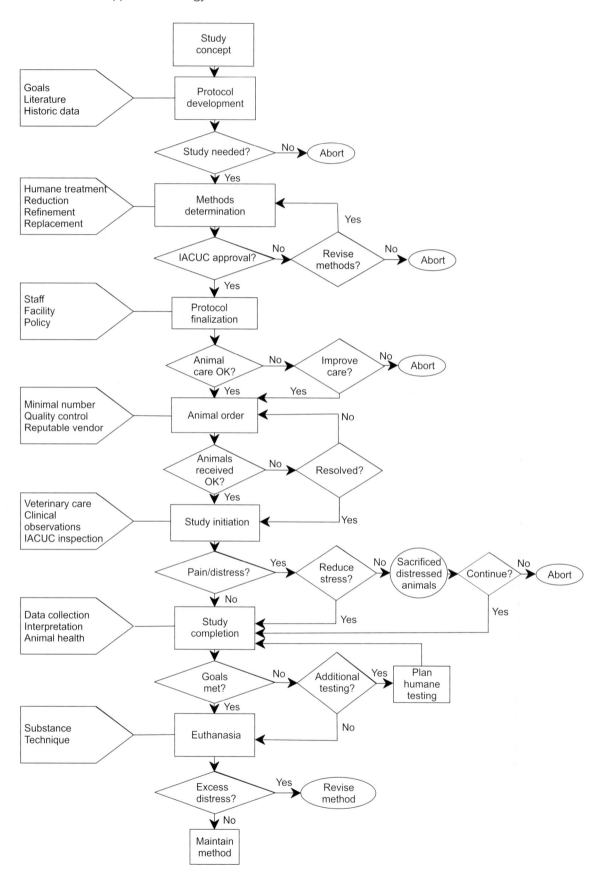

Figure 4 The schematic diagram for humane treatment of animals in the toxicology laboratory shows the complexities of the decision processes. The central portion indicates the basic steps and decisions regarding animal use to be considered during a research project. Influencing factors appear on the left; options and secondary decisions are given on the right.

of the groups, it is desirable to include members from diverse backgrounds among scientific and non-scientific disciplines. Outside experts may also serve as consultants. There may be need for subcommittees to carry out the many functions of the IACAC.

As noted in the 'Guide', the IACUC oversees and assesses the animal care programme and the use of animals in research. At least every 6 months, it inspects the facility (with emphasis on all animal housing, testing and supply areas), reviews protocols and carefully records all findings. A written report (containing meeting minutes, documents reviewed, areas inspected and items discussed) signed by most or all members is issued to principle investigators and facility management detailing any deficiencies. Specifically, protocols, and subsequent animal use and euthanasia are evaluated on the following bases (the 'Guide'):

- Rationale of proposed animal use.
- Justification of the species used.
- Justification of the number of animals used.
- Availability of alternative methods.
- Adequacy of staff training and experience.
- Atypical housing or husbandry requirements.
- Consideration of sedation, analgesia and anaesthesia.
- Unnecessary duplication of testing.
- Use of repeated and/or major surgical techniques.
- Criteria for excessive pain or distress.
- Process for relieving excessive pain or distress.
- Method of euthanasia.

Standardized procedures in addition to specialized research projects must be considered by the IACUC. Standardized protocols should not require a full review each time they are employed, but any revisions affecting animal use must be considered by the IACUC. Specialized protocols should each be reviewed by the IACUC. There should be a review/approval form for each project, which should be maintained as part of study records. These records should also be maintained in facility files, available for independent review, such as a USDA inspection. The IACUC report must reflect adherence to the Animal Welfare Act, with minor and major deviations being noted. A major deficiency is one that threatens the health, well being or safety of the animals.

Identification of animal welfare deficiencies need not only originate from formal inspections, however. Any staff member should be encouraged to present concerns to the IACUC. Technical or non-technical personnel, for example, should be free (without any negative consequences) to inform a direct supervisor or an IACUCC member of any excessive pain/distress witnessed during the course of a toxicology project. Such information may be kept confidential, but careful documentation must be made. It then becomes the responsibility of site management and/or the IACUC to investigate and take appropriate corrective action as warranted. This process is discussed by Silverman (1994).

There must be a reasonable and specific plan, with an outlined schedule, for the correction of significant deficiencies. Resolution of any major deviation should occur through a joint effort of the researcher, facility management officials of the area of concern (animal care supervisor, environmental or maintenance staff, purchasing agent, etc.), veterinary staff, along with the IACUC. If major deficiencies are not resolved according to the plan and schedule, the remaining deficiencies 'shall be reported in writing by the IACUC, through the Institutional official, to APHIS and any Federal agency funding that activity' (the 'Act'). The IACUC will also withhold approval and now is postponed until at least June 2000 for the specific studies affected until concerns are resolved. Of course, conflicts may occur among staff, researchers, management and study sponsors. These will have to be resolved in the light of the principles presented in the Introduction—ethics, science, social pressures and legal requirements.

Secondary responsibilities of the IACUC are training staff members, providing information on animal use, interacting with other personnel (health and safety officers, managers, legal staff, etc.), developing a liaison with outside organizations promoting humane research and engaging in public education (Dell, 1994). Any complaints or charges of animal misuse made by the public or the media should be investigated by the IACUC. This should aid facility management in arriving at an appropriate response.

FUTURE DIRECTIONS

It is apparent that the issue of animal welfare will not lessen in importance in the years to come. Animal rights groups continually question the value and humaneness of animal research. They are well funded, highly visible and often associated with the 'politically correct' among celebrities and government officials. In turn, government legislation will continue the attempts to ban or, at least, severely limit certain types of research. In 1992 the European Community's Council of Ministers voted to prohibit sales of cosmetics containing ingredients tested on animals after 1 January 1998 (Zurlo et al., 1993). This was done with the assumption that suitable alternatives would be available and now is postponed until at least June 2000. Over the last several years, groups in the USA such as the Soap and Detergent Association and the Cosmetic, Toiletry and Fragrance Association have substantially reduced animal use in product safety testing and have begun increased reliance on alternative methodologies.

A number of research centres have been established for the sole purpose of developing alternatives to animal testing. One well known facility in the USA is the Johns Hopkins Center for Alternatives to Animal Testing (CAAT). It is funded by several major chemical and health product companies, food and cosmetic companies, animal welfare groups and Federal agencies. For the most part, such organizations recognize that whole animal research will continue to be needed. Their goals are to develop and validate more fully *in vitro* computer modelling and other methods of toxicological research (Johns Hopkins CAAT, 1994). They serve as information sources for alternative methods, with data on advantages and disadvantages. In Europe, the European Centre for the Validation of Alternative Methods (ECVAM) spends millions of dollars on alternative research (Zurlo *et al.*, 1993). In the UK, FRAME (Fund for the Replacement of Animals in Medical Experiments) has been active for many years in the development/validation of alternative methods. These and comparable organizations worldwide are expected to provide new directions and new options over the years to come.

All individuals and organizations involved with animal research will be compelled to be increasingly vigilant in their approach to animal research, staying current with new legislation, new methodologies and changing public perceptions as they develop in the future. The basic need for animal research is not likely to disappear for many years. The approaches and attitudes toward animal welfare will need to evolve as new standards and technologies become available.

SUMMARY AND CONCLUSIONS

Because of ethical reasons, good scientific practice, social pressures and legal considerations, toxicological research must be humanely conducted. Additionally, animals must receive adequate care. Historically, the trend toward these ends by government, business, academics and society in general has been inexorable. Nations around the world have responded with specific legislation, such as the Animal Welfare Act in the USA. The 'Act' specifies facility construction, primary enclosure space, feed, water, temperature, lighting, humidity, sanitation and staff requirements for maintaining animal health. A convenient document for reviewing these requirements is the 'Guide for the Care and Use of Laboratory Animals'. For technical personnel, experience and training should be confirmed by AALAS (or equivalent) certification. The animal research facility itself should be certified in the appropriate care and use of animals by an agency such as AAALAC International.

Humane research in animals should be guided by close attention to the 'three Rs'. A *reduction* in numbers of test animals can be achieved through better statistical design,

shared controls and the use of only sufficient animals to obtain the required data. Animal research *refinement* toward less pain or distress involves the consideration of less stressful end-points or less intrusive techniques. Collection of more and better data from treated animals is desirable, as are better instrumentation and improved pain control (including euthanasia). The third 'R', *replacement*, means that alternatives to whole-animal models will be used whenever possible. These generally can be divided into simple living systems (cell cultures, microorganisms and various lower life forms), non-living systems (chemicals and synthetic tissues) and computer modelling.

A fourth 'R' could be *responsibility*. Each individual involved in animal research, from the animal care technician to the facility director, and from the researcher to the legislator, must be cognizant of standards for humane animal research. In addition to a commitment to good scientific process, there must be a thoughtful, considerate attention to animal welfare. To aid in this process, the IACUC oversees all animal issues in the facility, including justification of testing, adequacy of the facility and staff, presence of excess animal pain or suffering and response to internal or external concerns about animal treatment. Conflicts among all individuals or agencies must be resolved through a balance between study goals and animal welfare. Animal research will be crucial to the field of toxicology for the foreseeable future, but there are numerous specific practices to ensure that it can be conducted without unreasonable animal distress.

ACKNOWLEDGEMENTS

I would like to express my gratitude to Ms Veronica Phipps for text and figure preparation and to Harlan Sprague Dawley, Inc. (Indianapolis, IN) for providing photographs of animal-related activities.

REFERENCES

American Association for Laboratory Animal Science (1997). *AALAS Technician Certification Program—Candidate Bulletin*. AALAS, Cordova, TN.

American Veterinary Medical Association (AVMA) Panel on Euthanasia (1993). 1993 Report of the AVMA Panel on Euthanasia. *J. Am. Vet. Med. Assoc.*, **202**, 229–249.

Ames, B. N., McCann, J. and Yamasaki, F. (1975). Methods for detecting carcinogens and mutagens with the *Salmonella/mammalian-microsome* mutagenicity test. *Mutat. Res.*, **31**, 347–364.

Association for Assessment and Accreditation of Laboratory Animal Care International (1997a). Move to develop worldwide principles for care and use started as far back as '83. *AAALAC Int. Connection*, August, 11.

Association for Assessment and Accreditation of Laboratory Animal Care International (1997b). Snapshots of animal research regulations across Europe. *AAALAC Int. Connection*, August, 11.

Association for Assessment and Accreditation of Laboratory Animal Care International (1997c). U.S. and European guidelines more alike than different: a side-by-side comparison. *AAALAC Int. Connection*, August, 11.

Association for Assessment and Accreditation of Laboratory Animal Care International (1997d). *History Abstract, Accreditation Program, and Rules of Accreditation*. AALAC International, Rockville, MD.

Australian Council for the Care of Animals in Research and Teaching (1990). Australian code of practice for the care and use of animals for scientific purposes. *ACCART News*, **3**, No. 2, 1–5.

Ballantyne, B. (1986). Applanation tonometry and corneal pachymetry for prediction of eye irritating potential. *Pharmacologist*, **28**, 173.

Ballantyne, B. (1993). Ophthalmic toxicology. In Ballantyne, B., Marrs, T. C., and Turner, P. (Eds), *General and Applied Toxicology*, Vol. 1. Macmillan, Basingstoke, pp. 567–593.

Bennett, B. T. (1994). Alternative methodologies. In Bennett, B. T., Brown, M. J., and Schofield, J. C., *Essentials for Animal Research—A Primer for Research Personnel*, 2nd edn. National Agricultural Library, Beltsville, MD, pp. 9–17.

Bliss, C. (1935). The calculation of the dose–mortality curve. *Anal. Appl. Biol.*, **22**, 134–167.

Bruce, R. D. (1985). An up-and-down procedure for acute toxicity testing. *Fundam. Appl. Toxicol.*, **5**, 151–157.

Chu, I. and Toft, P. (1993). Recent progress in the eye irritation test. *Toxicol. Ind. Health*, **9**, 1017–1025.

Cohoon, D. R., Swanson, R. J. and Young, R. J. (1998). Using invariants of swimming motion in biotoxicity testing via computerized microscopy. In Salem, H. and Katz, S. A. (Eds), *Advances in Animal Alternatives for Safety and Efficacy Testing*. Taylor and Francis, Washington, DC, pp. 125–158.

Cooper, J. E. (1990a). Management, health and welfare of laboratory animals in developing countries. *SCAW News.*, **13**, No. 1, 14–15.

Cooper, J. E. (1990b). Management, health and welfare of laboratory animals in developing countries (Part Two). *SCAW Newsl.*, **13**, No. 2, 12–14.

Deichmann, W. B. and LeBlanc, T. J. (1943). Determination of the approximate lethal dose with about six animals. *J. Ind. Hyg. Toxicol.*, **25**, 415–417.

Dell, R. B. (1994). Interacting with the IACUC. *Lab. Anim.*, **23**, 34–35.

DePass, L. R. (1989). Alternative approaches in median lethality (LD_{50}) and acute testing. *Toxicol. Lett.*, **49**, 159–170.

DePass, L. R., Myers, R. C., Weaver, E. V. and Weil, C. S. (1984). An assessment of the importance of number of dosage levels, number of animals per dosage level, sex and method of LD_{50} and slope calculation in acute toxicity studies. In Goldberg, A. M. (Ed.), *Acute Toxicity Testing: Alternative Approaches*, Vol. 2. Mary Ann Liebert, New York.

Derelanko, M. J., Finegan, C. E. and Dunn, B. J. (1993). Reliability of using fewer rabbits to evaluate dermal irritation potential of industrial chemicals. *Fundam. Appl. Toxicol.*, **21**, 159–163.

Draize, J. H., Woodard, G. and Calvery, H. O. (1944). Method for the study of irritation and toxicity of substances applied topically to the skin and mucous membranes. *J. Pharmacol. Exp. Ther.*, **82**, 337–390.

Ehrich, M. (1998). Cell cultures for screening of antiesterase compounds. In Salem, H. and Katz, S. A. (Eds), *Advances in Animal Alternatives for Safety and Efficacy Testing*. Taylor and Francis, Washington, DC, pp. 229–234.

Enslein, K. (1988). An overview of structure–activity relationships as an alternative to testing in animals for carcinogenicity, mutagenicity, dermal and eye irritation, and acute oral toxicity. *Toxicol. Ind. Health*, **4**, 479–498.

Erb, N. E. (1990). A statistical approach for calculating the minimum number of animals needed in research. *ILAR News*, **32**, 11–16.

Finney, D. J. (1971). *Probit Analysis*, 3rd edn. Cambridge University Press, New York.

Gad, S. C. and Chengelis, C. P. (1988a). Lethality testing. In *Acute Toxicology Testing Perspectives and Horizons*. Telford Press, Caldwell, NJ, pp. 141–181.

Gad, S. C. and Chengelis, C. P. (1988b). Inhalation toxicology. In *Acute Toxicology Testing Perspectives and Horizons*. Telford Press, Caldwell, NJ, pp. 385–448.

Gad, S. C., Smith, A. C., Cramp, A. L., Gavigan, F. A. and Derelanko, M.J. (1984). Innovative designs and practices for acute systemic toxicity studies. *Drug Chem. Toxicol.*, **7**, 423–434.

Gordon, V. C., Mirhashemi, S. and Wei, R. (1998). Evaluation of the CORROSITEX method to determine the corrosivity potential of surfactants, surfactant-based formulations, chemicals, and mixtures. In Salem, H. and Katz, S. A. (Eds), *Advances in Animal Alternatives for Safety and Efficacy Testing*. Taylor and Francis, Washington, DC, pp. 309–329.

Johns Hopkins Center for Alternatives to Animal Testing (1994). *CAAT Newsl.*, **11**, 1–12.

King, L. R. and Stephens, K. M. (1991). Politics and the animal rights movement in the United States. Presented at the November 7–9 Annual Meeting of the Southern Political Science Association, Tampa, FL.

Laboratory Animal Welfare Act (1966). United States P.L. 89–544, amended by the Animal Welfare Act of 1970 (P.L. 91–597), 1976 (P.L. 94–279), 1985 (P.L. 99–198) and 1990 (P.L. 101–624).

Life Magazine (1966). Concentration camp for dogs. *Life Mag.*, **60**, No. 5 (February 4).

Lipnick, R. L., Cotruvo, J. A., Hill, R. N., Bruce, R. D., Stitzel, K. A., Walker, A. P., Chu, I., Goddard, M., Segal, L., Springer, J. A. and Myers, R.C. (1995). Comparison of the up-and-down, conventional LD_{50}, and fixed dose acute toxicity procedures. *Food Chem. Toxicol.*, **33**, 223–231.

McCance, I. (1989). The number of animals. *NIPS*, **4**, 172–176.

Mroczek, N. S. (1992). Recognizing animal suffering and pain. *Lab. Anim.*, **21**, 27–31.

Myers, R. C. and DePass, L. R. (1993). Acute toxicity testing by the dermal route. In Wang, R. G. M., Knaak, J. B. and Maibach, H. I. (Eds), *Health Risk Assessment—Dermal and Inhalation Exposure and Absorption of Toxicants*. CRC Press, Boca Raton, FL, pp. 167–199.

Myers, R. C., Ballantyne, B. Christopher, S. M. and Chun, J. S. (1998). Comparative evaluation of several methods and conditions for the *in vivo* measurement of corneal thickness in rabbits and rats. *Toxicology Methods*, **8**, 219–231.

National Research Council (1992). *Recognition and Alleviation of Pain and Distress in Laboratory Animals*. National Academy Press, Washington, DC.

National Research Council (1996). *Guide for the Care and Use of Laboratory Animals*. National Academy Press, Washington, DC.

Netherlands Animal Welfare Society (1991). Dutch animal welfare office makes progress. *ATLA News Views*, **19**, 389.

Office for Protection from Research Risks (1996). *Public Health Service Policy on Humane Care and Use of Laboratory Animals*. National Institutes of Health, Rockville, MD.

Organization for Economic Cooperation and Development (1981). *OECD Principles of Good Laboratory Practice*. OECD Document C(81)30, Annex 2.

Organization for Economic Cooperation and Development (1992). *OECD Guideline for Testing of Chemicals*. OECD Guideline 404, Acute Dermal Irritation/ Corrosion.

Rheins, L. A., Donnelly, T. A. and Edwards, S. M. (1998). SKIN^2: an *in vitro* tissue model for assessment of cutaneous safety and efficacy needs. In Salem, H. and Katz, S.A. (Eds), *Advances in Animal Alternatives for Safety and Efficacy Testing*. Taylor and Francis, Washington, DC, pp. 89–98.

Rowsell, H. C. (1991). The Canadian Council on Animal Care—its guidelines and policy directives: the veterinarian's responsibility. *Can. J. Vet. Res.*, **55**, 205.

Russell, W. M. S. and Burch, R. L. (1959). *The Principles of Humane Experimental Technique*. Methuen, London.

Salem, H. and Katz, S. A. (1998). *Advances in Animal Alternatives for Safety and Efficacy Testing*. Taylor and Francis, Washington, DC.

Schlede, E., Mischke, U., Diener, W. and Kayser, D. (1994). The international validation study of the acute-toxic-class method (oral). *Arch. Toxicol.*, **69**, 659–670.

Silverman, J. (1994). IACUC handling of mistreatment or non-compliance. *Lab. Anim.*, **23**, 30–32.

Singer, P. (1975). *Animal Liberation*. Random House, New York.

Sklarew, M. (1993). Toxicity tests in animals: alternative methods. *Environ. Health Perspect.*, **101**, 288–291.

Thompson, W. R. (1947). Use of moving averages and interpolation to estimate median effective dose. *Bacteriol. Rev.*, **11**, 115–145.

USDA (1995). Subchapter A—Animal Welfare. *9 CFR Ch. 1*, 1.1–4.11. United States Department of Agriculture, Washington, DC.

USDA (1996). Animal welfare enforcement—Fiscal Year 1996. *Animal and Plant Health Inspection Service 41–35–049*. United States Department of Agriculture, Washington, DC.

US Department of Transportation (1991). Method of testing corrosion to the skin. *49 CFR Part 173*, Appendix A.

US Environmental Protection Agency (1989a). Toxic Substances Control Act (TSCA); good laboratory practice standards. *Fed. Regist.*, **54**, 40 CFR 792, 34034–34050.

US Environmental Protection Agency (1989b). Federal Insecticide, Fungicide, and Rodenticide Act (FIFRA); good laboratory practice standards. *Fed. Regist.*, **54**, 40 CFR 160, 34067–34074.

US Food and Drug Administration (1978). Non-clinical laboratory studies; good laboratory practice regulations. *Fed. Regist.*, **43**, December 22, Part II, 59986–60026.

van den Heuvel, M. J., Clark, D. G., Fielder, R. J., Koundakjian, P. P., Oliver, G. J. A., Pelling, D., Tomlinson, N. J. and Walker, A. P. (1990). The international validation of a fixed-dose procedure as an alternative to the classical LD$_{50}$ test. *Food Chem. Toxicol.*, **28**, 469–482.

Wang, W.- D., Sun, T. S. C. and Stahr, H. M. (1998). Continued evaluation and application of a bioluminescent bacterial genotoxicity test. In Salem, H. and Katz, S. A. (Eds), *Advances in Animal Alternatives for Safety and Efficacy Testing*. Taylor and Francis, Washington, DC, pp. 181–190.

Weil, C. S., Carpenter, C. P. and Smyth, H. F. (1953). Specifications for calculating the median effective dose. *Am. Ind. Hyg. Assoc. Q.*, **14**, 200–206.

Zurlo, J., Rudacille, D., Goldberg, A. M. and Frazier, J. M. (1993). Current concepts in *in vitro* toxicity testing. *Lab. Anim.*, **22**, 24–33.

ADDITIONAL RESOURCES

American Association for Accreditation
of Laboratory Animal Care
11300 Rockville Pike, Suite 121,
Rockville, MD 20852–3035, USA

American Association of Laboratory
Animal Science
70 Timber Creek Drive, Suite 5,
Cordova, TN 38018, USA

American College of Toxicology
9650 Rockville Pike,
Besthesda, MD 20814–3998, USA

American Society of Primatologists
Regional Primate Center,
University of Washington,
Seattle, WA 98195, USA

American Veterinary Medical Association
1931 North Meacham Road, Suite 100,
Schaumburg, IL 60173–4360, USA

Animal and Plant Health Inspection Service
US Department of Agriculture,
4700 River Road, Unit 84,
Riverdale, MD 20737–1234, USA

Animal Welfare Information Center
National Agricultural Library,
US Department of Agriculture,
10301 Baltimore Boulevard, Room 205,
Beltsville, MD 20705, USA

Australian and New Zealand Council for the
Care of Animals in Research and Teaching, Limited
P.O. Box 19, Glen Osmond, SA 5064, Australia

Canadian Association for Laboratory Animal Science
CALAS National Office,
Biosciences Animal Service,
University of Alberta,
Edmonton, Alberta T6G 2E9, Canada

Canadian Council on Animal Care
Constitution Square,
350 Albert Street, Suite 315,
Ottawa, Ontario K1R 1B1, Canada

European Center for Validation of Alternative Methods
TP 580, JRC Environmental Institute,
21020 Ispra (VA), Italy

Foundation for Biomedical Research
818 Connecticut Avenue NW, Suite 303,
Washington, DC 20006, USA

Institute for Laboratory Animal Resources
National Academy of Sciences,
2101 Constitution Avenue NW,
Washington, DC 20418, USA

Institute of Laboratory Animal Science
University of Zürich,
Winterthurerstrasse 190,
8057 Zürich, Switzerland

International Council for Laboratory Animal Science
University of Kuopio,
SF-70211 Kuopio 10, Finland

Public Responsibility in Medicine and Research
132 Boylston Street, Fourth Floor,
Boston, MA 02116, USA

Scientists Center for Animal Welfare
Golden Triangle Building One,
7833 Walker Drive, Suite 340,
Greenbelt, MD 20770, USA

Society of Toxicology
1767 Business Center Drive,
Suite 302,
Reston, VA 20190–5332, USA

The Johns Hopkins Center for Alternatives to Animal Testing
111 Market Place, Suite 840,
Baltimore, MD 21202–6709, USA

Universities Federation for Animal Welfare
8 Hamilton Close,
South Mimms, Potters Bar,
Hertfordshire EN6 3QD, UK

Chapter 25

Occupational Hazards in the Toxicology Laboratory

Bryan Ballantyne

C O N T E N T S

- General Considerations
- Routes and Nature of Hazardous Exposures
- Latex Allergy
- Laboratory Animal Allergy
- Zoonoses
- Specific Considerations
- Protection, Precaution and Management
- References
- Further Reading

GENERAL CONSIDERATIONS

Many of the occupational hazards in the toxicology laboratory are common to those of laboratories specializing in other branches of science and technology. These cover a kaleidoscope of situations, including the handling of flammable and explosive materials, heating equipment, electrical devices, sharp instruments, glassware, lasers, etc. These general aspects of laboratory safety have been discussed in detail in various monographs (National Research Council, 1981; Fawcett, 1988; Armour, 1991).

In toxicology laboratories there are specific biological and chemical hazards, and special protective procedures and management protocols are required. Thus, there are exposures to a very wide range of materials, many at the research and development stage, whose human health hazards are unknown. Indeed, of course, the reason for conducting investigations on test chemicals is to determine various aspects of their toxicity and potential health hazards. A knowledge of the physicochemical properties of materials to be investigated, and of any relevant structure–biological activity relationships, should be considered in order to allow the most appropriate guidance on safe-handling practices. However, considerable caution is required, since many aspects of toxicity are not predictable. Some materials may have a relatively well defined acute toxicological profile, but other special aspects of toxicity are being investigated in the laboratory, e.g. long-term, reproductive or metabolism. Because of the potential for repeated exposure to these substances in the laboratory, specific protective and precautionary measures may be necessary. Also,

certain materials of high biological activity are used as positive controls, e.g. in genotoxicity, developmental toxicity, and sensitization studies. Clearly, for such materials the most stringent of storage and handling procedures are required. Additionally, there is a potential for exposure to chemicals used routinely in laboratory procedures, e.g. in the histology laboratory. Since the toxicology and potential human health hazards of these materials are usually well documented, most protective and precautionary procedures necessary should be known.

Physical injury can occur during the handling of animals and from instruments such as scalpels, scissors and needles. Exposure to, and handling of, laboratory animals may cause physical injury, infections and irritant and allergic reactions. This aspect of toxicology laboratory practice, considered later, may be a significant cause of morbidity.

Risk factors may be somewhat greater for certain groups of workers than for others, e.g. animal cage cleaners are exposed to chemicals, mechanical equipment, high-pressure water and high temperatures.

ROUTES AND NATURE OF HAZARDOUS EXPOSURES

Exposure may occur by various routes and involve different processes. In general, containment of chemicals for acute studies can be accomplished more easily than for chronic studies because of the smaller number of animals used in acute studies, thus allowing the work to be conducted in exhaust hoods, which is not feasible with the larger number of animals used in repeated exposure studies (Snellings, 1992).

During the dosing of animals there may be exposure to the test chemical. For example, whilst incorporating test material into feeds for peroral studies a dust may be created during milling and for mixing operations, and also during transfer of test diets. This could result in respiratory and cutaneous exposure. Test material applied to the skin of experimental animals may be disseminated by handling of animals, reclipping of hair, changing of bedding and sweeping the animal room floor (Darlow et al., 1969). Exposure to vapour may occur during application of volatile test material to the skin. With exposure to airborne materials there may be a potential for fire or explosion. Some chemicals, such as pyrophorics, must be diluted with nitrogen before mixing with air. Exposure to test material may occur from leaking chambers or from the handling of animals just removed from a chamber, particularly if exposed to dust or aerosol. Chemical exposure may also occur from contaminated protective clothing. Also, although gloves may give protection against test chemicals, they may be a source of allergic reactions (see later).

Some health hazards in the toxicology laboratory are clear and well known. These include irritant and allergic reactions to chemicals, animals and gloves. For other effects the evidence may be suggestive but unproven. Thus, there is limited evidence for an increased cancer incidence in laboratory workers (Nenzan, 1990; Summary, 1991) and for adverse reproductive effects (Heidam, 1984; Legge, 1986). Possible influences on reproductive performance and effects on the developing conceptus have been considered, but with variable findings. Thus, in some studies the risk of abortion or congenital malformation was not increased in laboratory workers (Baltzar et al., 1979; Olsen, 1983; Ayelsson et al., 1984; Heidam, 1984), but in others there have been indications of increased abortions (Strandberg et al., 1970; Lindbohm et al., 1984), or an increased risk of malformations (Meirik et al., 1979; Ericson et al., 1982, 1984). In a retrospective case report study, Taskinen et al. (1994) found a possible association between exposure to toluene, xylene and formalin/formaldehyde during early pregnancy and an increased risk of abortion, but cautioned that the findings need careful interpretation because of frequent simultaneous chemical exposures.

LATEX ALLERGY

Allergens present in latex (Turjanmaa, 1987; Alenius et al., 1991), may result in the production of IgE antibodies and/or initiate T cell-mediated reactions following exposure (Frosch et al., 1986). As a consequence, reactions to latex glove materials that have been documented include urtuaria, contact dermatitis, conjunctivitis, rhinitis and asthma (Seaton et al., 1986; Turjanmaa, 1987; Shama, 1991; Zotti et al., 1992). Thus, the clinical syndromes which result from latex hypersensitivity may be variable, and include both Type I- and Type IV-mediated responses. Overall, the prevalence of latex allergy may differ considerably for various exposure populations. For example, cited prevalences of latex allergy for health care workers in general in reliable series are 7.0% (Turjanmaa, 1987) and 12.1% (Liss et al., 1997). In one large detailed study of 741 nurses, the overall prevalence of latex sensitization, based on seropositivity for anti-latex IgE, was 8.9% (Grzybowski et al., 1996). In another study, 21 out of 384 hospital nurses (5.5%) were positive for the presence of latex-specific IgE antibodies (Kaczmarck et al., 1996). It is recognized that atopy is a high risk factor for the development of latex allergy (Kam et al., 1997; Liss et al., 1997).

Allergic contact dermatitis is a well documented type IV hypersensitivity reaction associated with latex exposure. Typical incidences are 7% in health care workers generally (Fisher, 1992) and 22% in dental workers (Katelaris et al., 1996). Contact urticaria, a Type 1 reaction, may occur within 5–60 min after cutaneous exposure, and be clinically present as erythema, hives, pruritis, and eczema. Rhinitis, conjunctivitis and peri-orbital oedema may also be present (Kam et al., 1997).

Asthma occurs in a small population of those exposed to latex. Respiratory exposure to latex allergen is usually related to the use of powdered gloves, with allergens being transferred from gloves to powder, which may then become airborne as gloves are handled (Swanson et al., 1992). In one series in which airborne latex was measured in a health care institution, the latex aeroallergen concentrations ranged 5 to 618 mg m^{-3} (Liss et al., 1997). Bronchial provocation testing has shown that airborne latex allergens produced a late asthmatic response. In one series latency was 4–16 h post-exposure, and with a duration of 3–48 h (Brugnami et al., 1994).

For laboratory workers with established dermatitis, suspected of being caused by the gloves being used, patch testing with the glove rubber may be useful for diagnostic purposes. The possible contribution of glove powder to delayed onset cutaneous hypersensitivity may be assessed by patch testing with epichlorhydrin and preservatives, including isothiazolin-3-one (Hesse et al., 1991). Localized urticaria may also be investigated by skin prick tests. Radioallergosorbent tests (RAST), enzyme-linked immunosorbent assays (ELISA) and Western blot tests may be useful, but apparently have a low sensitivity in health care workers (Holzman, 1993; Slater, 1994). The possible contribution of latex to occupational asthma requires, initially, confirmation of the presence of asthma by appropriate respiratory function tests, followed by challenge tests with monitoring of peak expiratory flow rate (PEFR) and forced expiratory volume in 1-see (FEV$_1$) (Marcos et al., 1991; Vandenplas et al., 1996). However, it should be borne in mind that provocation tests must be undertaken with considerable care and under skilled medical supervision, since severe systemic reactions, including anaphylaxis, may be induced (Pisati *et al.*, 1994). Clearly, laboratory workers presenting with respiratory tract hypersensitivity reactions should also be investigated for the possible contribution of LAA. Hamilton and Adkinson (1998) in a multicentre study found that the Grear NAL (non-amminated latex allergen preparation) skin test reagent at $100 \mu g \ ml^{-1}$ is a safe and effective way for confirmation of latex allergy.

With respect to pre-employment screening of laboratory animal workers, a complete history should be obtained which includes factors that may indicate atopy. Physical examinations should include respiratory function tests and, possibly, skin patch tests. For those with established allergic contact dermatitis, cotton liners and barrier creams may be effective, but the use of alternative forms of gloves is probably the best corrective measure. For those with established respiratory sensitization, a change in work conditions may be necessary.

LABORATORY ANIMAL ALLERGY

Laboratory animal allergy (LAA) has been recognized for several decades as a health-related problem in those handling animals in various types of biological laboratories. Its high incidence and severity are such that a change of employment may be necessary. In the UK, LAA is a prescribed industrial disease under the Social Security Act of 1975. The prevalence of LAA in several surveys is shown in **Table 1**, where the range is 19.2–56.0%. It is therefore a factor of considerable occupational health concern in toxicology laboratories, particularly with respect to precautionary and protective measures. Lutsky (1987) surveyed 252 laboratory animal facilities in 21 nations, and concluded that LAA is a world-wide occupational disease.

In addition to direct health consequences, those with LAA may be more susceptible to life-threatening anaphylaxis secondary to rodent bites (Teasdale and Davies,

1983; Hesford *et al.*, 1995) or to minor injuries from needles used in animal procedures (Watt and McSharry, 1996).

The rat and mouse are most frequently cited as causes of LAA, but hamsters, guinea pigs, rabbits and cats have also been implicated (Sjostedt *et al.*, 1995). Antigens responsible for LAA are usually associated with animal hair, dander and urinary protein. Two allergens have been identified in rat urine, saliva and pelt. Originally described were Rat n 1A, believed to be a prealbumin, and Rat n 1B, an α_{2u}-globulin (Newman Taylor *et al.*, 1977; Eggleston *et al.*, 1989). More recent studies, confirming nucleotide and amino acid sequences, have shown that both allergens are variants of α_{2u}-globulin (Bush *et al.*, 1998). In addition to the physiological proteinuria in rats, a raised excretion of urinary protein occurs in sexually mature male rats due to nephritis (Longbottom, 1984; Schumacher, 1987). Three mouse allergens have been identified (Sirayanian and Sandberg, 1979; Schumacher, 1980; Price and Longbottom, 1987). The major allergen, Mus m 1, previously referred to as Ag1, is a prealbumin found in urine, hair follicles and dander. As a result of testosterone-dependent gene expression, the concentrations in urine and serum are four times greater in male than female rats. The second mouse allergen, Mus m 2, is a glycoprotein in hair follicles and dander, but not urine. The third mouse allergen is albumin (Price and Longbottom, 1987). Airborne mouse allergens appear to be present in direct relationship to the number of mice present, and the degree of work activity in animal rooms or laboratories (Twiggs *et al.*, 1982).

In guinea pigs, two allergens (Cau p I and Cau p II) have been proposed (Schou, 1993), which are probably concentrated in the fur, possibly explaining the higher allergenic potency in dander from guinea pigs compared with urine and saliva (Sjostedt *et al.*, 1995). In the cat, the major allergen (Fed d 1) occurs principally in the pelt and sebaceous and mucous salivary glands, but not serum and urine (Anderson and Baer, 1981; Brown *et al.*, 1984). Fed d 1 is produced in sebaceous glands and transferred to fur by licking. At least 12 cat proteins have been

Table 1 Prevalence of laboratory animal allergy, based on clinical effects, noted in various surveys

Country	Group Size	Incidence (%)	Reference
Japan	5641	23.1	Aoyama *et al.* (1992)
UK	138	44.0	Venables *et al.* (1988a)
UK	146	30.0	Slovak and Hill (1981)
UK	9	22.9	Beeson *et al.* (1983)
Sweden	101	32.0	Willers *et al.* (1992)
Sweden	146	41.0	Agrup *et al.* (1986)
Sweden	110	20.9	Weissenbach *et al.* (1988)
The Netherlands	99	19.2	Kruize *et al.* (1997)
Australia	228	56.0	Bryant *et al.* (1995)
Australia	121	32.0	Schumacker *et al.* (1981)

determined to be allergenic, but Fed d 1 is the major one (Charpin *et al.*, 1991; Warner and Longbottom, 1991; Kleine-Tebbe *et al.*, 1993; Bush *et al.*, 1998). In the dog, the most important antigenic protein is Can f 1, a polypeptide present in hair, dander and saliva (Schou *et al.*, 1991; Bush *et al.*, 1998).

In general, animal aeroallergens are associated with relatively small particles, which can remain suspended in the air for long periods and have a respirable fraction. Airborne mouse allergen is in particles in the size range 3–18 μm (Price and Longbottom, 1990; Ohman *et al.*, 1994). Rat allergens are in particles in the size range from < 1 to > 20μm, with the majority being < 7μm in diameter (Platts-Mills *et al.*, 1986; Corn *et al.*, 1988).

Clinical Presentation

Commonly affected sites are the respiratory tract, eye and skin. Typical combinations of signs and symptoms for these sites are shown in **Figure 1** (Aoyama *et al.*, 1992). Rhinitis and conjunctivitis are common (Agrup *et al.*, 1986; Venables *et al.*, 1988a; Aoyama *et al.*, 1992), as are cough, dyspnoea and wheezing. Rhinoconjunctivitis is usually the presenting symptom complex, with nasal congestion, rhinorrhoea, sneezing and itching eyes with excess lacrimation. Asthma occurs in the more serious cases, with reported incidences in the range 17–71% (Kruize *et al.*, 1987; Hunskaar and Fosse, 1990). Urticaria and angio-oedema may be present. Slovak and Hill (1981) have described two distinguishable forms: regional LAA with classical rhinitis and negative pinprick tests, and progressive LAA with rhinitis leading to asthma and positive pinprick tests.

Willers *et al.* (1992) found that those with LAA have a significant increase of trapped gas after pulmonary provocation with methacholine, and hence they associated LAA with small airway hyper-reactivity. However, pulmonary function testing does not reveal a decrement in FVC or FEV_1 (Agrup *et al.*, 1986; Willers *et al.*, 1992). In a prospective study, Sjostedt *et al.* (1998) found an increased methacholine responsiveness in FEV_1 at follow-up in skin prick positive subjects. They suggest that airways responsiveness may start in the smaller airways and subsequently affect the larger airways.

In the Aoyama *et al.* (1992) series, 70% of LAA subjects developed signs and symptoms within 3 years of exposure and 33% of these occurred within 1 year, particularly in those with respiratory symptoms. Agrup *et al.* (1986) found that first symptoms appeared within 1 year of the start of animal handling in 7 of 41 subjects: for the whole group the mean time to symptoms was 2.3 years (range 1 month – 7 years). Kruize *et al.* (1997) reported a mean time of development of LAA symptoms of 109 months in non-atopics and 45 months in atopics. A longer latency of 0.5–12.0 years was described by Davies *et al.* (1983).

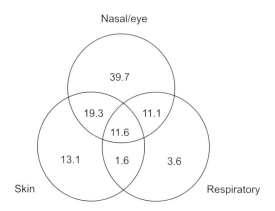

Figure 1 Combinations of symptoms in subjects with laboratory animal allergy in the survey by Aoyama *et al.* (1992). Reproduced with permission of the Editor of the *British Journal of Industrial Medicine*.

Predisposing Factors

Atopy

Predisposition of subjects (atopy) in most studies has been defined by a clinical history of allergy, positive skin prick tests against non-laboratory environmental allergens and increased concentrations of serum IgE. Atopy has been frequently correlated with the development of LAA (Agrup *et al.*, 1986; Kibby *et al.*, 1989; Aoyama *et al.*, 1992; Willers *et al.*, 1992; Bryant *et al.*, 1995; Fuortes *et al.*, 1996). However, not all cases are associated with atopy. For example, Gross (1980) found that prior allergies were more common in subjects with LAA (58%) in comparison with the general population (15%). Beeson *et al.* (1983) found the overall prevalence of atopy was 67% in LAA. The latency to onset of signs of LAA may be shorter in atopic than non-atopic subjects (Weissenbach *et al.*, 1988; Kruize *et al.*, 1997), and atopics may progress to a more severe form of the disease (Davies *et al.*, 1983). Also, atopy may be strongly associated with the more severe manifestations of LAA, notably asthma (Cockroft *et al.*, 1981; Slovak and Hill, 1987). In the study by Kruize *et al.* (1997), 13% of atopics with LAA had asthmatic symptoms compared with 6% non-atopics that had LAA.

Intensity of Exposure

The degree of exposure to allergens varies considerably and depends on, amongst other factors, stock density, tasks conducted, ventilation rates, cage design, bedding, air filtration and humidity. Although several studies have shown an association with the intensity of exposure expressed as concentration and/or duration of exposure (Cullinan *et al.*, 1994; Kruize *et al.*, 1997), others suggest that intensity of exposure may not be a significant factor in LAA. However, analysis is complicated by the possibility of a self-selection bias. Thus, Venables *et al.* (1988b) found an inverse relationship between the prevalence of LAA determined by symptoms and the duration of employment; they suggested that workers with LAA avoid exposure to animals. The available evidence indicates that environmental exposure is a strong determinant for the development of LAA, and that appropriate control measures may reduce morbidity (Bush *et al.*, 1998). In the study by Kruize *et al.* (1997), intensity as expressed by time of exposure was a clear determinant; thus, an increased relative risk for developing LAA was found for non-atopics exposed for more than 2 h per week, and an even higher relative risk for atopics with more than 2 h exposure per week.

Cigarette Smoking

Several studies have not shown an association between cigarette smoking and susceptibility to LAA (Agrup *et al.*, 1986; Willers *et al.*, 1992; Fuortes *et al.*, 1996; Kruize *et al.*, 1997). However, Venables *et al.* (1988a) examined data from three cross-sectional surveys of 296 laboratory workers exposed to small animals and found evidence for an association between smoking and occupational asthma and skin weals to animal urine extracts. They suggested that smoking may be a risk factor for LAA.

Clinical Confirmation

Skin prick tests are usually conducted with specific animal allergen extracts, but may not always be diagnostic. For example, Willers *et al.* (1992) noted a false positive incidence of 24% and a false negative incidence of 28%. Slovak and Hill (1987) found that 48% of those with LAA showed a positive skin reaction to allergens from the relevant species. They suggested that only those with a positive prick test develop progressive LAA (i.e. a strong correlation with asthma and a poor correlation with rhinitis only).

The radioallergosorbent test (RAST) is used to measure specific IgE antibodies to preparations from urine protein extracts or superficial skin scrapes. Beeson *et al.* (1983) found that in subjects with LAA, 53% had positive skin prick tests, and the RAST was also positive in 53%. Several groups (Vanto *et al.*, 1982; Davies *et al.*, 1983; Agrup *et al.*, 1986; Venables *et al.*, 1988a) have found that in those showing positive skin prick tests, there was a good correlation with the results from RAST. Weissenbach *et al.* (1988) and Willers *et al.* (1992) consider that skin tests are more sensitive than RAST. Cross reactions between various species may occur (Agrup *et al.*, (1986).

Recent studies have shown raised nitric oxide in exhaled air, increasing with symptom severity, suggesting this measurement may be a useful monitor in LAA (Adisesh *et al.*, 1999).

Workplace Management and Protective Measures

Lutsky *et al.* (1983) reviewed employer practices and concluded that, at that time, there were no consistent or formal policies for addressing LAA. Since then, however, there have been marked improvements (see below).

Pre-employment medical screens should include a history with particular, although not exclusive, reference to prior sensitization problems, personal habits, other occupational diseases and pulmonary and skin problems; respiratory function tests (including FVC, FEV_1 and PEFR; skin prick testing; and measurement of serum IgE. However, pre-employment medical screens need to be interpreted with caution. Some atopics will not develop LAA, and a history of atopy may not be sufficient to exclude from employment. Thus, Botham *et al.* (1995) found that if atopy or pre-existing sensitization had been used as an exclusion criterion, this would have resulted in incorrect decisions for about one-third of their population. They believe that skin prick tests and possibly RAST analysis should contribute to the pre-employment medical assessment. Also, they consider that atopics, and those already sensitized to laboratory animals, can be advised of their increased chances of developing LAA, but should not necessarily be excluded from employment. Greater consideration should be given to those with a history of LAA, chronic skin disease, asthma or cardiovascular diseases, since these appear to make individuals more susceptible to induction and consequences of LAA than either a history of atopy or the presence of IgE antibodies alone. Important factors are a history of allergy to environmental antigens (especially domestic animals), strong reactions to skin prick testing and high specific IgE to animal antigens. Fuortes *et al.* (1996) recommend that workers who are atopic or have respiratory symptoms should be placed in low-exposure situations.

Postplacement periodic medical evaluations are essential, and should include history, physical examination, respiratory function tests and possibly measurement of IgE as a potential indicator of the development of sensitization. In those developing LAA, the cause and possible progression of the disease should be carefully explained. With those who express a desire to continue working despite the development of symptoms, the prophylactic use of sodium cromoglycolate may provide some protection (Gross, 1980), but this should be regarded only as a temporary measure. In those with LAA, and particularly if asthma has developed, the only safe measure is one of job relocation where exposure to animal allergens does not occur.

Workplace management is the major way to control or prevent the development of LAA. The most important element is to reduce airborne allergen particles in workplaces and laboratories. For example, Gordon *et al.* (1992) demonstrated that rat urine aeroallergens can be significantly reduced by decreasing the stock density of rat housing areas and the use of filter cages or, when these cannot be employed, by replacing contact litter with non-contact absorbent litter. As noted previously, exposure concentrations of allergen vary considerably within the same facility, and between different facilities. Major determinants are stock density, tasks conducted, ventilation rates, cage design, bedding, air filtration and humidity. Clearly, attention should be directed at efficient extraction ventilation, handling procedures, personal protective equipment (including respiratory protective equipment), cage design and placement, the development of safe handling practices and worker education.

In the context of the number of laboratories using animals, there have been relatively few detailed measurements of aeroallergen exposure, but methods for measuring workplace aeroallergens have been described. These can be used not only to determine the degree of exposure, but also to assess the effectiveness of engineering and other controls to reduce exposure. Gordon *et al.* (1997a) have described a method for measuring urinary protein in personal air samples for assessment of occupational exposure. They found high exposures in laboratory technicians having direct handling contact with animals. Hollander *et al.* (1997) described the measurement of rat and mouse urinary aeroallergens in airborne dust samples by the use of a sandwich enzyme immunoassay, having a detection limit of 0.075 mg ml^{-1}. The highest levels of exposure were found during removal of contaminated bedding from cages. Nieuwenhuijsen *et al.* (1994), using a RAST procedure on specimens from personal air samples, found exposure concentrations to animal technicians over a workshift to be 32.4 μg m^{-3} (geometric mean). While handling rats the value was 68.0 μg m^{-3} and during cleaning out 53.6 μg m^{-3} They also detected low concentrations of rat urinary aeroallergen close to, but outside, animal facilities.

Gordon *et al.* (1997b), who measured air samples for rat and mouse urinary aeroallergens by RAST inhibition, found that there was a sevenfold reduction in concentrations when mice were housed in ventilated cages operated at positive pressure, compared with conventional caging. There was a twofold reduction in personal exposures when soiled litter was removed by vacuum. Rat urinary aeroallergens associated with handling rats were reduced 25-fold when performed in a ventilated cabinet, compared with handling on an open bench. They concluded that a significant reduction in exposure to aeroallergens can be obtained by the use of ventilation systems for housing and handling, but the removal of soiled litter was less effectively reduced by vacuum procedures, and thus respiratory protective equipment may be desirable for this operation. A one-way airflow ventilation system drawing airborne allergens from the working area has been reported to reduce airborne particulates significantly (Yamauchi *et al.*, 1989).

Fisher *et al.* (1998) described a comprehensive programme to reduce exposure to environmental allergens, which resulted in the incidence of LAA being reduced from 10% to zero. The programme included education and training; modification of work practices; engineering controls; the use of personal protective equipment, including respiratory protection (generally dust–mist respirators); a medical surveillance programme for symptom assessment; and RAST testing for animal allergies. The medical surveillance (including RAST), education and personal protective equipment instruction are performed annually and are mandatory for those working with laboratory animals. Engineering controls included filter-typed cages, high-efficiency particulate air-filtered room ventilation, increased room air exchanges and dust-free bedding. Reeb-Whitaker *et al.* (1999) found that for control of laboratory aeroallergen exposure, three strategies are the use of filter cage tops, operation of negatively pressurized cages, and the use of ventitated changing tables.

The value of protective and precautionary measures is also demonstrated by the study of Botham *et al.* (1987), who found that the first-year incidence of LAA fell from 37% in subjects who started work with animals in 1980–81 to 12% in those who started in 1984. This lower level of LAA was maintained in a subsequent study. The reduction coincided with the introduction of improved engineering controls and personal protective measures, including the use of educational programmes.

ZOONOSES

A concern about handling laboratory animals is the transmission from animals to the handler of viruses, bacteria or parasites through contact, a bite or inhalation. Examples for large animals include monkey virus B (Hull, 1973), tuberculosis from primates (Lennette, 1973) and Q fever from sheep (Lennette, 1973). Cat scratch disease is of presumed viral aetiology with the cat acting as a vector. There is regional lymphadenitis secondary to a primary cutaneous lesions; the disease is usually benign, with a good prognosis (Petersdorf, 1976). Rat bite fever may follow a bite from a rat, mouse or other rodent. The most common form, usually seen in laboratory workers, is caused by *Streptobacillus meliniformis*, a Gram-negative bacillus found in the oropharynx of more than 50% of healthy rats. It presents as a febrile illness with myalgia, weakness and vomiting, followed by rashes and arthralgias (Sandle, 1983).

Eradication programme have reduced the incidence of zoonotic disease. Most toxicology laboratories use only specific pathogen-free animals from suppliers with quality control programme. Details on the diagnosis, prevention and control of zoonoses were given by Acha and Szyfrei (1980).

SPECIFIC CONSIDERATIONS

In addition to the general physical and chemical hazards common to most laboratories of a toxicology facility, certain specialized sections may present particularly high-level concerns. In the pathology laboratory, personnel may be exposed to fixatives and solvents used in tissue preparation. For example, Kilburn et al. (1985) reported results of area sampling for formaldehyde, xylene and toluene in rooms where tissues and slides are processed. They determined the ranges to be formaldehyde 0.2–1.9, xylene 3.2–102 and toluene 8.9–12.6 ppm. They found that disturbances of memory, mood, equilibrium and sleep, that occurred simultaneously with headache and indigestion, were experienced more frequently in female histology technicians than in unexposed female clerical workers. Over a 4-year period, there was no evidence for cumulative effects (Kilburn and Warshaw, 1992). Formaldehyde has been shown to be carcinogenic in laboratory animals, but the currently available epidemiological information does not give any convincing evidence that it is tumourgenic in humans. Contact dermatitis from epoxy resin in immersion oil for microscopy has been described (Le Coz et al., 1999).

Several studies require positive control materials which are of high cytotoxicity, e.g. in genotoxicity, carcinogenesis and reproductive toxicity investigations. Although most studies on cytotoxic materials have been conducted on healthcare workers, the results are relevant to toxicology laboratory situations. Some studies on the effects of occupational exposure to cytostatic drugs have shown increases in urine mutagenicity, peripheral blood lymphocyte cytogenetics, and sister chromatic exchanges (Falck et al., 1979; Waksvik et al., 1981; Chrysostomou et al., 1986; Pohlova et al., 1986), but others have failed to demonstrate such effects (Gibson et al., 1984; Venitt et al., 1984). Differences are probably related to the degree of exposure and the protective measures used. In an animal toxicology study with cyclophosphamide, it was demonstrated that animal technicians can be exposed to the material (Sessink et al., 1993). Air filter samples showed < 0.1–1.0 μg day^{-1}; surface wipes showed cyclophosphamide in adjacent rooms (< 0.02–44 mg cm^{-2}); gloves were contaminated (2–99 μg per pair); and one of 87 urine samples from four animal technicians showed cyclophosphamide (0.7 μg).

The US Occupational Safety and Health Administration has published guidelines for handling antineoplastic drugs (OSHA, 1986). Many of the recommendations are applicable to the toxicology laboratory. Design features for a high toxicity laboratories have been published by DiBerardinis et al. (1993).

PROTECTION, PRECAUTION AND MANAGEMENT

Several texts on the design of toxicology laboratories, safety measures and routine safe practices have been written (Fawcett, 1983; Armour, 1991). Only representative examples of some of the more important features will be considered here.

The facets of particular relevance to laboratory design include the provision of adequate general ventilation and of specific ventilation for particular operations (e.g. laminar flow cabinets for high-toxicity materials) and the use of extractor lines or scavenger systems to prevent localized exposure of laboratory personnel to vapours, gases or dusts. The design of ventilation, scavenger systems and fume cupboards should be such that air from the work area is not carried up in front of the facial area of personnel. Systems should be designed with sufficient flexibility to allow for future laboratory modifications. The design of inhalation units for safe working conditions has been considered elsewhere (McClellan et al., 1984).

There should be sufficient storage space and shelving to avoid possible hazards from overcrowding of the bench. Separate appropriately illuminated, ventilated and temperature-regulated accessible storage is required in order that the quantities of test and working chemicals may be kept to a minimum in open laboratory conditions.

Protective clothing requires detailed consideration on an individual basis. However, because of the universal potential for breakage of glassware or splashing of chemicals, safety glasses should be worn routinely. Appropriate protective clothing is required when handling chemicals or animals, which may include laboratory coats, gown and gloves. Contaminated laboratory coats should be discarded. Front-buttoned laboratory coats may not give the same degree of protection as the wrap-around variety. Gloves should be chosen on the basis of known permeability characteristics. Although for widely used laboratory chemicals it is frequently known which is the most appropriate type of glove material, with unknown materials it may be appropriate to undertake permeability tests to ensure adequate protection. In some cases it may be necessary to wear two pairs of gloves to give extra protection. Smith and Grant (1988) found a six times lower puncture rate for the inner glove when two pairs of gloves were worn during surgery. In some situations differing glove requirements may be necessary. For example, during animal restraining procedures one technician may require to wear more physically protective gloves (e.g. leather) whilst restraining an animal, whilst the experimenter may require thinner gloves for palpation or procedures such as intravenous injections. It should be remembered that latex gloves themselves may be a source of adverse effects as discussed above. Also, severe uticaria has been documented following the use of glove powder (Van der Meeren and Van Erp, 1986). Respiratory protective devices should be made available for use when working with chemicals having an offensive smell or high vapour toxicity, or ready for use in strategic positions in case of spills or vapour leakage. In most cases cartridge respirators are used, although full-face air-supplied devices are preferable. Respirators should not be used at the expense of carefully controlled ventilation, since they restrict vision and may have medical problems associated with their use (Ballantyne, 1981). Choice of respirator is critical. For example, Sakaguchi *et al.* (1989) studied the use of respiratory protective equipment in animal facilities to protect against animal allergens. They found that most respirators designed for removal of particulates did eliminate a significant proportion of room air allergens; however, one had an efficacy of only 65%. The use of respirators requires a management programme to cover the following (Ballantyne, 1981):

■ Medical examination to eliminate those with medical conditions prohibiting or restricting their use;
■ Training programme for use and maintenance;
■ Routine inspection programmes;
■ Random audit programme.

Management, safety and training programmes should be in the form of carefully developed, readable and readily referenced protocols. For example, they should include factors such as the following. For all chemicals used, and all test materials, there should be a review of the known toxicity and occupational health problems in order that potential handling hazards can be determined and appropriate protective and precautionary measures undertaken. The Material Safety Data Sheet, if available, should help in this respect. Technical staff in training should handle materials and contaminated glassware, equipment and clothing under supervision. Safe methods should be developed for the legal disposal of hazardous materials without causing contamination of the environment (Pitt and Pitt, 1985). There should be strict laboratory regulations to prevent secondary routes of exposure, e.g. smoking, eating and drinking should be prohibited in working laboratories.

Before being assigned to a laboratory position, persons should have a full pre-employment medical examination to assess their physical, biochemical and physiological functions as a basis for future reference. Also, this examination should be sufficiently detailed to allow the exclusion or restriction of those with predisposing factors to the development of laboratory-associated adverse health effects, e.g. LAA, or those with existing medical conditions that could be exacerbated by exposure to chemical agents. Provision should be made for future periodic medical examinations with appropriate special investigations. Ideally these medical examinations should be conducted by a physician with experience in occupational medicine.

There should be adequate planning and facilities for the first-aid management of chemical and/or physical accidents. This should include the immediate access to rapid-release, high-volume showers and facilities for copiously washing the eye. A periodically maintained standard first-aid kit should be available and medical-grade oxygen accessible; these should be placed in a readily available and conspicuously marked area. If specific antidotes are available for chemicals used in the laboratory, these should also be readily available, e.g. cobalt edetate or nitrite/thiosulphate for cyanides and atropine/oximes for anticholinesterases. A number of laboratory personnel, available on an on-call basis, should be specially trained in first-aid procedures. Additionally, the designated safety officer should be sufficiently familiar with chemicals in the laboratory and able to offer relevant information to a treating physician. An active safety committee is essential for the development of policies, their oversight and the success of a safety programme.

REFERENCES

Acha, P. M. and Szyfrei, B. (1980). *Zoonoses and Communicable Diseases Common to Man and Animals. Scientific Publication No. 354*. World Health Organization, Washington, DC.

Adisesh, L. A., Kharitonov, S. A., Yates, D. H., Snashell, D. C., Newman-Taylor, A. J. and Barnes, P. J. (1998). Exhaled and nasal nitric oxide is increased in laboratory animal allergy. *Clin. Exp. Allergy*, **28**, 876–880.

Agrup, G., Belin, L., Sjostedt, K. and Skerfuing, S. (1986). Allergy to laboratory animals in laboratory technicians and animal keepers. *Br. J. Ind. Med.*, **43**, 192–198.

Alenius, H., Kurjanmaa, K., Paluoso, T., *et al.* (1991). Surgical latex glove allergy. Characterization of rubber protein allergens by immunoblotting. *Int. Arch. Appl. Immunol.*, **96**, 376–380.

Anderson, M. C. and Baer, H. (1981). Allergenically active components of rat allergen extracts. *J. Immunol.*, **127**, 972–975.

Aoyama, K., Ueda, A., Mando, F., *et al.* (1992). Allergy to laboratory animals: an epidemiological study. *Br. J. Ind. Med.*, **49**, 41–47.

Armour, M. A. (1991). *Hazardous Laboratory Chemical Disposal Guide*. CRC Press, Boca Raton, FL.

Ayelsson, G., Lutz, C. and Rylander, R. (1984). Exposure to solvents and outcome of pregnancy in university laboratory employees. *Br. J. Ind. Med.*, **41**, 305–312.

Ballantyne, B. (1981). Respiratory protection: an overview. In Ballantyne, B. and Schwabe, P. H. (Eds), *Respiratory Protection: Principles and Applications*. Chapman and Hall, London, pp. 3–38.

Baltzar, B., Ericson, A. and Kallen, B. (1979). Pregnancy outcome among women working in Swedish hospitals. *N. Engl. J. Med.*, **300**, 627–678.

Beeson, M. F., Deivdney, J. M. and Edwards, R. G., *et al.* (1983). Prevalence and diagnosis of laboratory animal allergy. *Clin. Allergy*, **13**, 433–442.

Botham, P. A., Davies, G. E. and Teasdale, E. L. (1987). Allergy to laboratory animals: a prospective study of its incidence and of the influence of atopy on its development. *Br. J. Ind. Med.*, **44**, 627–632.

Botham, P. A., Lamb, C. T., Teasdale, E. L., Bonner, S. M. and Tomenson, J. A. (1995). Allergy to laboratory animals: a follow up study of its incidence and of the influence of atopy and pre-existing sensitization on its development. *Occup. Environ. Med.*, **52**, 129–133.

Brown, P. R., Leitermann, K. and Ohman, J. L. (1984). Distribution of rat allergen I in cat tissues and fluids. *Int. Arch. Allergy Appl. Immunol.*, **74**, 67–70.

Brugnami, G., Marakini, A., Siracusa, A. and Appritti, G. (1994). Asma ritardata professionale da guanti in latice. *Arch. Sci. Lav.*, **10**, 593–596.

Bryant, D. H., Boscato, L. M., Mboloi, P. N. and Stuart, M. C. (1995). Allergy to laboratory animals among animal handlers. *Med. J. Aust.*, **163**, 415–418.

Bush, R. K., Wood, R. A. and Eggleston, P. A. (1998). Laboratory animal allergy. *J. Allergy Clin. Immunol.*, **102**, 99–112.

Charpin, C., Mata, P., Charpin, D., Lavaut, M., Allasia, C. and Vetvoet, D. (1991). Fed d 1 allergen distribution in cat fur and skin. *J. Allergy Clin. Immunol.*, **88**, 77–82.

Chrysostomou, A., Seshodri, R. and Morley, A. A. (1986). Mutation frequency in nurses and pharmacists working with cytostatic drugs. *Aust. N. Z. J. Med.*, **14**, 830–834.

Cockroft, A., Edwards, J., McCarthy, P. and Anderson, N. (1981). Allergy in laboratory animal workers. *Lancet*, **i**, 827–830.

Corn, M., Koegel, A., Hall, T., Scott, A., Newill, A. and Evans, R. (1988). Characteristics of airborne particles associated with animal allergy in laboratory workers. *Ann. Occup. Hyg.*, **32**, 435–436.

Cullinan, P., Lowson, D., Nieuwenhuijsen, M. J., Gordon, S., Tee, R. D., Venables, K. M., *et al.* (1994). Work related symptoms, sensitization, and estimated exposure to laboratory rats. *Occup. Environ. Med.*, **51**, 589–592.

Darlow, H. M., Simmons, D. J. and Roe, J. C. (1969). Hazards from experimental skin painting of carcinogens. *Arch. Environ. Health*, **18**, 883–893.

Davies, G. E., Thompson, A. V., Niewola, Z., *et al.* (1983). Allergy to laboratory animals: a retrospective and prospective study. *Br. J. Ind. Med.*, **40**, 442–449.

De Groot, H., DeJong, N. W., Duijster, E., van Wijk, R. G., Wermeulen, A., van Toorenenbergen, A. W., Geursen, L. and van Joost, T. (1998). Prevalence of material rubber latex allergy (Type I and Type IV) in laboratory workers in The Netherlands. *Contact Dermatitis*, **38**, 159–163.

DiBerardinis, L. J., Baum, J. S., First, M. W., *et al.* (1993). High-toxicity laboratory. *Guidelines for Laboratory Design*. Wiley, New York, Chapt. 5, pp. 133–138.

Eggleston, P. A., Newill, C. A., Ansori, A. A., *et al.* (1989). Task-related variation in airborne concentrations of laboratory animal allergens: studies with rats. *J. Allergy Clin. Immunol.*, **84**, 347–352.

Ericson, A., Kallen, B., Meirik, O. and Westerholm, P. (1982). Gastrointestinal atresia and maternal occupation during pregnancy. *J. Occup. Med.*, **24**, 515–518.

Ericson, A., Eriksson, M. and Zetterstrom, R. (1984). The incidence of congenital malformations in various socioeconomic groups in Sweden. *Acta Poedist. Scand.*, **73**, 664–666.

Falck, K., Grohn, P., Sorza, M., *et al.* (1979). Mutagenicity of urine in nurses handling cytostatic drugs. *Lancet*, **i**, 1250–1251.

Fawcett, H. H. (1983). Laboratory work. In Parmeggiani, L. (Ed.), *Encyclopedia of Occupational Health and Safety*, Vol. 2. International Labor Organization, Geneva, pp. 1177–1179.

Fisher, R., Saunders, W. B., Murray, S. J. and Stave, G. M. (1998). Prevention of laboratory animal allergy. *J. Occup. Environ. Med.*, **40**, 609–613.

Frosch, P. J., Wahl, R., Bahmer, F. A. and Maasch, H. J. (1986). Contact urticaria to rubber gloves is IgE-mediated. *Contact Dermatitis*, **14**, 241–245.

Fuortes, L. J., Weih, L., Jones, M. L., Burmeister, L. F., Thorme, P. S., Pollen, S. and Merchant, J. A. (1996). Epidemiologic assessment of laboratory animal allergy among university employees. *Am. J. Ind. Med.*, **29**, 67–74.

Gibson, J. F., Grampevtz, D. and Hedworth-Whitty, A. (1984). Mutagenicity from nurses handling cytotoxic drugs. *Lancet*, **i**, 100–101.

Gordon, S., Tee, R. D., Lowson, D., *et al.* (1992). Reduction of airborne allergenic urinary proteins from laboratory rats. *Br. J. Ind. Med.*, **49**, 416–422.

Gordon, S., Kiernan, L. A., Nieuwenhuijsen, M. J., Cook, A. D., Tee, R. D. and Newman Taylor, A. J. (1997a). Measurement of exposure to mouse urinary proteins in an epidemiological study. *Occup. Environ. Med.*, **54**, 135–140.

Gordon, S., Wallace, J., Cook, A. D., Tee, R. D. and Newman Taylor, A. J. (1997b). Reduction of exposure to laboratory animal allergens in the workplace. *Clin. Exp. Allergy*, **27**, 744–751.

Gross, N. J. (1980). Allergy to laboratory animals: epidemiologic, clinical and physiologic aspects, and a trial of cromolyn in its management. *J. Allergy Clin. Immunol.*, **66**, 158–165.

Grzybowski, M., Ownby, D. R., Peyser, P. A., Johnson, C. C. and Schork, M. A. (1996). The prevalence of anti-latex IgE antibodies among registered nurses. *J. Allergy Clin. Immunol.*, **98**, 535–544.

Hamilton, R. G. and Adkinson, N. F. (1998). Diagnosis of material rubber latex allergy: multicenter latex skin testing efficacy study. *J. Allergy Clin. Immunol.*, **102**, 482–490.

Heese, A., Hintzenstern, J. V., Peters, K. P., Kosh, H. V. and Horstein, O. P. (1991). Allergic and irritant reaction to rubber gloves in medical health services. *J. Am. Acad. Dermatol.*, **25**, 831–839.

Heidam, L. Z. (1984). Spontaneous abortions among laboratory workers: a follow up study. *J. Epidemiol. Community Health*, **38**, 36–41.

Hesford, J. D., Platts-Mills, T. A. E. and Edlich, R. F. (1995). Anaphylaxis after laboratory rat bite: an occupational hazard. *J. Emerg. Med.*, **13**, 765–768.

Hollander, A., Van Run, P., Spithoven, J., Heederik, D. and Doekes, G. (1997). Exposure of laboratory animal workers to airborne rat and mouse urinary allergens. *Clin. Exp. Allergy*, **27**, 617–626.

Holzman, R. S. (1993). Latex allergy: an emergency operating room problem. *Anesthes. Analgesia*, **76**, 635–641.

Hull, R. N. (1973). Biohazard associated with simian viruses. In Hellman, A., Oxman, M. N. and Pollack, R., (Eds), *Biohazards in Biological Research*. Cold Spring Harbor Laboratory Press, Cold Spring Harbor, NY.

Hunskaar, S. and Fosse, R. T. (1990). Allergy to laboratory mice and rats: a review of the pathophysiology, epidemiology and clinical aspects. *Lab. Anim.*, **24**, 358–374.

Kaczmarck, R. G., Silverman, B. G., Gross, T. P., Hamilton, R. G., *et al.* (1996). Prevalence of latex-specific IgE antibodies in hospital personnel. *Ann. Allergy Asthma Immunol.*, **76**, 51–56.

Kam, P. C. A., Lee, M. S. M. and Thompson, J. F. (1997). Latex allergy: an emerging clinical and occupational health problem. *Anaesthesia*, **52**, 570–575.

Katelaris, C. H., Widmer R. H. and Lazarus, R. M. (1996). Prevalence of latex allergy in a dental school. *Med. J. Aust.*, **164**, 711–714.

Kibby, T., Powell, G. and Cromer, J. (1989). Allergy to laboratory animals: a prospective and cross-sectional study. *J. Occup. Med.*, **31**, 842–846.

Kilburn, K. H. and Warshaw, R. (1992). Neurobehavioural effects of formaldehyde and solvents in histology technicians: repeated testing across time. *Environ. Res.*, **58**, 134–146.

Kilburn, K. H., Seidman, B. C. and Warshaw, R. (1985). Neurobehavioural and respiratory symptoms of formaldehyde and xylene exposures in histology technicians. *Arch. Environ. Health*, **40**, 229–233.

Kleine-Tebbe, J., Kleine-Tebbe, A., Jeep S., Schou, C., Locoenstein, H. and Kunkel, G. (1993). Role of the major allergen (Fed d 1) in patients sensitized to cat allergens. *Int. Arch. Allergy Immunol.*, **100**, 256–262.

Kruize, H., Post, W., Heederik, D., Martens, R., Hollander, A. and van der Beek, D. (1997). Respiratory allergy in laboratory animals workers: a retrospective cohort study using pre-employment screening data. *Occup. Environ. Med.*, **54**, 830–835.

Le Coz, C-J., Coninx, D., Van Rengen, A., El Aboudi, S., Ducombs, G., Benz, M-H., Boursier, S., Avenel-Audran, M., Verret, J-L., Erikstam, U., Bruze, M. and Goosens, A. (1999). An epidemic of occupational contact dermatitis from an immersion oil for microscopy in laboratory personnel. *Contact Dermatitis*, **40**, 77–83.

Legge, M. (1986). Reproductive hazards in laboratory environments. *Aust. J. Med. Lab. Sci.*, **7**, 44–47.

Lennette, E. H. (1973). Potential hazards posed by environmental agents. In Hellman, A., Oxman, M. N. and Pollack, R. (Eds), *Biohazards in Biological Research*. Cold Spring Harbor Laboratory Press, Cold Spring Harbor, NY.

Lindbohm, M.-L., Hemminki, K. and Kyyronen, P. (1984). Parental occupational exposure and spontaneous abortions in Finland. *Am. J. Epidemiol.*, **120**, 370–378.

Liss, G. M., Sussmenn, G. L., Deal, K., Brown, S., *et al.* (1997). Latex allergy: epidemiological study of 1251 hospital workers. *Occup. Environ. Med.*, **54**, 355–342.

Longbottom, J. L. (1984). Occupational allergy due to animal allergens. *Clin. Immunol. Allergy*, **4**, 19–36.

Lutsky, I. (1987). A world-wide survey of management practices in laboratory animal allergy. *Ann. Allergy*, **58**, 243–247.

Lutsky, I. I., Kalbfleisch, J. H. and Fink, J. N. (1983). Occupational allergy to laboratory animals: employer practices. *J. Occup. Med.*, **25**, 372–376.

Marcos, C., Lazara, M. and Fisj, J. (1991). Occupational asthma due to latex surgical gloves. *Ann. Allergy*, **67**, 319–323.

McClellan, R. O., Boecker, B. B. and Lopez, J. A. (1984). Inhalation toxicology: considerations on the design and operations of laboratories. In Tegeris, S. (Ed.), *Toxicology Laboratory Design and Management*. Karger, Basle, pp. 170–189.

Meirik, O., Kallen, B., Gauftin, U. and Ericson, A. (1979). Major malformations in infants born of women who worked in laboratories while pregnant. *Lancet*, **ii**, 91.

National Research Council (1981). *Prudent Practices for Handling Hazardous Chemicals in Laboratories*. National Academy Press, Washington, DC.

Nenzan, B. (1990). Cancer: a threat to laboratory personnel. *Arbetsmiljoe*, **3**, 10–12.

Newman Taylor, A., Longbottom, J. L. and Repys, J. (1977). Respiratory allergenicity to urine proteins of rats and mice. *Lancet*, **ii**, 847–849.

Nieuwenhuijsen, M. J., Gordon, S., Tee, R. D., Venables, K. M., McDonald, J. C. and Newman Taylor, A. J. (1994). Exposure to dust and rat urinary aeroallergens in research establishments. *Occup. Environ. Med.*, **51**, 593–596.

Ohman, J. L., Hayberg, K., MacDonald, M. R., Jones, R. R., Paigen, B. J. and Kacergis, J. B. (1994). Distribution of airborne mouse allergen in a major mouse breeding facility. *J. Allergy Clin. Immunol.*, **94**, 810–817.

Olsen, J. (1983). Risk of exposure to teratogens amongst laboratory staff and painters. *Dan. Med. Bull.*, **30**, 24–28.

OSHA (1986). *Work Practice Guidelines for Personnel Dealing with Cytotoxic (Antineoplastic) Drugs*. Department of Labor, Washington, DC.

Petersdorf, R. G. (1976). Cat scratch disease. In Isselbacher, K. J., Adams, R. D. and Braunwald, E. (Eds), *Harrison's Principles of Internal Medicine*. McGraw-Hill, New York, pp. 860–861.

Pisati, G., Baruffins, A., Bernabeo, F. and Stanizzi, R. (1994). Bronchial provocation testing in the diagnoses of occupational asthma due to latex surgical gloves. *Eur. Respir. J.*, **1**, 332–336.

Pitt, M. J. and Pitt, E. (1985). *Handbook of Laboratory Waste Disposal*. J Wiley, New York.

Platts-Mills, T. A. E., Heymann, P. W., Longbottom, J. L. and Wilkins, S. R. (1986). Airborne allergens associated with asthma: particle sizes carrying dust mite and rat allergens measured with a cascade impactor. *J. Allergy Clin. Immunol.*, **77**, 850.

Pohlova, H., Cerna, M. and Rossner, P. (1986). Chromosomal aberrations, sister chromatid exchanges and urine mutagenicity in workers occupationally exposed to cytostatic drugs. *Mutat. Res.*, **174**, 231–219.

Price, J. A. and Longbottom, J. L. (1987). Allergy to mice. I. Identification of two major mouse allergens (Ag 1 and Ag 3) and investigation of their possible origin. *Clin. Allergy*, **17**, 43–53.

Price, J. A. and Longbottom, J. (1990). Further characterization of two major mouse allergens (Ag 1 and Ag 3) and immunohistochemical investigations of their sources. *Clin. Exp. Allergy*, **20**, 71–77.

Reeb-Whitaker, C. K., Harrison, D. J., Jones, R. B., Kacegris, J. B., Myers, D. D. and Paigen, B. (1999). Control strategies for aeroallergens in an animal facility. *J. Allergy Clin. Immunol.*, **103**, 139–146.

Sakaguchi, M., Inouye, S., Miyazawa, H., *et al.* (1989). Evaluation of dust respirators for elimination of mouse aeroallergens. *Am. Assoc. Anim. Lab. Sci.*, **39**, 63–66.

Sandle, M. A. (1983). Rat bite fever. In Kaye, D. and Rose, L. F. (Eds), *Fundamentals of Internal Medicine*. C. V. Mosby, St Louis, pp. 266–267.

Schou, C. (1993). Review: defining allegens of mammalian origin. *Clin. Exp. Allergy*, **23**, 7–14.

Schou, C., Svendsen, V. G. and Lowenstein, H. (1991). Purification and characterization of the major dog allergen, Can f1. *Clin. Exp. Allergy*, **21**, 321–328.

Schumacher, M. J. (1980). Characterization of allergens from urine and pelts of laboratory mice. *Mol. Immunol.*, **17**, 1087–1095.

Schumacher, M. J. (1987). Clinically relevant antigens from laboratory and domestic small animals. *NER Allergy Proc.*, **8**, 225–231.

Schumacher, M. J., Tait, B. D. and Holmes, M. C. (1981). Allergy to murine antigens in a biological research institute. *J. Allergy Clin. Immunol.*, **68**, 310–318.

Seaton, A., Cherrie, B. and Turnbull, J. (1986). Rubber glove asthma. *Br. Med. J.*, **296**, 531–532.

Sessink, P., de Roos, J. H. C., Pierik, F. H., *et al.* (1993). Occupational exposure of animal caretakers to cyclophosphamide. *J. Occup. Med.*, **35**, 47–52.

Shama, S. K. (1991). Hand dermatitis from gloves. *Occup. Environ. Med. Rep.*, **5**, 45–48.

Sirayanian, R. and Sandberg, A. (1979). Characterization of mouse allergens. *J. Allergy Clin. Immunol.*, **63**, 435–442.

Sjostedt, L., Willers, S. and Orbeck, A. (1995). Laboratory animal allergy—a review. *Indoor Environ.*, **4**, 67–79.

Sjostedt, L., Willers, S., Orback, A. and Wollmer, P. (1998). A seven-year follow up study of lung function and methacholine responsiveness in sensitized and non-sensitized workers handling laboratory animals. *J. Occup. Environ. Med.*, **40**, 118–124.

Slater, J. E. (1994) Latex allergy. *J. Allergy Clin. Immunol.*, **94**, 139–149.

Slovak, A. J. M. and Hill, R. N. (1981). Laboratory animal allergy: a clinical survey of an exposed population. *Br. J. Ind. Med.*, **38**, 38–41.

Slovak, A. J. M. and Hill, R. N. (1987). Does atopy have any predictive value for laboratory animal allergy? *Br. J. Ind. Med.*, **44**, 129–132.

Smith, J. R. and Grant, J. M. (1988). Does two pairs of gloves protect against skin contamination? *Br. Med J.*, **297**, 1193.

Snellings, W. M. (1992). Toxicology laboratory hazards. In Sullivan, J. B. and Kriegers, G. R. (Eds), *Hazardous Materials Toxicology*. Williams and Wilkins, Baltimore, pp. 551–556.

Strandberg, M., Sandback, K., Axelson, O. and Sundell, O. (1970). Spontaneous abortion among women in hospital laboratories. *Lancet*, **i**, 384–385.

Summary (1991). Three workers in laboratory die of brain cancer. *Health Saf. Work*, **13**, 12.

Swanson, M. C., Bubak, M. E., Hunt, L. W. and Reed, C. E. (1992). Occupational respiratory allergic disease from latex. *J. Allergy Clin. Immunol.*, **87**, 227.

Taskinen, H., Kyyronen, P., Hemininki, K., Hoikkala, M., Lajunen, K. and Lindbohm, M.-L. (1994). Laboratory work and outcome. *J. Occup. Med.*, **36**, 311–319.

Teasdale, E. L. and Davies, G. E. (1983). Anaphylaxis after bites by rodents. *Br. Med. J.*, **286**, 1480.

Turjanmaa, K. (1987). Incidence of immediate allergy to latex gloves in hospital personnel. *Contact Dermatitis*, **17**, 270–275.

Turjanmaa, K., Laurila, K., Makinen-Kiljunen, S. and Reunala, T. (1989). Rubber contact urticaria. *Contact Dermatitis*, **19**, 362–367.

Twiggs, J. T., Agarwal, M. K., Dahlberg, M. J. E. and Yunginer, J. W. (1982). Immunochemical measurement of airborne mouse allergens in a laboratory animal facility. *J. Allergy Clin. Immunol.*, **69**, 522–526.

Vandenplas, O., Delwiche, J.-P., Evrard, G., Airmont, P., Van der Brempt, X. and Delaunois, L. (1995). Prevalence of occupational asthma due to latex among hospital personnel. *Am. J. Respir. Crit. Care Med.*, **151**, 54–60.

Vandenplas, O., Delwiche, J.-P. and Sibille, Y. (1996). Occupational asthma due to latex in 2 hospital administrative employees. *Thorax*, **51**, 452–453.

Van der Meeren, H. L. M. and Van Erp, P. E. J. (1986). Life threatening urticaria from glove powder. *Contact Dermatitis*, **14**, 190–191.

Vanto, T., Viander, M., Kosvikko, A., Schwartz, B. and Lowenstein, H. (1982). RAST in the diagnosis of dog dander allergy. *Allergy*, **37**, 75–85.

Venables, K. M., Upton, J. L., Hawkins, E. R., *et al.* (1988a). Smoking atopy, and laboratory animal allergy. *Br. J. Ind. Med.*, **45**, 667–676.

Venables, K. M., Tee, R. D., Hawkins, E. R., *et al.* (1988b). Laboratory animal allergy in a pharmaceutical company. *Br. J. Ind. Med.*, **45**, 660–666.

Venitt, S., Crofton-Sleigh, C., Hunt, J., *et al.* (1984). Monitoring exposure of pharmacy personnel to cytotoxic drugs. *Lancet*, **i**, 74–99.

Waksvik, H., Klepp, O. and Broggen, A. (1981). Chromosome analysis of nurses handling cytotoxic drugs. *Cancer Treat. Rep.*, **65**, 607–620.

Warner, J. A. and Longbottom, J. (1991). Allergy to rabbits. *Allergy*, **46**, 481–491.

Watt, A. D. and McSharry, C. P. (1996). Laboratory animal allergy: anaphylaxis from a needle injury. *Occup. Environ. Med.*, **53**, 573–574.

Weissenbach, T., Wuthrich, B. and Weihe, W. H. (1988). Laboratory animal allergies: an epidemiologic, allergologic study in industrial exposure to laboratory animals. *Schweiz. Med. Wochenschr.*, **118**, 930–938.

Willers, S., Hjortsberg, U., Wihl, J-A. and Orback, P. (1992). Sensitization to laboratory animals and small-airway hyperreactivity. *Indoor Environ.*, **1**, 82–87.

Yamauchi, C., Obara, T., Fukuyama, N. and Eudo, T. (1989). Evaluation of a one-way airflow system in an animal room based on counts of airborne dust particles and measurement of ammonia levels. *Lab. Anim.*, **23**, 7–15.

Zotti, R., de Larese, F. and Fiorito, A. (1992). Asthma and contact urticaria from latex gloves in a hospital nurse. *Br. J. Ind. Med.*, **49**, 596–598.

FURTHER READING

Brune, D. K. and Edling, C. (1989). *Occupational Hazards in the Health Professions*. CRC Press, Boca Raton, FL.

Charrey, W. and Schirmer, J. (1990). *Essentials of Modern Hospital Safety*. Lewis, Chelsea, MI.

Hall, S. K. (1994). *Chemical Safety in the Laboratory*. Lewis, Boca Raton, FL.

Laboratory Hazards Bulletin. Published monthly by the Royal Society of Chemistry Information Services, Cambridge.

Purchase, R. (1994). *The Laboratory Environment*. Royal Society of Chemistry, Cambridge.

Stricoff, R. S. and Walters, D. B. (1990). *Laboratory Health and Safety Handbook*. Wiley, New York.

PART THREE

TOXICITY BY ROUTES

Chapter 26
Parenteral Toxicity

David Walker

C O N T E N T S

INTRODUCTION

'Parenteral' is defined, for the purposes of this book, as the administration of a test substance by any route other than peroral, percutaneous and inhalational (including intranasal and intratracheal). In toxicity studies this is usually by injection but also includes infusion and implantation, either of which may or may not require surgical interference. The standard routes of injection in toxicology are intravenous, subcutaneous, intramuscular and intraperitoneal. Less frequently employed routes include intracutaneous, intra-arterial, intracerebral, intrapleural and intrathecal. Parenteral routes are commonly used to determine acute toxicity, especially of novel pharmaceutical products, whatever their intended clinical mode of administration. They are not so popular as oral dosing for repeat-dose experiments, particularly lifespan studies. Indications for, and disadvantages of, various routes of injection are discussed subsequently, but it is pertinent here to consider the relative merits in toxicology of oral and parenteral routes as a whole.

Ingestion is the most common, convenient and safest method of drug administration in the human subject. It is also the usual route of exposure to food additives and contaminants. Therefore, it is not surprising that it is the route most favoured in animal toxicology, particularly for long-term studies. Dietary inclusion is a convenient, economical method of dosing, more practical and less stressful than repeated injections in small rodents. Nevertheless, it has limitations such as chemical instability of the test substance in the diet, depression of palatability, erratic or incomplete absorption, inability of the rodent to vomit and physiological alterations which tend to confound estimations of no-effect levels. These include changes brought about in intestinal flora, laxation bulk or high osmotic load, caecal enlargement and retarded growth caused by high intake of non-digestible substances.

Parenteral injections provide the advantage of more rapid and predictable absorption. They are preferable when gastrointestinal absorption is poor and essential for polypeptide drugs and other compounds which are digested by intestinal enzymes or otherwise degraded and destroyed. On the other hand, parenteral formulations may necessarily include preservatives and other ingredients not required for oral drugs and these may introduce toxicological complications. Also, careful attention to technique is necessary to avoid artefacts. Parenteral injections should be aseptic and even so the direct introduction of exogenous substances into tissue is often irritant or necrogenic. Finally, no parenteral routes are very practical for the daily dosing of small rodents in lifespan carcinogenicity studies.

The contents of this chapter have been arranged in the following sequence of sections:

Indications. Although the intended clinical route determines, more than any other factor, that selected for prior toxicology, there are also indications for parenteral administration in toxicity studies on oral drugs, pesticides and industrial chemicals. Objectives include estimation of absorption, determination of mechanism and investigation of pathogenesis. The indications for the parenteral route described in this section are intended to illustrate the experimental benefits of facility and expediency which accrue from this approach.

Techniques. Injection technique is an art which by itself may determine the success or failure of an experiment. Animals are not usually cooperative subjects and, if over-restrained or under-conditioned, readily become stressed. At the stage of experimental design the toxicologist should contemplate carefully the practicality of route, site and frequency of injection with respect to the chosen species model. Some practical aspects of conventional injection technique are described in this section together with a consideration of infusion methods and a discussion on the possible introduction to toxicology of new routes reflecting novel systems of drug delivery.

Artefacts and Alterations. There are well known artefacts in toxicology resulting from errors in technique or imprudent selection of route. These include intravenous too-rapid or perivascular injection, intramuscular myodegeneration and subcutaneous sarcoma. Also, the introduction of exogenous substances into tissues may exert more subtle alterations which are primarily local effects and yet have a profound influence on systemic toxicity. These may not always be anticipated, appreciated or even discovered and it is the intention in this section to alert the unwary toxicologist to their potentially complicating properties.

Vehicles and Additives. Solvents and excipients often constitute a large proportion of the total volume of parenteral drug products. They are usually regarded as pharmacologically inert and conventionally in toxicity studies this is affirmed by an absence of findings in control groups. However, the vehicle is an important determinant of bioavailability and in large or repeated doses it may result in local or systemic toxicity *per se*. The attempt in this section is not to present a toxicological review of drug formulations but to remind the reader that sometimes findings may be ascribed to a constituent other than the active principle.

Quality Control Tests. Biological quality control tests for pyrogenicity, abnormal toxicity and local reactivity are performed usually, and often statutorily, on batch samples of finished pharmaceutical and medical products. They are included in this chapter because the specified routes of administration are almost invariably parenteral. In this section the common prescribed methods are described and subjected to critical appraisal. The descriptions have a historical flavour and one subsection is devoted to an *in vitro* technique which is currently replacing the rabbit pyrogen test, perhaps the best example in toxicology of a well validated alternative to animal use.

The theme of this chapter is an illustration of the various aspects of parenteral toxicity by a collation of published examples and personal experiences. There has been no intention to provide a comprehensive review and it may well be that some readers will recall examples of their own more apposite than those selected. To them the apology of omission or oversight is offered in advance.

INDICATIONS

The indications for parenteral toxicity are important because the selection of route in animal studies has not always been prudent or even applicable and a correct choice is essential to achieve experimental objectives. The indications for parenteral administration in animal toxicology are a simulation of the intended route in man and veterinary species, an estimation of absorption, a determination of intrinsic toxicity, an investigation of gastrointestinal target pathogenesis and a facilitation of certain bioassays for carcinogenicity.

Intended Route

For potential medical pharmaceutical products, the dose route in the animal model should be the same as that proposed clinically for the human patient. This concept is invariable in guidelines issued by regulatory authorities concerned with the assessment and registration of new drugs. There are two main indications for parenteral therapy in man: inadequate absorption of the active ingredient by the gastrointestinal tract after ingestion and a clinical requirement to confine or concentrate the desired pharmacological effect in a target organ or tissue. Examples of both reasons are listed in **Table 1**. Veterinary medicine adds a third, that of facility, because it is often easier to inject large animals than to dose them by mouth. Also, the oral route is contraindicated for antibiotics in several animals, such as ruminants and rabbits, because digestion in these species depends considerably on a normal gastrointestinal flora.

Table 1 Indications for parenteral therapeutic routes

Reason	Example
Inadequate absorption after oral dosing	
Large polar molecules excreted unchanged in the faeces	Aminoglycoside antibiotics (e.g. streptomycin)
Digestion by pancreatic or intestinal proteolytic enzymes	Polypeptide hormones (e.g. insulin)
Gastrointestinal inactivation and/or hepatic conjugation	Catecholamines (e.g. epinephrine)
Gastrointestinal irritation and/or emesis	Chemotherapeutic alkaloids (e.g. emetine)
Need to target pharmacological effect	
Prompt bactericidal action in life-threatening infections	Certain antibiotics (e.g. benzylpenicillin)
Rapid depression of the central nervous system	Barbiturate anaesthetics (e.g. thiopentone sodium)
Infiltration anaesthesia, nerve block and intrathecal injection	Local anaesthetics (e.g. lignocaine)
Reversal of disturbed body fluid volume or composition	Plasma volume expanders (e.g. dextran–saline)
Intra-arterial administration for local tumour delivery	Cytotoxic drugs (e.g. vincristine)

Patients are also exposed by parenteral routes to inserted or surgically implanted medical devices which may incorporate plasticizers to impart flexibility or clarity. Low levels of phthalate esters have been detected in the tissues of patients exposed to medical devices (Jaeger and Rubin, 1970). It follows that plasticizers and/or finished products should be tested by parenteral route toxicology. A good example of this was the demonstration of antifertility effects and mutagenicity in a dominant-lethal study on di-2-ethylhexyl phthalate injected subcutaneously in mice (Agarwal *et al.*, 1985). The oral route would have been not only inappropriate but also misleading because the compound is hydrolysed in the intestine. Medical devices may also incorporate heavy metals such as nickel, which is oxytocic, allergenic and increases coronary artery resistance. Potential sources of repeated nickel exposure include prostheses, indwelling intravenous needles and heater tanks for dialysis fluids (Sunderman, 1983).

Estimation of Absorption

Pharmacokinetics is an integral part of toxicology and few candidate drugs escape a parenteral study in animals, whatever their intended clinical route. Frequently acute toxicity manifests itself best by a parenteral route and intravenous injection is the most convenient procedure for determining half-life. Medical regulatory authorities invariably include, in their guidelines on testing for acute toxicity, a requirement to use at least one route which ensures systemic absorption, e.g. intravenous, intramuscular, subcutaneous. Availability has been expressed as the ratio in areas under the blood concentration–time curves of oral to intravenous routes after equivalent doses (Rowland, 1972). When the areas are equal, the drug is fully available. If the area ratio is less than unity, the drug is incompletely available because of poor absorption, metabolism on entry to the systemic circulation or a combination of both. Similarly, good gastrointestinal absorption is indicated by comparable LD_{50} values obtained in the same species by gavage and intraperitoneal injection, e.g. the cholinergic rodenticide phosacetim (Dubois *et al.*, 1967). Conversely, a higher parenteral LD_{50} value indicates poor availability from the injection site, e.g. subcutaneous trimethoprim (Honda *et al.*, 1973). Even intramuscular administration may occasionally provide absorption inferior to oral dosing, although this is the exception to the rule, e.g. aqueous chloramphenicol suspension in dogs (Watson, 1972).

It is well acknowledged that the absorption of drugs from diet mixtures is determined with difficulty and that comparable intravenous doses provide helpful information on first-pass gut–hepatic metabolism and biliary excretion. In the absence of a parenteral dose the presence of drugs or metabolites in the faeces following biliary excretion might be misinterpreted as incomplete absorption after oral administration (Smyth *et al.*, 1979). Parenteral dosing is also expedient in another context with respect to absorption after ingestion. That is the situation when good absorption from the gastrointestinal tract has been established in man but not in any of the commonly used laboratory animals. Then it is more practicable and economic to inject the compound into a rat than to continue searching for a species which absorbs it like man.

Tin compounds as a group illustrate well the close relation between absorption and toxicity (Winship, 1988). Only about 5% of inorganic tin salts are absorbed from the gastrointestinal tract and as a result their toxicities are low. On the other hand, many of the organotin compounds are toxic, especially trimethyltin and triethyltin, which are well absorbed after ingestion. Most of the other alkyl- and aryltin compounds are poorly absorbed from the gastrointestinal tract and are consequently less toxic by oral dosing than by parenteral administration.

Significant differences in toxicity, reflecting availability, have been demonstrated in repeat-dose studies between oral and parenteral routes even for readily absorbed compounds. Dietary inclusion often results in a rather flat blood level curve but intravenous or intraperitoneal injections cause high peaks followed by exponential declines. This difference was examined for lithium administered to rats over 22 weeks (Plenge *et al.*, 1981). Both functional and structural evidence of nephrotoxicity were more pronounced in the dietary group than in rats receiving daily intraperitoneal injections. It was postulated that regenerative processes were allowed to operate during the periods of very low serum lithium levels between injections which were continuously exceeded in the dietary inclusion group. These findings were correlated with therapeutic schedules, plasma lithium levels and diuresis in manic-depressive patients to propose that their twice-daily dose should be reduced in frequency and increased in amount.

Intrinsic Toxicity

The true toxic potential of a compound can only be assessed when it is administered in a form which is readily available for absorption and distribution to its target sites. Occupational exposure to many highly toxic industrial chemicals and pesticides is usually via oral, inhalational and percutaneous routes. Consequently, parenteral administration might be considered inappropriate to their toxicological evaluations. However, these occupational routes often minimize or preclude absorption, especially when the toxic compound is formulated in an inert fluid vehicle or powder carrier. Therefore, to determine intrinsic toxicity, an essential requirement despite low risk, a parenteral route of administration may be necessary. Also, for an expensive novel compound, low volume injections are more economical than large doses given by less absorptive routes.

Pyrethrins (pyrethrum) and their synthetic analogues (pyrethroids) have come to be regarded as one of the safest chemical classes of insecticides. Allergy to natural pyrethrum has long been known and contact facial parasthesia is an established occupational hazard of workers handling some of the cyano-pyrethroids. Otherwise, scientifically validated cases of human systemic toxicity following peroral, inhalational or percutaneous exposure to pyrethroids are rare. Nevertheless, they are extremely toxic in laboratory animals by intravenous injection. When the earliest analogues were synthesized their acute toxicities were compared by oral and intravenous routes in rats (Verschoyle and Barnes, 1972). The intravenous LD_{50} results, and those of natural pyrethrins, were usually well below 10 mg kg^{-1}, but corresponding oral values were several hundred times higher. Moreover, the intravenous effects were rapid and signs of toxicity following sublethal doses were short-lived in survivors. It was inferred that these compounds acted *per se* without metabolic activation to more toxic molecules.

Subsequently, it was shown that many pyrethroids are highly potent neurotoxins but that they are rapidly metabolized to less toxic compounds by hydrolysis of a central ester bond or by oxidative attack at several sites (Gray and Soderlund, 1985). It was confirmed that intrinsic toxicity was well demonstrated by intravenous administration which minimized metabolism and that the oral, and even intraperitoneal, routes hindered interpretation of pyrethroid toxicity by involving complex pharmacokinetic and pharmacodynamic factors. Furthermore, it was shown that an even more target-direct parenteral route, intracerebral, could elucidate structure–activity relations. Thus structural features which permitted rapid metabolism (e.g. *trans* substitution, possession of primary alcohol moiety) also conferred low intrinsic neurotoxicity and those which provided metabolic stability (e.g. *cis* substitution, possession of an (S)-α-cyano substituent) were more toxic.

Parenteral dosing has similarly been used to confirm the predicted property of environmental contaminants to cause toxic changes by providing doses exceeding those to which workers might be exposed or which would be impractical in animal models by the inhalational route. An example of this was the exposure of Fischer-344 rats in an inhalation chamber 20 h a day, 5 $\frac{1}{2}$ days a week, for 9 months to diluted diesel exhaust providing a maximum concentration of particulates at 1.5 mg m^{-3} (Chen and Vostal, 1981). This did not increase lung or liver microsomal activity of aryl hydrocarbon hydroxylase, which is known to be induced by polyaromatic hydrocarbons. The total mass of hydrocarbons deposited in the lung during the inhalation exposure was estimated and an equivalent dose (2 mg kg^{-1}) of extractable hydrocarbons was injected intraperitoneally daily for 4 days. Again this failed to induce the enzyme, but similarly administered doses 10–50 times higher did. Ambient concentrations were estimated at levels approximately 100 times lower than those to which the rats were exposed. Thus hazard was demonstrated and risk was determined to be negligible.

Gastroenteric Target Pathogenesis

Perhaps the most common clinical symptoms of drug toxicity in human patients, even at therapeutic dose levels, are nausea and vomiting. Occasionally these may be accompanied by pathological changes such as gastric and intestinal erosion or ulceration. Nausea following ingestion of a medicine may indicate local mucosal irritation, but frequently it is the result of a central effect after absorption or a combination of both mechanisms. It is well recognized in, and a considerable cause of discomfort to, cancer patients receiving intravenous cytotoxic drugs. Common culprits include cisplatin, dacarbazine, cyclophosphamide, doxorubicin and fluorouracil. Necrosis and desquamation of intestinal epithelium have been demonstrated in laboratory animals following parenteral administration of nitrogen mustards and their emetic property in patients has been attributed to stimulation of the central nervous system. Cyclophosphamide causes nausea and vomiting with equal frequency following intravenous injection or ingestion. Intravenous fluorouracil therapy may cause oral or colostomic stomatitis, proctitis and possible enteric injury at any level. These gastrointestinal effects of cytotoxic drugs have been summarized (Calabresi and Parks, 1975).

Another pharmaceutical class, the non-steroidal anti-inflammatory drugs, is notorious for its property to induce gastric ulceration and emesis. The nausea caused by salicylates involves receptors in both the gastric mucosa and in the brain medulla, the former stimulated by direct irritation. In man, centrally induced nausea and emesis appear at plasma salicylate concentrations of about 0.27 mg ml^{-1}, but the same effects may occur at much lower levels as a result of local irritation (Woodbury and Fingle, 1975).

It is most likely that many novel candidate oral drugs in these or other classes will possess similar undesirable properties and this poses a double problem for the toxicologist—their detection and pathogeneses. Detection is hindered by the inability of the rat to vomit and by its gastric differences from man, anatomical and chemical. The investigation of pathogenesis must necessarily involve a parenteral route if only to negate a purely local mechanism. Gastric ulceration caused by aspirin after oral dosing is well documented in man and rat and yet, despite prolonged and prolific use of the drug, the pathogenesis of its lesion is still incompletely understood. However, the parenteral route has made significant contributions. These include the demonstration that both aspirin and sodium salicylate, its hydrolysis product, cause gastric mucosal injury in rats by intravenous injection but only in the presence of luminal acid. Also, pre-treatment with exogenous prostaglandin, either by intraluminal instillation or by subcutaneous injection, has a protective effect which is complete against aspirin and incomplete against sodium salicylate (Rowe *et al.*, 1987).

Another example of gastrointestinal lesions evoked by either oral and parenteral routes has been provided from the acute toxicology of the trichothecene toxin T-2 (Fairhurst *et al.*, 1987). LD_{50} values in rats, mice and guinea-pigs by intravenous, intragastric, subcutaneous, intraperitoneal and intratracheal routes ranged between 1 and 14 mg kg^{-1}. Oral sublethal doses caused pigeons to vomit and produced lymphocytolysis and mucosal ulceration in the gastrointestinal tract of rats. The latter recalled similar descriptions in various species after parenteral dosing and so it was inferred that these changes in the gut were not due to the luminal presence of T-2. A possible explanation offered was biliary excretion of an active metabolite.

Carcinogenesis

Regulatory authorities require evidence of lifespan carcinogenicity studies in experimental animals, by the intended clinical routes, for new drugs which are to be given to man continuously or intermittently for prolonged periods or which have chemical structures suggestive of a carcinogenic potential. Most of these are formulated for ingestion, which minimizes practical difficulties of animal dosing. However, parenteral products in these categories create an experimental problem because the relatively small size of rodents, in which the majority of carcinogenicity studies are now conducted, limits the availability of injection sites and repetitive dosing is likely to lead to local intolerance. Fortunately, the intravenous route is required infrequently. For instance, it is unnecessary to test for carcinogenicity the cytotoxic drugs which may be given repetitively by this route. Also, the intraperitoneal route, not favoured in man, is inappropriate although it has been used in animals for carcinogenicity studies on poorly absorbed materials. The subcutaneous route is more popular but may provide sarcomas which do not represent true carcinogenic potential (see below). The intramuscular route is compromised by the limited availability of sites and the probability of local reaction following repetitive injections (see below). This might be avoided by a restriction of dosing to twice weekly or the use of a larger species such as the dog, but the latter is not a serious alternative. Remote tumours in the dog have been induced by parenteral injections, but its routine use as a model for carcinogenesis is precluded by a prolonged latent period

of up to 10 years and the prohibitive cost which this would incur (Bonser, 1969).

Although parenteral routes are not easily incorporated in routine or standard protocols for carcinogenicity, they have been invaluable in the investigation of mechanisms. This applies particularly to the polycyclic hydrocarbons, which require relatively few administrations to exert their effects and are characterized by short periods of latency. For example, in the Syrian hamster a genetic influence was discovered by the difference in mean latency from 9 to 15–16 weeks between various inbred strains simply by single subcutaneous injections of 9, 10-dimethyl-1, 2-benzanthracene (Homburger, 1972). Also, in the same species and by the same route, an inverse relationship was demonstrated between mean induction time of nasal or laryngeal tumours and dose of diethylnitrosamine after only 12 weekly injections (Montesano and Saffiotti, 1968).

Another popular experimental application of the parenteral route is the expediency of localizing carcinogens to their target tissues with the objectives of confining tumours to the organ under study, increasing yields and foreshortening latent periods. Thus, via surgical intervention in rats, local adenocarcinomas have been induced by direct implantation of 7, 12-dimethylbenzanthracene crystals in the pancreas (Dissin *et al.*, 1975) and squamous cell carcinomas have been produced in the lung by intrapulmonary injection of 3-methylcholanthrene in beeswax pellets (Hirano *et al.*, 1974).

A similar target approach via parenteral methods was used to investigate the effects of asbestos and so circumvent the technical demands of inhalation toxicology. Mesotheliomas were first induced in the rat by direct intrapleural application of dusts (Wagner, 1962). Then it was discovered, almost fortuitously, that two subcutaneous injections in mice of 10 mg of asbestos suspended in 0.4 ml of saline, one in each flank and repeated twice at intervals of 5 weeks, produced extensive inflammatory and proliferative changes in the pleural and peritoneal serosas within two years (Roe *et al.*, 1967). These were much more conspicuous than local inflammatory and neoplastic reactions at the administration sites, which the experiment was designed to investigate. Thus the unexpected transport of fibres from subcutis to serosa facilitated further the study of asbestos pathogenesis. Other workers in this field reverted to direct implantation of the rat visceral pleura with asbestos carried on fibrous glass pledgets and, after numerous experiments by this technique, inferred that the carcinogenicity was primarily related to structural shape rather than physicochemical properties (Stanton and Wrench, 1972).

Parenteral carcinogenicity testing would be incomplete without a mention of the once-fashionable, now almost obsolete, neonatal mouse test. A small dose of the test substance was injected, into subcutaneous tissues or into the peritoneal cavity, once within 24 h of birth and the mice were allowed to live for about 1 year. Sometimes supplementary injections were administered over the first week or two. The appeal of this assay was the small quantity of compound required, the restricted dosing and a reduction in the adult study duration. There was a common belief that newborn animals were more responsive to carcinogens than adults but a review of 30 studies, mostly on genotoxic agents, did not confirm this unequivocally (Toth, 1968). Despite some enthusiasm for the method and its application to food additives, with the attribution of hepato-carcinogenicity to safrole (Epstein et al., 1970), doubts about its value and validity grew. An increased incidence of liver cell tumours in mice parenterally exposed at birth was regarded as unreliable evidence of carcinogenic potential (Roe, 1975). Finally, it was concluded that the range of neoplasms produced was restricted, that induction of common tumours was not a good indication of carcinogenicity and that the neonate might react differently to the adult because of its immunological and enzymatic immaturity (Grasso and Grant, 1977). Now it would appear that the neonatal mouse test has fallen into disuse.

TECHNIQUES

The common parenteral routes in toxicology are intravenous, subcutaneous, intraperitoneal and intramuscular. It is not intended here to describe in detail the numerous techniques for these routes in the various species of animal used in toxicity studies because there is a plethora of relevant scientific publications. Moreover, most of them have been collated in several standard texts on laboratory animals to which the interested reader is referred. These include the rabbit (Bivin and Timmons, 1974), the rat (Kraus, 1980) and most other species, with good illustrations (Green, 1979) and useful tabular summaries of injection sites, needle sizes and suggested maximum volumes (Flecknell, 1987). These texts describe techniques applicable to all scientific procedures or to anaesthetization. The following remarks apply specifically to toxicology.

Injection Technique

Intravenous

Numerous veins have been suggested for intravenous injections in the various laboratory species but some of them, in small rodents, necessitate sedation or anaesthesia and surgical exposure. As such they are unsuitable for routine toxicology where the important criteria of technique are simplicity, often repeatability, and always avoidance of undue stress. In conscious animals the author's preferred veins for repeated injections are lateral caudal in mice and rats, marginal ear in rabbits and

guinea-pigs, cephalic in dogs, saphenous in marmosets and alar in chickens. Injection may be facilitated in rodents by warming the animal or its tail to promote vasodilation and by simple restraint systems, all of which are well described in publication on animal technology. Successful intravenous injections rely on simple preparations such as clipping or shaving fur, good illumination, slight magnification, sharp needles and swabbing with surgical spirit, which not only provides asepsis but also renders veins more conspicuous. A series of injections into a frequently used vein should follow a cycle of distal to proximal. In this way it is possible to deliver large volumes (over 40 ml) into the same vein of pyrogen test rabbits twice a week almost indefinitely. The administration of large volumes to fractious or frightened animals may be facilitated by a break in the needle, connecting the cut ends with flexible polythene tubing (Nicholls, 1970). The speed of intravenous injection has a profound effect on acute toxicity (see below).

Subcutaneous

Injections into the subcutaneous tissues are considerably easier, even in small rodents. The advised site in all toxicology species is the dorsal neck or back. The technique is to pick up a tent of loose skin and to inject into it, but care is necessary to avoid passing the needle through the two layers. The injected area is usually massaged and large volumes can be divided to multiple sites. It should be noted that absorption may vary with site because different LD_{50} values have been reported for dorsal and ventral subcutaneous injections in mice (Balazs, 1970).

Intraperitoneal

The intraperitoneal route is sometimes regarded as hazardous because there is a risk of penetrating viscera such as liver, intestines or urinary bladder. In practice, with the subject firmly restrained in dorsal recumbency and the use of a small needle carefully inserted, such errors are infrequent. The risk may be reduced further by prior starvation but great care is necessary injecting viscous or oily fluids which require heavy pressure on the plunger of the syringe. Probably of more concern to the toxicologist is the extreme sensitivity of the peritoneum, which may react to some compounds by acute shock or severe local reaction, so confounding systemic toxicity. The intraperitoneal route is preferred to intravenous injection in neonatal rats since their veins are so small. It is a hazardous technique, although an unconventional dorsal approach claims safety (Hornick, 1986).

Intramuscular

The usual sites for intramuscular injection are the same for virtually all laboratory animals used in toxicology. They are the posterior thigh muscles and the quadriceps.

The former, usually providing the larger muscle mass, is favoured more frequently but is disadvantageous because there is a risk of hitting the sciatic nerve or delivering the injected material into a fascial plane. These pitfalls may be avoided by careful consideration of anatomy or by injecting into the quadriceps, although this approach seems to be more painful. Intramuscular injections may penetrate blood vessels but the risk of this is difficult to estimate. The simple precaution of withdrawing the plunger of the syringe before depressing it is not always reliable when fine needles enter small blood vessels. Local reaction to intramuscular injection merits much attention in veterinary medicine (see below).

Other Routes

Less frequently used routes of injection used in toxicology include intrapleural, intra-arterial, intrathecal, intracerebral and intracerebroventricular. These are not common in standard protocols and are more frequently employed in studies on mechanisms. Anaesthesia and surgical exposure are usually necessary. Surgery may be avoided for intra-arterial injection of rabbits by the use of the neuroleptanalgesic combination of fentanyl citrate and fluanisone, which provides good visualization of the middle pinnal artery. Actual techniques for these less frequently used routes are often described in the methods sections of papers on relevant toxicity studies.

Infusion systems

One prime objective of clinical pharmacology is the maintenance of a fairly constant blood concentration of the drug within an established therapeutic range. Blood levels below this are ineffectual and those above it may be toxic. This objective is not difficult to achieve with drugs which have a prolonged half-life, but compounds which are rapidly excreted may thwart it. Necessarily they have to be administered by inconvenient regimes with short intervals between doses, and this may result in unacceptibly high peaks in blood levels. The problem is exaggerated in some animal models in which the half-life of certain drugs may be more than an order of magnitude less than that in man (Nau, 1983).

Attempts to avoid excessive fluctuations in blood level have been the main thrust in the emergence, over the last decade or more, of a whole new industry developing novel delivery, particularly rate-controlled, systems (Urquhart, 1982). Examples of their application in human therapy include insulin for diabetic ketoacidosis, cisplatin for solid tumours, nitroglycerine for angina and scopolamine for motion sickness. Even veterinary medicine has been influenced, with slow or pulsed release of anthelmintics and trace elements from glass bullets or corrosive devices residing in the ruminant stomach. The rate-controlled methods are mainly conventional infu-

sion systems and implanted devices. It is reasonable to expect that drugs intended for these systems should be tested for toxicity in similar animal models, but such methods at present are not common in routine toxicology. Presumably cost and impracticability are deterrents. Nevertheless, they offer attractive features, not the least of which is the means by which steady states of rapidly excreted compounds may be achieved.

The basic components of an intravenous infusion system in laboratory animals are a flexible, indwelling, securely anchored cannula, an extension line usually burrowed subcutaneously to a convenient point of exit, an electrically operated infusion pump and a mechanical contrivance to permit movement and prevent self-mutilation. Clinical microprocessor-controlled pumps may be used despite their large size because they will deliver as little as 0.1 ml h^{-1}. Like injection techniques and choice of veins, infusion systems in laboratory animals are the subject of many publications, although few of them apply to toxicology. Most suffer to varying extents from the disadvantages of anaesthesia, surgical exposure and post-operative complications of leakage and stress. Favoured veins in the rat are the jugular, femoral and caudal. At least one non-surgical method has been described in this species, providing continuous infusion for a week via the lateral caudal vein (Rhodes and Patterson, 1979).

Presumably the impracticality of conventional infusion systems in laboratory animals will always preclude their routine use in toxicology, but they have permitted valuable insights into mechanisms, particularly of cytotoxic drugs, because they provide the means by which protracted delivery may be compared with bolus injection. Some comparative studies with this objective have shown little difference in host toxicity between the two methods, e.g. for doxorubicin, cytosine arabinoside and neocarzinostatin in a rat model of acute myelogenous leukaemia (Ensminger et al., 1979). In others toxicity was reduced by continuous infusion, e.g. the pulmonary fibrogenesis of bleomycin, the cardiac toxicity of doxorubicin and the myelosuppression of fluorouracil (Carlson and Sikic, 1983). Similarly, infusion LD_{50} values of alkylating agents were lowered by bolus injections, e.g. mechlorethamine, phenylalanine mustard and carmustine (Valeriote and Vietti, 1985). However, it should not be assumed that infusion is invariably less toxic. A 24 h infusion of fenoldopam mesylate administered at a rate of 0.005 mg kg^{-1} min^{-1} (total 7.2 mg^{-1} kg^{-1}) caused medial necrosis in the splanchnic arteries of rats, but daily intravenous injections of 20 mg kg^{-1} for 12 days had no effect (Yuhas et al., 1985). Presumably these differences are functions of variable rates of enzyme induction and detoxification.

Intravenous infusion systems have also proved their worth in the toxicology of addictive drugs by providing the means for self-administration through lever activation. By this method cocaine was found to be considerably more toxic than heroin to rats (Bozarth and Wise, 1985).

Osmotic Minipumps

An attractive alternative to intravenous infusion is the subcutaneous implantation of self-powered miniature diffusion cells (Pinedo *et al.*, 1976) or osmotic minipumps (Ray and Theeuwes, 1987). Some of these devices are small enough to implant in mice. The necessary surgery is simple and the duration of anaesthesia is brief.

A range of Alzet miniature osmotic pumps are commercially available. The smallest, which is suitable for mice, measures 17×6 mm, has a reservoir capacity of 0.1 ml and pumps at a rate of 0.001 ml h^{-1} for 3 days. Larger versions, for dogs, will deliver either 0.005 ml h^{-1} for 2 weeks or 0.0025 ml h^{-1} for 1 month. Each pump consists of a collapsible impermeable reservoir surrounded by concentrated sodium chloride invested by a semipermeable membrane **(Figure 1)**. The reservoir is filled with the test substance by injection, capped with the flow moderator and then the pump is implanted. The osmotic agent imbibes tissue water, which gradually compresses the reservoir and displaces its contents through the delivery portal. Rate and duration of delivery are pre-set at manufacture. Duration may be extended by serial implantation. Osmotic minipumps are usually implanted subcutaneously or intraperitoneally but can be fitted with simple catheters for delivery to remote target sites,

e.g. intravenous, intracerebroventricular, or into solid organs. They are produced in sterile packs and manufactured from tissue-compatible components. The wall of the elastomeric reservoir is inert to most aqueous drug formulations, dilute acids, bases and alcohols, but is incompatible with natural oils.

Osmotic minipumps are advantageous over infusion systems by their simplicity of insertion, particularly an absence of any cumbersome external connections, so that the test animal is unrestricted and less stressed. Nevertheless, their use in toxicology is not widespread. Probable reasons for this include cost, necessity for serial implantation and incompatibility with oily vehicles. However, it would not be surprising if their popularity improved in the future because it is becoming increasingly appreciated that drug toxicity is not only dose-related but also regimen-dependent. The osmotic minipump provides the means by which constant availability could be achieved for drugs with short half-lives and whose conventional administration results in a cycle of high, possibly toxic, blood levels and low sub-therapeutic troughs.

This concept was applied to the embryotoxicology of valproic acid, an antiepileptic drug which has a half-life of 8–16 h in man but only 48 min in the mouse (Nau, 1983). Effects of the same total dose were compared in pregnant mice between daily subcutaneous injections from gestational day 7 to day 14 and constant delivery from a subcutaneous osmotic minipump. The intermittent bolus administration produced high rates of resorption and exencephaly. To achieve comparable embryolethality by the steady-state system, the dose had to be increased by a factor of 10 and even then exencephaly barely exceeded control values. Similar results were obtained in pregnant rats with sodium salicylate (Gabrielsson *et al.*, 1985). Unlike valproic acid, this drug is pharmacokinetically similar in man and rodent. Its foetal adverse effects following daily intravenous injections were reduced by constant delivery into the jugular vein via an indwelling catheter from a subcutaneous osmotic minipump. The difference was more evident at the lower analgetic dose of 75 mg kg^{-1} day^{-1} than at the higher antirheumatic level of 150 mg kg^{-1} day^{-1}.

These examples may illustrate the most apposite application of osmotic minipumps to toxicology because conventional bolus dosing at a brief time of embryo susceptibility could exaggerate teratological properties. However, other applications have been described. The pulmonary fibrogenic effect of bleomycin injected into tumour-bearing mice was significantly reduced by continuous infusion of the same total dose from an osmotic minipump (Sikic *et al.*, 1978). Conversely, lung damage in rats injected subcutaneously with paraquat was increased by a similar dose delivered from an osmotic minipump (Dey *et al.*, 1982). Obviously the effect of dosing regime on toxicity is drug specific and the contrivance of steady-state availability may increase or

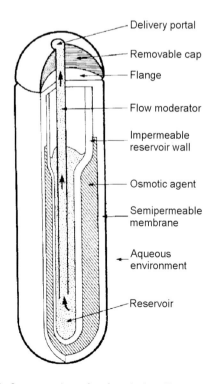

Figure 1 Cross-section of a functioning Alzet osmotic minipump. Reproduced by permission of Charles River UK Ltd.

Delivery portal

Removable cap

Flange

Flow moderator

Impermeable reservoir wall

Osmotic agent

Semipermeable membrane

Aqueous environment

Reservoir

decrease it. The future contribution to toxicology of rate-control systems such as osmotic minipumps and trans-dermal devices is difficult to predict. Suffice it to say that any means of improving species bioequivalence which circumvents differences in metabolism, absorption and excretion must improve the model.

ARTEFACTS AND ALTERATIONS

Many sequelae of parenteral injections are the effects of technique or local perturbation which either modify systemic toxicity of the test substance or completely misrepresent it. Obviously the toxicologist must be fully aware of such potential artefacts and alterations. The common examples are intravenous rapid injection, subcutaneous sarcoma, intramuscular reaction and intraperitoneal sensitivity. There are also other more subtle changes which are not always anticipated or even considered in the determination and description of toxic effects.

Intravenous

One of the therapeutic, and consequently toxicological, reasons for intravenous injection is the introduction into the bloodstream of hypertonic, irritant or even vesicant solutions because the endothelium is relatively refractory and the drug is rapidly and greatly diluted. It follows that careful technique is necessary to avoid partial perivascular injection with its possible consequences of local inflammatory reaction in and around the sensitive venous adventitia. This might not influence acute toxicity but it could end prematurely the experimental life of affected animals in repeat-dose studies or pyrogen testing laboratories. Lesions at the caudal vein site of administration were found in over 50% of 1422 rats injected daily for 4 weeks with a variety of test articles (Kast and Tsunenari, 1983). They included periphlebitis, phlebitis, cushion-like swellings of the intima and thrombosis with hair penetration of the caudal vein wall.

The physico-chemical properties of intravenously administered substances are important considerations. Oily vehicles are contraindicated and drugs which either precipitate blood constituents or haemolyse erythrocytes should not be injected by this route. Nevertheless, emulsions of vegetable oil, lecithin and water or saline have been given intravenously to the dog. Other considerations include total volume, osmolarity and acidity (Balazs, 1970). Overwhelming volumes should be avoided and hypotonicity may increase toxicity, but a wide range of pH is permissible for slowly administered solutions. Concentrated solutions of compounds with low aqueous solubility may precipitate in the blood. The effect of this on toxicity was described for the pyre-

throid cismethrin in rats (Gray and Soderlund, 1985). Its intravenous injection in a concentrated form reduced acute toxicity and delayed its onset. This was attributed to initial precipitation in the pulmonary capillaries and subsequent slow release into the bloodstream before final distribution to target nervous tissue.

Pulmonary embolism of hair and skin fragments is another pathological artefact of intravenous injection which has been recognized in experimental mice, rats, rabbits and dogs. Pulmonary thromboarteritis and/or giant cell granulomas with hair or skin particles were discovered in over 25% of 1422 rats after daily injections in the caudal vein for 1 month (Kast and Tsunenari, 1983). Pathologists should note that this incidence was derived from the examination of single left lobe sections so that the true percentage of affected rats was probably higher. Findings were similar in rabbits injected through an ear vein but the incidence was lower.

Regimen dependence and differences in toxicity between bolus dosing and continuous infusion have been discussed above. One determinant of these differences is the actual delivery speed of administration and the effect this has on activating detoxification or compensatory mechanisms. It is well recognized that the rapidity with which many compounds are injected intravenously profoundly influences their acute toxicities. This is one reason why the intravenous median lethal dose is almost as much a function of technique as it is of a compound's inherent toxicity. Despite this, it is surprising how few reports on acute toxicity are qualified by any mention of injection speed, let alone its measurement. Generally intravenous administration should be slow, but this is subject to wide interpretation. Slow has been defined as not more than $0.02 \, \text{ml s}^{-1}$ with concomitant advice for a limit on total volume of 0.1–0.5 ml for rodents and 2 ml for larger laboratory animals (Balazs, 1970). However, it should be considered that, for some drugs, a slow infusion might equilibrate with the rate of detoxification and so nullify a toxic response. Moreover, there are exceptional indications for rapid injection. One such was the requirement to simulate the clinical accident of injecting local anaesthetics intravenously. For this a dog model was used (Liu et al., 1983). It was demonstrated that the toxicities of lignocaine (lidocaine), etidocaine, bupivacaine and tetracaine for the canine central nervous system were directly proportional to their human anaesthetic potencies.

There are probably numerous examples of too-rapid intravenous injection in toxicology, mostly unpublished. Pyrogen test technicians are very familiar with the lethal consequences in rabbits of injecting adrenaline, potassium salts and other products too fast. The author was once requested to investigate the death of a racehorse after the reputedly rapid intravenous injection of a veterinary multivitamin preparation (Walker, 1981). Injection of the diluted product into the caudal vein of mice at a volume rate of $12.5 \, \text{ml kg}^{-1}$ had no effect when the speed of delivery was timed at 0.025 ml s^{-1}. When this was increased to 0.167 ml s^{-1} the same dose approximated the LD$_{50}$.

Similarly with infusions, it might be expected that acute toxicity would relate positively to the time rate of delivery. Probably for many drugs this holds, but sometimes results are confusing if not anomalous. Thus, in mice perfused via a caudal vein with phytic acid at a total constant dose of 0.28 mg g^{-1} convulsive deaths occurred when the delivery rate was approximately 0.03 mg g^{-1} min^{-1} but not when it was reduced to < 0.02 mg g^{-1} min^{-1} or increased to > 0.05 mg g^{-1} min^{-1} (Gersonde and Weiner, 1982). The observed toxicity was consistent with the ability of phytic acid to bind calcium and the seemingly anomalous result was tentatively ascribed to the rapidity with which hypocalcaemia elicited the compensatory response of parathyroid hormone secretion.

By a completely different mechanism, mechanical rather than pharmacological, the delivery rate of an intra-arterial infusion may determine its toxicity, particularly its topographical distribution. The cerebral distribution of ^{14}C-labelled iodoantipyrine was investigated in rhesus monkeys infused via the cervical segment of the internal carotid artery (Blacklock *et al.*, 1986). After a slow infusion of 0.4 ml min^{-1}, isotope deposition in the ipsilateral hemisphere was markedly heterogeneous, but a fast rate of 4 ml min^{-1} and retrograde needle direction to promote mixing produced uniform distribution. The authors attributed the heterogeneous deposition to drug streaming within the internal carotid artery and its branches. They suggested that this might be the cause of focal cerebral and retinal toxicity sometimes observed in patients treated for brain tumours by slow intra-arterial chemotherapeutic infusion.

Subcutaneous

Clinically the subcutaneous route is used for non-irritant drugs. It provides a reasonably even, slow rate of absorption which may be retarded further by various techniques such as the combination of zinc and protamine with insulin or the incorporation of vasoconstrictor agents in formulations of local anaesthetics. In toxicology it is the route of choice for drugs which are intended for subcutaneous administration and is also used for oral compounds which are poorly absorbed from the gastrointestinal tract of the animal model. The subcutaneous tissues of rats and other animals readily react to the introduction of an irritant with the formation of a sterile abscess, particularly when the formulation is designed to provide a depot. This type of abscess is the result of necrotic tissue attracting a purulent exudate. It may occur even after intraperitoneal injection when an irritant such as oxytetracycline leaks into the subcutis from the needle as it is advanced through the body wall (Porter *et al.*, 1985). Subcutaneous infection is not so common

even though aseptic technique is sometimes disregarded in toxicology. Nevertheless, it has been recorded as, for example, in dogs which received a daily subcutaneous injection of suspended cortisone acetate for 3–4 weeks (Thompson *et al.*, 1971).

The most notorious artefact of subcutaneous injections in toxicology is the sarcoma of carcinogenicity studies, particularly those conducted in the rat. The subcutaneous method came into fashion 50 years ago to demonstrate the carcinogenicity of substances whose chemical structure suggested this property but which failed to exhibit it when applied topically, such as the coal-tar derivatives. Then it became used to screen drugs, food additives and other chemicals for carcinogenicity. Eventually it was realized that numerous substances which induced subcutaneous sarcomas in rodents, after repeated injections of high doses, were not intrinsically carcinogenic. The method fell into disrepute and is now used less frequently and with more caution in its interpretation.

The unravelling of this phenomenon and the postulation of a pathogenesis constituted a comprehensive review which cited numerous subcutaneous studies (Grasso and Golberg, 1966). Most of the following remarks are excerpts from this thorough publication. The authors defined three physical categories of materials which had been shown to induce subcutaneous sarcoma: water-soluble compounds, substances which dissolved initially and then came out of solution at the injection site and implanted solids. The water-soluble compounds included hypertonic solutions of various sugars and saline, food colours and aldehydes, although some positive results from earlier studies were not confirmed by later work. The tumorigenic water-soluble substances exhibited three common factors: neoplasms were restricted to local sarcomas, they resulted from the frequent administration of high doses and had latent periods of about 40 weeks. Examples of materials which came out of solution to accumulate at the injection site as foreign bodies were carboxymethylcellulose and iron–dextran. Examples of implanted solids included many plastics and other materials which appeared to produce sarcomas irrespective of their chemical composition. Their tumorigenic property seemed to depend more on physical characteristics such as shape and size.

Pathogenetic studies on the reaction to implanted solids were particularly enlightening. The gradual development of a thick connective tissue capsule invariably preceded tumour formation by several months. This was an essential step in tumorigenesis because sarcomas did not appear if the capsule failed to develop or if it was surgically excised. Moreover, once the capsule had fully formed, removal of the implant did not prevent the malignant outcome. It was suggested that a similar mechanism operated in the induction of sarcomas by repeated injections of fluid. It was postulated that frequent repetitive trauma of young fibroblasts at the injection site impeded normal repair and eventually disrupted the homeostatic forces controlling these cells so that their autonomous proliferation ensued.

The problem was, and still is, a distinction between the consequence of this 'indirect' mechanism and the effects of 'true' carcinogens which act directly on intracellular receptors at the injection site. Interpretation is facilitated when true carcinogens induce remote tumours. When local tumours alone develop it is necessary either to confirm carcinogenicity by demonstrating dose dependence or to refute it by establishing the nature of an indirect mechanism as described above.

The authors of this review concluded that malignant transformation of subcutaneous fibroblasts could be induced by implanted or repeatedly injected materials either by virtue of their carcinogenic properties or through non-specific physical or physicochemical factors. They further inferred that the neoplastic outcome of physico-chemical insults which derange normal fibrosis did not constitute a carcinogenic property. These conclusions were soon affirmed in a WHO publication which recommended· that the routine testing of food additives and contaminants by subcutaneous injection should be considered inappropriate unless this was necessary to circumvent poor gastrointestinal absorption (World Health Organization, 1967). This recommendation would seem to be equally appropriate to the testing of drugs and indeed a subsequent WHO publication addressed the potential invalidity of pharmaceutical studies which resulted in local sarcomas alone (World Health Organization, 1969). The conclusions of the review authors have stood the test of time, now over 20 years, and remain basically unchanged (P. Grasso, personal communication).

Intramuscular

After intramuscular injection, aqueous drugs are soon available but absorption from oils and repository suspensions is protracted. Isotonic and slightly hypertonic solutions are better tolerated than hypotonic formulations and even irritant compounds, precluded from the subcutaneous route, may be injected into muscle. The intramuscular route is well used in human patients but is more favoured by veterinary practice because of its practicality in large animals. It has been claimed that actual site of intramuscular deposition is an important determinant of bioavailability but, although differences between muscles have been demonstrated for a few drugs in some species, this is not invariable. For example, gentamicin is equally absorbed from the longissimus dorsi and biceps femoris muscles of dogs (Wilson et al., 1989). In toxicology intramuscular administration is indicated for the study of novel drugs intended by this route but the relatively small mass of muscle available in rats and rabbits

limits the frequency of injection, even of non-irritant drugs. This is one reason why it has not been widely adopted for carcinogenicity studies, although it should be noted that rhabdomyosarcomas have been induced in rats by this route following single injections of cobalt salts and repeated doses of triphenylmethane food dyes (Magee, 1970).

Those well recognized artefacts of intramuscular injection, accidental intravascular injection and trauma of the sciatic nerve have already been mentioned in the section on technique (see above). Both occur in clinical, especially veterinary, medicine. The high risk of injecting the sciatic nerve by over-penetrating the posterior thigh muscles has been emphasized in the cat (Baxter and Evans, 1973) and in the weanling pig (Van Alstine and Dietrich, 1988), with consequent advice to prefer the quadriceps and neck sites, respectively.

There is a similar danger of nerve damage in most laboratory species used for toxicology. The author gave rats single injections of licensed tetracycline into the posterior thigh muscles at a high dose rate of 50 mg kg^{-1} (D. Walker, unpublished data). Paralysis was almost immediate, characterized by flexion of the lateral digits, and subsequently improved but was still evident 1 week later when histopathology of the injection sites revealed necrotic foci surrounded by inflammatory cells and regenerating muscle fibres. This reaction is typical of myonecrogenic drugs, irrespective of damage to the sciatic nerve. The rabbit, with its relatively large dorsal mass of lumbar muscle, is preferable for local toxicology. This model was used to predict human tolerance to different esters of clindamycin by single injections of 50 mg in 1 ml (Gray et al., 1974). Within 24 h the normal range of serum creatine phosphokinase (62 ± 19 iu l^{-1}) was markedly elevated by clindamycin 2-phosphate (to 1500 iu l^{-1}) and clindamycin hydrochloride (to 4100 iu l^{-1}). The authors inferred that an activity of > 3000 iu l^{-1} in the rabbit test would be too irritant in the human and that values < 2000 iu l^{-1} would be clinically tolerable. They emphasized the sensitivity of this assay by advice to handle the animals carefully.

Allusion has been made to the prominence of the intramuscular route in veterinary therapeutics. This merits special attention not only because it so often results in muscle damage but also because there is a related aspect of drug residues in food animals, a matter of considerable current concern to consumer and legislator. Consequently, the rest of this subsection is apportioned entirely to the clinical toxicology of local intramuscular reaction caused by veterinary pharmaceutical products.

A myonecrogenic property is common in licensed veterinary parenteral antibiotics and has been well documented, especially by Danish workers. It has been shown that most preparations of penicillin, streptomycin and their combinations are relatively innocuous after intramuscular injection of pigs and cattle, but tetracycline, oxytetracycline, erythromycin and tylosin cause severe local reaction: necrosis within 6 days and scarring at 3 weeks (Rasmussen and Hogh, 1971). These findings were confirmed in a subsequent histopathological study which revealed, on the sixth day, fibrovascular proliferation and myoregeneration after penicillin and streptomycin but necrosis surrounded by demarcating reaction after the other antibiotics (Svendsen, 1972). In the porcine sites there were foreign body giant cells and, when the vehicle was oily, cyst formations in the demarcating zones. After 3 weeks the more severe reactions had become thick layers of scar tissue surrounding residual foci of necrosis. Subsequent studies provided similar findings in the hen (Blom and Rasmussen, 1976) and added sulphonamides, trimethoprim and their potentiating combinations to the list of myonecrogenic products (Rasmussen and Svendsen, 1976). More recently the fluoroquinolones have been similarly incriminated: enro-floxacin by its effect on serum creatine phosphokinase activity (Pyörälä et al., 1994) and difloxacin by histopathological examination (D. Walker, unpublished data).

Local reaction is not confined to antibiotics and chemotherapeutic agents. It has also been ascribed to vaccines, vitamins, metallic salts and other compounds. Iron in various formulations is commonly injected into the ham muscle of piglets a few days old to prevent anaemia, although modern recommendations are for the use of alternative sites. The local reaction to some of these preparations is, within 24 h, acute inflammation, hyaline myodegeneration and siderophagocytosis, but there are claims that careful attention to injection technique, particularly direction of delivery towards the popliteal lymph node, is mitigating (Schmitz et al., 1976). Acute myodegeneration and fatal hyperkalaemia may also occur in vitamin E-deficient piglets injected by the intraperitoneal route with iron–dextrose, but this is an entirely different pathogenesis, possibly peroxidation (Patterson et al., 1971).

Another metal commonly used in veterinary medicine which forms irritant salts is copper. The sheep is particularly susceptible to its deficiency and toxicity. The pharmaceutical search for suitable parenteral compounds to prevent swayback in lambs provided a choice between soluble but systemically toxic salts and safer but less efficacious complexes (Suttle, 1981). An example of the latter was the copper salt of methionine, which causes undesirable reactions in sheep and cattle. The pathogenesis of these lesions was investigated by the author (D. Walker, unpublished data). Single 0.02 ml injections were administered into the posterior thigh muscles of rats providing a dose rate of 2 mg kg^{-1} (Cu), about twice the ovine recommendation. Within 3 days the reaction was a central blue focus of unabsorbed copper methionine surrounded by necrotic tissue. On the fourth day this changed strikingly to liquefaction, which progressed for 2 weeks as necrotic tissue became copious sterile pus. Then the abscess resolved to leave a

small dry residual nodule of large vacuolated histiocytes and foreign material. Eventually this disappeared completely and the absence of scar tissue was remarkable in contrast with the effects of antibiotics described above.

Intraperitoneal

Although the peritoneal cavity provides a large surface area through which drugs may be readily absorbed, it is not a common parenteral route in human medicine. Reasons for this include its sensitivity to irritants, a danger of infection and a proclivity to form adhesions. Even so, it is a valuable route for dialysis in the treatment of drug overdosage and for total parenteral nutrition when intravenous feeding is compromised by catheter sepsis or venous thrombosis. A rabbit model has been used to evaluate intraperitoneal nutrition (Stone et al., 1986). In toxicology the intraperitoneal route is used more frequently than intended clinical administration might dictate, probably because it may achieve comparable absorption to intravenous injection and is technically simpler. It has not been widely adopted for carcinogenicity studies because it does not correspond with the usual exposures to drugs, food additives and pesticides. However, it has found application in the study of genotoxic carcinogens and in the determination of promoting activity. It has been shown, for example, that the antioxidant butylated hydroxytoluene enhances the formation of lung tumours in mice after a single dose of ethyl carbamate irrespective of route, intraperitoneal or oral (Witschi, 1981).

The accidental risk of penetrating viscera by the intraperitoneal route has been mentioned above in the section on techniques (see above). This error in rats was investigated by injecting viscous oily iodinated radiopaque media into the left caudal quadrant of the peritoneal cavity (Lewis et al., 1966). Radiographs revealed that some of the contrast medium was not injected into the peritoneal cavity in 20% of animals. Misdirected material was discovered mainly in the gastrointestinal tract but also in retroperitoneal, subcutaneous and intravesical sites. Insoluble materials injected into the peritoneal cavity rapidly elicit focal granulomatous plaques on visceral and parietal surfaces. Foreign-body granulomas so caused by single injections in young rodents may persist for life. However, the artefact of most concern to the toxicologist is acute peritonitis.

The typical inflammatory reaction of the rat peritoneum to the introduction of an irritant was observed by the author determining the acute toxicity of copper methionine by this route (D. Walker, unpublished data). Within hours of a single injection, peritoneal fluid was increased and in survivors 1 week later adhesions of the liver lobules were invariable. Acute peritonitis may be so severe that it contributes to lethality. This occurred following the intraperitoneal injection of sterigmatocystin in rats (Purchase and van der Watt, 1969). Then the investigator is presented with a dilemma of interpretation: should the lethal contribution be regarded as an integral feature of toxicity or should it be disregarded as an artefact of administration? The dilemma may be resolved by injecting another group intravenously to accord a gratuitous effect to the intraperitoneal route.

This was strikingly illustrated by the injection of copper acetate in chicks (McCormick and Fleet, 1988). Mortality following a single dose of 1.84 mg kg^{-1} (Cu) was 46% by intraperitoneal injection but only 4% by intravenous administration even though the accumulation of copper at 24 h in total hepatic tissue and cytosol was comparable for both routes. Copious peritoneal fluid, equivalent to 41% of total plasma volume, was observed 1–3 h after intraperitoneal injections but not after intravenous administrations. The peritoneal fluid was assumed to be plasma because it was clear, was amber-coloured and lacked red blood cells. The authors were impressed by the extent and rapidity with which this fluid formed, postulated its pathogenesis by increased permeability of peritoneal capillaries, and inferred that death was caused by haemoconcentration not by hepatotoxicity.

Another difference between these routes was demonstrated by the administration of lead acetate to mice (Maintani et al., 1986). Following a single dose of 30 mg kg^{-1} (Pb), the intraperitoneal injection induced twice as much metallothionein in the liver than the intravenous administration despite a lower hepatic concentration of the metal. This difference prompted the authors to suggest a role of leucocytic endogenous mediator or interleukin 1, produced by peritoneal leucocytes, for metallothionein induction.

The intrapleural route has often been used in toxicology to circumvent inhalation exposure but, like the peritoneum, the pleura is highly sensitive. This was shown in anaesthetized rats by the intrapleural instillation, via a surgical incision, of 2 μm inert polystyrene microspheres suspended in sterile phosphate-buffered saline (Valdez and Lehnert, 1988). Lavage of the intrapleural space, 24 h after instillation, revealed a threefold increase in the population of free cells, particularly polymorphonuclear leucocytes but also mononuclear phagocytes. Even the saline vehicle alone caused a 40% increase in the number of pleural cells.

VEHICLES AND ADDITIVES

Basically a parenteral drug is a sterile solution, suspension or emulsion of an active constituent in a carrier described as a vehicle or excipient. The formulation may also include other ingredients such as suspending or emulsifying agents, preservatives, antioxidants, buffers and chelating compounds. Usually these additives are incorporated in such small amounts that they have no toxic effects either experimentally or clinically. Therefore, there is no attempt here to list them or to review their inherent toxicities. Vehicles, on the other hand, often constitute a considerable proportion of the formulation, are vital determinants of bioavailability, and consequently merit more attention. It is assumed that their pharmacological activity is minimal and this is usually confirmed by negative findings in control groups conventionally dosed with the vehicle alone. However, the examples cited in this section should alert toxicologists to the potential influences which vehicles may exert on systemic or local toxicity.

Ideally the vehicle should be compatible with the active constituent and should possess no toxic effects at the recommended clinical dose. Also, novel drugs should be tested for toxicity in the vehicle proposed for the final product. Sometimes initial studies may suggest a change in formulation. If this involves vehicle substitution then bioavailability and toxicity studies must be repeated because such a change can have profound effects on the release pattern of the active constituent. For example, when a lyophilized water-soluble glycinate salt of chloramphenicol became available in veterinary medicine to replace the customary solution of propylene glycol, it was found that both the duration and magnitude of plasma antibiotic concentrations were significantly increased in dogs after intramuscular injection (Bergt and Stowe, 1975).

Excipient Solvents

The term excipient is usually defined as any more or less inert substance included in a formulation in order to confer a suitable consistency or form to the product. It also has a wider application to embrace substances with slight pharmacological activity and probably this is more apposite in toxicology. Even water, the essential or true excipient of aqueous solutions, influences toxicity by its effect on osmolarity. The intravenous injection of rats with distilled water, at a volume rate of 1 ml kg^{-1}, induces hypotensive bradycardia and its LD$_{50}$ value in mice is 44 ml kg^{-1} compared with 68 ml kg^{-1} for isotonic saline (Balazs, 1970). Thus the intravenous injection of 1 ml of hypotonic solution might kill a mouse simply because of its excipient. Moreover, such overwhelming volumes should be avoided, even by intravenous infusion, because excessive hydration may alter renal clearance.

Aqueous excipients also have local effects, albeit more detectable biochemically than morphologically. Thus single 1 ml injections of normal saline and sterile water into the dorsal muscles of rabbits raised, within 24 h, serum creatine phosphokinase activities from a normal level of 62 ± 19 iu 1^{-1} to 223 and 537 iu 1^{-1}, respectively (Gray et al., 1974).

Among the non-aqueous solvents, vegetable oils and polyethylene glycol are probably the most pharmacologically inert. Mineral oils, because of their intolerable effects at the injection site, have now been abandoned as vehicles except as inflammatory adjuvants for experimental vaccines. Vegetable oils are common vehicles for intramuscular injections and polyethylene glycols are used for subcutaneous and intravenous routes. The solubility of water-insoluble components often increases exponentially with increasing concentration of solvent in water. Thus, to reduce dose, the concentration of a non-aqueous solvent may be kept up to 40%. However the dose of such a solvent should not exceed 20% of its LD_{50} value (Balazs, 1970). Compatibility of solutions incorporating non-aqueous solvents with plasma should be investigated in vitro before definitive formulation.

Glycerol formal is another common organic solvent for experimental drugs and provides a good example of the variable influence which a vehicle may confer on toxicity according to its application and route of administration. Generally it is regarded as rather inert and this was illustrated by its negligible effect in dose volumes of up to 0.2 ml kg^{-1} on the acute intravenous toxicities of various pyrethrins and pyrethroids in rats (Verschoyle and Barnes, 1972). Moreover, by the intraperitoneal route, it increased the LD_{50} value of cismethrin above that determined by oral dosing, a contrary expectation for pyrethroids (Gray and Soderlund, 1985). On the other hand, glycerol formal administered intramuscularly to the pregnant rat was embryotoxic and teratogenic in positive relation to doses from 0.25 to 1.0 ml kg^{-1} per day (Aliverti et al., 1978). This prompted the authors to recommend more teratology on solvents proposed for toxicity studies.

Another undesirable property of glycerol formal, which it shares with other vehicles such as propylene glycol, is local irritancy. Propylene glycol is completely miscible with water and dissolves in many oils. It used to be a common vehicle for veterinary antibiotics such as chloramphenicol and oxytetracycline. The well known painful response by animals to intramuscular injections of these formulations was attributed, at least in part, to the propylene glycol base (Bergt and Stowe, 1975). Glycerol formal, which contributes 75% of the vehicle for certain potentiated sulphonamides, has been similarly implicated. Both of these solvents cause intramuscular necrosis. This was demonstrated in pigs 6 days after injections with 5 ml doses of 33% glycerol formal and 40% propylene glycol (Rasmussen and Svendsen, 1976). Loss of creatine phosphokinase from the intramuscular site of rabbits injected with propylene glycol or glycerol formal has been proposed as a predictive tool for local toxicity (Svendsen et al., 1978).

Oily Vehicles

Parenteral drugs with a poor aqueous solubility are commonly formulated in vegetable oils as solutions, suspensions or emulsions. Oil is slowly absorbed from an intramuscular or subcutaneous injection site and the duration of pharmacological action of drugs dissolved or emulsified in oily vehicles is prolonged by comparison with that of aqueous formulations. When a drug dissolved entirely in an oily solvent is injected into muscle it is partitioned between the oil and the surrounding aqueous tissue phase and then absorption occurs mainly via the latter followed by diffusion through capillaries. The absorption rate of the oily solvent itself, such as methyl oleate, is much slower than that of the drug dissolved in it (Tanaka et al., 1974).

It has been assumed that the fate of injected oil was a local metabolic degradation, phagocytosis and absorption into the blood. It is now known that some of it is absorbed into the lymphatic system, although this may be a minor pathway. The first human case history of lymphadenopathy following repeated oil-based injections was a 17-year-old male who presented with an enlarged left inguinal lymph node (Ahmed and Greenwood, 1973). The lymphadenopathy was a foreign body giant cell reaction to cystic spaces which contained neutral fat and it was attributed to therapy for diabetes insipidus by regular self-administered injections of pitressin tannate in arachis oil into the left thigh.

Then a comprehensive study was performed in dogs, rabbits and rats on the fate of vegetable oils after intramuscular injection (Svendsen and Aaes-Jorgensen, 1979). The vehicles tested were sesame oil, containing mainly long-chain saturated and unsaturated fatty acids such as oleic and linoleic acid, and a commercial product, composed only of short-chain fatty acids, particularly caprylic and capric acid. In different experiments administration was single or repeated, sometimes ^{14}C-labelled, and detection of oil was by histology including frozen sections, liquid scintillation counting and autoradiography. Pulmonary oil microembolism occurred in dogs injected with either vehicle intramuscularly once a week for 6 months at a volume dose rate of 0.45 ml kg^{-1}. The iliac lymph nodes in the sesame group were enlarged and cystic due to the presence of oil. Pulmonary microembolism was also detected in rabbits and rats injected three times a week for 2 and 5 weeks, respectively. The authors concluded that both vehicles caused pulmonary microembolism by a lymphogenic pathway despite different absorption characteristics. However, the doses were considerably higher than those recommended clinically for most depot preparations and were administered more frequently.

Apart from its own fate, the oil used as a drug vehicle may exert secondary or remote effects which the unwary toxicologist could miss. In a 74 week study on progesterone, beagles were injected subcutaneously and aseptically daily in different dorsal sites with the hormone dissolved in 90% ethyl oleate, 7% ethanol and 3% benzyl alcohol (Capel-Edwards *et al.*, 1973). The vehicle volume dose rate was $0.07 \, \text{ml kg}^{-1}$ up to week 36 and $0.2 \, \text{ml kg}^{-1}$ thereafter. Reactions at the injection sites occurred in all dogs, including controls injected with the vehicle alone, especially after the increase in dose volume at 37 weeks. They included sterile abscesses which ulcerated and healed. The ensuing haematological changes included neutrophil leucocytosis, increased erythrocyte sedimentation rate, mild anaemia, haemosiderosis and thrombocytosis. These were interpreted as representing a low-grade chronic inflammatory condition and, since they occurred in both control and progesterone-treated animals, were regarded as secondary effects of the subcutaneous reaction caused by the oily vehicle.

Other Ingredients

Examples of some common non-vehicular ingredients of parenteral drug formulations are as follows: the preservatives chlorocresol, benzoic acid, sorbic acid, phenol, benzethonium chloride and the esters of *p*-hydroxybenzoic acid; the antioxidants sodium metabisulphite and formaldehyde sulphoxylates; and the chelating agents citric acid and disodium ethylenediaminetetraacetic acid. Many of these compounds are toxic but they rarely increase pharmaceutical toxicity because of their low inclusion rates. Moreover, dilution may decrease toxicity. For example, the intraperitoneal LD_{50} values determined in the rat for sodium metabisulphite, an antioxidant added to solutions for peritoneal dialysis, were 498, 650 and $740 \, \text{ml kg}^{-1}$ for 25, 5 and 1.25% solutions, respectively (Wilkins *et al.*, 1968). However, the toxicologist should not disregard minor ingredients of novel formulations and should always consider their potential roles in unexpected circumstances. For instance, the consumption of a single meal containing only 1% benzoic acid may be fatal to the cat (Clarke, 1975). Also, it should be noted that autoclaving parenteral solutions may alter the relative proportions of constituents.

The author encountered one case of preservative toxicity, albeit in a statutory quality control test without clinical repercussions (Walker, 1979). The test, on allergen extracts, required no deaths in five mice, each weighing approximately 20 g, within 24 h of 1 ml intraperitoneal injections of the final product. Infrequently, but expensively, batches failed and phenol, incorporated in the product at a 0.4% concentration, was thought to be responsible. An intraperitoneal LD_1 for phenol was determined as $190 \, \text{mg kg}^{-1}$. This suggested that one in every 100 mice might die from phenol toxicity *per se*, i.e. one in 20 batches of extract would fail irrespective of any allergen toxicity. As a result, the test dose was reduced.

QUALITY CONTROL TESTS

Biological quality control tests are conducted routinely, and usually statutorily, on batch samples of finished pharmaceutical and biological products and on medical devices or extracts prepared from them. They are also performed on drugs and materials undergoing development, but less frequently. The statutory obligations are in compliance with pharmacopoeial methods or other official standards. These tests are designed to provide a broad screen for the detection of microbiological, endotoxic or chemical contamination and misformulation which might result in overdosage. Their objectives are in variously described as verifications of freedom from 'unexpected or unacceptable biological reactivity' and 'abnormal or undue toxicity'. Collectively and historically they have probably been of considerable benefit in the protection of patients from contaminated parenteral injections and tissue implantations but conceivably their future role will diminish as chemical analyses and microbiological assays become increasingly sophisticated by good manufacturing practice. For each type of test there are numerous variations on a theme which include differences between national pharmacopoeias and modifications of these official methods by the quality control departments of the manufacturers. Most biological quality control tests may be distinguished from other more or less standard toxicological protocols by their dependence on numerical pass–fail criteria, either of magnitude (e.g. temperature response in pyrogen tests) or frequency (e.g. lethality in safety tests). Usually, but not invariably, their interpretation does not require toxicological or pathological expertise. Nevertheless, they are included in this chapter because almost invariably their methods involve parenteral routes.

The most commonly conducted biological quality control tests are for pyrogenicity of parenteral products in rabbits, abnormal toxicity of pharmaceuticals in mice, safety of biologicals in guinea-pigs, muscle implantation of medical devices in rabbits and intracutaneous reactivity of rubber or plastic extracts in rabbits. These tests are described and evaluated below. There are other tests in this broad category which, because of their relatively infrequent use, are not appraised here. These include blood pressure response to depressor substances in cats and anaphylaxis of potential allergens in guinea-pigs. Few regulatory authorities now seem to require the traditional methods of antigenicity testing (Ronneberger, 1977).

The Pyrogen Test

The rabbit pyrogen test has been used extensively now for 50 years, principally to detect bacterial endotoxins in finished pharmaceutical parenteral products. In fact, the method is probably the oldest and most frequently used protocol in animal toxicology. Even so its demise is approaching by the increasing adoption of an alternative *in vitro* technique. Most pyrogens are bacterial endotoxins, lipopolysaccharide components of Gram-negative bacteria. They are potent ubiquitous substances, resistant to steam sterilization, and readily contaminate parenteral solutions from inadequately treated water and raw materials.

A positive response in the rabbit test may be obtained with tap water. The necessity for high-quality water to carry parenteral drugs was recognized by the detection of pyrogens in rabbits and the attribution of a microbiological origin to them (Seibert, 1923). This led to the design and adoption of the rabbit pyrogen test in a standard protocol which was first officially recognized in the US Pharmacopeia in 1942.

The suitability of the rabbit model was thoroughly investigated by a direct comparison of response between man and and animal following the intravenous injection in both species of purified endotoxins in various doses. The endotoxins were prepared from *Salmonella typhosa*, *Escherichia coli* and *Pseudomonas* (Greisman and Hornick, 1969). Human volunteers were inmates of a house of correction. The experimental design included a recognition of differences between the species such as circadian influence in man and emotional lability in the rabbit. It was found that, on a unit bodyweight basis, rabbit and man were similarly sensitive to threshold pyrogenic quantities of endotoxin. This work, preceded and succeeded by thousands of pyrogen tests on numerous products, validated the rabbit model.

The objective of the rabbit pyrogen test is the measurement of temperature rise following intravenous aseptic injection of sterile test substance. Official methods are well described in current editions of pharmacopoeias (e.g. British Pharmacopoeia, 1993; European Pharmacopoeia, 1997; United States Pharmacopeia, 1995). Dose rates for licensed products are prescribed in the pharmacopoeial monographs and those for developmental compounds are usually determined by the clinical intention or an increase on this below the level of acute intravenous toxicity. Other protocols include limitations on the re-use of rabbits previously exposed to antigenic materials or cytotoxic drugs (Personeus, 1969) and extraction procedures for medical devices (e.g. International Organization for Standardization, 1992).

All methods require the initial use of three rabbits preconditioned to the technique. Minimum weights are stipulated but neither sex nor breed is specified. Injections are administered in a marginal ear vein at volume rates of between 0.5 and 10 ml kg^{-1}. Temperatures are recorded by rectal thermocouple or thermister probe thermometers at intervals for up to 90 min before injection (to derive the baseline: initial or control) and for 3 h after (to determine the maximum). The difference between the maximum and the initial (British Pharmacopoeia and European Pharmacopoeia) or control (US Pharmacopeia) is the response. Differences between the British or European and American methods comprise rabbit conditioning before definitive use, rabbit qualification according to previous use, rabbit eligibility with respect to baseline temperature, pass–fail criteria of summed or individual response and re-test requirements following an inconclusive result. The prolonged perpetuation of these differences has little to commend it since the specifications were set arbitrarily and each method has been used extensively to test numerous identical products. Fortunately, both methods address the biological vagaries of the rabbit model. Thus environmental conditions are specified to allay excitement, conditioning is obligatory and re-use, which improves the reliability of response (Weary and Wallin, 1973), is neither discouraged nor permitted so frequently that it might influence sensitivity (Webb, 1969). Also, immature rabbits, which are significantly more resistant than mature animals to endotoxic pyrogens (Greisman and Hornick, 1969) are precluded from use.

The rabbit pyrogen test has been managed traditionally in some laboratories by quality control chemists or microbiologists, not toxicologists, and this may be one reason why some of its limitations and contraindications are not always recognized. Several substances and even whole drug classes thwart the test objective by their inherent pharmacological, toxicological or antigenic properties. Examples compiled from relevant publications (Personeus, 1969; Cooper *et al.*, 1971) and the author's own experience are listed in **Table 2**.

Table 2 Pharmacological and iatrogenic interference with the rabbit pyrogen test

Drug class	Example	Complicating effect on pyrogen test
Antipyretic analgesics	Certain steroids	Reversal of pyrogenic response
Hypnotics and anaesthetics	Phenothiazines	Hypothermia decreasing normal temperature
Antigenic agents	Plasma proteins	Potential anaphylactic reaction on re-use
Cytotoxic drugs	Mitozantrone	Progressive nephropathy with re-use
Acutely toxic substances	Potassium salts	Death by too-rapid injection
Miscellaneous	Amphotericin B	Hyperthermia increasing normal temperature

The LAL Test

Injection fever, a hazard of parenteral administration first recognized in the latter part of the nineteenth century, is now part of medical history. The occurrence in patients of febrile reactions to injections has been eliminated by a combination of decontaminating parenteral water, batch pyrogen testing of finished products and aseptic administration technique. The contribution of the rabbit test is difficult to assess but it has probably been considerable. Now, though, it is becoming replaced by an *in vitro* technique.

The search for an alternative method was prompted by the high cost of the rabbit test in labour and time; its shortcomings which have been tabulated; its non-quantitative nature; and perhaps latterly by a modern inclination to avoid the use of live laboratory animals. However, the precipitant factor for this search was the inapplicability of the rabbit test to short-lived radiopharmaceuticals. This led directly to the first successful application of an *in vitro* alternative (Cooper *et al.*, 1971). It was based on the discovery by previous workers that a lysate of circulating amoebocytes from the horseshoe crab, *Limulus polyphemus*, reacted in aqueous media with picogram quantities of endotoxin to form a gel. Limulus amoebocyte lysate (LAL) became commercially available and its use to test a variety of parenteral products was soon investigated. Excellent correlation was obtained with results by the rabbit test after due allowance was made for the greater sensitivity of the LAL method (Eibert, 1972).

In 1973, the US Food and Drug Administration declared LAL a biological product, subject to licensing requirements, which could be used voluntarily by pharmaceutical manufactures for the in-process testing of drugs but which was not suitable to replace the rabbit test. This provided the means of gaining experience in the use of LAL and establishing a database. Its production was improved considerably and modern yields of LAL now consistently exceed 100 times the original endotoxin sensitivity. More extensive correlations with the rabbit test were recorded (Mascoli and Weary, 1979) and in 1980 recognition by the US Pharmacopeia was a significant benchmark. In 1987 a guideline was published on the validation of LAL testing on end-products for human and veterinary drugs, biological products and medical devices (US Food and Drug Administration, 1987). These set forth acceptable conditions for its use in lieu of the rabbit test.

The LAL test was not described in the 1988 British Pharmacopoeia although its use was suggested for radiopharmaceuticals intended for administration into cerebrospinal fluid (British Pharmacopoeia, 1988). However, an edited version of the European method appeared in the 1989 Addendum (British Pharmacopoeia, 1989). The introduction to this stated 'It is expected that this *in vitro* test will find progressive application in appropriate monographs of both the British and European Pharmacopoeias in place of the *in vivo* test for pyrogens'.

This expectation has been borne out between the publications of the first and second editions of this textbook. In the 1993 British Pharmacopoeia a substitution of the rabbit pyrogen test by a test for bacterial endotoxins was introduced (e.g. Water for Injections, Sodium Chloride, Oxytocin, Oxytetracycline), although the former specification persisted in many monographs, particularly those for antibiotics (British Pharmacopoeia, 1993). By 1997 the substitution was more extensive and now (European Pharmacopoeia, 1997) includes more antibiotics (e.g. Cloxacillin, Gentamicin, Streptomycin, Tetracycline). Moreover, it was stated in this pharmacopoeia that the test for bacterial endotoxins could be considered for a product that is defined in a monograph prescribing compliance with the rabbit pyrogen test, although validations would be required. Between these dates the American preference for the LAL test became even more comprehensive so that currently (United States Pharmacopeia, 1995) monographs which still specify the pyrogen test are now relatively rare (e.g. Polymyxin B). Each monograph which now includes the *in vitro* test specifies the concentration of bacterial endotoxin which must not be exceeded. Whereas the result of the rabbit test depends on the dose of pyrogen, that of the LAL test depends on the concentration of endotoxin in the reaction mixture.

Thus we are now observing a considerable substitution of the long established rabbit test by an *in vitro* technique which must be one of the best validated alternatives of all those introduced to toxicology during the last two decades. The regulatory authorities were prudent to insist on a prolonged delay before its official adoption and even now it is not certain that the LAL test will replace the rabbit method completely. It will not, for example, detect non-endotoxic pyrogenicity attributable to chemical contamination, particulate matter and live Gram-positive bacteria, although these exclusions may be largely overcome by good manufacturing practice. Other limitations of the LAL test have been identified (Assal, 1989) and it seems likely that a minority of substances will require the rabbit method for some time yet.

Abnormal Toxicity Tests

The abnormal toxicity or safety test is, by modern toxicological standards, a relatively crude assay, simple and cheap to conduct but completely non-specific in its objective. A typical method for general pharmaceuticals (method A) is the intravenous injection of five mice and their subsequent observation for one or two days. If no mouse dies the batch is released. Traditionally for biological products, two guinea-pigs also are injected, by the intraperitoneal route (method B). Extracts prepared

Table 3 Summary of British, European and American tests for abnormal toxicity or safety

Reference[a]	Title of test	Number and species	Dose and route[b]	Test duration	Pass criteria
General pharmaceuticals					
BP 1993, p. A174	Abnormal Toxicity Method A	5 mice	0.5 ml iv	24 h	No deaths
EP 1997, p. 81	Abnormal Toxicity General	5 mice	0.5 ml iv	24 h	No deaths
USP 1995, p. 1703	Safety (general)	5 mice	0.5 ml iv	48 h	Neither deaths (0/5) nor toxicity ($\leqslant 1/5$)
Biological products					
BP 1993, p. A174	Abnormal Toxicity Method B	5 mice	$\leqslant 1$ ml ip	7 days	Neither deaths nor
		2 guinea pigs	$\leqslant 5$ ml ip	7 days	signs of ill-health
EP 1997, p. 81	Abnormal Toxicity Human Use Immunosera and Vaccines	5 mice	$\leqslant 1$ ml ip	7 days	Neither deaths nor
		2 guinea pigs	$\leqslant 5$ ml ip	7 days	signs of ill-health
EP 1997, p. 82	Abnormal Toxicity Veterinary Use Immunosera and Vaccines	5 mice	0.5 ml sc	7 days	Neither deaths nor significant local
		2 guinea pigs	$\geqslant 2$ ml ip	7 days	or systemic reaction
USP 1995, p. 1703	Safety (biologics)	$\geqslant 2$ mice	0.5 ml ip	7 days	No loss of weight,
		$\geqslant 2$ guinea pigs	5 ml ip	7 days	unexpected responses or deaths
Extracts of solids					
USP 1995, p. 1701	Systemic Injection (elastomeric plastics)	5 mice x 2 groups	50 ml/kg iv/ip[c]	72 h	No reaction to sample significantly greater than that to blank
ISO 10993–11	Systemic Toxicity (medical devices)	Refers to USP for recommended test method			

[a] BP = British Pharmacopoeia (1993); EP = European Pharmacopoeia (1997); USP = United States Pharmacopeia (1995); ISO = International Organization for Standardization (1993).
[b] iv = intravenous; ip = intraperitoneal; sc = subcutaneous.
[c] Route of injection in the tests for medical devices depends on the extractant (and therefore the extract): iv for polar (e.g. saline, alcohol in saline): ip for non-polar (e.g. vegetable oil, polyethylene glycol 400).

from medical devices are tested in two groups of mice: test or sample (extract) and control or blank (extractant). For each of these three product categories there are slight, but incongruous, differences in the national method specifications (**Table 3**). The quantity of test substance to be injected is specified by the individual monograph except that the dose for a biological product may be the label recommendation subject to a maximum volume, as tabulated. Bodyweights, when stipulated, are very approximately 20 g for mice and 300 g for guinea-pigs. The delivery rate for intravenous injections in mice, unless otherwise prescribed, is 0.02–0.03 ml s^{-1}. In most specifications there is a provision for re-test when results are inconclusive and usually the American versions require more animals than the initial number tested.

National variations in the methods probably have minimal influence on the outcome, but there is little merit in their perpetuation and they frustrate laboratories routinely testing to international specifications. The value of the abnormal toxicity test is difficult to assess but almost certainly it has detected contamination or misformulation. However, in the author's experience, failures are extremely rare and usually attributable to faulty technique or intentional over-concentration of active ingredient or preservative to validate the method. The test does not seem to have attracted much scientific appraisal. Good injection technique is essential to avoid spurious results and the importance of animal acclimatization or conditioning has been emphasized by its effect

on bodyweight which, in some specifications, must not decrease over the test duration (Prasad *et al.*, 1978).

The abnormal toxicity test, like the rabbit pyrogen test, is disappearing from pharmacopoeial monographs. Although largely retained (method B) for blood products and biologicals (antisera and vaccines), it is now only required (method A) for other pharmaceuticals derived from bacterial sources (e.g. Bacitracin Zinc, Polymyxin B, Streptokinase) or from human urine (e.g. Chorionic Gonadotrophin, Menotrophin, Urokinase) (British Pharmacopoeia, 1993).

Local Reaction Tests

Intracutaneous tests in rabbits on polar and non-polar extracts of medical devices and plastics are the local equivalents of the systemic toxicity or systemic injection methods in mice. Specified methods of extraction and extractants (**Table 3**, footnote) are identical. Two rabbits are used for each type of extractant and five intracutaneous injections of 0.2 ml are administered in the clipped dorsal skin. The effects of the injections are compared after 24, 48 and 72 h between the sample extract on one side of the spinal column and the blank extractant on the other (United States Pharmacopeia, 1995) or between anterior test and posterior control sites (International Organization for Standardization, 1995). In both methods the local effects of erythema and oedema are accorded standard numerical ratings and the mean difference between test and control sites determines the outcome.

Implantation tests in rabbits are also required for medical devices and plastics, but in this case to evaluate the local effects of direct contact between solid samples and muscle tissue. The international specification (International Organization for Standardization, 1994) applies to externally communicating devices and implants in soft tissue, bone and blood. The American specification (United States Pharmacopeia, 1995) is for plastic materials and other polymers in direct contact with living tissue. The American method stipulates the aseptic implantation of four sterile smooth sample strips, each measuring 10×1 mm, at intervals on one side of the spinal column and two similar negative control strips on the opposite side. Implantation is via wide-bore hypodermic needles into the paravertebral muscles of two healthy adult rabbits. The animals are killed after a minimum period of 120 h and, following a delay for bleeding to cease, the implantation sites are dissected. Reactions, particularly encapsulations, are graded and pass–fail criteria are numerical, based on differences between mean scores for sample and control sites. The international method is similar but specifies not less than three rabbits, four negative control strips, additional implantation of positive control specimens, a minimum duration of 7 days and histology of the sites. It also advocates a less objective assessment of the results. Type of anaesthetic is not suggested but the author advocates the reversible neuroleptanalgesic combination of fluanisone and fentanyl citrate.

The international standard (International Organization for Standardization, 1994) is more comprehensive than the US Pharmacopeia. It is not confined to the short study durations just described, suggests various test systems in addition to the rabbit and also provides protocols for subcutaneous and osseous implantation in addition to the intramuscular route. Evaluation in all cases is a comparison between test and control material according to macroscopic and histopathological responses as a function of time; it is not, unlike the American protocol for muscle, a simple numerical difference and implies interpretation by a toxicologist or pathologist.

In the author's experience, one problem with the muscle implantation test is a tendency for the strips to migrate from their implantation sites, even to subcutaneous positions, and this often prolongs the search for them. Nevertheless, it is an effective detection system for toxic ingredients of solid materials which leach in contact with tissue fluid. It is important to recognize the microscopic effects of the standard negative control strips (additive-free polyethylene). These are typical of skeletal muscle in contact for 1 week with a foreign body and comprise mild mononuclear cell infiltration, multinucleated giant cell formation, fibroplasia, slight dystrophic calcification, muscle fibre atrophy and

centripetal migration of sarcolemmal nuclei. Also, traumatic haemorrhage is common. Positive reactions are similar but more pronounced and additionally include focal necrosis and exudation, particularly of heterophils. It is a useful test, not only for finished products but also to identify unacceptable changes in formulation or manufacturing process such as the introduction of chlorinating cycles to remove bloom on latex catheters (D. Walker, unpublished data).

REFERENCES

Agarwal, D. K., Lawrence, W. H. and Autian, J. (1985). Antifertility and mutagenic effects in mice from parenteral administration of di-2-ethylhexyl phthalate. *J. Toxicol. Environ. Health*, **16**, 71–84.

Ahmed, A. and Greenwood, N. (1973). Lymphadenopathy following repeated oil-based injections. *J. Pathol.*, **111**, 207–208.

Aliverti, V., Bonanomi, L. and Mariani, L. (1978). Teratogenic evaluation of glycerol formol in the rat. *Proc. 20th Congr. Eur. Soc. Toxicol., Berlin*, Abstract No. 84

Assal, A. N. (1989). Comments on pyrogen testing methods. *Anim. Tech.*, **40**, 129–131.

Balazs, T. (1970). In Paget, G. E. (Ed.), *Methods in Toxicology*, Blackwell, Oxford, pp. 49–81.

Baxter, J. S. and Evans, J. M. (1973). Intramuscular injection in the cat. *J. Small Anim. Pract.*, **14**, 297–302.

Bergt, G. and Stowe, C. M. (1975). Comparison of bioavailability of two chloramphenicol preparations in dogs after intramuscular injection. *Am. J. Vet. Res.*, **36**, 1481–1482.

Bivin, W. S. and Timmons, E. H. (1974). In Weisbroth, S. H., Flatt, R. E. and Kraus, A. L. (Eds.), *The Biology of the Laboratory Rabbit*. Academic Press, New York, pp. 76–77.

Blacklock, J. B., Wright, D. C., Dedrick, R. L., Blasberg, R. G., Lutz, R. J., Doppman, J. L. and Oldfield, E. H. (1986). Drug-streaming during intra-arterial chemotherapy. *J. Neurosurg.*, **64**, 284–291.

Blom, L. and Rasmussen, F. (1976). Tissue damage at the injection site after intramuscular injection of drugs in hens. *Br. Poult. Sci.*, **17**, 1–4.

Bonser, G. M. (1969). How valuable the dog in the routine testing of suspected carcinogens? *J. Natl. Cancer Inst.*, **43**, 271–274.

Bozarth, M. A. and Wise, R. A. (1985). Toxicity associated with long-term intravenous heroin and cocaine self-administration in the rat. *J. Am. Med. Assoc.*, **254**, 81–83.

British Pharmacopoeia (1988). *British Pharmacopoeia 1988*, Vol. II. HMSO, London, pp. A183–A185.

British Pharmacopoeia (1989). *British Pharmacopoeia, Addendum (1989)*. HMSO, London, p. A132

British Pharmacopoeia (1993). *British Pharmacopoeia 1993*, Vol. II. HMSO, London, pp. A171–174

Calabresi, P. and Parks, R. E. (1975). In Goodman, L. S. and Gilman, A. (Eds.), *The Pharmacological Basis of Therapeutics*, 5th edn. Macmillan, New York, pp. 1248–1307.

Capel-Edwards, K., Hall, D. E., Fellowes, K. P., Vallance, D. K., Davies, M. J., Lamb, D. and Robertson, W. B. (1973).

Long-term administration of progesterone to the female beagle dog. *Toxicol. Appl. Pharmacol.*, **24**, 474–488.

Carlson, R. W. and Sikic, B. I. (1983). Continuous infusion or bolus injection in cancer chemotherapy. *Ann. Intern. Med.*, **99**, 823–833.

Chen, K. C. and Vostal, J. J. (1981). Aryl hydrocarbon hydroxylase activity induced by injected diesel particulate extract vs inhalation of diluted diesel exhaust. *J. Appl. Toxicol.*, **1**, 127–131.

Clarke, E. G. C. (1975). *Poisoning in Veterinary Practice*. Association of the British Pharmaceutical Industry, London, p. 10.

Cooper, J. F., Levin, J. and Wagner, H. N. (1971). Quantitative comparison of *in vitro* and *in vivo* methods for the detection of endotoxin. *J. Lab. Clin. Med.*, **78**, 138–148.

Dey, M. S., Breeze, R. A., Dey, R. A., Kreiger, R. I., Naser, L. J. and Renzi, B. E. (1982). Disposition and toxicity of paraquat delivered subcutaneously by injection and osmotic pump in the rat. *Toxicologist*, **2**, 96.

Dissin, J., Mills, L. R., Mains, D. L., Black, O. and Webster, P. D. (1975). Experimental induction of pancreatic adenocarcinoma in rats. *J. Natl. Cancer Inst.*, **55**, 857–864.

Dubois, K. P., Kinoshita, F. and Jackson, P. (1967). Acute toxicity and mechanism of action of a cholinergic rodenticide. *Arch. Int. Pharmacodyn.*, **169**, 108–116.

Eibert, J. (1972). Pyrogen testing: horseshoe crabs vs rabbits. *Bull. Parenter. Drug Assoc.*, **26**, 253–260.

Ensminger, W. D., Greenberger, J. S., Egan, E. M., Muse, M. B. and Moloney, W. C. (1979). Technique for preclinical evaluation of continuous infusion chemotherapy with the use of WF rat acute myelogenous leukaemia. *J. Natl. Cancer Inst.*, **62**, 1265–1268.

Epstein, S. S., Fujii, K., Andrea, J. and Mantel, N. (1970). Carcinogenicity testing of selected food additives by parenteral administration to infant Swiss mice. *Toxicol. Appl. Pharmacol.*, **16**, 321–334.

European Pharmacopoeia (1997). *European Pharmacopoeia 1997*, 3rd edn. Council of Europe, Strasbourg, pp. 80–82, 89–95.

Fairhurst, S., Marrs, T. C., Parker, H. C., Scawin, J. W. and Swanston, D. W. (1987). Acute toxicity of T2 toxin in rats, mice, guinea pigs and pigeons. *Toxicology*, **43**, 31–49.

Flecknell, P. A. (1987). In Tuffery, A. A. (Ed.), *Laboratory Animals: an Introduction for New Experimenters*, Wiley, Chichester, pp. 225–246.

Gabrielsson, J., Paalzow, L., Larsson, S. and Blomquist, I. (1985). Constant rate of infusion—improvement of tests for teratogenicity and embryotoxicity. *Life Sci.*, **37**, 2275–2282.

Gersonde, K. and Weiner, M. (1982). The influence of infusion rate on the acute intravenous toxicity of phytic acid, a calcium-binding agent. *Toxicology*, **22**, 279–286.

Grasso, P. and Grant, D. (1977). In Ballantyne, B. (Ed.) *Current Approaches in Toxicology*. Wright, Bristol, pp. 219–220.

Grasso, P. and Goldberg, L. (1966). Subcutaneous sarcoma as an index of carcinogenic potency. *Food Cosmet. Toxicol.*, **4**, 297–320.

Gray, A. J. and Soderlund, D. M. (1985). In Hutson, D. H. and Roberts, T. R. (Eds.), *Insecticides*, Wiley, Chichester, pp. 193–248.

Gray, J. E., Weaver, R. N., Moran, J. and Feenstra, E. S. (1974). The parenteral toxicity of clindamycin 2-phosphate in laboratory animals. *Toxicol. Appl. Pharmacol.*, **27**, 308–321.

Green, C. J. (1979). *Animal Anaesthesia*, Laboratory Animals, London, pp. 135–205.

Greisman, S. E. and Hornick, R. B. (1969). Comparative pyrogenic reactivity of rabbit and man to bacterial endotoxin. *Proc. Soc. Exp. Biol.*, **131**, 1154–1158.

Hirano, T., Stanton, M. and Layard, M. (1974). Measurement of epidermoid carcinoma development induced in the lungs of rats by 3-methylcholanthrene-containing beeswax pellets. *J. Natl. Cancer Inst.*, **53**, 1209–1219.

Homberger, F. (1972). In Homberger, F. (Ed.), *Progress in Experimental Tumor Research. Pathology of the Syrian Hamster*, Karger, Basle, pp. 165–166.

Honda, K., Matuyama, D., Mitarai, H., Nakamura, T., Ota, E. and Tejima, Y. (1973). Toxicological studies on sulphamethoxazole–trimethoprim combination—acute and subacute toxicities. *Chemotherapy*, **21**, 175–186.

Hornick, P. (1986). A new method of giving repetitive intraperitoneal injections to neonatal rats. *Lab. Anim.*, **20**, 14–15.

International Organization for Standardization (1992). *Biological Evaluation of Medical Devices: Sample Preparation and Reference Materials*, ISO 10993–12. ISO, Geneva.

International Organization for Standardization (1993). *Biological Evaluation of Medical Devices: Tests for Systemic Toxicity*, ISO 10993–11. ISO, Geneva.

International Organization for Standardization (1994). *Biological Evaluation of Medical Devices: Tests for Local Effects after Implantation*, ISO 10993–6. ISO, Geneva.

International Organization for Standardization (1995). *Biological Evaluation of Medical Devices: Tests for Irritation and Sensitization*, ISO 10993–10. ISO, Geneva.

Jaeger, R. J. and Rubin, R. J. (1970). Plasticizers from plastic devices: extraction, metabolism and accumulation in biological systems. *Science*, **170**, 460–461.

Kast, A. and Tsunenari, Y. (1983). Hair embolism in lungs of rat and rabbit caused by intravenous injection. *Lab. Anim.*, **17**, 203–207.

Kraus, A. L. (1980). In Baker, H. J., Lindsey, J. R. and Weisbroth, S. H. (Eds.), *The Laboratory Rat. Research Applications*, Academic Press, New York, pp. 20–22.

Lewis, R. E., Kunz, A. L., and Bell, R. E. (1966). Error of intraperitoneal injections in rats. *Lab. Anim. Care*, **16**, 505–509.

Liu, P. L., Feldman, H. S., Giasi, R., Patterson, M. K. and Covino, B. G. (1983). Comparative CNS toxicity of lidocaine, etidocaine, bupivacaine and tetracaine in awake dogs following rapid intravenous administration. *Anesth. Analg.*, **62**, 375–379.

Magee, P. N. (1970). In Paget, G. E. (Ed.) *Methods in Toxicology*, Blackwell, Oxford, p. 173.

Maintani, T., Watahiki, A. and Suzuki, K. T. (1986). Induction of metallothionein after lead administration by three injection routes in mice. *Toxicol. Appl. Pharmacol.*, **83**, 211–217.

Mascoli, C. C. and Weary, M. E. (1979). Limulus amebocyte lysate (LAL) test for detecting pyrogens in parenteral injectable products and medical devices: advantages to manufacturers and regulatory officials. *J. Parenter. Drug Assoc.*, **33**, 81.

McCormick, C. C. and Fleet, J. C. (1988). The toxicity of parenteral copper in the chick: dependence on route of administration. *J. Nutr.*, **118**, 1398–1402.

Montesano, R. and Saffiotti, U. (1968). Carcinogenic response of the respiratory tract of Syrian golden hamsters to different doses of diethylnitrosamine. *Cancer Res.*, **28**, 2197–2210.

Nau, H. (1983). The role of delivery systems in toxicology and drug development. *Pharm. Int*. **4**, 228–231.

Nicholls, P. J. (1970). Trouble-free intravenous injection of rabbits. *J. Inst. Anim. Tech*., **21**, 12.

Patterson, D. S. P., Allen, W. M., Berrett, S., Sweasy, D. and Done, J. T. (1971). The toxicity of parenteral iron preparations in the rabbit and pig with a comparison of the clinical and biochemical responses to iron–dextrose in 2 days old and 8 days old piglets. *Zbl. Vet. Med. A*., **18**, 453–464.

Personeus, G. R. (1969). Pyrogen testing of biologicals and small volume parenterals. *Bull. Parenter. Drug. Assoc*., **23**, 201–207.

Pinedo, H. M., Zaharko, D. S. and Dedrick R. L. (1976). Device for constant sc infusion of methotrexate: plasma results in mice. *Cancer Treat. Rep*., **60**, 889–893.

Plenge, P., Mellerup, E. T. and Norgaard, T. (1981). Functional and structural rat kidney changes caused by peroral or parenteral lithium treatment. *Acta Psychiat. Scand*., **63**, 303–313.

Porter, W. P., Bitar, Y. M., Strandberg, J. D. and Charache, P. C. (1985). A comparison of subcutaneous and intraperitoneal oxytetracycline injection methods for control of infectious disease in the rat. *Lab. Anim*., **19**, 3–6.

Prasad, S., Gatmaitan, B. R. and Oconnell, R. C. (1978) Effect of a conditioning method on general safety test in guinea pigs. *Lab. Anim. Sci*., **28**, 591–593.

Purchase, I. F. H. and van der Watt, J. J. (1969). Acute toxicity of sterigmatocystin to rats. *Food Cosmet. Toxicol*., **7**, 135–139.

Pyörälä, S., Manner, L., Kesti, E. and Sandholm, M. (1994). Local tissue damage in cows after intramuscular injections of eight antimicrobial agents. *Acta Vet. Scand*., **35**, 107–110.

Rasmussen, F. and Hogh, P. (1971). Irritating effect and concentrations at the injection site after intramuscular injection of antibiotic preparations in cows and pigs. *Nord. Vet.-Med*., **23**, 593–605.

Rasmussen, F. and Svendsen, O. (1976). Tissue damage and concentration at the injection site after intramuscular injection of chemotherapeutics and vehicles in pigs. *Res. Vet. Sci*., **20**, 55–60.

Ray, N. and Theeuwes, F. (1987) In Johnson and Lloyd-Jones (eds.), *Drug Delivery Systems*, Ellis Horwood, Chichester, pp. 120–138.

Rhodes, M. L. and Patterson, C. E. (1979). Chronic intravenous infusion in the rat: a nonsurgical approach. *Lab. Anim. Sci*., **29**, 82–84.

Roe, F. J. C. (1975). In Butler, W. H. and Newberne, P. M. (Eds.), *Mouse Hepatic Neoplasia*, Elsevier, Amsterdam, pp. 133–142.

Roe, F. J. C., Carter, R. L., Walters, M. A. and Harington, J. S. (1967). The pathological effects of subcutaneous injections of asbestos fibres in mice: migration of fibres to submesothelial tissues and induction of mesotheliomata. *Int. J. Cancer*, **2**, 628–638.

Ronneberger, H. (1977). In Duncan, W. A. M. and Leonard, B. J. (Eds.), *Clinical Toxicology*, Excerpta Medica, Amsterdam, pp. 141–142.

Rowe, P. H., Starlinger, M. J., Kasdon, E., Hollands, M. J. and Silen, W. (1987). Parenteral aspirin and sodium salicylate are equally injurious to the rat gastric mucosa. *Gastroenterology*, **93**, 863–871.

Rowland, M. (1972). Influence of route of administration on drug availability. *J. Pharm. Sci*., **61**, 70–74.

Schmitz, H., Schaub, E. and Müller, A. (1976). Intramuscular iron therapy. *Schweiz. Arch. Tierheilk*., **118**, 441–479.

Seibert, F. B. (1923). Fever-producing substance found in some distilled waters. *Am. J. Physiol*., **67**, 90.

Sikic, B. I., Collins, J. M., Mimnaugh, E. G. and Gram, T. E. (1978). Improved therapeutic index of bleomycin when administered by continuous infusion in mice. *Cancer Treat. Rep*., **62**, 2011–2017.

Smyth, R. D., Gaver, R. C., Dandekar, K. A., Van Harken, D. R. and Hottendorf, G. H. (1979). Evaluation of the availability of drugs incorporated in rat laboratory diet. *Toxicol. Appl. Pharmacol*., **50**, 493–499.

Stanton, M. F. and Wrench, C. (1972). Mechanisms of mesothelioma induction with asbestos and fibrous glass. *J. Natl. Cancer Inst*., **48**, 797–821.

Stone, M. M., Mulvihill, S. J., Lewin, K. J. and Fonkalsrud, E. W. (1986). Long-term total intraperitoneal nutrition in a rabbit model. *J. Pediatr. Surg*., **21**, 267–270.

Sunderman, F. W. (1983). Potential toxicity from nickel contamination of intravenous fluids. *Ann. Clin. Lab. Sci*., **13**, 1–4.

Suttle, N. F. (1981). Comparison between parenterally administered copper complexes of their ability to alleviate hypocupraemia in sheep and cattle. *Vet. Rec*., **109**, 304–307.

Svendsen, O. (1972). Histologic changes after intramuscular injections with antibiotic preparations. *Nord. Vet.-Med*., **24**, 181–185.

Svendsen, O. and Aaes-Jorgensen, T. (1979). Studies on the fate of vegetable oil after intramuscular injection into experimental animals. *Acta Pharmacol. Toxicol*., **45**, 352–378.

Svendsen, O., Rasmussen, F., Nielsen, P. and Steiness, E. (1978). The loss of creatine phosphokinase (CPK) from the intramuscular injection site of rabbits as a predictive tool for local toxicity. *Proc. 20th Congr. Euro. Soc. Toxicol., Berlin*, Abstract No. 56.

Tanaka, T., Kobayashi, H., Okumura, K., Muranishi, S. and Sezaki, H. (1974). Intramuscular absorption of drugs from oily solutions in the rat. *Chem. Pharm. Bull*., **22**, 1275–1284.

Thompson, S. W., Sparano, B. M. and Diener, R. M. (1971). Vacuoles in the hepatocytes of cortisone-treated dogs. *Am. J. Pathol*., **63**, 135–145.

Toth, B. (1968). A critical review of experiments in chemical carcinogenesis using newborn animals. *Cancer Res*., **28**, 727–738.

US Food and Drug Administration (1987). *Guideline on Validation of the Limulus Amebocyte Lysate Test as an End-Product Endotoxin Test for Human and Animal Parenteral Drugs, Biological Products, and Medical Devices*. US Food and Drug Administration, Rockville.

United States Pharmacopeia, (1995). *United States Pharmacopeia, MD. 23rd Revision*. US Pharmacopeia Convention, Rockville, MD, pp. 1696–1697, 1701–1703, 1718.

Urquhart, J. (1982). Rate-controlled drug dosage. *Drugs*, **23**, 207–226.

Valdez, Y. E. and Lehnert, B. E. (1988). A procedure for instilling agents into the pleural space compartment of the rat without co-administration into the lung compartment. *Anim. Tech*., **39**, 1–8.

Valeriote, F. and Vietti, T. (1985). Comparison of cytotoxicity of single dose and infusion of alkylating agents. *Cancer Drug Delivery*, **2**, 11–18.

Van Alstine, W. G. and Dietrich, J. A. (1988). Porcine sciatic nerve damage after intramuscular injection. *Comp. Food Anim.*, **10**, 1329–1332.

Verschoyle, R. D. and Barnes, J. M. (1972). Toxicity of natural and synthetic pyrethrins to rats. *Pestic. Biochem. Physiol.*, **2**, 308–311.

Wagner, J. C. (1962). Experimental production of mesothelial tumours of the pleura by implantation of dusts in laboratory animals. *Nature*, **196**, 180–181.

Walker, D. (1979). Acute toxicity: how and why? *Proc. Symp. Assoc. Vet. Indu., London*, 7–16.

Walker, D. (1981). An alternative to the LD_{50}: the study of acute sublethal effects. *Proc. Symp. Dutch Soc. Toxicol., Utrecht*, 60–73.

Watson, A. D. J. (1972). Chloramphenicol plasma levels in the dog: a comparison of oral, subcutaneous, and intramuscular administration. *J. Small Anim. Pract.*, **13**, 147–151.

Weary, M. E. and Wallin, R. F. (1973). The rabbit pyrogen test. *Lab. Anim. Sci.*, **23**, 677–681.

Webb, F. W. (1969). In Brown, A. M. (Ed.), *Uniformity*, Carworth Europe, Huntingdon, pp. 11–32.

Wilkins, J. W., Greene, J. A. and Weller, J. M. (1968). Toxicity of intraperitoneal bisulfite. *Clin. Pharmacol. Ther.*, **9**, 328–332.

Wilson, R. C., Duran, S. H., Horton, C. R. and Wright, L. C. (1989). Bioavailability of gentamicin in dogs after intramuscular or subcutaneous injections. *Am. J. Vet. Res.*, **50**, 1748–1750.

Winship, K. A. (1988). Toxicity of tin and its compounds. *Adverse Drug React. Acute Poisoning Rev.*, **7**, 19–38.

Witschi, H. P. (1981). Enhancement of tumor formation in mouse lung by dietary butylated hydroxytoluene. *Toxicology*, **21**, 95–104.

Woodbury, D. M. and Fingle, E. (1975). In Goodman, L. S. and Gilman, A. (Eds), *The Pharmacological Basis of Therapeutics*, 5th edn. Macmillan, New York, p. 328.

World Health Organization (1967). Procedures for investigating intentional and unintentional food additives. *WHO Tech. Rep. Ser.*, 348.

World Health Organization (1969). Principles for the testing and evaluation of drugs for carcinogenicity. *WHO Tech. Rep. Ser.*, 426.

Yuhas, E. M., Morgan, D.G., Arena, E., Kupp, R. P., Saunders, L. Z. and Lewis, H. B. (1985). Arterial medial necrosis and hemorrhage induced in rats by intravenous infusion of fenoldopam mesylate, a dopaminergic vasodilator. *Am. J. Pathol.*, **119**, 83–91.

Chapter 27
Peroral Toxicity

Tipton R. Tyler

CONTENTS

INTRODUCTION

In assessing the toxic properties of any substance, careful consideration must be given to the manner in which it is introduced into the animal. A rapid review of the toxicological literature will quickly reveal that the peroral route is certainly the most common method of administration encountered. There are a number of reasons for this, not the least of which is the ease and quantitative determination of dose administration. It is a route by which a large number of substances gain entrance into the animal body, i.e. many pharmaceutical preparations are designed to be administered orally. Environmental contaminants that enter drinking water supplies will be inadvertently ingested. It is virtually impossible to avoid ingestion of traces of chemical residues used on field crops, used in animal husbandry and used in food processing or in food packaging. Ingestion of chemicals adsorbed on soil particles associated with landfills needs to be considered in assessing potential risks. In addition, it is often important to gain toxicological information on substances which could be accidentally swallowed or swallowed in suicidal or homicidal incidents.

At times the peroral route of administration is used to study the toxic effects of a material when the primary concern is by some other mode of exposure, e.g. inhalation or dermal exposure. Often this is done because it is far easier to obtain a quantitative estimate of dose when delivered perorally. In some instances where a chemical might have a low vapour pressure, inhalation studies cannot be conducted at vapour concentrations high enough to assess toxic properties even though inhalation would be considered the most likely route of exposure. In other instances certain end-points may be technically difficult to measure when the most appropriate route of exposure is considered, for instance conducting motor activity or behavioural studies while animals are being treated by occluded dermal application.

Route to route extrapolation requires an in-depth knowledge of a number of biological, chemical and physical processes, including an understanding of the anatomy, physiology and the pharmacodynamics and pharmacokinetics of the test substance. It should be remembered that a major consideration in toxicological assessment of test substances is the route of administration. When technically feasible, the route of administration should be appropriate to realistic exposure scenarios. This is particularly important in the field of risk assessment where route to route extrapolations add to the uncertainty already inherent in the imprecise approximations and assumptions used to obtain the risk estimates. However, where the nature of the testing requires alternative modes of dosing, physiologically based pharmacokinetic (PBPK) modelling has proved useful as this methodology does incorporate much of the known physiological and biological information concerning the absorption distribution and excretion in various animal species.

This chapter will review techniques used in peroral administration studies, discuss variables in the design of peroral studies which may influence the expression of toxicological responses and point out some specific characteristics of peroral administration which must be carefully considered when attempting route to route extrapolation. Initially, however, it is important to review some anatomical features and physiological processes that can affect toxicological responses of perorally administered chemical substances.

ANATOMICAL CONSIDERATIONS

Anatomical features that can affect the toxic manifestations of ingested substances both between various animal species and within the same species include:

- The structure of the gastro-intestinal (GI) tract, particularly the upper portion of the tract which is often involved when dosing animals by gavage or intubation.
- The type of cellular lining in various parts of the GI tract.
- The location and nature of glands which empty secretions into the tract.
- The blood supply and drainage patterns from various parts of the tract.
- The innervation of the tract.

Morphology

The arrangement of the pharynx, epiglottis and oesophagus determines the ease with which substances can be administered to animals by gavage or intubation. In rats and mice these structures are relatively straight and unobstructed by folds of tissue. Grasping these animals by folds of skin on the dorsal aspect of the head and neck with gentle extension of the neck allows for easy passage of an animal feeding needle into the oesophagus and stomach. Accomplished technicians can dose several animals per minute by this method with amazingly few errors; errors in which the material inadvertently gains entrance to the trachea (lunging the animal). The structure in guinea pigs and rabbits, on the other hand, is complicated by folds of tissue which impede the direct entrance of rigid feeding needles and often flexible tubing is employed in dosing rather than stainless-steel needles. This procedure generally requires more time. In general, technical considerations including animal size require the use of flexible intubation for dogs, monkeys and other larger mammals.

The GI tract is exposed to wide variety of chemical and physical conditions, some of which are hostile or incompatible with life. Organisms, therefore, have developed resistant cellular linings of this tube to protect the surrounding visceral elements from the GI tract contents. The mouth and oesophagus of rodents are lined with keratinized stratified squamous epithelium, while that of primates and man is of the non-keratinized type (Ham and Cormack, 1979). In both cases the cellular lining is designed primarily for protection against mechanical abrasion and chemical corrosion rather than for absorptive function. The cells undergo continual renewal with mitotic division taking place in the deepest 2–3 layers, the older cells being displaced toward the lumen.

All rodents have two distinct areas of the stomach, the non-glandular or forestomach and the glandular stomach (**Figure 1**). The forestomach is developed to the greatest degree in ruminant species (consisting of the rumen and abomasom), to different degrees in various rodent species and is not present in man or primates. The function of this organ is generally believed to be for the storage of food, although in ruminants and some other species (Bauchop and Martucci, 1968; Dellow *et al.*, 1983; Grajal *et al.*, 1989) it acts as a fermentation vessel from which the animal derives a major portion of its energy needs. The cellular lining of the forestomach is a continuation of the oesophageal keratinized squamous epithelium. There are relatively few glands scattered in the submucosa of the oesophagus and forestomach; those that are present secrete mucus, primarily for the purpose of lubrication to assist in the passage of food.

In rodents, the true or glandular stomach is separated from the forestomach by elevated border, the dividing or limiting ridge (**Figure 1**). This distinct structure assists in maintaining some degree of separation of the stomach contents between the forestomach and the true or glandular stomach. In contrast to the forestomach, the

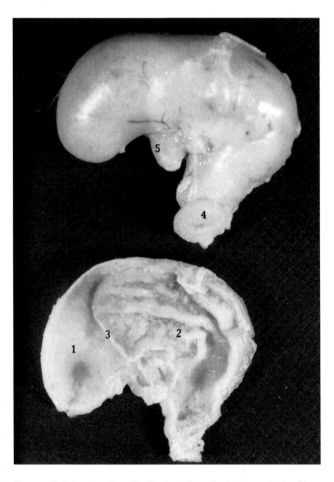

Figure 1 Intact and longitudinal section of rat stomach. 1 = Non-glandular or forestomach; 2 = glandular stomach; 3 = limiting ridge; 4 = pylorus; 5 = oesophagus.

mucosal lining of the true stomach is thicker and characterized by a columnar lining which form numerous tubular glands or gastric pits. Three types of secreting cells are found in this lining: neck cells, which secrete mucous, which acts to protect the lining from the hostile, acidic environment; parietal cells, which secrete hydrochloric acid; and chief cells, which secrete digestive proenzymes, including pepsinogen.

The flow of gastric contents from the stomach to the duodenum is controlled by the pyloric sphincter. This structure normally remains closed, limiting the flow of stomach contents to the small intestine. The sphincter is controlled by both hormones and nervous impulses and is influenced by factors such as the degree of distention of the duodenum, the degree of irritation to the duodenal mucosa, the acidity of the duodenal chyme, the degree of osmolality of the chyme and the presence of products of digestion, particularly those of meat and to a lesser extent fat (Guyton, 1981).

The epithelium of the small intestine is designed to perform efficient absorptive functions but, in addition, performs some secretory functions. The walls of the small intestine are highly convoluted in nature. The mucosal lining is arranged in tiny projections known as intestinal villi. The epithelial cells lining the luminal surface and forming the intestinal villa are characterized by possessing numerous microvilli. The entire structure, therefore, possesses a tremendous surface area through which absorption can occur. The columnar cells lining the small intestine are in a process of continual renewal; it is estimated that the entire intestinal epithelium is renewed every third day (Ham and Cormack, 1979).

In addition to the epithelial cells lining the tract, glandular structures are also present. The ducts of the exocrine glands, the liver and pancreas, empty into the small intestine in the very upper portion of the duodenum. Brunner's glands, composed of goblet cells, are also found in great number, primarily in the submucosa of the proximal portion of the duodenum. These glands secrete mucous into the lumen that acts both as a protective coating of the lining and to serve in a lubricating role. Various digestive enzymes are secreted from the crypts of Lieberkühn.

The primary function of the large intestine is to absorb water. The epithelial lining differs from that of the small intestine in that no villi are present. The secretory cells of the crypts of Lieberkühn are primarily goblet cells that secrete mucous for lubricating and protective purposes. As the chyme passes through the large intestine, therefore, the liquid aqueous phase is absorbed and the solid material becomes more concentrated. The external and internal anal and sphincters control the flow of semisolid faecal material from the tract. In some species the caecum is well developed and serves as a vessel in which digestion occurs through fermentation.

Circulation

The circulatory pattern of the GI tract is a particularly important consideration when extrapolating toxicological data obtained from peroral studies to other routes of exposure. Arterial blood is supplied by a number of arteries. However, the veins draining the tract, from the lower oesophagus to the very distal portion of the rectum, flow into a single vein, the portal vein. All portal vein blood empties into the sinusoids of the liver; thus all material absorbed from the lower portion of the oesophagus to the rectum is delivered to the liver prior to entering the general systemic circulation. During this 'first pass' the liver, being the major organ for the metabolism of most xenobiotic substances and many other endogenous chemicals, may modify, through metabolic processes, a significant portion of an absorbed nutrient or toxicant. Thus, a major portion of an absorbed chemical can be metabolized prior to being delivered to the potential target organ through systemic circulation. This can lead to either enhancement of toxicity in the case of metabolic activation, or moderation of the toxicity in the case of detoxification, over what might occur by another route of administration where the liver is not the first organ encountered, e.g. pulmonary or dermal exposure. Expressions of toxic responses moderated by the hepatic portal pattern of blood circulation are often referred to as the 'first pass effects'.

In contrast to the portal venous drainage of the major portion of the GI tract, the drainage of the buccal cavity, the mouth and the tongue, is into the jugular vein and hence directly enters the general systemic circulation, bypassing the hepatic–portal loop. This is the reason why certain drugs that are rapidly metabolized by liver enzymes are administered by buccal absorption, e.g. nitroglycerin. An analogous pattern exists at the juncture of the rectum and anus. Here there is an anastomosis of veins of the hepatic portal system and the systemic system (Johnson, 1981). This pattern of circulation allows a portion of a pharmaceutical rectal suppository preparations to be absorbed directly into the systemic circulatory system.

Innervation

Movement of contents through the GI tract is controlled by peristaltic contractions of the smooth muscle fibres within the structural portion of the walls of the tube. The contractions of these muscle fibres are mediated by the autonomic nervous system and, to some extent, by hormonal secretions. The GI tract has an intrinsic nervous system that extends from the oesophagus to the anus. This intrinsic system is under the control of both parasympathetic and sympathetic signals from the brain. With the exception of the very proximal and distal portion of the tract, parasympathetic innervation arises from the vagus nerve. The sympathetic innervation arises from the spinal cord between segments T-8 and L-3, preganglionic fibres passing down the spinal cord to various ganglia, and postganglionic fibres accompanying the blood vessels to the various parts of the tract. In general, stimulation of the parasympathetic system increases strength and frequency of mixing and propulsive contractions of the smooth muscles of the GI tract wall, thereby leading to an increased movement of contents through the tract. Sympathetic stimulation, on the other hand, has an opposite effect and strong sympathetic stimulation can completely block the movement of the contents through the tract.

Afferent nerve fibres also arise in the gut wall and are stimulated by processes such as irritation of the mucosa and distention of the wall of the tract. Signals from these fibres are processed in the medulla and contribute to overall control of the movement of contents through the tract. In addition, in some species these afferent fibres send signals to the vomiting centre in the medulla, leading to emesis or the expulsion of gastric and intestinal contents (Smith, 1986). The vomiting reflex can be initiated by various stimuli on the GI tract, e.g. irritation or distention of various segments of the tract, and also by direct action of agents on an area known as the chemoreceptor trigger zone of the vomiting centre in the medulla itself, e.g. chemical emetics such as ipecac (Venho, 1986). Not all mammalian species are capable of vomiting; in general, rodents and rabbits are believed to be incapable of expressing the vomiting reflex, whereas dogs, cats, monkeys and man certainly exhibit the reflex when stimulated. The fact that an animal may exhibit the reflex can cause problems in administering certain test substances by the peroral route.

PHYSIOLOGICAL CONSIDERATIONS

Physiological factors that affect the absorption of both nutrients and exogenous chemical substances include:

- The concentration of the substance in the GI tract contents;
- The pH of the GI tract contents;
- The ionic concentration of the GI tract contents;
- The rate of passage of the contents through the tract;
- The surface area available for absorption;
- The blood supply to the serosal side of the GI tract wall.

Factors Affecting pH and Volume

The pH of the milieu is particularly important in the case of ionic materials, as they are absorbed almost entirely in the non-charged state, i.e. as free acids or free bases. Crouthamel *et al.* (1971) demonstrated that the non-ionized forms of the drugs sulfaethidole and barbital were absorbed 3–5 times faster from either the stomach or the intestine of the rat than the ionized forms. Schanker *et al.* (1957) demonstrated that acids having a pK_a value greater than 2 were, in general, well absorbed from the stomach of rats when introduced in a 0.1 M HCl solution. Strong acids such as sulphonic acids, phenolsulphonphthalein and 5-sulphosalicylic acid were not absorbed under these conditions, nor were organic bases having a pK_a greater than 2.5. On the other hand, the absorption of acids was distinctly depressed when they were introduced into the rat stomach in 0.15 M sodium bicarbonate solution, while a marked increase in the absorption of bases was noted under these conditions.

The pH and volume of GI tract contents are controlled by a number of hormonal and neurological mechanisms, and vary in accordance with the feeding cycle. In the postprandial state the stomach secretes HCl at only a fraction of the maximal rate. The empty stomach, therefore, contains a relatively small volume of acidified fluid. HCl is secreted by the parietal cells of the glandular stomach, secretion being primarily under the control of the hormone gastrin and the parasympathetic mediator acetylcholine. Other mediators of HCl secretion include histamine and perhaps an intestinal-derived hormone, enterooxyntin (Johnson, 1985). Gastric secretion is stimulated by the anticipation of feeding and by tasting, smelling, chewing and swallowing food. These stimuli to gastric secretion are mediated through the nervous system, and in particular by impulses delivered by the vagus nerve. In addition to the neurological stimulation of the secretory pathways, distention of the stomach and the presence of specific molecular species such as amino acids and peptides stimulate the secretion of gastrin and subsequently HCl.

Ingestion of food will dilute the acidic fluid in the empty stomach, resulting in the release of gastrin and the subsequent production of HCl by the parietal cells. As the digestion process continues, the release of HCl eventually overwhelms the buffering capacity of the chyme. Gastrin secretion is inhibited at pH values below 3 and blocked at pH values of 2 and less. Therefore, by a classical feedback mechanism, further gastrin release and consequently HCl secretion are prevented.

Secretions from the cells of the intestinal lining tend to neutralize chyme flowing from the stomach. The secretion of fluid and bicarbonate by the mucosal cells of the duodenum is controlled by the quantity of acid which flows through the cardiac valve (Johnson, 1985). These secretions, both enzymes and bicarbonate, are secreted from the acinar cells. It is the pancreatic secretions, however, which account for the major portion of neutralization of acid coming from the stomach. Pancreatic secretions are not only under the control of the acid environment, but also respond to nervous stimuli arising primarily from the vagus nerve. Pancreatic secretions are also under hormonal control, being stimulated by release of secretin and cholecystokinin. Secretin appears to control the release of the alkaline component of the pancreatic and intestinal secretions, water and bicarbonate, while cholecystokinin stimulates the release of the enzymatic component, i.e. pepsin, amylases and lipases.

Factors Affecting Movement of Contents

Mixing and movement of contents down the intestinal tract occur by the rhythmic contractions, peristalsis, of the stomach and intestine. The contractions are produced by the layers of smooth muscle, which comprise the outer layer of the GI tract walls. In the stomach nervous impulses arise primarily from the vagus nerve bringing about strong contractions of the smooth muscle layers. In the small intestine the contractions are controlled by activities of the smooth muscle cells themselves in addition to being initiated by nervous impulses (Weisbrodt, 1985). Humeral substances, endogenous and exogenous chemicals, and physical distention affect the motility of the GI tract. Epinephrine inhibits whereas serotonin stimulates contractions. Gastrin, cholecystokinin and other hormones, e.g. motilin, stimulate contractions whereas secretin has an inhibitory action.

Under normal conditions, the contractions of the stomach result in mixing of ingested food with the gastric secretions. The peristaltic activity within the small intestine occurs in relatively short segments, primarily leading to mixing action allowing for maximum contact with the vast surface area of the intestinal lining. The small and large intestine are capable of undergoing coordinated contractions which can cause the movement of the chyme through the entire tract in a relatively short period of time. In addition, there appear to be other mechanisms which promote the rapid movement of certain materials throughout the upper GI tract. Frederick *et al.* (1992), for instance, demonstrated that in rats up to 15% of a gavage dose of ethyl acrylate administered in corn oil can be recovered from the duodenum and 3% in the ileum within 1–2 min after administration.

The effect of the rate of passage of GI tract contents can be complex. Upon first consideration, the longer a solute remains in contact with an absorptive surface, the greater is the likelihood of absorption. Thus, physiological states or conditions that impede transport through the intestinal tract would be expected to increase the amount of material absorbed. There are conditions, however, where prolonged retention in parts of the tract may lead to decreased absorption and a reduction in the potency of a toxicant or the efficacy of a pharmaceutical preparation. Thus, retention of acid-labile penicillin or erythromycin in the stomach can lead to drug degradation and a lowering of the efficacy of these antibiotics (Welling, 1984).

Factors Affecting Circulation

An increase in blood flow to the GI tract accompanies the postprandial increase in GI tract secretions and motility. The increase in blood flow is relatively greater to the gastric and intestinal mucosa and pancreas than to the GI tract musculature. Blood flow increases are mediated by hormones secreted from the intestinal mucosa; glucagon and cholecystokinin act to increase the blood flow to the intestine and pancreas and gastrin to the gastric mucosa. Presumably the blood flow to the GI tract tissue results from vasodilatation caused by the indirect release of local vasodilator metabolites along with direct stimulatory action of cholecystokinin and acetylcholine released by vagal discharge.

ABSORPTION MECHANISMS

There are five different means by which nutrients and exogenous materials can pass from the mucosal side of the GI tract across to the serosal side:

- Passive diffusion through a lipid membrane;
- Diffusion through pores;
- Active energy-dependent transport;
- Absorption through lymphatics;
- Absorption of macromolecules by pinocytosis.

Effects of pH and Volume

A number of barriers are present to impede the simple diffusion of molecules across the membranes of the epithelial cells lining the tract. First, the molecules must transverse the unstirred layers of fluid lying immediately adjacent to the membrane, then cross the mucus layer coating the membrane and finally cross the bilipid membrane itself into the cell. Once within the cytoplasm of the cell, the molecule must pass through the cytoplasm and then through the basement membrane and the capillary or lymphatic wall membranes. The bilipid structure of the cell membrane greatly favours the absorption of hydrophobic species over hydrophilic species. This accounts for the greater absorption rate of non-ionized species over ionized species, as demonstrated by Crouthamel *et al.* (1971) and Schanker *et al.* (1957). The fact that ionized forms are absorbed to a slight degree may be the result of microenvironments of lower pH in the unstirred layers immediately adjacent to the membrane, or to the acidity of the membrane itself.

The process of diffusion is driven by the concentration gradient across the membrane, and thus the fluid volume in the tract can have a major influence on the rate at which an ingested material may appear in the bloodstream. Presumably, the greater volumes of fluid dilute the various solutes. Herein lies the basis for the oft given advice in poisoning cases of 'give two glasses of water' in order to dilute the poison. As it turns out, this is not always appropriate advice. For instance, dilution of glutaraldehyde in water actually increases its peroral toxicity, the LD_{50} of the material being reduced from 1.3 mg kg^{-1} in the rat when administered as a 50% solution to 12 mg kg^{-1} as a 1% solution (Tyler and Ballantyne, 1988). As discussed above, ingestion of food is a powerful stimulant for both the secretion of gastric and intestinal secretions and the release of acid in the stomach. Therefore, it would be expected that the effects, particularly acute effects, of an orally administered toxicant might be greatly influenced by the prandial state of the animal.

The transport of an absorbed molecule into the bloodstream is driven by a large concentration gradient between the luminal side and the serosal side of the intestine. Because of the rapid blood flow and concomitant rapid removal of absorbed solutes into the general systemic circulation, concentration gradients are invariably favourable for movement from the gut into the circulatory system. The major impediment to absorption of nutrients and exogenous chemicals, then, is the initial movement across the mucosal cell membrane.

It is believed that a major portion of the water present in the GI tract is reabsorbed through pores that are present in the apical junctions of the epithelial cell lining. These pores are large enough to allow penetration of small molecules, particularly small ionized species. The net direction of flow of water is either from the GI tract into the serosal fluid, as is generally the case when the contents are either iso-osmotic or hypotonic, or into the GI tract, as might occur when the gastro-intestinal contents are hyper-osmotic or in certain pathological states. Vogel *et al.* (1975) studied the effect of water flow on the toxicity of atropine, an azoniaspiro compound, phenoabarbitol and nicotine by infusing solutions of these substances into the duodenum of rats. Mannitol was concomitantly infused to adjust the osmotic concentration of the contents and thus the flow of water from the serosal side to the mucosal side of the GI tract. Toxic effects were increased by a factor of 2–4 with a decrease in osmotic concentration from triple isotonicity to isotonicity for three of the four materials, the only exception being with the azoniaspiro compound. No explanation for this latter discrepancy was given. The presumptive depression of absorption of solutes resulting from the flow of water from the serosa into the lumen of the intestine has been termed solvent drag. As demonstrated by the work of Vogel *et al.* (1975), this process can play an important role in evoking toxic responses of certain compounds, primarily small water-soluble ions.

Active Transport

The active transport or energy-dependent transport mechanisms of absorption are primarily reserved for

nutrients, i.e. amino acids, sugars, essential vitamins and minerals, etc. There are examples where specific exogenous substances can also be absorbed from the GI tract using these same transport systems. For instance, pyrimidines and amino acids are absorbed by active transport systems. 5-Fluorouracil and 5-bromouracil are actively transported across the rat intestinal epithelium by the process which transports natural pyrimidines (Schanker and Jeffrey, 1961), and penicillamine and levodopa utilize an active transport mechanism for natural amino acids. Processes designed for the transport of essential metals are also responsible for the absorption of some toxic metals such as lead and aluminium. Chlorothiazide has been demonstrated to be absorbed by a non-saturable active absorption process (Welling, 1984).

Lymphatics

Absorption by way of the lymphatics is limited to non-polar materials and occurs by mechanisms analogous to that which absorbs fatty acids. Bile salts play an important role in dispersing triglycerides and other fat-soluble molecules and are critical in the formation of micelles that allow dissolution of the fatty materials within the chyme. The fact that rats do not possess a gall bladder may lead to differences in their ability to absorb materials efficiently by way of the lymphatics. Fatty acids, derived from the hydrolysis of triglycerides by various lipases, migrate to the brush border of the mucosal cells and readily diffuse through the mucosal membrane into the cytosol of the cell. Once in the cell, the fatty acids are reincorporated into triglycerides within the endoplasmic reticulum and packaged into chylomicrons, a conglomerate of triglycerides, cholesterol and phospholipids encased in a protein coat. The highly non-polar nature of the interior of the chylomicron provides an ideal environment to entrain other lipid-soluble molecules. The protein coat provides a hydrophilic exterior to the conglomerate that is extruded from the cell into the serosal fluid and into the central lacteals of the villi. The chylomicrons are pumped through the lymphatic system and empty into the systemic circulatory system at the entrance of the thoracic duct in the veins of the neck. In this manner, fatty lipophilic materials avoid entering the hepatic portal circulatory system and possible first-pass effects of metabolism by liver enzymes. Sieber (1976) has shown that p,p'-DDT and some structurally related analogues are absorbed through the lymphatics. The extent of lymphatic absorption is limited, however, presumably because of the relatively slow rate of movement of lymph through the lymphatics as compared with movement of blood through the general circulatory system. The extent of absorption may also vary greatly, depending on the vehicle in which a test substance is administered. Thus, Sieber (1976) recovered only 15% of a dose of p,p'-DDT in the lymph when administered in ethanol compared with 34% when administered in corn oil.

p-Aminosalicylic acid (PAS) and tetracycline have also been demonstrated to be absorbed by way of the lymphatics; however, both of these drugs are also rapidly distributed throughout the extracellular fluid, including lymph, when administered by the intravenous route (DeMarco and Levine, 1969). This finding suggests that care must be taken in interpretation of data in which accountability of a substance in lymph is used to determine absorption through lymphatics after peroral dosing. Other materials shown to be absorbed by way of the lymphatics include 3-methylcholanthrene, polychlorinated biphenyls and benzpyrene.

Macromolecules

The direct absorption of macromolecules from the GI tract is well established and has grave toxicological implications in some instances, e.g. the absorption of *Botulinum* toxins, which are proteins of molecular weight ranging from 200 000 to 400 000. Macromolecules are believed to be absorbed by pinocytosis. Intestinal mucosa in the area of the Peyer's patches, lymphoid follicle aggregates, are believed to be particularly active in this respect (Aungst and Shen, 1986). Peyer's patches are the site of lymphoid follicle-associated epithelium which contain M cells capable of transporting antigens and microorganisms (Kerneis *et al.*, 1997). Mucosa-associated lymphoid tissue is separated from the lumen of the intestine by lymphoid follicle-associated epithelium. Macromolecules and microorganisms can exploit the M cells of the follicle-associated epithelium to cross the digestive tract.

The ability of macrostructures to cross the epithelium lining, particularly in the area of Peyer's patches, has been explored for use in the delivery of pharmaceutical and molecular biological preparations. Polyanhydride copolymers of fumaric and sebacic acid have demonstrated high biological adhesive properties (Mathiowitz *et al.*, 1997). Microspheres of this copolymer with diameters ranging from 0.1 to 10 μm and fed to rats were observed by histological procedures to transverse both the mucosal epithelium, through and between individual cells, and the follicle-associated epithelium covering the lymphatic elements of Peyer's patches. These degradable copolymers were then used to deliver three model pharmaceutical preparations: dicumarol (a poorly absorbed anticoagulant), insulin and plasmid DNA. Neither of the last two materials exhibits activity when administered orally. However, when encapsulated in these copolymer microspheres and given by gavage, definitive enhanced systemic uptake was observed for all three model compounds. This study demonstrates the possibilities of transport of labile and/or relatively large particles through the intestinal mucosa, predominantly in areas of rich lymphoid activity.

Once taken into the mucosal cells, the macromolecules are transported to the general circulation by way of the lymphatics. The process is age dependent, the ability to absorb large molecules decreasing with age. In this respect it should be recalled that newborns are able to obtain immunity to disease states through the absorption of immunoglobulins in the cholestrum of milk.

PRACTICAL IMPLICATIONS

Procedures Used for Peroral Dosing

Generally, the procedures used in administering test substances to animals can be grouped into one of two categories: those procedures in which the material is administered as a bolus and those in which it is administered more or less on a continuous basis. In the first category, the most common means of administration, at least in rodents, is by gavage. In this procedure, described previously, the material is fed through an animal feeding needle directly into the animal's stomach. A similar procedure using a flexible tube is often used for dogs, monkeys and farm animals. In these larger species gelatin capsules filled with the test substance are also commonly used; in this case, however, the test substance is generally in a solid form. Sometimes gelatin capsule administration can be used to overcome problems of emesis.

Gavage administration of test materials can be accomplished fairly rapidly and automated systems have been adapted from equipment designed for cutaneous application in which animals are weighed, the weights down loaded in real time to a computer and the dosing volume for each individual animal, based on body weight, automatically calculated. The animal handler then inserts the feeding needle into the animal's stomach and the dosing volume is automatically dispensed (Wilson *et al.*, 1991).

The gavage procedure is fairly labour intensive and can represent a major cost factor in large studies. To appreciate the magnitude of the problem, consider that in a 2 year study generally 50 animals of each species and each sex are used in each dosage group. In addition, 30 or more additional animals of each sex may be included in each dosage group for satellite studies, interim sacrifices or recovery groups. Thus, in a two-species study with three dosage groups and two control groups (vehicle control and naive control), more than 1500 animals may have to be dosed every day, 5–7 days a week for 24 or more months.

Alternatively, studies are carried out in which the test material is incorporated into the feed or dissolved in the animal's drinking water. When incorporated into feed, care must be taken to produce a uniform dispersion of the material. Differences in density and or particle size can lead to the non-homogeneous mixing or the settling out of the test substance in the fines. In addition, test substances may degrade in these medias. Good laboratory practice requires that homogeneity studies and stability studies be conducted prior to study initiation in order to ensure the validity of the studies.

Animals may refuse to eat feed in cases where the test chemical imparts unacceptable taste. Rodents often waste material, tossing the feed out of the feed cups and thus making it impossible to determine feed consumption accurately and, therefore, impossible to obtain an accurate estimate of dose.

Although dispersion is not a problem with soluble test materials administered in drinking water, as mentioned above, stability often is. As an example, the decomposition rate of vinyl acetate in water was found to be approximately 8.5% per day at room temperature and 5% per day at 4°C (Lijensky and Reuber, 1983). A chronic drinking water study was conducted with the ester in rats using a procedure in which solutions were prepared on a weekly basis. It was estimated that the animals received at least half the nominal dose. The affect of the decomposition products was not considered in the evaluation of the results of the study. In a subsequent chronic study with the material, drinking water was prepared daily, a labour-intensive procedure, to reduce the influence of the hydrolysis products. In addition, the drinking water was over-formulated by 5% to compensate for the daily rate of hydrolysis (Bogdanffy *et al.*, 1994).

In addition to instability, volatile materials may evaporate from the water into room air. Evaporation will occur at the tip of the drinking water tube and can lead to an overestimate of the actual dose to the animal. The volatilization of the test substance may also lead to appreciable inhalation exposure that should be monitored. As with feeding studies, animals will refuse to drink and/or waste water containing chemicals that impart an unpalatable taste.

Under ideal conditions, the choice of dosing procedures should be dictated by the type of exposure anticipated in normal use or as encountered in the environment. If, in its end use, a material will be administered in bolus form, as is the case with many drugs that are designed to be administered by capsule, then certainly administration by gavage is appropriate. On the other hand, when data from a study will be used to estimate the risk from chronic exposure of a contaminant in food or water, a feeding or drinking water study would be more appropriate. A material entering the GI tract as a bolus, in contrast to the more uniform pattern when ingested in feed or water, will affect both the rate of absorption and peak plasma concentrations in both the hepatic–portal and the systemic circulatory systems. In the case of bolus administration, hepatic metabolic enzyme systems may become saturated, allowing higher concentrations of unmetabolized chemical to enter the

systemic circulation, possibly influencing toxic responses. Often animals will tolerate higher daily dosages when a material is given in feed or water as opposed to gavage. Presumably this relates to the higher peak plasma concentrations attained in bolus administration.

More often than not, the physical and/or chemical properties of a test substance dictate the manner in which it will be administered. Chemicals that are insoluble in water cannot be administered in drinking water. Volatile chemicals are not suited for feeding studies. Reactive materials will not maintain the degree of purity required for testing when formulated in feed or water. Under these conditions, gavage administration is sometimes the only rational alternative available. 2-Ethylhexanol (2-EH) is a case in point. This chemical was nominated for chronic testing under the provisions of Section 4 of the Toxic Substances Control Act (US EPA, 1990). The concern arose from possible exposure to the chemical in the environment owing to its high production volume. The proposed Test Rule required a chronic study to be conducted by the oral route. The material is an industrial chemical intermediate, and considering its noxious nature it would be highly unlikely that repeated exposure would occur as a result of swallowing bolus doses. Therefore, a means of more uniform administration was sought. Although this alcohol has a relatively low vapour pressure, 0.05 mmHg at 20 °C, it was found to evaporate rapidly when formulated in feed. The maximum solubility in water is approximately 0.06%. A short-term repeated (11 day) exposure study was conducted with water saturated with 2-EH, the maximum dosage achieved being about 160 mg kg^{-1} day^{-1}. At this dose, no toxic effects were noted in either rats or mice. Oral dosing, therefore, proved to be unacceptable for a guideline study, which requires demonstration of toxicity. A similar situation existed for inhalation exposure where maximum air concentrations were without appreciable toxic effects.

Interest was expressed in conducting a feeding experiment with microencapsulated 2-EH. Microencapsulation is a process whereby the test material is uniformly coated with a degradable but impervious material (Melnick *et al.*, 1987a). Microencapsulation has been used in feeding studies to prevent evaporation of volatile materials and to mask objectionable tastes (Melnick *et al.*, 1987b; Aida *et al.*, 1989; Yuan *et al.*, 1991). Microcapsules of 2-EH were prepared using food-grade modified cornstarch as the coating medium. Again, a short-term repeated study was conducted with this material in rats and mice. Using this technique, 2-EH was shown to remain stable in the feed. In rats dosages of up to 2700 mg kg^{-1} day^{-1} were achieved and produced toxic effects as expected. In contrast, dosages of greater than 5000 mg kg^{-1} day^{-1} were attained in mice, this being in the range of the single dose LD$_{50}$ of between 3.2 and 6.4 mg kg^{-1} for this species. Even at this dose no appreciable toxicity was noted, suggesting that microencapsulated 2-EH may not be appropriate for chronic feeding studies in mice. After conducting several more short-term repeated studies using various dosing vehicles, the only feasible procedure for conducting the chronic study was by gavage using an aqueous emulsifier for the dosing vehicle.

Decreases in toxic responses in mice to microencapsulated test material do not appear to be confined to 2-EH. Dieter et al. (1993) administered citral (3,7-dimethyl-locta-2, 6-dien-1-al) to rats and mice both in an encapsulated form and by gavage. Mice received microencapsulated test material at doses of 0,534, 1065, 2137, 4275 and 8550 mg kg^{-1} for 14 days. At these doses no mortality was observed and toxicity was confined to decreases in body weight at the highest dosage. In contrast, complete mortality was noted when the mice were dosed by gavage with 2137 mg kg^{-1} and in two out of five males at 1068 mg kg^{-1}. In addition, cytoplasmic vacuolization of hepatocytes occurred at doses of 1068 mg kg^{-1} and above and forestomach lesions were noted at doses of 1068 mg kg^{-1} and above. Rats receiving 1140 and 2280 mg kg^{-1} citral in microcapsules experienced decreased weight gain and decreased absolute weights of the liver, kidney and spleen. When doses of 2280 mg kg^{-1} were given by gavage, minimal toxicity to the fore-stomach was observed in the rat. Thus, whereas mice appear to have had a differential response when citral was administered by microcapsules as compared with gavage, little difference in response was noted with mode of administration in rats.

Dosing Vehicles

It is often necessary, when conducting studies by gavage, to dilute the test substance in a dosing vehicle. Generally an aqueous vehicle is preferred, but often materials are insoluble in water and a less polar medium is required. For such materials corn oil is generally the vehicle of choice. Administering test substances in corn oil can have a profound influence on the toxicity observed. For instance, Farooqui et al. (1995) investigated the effect of a series of various vegetable oils, mineral oil and an ethoxylated fatty acid emulsifying agent (Tween-20) on the acute toxicity of a series of unsaturated aliphatic nitriles. In all cases, the dosing vehicles exacerbated the toxicity of these materials over that when administered in saline. This result was not entirely unexpected considering that these chemicals are sparingly soluble in water and solutions in oil or emulsion would probably enhance the absorption across the GI mucosa.

Kim et al. (1990) found that carbon tetrachloride at single doses of 10 and 25 mg kg^{-1} in corn oil caused less severe hepatic injury than when given at these same dosages either undiluted or as an aqueous emulsion to rats. Although clearly affecting the severity of the injury,

the formulations appeared to have little affect on the time course of hepatic injury as evaluated by serum enzyme activities and histopathological examination. In contrast, the hepatotoxicity of chloroform in mice was shown to be enhanced by formulation in corn oil over that when administered as an aqueous emulsion (Bull et al., 1986). Both the corn oil and aqueous emulsion formulations produced significantly decreased body weights and increased liver weights when given to B6C3F1 mice at dosages from 60 up to 270 mg kg^{-1} day^{-1} for 90 days. The effect in corn oil, however, was greatly enhanced over that when administered as an emulsion. Further, the mice receiving the corn oil formulation demonstrated clear pathological changes in the liver. Similar lesions were not seen in animals administered corn oil without chloroform or in animals receiving chloroform at similar dosages in the emulsion. Jorgenson et al. (1985) postulated that differences in carcinogenic response in female mice obtained in two bioassays with chloroform might be explained by the formulation. These workers could not confirm a previous finding that chloroform induced hepatocellular carcinomas in female B6C3F1 mice (Reuber, 1979).

In the NCI study, an 80% incidence of hepatocellular carcinomas was observed when the chlorinated hydrocarbon was administered in corn oil at a dosage level of 238 mg kg^{-1} day^{-1}, 7 days a week for 78 weeks. Jorgenson et al. (1985) found only a 2% incidence of hepatocellular carcinoma when they administered the chemical in drinking water at a dosage level of 263 mg kg^{-1} day^{-1}. They suggested that either the dosing regimen, bolus vs the more gradual dosing via drinking water, or the dosing vehicle might have accounted for the discrepancies in the two bioassays.

Other examples of the effect of vehicle on absorption and subsequent toxicity include 1,1-dichloroethylene, which when given to fasted rats in corn oil or mineral oil has been shown to enhance hepatic injury compared with when given as an aqueous emulsion (Chieco et al., 1981). The dosing vehicle had little effect on subsequent liver injury when 1, 1-dichloroethylene was given by gavage to fed animals. Administering corn oil formulations of methylene chloride, dichloroethane, trichloroethylene and chloroform decreased the rate and extent of uptake, as measured by the area under the blood concentration–time curve and peak plasma concentrations, compared with those when administered in aqueous solution (Withey et al., 1983). Thus, with the exception of carbon tetrachloride, corn oil formulations of chlorinated hydrocarbons appears to enhance the toxic response to the liver. Perhaps the anomalous behaviour of carbon tetrachloride results from a different mechanism of hepatic toxicity, that believed to occur through the formation of free radicals, a mechanism which, perhaps, is enhanced by more rapid uptake and corresponding higher peak plasma concentrations.

Ingestion of significant quantities of corn oil will clearly increase the flow of lymph. As described previously, this can lead to an increase in the quantity of lipophilic material, e.g. p,p'-DDT and analogues, absorbed through the lymphatics (Sieber, 1976). This mechanism may also account for the enhancement of maximum plasma levels and bioavailability and an increase in the duration of the absorption time of the refractory antibiotic griseofulvin when administered in a corn oil emulsion compared with administration as an aqueous suspension (Bates and Carrigan, 1975).

Prandial State

The presence of food or, for that matter, even the anticipation of the presence of food, can have a profound effect on the physiological state of the GI tract. The manner in which the ionic milieu, the pH and the fluid volume affect the absorption and subsequently the toxicity of drugs and chemicals can be complex. Common advice has suggested that 'gastric absorption is favoured by an empty stomach in which the drug, in undiluted gastric juice, will have good access to the mucosal wall' and that 'only when a drug is irritating to the gastric mucosa is it rational to administer it with or after a meal' (Goldstein et al., 1974). This advice clearly is not universal for all drugs, and does not reflect the effect of prandial state on the known toxicity of many chemicals.

Perhaps the most familiar example of the effect of prandial state on toxicological response is that of ethanol. It has been commonly experienced that drinking comparable quantities of ethanol on an empty stomach in contrast to drinking with or immediately after a meal results in a stronger and more prolonged pharmacological response. The effect of prandial state on the pharmacokinetics of ethanol has been studied in man (Jones and Jönsson, 1994). Volunteers were administered ethanol [80 mg (kg body weight)$^{-1}$] in a fasted condition or immediately after a standardized meal. Without exception, when injected after eating, ethanol blood concentrations were reduced throughout the absorption and elimination phase and had a lower C_{max} and a smaller area under the curve. It has been postulated that either first-pass metabolism is increased immediately after eating, resulting in the observed changes in kinetic behaviour, or that the ethanol is adsorbed on food particles, decreasing its availability and slowing its absorption into the hepatic portal circulation.

Welling (1977) reviewed the effect of food and diet on GI absorption, grouping a series of drugs into four different categories:

- Drugs whose absorption may be reduced by food;
- Drugs whose absorption may be delayed by food;
- Drugs whose absorption may be unaffected by food;
- Drugs whose absorption may be increased by food.

The first category was represented by members of the penicillin family, tetracycline, aspirin and several other materials. The second group contains many of the sulpha and cephalosporin drugs. Drugs which appeared to be unaffected by the prandial state included theophylline and prenisone, and those which were enhanced by the presence of food in the GI tract included griseofulvin, nitrofurantoin, propoxyphene and a few others. No generalizations could be made as to what structural or other features contributed to either a depression or an enhancement of absorption in the presence or absence of food. In a later paper, however, Welling (1984) discussed the effects of stomach emptying time, which could enhance the absorption of drugs, particularly basic drugs, by increasing the percentage dissolved prior to passing into the small intestine and by prolonging the time during which the drug comes into contact with the absorptive surface, the mucosal wall. In addition, food interactions can affect the absorption of specific molecules, for instance the absorption of penicillamine and tetracyclines is impeded by chelation with heavy metals and complex formation with proteins.

In addition to the effect of dosing vehicle, the effect of prandial state on the absorption of chlorinated hydrocarbons has been studied. Chieco et al. (1981) demonstrated that the hepatotoxicity of 1, 1-dichloroethylene was diminished in fasted animals when administered in aqueous suspension. The metabolism of vinylidene chloride was shown to be diminished in fasted rats (McKenna et al., 1978). A 50% increase in the amount of parent compound was eliminated in exhaled air of fasted rats compared with fed rats receiving a single 50 mg kg^{-1} oral dose of ^{14}C-labelled chemical. In addition, fasting also resulted in an increased concentration of covalently bound metabolites in the liver and, contrary to the experience with 1, 1-dichloroethylene, led to an enhancement of hepatotoxicity. The increased covalent binding and hepatotoxicity may have resulted from depleted concentrations of glutathione in the livers of the fasted animals.

The acute peroral toxicity of epoxidized soybean oil and polypropylene glycol were both shown to be widely divergent depending on whether or not rats were fed or fasted when dosed (Tyler and Ballantyne, 1988). The LD$_{50}$ values obtained under the two prandial states are shown in **Table 1**. In this case the prandial state has opposite effects on the toxicity of these two dissimilar materials. The reasons for this discrepant behaviour are not understood. In contrast to the effects of prandial state with these chemicals, Bates and Carrigan (1975) found no effect on the absorption, maximum plasma concentrations or bioavailability when griseofulvin was given orally in corn oil emulsion to either fed or fasted rats.

Results obtained in studies in which animals have been fasted for prolonged periods of time, over 20 h, may reflect functional changes in the intestinal mucosa

Table 1 Effect of feeding and fasting on the acute oral LD_{50} in rats

Material	Prandial state	LD_{50} mg kg^{-1}
Epoxidized soybean oil	Fasted	64 000
	Fed	19 000
Polypropylene glycol	Fasted	800
	Fed	4 000

Table 2 Effect of prandial state on acute toxicity (LD_{50}) of a series of glycol ethers[a]

Glycol ether	LD_{50} (mmol kg^{-1})			
	Rats		Mice	
	Fasted	Fed	Fasted	Fed
Ethylene glycol monomethyl ether	30	52	52	59
Ethylene glycol monoethyl ether	39	90	27	59
Ethylene glycol monopropyl ether	30	59	17	30
Ethylene glycol monobutyl ether	15	15	13	17
Diethylene glycol monomethhyl ether	59	100	59	68
Diethylene glycol monoethyl ether	78	120	45	45
Diethylene glycol monopropyl ether	45	65	26	39
Diethylene glycol monobutyl ether	45	59	15	34
Ethylene glycol mono-2-ethylhexyl ether	45	30	42	22

[a] Unpublished data obtained from the Eastman Kodak Company, Rochester, NY.

(Doluisio *et al.*, 1969). Although fasting for up to 20 h had little effect on intestinal absorption of salicylic acid, barbital, haloperidol or chlorpromazine in a surgical preparation, significant decrements in the absorption rate were noted when trials were conducted with rats fasted for over 20 h. Krasavage and Terhaar (1981) investigated the effect of prandial state on a series of glycol ethers (**Table 2**). These chemicals, monoethers of ethylene glycol, are solvents that are soluble in water and have appreciable solubility in less polar solvents. The ethylene glycol monoethers are in general more toxic than the diethylene glycol monoethers. However, prandial state also appears to play a moderating role in the toxicity of these solvents, animals dosed in the fed state universally demonstrating resistance to the toxic effects of the chemicals. The mechanism of the toxicity of monobutyl and monopropyl ethers in rodents differs from that of the lower homologues, the methyl and ethyl ethers, the former producing toxic responses primarily through effects on red blood cells leading to haemolysis. The moderating effect of feeding appears to have a lesser influence on this toxic activity than it does on the toxicity of the lower homologues. In addition, the moderating effects of feeding appear to be accentuated in rats compared with mice.

Effects of Direct Contact

Severely irritating and corrosive materials can produce toxic effects by direct contact with the oesophageal and stomach tissues. Such effects are encountered in accidental swallowing but occasionally these effects can complicate the interpretation of animal studies when administration of test materials is by gavage. In humans, particularly in the case of accidental poisonings in children caused by swallowing caustic materials, severe injury and fatalities may result from oesophageal perforation and resulting systemic complications. More commonly oesophageal burns occur leading later to the development of strictures and possible infection. The development of strictures appears to be directly correlated with the severity of the burn, third-degree burns, defined by ulcerations, white plaques and sloughing of the mucosa in a circumferential pattern leading to a high incidence of stricture formation, requiring surgical correction (Anderson *et al.*, 1990). In cases where caustics happen to reach the stomach with minimal oesophageal injury, regurgitation may result in further injury to the oesophagus and exacerbate an already critical condition. This is the basis therefore of the first-aid advice not to induce vomiting in cases of swallowing caustic or severely irritating chemicals.

In studies where irritating materials are given to animals by gavage, little opportunity exists for irritation or corrosive injury to the oesophagus since the test material is injected through an animal feeding needle or a tube directly into the stomach. Rodents are believed to lack the vomiting response and therefore regurgitation of materials back into the oesophagus is not ordinarily encountered. However, in practical situations, oesophageal perforation or tears can occur in a dosage-related manner, suggesting that materials do come into contact with the oesophageal tissue, particularly in the area of the gastro–oesophageal junction. Such dose-related injury has been seen in rats repeatedly administered diethylene glycol monobutyl ether by gavage (Hobson *et al.*, 1987) and when propan-2-ol was administered to rats by gavage in a repeated dose reproductive probe study (**Table 3**). Presumably the oesophageal injury was exacerbated by repeated direct exposure to the irritating properties of these materials through some sort of regurgitating process in the area of the gastro–oesophageal junction.

A second type of direct irritation to the rodent GI tract occurs in the forestomach. A number of chemicals have been shown to produce severe irritation to forestomach tissue when given by gavage, including butylated

Table 3 Treatment-related oesophageal injury produced by gavage of propan-2-ol to rats

Dose[a] (mmol kg^{-1})	Dead with oesophageal injury (%)
0	0
0.1	0
0.5	0
1.0	57
1.75	8
2.5	25

[a] Given as an aqueous solution at a dosage volume of 5 ml kg^{-1}.

hydroxyanisole, propionic acid, ethyl acrylate, diglycidylresorcinol ether, epichlorohydrin, methyl acrylamidoglycolate methyl ether, aristolochic acid and citral.

Ethyl acrylate, has been shown to cause forestomach tumours in rats and mice when administered in corn oil by gavage (NTP, 1986). In that study there was no increase in the incidence of tumours in any other organ or tissue. In addition, a 27 month bioassay in rats and mice by inhalation was without a carcinogenic response (Miller *et al.*, 1985), a lifetime mouse skin painting study did not result in the induction of skin tumours at the site of contact (DePass *et al.*, 1984), a 2 year drinking water study in rats did not result in forestomach tumours or an increase in any other tumour type and a study in which dogs, which do not posses a forestomach, were administered ethyl acrylate by capsule for a 2 year period did not induce a carcinogenic response (Borzelleca *et al.* 1964). The relationship between the irritant response and forestomach tumours is not clear; however, Ghanayem *et al.* (1991) have shown that administration of ethyl acrylate to rats in corn oil for 13 weeks results in severe epithelial hyperplasia of the forestomach without involvement of the glandular stomach or the liver. There was a significant decrease in the incidence and severity of forestomach mucosal hyperplasia in animals treated in a similar manner for 13 weeks and sacrificed 8 weeks later. An even greater decline in the severity of the response was noted in animals allowed a 19 month recovery period, with no tumours developing in the forestomach of these animals. In a following study, these workers demonstrated that repeated oral gavage administration of ethyl acrylate in corn oil to rats for either 6 or 12 months produced extensive mucosal cell proliferation in the forestomach (Ghanayem *et al.*, 1993). In animals dosed for 6 months there was a significant time-dependent regression in cell proliferation at 15 months after cessation of dosing with no evidence of neoplasia. In those rats dosed for 12 months, on the other hand, squamous cell carcinomas or papillomas were seen in four of 13 animals at 9 months after dosing had been discontinued. These data suggest that local effects of irritation produced by gavage administration can have a profound influence on the toxicity of a material. In addition, the length of time over which the irritation takes place is a critical factor in eliciting the toxic response, particularly as related to neoplastic events associated with chronic irritation.

CONSIDERATIONS IN HAZARD EVALUATION AND RISK ASSESSMENT

From the forgoing discussion, it is abundantly clear that once ingested, there are numerous factors which affect the manner in which chemical toxicants pass through and are absorbed from the GI tract. It is equally clear that differences exist between animal species with regard to both anatomical structure and physiological function. In addition, hepatic–portal circulation and potential absorption through the central lacteals of the intestinal villa with subsequent lymphatic absorption provide unique differences in the uptake and disposition of toxicants from the GI tract as compared with uptake by other typical routes of exposure to environmental chemicals, e.g. the skin and respiratory tract, or by intravenous administration of pharmaceutical preparations or social poisons. A clear understanding of and accountability for these factors and differences are essential when attempting to extrapolate hazards and risks from studies which have been conducted by oral administration in laboratory animals to exposure in humans, either by ingestion or by other routes.

Anatomical and Physiological Considerations

As pointed out above, one of the more obvious distinguishing anatomical differences between the GI tract of humans and that of rodents is the presence of a food storage compartment in the stomach, the forestomach. The epithelial lining of this structure is very similar to that of the human oesophagus; however, the residence time of food in the oesophagus is transient whereas that in the forestomach may be prolonged. Other, less obvious, differences exist between common laboratory animals and man which can influence passage and absorption and subsequently the toxicity of environmental chemicals and drugs. **Table 4**, for instance, demonstrates the proportional differences between lengths of various segments of the intestinal tract of humans and rats. In the rat the jejunum accounts for approximately 88% and the ileum only 4% of the length of the small intestine, whereas the corresponding proportions in humans are 38% and 57%, respectively. In addition to differences in the length of various segments of the small intestine, there are differences in the mucosal structure, e.g. the intestinal villi of rats are about twice as long as those of man and other non-rodents (DeSesso and Mavis, 1989).

Table 4 Comparison of lengths of intestinal segments between humans and rats[a]

Segment	Humans		Rats	
	Length (cm)	% of total	Length (cm)	% of total
Small intestine	500	–	125	–
Duodenum	25	5	10	8
Jejunum	190	38	110	88
Ileum	285	57	5	4
Large intestine	170	–	24	–
Caecum	7	4	6	25
Colon	108	64	10	42
Rectum	55[b]	32	8	33

[a] Adapted from DeSesso and Mavis (1989).
[b] Includes both sigmoid colon and rectum.

In addition to species differences in the structure of the GI tract, differences also exist in physiological function. For most mammalian species, both rodent and non-rodent, the anterior portion of the stomach is generally less acidic than the posterior portion, ranging in pH from about 4.3 in the pig to 6.9 in the hamster, a species with a prominent limiting ridge (Calabrese, 1983). Posterior gastric pH also can very widely, ranging from about 2.2 in the pig to 4.2 in the cat. The rabbit, on the other hand, is an exception to this pattern, producing notably acidic gastric fluid and demonstrating little difference in the pH between the two portions of the stomach, fluid in both the anterior and posterior parts having a pH range of around 1.9. The distribution and kinds of microflora may also differ between animal species. Although the gastric contents of most species contain few micro-organisms, the forestomach and upper small intestine of the rat support a considerable population of micro-flora.

'First-pass' Effect Considerations

The hepatic–portal circulatory pattern, which is unique to the GI tract, requires special consideration when attempting to extrapolate quantitatively or qualitatively effects encountered by oral administration to other routes of exposure. As has been pointed out previously, all material absorbed from the distil portion of the oeso-phagus to the distal rectum are transported by way of the portal vein to the liver. The liver, being a primary organ of metabolism, can have a major influence on the con-centrations of parent toxicant and metabolites that enter the general circulatory system. The bioavailability of the anti-inflammatory drug diclofenac sodium, for instance, can be reduced by extents ranging from 50 to 60% when given orally (Peris-Ribera et al., 1991). Propranolol and lidocaine are two other drugs that have been shown to be rapidly metabolized by the liver and exhibit differences in plasma time–concentration patterns when administered orally compared with methods in which they directly enter the systemic circulation.

Considerations of Bolus versus Continuous Dosing

Bolus administration can also affect the concentration–time pattern of ingested chemicals and therefore affect potential toxic responses. **Table 5** demonstrates the effect of bolus dosing on the developmental toxicity of ethylene glycol in mice. Acute toxic responses may be elicited by high peak concentrations and thus toxicity accentuated by gavage dosing, diminished when given in feed or water. High portal vein concentrations of chemicals that are substrates for high-affinity, low-capacity meta-bolic enzymes can saturate these enzymes, resulting in breakthrough of the chemical into the systemic circula-tion. Cumulative toxicity, on the other hand, may be uninfluenced or diminished by bolus doses, particularly if maximum tolerated doses are appreciably lower than when administered in a more continuous manner, e.g. feeding or drinking water. Dosing chemicals in corn oil vehicle may increase the amount absorbed by way of the lymphatics, reducing the effect of hepatic portal circula-tion, since corn oil will stimulate the flow of lymph. Careful consideration must be given to these variables when, as so often is the case, oral toxicity data are the only data available, and extrapolation is attempted to predict what air concentration of a chemical will produce similar toxic effects from exposure by inhalation.

Table 5 Effect of bolus vs continuous dosing of ethylene glycol on developmental effects in mice

Procedure	Minimum effect level (mg kg^{-1})	NOEL[c] (mg kg^{-1})
Gavage[a]	500	150
Drinking water[b]	2000	1000

[a] Tyl et al. (1989).
[b] NTP (1984).
[c] No observed effect level.

Enterohepatic Circulation

Higher molecular weight xenobiotics which are absorbed into the systemic circulation are preferentially cleared by way of biliary excretion. This route of elimination is a major consideration for materials with molecular weights of 300–500 and higher. There is considerable variability between species in the ability to excrete che-micals through bile; the rat, dog and hen are considered 'good' biliary excretors whereas rabbits, guinea pigs, rhesus monkeys and man are grouped as 'poor' biliary excretors (Williams, 1971). The molecular weight cut-off for excretion via this route appears to decrease with increased biliary elimination ability. Thus, for the 'good' eliminators, bile becomes a primary route for materials of molecular weight 300 and greater, whereas higher molecular weight materials tend to be required before becoming a major pathway in 'poor' eliminators.

Conjugates, particularly glucuronide conjugates, appear to enhance the opportunity for biliary excretion. Conjugation not only increases molecular weight but also increases polarity, both properties enhancing the ability for excretion in bile. The excretion of conjugates by way of bile leads to the interesting and in some cases toxicologically significant phenomenon of enterohepatic circulation. Higher molecular weight materials absorbed into the systemic circulation eventually make their way to the liver by way of the hepatic portal circulation. These materials can be metabolically converted into glucuronide conjugates and subsequently discharged into the duodenum. Although mammalian tissue levels of β-glucuronidases are low, intestinal microflora have considerable capacity to hydrolyse the conjugate, yielding the parent material (aglycone). This material may then be reabsorbed into the hepatic portal circulation and recycle in the same manner.

Enterohepatic circulation can result in extending the half-lives of materials for considerable periods as materials are recycled through the intestine, portal vein, liver and bile. In some instances this may lead to enhanced liver or intestinal toxicity. The intestinal carcinogenicity of aromatic amines maybe manifested through biliary excretion as glucuronide conjugates of o-hydroxyamines formed in the liver with subsequent intestinal hydrolysis of these conjugates to form carcinogenic free o-hydroxyamines (Plaa, 1971). Differences in ability to eliminate chemicals by way of bile may also be a major reason for species differences in toxicity. In the rat, for instance, 60% of a dose of morphine is eliminated through bile whereas in man only 7% of the dose is so eliminated (Williams, 1971).

Localized Effect Considerations

The forestomach has been shown to be the site of both neoplastic and non-neoplastic lesions possibly associated with an irritant response and associated cellular hyperplasia. It is important to note the difference in anatomical structure and function of the stomach between rodents and humans when attempting rodent to human extrapolation. Thus, it is difficult to evaluate the significance of a chemically induced tumourigenic response in the forestomach particularly when the chemical produces no similar carcinogenic response in other organs or tissues and does not exhibit genotoxic activity. In addition, irritation, hyperplasia and eventual tumour formation appear to be more related to the concentration

of test substance in the dosing solution than to total dose administered (Davis et al., 1986; Clayson et al., 1990). Although consideration has been given to the use of the forestomach as a model for the human oesophagus, attempts to demonstrate similar reactivities for the oesophageal and forestomach mucosa in various species have been unsuccessful (Wester and Kroes, 1988). Taken as a whole, critical evaluation is required in determining appropriate classification of chemicals that produce a carcinogenic response in the forestomach of rodents alone, and without evidence of genotoxic activity.

Consideration of Gastro-intestinal Parameters in Modelling

Current efforts in attempts to extrapolate toxicity data between species and routes of administration centre around the use of physiologically based pharmacokinetic models. These models, which are based on realistic anatomical and physiological concepts, account for major differences encountered in route to route extrapolations, such as the hepatic–portal circulation, and species to species extrapolations, such as proportional differences in organ perfusion. On the other hand, the effect of dosing vehicle, differences in epithelial cell type, effects of prandial state and local effects of chemical insult prove harder to take into account in these models. Staats et al. (1991) attempted to explain differences in the GI absorption of trichloroethylene when administered to rats by gavage in either water or corn oil. A physiologically based pharmacokinetic model that incorporated a two-compartment GI tract simulated blood concentrations time-course data more accurately than did a model incorporating a one-compartment description. Curiously, although the physiologically based pharmacokinetic approach is usually based on specific anatomical and physiological considerations, in this case the selection of the compartments was arbitrary. Although the authors suggested that the compartments might represent the stomach and small intestine, respectively, no terms specific for these two distinct portions of the tract were incorporated into their model to account for physiological differences or transport.

Frederick et al. (1992), on the other hand, developed a physiologically based pharmacokinetic model that includes a description of the interaction of ethyl acrylate on the tissues of the entire GI tract. The model was designed to describe the effects resulting from tissue contact as measured by glutathione depletion, this being an important factor in understanding the mechanism of toxicity of this chemical. This model incorporated both portions of the rodent stomach, the forestomach and the glandular stomach, the duodenum and remainder of the small intestine and the caecum, large intestine and colon.

An attempt to model the lymphatic uptake of lipophilic substances from the GI tract has been undertaken by Roth *et al.* (1993). This model emphasizes the role of chylomicron production and transport in the uptake of lipophilic materials. In addition, such factors as the shedding of epithelium into the intestinal lumen is taken into account. The model was validated with studies conducted in rats using hexachlorobenzene. Enterohepatic circulation, characterized by the biliary uptake of hexachlorobenzene from the hepatic–portal circulation, with subsequent flow into the small intestine, followed by resorption from the colon back into the hepatic-portal circulation, was accurately characterized in this model.

These models, taken in total, demonstrate the complexity and difficulties involved in addressing anatomical, physiological and mechanistic details in attempts to extrapolate toxicological information obtained in peroral studies in one species to health risks by other routes of exposure in other species.

SUMMARY

From the above discussion, it is clear that numerous factors which affect the passage of drugs and chemicals through and absorption from the GI tract. These factors involve both anatomical features, which can differ between species, and physiological features, the function which can be influenced by conditions under which a material is administered. Any attempt to extrapolate toxic effects of chemicals obtained after oral dosing of animals must take into consideration anatomical and physiological differences between the species of comparison, including factors such as:

- The presence of a fore-stomach;
- pH differences between various segments of the GI tract;
- The presence or absence of microflora in various parts of the GI tract;
- Other factors that may be specific to the chemical under study, e.g. length of intestinal segments, presence or absence of a gall bladder, prevalence of Peyer's patches.

Physiological differences between routes of administration must also be considered including:

- Hepatic – portal circulation;
- Lymphatic absorption;
- Possible pharmacological effects of the chemical on the function of the GI. tract, e.g. possible effects on gastric motility or blood circulation;
- The influence of conditions under which a material was administered;
- The prandial state of the animal;

- Mode of dosing – more or less continuous as opposed to bolus dosing;
- Possible effects of dosing vehicle on absorption and metabolism;
- Direct effects of the chemical at the site of contact.

All such factors will influence the extrapolation of results obtained from animal testing, particularly as it applies to extrapolation between rodents and humans and between the peroral route of administration and other common routes of exposure, including inhalation and skin absorption.

REFERENCES

Aida, Y., Ando, M., Takada, K., Momma, J., Yoshimoto, H., Nakaji, Y., Kurokawa, Y. and Tobe, M. (1989). Practical application of microcapsulation for toxicity studies using bromodichloromethane as a model compound. *J. Am. Coll. Toxicol.*, **8**, 1177–1187.

Anderson, K. D., Rouse, T. M. and Randolph, J. G. (1990). A controlled trial of corticosteroids in children with corrosive injury on the esophagus. *N. Engl. J. Med.*, **323**, 637–640.

Aungst, B. and Shen, D. D. (1986). Gastrointestinal absorption of toxic agents. In Rozman, K. and Hänninen, O. (Eds), *Gastrointestinal Toxicology*. Elsevier, New York, pp. 35–36.

Bates, T. and Carrigan, P. (1975). Apparent absorption kinetics of micronized griseofulvin after its oral administration on single- and multiple-dose regimens to rats as a corn oil-in-water emulsion and aqueous suspension. *J. Pharm. Sci.*, **64**, 1475–1481.

Bauchop, T. and Martucci, R. W. (1968). Rumen-like digestion of the langur monkey. *Science*, **161**, 698–700.

Bogdanffy, M. S., Tyler, T. R., Vinegar, M. B., Rickard, R. W., Carpanini, F. M. B. and Cascier, T. C. (1994). Chronic toxicity and oncogenicity study with vinyl acetate in the rat: *in utero* exposure in drinking water. *Fundam. Appl. Toxicol.*, **23**, 206–214.

Borzelleca, J. F., Larson, P. S., Hennigar, G. R., Jr. Huf, E. G., Crawford, E. M. and Smith, R. B., Jr (1964). Studies on the chronic oral toxicity of monomeric ethyl acrylate and methyl methacrylate. *Toxicol. Appl. Pharmacol.*, **6**, 29–36.

Bull, R. J., Brown, J. M., Meierhenry, E. A., Jorgenson, T. A., Robinson, M. and Stober, J. A. (1986). Enhancement of the hepatotoxicity of chloroform in B6C3F1 mice by corn oil: implications for chloroform carcinogenesis. *Environ. Health Perspect.*, **69**, 49–58.

Calabrese, E. J. (1983). Absorption – interspecies differences. In *Principles of Animal Extrapolation*, Wiley, New York, Chapt. 2, pp. 45–47.

Chieco, P., Moslen, M. T. and Reynolds, E. S. (1981). Effect of administrative vehicle on oral 1,1-dichloroethylene toxicity. *Toxicol. Appl. Pharmacol.*, **57**, 146–155.

Clayson, D. B., Iverson, F., Nera, E. A. and Lok, E. (1990). The significance of induced forestomach tumors. *Annu. Rev. Pharmacol. Toxicol.*, **30**, 441–463.

Crouthamel, W. G., Tan, G. H., Dittert, L. W. and Doluisio, J. T. (1971). Drug absorption IV. Influence of pH on absorption kinetics of weakly acidic drugs. *J. Pharm. Sci.*, **60**, 1160–1163.

Davis, R. A., Siglin, J. C., Becci, P. J. and Friedman, M. A. (1986). Concentration dependence and reversibility of gastric lesions induced by repeated gavage of acrylic monomers. *Toxicologist*, **6**, 188.

Dellow, D. W., Nolan, J. V. and Hume, I. D. (1983). Studies on the nutrition of macropodine marsupials. V. Microbial fermentation in the forestomach of *Thyogale thetis* and *Macropus eugenii*. *Aust. J. Zool.*, **31**, 433–443.

DeMarco, T. J. and Levine, R. R. (1969). Role of the lymphatics in the intestinal absorption and distribution of drugs. *J. Pharmacol. Exp. Ther.*, **169**, 142–151.

DePass, L. R., Fowler, E. H., Meckley, D. R. and Weil, C. S. (1984). Dermal oncogenicity bioassays of acrylic acid, ethyl acrylate and butyl acrylate. *J. Toxicol. Environ. Health*, **14**, 115–120.

DeSesso, J. M. and Mavis, R. D. (1989). *Identification of Critical Biological Parameters Affecting Gastrointestinal Absorption*. Report No. MTR-89W00223. MITRE Corporation, McLean, VA.

Dieter, M. P., Goehl, T.J., Jameson, C. W., Elwell, M. R., Hilderbrandt, P. K. and Yuan, J. H. (1993). Comparison of the toxicity of citral in F344 rats and B6C3F1 mice when administered by microencapsulation in feed or by corn-oil gavage. *Food Chem. Toxicol.*, **31**, 463–474.

Doluisio, J. T., Tan, G. H., Billups, N. F. and Diamond, L. (1969). Drug absorption. II: effect of fasting on intestinal drug absorption. *J. Pharm. Sci.*, **58**, 1200–1201.

EPA (1990). Part 799: Identification of specific chemical substance and mixture testing requirements – 2-ethylhexanol. *Code of Federal Regulations*, Part 40, 605–606.

Farooqui, M. Y. H., Ybarra, B., Piper, J. and Tamez, A. (1995). Effect of dosing vehicle on the toxicity and metabolism of unsaturated aliphatic nitriles. *J. Appl. Toxicol.*, **15**, 411–420.

Frederick, C. B., Potter, D. W., Chang-Mateu, M. I. and Andersen, M. E. (1992). A physiologically-based pharmacokinetic and pharmacodynamic model to describe the oral dosing of rats with ethyl acrylate and its implications for risk assessment. *Toxicol. Appl. Pharmacol.*, **114**, 246–260.

Ghanayem, B. I., Matthews, H. B. and Marenpot, R. R. (1991). Sustainability of forestomach hyperplasia in rats treated with ethyl acrylate for 13 weeks and regression after cessation of dosing. *Toxicol. Pathol.*, **19**, 273–279.

Ghanayem, B. I., Sanchez, I. M., Maronpot, R. R., Elwell, M. R. and Matthews, H. B. (1993). Relationship between time of sustained ethyl acrylate forestomach hyperplasia and carcinogenicity. *Environ. Health Perspect.*, **101**, Suppl. 5, 277–280.

Goldstein, A., Aronow, L. and Kalman, S. M. (1974). Principles of drug action. In *The Basis of Pharmacology*, 2nd edn. Wiley, New York, Chapt. 2.

Grajal, A., Strahl, S. D., Parra, R., Dominguez, M. G. and Neher, A. (1989). Foregut fermination in the hoatzin, a neotropical leaf-eating bird. *Science*, **245**, 1236–1238.

Grouthamel, W. G., Tan, G. H., Dittert, L. W. and Doluisio, J. T. (1971). Drug absorption. IV. Influence of pH on absorption kinetics of weakly acidic drugs. *J. Pharm. Sci.*, **60**, 1160–1163.

Guyton, A. C. (1981). *Textbook of Medical Physiology*, 6th edn. W. B. Saunders, Philadelphia, PA, Chapt. 63–66.

Ham, A. W. and Cormack, D. H. (1979). The digestive system. In *Histology*, 8th edn. J. B. Lippincott, Philadelphia, PA, Chapt. 2, pp. 645–693.

Hobson, D. W., Wyman, J. F., Lee, L. H., Bruner, R. H. and Uddin, D. E. (1987). *The Subchronic Toxicity of Diethylene Glycol Monobutyl Ether Administered Orally to Rats*. Naval Medical Research and Development Command, NMRI 87-48. NTIS, Springfield, VA.

Johnson, F. R. (1981). The digestive system. In Romanes, G. J. (Ed.), *Cunningham's Textbook of Anatomy*, 12th edn. Oxford University Press, New York, Chapt. 6, pp. 411–489.

Johnson, L. R. (1985). Gastric secretion and pancreatic secretion. In Johnson, L. R. (Ed.), *Gastrointestinal Physiology*, 3rd edn. C. V. Mosby, St Louis, MO, Chapt. 8 and 9.

Jones, A. W. and Jönsson, K. Å (1994). Food-induced lowering of blood-ethanol profiles and increased rate of elimination immediately after a meal. *J. Forensic Sci.*, **39**, 1084–1093.

Jorgenson, T. A., Meierhenry, E. F., Rushbrook, C. J., Bull, R. J. and Robinson, M. (1985). Carcinogenicity of chloroform in drinking water to male Osborne–Mendel rats and female B6C3F1 mice. *Fundam. Appl. Toxicol.*, **5**, 760–769.

Kerneis, S., Bogdanova, A., Kraehenbuhl, J.-P. and Pringault, E. (1997). Conversion by Peyer's patch lymphocytes of human enterocytes into M cells that transport bacteria. *Science*, **277**, 949–952.

Kim, H. J., Odend'hal, S. and Bruckner, J. V. (1990). Effect of dosing vehicles on the acute hepatotoxicity of carbon tetrachloride in rats. *Toxicol. Appl. Pharmacol.*, **102**, 34–49.

Krasavage, W. J. and Terhaar, C. J. (1981). *Comparative Toxicity of Nine Glycol Ethers: I. Acute Oral LD50*. Eastman Kodak, Health Safety and Human Factors Laboratory, Rochester, NY.

Lijensky, W. and Reuber, M. D. (1983). Chronic toxicity studies of vinyl acetate in Fischer rats. *Toxicol. Appl. Pharmacol.*, **68**, 43–53.

Mathiowitz, E., Jacob, J. S., Jong, Y. S., Carino, G. P., Chickering, D. E., Chaturvedi, P., Santos, C. A., Vijayaraghavan, K., Montgomery, S., Bassett, M. and Morrell, C. (1997). Biologically erodable microspheres as potential oral drug delivery systems. *Nature*, **386**, 410–414.

McKenna, M. J., Zempel, J. A., Madrid, E. O., Braun, W. H. and Gehring, P. J. (1978). Metabolism and pharmacokinetic profile of vinylidene chloride in rats following oral administration. *Toxicol. Appl. Pharmacol.*, **45**, 821–835.

Melnick, R. L., Jameson, C. W., Goehl, T. J. and Kuhn, G. O. (1987a). Applications of microencapsulation for toxicology studies. I. Principles and stabilization of trichloroethylene in gelatin–sorbitol microcapsules. *Fundam. Appl. Toxicol.*, **8**, 425–431.

Melnick, R. L., Jameson, C. W., Goehl, T. J., Maronpot, R. R., Collins, B. J., Greenwell, A., Harrington, F. W., Wilson, R. E., Tomaszewski, K. E. and Agarwal, D. K. (1987b). Application of microencapsulation for toxicology studies. II. Toxicity of microencapsulated trichloroethylene in Fischer 344 rats. *Fundam. Appl. Toxicol.*, **8**, 432–442.

Miller, R. R., Young, J. T., Kociba, R. J., Keyes, D. G., Bodner, K. M., Calhoun, L. L. and Ayres, J. A. (1985). Chronic toxicity and oncogenicity bioassay of inhaled ethyl acrylate in Fischer 344 rats and B6C3F1 mice. *Drug Chem. Toxicol.*, **8**, 1–42.

NTP (1984). *Final Report—Ethylene Glycol: Fertility Assessment in CD-1 Mice When Administered in Drinking Water*. Report No. NTP-82-FACB-015. National Institute of Environmental Health Sciences, Research Triangle Park, NC.

NTP (1986). *Carcinogenesis Studies of Ethyl Acrylate in F344/N Rats and B6C3F1 Mice (Gavage Studies)*. NIH Publication No. 87–2515. NTP Public Information Office, National Toxicology Program, Research Triangle Park, NC.

Peris-Ribera, J.-E., Torres-Molina, F., Garcia-Carbonell, M. C., Aristorena, J. C. and Pla-Delfina, J. M. (1991). Pharmacokinetics and bioavailability of diclofenac in the rat. *J. Pharmacokinet. Biopharm.*, **19**, 647–664.

Plaa, G. L. (1971). Biliary and other routes of excretion of drugs. In LaDu, B. N., Mandel, H. G., and Way, E. L. (Eds), *Fundamentals of Drug Metabolism and Drug Disposition*, Williams and Wilkins, Baltimore, Chapt. 9, pp. 134–136.

Reuber, M. D. (1979). Carcinogenicity of chloroform. *Environ. Health Perspect.*, **31**, 171–182.

Roth, W. L., Freeman, R. A. and Wilson, A. G. E. (1993). A physiologically based model for gastrointestinal absorption and excretion of chemicals carried by lipids. *Risk Anal.*, **13**, 531–543.

Schanker, L. S. and Jeffrey, J. J. (1961). Active transport of foreign pyrimidines across the intestinal epithelium. *Nature*, **190**, 727–728.

Schanker, L. S., Shore, P. A., Brodie, B. B. and Hogben, C. A. (1957). Absorption of drugs from the stomach, I. The rat. *Pharmacol. Exp. Ther.*, **120**, 528–539.

Sieber, S. M. (1976). The lymphatic absorption of *p,p'*-DDT and some structurally-related compounds in the rat. *Pharmacology*, **14**, 443–454.

Smith, P. L. (1986). Gastrointestinal physiology. In Rozman, K. and O. Hanninen (Eds) *Gastrointestinal Toxicology*. Elsevier, New York, Chapter. 1, pp. 1–28.

Staats, D. A., Fisher, J. W. and Connolly, R. B. (1991). Gastrointestinal absorption of xenobiotics in physiologically based pharmacokinetic models: a two-compartment description. *Drug Metab. Dispos.*, **19**, 144–148.

Tyl, R. W., Fisher, L. C., Kubena, M. F., Losco, P. E. and Vrbanic, M. A., (1989). Determination of a developmental toxicity 'no observable effect level' for ethylene glycol (EC) by gavage in CD-1 mice. *Teratology*, **39**, 487.

Tyler, T. R. and Ballantyne, B. (1988). Practical assessment and communication of chemical hazards in the workplace. In Ballantyne, B. (Ed.), *Perspectives in Basic and Applied Toxicology*. Wright, Bristol, Chapt. 14.

Venho, V. M. K. (1986). Toxicants in the gastrointestinal tract: drugs. In Rozman, K. and O. Hanninen (Eds), *Gastrointestinal Toxicology*. Elsevier, New York, Chapt. 13, pp. 367–368.

Vogel, G., Becker, U. and Ulbrich, M. (1975). The relevance of the osmolarity of the intestinal fluid to the effectiveness and toxicity of drugs given by the intraduodenal route–solvent drug influence on the intestinal absorption of drugs. *Arzneim.–Forsch.*, **25**, 1037–1039.

Weisbrodt, N. W. (1985). Motility of the small intestine. In Johnson, L. R. (Ed.), *Gastrointestinal Physiology*, 3rd edn., C. V. Mosby, Princeton, NJ, Chapt. 5, pp. 39–45.

Welling, P. G. (1977). Influence of food and diet on gastrointestinal drug absorption: a review *J. Pharmacokinet. Biopharm.*, **5**, 291–334.

Welling, P. G. (1984). Interactions affecting drug absorptions. *Clin. Pharmacokinet.*, **9**, 404–434.

Wester, P. W. and Kroes, R. (1988). Forestomach carcinogens: pathology and relevance to man. *Toxicol. Pathol.*, **16**, 165–171.

Williams, R. T. (1971). Species variation in drug metabolism. In LaDu, B. N., Mandel, H. G. and Way, E. L. (Eds) *Fundamentals of Drug Metabolism and Drug Disposition*. Williams and Wilkins, Baltimore, Chapt. 11, pp. 201–203.

Wilson, R. E., Fisher, L. C. and Van Miller, J. P. (1991). Dosing developmental cutaneous toxicity studies using an automated dual delivery system. *Toxicologist*, **11**, 342.

Withey, J. R., Collins, B. T. and Collins, P. G. (1983). Effect of vehicle on the pharmacokinetics and uptake of four halogenated hydrocarbons from the gastrointestinal tract of the rat. *J. Appl. Toxicol.*, **3**, 249–253.

Yuan, J., Jameson, C. W. Goehl, T. J. and Collins, B. J., (1991). Molecular encapsulator: a novel vehicle for toxicology studies. *Toxicol. Methods*, **1**, 231–241.

Chapter 28

Role of Gastro-intestinal Microflora in the Metabolic and Toxicological Activities of Xenobiotics

Ian R. Rowland and Sharat D. Gangolli

CONTENTS

INTRODUCTION

The microflora of the mammalian gastro-intestinal tract, particularly that of the large intestine, interacts with its host both at the local (intestinal mucosa) level and systemically, exerting an extremely diverse range of immunological, physiological and metabolic effects. From the point of view of the host, these effects have consequences, both beneficial and detrimental, for nutrition, infections, xenobiotic metabolism, toxicity of ingested chemicals and cancer.

The microflora relies totally on its host for nutrients, which are provided in the form of undigested dietary residues (especially indigestible carbohydrates such as dietary fibre, resistant starch and non-digestible oligosaccharides), host secretions (intestinal mucins, enzymes, gut hormones, and sloughed mucosal cells. The host animal receives some nutrients from the microflora in the form of vitamins and short chain fatty acids (acetic, propionic and butyric acid) which are absorbed and used as energy sources by the liver and other tissues, including the colonic epithelium (Cummings, 1997).

The gut microflora is a source of infection for wounds and for the urogenital tract and furthermore some members of the microflora can generate potent toxins. However, the microflora plays a very important role in preventing infections of the gut by enteric pathogens such as *Salmonella* and *Shigella* species. This process, which is thought to be a consequence of competition for nutrients and receptors sites, and also the production

by the commensal organisms of inhibitory products, is known as colonization resistance and is a major beneficial effect of the normal gut microflora (Van der Waaij, 1984). In relation to its role in toxic events and carcinogenesis, the gut microflora can have both beneficial and detrimental effects. In general, as will be seen below, the microflora exerts these effects via metabolism, namely by conversion of an ingested chemical to a form that is more or less toxic than the parent compound, resulting in activation or detoxification. There are instances, however, where the microflora has indirect effects on the toxicity of chemicals, for example by modifying mammalian metabolic processes that participate in activation or detoxification.

Before reviewing the role of the gut microflora in the toxicology and carcinogenesis, it is necessary to provide an introduction to the types of bacteria present, their distribution in the gut and the main factors influencing the ecology of the gut.

THE BACTERIAL FLORA OF THE GASTRO-INTESTINAL TRACT OF HUMANS AND LABORATORY ANIMALS

The Microflora of the Mouth

The wide range of surfaces in the oral cavity provides diverse ecological niches and results in a diversity of microfloras both in health and in disease states. The subject has been extensively investigated particularly in relation to dental caries and has been reviewed by Theilade (1990).

From the point of view of toxicology, the saliva flora is of importance because many ingested foreign compounds are secreted in saliva. The salivary flora is dominated by Gram-positive rods and cocci, e.g. actinomyces, lactobacilli, streptococci, micrococci and enterococci. Gram-negative cocci (*Veillonella* spp. and *Neisseria* spp.) are also found (Theilade, 1990).

The salivary flora is of particular importance in the metabolism of nitrate. Ingested nitrate is rapidly absorbed from the proximal small intestine and is then actively secreted in saliva. It has been estimated that about 25% of ingested nitrate is recirculated in saliva (Spiegelhalder *et al.*, 1976). Several of the bacterial species in saliva possess nitrate reductase activity and the level of carriage of these organisms and the specific activity of their enzyme are important factors governing the level of conversion of nitrate to nitrite in saliva in individuals (Packer *et al.*, 1989). Salivary nitrite is the primary source of nitrite in the normal acidic stomach, where it can react with amines, amides and analogous substances to generate *N*-nitroso compounds.

The Microflora of the Stomach

The presence of bacteria in the stomach is largely determined by the pH of the contents. At pH values below 3, bacteria capable of living as commensals in the gut are rapidly killed. Since the pH of the gastric contents of the fasting normal human is usually less than 3, such samples are invariably sterile (Drasar, 1988). However, during a meal, the gastric acid is buffered, which permits bacteria swallowed with food to survive at least until the pH drops. Thus, under such conditions, the gastric flora can only be considered transient. However, where gastric acid secretion is impaired, allowing the pH to remain above 3, bacteria can survive longer and even proliferate. Reduced gastric acid secretion (hypochlorhydria) occurs naturally with ageing and is common after gastric surgery and certain diseases such as pernicious anaemia and hypogammaglobulinaemia. In the latter two cases, subjects are often achlorhydric, which results in the gastric pH rising to 7 and above (Hill, 1995). This allows a diverse flora with up to 10^9 organisms per gram to establish, consisting usually of species of salivary bacteria of the genera *Streptococcus, Neisseria, Staphylococcus* and *Veillonella*, although *Bacteroides, Lactobacillus* and *Escherichia* species are also found (Hill, 1995). Hypochlorhydria is also common in patients with atrophic gastritis associated with chronic *Helicobacter pylori* infection.

The gastric flora of hypochlorhydric individuals has toxicological significance since it increases the likelihood

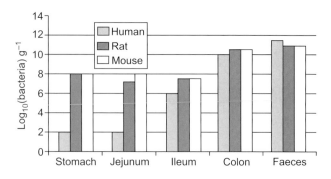

Figure 1 Distribution of bacteria in the gastro-intestinal tracts of man and laboratory animals. Data from Drasar (1988).

of xenobiotic metabolism by the bacteria, particularly since the gastric emptying time of such patients may be up to 5 h (Hill, 1995). It has been suggested that the increased gastric cancer risk of achlorhydric patients is linked to increased formation of *N*-nitroso compounds by their gastric bacteria flora (Hill, 1988). It is important to note that the pH of the gastric contents of the rat and mouse is usually about 5 and not surprisingly, therefore, these animals harbour a substantial microflora in their stomachs **(Figure 1)**. There is therefore an increased potential for bacterial metabolism at this site in comparison with humans, although the relatively short residence time of material in the rodent stomach may mitigate this.

The Microflora of the Small Intestine

The normal human small intestine harbours only a sparse, transient flora due to the bactericidal activity of many of the biliary and pancreatic secretions and the relatively rapid movement of the contents by peristalsis. In some populations, notably in India and South America, small intestinal colonization is common and appears to be associated with malnutrition (Bhat *et al.*, 1972). As the gut contents reach the terminal ileum, the rate of transit slows and a more permanent flora begins to develop, assisted by reflux of caecal material **(Figure 1)**.

The Microflora of the Large Intestine

The microbial community that inhabits the human large intestine is an exceedingly complex ecological system. Studies of the ecology and metabolism of the microflora poses a number of technical problems:

1. *Predominance of strictly anaerobic bacteria.* Over 99% of the bacteria in the large intestine are highly fastidious anaerobes many of which are killed by even brief exposure to air **(Table 1)**. Over the last 25 years, sophisticated methods have been developed to culture these organisms, initially using roll tubes in which agar is spread as a layer on the inside of tubes

Table 1 The bacterial flora of human faeces. Data from Mitsuoka (1982); Drasar (1988); Hill (1995)

Bacterial group	Log (bacteria) g^{-1} faeces
Strict anaerobes	
Bacteroides	10–11
Eubacteria	9–10
Bifidobacteria	10–11
Propionibacteria	9–10
Peptococci	9–10
Clostridia	6–9
Fusobacteria	5–10
Microaerophiles	
Lactobacilli	4–10
Facultative organisms	
Enterococci	7–8
Enterobacteria	7–9

that are flushed with anaerobic gases (Holdeman and Moore, 1973). More recently, anaerobic cabinets have become commercially available, which comprise large Perspex cabinets that are flushed with an anaerobic gas mixture (usually nitrogen, carbon dioxide and hydrogen) and contain palladium catalysts that remove any traces of oxygen. These cabinets facilitate the handling of faecal samples and allow the use of the conventional plating techniques of serial dilution and spreading of samples on Petri dishes. Materials can be placed inside the cabinets via an airlock and the operator gains access and manipulates the samples using gloves. Anaerobic cabinets can also be used for incubating faecal samples or faecal organisms in studies of xenobiotic metabolism.

An associated problem, which is a consequence of the presence of strict anaerobes in the microflora, is that samples of gut contents and faeces need to be processed quickly after collection to ensure viability of the organisms is retained. The gut organisms are differentially sensitive to freezing, so quantitative studies are not feasible with frozen samples. It should also be noted that studies of reductive bacterial metabolism cannot be performed on frozen samples owing to inactivation of bacteria and/or enzymes and cofactors (Coates *et al.*, 1988).

2. *Identification of predominant organisms in the gut.* In addition to requiring strict anaerobic conditions for their culture, faecal bacteria need complex growth media containing many rich supplements including minerals, vitamins and blood (Holdeman and Moore, 1973). More importantly, there are few reliable selective agars for initial isolation of the main groups of anaerobes. Identification of such bacteria to even the genus level requires laborious 'picking off' of colonies from non-selective agars, purification and screening for a range of biochemical markers (Holdeman and Moore, 1973). The availability of commercial, semi-automated rapid screening systems

such as API has speeded up the process but these classical methods make comparisons of microfloras of different people, or studies of dietary effects, very time consuming and expensive. Molecular methods incorporating DNA probes, 16sRNA, and pulsed field gel electrophoresis are now being developed which will permit much more rapid and accurate quantitation and identification of gut bacteria and additionally allow the use of frozen samples (Vandamme *et al.*, 1996).

3. *Sampling of colonic contents.* Most data on the composition of the human large intestinal microflora and its metabolic activities have been derived from analyses of faecal samples. How representative the faecal flora is of the colonic flora is debatable. Alternative methods of varying degrees of complexity and unpleasantness for the subject have been used for obtaining samples of colon contents, but these also have disadvantages and do not necessarily provide representative samples (reviewed by Hill, 1995; Coates *et al.*, 1988).

It has been estimated that the human colon harbours over 400 species of bacteria (Mitsuoka 1982; Drasar, 1988). The faecal flora is dominated by strictly anaerobic rod-shaped bacteria of the genera *Bacteroides*, *Eubacterium*, *Fusobacterium*, *Bifidobacterium* and *Propionibacterium* (**Table 1**). Other genera found in large numbers include *Clostridium* and various anaerobic cocci. Less numerous are lactobacilli, which are microaerophilic, and the main facultative organisms (i.e. those that can grow in the presence or absence of oxygen), namely enterococci and enterobacteria.

Because of the technical difficulties in enumerating the faecal microflora, comparisons of the microflora of populations from different countries have yielded equivocal results (Aries *et al.*, 1969; Drasar and Hill, 1974; Finegold *et al.*, 1983). It is often considered that the microflora is very stable, but this may be so only at a superficial (main bacterial group) level. A recent, highly detailed, study of the faecal lactic acid bacteria of two individuals has revealed enormous day to day variation at the species and strain level (McCartney *et al.*, 1996).

Although it appears that the main groups of anaerobes found in faeces of rats and mice are similar to those in humans (reviewed by Drasar, 1988), there may be large differences in genera and species. Certainly major differences in metabolic activity have been detected among laboratory animals and humans (see below).

In view of the importance of intestinal bacterial metabolism in mediating toxicological events, some general points need to be made to provide an introduction to the more detailed discussions of specific reactions described below.

Little is known about the ability of the individual species that comprise the microflora to metabolize nutrients and foreign compounds. Even if it were, it would be difficult to predict whether a reaction that occurred *in vitro* with a pure culture of a gut organism would proceed when that organism was surrounded by other members of the ecosystem within the mammalian gut. Indeed, marked differences have been reported in the metabolic activity of a gut anaerobe when measured *in vitro* and when the same organism was mono-associated with a gnotobiotic rat (Cole *et al.*, 1985). Information on the reactions performed by the individual species that constitute the flora is therefore usually of little use.

A more valid and useful approach for understanding the role of the microflora in toxic events in man is to consider the flora as an additional 'organ' within the host, ignoring its multi-organism composition. (Midtvedt, 1989; Rowland, 1989).

The reactions catalysed by the gut microflora are limited by the prevailing conditions in the lumen of the intestinal tract, notably the low redox potential and the lack of oxygen. Consequently, oxidative reactions are rare. It should be noted, however, that the physicochemical conditions, particularly in oxygen tension, in the region close to the intestinal mucosa are likely to be very different from those in the lumen and may permit very different types of reactions to occur, although these have not been studied.

An important factor to be taken into account when considering foreign compound metabolism by gut bacteria is the location of the main population in the alimentary tract. The colon is the region of the gut that harbours the greatest number of bacteria, indeed other areas of the human gastro-intestinal tract are very sparsely populated. This does not mean, however, that only poorly absorbed chemicals encounter the colonic flora. Substances, and their metabolites, may enter the colon across

Table 2 Toxicological implications of gut microflora activities

1. Activation to toxicants, mutagens, carcinogens
   Azo compounds
   Nitro compounds
   Plant glycosides
   IQ
2. Synthesis of carcinogens
   N-Nitroso compounds
   Fecapentaenes
3. Synthesis of promoters
   Bile acids
   Protein breakdown products (ammonia, phenols, cresols)
   Fecapentaenes
4. Enterohepatic circulation and deconjugation
   Steroid hormones and drugs
   Carcinogens
5. Detoxification/protection
   Methyl mercury
   Phyto-oestrogens
   Flavonoids
   Carcinogen binding

the intestinal wall from the blood or may reach the colon after excretion in the bile. Thus there is ample opportunity for a wide variety of materials in diet to encounter and be metabolized by the colonic microflora.

Metabolism of foreign or endogenously produced substances by the colonic microflora can have wide-ranging implications for human health with both beneficial and detrimental consequences. These are summarized in **Table 2** and are considered in more detail below.

ACTIVATION OF CHEMICALS TO TOXIC, MUTAGENIC AND CARCINOGENIC DERIVATIVES

Azo Compounds

A major proportion of colouring agents used in production of food, cosmetics, textiles, rubber products, pharmaceuticals, plastics, leather and printing inks are based on azo compounds (Collier *et al.*, 1993). These azo dyes contain one or more R–N=N–R′ bonds, which, after consumption of the dye, can be reductively cleaved by azoreductase enzymes to yield aromatic amines. Although for some azo dyes their toxicity is a consequence of the interaction of the parent compound with certain cytosolic receptors, in particular the *Ah* receptor (Lubet *et al.*, 1983), for others toxicity is mediated by arylamines and free radicals formed during azo reduction (Collier *et al.*, 1993). Azoreduction can be catalysed by mammalian reductases in the liver and by bacterial activity in the gut; however, the latter is considered to play a more important role than the hepatic enzymes (Brown, 1981; Rafii *et al.*, 1995).

One of the best illustrations of the importance of gut bacterial azo reduction is the metabolism of Direct Black 38. Workers exposed to Direct Black 38, a dye used in the leather and textile industry, have an elevated risk of bladder cancer, which has been attributed to the reduction of the dye by the gut microflora to benzidine, a proven human bladder carcinogen (Cerniglia *et al.*, 1982). Incubation of Direct Black 38 with cultures of human intestinal bacteria results in the rapid formation of benzidine, indicating that the microflora is the major site of metabolism of the dye. Studies with more sophisticated, continuous culture systems have revealed that several of the other urinary metabolites of the dye, including the *N*-acetylated derivative, can be attributed to gut microflora metabolism (Manning *et al.*, 1985). Since acetylation is a crucial step in the activation of aromatic amines to their ultimate carcinogenic metabolite, these studies implicate the gut microflora not only in the overall metabolism in the body of benzidine-based azo dyes but also in the generation of the reactive, carcinogenic species.

Other azo dyes exhibiting carcinogenic effects, or generating carcinogens after reduction, include Butter Yellow and Methyl Red (both reduced to 4-aminodimethylaniline), Trypan Blue (reduced to the bladder carcinogen *o*-tolidine) and Orange II (converted to 1-amino-2-naphthol) (Hartman *et al.*, 1978; Chung *et al.*, 1992).

The Ames mutagenicity assay, modified to include a reduction step with gut bacteria (mixed or pure cultures) prior to exposure to the *Salmonella* strains, has been extensively used in studies on azo dyes (Garner and Nutman, 1977; Haveland-Smith and Combes, 1980; Dillon *et al.*, 1994; Rafii *et al.*, 1997). The majority of the azo dyes shown to be mutagenic are benzidine-based and are not used in foods, cosmetics or pharmaceuticals. Structure–activity investigations have revealed that at least two amino or nitro groups are necessary for mutagenicity (Garner and Nutman, 1977). The azo dyes currently approved for food use by FDA do not exhibit mutagenicity (Rafii *et al.*, 1997). D & C Red No. 9, which until recently had a provisional FDA listing for use in cosmetics and drugs, has been shown to induce splenic sarcomas and liver nodules in rats and to be mutagenic after an extensive period of reduction (Dillon *et al.*, 1994). Although not detected in the reduction mixture, 1-amino-2-naphthol was presumed to be the mutagenic metabolite.

Azo reduction by intestinal bacteria is exploited for the clinical effects of some drugs such as the early antibiotic agents prontosil rubrum and neoprontosil, which are azo derivatives of sulphonamides. One of the most important of these azo drugs is sulphasalazine (salicylazosulphapyridine), commonly used to treat patients with ulcerative colitis. The drug is activated by azoreductase in the colon to yield sulphapyridine and 5-aminosalicylic acid, which suppresses mucosal inflammation (Peppercorn and Goldman, 1972).

Nitro Compounds

There is extensive human exposure, both deliberate and accidental, to nitro compounds. For example, heterocyclic and aromatic nitro compounds are extensively used in industry as important intermediates in the manufacture of consumer products and comprise an important class of drugs with uses as antibiotic, anti-parasitic and radiosensitizing agents. In addition, nitroaromatics are ubiquitous environmental contaminants derived from diesel exhaust, cigarette smoke and airborne particulates. These compounds often possess toxic, mutagenic and carcinogenic activity and so may contribute to the environmental cancer risk in man.

Reduction of the nitro group to an amine occurs via nitroso and hydroxylamino intermediates and is usually required for the pharmacological and toxicological activity of these compounds to be expressed. For example,

reduction is a crucial step in the anti-trichomonad activity and mutagenicity of metronidazole (Lindmark and Muller, 1976) and in the induction of methaemoglobinaemia by nitrobenzenes (Reddy *et al.*, 1976). The nitro group on nitroaromatic compounds can be reduced by both hepatic and gut microflora-associated reductases, but in most cases the latter appear to be the more important. Evidence for the importance of bacterial reductases in the induction of methaemoglobinaemia by nitrobenzene has been obtained by exposing conventional flora, antibiotic-treated and germ-free rats to the compound. Methaemoglobin levels of 30–40% were induced in the conventional rats, whereas no increase was detected in the animals without a gut flora (Reddy *et al.*, 1976). Levin and Dent (1982) demonstrated that nitrobenzene was readily reduced by caecal contents to aniline, via nitrosobenzene and phenylhydroxylamine (the presumed methaemoglobinogenic metabolites). Although aniline was also produced in the presence of liver microsomes, the rate of reduction was less than 1% of that in the presence of bacteria. There is conclusive evidence, therefore, that the intestinal microflora is a major determinant of both the metabolism and acute toxicity of nitrobenzene.

The toxicity of the important chemical intermediates, dinitrotoluenes, has been shown to be similarly dependent on the reductive activity of the intestinal microflora. In this case, genotoxicity and the ability to bind covalently to macromolecules (a critical early step in tumorigenesis) were lower in germ-free than in conventional rats (Mirsalis and Hamm, 1982). Studies in germ-free and conventional microflora rats and in *in vitro* cultures have demonstrated the crucial role of gut microflora-mediated reduction in the metabolism of nitrated polycyclic aromatic hydrocarbons, such as 1-nitropyrene and 6-nitrochrysene (El-Bayoumy *et al.*, 1983; Manning *et al.*, 1988). It is significant that 6-aminochrysene is known to induce liver and lung tumours in mice, suggesting that nitroreduction by the gut microflora plays an important role in the activation and tumorigenesis by nitrochrysene.

Plant Glycosides

Plants glycosides comprise a wide variety of low molecular weight substances linked to sugar moieties (Brown, 1988). They are widely distributed in fruits and vegetables and in beverages, such as tea and wine, derived from plants. Estimates of human intake of plant glycosides range from 50 to 1000 mg per day (Brown, 1988). In their glycosidic form most of these substances are relatively harmless. It is usually assumed that they are poorly absorbed from the gut and thus pass intact into the colon; however, there is some evidence that flavonoid glycosides may be at least partially absorbed (Hollman *et al.*, 1995). Glycosides reaching the colon are subjected to the action of β-glycosidases associated with the resident microbial flora, which cleave the sugar moiety releasing aglycones, which have a variety of biological activities including toxicity, mutagenicity and carcinogenicity. Amygdalin, a glycoside found in several drupes and pomes, is hydrolysed to mandelonitrile, which subsequently decomposes to cyanide. After oral exposure to amygdalin, germ-free rats, in contrast to rats with a conventional microflora, have lower thiocyanate levels in the blood and do not exhibit cyanide toxicity. Cyanogenic glycosides are also present in cassava, a staple crop in many countries in the tropics. In periods of food shortage, the plants are sometimes consumed without appropriate treatments for removing the glycosides, leading to cyanide exposure and acute poisoning or chronic neurological disease (Brown, 1988).

Cycasin (a glycosidic component of cycad nuts) is hydrolysed by bacterial β-glucosidase in the colon of conventional flora rats releasing the aglycone methylazoxymethanol (MAM), which induces colon tumours. No such tumours are found in germ-free rats fed the glycoside.

Many of the plant glycosides are mutagenic after hydrolysis by bacterial glycosidases. Some of the most common of these are the glycosides of quercetin, including rutin (quercetin-O-rutinoside) and quercetrin (qercetin-O-rhamnoside), which are found in lettuce and many other edible plants. When tested for mutagenicity using the *Salmonella*/microsome assay, mutagenic activity in these plant materials can only be detected when a faecal bacterial extract is added to the incubation mixture (Van der Hoeven *et al.*, 1983). Similarly, potent mutagenic activity can be detected in red wine and tea when the beverages are incubated with an extract of human faeces, a finding attributed to the presence of plant glycosides. Apart from cycasin, plant glycosides do not appear to be carcinogenic, despite their demonstrable mutagenic activity. Quercetin has been investigated for carcinogenicity in a number of animal models and in general has been found not to exhibit tumorigenic properties (Brown, 1988). In two-stage carcinogenicity studies in rats with quercetin, no evidence was found for initiating activity for liver tumours (using phenobarbital and partial hepatectomy as promoters) or for tumour-promoting activity (using MAM as an initiator). A similar lack of initiating and promoting activity towards rat bladder carcinogenesis has been reported. Assessment of the toxicological significance of glycoside hydrolysis by intestinal microflora is complicated by reports of potential anti-carcinogenic and anti-mutagenic effects of flavonoid aglycones (see below).

It is clear, therefore, that hydrolysis of plant glycosides in the gut can lead, potentially, to both adverse and beneficial consequences for man. Further studies are needed to establish the repercussions for colon cancer of flavonoid release from glycosides by β-glycosidases in the gut.

IQ

2-Amino-3-methyl-3H-imidazo[4,5-f]quinoline (IQ) is one of several heterocyclic amine compounds formed in small quantities when meat and fish are grilled or fried. It induces tumours at various sites in rodents, including the large intestine, suggesting that it may play a role in the aetiology of colon cancer in man (Ohgaki *et al.*, 1991).

Incubation of IQ with a human faecal suspension yields the 7-keto derivative, 2-amino-3,6-dihydro-3-methyl-7H-imidazo[4,5-f]quinolin-7-one (7-OHIQ). The 7-keto metabolite has been found in faeces of individuals consuming a diet containing a high level of fried meat indicating that the formation of 7-OHIQ can occur *in vivo* in man (Carman *et al.*, 1988). Unlike IQ itself, the bacterial metabolite is a direct-acting and potent mutagen in *Salmonella typhimurium* and induces DNA damage in colon cells *in vitro* (Carman *et al.*, 1988; Rumney *et al.*, 1993; Rowland and Pool-Zobel, unpublished observation, 1996). Thus there is strong evidence for the bacterial formation in the human gut of a directly genotoxic derivative of a dietary carcinogen.

Dechlorination Reactions

The metabolism of trichloroethylene and its main metabolite (trichloroacetic acid) (TCA) by gut microflora has been studied *in vitro* and *in vivo* in rodents. Anaerobic incubations of rat or mouse caecal contents did not reveal any metabolism of trichloroethylene, but TCA was converted to dichloroacetic acid under these conditions (Moghaddam *et al.*, 1996). Metabolism was inhibited under aerobic conditions, suggesting that strict anaerobes were responsible for the dechlorination process. A follow-up study of trichloroethylene metabolism in normal mice and in mice with a depleted microflora indicated that although dichloroacetic acid was formed, there was no evidence for a role for the gut microflora (Moghaddam *et al.*, 1997).

Several genera of gut bacteria, including bacteroides, clostridia and coliforms, have been shown to dechlorinate p, p-DDT reductively to p, p-TDE (Braunberg and Beck, 1968). In this case, *in vivo* studies in rats supported the *in vitro* evidence. When p, p-DDT was given orally, p, p-TDE was detected in the liver, whereas only DDT was found after intraperitoneal administration (Mendel and Walton, 1966).

SYNTHESIS OF CARCINOGENS

Nitrate Reduction and *N*-Nitroso Compound Synthesis

Nitrate, ingested via the diet and drinking water, is readily converted by the nitrate reductase activity of the intestinal microflora to its more reactive and toxic reduction product, nitrite. Nitrite reacts with nitrogenous compounds such as amines, amides and methylureas in the body to produce N-nitroso compounds, many of which are highly carcinogenic. The reaction can occur chemically in the acidic conditions prevalent in the human stomach and can also be catalysed at neutral pH by gut bacteria. To assess the significance of the gut microflora in nitrosation reactions in the body, Massey *et al.* (1988) investigated the concentration of N-nitroso compounds in tissues and gut contents of germ-free and conventional microflora rats. The compounds were detected in significant amounts only in gut contents of the conventional flora rats, with the largest quantities being found in the colon contents. In contrast, in the germ-free rats, little or no nitroso compounds were detected in the gut contents. The enzyme involved in the nitrosation process has not been isolated, but from studies in pure cultures of bacteria, it has been suggested that nitrosation may be associated with the activity of nitrate and nitrite reductases (Leach, 1988). Subsequently, the investigations have been extended to man. N-Nitroso compounds were detectable at concentrations up to 590 mg kg^{-1} in faeces of male and female volunteers (Rowland *et al.*, 1991). The importance of ingested nitrate to the level of faecal nitroso compounds was demonstrated by providing the volunteers with nitrate-free food and water. Under these dietary conditions, the concentrations of faecal nitroso compounds decreased to almost undetectable values over a period of 5 days. When nitrate was added to the drinking water, a rapid rise in faecal nitroso compound concentration was seen, reaching a level similar to that recorded for the volunteers on their own diets.

Subsequently, Bingham *et al.* (1996) studied the effect of meat consumption on levels of faecal N-nitroso compounds in human volunteers. When red meat (beef, lamb and pork) intake was increased from 60 to 600 g day^{-1}, subjects excreted approximately three times more N-nitroso compounds in faeces. In two volunteers, white meat intake was increased to 600 g day^{-1} without any increase in faecal N-nitroso compound level. There is weak epidemiological evidence to suggest that red meat but not white meat intake is associated with colon cancer risk.

Fecapentaenes

Using the Ames *Salmonella* assay, mutagenic activity has been detected in human faecal samples. Faeces from individuals excreting large amounts of mutagenic activity have been extracted and the mutagenic agents purified. Structural analysis revealed a glyceryl ether compound containing a pentaene moiety with a chain length of 12 or 14 (Bruce *et al.*, 1982; Hirai *et al.*, 1982). They have been termed fecapentaene-12 or -14 (FP12, FP14). Both types are found in faeces although the ratio

varies considerably. The gut microflora has been implicated in their synthesis by the demonstration of fecapentaene production *in vitro* by faecal suspensions under anaerobic conditions and the inhibition of that synthesis by antibiotics and heat sterilization (Hirai *et al.*, 1982).

Although FP occur in faeces of the majority of Western populations, more detailed epidemiological studies have revealed some anomalies. For example, lower FP levels were found in faeces from colorectal cancer patients than in controls and faecal excretion of FP is higher in vegetarians, a population at low risk from colon cancer (Schiffman *et al.*, 1989; de Kok *et al.*, 1992). These and other studies suggest that there is an inverse correlation between FP excretion and risk of colon cancer. This has a certain logic in that FP is a very potent direct-acting mutagen and would be expected to react extremely rapidly with DNA and other macromolecules in the colonic mucosa. Thus increased faecal excretion may reflect lower endogenous exposure to the genotoxin. At low concentrations (0.6–10 μg ml^{-1}), fecapentaene-12 induces single-strand DNA breaks, gene mutations, chromosome aberrations, sister chromatid exchanges and unscheduled DNA synthesis in human fibroblasts *in vitro* (Plummer *et al.*, 1986). Results of *in vivo* studies have yielded more equivocal results. Fecapentaene-12 increased the proliferation of mucosal cells and DNA single-strand breaks when it was instilled into rat colon (Hinzman *et al.*, 1987). Similarly, intrarectal administration to mice increased mitosis, but not nuclear aberrations, in colonic crypt cells. Rodent bioassays have indicated that fecapentaene-12 does not have carcinogenic or tumour-initiating activity (Ward *et al.*, 1988; Weisburger *et al.*, 1990; Shamsuddin *et al.*, 1991). However, Zarkovic *et al.*, (1993) have provided evidence for tumour-promoting activity of fecapentaene and this is consistent with some of the data described above, which indicates that the compound induces mucosal cell proliferation in the colon.

SYNTHESIS OF TUMOUR PROMOTERS

Investigations of possible tumour promoters generated by bacterial activity in the colon have focused on bile acids and protein breakdown products and have been extensively reviewed (Hill, 1988; Clinton, 1992), so only a brief summary will be provided here.

Secondary Bile Acids

The liver secretes two major bile acids—cholic and chenodeoxycholic acid—that are subject to extensive metabolism by the intestinal microflora (MacDonald *et al.*, 1993). Of particular importance *in vivo* is 7-α-dehydroxylation, which converts cholic to deoxycholic acid and chenodeoxycholic to lithocholic acid. These two secondary bile acids, which comprise over 80% of faecal bile acids, are postulated to play an important role in the aetiology of colon cancer by acting as promoters of the tumorigenic process. There is considerable evidence to indicate that acid steroids, in particular secondary bile acids, can exert a range of biological effects. They induce cell necrosis, hyperplasia, metabolic alterations and DNA synthesis in intestinal mucosal cells, enhance the genotoxicity of a number of mutagens in *in vitro* assays, and exhibit tumour-promoting activity in the colon (reviewed by Rowland *et al.*, 1985). There is also some recent evidence that secondary bile acids, albeit at relatively high concentrations, can induce DNA damage in colon cells in culture (Venturi *et al.*, 1997).

Protein and Amino Acid Metabolites.

Epidemiological studies indicate a link between high intake of protein and incidence of colon cancer. These studies together with investigations *in vitro* and in laboratory animals have led to the hypothesis that colonic ammonia, produced by bacterial catabolism of amino acids and other nitrogenous compounds, may participate in tumour promotion (Clinton, 1992). Increasing the protein content of the diet increases the colonic luminal ammonia concentration. Ammonia exhibits a number of effects that suggest that it may be involved in promotion including increasing mucosal cell turnover and altering DNA synthesis. More definitively, it has been shown to increase the incidence of colon carcinomas induced by *N*-methyl-*N*-nitro-*N*-nitrosoguanidine in rats. Less well studied than ammonia has been the formation of phenols and cresols by bacterial deamination of certain aromatic amino acids in the colon. The generation of phenols is higher when high protein diets are consumed and there is some evidence for tumour-promoting activity, albeit in a mouse skin assay (Hill, 1988).

Fecapentaenes

Evidence has been obtained that fecapentaenes may possess tumour-promoting activity in a rat colon carcinogenesis model using *N*-methyl-*N*-nitrosurea (MNU) as an initiating agent (Zarkovic *et al.*, 1993). The number of carcinoma-bearing rats and the number of carcinomas per rat were significantly higher in the animals given MNU and fecapentaene compared with those given MNU alone.

β-GLUCURONIDASE AND ENTEROHEPATIC CIRCULATION

Many toxic and carcinogenic compounds and also endogenously produced compounds such as steroids are oxidized in the liver by cytochrome P450-dependent enzymes and then conjugated by 'Phase II enzymes' to glucuronic acid, sulphate, glutathione or amino acids. Because of the high molecular weight and polar nature of these of these conjugates, they are extensively excreted via the bile into the small intestine. In the colon, the bacterial activities such as β-glucuronidase, sulphatase and C–S lyase, can hydrolyse the conjugates releasing the parent compound, or its hepatic metabolite. Since the deconjugated compounds are usually more easily absorbed, deconjugation may result in an enterohepatic circulation as the compound is reabsorbed, returning to the liver where it can be subjected to further metabolism and conjugation. Enterohepatic circulation is responsible for conservation and reutilization of endogenous substrates such as steroids and bile acids. Enterohepatic cycling is useful for some drugs by helping to maintain therapeutic levels in plasma. However, it also results in xenobiotics being retained in the body, thus potentiating their pharmacological, physiological and toxic effects (Larsen, 1988).

The critical role of the intestinal microflora is evident from studies on antibiotic-treated animals and by the use of the β-glucuronidase inhibitor D-saccharic acid-1,4-lactone. For example, antibiotic suppression of the gut microflora decreases enterohepatic circulation of oestrodiol, mestranol and morphine (Chipman and Coleman, 1995). A selective list of compounds known to undergo enterohepatic circulation is given in **Table 3**.

Oestrogen Conjugates

Enterohepatic circulation appears to be of particular importance in the absorption and metabolism of endogenously produced and synthetic steroids. Most natural and synthetic steroids, including oestrogens, are conjugated with glucuronic and/or sulphuric acid in the liver prior to excretion in urine or bile. Glucuronidation can also occur in several other tissues, including the intestinal wall. Bacterial β-glucuronidase and sulphatase acting on the conjugates of these steroids can thus affect hormonal activity and bioavailability of these steroids and their metabolites (Eyssen and Caenepeel, 1988). For example, absorption of oestrone-3-sulphate from intestinal loops is more efficient in rats with a microflora than in germ-free rats. Hydrolysis of oestrogen sulphate conjugates has been demonstrated in *in vitro* incubations with pure cultures of gut bacteria from humans. The organisms included strains of *Clostridium*, *Peptostreptococcus*, *Peptococcus* and *Eubacterium* spp. Similarly, hydrolysis of steroid glucuronides, including oestrone-3-glucuronide and oestradiol-17-glucuronide, has been shown to occur in the presence organisms such as *Escherichia coli* and *Peptostreptococcus productus*.

Table 3 Examples of compounds that undergo enterohepatic circulation

Type of compound	Example	Conjugate[a]
Antibiotic	Chloramphenicol	Gluc
	Griseofulvin	
	Metronidazole	Gluc
Neuroactive agent	Morphine	O-gluc
	Phenobarbital (phenobarbitone)	Gluc
Analgaesic	Acetaminophen (paracetamol)	Glut
	Phenacetin	Gluc
Carcinogen	Benzo[a]pyrene	Gluc/sulphate
	Benzidine	Gluc/glut
	Aflatoxin B$_1$	Glut
	Safrole	Gluc/glut
Pesticide	Propachlor	Gluc/glut/cyst
	3-Phenoxybenzoic acid	
Metal	Methylmercury	Glut
Endogenous compound	Bile acids	Glycine/taurine
	Oestradiol	Gluc
	Testosterone	
Synthetic hormone	Diethylstilboestrol	Gluc
	Ethinyloestradiol	O-Gluc/sulphate
Circulatory system drug	Digoxin	
	Warfarin	Sulphate/O-gluc
Industrial chemicals	Dinitrotoluenes	Gluc
	Hexachlorobutadiene	Glut
	Phenol	Gluc

[a] Gluc = glucuronide; Glut = glutathione.
Source: after Larsen (1988) and Chipman and Coleman (1995).

Other Conjugates

A number of drugs, such as chloramphenicol, diflunisal, fenclofenac, phenacetin and phenobarbital, also undergo enterohepatic circulation, which influences their pharmaceutical and toxicological effects. For example, chloramphenicol is excreted as a glucuronide conjugate in the bile of rats, and is subsequently hydrolysed in the gut and reduced to an arylamine. This is then reabsorbed and exerts a toxic effect on the thyroid (Larsen, 1988).

In the case of carcinogens and mutagens, the activity of β-glucuronidase in the colon may increase the likelihood of tumour induction. For example, with the colon carcinogen 1,2-dimethylhydrazine (DMH), small amounts of procarcinogenic glucuronide conjugates of the activated metabolite (methylazoxymethanol; MAM) formed in the liver are excreted in the bile. Hydrolysis of the conjugates by colonic bacteria releases the MAM in the colon. As might be expected, germ-free rats have fewer colon tumours after treatment with DMH or with MAM–glucuronic acid conjugate than do conventional flora animals (Reddy et al., 1974). The carcinogen benzo[a]pyrene (BaP), a common contaminant of the human diet, undergoes a similar sequence of reactions to that of DMH. Polar conjugates, including the glucuronide (about 35% of the dose), are excreted in bile following administration of BaP to rodents and are hydrolysed to BaP and BaP diols by gut bacteria (Chipman et al., 1983). These products, unlike the conjugates from which they are derived, bind to DNA and are mutagenic in in vitro assays. It is possible, therefore, that bacterial metabolites of BaP formed in the colon may be initiators of carcinogenesis. Other carcinogens for which β-glucuronidase activity is important for their action include benzidine, nitropyrene and dinitrotoluenes.

DETOXIFICATION AND PROTECTIVE EFFECTS OF THE MICROFLORA

Demethylation of Methylmercury

The high neurotoxicity of methylmercury (MeHg) is due to a combination of its efficient absorption from the gut, its long retention time in the body and its ability to penetrate the blood–brain barrier.

Because of its rapid and virtually complete absorption from the gut, the body burden of mercury after methylmercury (MeHg) exposure is determined largely by its rate of elimination, the main route of which is the faeces (Clarkson, 1979). In rats and mice given MeHg, the majority (50–90%) of the mercury in faeces is in the mercuric form, and therefore demethylation of MeHg would appear to be an important step in the excretion of the organomercurial from the body. The role of the gut microflora in this process has been reviewed recently (Rowland, 1995), so will be discussed only briefly below.

Ingested MeHg undergoes enterohepatic circulation and reaches the gut flora as an MeHg–glutathione complex in bile. Incubation of methylmercuric chloride (or its glutathione complex) with gut contents from the rat or mouse, or with suspensions of human faeces, results in extensive metabolism of the organomercurial with a variety of metabolites being produced, including elemental mercury and mercuric ion. Studies in germ-free rodents and animals treated with antibiotics to suppress their gut bacteria provide further evidence for the importance of gut bacteria in demethylation *in vivo*. Suppression or absence of the gut microflora was associated with decreased excretion of total mercury, lower amounts of mercuric ion in faeces, and significantly higher body burdens of mercury in comparison with conventional flora animals. The concentration of mercury in the brain after MeHg exposure was found to be 25–45% greater in germ-free or antibiotic-treated animals than in controls and was associated with a higher incidence of neurotoxicity and neuropathological damage.

Changes in gut microflora with age may influence susceptibility to *MeHg toxicity. Suckling mice absorb and retain the majority of an oral dose of MeHg (half-time of mercury elimination, $t_{1/2}$, greater than 100 days)* whereas older mice excrete the mercurial much more rapidly ($t_{1/2}$ 6–10 days). This developmental change in rate of excretion coincides with an increase in the demethylation activity of the gut microflora during weaning. Corresponding developmental changes in demethylating capacity occur in the human gut microflora. The virtual absence of demethylating capacity in faecal suspensions from unweaned human babies implies that they would absorb and retain more of an oral dose of MeHg than adults, making them more susceptible to MeHg neurotoxicity.

Phytoestrogens

Two groups of diphenolic hormone-like compounds, the isoflavonoids and lignans, are considered to be potential cancer-preventing agents because of their abundance in the plasma of subjects living in areas with low cancer incidence.

Genistin and daidzin and their aglycones genistein and daidzein are isoflavonoid phyto-oestrogens found almost exclusively in soybean products. The lignans are more widely distributed, being found in cereal brans, especially rye, fruits and berries and flaxseed. The major lignans are matairesinol and secoisolariciresinol, usually found as the glycosides and diglycosides.

The isoflavonoids and lignans undergo extensive metabolism in the human body with the intestinal flora being the major site of biotransformation (Rowland *et al.*, 1999). The glycosides of both isoflavonoids and lignans are rapidly hydrolysed by gut bacteria. It is thought that hydrolysis is necessary for their absorption from the gut; however, there is some evidence that glycosides of the related flavonoids may be absorbed intact.

The aglycones undergo further metabolism by gut bacteria. Genistein may be converted to the hormonally inert *p*-ethylphenol, whilst daidzein can be reduced to the isoflavan equol and *O*-desmethylangolensin (*O*-Dma) (Setchell and Adlercreutz, 1988). The lignans undergo similar bacterial metabolism with matairesinol being converted to enterolactone and secoisolariciresinol to enterodiol. Enterodiol may then be converted to enterolactone in the gut. The various bacterial metabolites can be detected in both urine and faeces (Setchell and Adlercreutz, 1988).

Studies in human subjects have shown that there are considerable inter-individual differences in isoflavone and lignan metabolism. For example, it has been reported that 35% of the population are able to produce equol after a soy challenge (Lampe *et al.*, 1998; Rowland *et al.*, 1999). The individual variation in metabolism may have important physiological and health implications which have not been fully assessed. There have been extensive investigations into the biological activities of the phyto-oestrogens and some of their urinary metabolites, particularly in relation to their oestrogenic and anti-oestrogenic activity and also antioxidant properties (reviewed by Rowland *et al.*, 1999). Although these investigations suggest that, certainly for the isoflavonoids, there may be differences in biological activity between parent compounds and bacterial metabolites, most do not provide direct comparisons within the same study. There is evidence, however, that equol has more potent biological effects than daidzein, both *in vitro* and *in vivo*, in relation to potential cancer-preventing properties. Markiewicz *et al.* (1993) showed, in an *in vitro* assay, that the oestrogenic potency of equol was about three times greater than that of daidzein. This is consistent with a subsequent study in the MCF-7 oestrogen-dependent breast tumour cell line. In the latter cells, equol was 100 times more potent than daidzein in eliciting an oestrogenic response and was more effective in competing with oestradiol for binding to the oestrogen receptor. There is also evidence that equol and daidzein exhibit different antioxidant activities. Equol was more potent than daidzein in inhibiting lipid peroxidation in liposomes induced by Fe(II) or Fe(III) (Arora *et al.*, 1998) A recent epidemiological case control study in breast cancer patients provides evidence that a high urinary excretion of both equol and enterolactone was found to be associated with a significant decrease in breast cancer risk (Ingram *et al.*, 1997). For equol the reduction was almost fourfold between the lowest and highest quartiles of excretion and for enterolactone there was a threefold decrease. Importantly, the decrease in risk associated with daidzein excretion was not significant.

Studies in laboratory animals have yielded equivocal results. Supplementation of a high-fat diet with 5% flaxseed flour, a rich source of lignans, which resulted in a large increase in urinary enterolactone and enterodiol concentration, reduced cell proliferation and nuclear aberrations (considered to be early markers for carcinogenesis) in rat mammary gland, although no consistent influence on tumour incidence was detected (Serraino and Thompson, 1991a, b). Evidence that lignans may be protective against colon cancer has been obtained from a study in which rats, treated with azoxymethane as an inducer of colon tumours, were fed a basal diet with or without supplementation with flaxseed oil (Serraino and Thompson, 1992). The incidence of aberrant crypt foci (an early marker of neoplasia) in the colons of the rats after 4 weeks was reduced by about 50% in the rats fed the flaxseed oil diet.

There is clearly an urgent need for further studies in this area, in particular to elucidate the importance of the microbial metabolites in the beneficial effects.

Plant Flavonoids

In addition to the capacity of flavonoid glycosides to exert toxic and genotoxic effects after hydrolysis by gut microbial enzymes (see Plant Glycosides), there is evidence that they may also afford protection against genotoxic and carcinogenic activity of other chemicals. Quercetin has been shown to antagonize tumour induction by carcinogens such as benzo[*a*]pyrene and 4-dimethylaminoazobenzene, and inhibits the mutagenic activity of benzo[*a*]pyrene and its diol-epoxide metabolite. Quercetin, myricetin and morin exhibit potent antimutagenic effects *in vitro* against a range of heterocyclic amine carcinogens in the human diet, including IQ, MeIQ and MeIQx (Alldrick *et al.*, 1986). The mechanism of action of the flavonoids appears to be inhibition of the activity of the hepatic enzymes responsible for activating the amines to their ultimate genotoxic species. The enzymes involved, cytochrome P450 IA-dependent mixed function oxidases, in addition to being present in the liver are also found in the intestinal tract. It is possible, therefore, that flavonoids released from their glycosidic forms by β-glucosidases in the gut may inhibit the bioactivation, by gut mucosal oxidases, of dietary carcinogen precursors to their reactive species. Indeed, quercetin and rutin (a glycosidic derivative) have been

shown to decrease the incidence of colon tumours induced by azoxymethane in mice, although the effect appeared to be on the promotional phase of the carcinogenic process possibly by decreasing gut mucosal cell proliferation (Deschner *et al.*, 1991).

Binding of Carcinogens

There are a number of reports describing the binding, by freeze-dried preparations of intestinal bacteria and particularly lactic acid-producing bacteria (LAB), of a variety of dietary carcinogens including the heterocyclic amines formed during cooking of meat, the fungal toxin aflatoxin B_1 (AFB1) and the food contaminant AF2 (Morotomi and Mutai, 1986). The extent of the binding was dependent on the mutagen and on the bacterial strain used. Significant binding ability was observed towards the heterocyclic amines 3-amino-1, 4-dimethyl-5*H*-pyrido[4,3-*b*]indole (Trp-P-1) and 3-amino-1-methyl-5*H*-pyrido[4,3-*b*]indole (Trp-P-2), and the least binding was observed with AF2 and AFB1. In some studies, binding was associated with a concomitant decrease in mutagenic activity *in vitro* (Morotomi and Mutai, 1986; Orrhage *et al.*, 1994). The binding of carcinogens to bacteria was reported to be pH dependent and to occur with dead cells. These results indicate that the binding is a physical phenomenon, mostly due to a cation-exchange mechanism involving cell wall peptidoglycans and polysaccharides (Zhang and Ohta, 1991).

Carcinogen binding has important implications for carcinogenesis, since it could lead, in theory, to a decrease in the bioavailability of ingested carcinogens in the gut, reducing their capacity to damage the intestinal mucosa and decreasing their absorption into the blood and hence their interaction with other tissues in the body. There is some experimental evidence in rats that administration of lactic acid bacteria decreases the amount of orally administered carcinogens reaching the blood (Zhang and Ohta, 1993). However, the animals were probably in an abnormal physiological state having been starved for 4 days. More recently, Bolognani *et al.* (1997) reported no effect of consumption of lactic acid bacteria on absorption or genotoxic activity *in vivo* of carcinogens in normally fed rats. The results of this study suggest that although LAB may bind carcinogens *in vitro*, this has little biological significance *in vivo* either for absorption and distribution of carcinogens in the body, or for their genotoxic activity in the liver.

FACTORS AFFECTING GUT MICROFLORA METABOLISM AND TOXICITY

A large number of factors can influence both the metabolism of the gut microflora and its involvement in toxic events. Such factors include age, drugs, diet and species differences and have been reviewed previously (Mallett and Rowland, 1988).

Species Differences in Gut Flora Metabolism

Although laboratory animals are very convenient for studying metabolism and toxic events and permit the monitoring of the flora in different gut regions and faeces, their use as models for the human faecal microflora and its metabolism is questionable. Differences exist in the bacterial composition of the gut floras of animals and man (Drasar, 1988) and, more importantly, in gut microbial enzymic activity (Rowland et al., 1986). Marked differences are apparent in azoreductase, nitroreductase, nitrate reductase, β-glucuronidase and β-glucosidase activities in gut contents of rat, mouse, hamster, guinea pig, rabbit, marmoset and man, with no animal species providing a similar enzyme profile to that of man. Consequently, although they are more difficult and expensive to perform, studies using human volunteer or germ-free animals associated with a complete human microflora provide more relevant data (Rumney and Rowland, 1992)

The Effect of Age on Microbial Metabolism

During weaning, a major change in microbial population occurs in the mammalian gut and there is a concomitant change in various xenobiotic-metabolizing enzymes (Brennan-Craddock et al., 1992). In mice aged 2–12 weeks, nitrate reductase activity tended to decrease with age, whilst nitroreductase and β-glucuronidase activities increased sharply between 2 and 4 weeks. Increases in the rate of bacterial demethylation of methylmercury at the time of weaning have also been reported, which may have important implications for the susceptibility of infants to neurotoxic damage by the organomercurials (see Demethylation of Methylmercury).

Drugs

Treatment of animals and man with antibiotics, particularly via the oral route and with poorly absorbed drugs, often results in suppression of some of the components of the gut microflora and is associated with diarrhoea. The extent of the suppression of the flora depends partly on the spectrum of activity of the antibiotic and partly on the resistance of the gut bacteria. Perturbation of the flora by antibacterial drugs can lead to loss of colonization resistance of the gut, that is, the ability of the micro-

bial population to prevent colonization by enteric pathogens. For example, the susceptibility of mice to *Salmonella* infection is greatly increased by administration of streptomycin (Miller and Bohnhoff, 1962). The suppressive effects of antibiotics on the microflora have been exploited in toxicology to provide evidence for a role for the microflora in xenobiotic metabolism. In such studies, mixtures of broad-spectrum antibiotics are used to suppress virtually all the bacteria in the gut. Examples of the use of such combinations have been given by Coates et al. (1988).

Drugs that affect the physiology of the gastro-intestinal tract can influence the resident microbial population. Cimetidine and ranitidine, which inhibit gastric acid secretion, elevate the stomach pH and allow bacteria to proliferate. The major toxicological concern of such events has been the possibility of bacterial nitrate reduction to nitrite and subsequent N-nitroso compound formation as with hypochlorhydric individuals (Stockbruegger et al., 1982).

Diet

The influence of diet on the gut microflora has been extensively studied, particularly the non-digestible carbohydrates such as dietary fibre components. In general, diet has been found to have little influence on the bacterial composition of the faecal microflora, although this may be due to the technical difficulties of analysing the flora. The exceptions are the non-digestible oligosaccharides (NDO) and the resistant starches. NDO are low molecular weight sugars (degree of polymerization 2–10) that are poorly digested in the upper gut and so reach the colon, where they are fermented and selectively stimulate numbers of bifidobacteria and lactobacilli (Rowland and Tanaka, 1993; Gibson et al., 1995). Resistant starch, which is poorly digested by amylase in the small intestine, appears to have similar modulatory effects on the faecal microflora to NDO, in that lactic acid bacteria are stimulated (Silvi et al., 1999). Despite the apparent lack of effect of diet on the gut flora, major changes in gut bacteria metabolism and on bacterial enzyme activities have been observed in animals fed diets containing fibre or other non-digestible carbohydrates. Altering the fat content of the diet also appears to modulate bacterial metabolic processes in the gut. Examples of these effects are given in Table 4 and have been discussed in more detail by Mallett and Rowland (1988).

There are some examples of modification of toxicity of xenobiotics due to dietary modulation of gut flora metabolism. Rats given pectin exhibited increased nitrate reductase activity in the gut and showed a 10-fold increase in blood methaemoglobin after a nitrate challenge (Wise et al., 1982). Similarly, rats fed a pectin diet and given nitrobenzene showed marked methaemoglobinaemia compared with rats fed a pectin free diet

Table 4 Modification of gut bacterial metabolism by some dietary components

Dietary component	Species	Observation[b]
Cellulose	Rat	Decreased activities of many gut flora enzymes, e.g. GN, NR, NT
Pectin	Rat, mouse	Increased activities of NT, NR and GN
Carrageenan	Rat	Markedly decreased activities of most bacterial enzymes
NDO[a]	Rat	Decreased activity of GN, IQ metabolism, ammonia production
Resistant starch	Rat	Decreased ammonia production, lower GN, increased GS activity
Fat	Rat	Increased GN activity, increased IQ metabolism
Meat	Rat, man	Increased GN activity
Cyclamate	Rat, man	Increased sulphamatase activity

[a] NDO = non-digestible oligosaccharides.
[b] GN β-glucuronidase; NT = nitrate reductase; NR = nitroreductase; GS β-glucosidase.
Source: after Mallett and Rowland (1988).

(Goldstein et al., 1984). The reductive metabolism of nitrobenzene in vitro differed both qualitatively and quantitatively for the two treatments.

REFERENCES

Adlercreutz, H. (1993). Dietary lignans and isoflavonoid phytoestrogens and cancer. *Klin. Lab.*, **2a**, 4–12.

Alldrick, A. J., Flynn, J. and Rowland, I. R. (1986). Effect of plant derived flavonoids and polyphenolic acids on the activity of mutagens from cooked food. *Mutat. Res.*, **163**, 225–232.

Aries, V., Crowther, J. S., Drasar, B. S., Hill, M. J. and Williams, R. E. O. (1969). Bacteria and the aetiology of cancer of the large bowel. *Gut*, **10**, 334–335.

Arora, A., Nair, M. G. and Strasburg, G. M. (1998). Antioxidant activities of isoflavones and their biological metabolites in a liposomal system. *Arch. Biochem. Biophys.*, **356**, 133–141.

Bhat, P., Shantakumari, S. and Rajan, D. (1972). Bacterial flora of the gastrointestinal tract in Southern India control subjects and patients with tropical sprue. *Gastroenterology*, **62**, 11–15.

Bingham, S. A., Pignatelli, B., Pollock, J., Ellul, A., Mallaveille, C., Gross, G., Runswick, S., Cummings, J. H. and O'Neill, I. K. (1996). Does increased formation of of endogenous N-nitroso compounds in the human colon explain the association between red meat and colon cancer? *Carcinogenesis*, **17**, 515–523.

Bolognani, F., Rumney, C. J. and Rowland, I. R. (1997). Influence of carcinogen binding by lactic acid-producing

bacteria on tissue distribution and *in vivo* mutagenicity of dietary carcinogens. *Food Chem. Toxicol.*, **35**, 535–545.

Braunberg, R. C. and Beck, V. (1968). Interaction of DDT and the gastrointestinal flora of the rat. *J. Agric. Food Chem.*, **16**, 451–453.

Brennan-Craddock, W. E., Mallett, A. K., Rowland, I. R. and Neale, S. (1992). Developmental changes to gut microflora metabolism in mice. *J. Appl. Bacteriol.*, **73**, 163–167.

Brown, J. P. (1981). Reduction of polymeric azo and nitro dyes by intestinal bacteria. *Appl. Environ. Microbiol.*, **41**, 1283–1286.

Brown, J. P. (1988). Hydrolysis of glycosides and esters. In Rowland, I. R. (Ed.), *Role of the Gut Flora in Toxicity and Cancer*, Academic Press, London, pp. 109–144.

Bruce, W. R., Baptista, J., Che, T., Furrer, R., Gingerich, J. S., Gupta, I., Krepinski, J. J., Grey, A. A. and Yates, P. (1982). General structure of 'fecapentaenes', the mutagenic substances in human feces. *Naturwissenschaften*, **69**, 557–558.

Carman, R. J., Van Tassell, R. L., Kingston, D. G. I., Bashir, M. and Wilkins, T. D. (1988). Conversion of IQ, a dietary pyrolysis carcinogen, to a direct-acting mutagen by normal intestinal bacteria of human. *Mutat. Res.*, **206**, 335–342.

Cerniglia, C. E., Freeman, J. P., Franklin, W. and Pack, L. D. (1982). Metabolism of benzidine and benzidine-congener based dyes by human, monkey and rat intestinal bacteria. *Biochem. Biophys. Res. Commun.*, **107**, 1224–1229.

Chipman, J. K. and Coleman, R. (1995). Mechanism and consequences of enterohepatic circulation. In Hill, M. J. (Ed.), *Role of Gut Bacteria in Human Toxicology and Pharmacology*. Taylor and Francis, London, pp. 245–259.

Chipman, J. K., Millburn, P. and Brooks, T. M. (1983). Mutagenicity and *in vivo* disposition of biliary metabolites of benzo[a]pyrene. *Toxicol. Lett.*, **17**, 233–240.

Chung, K. -T., Stevens, S. E. and Cerniglia, C. E. (1992). The reduction of azo dyes by the intestinal microflora. *Crit. Rev. Microbiol.*, **18**, 175–190.

Clarkson, T. W. (1979). General principles underlying the toxic action of metals. In Friburg, L., Nordbcry, G. F. and Vouk, V. B. (Eds), *Handbook on Toxicology of Metals*. Elsevier, Amsterdam, pp. 99–117.

Clinton, S. K. (1992). Dietary protein and carcinogenesis. In Rowland, I. R. (Ed.), *Nutrition, Toxicity, and Cancer*, CRC Press, Boca Raton, FL, pp. 455–475.

Coates, M. E., Drasar, B. S., Mallett, A. K. and Rowland, I. R. (1988). Methodological considerations for the study of bacterial metabolism. In Rowland, I. R. (Ed.), *Role of the Gut Flora in Toxicity and Cancer*. Academic Press, London, pp. 1–21.

Cole, C. B., Fuller, R., Mallett, A. K. and Rowland, I. R. (1985). The influence of the host on expression of intestinal microbial enzyme activities involved in metabolism of foreign compounds. *J. Appl. Bacteriol.*, **58**, 549–553.

Collier, S. W., Storm, J. E. and Bronough R. L. (1993). Reduction of azo dyes during in vitro percutaneous absorption. *Toxicol. Appl. Pharmacol.*, **118**, 73–79.

Cummings, J. H. (1997). *The Large Intestine in Nutrition and Disease*. Institute Danone, Brussels.

de Kok, T.M.C.M., van Faasen, A., ten Hoor, F. and Kleinjans, J. C. S. (1992). Fecapentaene excretion and fecal mutagenicity in relation to nutrient intake and fecal parameters in humans on omnivorous and vegetarian diets. *Cancer Lett.*, **62**, 11.

Deschner, E. D., Ruperto, J., Wong, G., and Newmark, H. L. (1991). Quercetin and rutin as inhibitors of azoxymethanol-induced colonic neoplasia, *Carcinogenesis*, **12**, 1193.

Dillon, D., Combes, R. and Zeiger, E. (1994). Activation by caecal reduction of the azo dye D & C Red No. 9 to a bacterial mutagen. *Mutagenesis*, **9**, 295–299.

Drasar, B. S. (1988). The bacterial flora of the intestine. In Rowland, I. R. (Ed.), *The Role of the Gut Flora in Toxicity and Cancer*, Academic Press, London, pp. 23–38.

Drasar, B. S. and Hill, M. J. (1974). *Human Intestinal Flora*. Academic Press, London.

El-Bayoumy, K., Sharma, C., Louis, Y. M., Reddy, B., and Hecht, S. S. (1983). The role of intestinal microflora in the metabolic reduction of 1-nitropyrene to 1-aminopyrene in conventional and germfree rats and in humans. *Cancer Lett.*, **19**, 311.

Eyssen, H. and Caenepeel, P. (1988). Metabolism of fats, bile acids and steroids. In Rowland, I. R. (Ed.), *Role of the Gut Flora in Toxicity and Cancer*. Academic Press, London, pp. 263–286.

Finegold, S. M., Sutter, V. L. and Mathisen, G. E. (1983) Normal and indigenous intestinal flora. In Hentges, D. J. (Ed.), *Human Intestinal Microflora in Health and Disease*. Academic Press, New York, pp. 3–31.

Garner, R. C. and Nutman, C. A. (1977). Testing of some azo dyes and their reduction products for mutagenicity using *Salmonella typhimurium* TA 1538. *Mutat. Res.*, **44**, 9–19.

Gibson, G. R., Beatty, E. M., Wang, X. and Cummings, J. H. (1995). Selective stimulation of bifidobacteria in the human colon by oligofructose and inulin. *Gastroenterology*, **108**, 975–982.

Goldstein, R. S., Chism, J. P., Sherrill, J. M. and Hamm, T. E. (1984). Influence of dietary pectin on intestinal microfloral metabolism and toxicity of nitrobenzene. *Toxicol. Appl. Pharmacol.*, **75**, 547–553.

Hartman, C. P., Fulk, G. E. and Andrews, A. W. (1978). Azo reduction of trypan blue to a known carcinogen by a cell free extract of a human intestinal anaerobe. *Mutat. Res.*, **58**, 125–132.

Haveland-Smith, R. B. and Combes R. D. (1980). Screening of food dyes for genotoxic activity. *Food Cosmet. Toxicol.*, **18**, 215–221.

Hill, M. J. (1988). Gut flora and cancer in humans and laboratory animals. In Rowland, I. R. (Ed.), *The Role of the Gut Flora in Toxicity and Cancer*. Academic Press, London, pp. 461–502.

Hill, M. J. (1995). The normal gut bacterial flora. In Hill, M. J. (Ed.), *The Role of Gut Bacteria in Human Toxicology and Pharmacology*. Taylor and Francis, London, pp. 3–17.

Hinzman, M. J., Novotny, C., Ullah, A. and Shamsuddin, A. M. (1987). Fecal mutagen fecapentaene-12 damages mammalian colon epithelial DNA. *Carcinogenesis*, **8**, 1475.

Hirai, N., Kingston, D. G. I., van Tassell, R. L. and Wilkins, T. D. (1982). Structure elucidation of a potent mutagen from human feces. *J. Am. Chem. Soc.*, **104**, 6149–6150.

Holdeman, L. V. and Moore, W. E. C. (1973). *Anaerobe Laboratory Manual*, 2nd edn. Anaerobe Laboratory, Blacksburg, VA.

Hollman, P. C. H., de Vries, J. M. H., van Leeuwen, S. D., Mengeles, M. J. B. and Katan, M. B. (1995). Absorption of dietary quercetin glycosides and quercetin in healthy ileostomy volunteers. *Am. J. Clin. Nutr.*, **62**, 1276–1282

Ingram, D., Sanders, K., Kolybaba, M. and Lopez, D. (1997). Case control study of phytoestrogens and breast cancer. *Lancet*, **350**, 990–994.

Lampe, J. W., Karr, S. C., Hutchins, A. M. and Slavin, J. L. (1998). Urinary equol excretion with a soy challenge: influence of habitual diet. *Proc. Soc. Exp. Biol. Med.*, **217**, 335–339.

Laqueur, G. L. and Spatz, M. (1968). The toxicology of cycasin. *Cancer Res.*, **28**, 2262.

Larsen, G. L. (1988). Deconjugation of biliary metabolites by microfloral β-glucuronidases, sulphatases and cysteine conjugate β-lyases and their subsequent enterohepatic circulation. In Rowland, I. R. (Ed.), *Role of the Gut Flora in Toxicity and Cancer*. Academic Press, London, pp. 79–107.

Leach, S. (1988). Mechanisms of endogenous *N*-nitrosation. In Hill, M. J. (Ed.), *Nitrosamines Toxicology and Microbiology*. Ellis Horwood, Chichester, pp. 69–87.

Levin, A. A. and Dent, J. G. (1982). Comparison of the metabolism of nitrobenzene by hepatic microsomes and cecal microflora from Fischer-344 rats *in vitro* and the relative importance of each *in vivo*. *Drug Metab. Dispos.*, **10**, 450–454.

Lindmark, D. G. and Muller, M. (1976). Antitrichomonad action, mutagenicity, and reduction of metronidazole and other nitroimidazoles. *Antimicrob. Agents Chemother.*, **10**, 476.

Lubet, R. A., Connolly, G., Kouri, R. E., Nebert, D. W. and Bigelow, S. W. (1983). Biological effects of the Sudan dyes: role of *Ah* receptor. *Biochem. Pharmacol.*, **32**, 3053–3058.

MacDonald, I. A., Bokkenheuser, V. D., Winter, J., McLernon, A. M. and Mosbach, E. H. (1993). Degradation of steroids in the human gut. *J. Lipid Res.*, **24**, 675–700.

Mallett, A. K. and Rowland, I. R. (1988). Factors affecting the gut microflora. In Rowland, I. R. (Ed.), *Role of the Gut Flora in Toxicity and Cancer*. Academic Press, London, pp. 348–382.

Manning, B. W., Cerniglia, C. E. and Federle, T. W. (1985). Metabolism of the benzidine-based azo dye Direct Black 38 by human intestinal microbiota. *Appl. Environ. Microbiol.*, **50**, 10.

Manning, B. W., Campbell, W. L., Franklin, W., Declos, K. B. and Cerniglia, C. E. (1988). Metabolism of 6-nitrochrysene by intestinal microflora. *Appl. Environ. Microbiol.*, **54**, 197.

Markiewicz, L., Garey, J., Adlercreutz, H. and Gurpide, E. (1993). *J. Steroid Biochem.*, **45**, 399–405.

Massey, R. C., Key, P. E., Mallett, A. K. and Rowland, I. R. (1988). An investigation of the endogenous formation of apparent total *N*-nitroso compounds in conventional microflora and germ-free rats. *Food Chem. Toxicol.*, **26**, 595–600.

McCartney, A. L., Wang, W. Z. and Tannock, G. W. (1996). Molecular analysis of the composition of the bifidobacterial and lactobacillus microflora of humans. *Appl. Environ. Microbiol.*, **62**, 4608–4613.

Mendel, J. L. and Walton, M. S. (1966). Conversion of *p, p*-DDT to *p, p*-DDD by intestinal flora of the rat. *Science*, **151**, 1527–1528.

Midtvedt, T. (1989). Monitoring the functional state of the microflora. In Hattori, T., Ishida, Y., Maruyama, Y., Morita, R. Y. and Uchida, A. (Eds), *Recent Advances in Microbial Ecology*. Japan Scientific Societies Press, Tokyo, pp. 515–519.

Miller, C. P. and Bohnhoff, M. (1962). A study of experimental *Salmonella* infection in the mouse. *J. Infect. Dis.*, **111**, 107–116.

Mirsalis, J. C., Hamm, T. E., Sherrill, J. M. and Butterworth, B. E., (1982). Role of gut flora in genotoxicity of dinitrotoluene. *Nature*, **295**, 322–323.

Mitsuoka, T. (1982). Recent trends in research on intestinal flora. *Bifidobacteria Microflora*, **3**, 3–24.

Moghaddam, A. P., Abbas, R., Fisher, J. W., Stavrou, S. and Lipscomb, J. C. (1996). Formation of dichloroacetic acid by rat and mouse gut microflora, an *in vitro* study. *Biochem. Biophys. Res. Commun.*, **228**, 639–645.

Moghaddam, A. P., Abbas, R., Fisher, J. W., Stavrou, S. and Lipscomb, J. C. (1997). The role of mouse intestinal microflora in the metabolism of trichloroethylene, an *in vivo* study. *Hum. Exp. Toxicol.*, **16**, 629–635.

Morotomi, M. and Mutai, M. (1986). *In vitro* binding of potent mutagenic pyrolyzates to intestinal bacteria, *J. Natl. Cancer Inst.*, **77**, 195–201.

Ohgaki, H., Takayama, S. and Sugimura, T. (1991). Carcinogenicities of heterocyclic amines. *Mutat. Res.*, **259**, 399–411.

Orrhage, K., Sillerstrom, E., Gustafsson, J. A., Nord, C. E. and Rafter, J. (1994). Binding of mutagenic heterocyclic amines by intestinal and lactic acid bacteria. *Mutat. Res.*, **311**, 239–248.

Packer, P. J., Leach, S. A., Duncan, S. N., Thompson, M. H. and Hill, M. J. (1989). The effect of different sources of nitrate exposure on urinary nitrate recovery in humans and its relevance to the methods for estimating nitrate exposure in epidemiological studies. *Carcinogenesis*, **10**, 1989–1996.

Peppercorn, M. A. and Goldman P. (1972). *J. Pharmacol. Exp. Ther.*, **181**, 555.

Plummer, S. M., Grafstom, R. C., Yang, L. L., Curren, R. D., Linnainmaa, K. and Harris, C. C. (1986). Fecapentaene-12 causes DNA damage and mutations in human cells. *Carcinogenesis*, **7**, 1607–1609.

Rafii, F., Moore, J. D., Ruseler-Van-Embden, J. G. H. and Cerniglia, C. E. (1995). Bacterial reduction of azo dyes used in food and drugs and cosmetics. *Microecol. Ther.*, **25**, 147–156.

Rafii, F., Hall, J. D. and Cerniglia, C. E. (1997). Mutagenicity of azo dyes used in foods, drugs and cosmetics before and after reduction by *Clostridium* species from the human intestinal tract. *Food Chem. Toxicol.*, **35**, 897–901.

Reddy, B. G., Pohl, L. R. and Krishna, G. (1976). The requirement of the gut flora in nitrobenzene-induced methemoglobinemia in rats. *Biochem. Pharmacol.*, **25**, 1119–1122.

Reddy, B. S., Weisburger, J. H., Narisawa, T. and Wynder, E. L. (1974). Colon carcinogenesis in germfree rats with 1,2-dimethylhydrazine and *N*-methyl-*N*-nitro-*N*-nitrosoguanidine. *Cancer Res.*, **74**, 2368–2372.

Rowland, I. R. (1989). Metabolic profiles of intestinal floras. In Hattori, T., Ishida, Y., Maruyama, Y., Morita, R. Y. and Uchida, A. (Eds), *Recent Advances in Microbial Ecology*. Japan Scientific Societies Press, Tokyo, pp. 510–514.

Rowland, I. R. (1995). Interaction of the gut flora with metal compounds. In Hill, M. J. (Ed.), *Role of Gut Bacteria in Human Toxicology and Pharmacology*. Taylor and Francis, London, pp. 197–211.

Rowland, I. R. and Tanaka, R. (1993). The effects of transgalactosylated oligosaccharides on gut flora metabolism in rats associated with a human faecal microflora. *J. Appl. Bacteriol.*, **74**, 667–674.

Rowland, I. R., Mallett, A. K. and Wise, A. (1985). The effect of diet on the mammalian gut flora and its metabolic activities. *CRC Crit. Rev. Toxicol.*, **16**, 31–103.

Rowland, I. R., Granli, T., Bockman, O. C., Key, P. E. and Massey, R. C. (1991). Endogenous *N*-nitrosation in man assessed by measurement of apparent total *N*-nitroso compound in faeces. *Carcinogenesis*, **12**, 1395–1401.

Rowland, I. R., Mallett, A. K., Bearne, C. A. and Farthing, M. J. G. (1986). Enzyme activities of the hindgut microflora of laboratory animals and man. *Xenobiotica*, **16**, 519–523.

Rowland, I., Wiseman, H., Sanders, T., Adlercreutz, H. and Bowey, E. (1999). Metabolism of oestrogens and phytoestrogens: the role of the gut microflora. *Biochem. Soc. Trans.*, **27**, 304–308.

Rumney, C. J. and Rowland, I. R. (1992). *In vivo* and *in vitro* models of the human colonic flora. *Crit. Rev. Food Sci. Nutr.*, **31**, 299–331.

Rumney, C. J., Rowland, I. R. and O'Neill, I. K. (1993). Conversion of IQ to 7-OHIQ by gut microflora. *Nutr. Cancer*, **19**, 67–76.

Schiffman, M. H., Van Tassell, R. L., Robinson, A., Smith, L., Daniel, J., Hoover, R. N., Weil, R., Rosenthal, J., Nair, P. P., Schwarz, S., Pettigrew, H., Curale, S., Batist, G., Block, G. and Wilkins, T. D. (1989). Case control study of colorectal cancer and fecapentaene excretion. *Cancer Res.*, **49**, 1322.

Serraino, M. and Thompson, L. U. (1991a). The effect of flaxseed supplementation on the initiation and promotional stages of mammary tumorigenesis. *Nutr. Cancer*, **17**, 153.

Serraino, M. and Thompson, L. U. (1991b). The effect of flaxseed supplementation on early risk markers for mammary carcinogenesis. *Cancer Lett.*, **60**, 135.

Serraino, M. and Thompson, L. U. (1992). Flaxseed supplementation and early markers of colon carcinogenesis, *Cancer Lett.*, **63**, 159.

Setchell, K. D. R. and Adlercreutz, H. (1988). Mammalian lignans and phyto-oestrogens. Recent studies on their formation, metabolism and biological role in health and disease. In Rowland, I. R. (Ed.), *Role of the Gut Flora in Toxicity and Cancer*. Academic Press, London, pp. 315–345.

Shamsuddin, A. M., Ullah, A., Baten, A. and Hale, E. (1991). Stability of fecapentaene-12 and its carcinogenicity in F344 rats. *Carcinogenesis*, **12**, 601.

Silvi, S., Rumney, C. J., Cresci, A. and Rowland, I. R. (1999). Resistant starch modifies gut microflora and microbial metabolism in human flora associated rats inoculated with faeces from Italian and UK donors. *J. Appl. Microbiol.*, in press.

Spiegelhalder, B., Eisenbrand, G. and Preussman, R. (1976). Influence of dietary nitrate on nitrite content of human saliva: possible relevance to *in vivo* formation of *N*-nitroso compounds. *Food Cosmet. Toxicol.*, **14**, 545–548.

Stockbruegger, R. W., Cotton, P. B., Eugenides, N., Bartholomew, B. A., Hill, M. J. and Walters, C. L. (1982). Intragastric nitrites, nitrosamines and bacterial overgrowth during cimetidine treatment. *Gut*, **23**, 1048–1054.

Theilade, E. (1990). Factors controlling the microflora of the healthy mouth. In Hill, M. J. and Marsh, P. D. (Eds), *Human Microbial Ecology*. CRC Press, Boca Raton, FL, pp. 1–35.

Vandamme, P., Pot, B., Gillis, M., deVos, P., Kersters, K. and Swings, J. (1996). Polyphasic taxonomy, a consensus approach to bacterial systematics. *Microbiol. Rev.*, **60**, 407–438.

Van der Hoeven, J. C., Lagerweij, W. J., Bruggeman, I. M., Voragen, F. G. and Koeman, J. H. (1983). Mutagenicity of extracts of some vegetables commonly consumed in the Netherlands, *J. Agric. Food Chem.*, **31**, 1020.

Van der Waaij, D. (1984). Colonization resistance of the digestive tract. In Coates, M. E. and Gustafsson, B. E. (Eds), *The Germ Free Animal in Biomedical Research*. Laboratory Animals, London, p. 155.

Venturi, M., Hambly, R. J., Glinghammar, B., Rafter, J. J. and Rowland, I. R. (1997). Genotoxic activity in human faecal water and the role of bile acids: a study using the Comet assay. *Carcinogenesis*, **18**, 2353–2359.

Ward, J. M., Anjo, T., Ohannesian, L., Keefer, L. K., Devor, D. E., Donovan, P. J., Smith, G. T., Henneman, J. R., Streeter, A. J., Konishi, N., Rehm, S., Reist, E. J., Bradford, W. W. and Rice, J. M. (1988). Inactivity of fecapentaene-12 as a rodent carcinogen or tumor initiator. *Cancer Lett.*, **42**, 49.

Weisburger, J. H., Jones, R. C., Wang, C. X., Backlund, J. Y. C., Williams, G. M., Kingston, D. G. I., Van Tassell, R. L.,

Keyes, R. F., Wilkins, T. D., De Wit, P. P., Van der Steeg, M. and Van der Gen, A. (1990). Carcinogenicity tests of fecapentaene-12 in mice and rats. *Cancer Lett.*, **49**, 89.

Wise, A., Mallett, A. K. and Rowland, I. R. (1982). Dietary fibre, bacterial metabolism and toxicity of nitrate in the rat. *Xenobiotica*, **12**, 111–118.

Zarkovic, M., Qin, X., Nakatsuru, Y., Oda, H., Nakamura, T., Shamsuddin, A. M. and Ishikawa, T. (1993). Tumor promotion by fecapentaene-12 in a rat colon carcinogenesis model. *Carcinogenesis*, **14**, 1261.

Zava, D. T. and Duwe, G. (1997). Estrogenic and antiproliferative properties of genistein and other flavonoids in human breast cancer cells *in vitro*. *Nutr. Cancer*, **27**, 31–40.

Zhang, X. B. and Ohta, Y. (1991). Binding of mutagens by fractions of the cell wall skeleton of lactic acid bacteria. *J. Dairy Sci.*, **74**, 1477–1481.

Zhang, X. B. and Ohta, Y. (1993). Microorganisms in the gastrointestinal tract of the rat prevent absorption of the mutagen-carcinogens 3-amino-1,4-dimethyl-5*H*-pyrido [4, 3–*b*] indole. *Can. J. Microbiol.*, **39**, 841–845.

Chapter 29
Percutaneous Toxicity

Hon-Wing Leung and Dennis J. Paustenbach

CONTENTS

INTRODUCTION

Traditionally, evaluation of human exposure to chemicals has been focused on the inhalation and oral routes. However, the skin is also an important portal of entry. In fact, in certain occupations such as farm workers applying pesticides, and in certain populations such as children playing on contaminated ground, absorption through the skin may be the predominant route. The percutaneous route is the most complex of the three primary exposure routes (percutaneous, peroral and inhalation), and the most difficult to quantify. While the percutaneous absorption of many industrial chemicals in the liquid state has been determined, only a few chemicals in other physical states, e.g. gas or vapour, and those associated with other environmental matrices, e.g. soil, have been studied. The kinetic behaviour of chemicals in such physical forms can be very different from that of neat chemicals. Furthermore, most laboratory studies on percutaneous absorption have been performed with chemicals at high concentrations. These experimental data may not be applicable for the low concentrations usually encountered in the environment. Recent developments in various mathematical models may provide a means to address these limitations. These mathematical models permit the simulation of percutaneous absorption over a wide range of exposure conditions. In addition, they can be used to examine the influence of various factors governing the skin uptake of matrix-associated chemicals.

FACTORS AFFECTING PERCUTANEOUS ABSORPTION

Structure of the Skin

The skin behaves as a rate-limiting barrier which allows a relatively slow penetration of chemicals. The barrier function of the skin is believed to reside almost entirely in the stratum corneum (Scheuplein and Blank, 1985). The stratum corneum typically mimics the characteristics of a lipophilic structure (Raykar *et al.*, 1988). Fatty chemicals tend to accumulate in the stratum corneum, which behaves as a storage site and releases these chemicals slowly over a long period of time, a phenomenon known as a reservoir effect (Vickers, 1963). Percutaneous absorption will be affected if there is a loss of barrier function of the stratum corneum through disease or damage. Absorption can be increased almost twofold if all the barrier function is removed. Some solvents such as dimethyl sulphoxide actually dissolve lipids, thus destroying the barrier function and allowing the chemical to penetrate the skin rapidly into the bloodstream. In addition, damage to the skin due to occupations such as bricklaying, cement working or degreasing can significantly increase the absorption of chemicals. The site of application of a chemical can markedly affect the rate of percutaneous absorption. For example, compared with the palm and forearm, the abdomen and dorsum of the hand are twice as permeable, the scalp, angle of the jaw, and forehead are four times as permeable and the scrotum is almost 12 times as permeable (**Table 1**). These regional variations in the percutaneous absorption may be related in part to the thickness of the stratum corneum. The living cells of the epidermis are more permeable and do not represent the rate-limiting step under most circumstances. Although chemicals may be absorbed through hair follicles and sweat ducts (transappendageal route), their total area is relatively small in humans, and for most chemicals absorption through the general skin surface (transepidermal route) is the preferred route (Dugard, 1983). In short, for humans, hairy skin seems to be no more permeable than non-hairy skin. However, in the case of some molecules that penetrate the bulk of the stratum corneum slowly, such as electrolytes and polar molecules, the transappendageal

Table 1 Regional differences in the percutaneous absorption of parathion in humans *in vivo*

Anatomical region	Dose absorbed (%)	Thickness of stratum corneum (μm)
Forearm	8.6	16.0
Palm	11.8	400.0
Ball of foot	13.5	600.0
Abdomen	18.5	15.0
Dorsum of hand	21.0	49.0
Fossa cubitalis	28.4	
Scalp	32.1	
Jaw angle	33.9	
Forehead	36.3	13.0
Ear canal	46.6	
Axilla	64.0	
Scrotum	101.6	5.0

route may predominate (Menon and Elias, 1997). In humans the capacity of these shunts to facilitate transfer is limited by the small fraction of skin area that consists of shafts and pores (Scheuplein, 1967). However, for mouse skin, hair follicles appear to contribute significantly to overall percutaneous absorption (Kao *et al.*, 1988). The skin contains many of the enzymes as in the liver; thus, metabolism by the skin may affect absorption. The metabolizing potential of skin has been estimated to be about 2% of that of the liver, with most of the enzyme activity localized in the epidermal layer (Pannatier *et al.*, 1978). The more slowly a chemical is absorbed through the skin, the greater is the opportunity for some metabolism to occur. However, metabolism by the skin is probably too small to be worthy of consideration for most chemicals.

Other Environmental and Physical Factors

The concentration of the applied chemical and the surface area of contact are the two most important factors affecting absorption of a chemical through the skin. The greatest potential for absorption occurs when a high concentration of a chemical is spread over a large surface area of the body (Wester and Noonan, 1980). However, the relationship between the concentration of an applied chemical and the efficiency of its absorption is not necessarily linear. The rate of percutaneous absorption can either decrease or increase with increasing dose, depending on the chemical. Usually, percutaneous uptake will increase if the skin has been damaged by the chemical. Occlusion of the skin, as with bandaging or putting on clothing after exposure, which changes the hydration and temperature of the skin and prevents loss through wiping or evaporation, can markedly increase the absorption of chemicals. The frequency of applica-

tion is another factor which will often affect the degree of percutaneous absorption. This is possibly because the initial chemical application may have damaged the barrier function of the stratum corneum, resulting in increased absorption for subsequent applications (Wester *et al.*, 1980).

DETERMINATION OF PERCUTANEOUS ABSORPTION

Percutaneous absorption is defined as the transport of externally applied chemicals through the cutaneous structures and the extracellular medium to the bloodstream. This consists of two consecutive processes: (1) a penetration phase, i.e. the passage of a chemical through the superficial skin structures, the stratum corneum and the epidermis, to the extracellular medium; and (2) a resorption phase, during which rapid diffusion occurs from the extracellular fluid to the blood via the cutaneous circulation.

The simplest way to model the rate of skin absorption is to assume that Fick's first law of diffusion at steady state is applicable:

$$J = \mathrm{d}Q/\mathrm{d}t = D \cdot k/e \cdot \Delta C \approx D \cdot k/e \cdot C$$

where J = flux, $\mathrm{d}Q/\mathrm{d}t$ = rate of absorption of chemical, D = diffusion constant in the stratum corneum, k = stratum corneum–vehicle partition coefficient of the chemical, e = thickness of the stratum corneum, ΔC = concentration gradient, and C = applied chemical concentration. The concentration gradient is equal to the difference between the concentration above and that below the stratum corneum. Since the concentration below is usually negligible relative to the concentration above, the concentration gradient can be approximated as equal to the applied chemical concentration.

The above equation describes the kinetics of penetration through the skin at the steady state. It must be emphasized that it is an oversimplification and is an approximation for most *in vivo* exposure situations, where true steady-state conditions are rarely attained. None the less, this equation includes the most salient factors which account for the percutaneous absorption of chemicals. The two factors which strongly influence the transfer rate are the partition coefficient and the diffusion coefficient of the stratum corneum (Borsadia *et al.*, 1992). The partition coefficient in the diffusion equation illustrates the importance of solubility characteristics for a chemical to penetrate the skin (Surber *et al.*, 1990). Lipophilic chemicals tend to accumulate in the stratum corneum and a high concentration of the chemical is achieved at the point of contact. Assuming that the chemical is at least slightly soluble in water, penetration at this level will be fairly rapid, owing to migration into

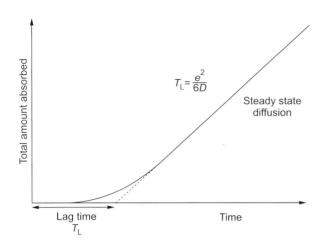

Figure 1 Typical time course of chemical diffusion through the intact human skin. T_L = lag time; e = thickness of the membrane; D = diffusion constant.

Table 2 Relative ranking of the skin permeability in different animal species

Ranking	Animal species	Thickness of stratum corneum (μm)	Epidermis (μm)	Whole skin (mm)
Most permeable	Mouse	5.8	12.6	0.84
	Guinea pig			
	Goat			
	Rabbit			
	Horse			
	Cat			
	Dog			
	Monkey			
	Pig	26.4	65.8	3.43
	Man	16.8	46.9	2.97
Least permeable	Chimpanzee			

Table 3 *In vivo* human percutaneous absorption rates of some neat chemical liquids

Chemical	Percutaneous absorption rate (mg cm^{-2} h^{-1})
Aniline	0.2–0.7
Benzene	0.24–0.4
2-Butoxyethanol	0.05–0.68
2-(2-Butoxyethoxy)ethanol	0.035
Carbon disulphide	9.7
Dimethylformamide	9.4
Ethylbenzene	22–33
2-Ethoxyethanol	0.796
2-(2-Ethoxyethoxy)ethanol	0.125
Methanol	11.5
2-Methoxyethanol	2.82
Methyl *n*-butyl ketone	0.25–0.48
Nitrobenzene	2
Styrene	9–15
Toluene	14–23
Xylenes (mixed)	4.5–9.6
m-Xylene	0.12–0.15

the intercellular spaces. With purely lipophilic chemicals, however, penetration may not extend beyond the stratum corneum. For these chemicals the stratum corneum behaves as a storage site, and the chemicals may be released over a long period of time. This phenomenon, known as the 'reservoir effect', may explain why sometimes a single exposure to certain chemicals in the skin can lead to prolonged effects (Rougier *et al.*, 1985). Accordingly, the stratum corneum is an effective barrier for hydrophilic substances, which therefore have very low skin absorption rates.

As the stratum corneum has a non-negligible thickness, there is a period of transient diffusion during which the rate of transfer through the skin rises to reach a steady state (**Figure 1**). The steady state is maintained indefinitely thereafter, provided that the system remains constant. The common method of analysing kinetic profiles such as that depicted in **Figure 1** is to determine the lag time by extrapolating the linear portion of the curve to the *x* axis. Depending on the type of chemicals, the lag time can sometimes be as long as several hours or even days. From an exposure assessment standpoint, if the exposure time is shorter than the lag time, it is unlikely that there will be significant systemic absorption and accumulation (Flynn, 1990).

Since it is difficult to measure a skin–vehicle partition coefficient, it is often combined with the diffusion constant and stratum corneum thickness to form the permeability coefficient, K_p:

$$J = D \cdot k/e \cdot C = K_p \cdot C$$

In Vivo Studies

Historically, absorption of a chemical through the skin has most often been studied in humans. More recently, studies have also been performed with a variety of laboratory animals. The use of the hairless mouse is increasingly being explored as a relevant animal model of percutaneous absorption in man (Simon and Maibach, 1998). In addition, some studies have used athymic rodents grafted with human skin (Reifenrath *et al.*, 1984). Certainly, percutaneous absorption studies in which the chemical is applied to human skin *in vivo* yield the most relevant information for human exposure assessment. However, owing to the potential toxicity of many chemicals, *in vivo* human percutaneous absorption studies have been largely supplanted by experiments with laboratory animals. Unfortunately, there are a number of difficulties associated with the extrapolation of animal data to humans, e.g. different sites of application, differences between shaved versus unshaved skin and difference in skin metabolism (or lack of). Based on studies with organophosphate pesticides, Marzulli *et al.* (1969) ranked, from highest to lowest, the relative permeability of the skin in several animal species (**Table 2**). In general, the penetration of chemicals through the human skin is similar to that of the pig, but much slower than that of the guinea pig and mouse. There appears to be a weak correlation between the absorption rates and the thickness of skin. Undoubtedly factors other than skin thickness also play a role. The species differences in skin permeability suggest that results must be carefully interpreted within the scope of the methods and species used, and some adjustment should be applied when extrapolating animal data to predict the human response. **Table 3** presents the percutaneous absorption rates of chemicals that have been determined for humans *in vivo*.

In Vitro Studies

Starting in the 1980s, *in vitro* studies using human skin were conducted more frequently for estimating percutaneous absorption. In these studies a piece of excised human skin is attached to a diffusion apparatus (**Figure 2**) which has a top chamber to hold the applied dose of a chemical, an O-ring to hold the skin in place and a temperature-controlled bottom chamber containing saline or other fluids (plus a sampling port to withdraw fractions for analysis). Although human forearm skin is optimal, it is difficult to obtain, so it is common practice to use abdominal skin. It is generally believed that properly conducted *in vitro* tests using human skin, for most classes of chemicals, can be a reasonably good predictor of the absorption rate in humans *in vivo* (Bronaugh *et al.*,

1982). **Table 4** shows the *in vitro* human skin permeability coefficients of some industrial chemicals.

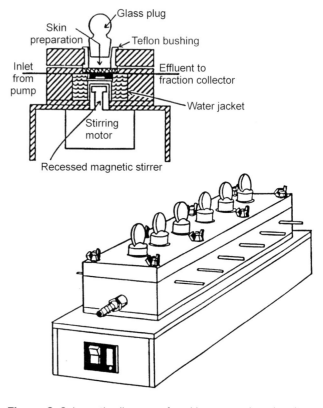

Figure 2 Schematic diagram of a skin penetration chamber. Above, side view of an individual media well; below, entire assembled chamber.

Table 4 *In vitro* human percutaneous permeability coefficients of aqueous solutions of some industrial chemicals

Organic chemical	K_p (cm h^{-1})	Organic chemical	K_p (cm h^{-1})	Inorganic chemical	K_p (cm h^{-1})
2-Amino-4-nitrophenol	0.00066	2-Ethoxyethanol	0.0003	Cobalt chloride	0.0004
4-Amino-2-nitrophenol	0.0028	*p*-Ethylphenol	0.035	Mercuric chloride	0.00093
Benzene	0.11	Heptanol	0.038	Nickel chloride	0.0001
p-Bromophenol	0.036	Hexanol	0.028	Nickel sulphate	<0.000009
Butane-2,3-diol	<0.00005	Methanol	0.0016	Silver nitrate	<0.00035
n-Butanol	0.0025	Methyl hydroxybenzoate	0.0091		
Butan-2-one	0.0045	β-Naphthol	0.028		
Chlorocresol	0.055	3-Nitrophenol	0.0056		
o-Chlorophenol	0.033	4-Nitrophenol	0.0056		
p-Chlorophenol	0.036	Nitrosodiethanolamine	0.0000055		
Chloroxylenol	0.059	Nonanol	0.06		
m-Cresol	0.015	Octanol	0.061		
o-Cresol	0.016	Pentanol	0.006		
p-Cresol	0.018	Phenol	0.0082		
Decanol	0.08	Propanol	0.0017		
2,4-Dichlorophenol	0.06	Resorcinol	0.00024		
Diethanolamine	0.000034	Thymol	0.053		
Diethyl ether	0.016	Toluene	1.01		
1,4-Dioxane	0.00043	2,4,6-Trichlorophenol	0.059		
Ethanol	0.0008	3,4-Xylenol	0.036		
Ethanolamine	0.000043				

Bioavailability

Cutaneous bioavailability is defined as the percentage of an applied dose of a chemical absorbed through the skin into the bloodstream. This is usually determined by measuring the total radioactivity in blood or excreta following a topical application of a radiolabelled compound. The amount of radioactivity retained in the body or excreted through expiration or sweat can be determined by measuring the amount of radioactivity excreted following an intravenous injection. Three indirect methods for estimating the bioavailability of a chemical following topical application can be used:

(1) If an intravenous dose is assumed to have maximum bioavailability (i.e. 100%), the extent of absorption following a cutaneous dose can be estimated by comparing the total quantity in the body compartment after giving equivalent doses by both the intravenous and cutaneous routes (Andersen and Keller, 1984). The total dose can be represented as the concentration–time integral carried out to infinite time, i.e. the area under the plasma concentration–time curve (AUC_∞):

$$\text{bioavailability} = \frac{AUC_\infty(\text{cutaneous})}{AUC_\infty(\text{intravenous})}$$

The radioactivity in the blood or excreta consists of a mixture of the parent compound and any metabolite(s). Since a radiolabel does not distinguish between the parent chemical and its metabolite(s), the bioavailability determined with this methodology actually represents the composite absorption of the parent chemical and its metabolite(s). Specific chemical assays are necessary to quantify the absolute bioavailability of chemicals which undergo metabolism as they are absorbed through the skin.

(2) This method calculates the extent of absorption by monitoring the cumulative amount of the chemical in all routes of excretion (urine, faeces, exhaled air, etc.) over infinite time following topical dosing. Thus:

$$\text{bioavailability} = \frac{\text{total amount in excreta}}{\text{applied dose}}$$

In reality, the duration of excreta collection is only for a finite time, since collection of excreta over an extremely prolonged period is impractical. For certain chemicals, especially those which have low whole-body clearance, there may be a considerable portion of the absorbed dose remaining in the body at the cessation of the collection period. Hence the total amount recovered in the excreta does not represent the total dose absorbed. This residual amount and any material excreted in routes not assayed can be estimated by determining the amount excreted following an intravenous administration (Wester and Maibach, 1985). Thus:

$$\text{bioavailability} = \frac{\text{total excreted (cutaneous)}}{\text{total excreted (intravenous)}}$$

(3) This method, which is the most expedient but also the least reliable, consists of quantifying the amount of a chemical recovered from the skin surface after topical application:

$$\text{bioavailability} = \frac{\text{applied dose} - \text{dose remaining on skin}}{\text{applied dose}}$$

The limitation of this surface recovery method is that it is prone to inaccuracies. Losses of the chemical from the skin may occur as a result of evaporation, and total recovery from the skin is difficult to ascertain with high confidence.

Mathematical Models

In addition to the methods discussed above to determine percutaneous absorption, many mathematical modelling approaches have been developed. Unlike empirical studies, mathematical models can readily be used not only to simulate a wide range of exposure conditions, including those at non-steady state, but also to evaluate the influence of various biological or physicochemical factors, such as contact area, membrane thickness, molecular size, lipophilicity or volatility on percutaneous absorption. However, their use to predict the rates of percutaneous absorption is limited owing to insufficient validation.

Models Based on Physicochemical Properties

Berner and Cooper (1987) envisioned two parallel pathways of diffusion for the cutaneous transport of chemicals. The flux of polar molecules at constant concentration is independent of the partition coefficient in the stratum corneum [for simplicity, the *n*-octanol–water partition coefficient (K_{ow}) is commonly used as a substitute]. This pathway is referred to as the polar or aqueous pathway. With lipophilic substances the flux becomes a function of the partition coefficient, and this pathway is referred to as the non-polar or lipophilic pathway. On the basis of this concept, Fiserova-Bergerova *et al.* (1990) proposed a model to evaluate the percutaneous absorption potential of industrial chemicals. The flux of a chemical across the skin can be related to its physicochemical properties, as shown in the following empirical equation:

$$J = (C/15)(0.038 + 0.153K_{ow})e^{-0.016MW}$$

where J = flux of the chemical across the skin, C = saturated aqueous solution concentration of the chemical, K_{ow} = n-octanol–water partition coefficient and MW = molecular weight of the chemical. The critical flux is determined by comparing the skin uptake rate with the inhalation uptake rate during exposure to the ambient occupational exposure limit. The critical flux assumes an exposure of 2% of the body surface area (equivalent to the stretched palms and fingers) to a saturated aqueous solution of the chemical. The chemical is classified as having cutaneous absorption or cutaneous toxicity potential if the flux exceeds the critical flux by 30 or 300%, respectively. Later, Guy and Potts (1993), contending that the flux predictions were overly conservative, simplified the model by considering that the stratum corneum could be adequately characterized as a simple lipophilic barrier alone. The simplified model resulted in significantly lower estimates of maximum percutaneous penetration fluxes.

McKone (1990) described a model for predicting the uptake fraction of chemicals adsorbed on soil. The model is used to estimate the amount of chemical that crosses the stratum corneum into the underlying tissue layer. It is referred to as an uptake fraction to differentiate it from a process that includes transport into blood. The approach is based on the concept of fugacity, which is directly related to concentration, and measures the tendency of a chemical to move from one phase to another. Since the skin contains about 10% fat, and soil has an organic carbon content of only about 1–4%, a chemical in a soil matrix placed on the skin will ultimately move from the soil to the underlying adipose layers of the skin. However, the rate at which this occurs will determine whether there will be any appreciable uptake during the period of time between deposition on the skin and removal by evaporation, washing or other processes. It is the mass-transfer coefficients of the soil–skin layer and the soil–air layer that define the rates at which these competing processes occur.

McKone's model predicts that the uptake fraction of a chemical in soil is particularly sensitive to the values of the n-octanol–water partition coefficient (K_{ow}), the air–water partition coefficient (K_h) and the mass of soil deposited on the skin (I_s). When K_h is very small (< 0.001), i.e. there is little vapour loss, the only loss mechanisms are mass transfer and wash-off. Under this condition, the uptake fraction is inversely proportional to K_{ow} and I_s. When $I_s = 10$ mg cm^{-2} and $K_{ow} \leqslant 10^4$, the uptake is almost complete in 12 h. When $K_h > 0.001$, there is competition between vapour loss and diffusion as removal mechanisms, and vapour loss becomes more important in controlling uptake fraction. Under such conditions, the model predicts that the uptake fraction decreases strongly when K_{ow} is large, but is less sensitive to soil loading when K_{ow} is small. Furthermore, the model reveals that the efficiency of uptake depends strongly on the amount of soil on the skin surface.

When the soil loading is < 1 mg cm^{-2}, a fairly high uptake fraction, sometimes approaching unity, is predicted. With 20 mg cm^{-2} of soil, an uptake of only 0.5% is predicted. Overall, a few generalizations can be made from McKone's model: (1) for chemicals with $K_{ow} \leqslant 10^6$ and $K_h < 0.001$, it is not unreasonable to assume 100% uptake in 12 h; (2) for chemicals with $K_h \geqslant 0.01$, the uptake fraction is unlikely to exceed 40% in 12 h and will be well below that when $K_{ow} > 10$; and (3) for chemicals with $K_h \geqslant 0.1$, one can expect $\leqslant 3\%$ uptake in 12 h. In most occupational settings, contaminated soil will rarely be in contact with the skin for more than 4 h before it is washed off. Consequently, this should be accounted for when conducting a risk assessment.

Pharmacokinetic Models

An example of a pharmacokinetic model to describe the percutaneous absorption of chemicals is that of Guy et al. (1982). In this model, movement of a chemical through the various compartments representing the skin structures is described by first-order rate constants: K_1 describes diffusion from the skin surface through the stratum corneum; K_2 relates to diffusion through the epidermis; and K_3 measures the back-diffusion from the epidermis to the stratum corneum. The ratio K_3/K_2 therefore, may be regarded as the relative affinity or the partition coefficient of the chemical for the stratum corneum compared with the epidermis. The larger the value of K_3, the higher is the affinity for the stratum corneum and therefore the larger is the reservoir effect. Finally, K_4 measures the clearance from the capillary blood. This model can be used to evaluate vehicle effects when it is configured with an input rate constant to the skin surface. It has been successfully used to estimate the absorption rates of a variety of steroid compounds (Guy et al., 1983).

Zatz (1985) developed a model that treated the barrier membrane as a series of spaces filled with immiscible liquids and assumed that transport from one space to another is a first-order process. The advantage of this model is that it is possible to study conditions under which Fick's law does not apply, i.e. non-steady-state conditions. Two general types of experimental conditions were studied. The first, referred to as the 'infinite dose' situation, requires that the amount of chemical lost by penetration be too small to alter the concentration of the chemical on the skin surface. The second, referred to as the 'finite dose' situation, describes the condition in which the concentration decreases during the experiment. In the infinite dose condition, the model predicts that the concentration profile is essentially linear once steady state has been reached. Increasing the number of compartments, which is analogous to increasing the membrane thickness, has the effect of decreasing the steady-state flux. In the finite dose condition, the chemical is applied as a thin film. All other model parameters being the same, penetration is reduced under the finite dose condition. This is because the chemical concentration is continuously reduced, which results in a decrease in the gradient across the membrane.

A physiologically based pharmacokinetic model was recently developed to describe the percutaneous absorption of volatile organic contaminants in dilute aqueous solutions (Shatkin and Brown, 1991). The model contained three body compartments: stratum corneum, viable epidermis and blood. Physiological parameters such as volume of the body compartments and blood flow-rates were obtained directly from the literature. Partition coefficients between compartments were estimated from the n-octanol–water partition coefficients. The exposure scenario modelled was either hand or full-body immersion in a vessel of solute-contaminated water of a known volume. Sensitivity analyses of the various model parameters suggested that the uptake of chemicals in aqueous solutions was most markedly influenced by epidermal blood flow-rates, followed by epidermal thickness and the fat content in the stratum corneum. In general, thicker and fattier skin would provide better barriers to percutaneous penetration of chemicals.

CALCULATIONS OF PERCUTANEOUS ABSORPTION

To calculate the percutaneous absorption of a chemical, one needs to know, in addition to the percutaneous absorption rate and bioavailability, the area of exposed skin, the concentration of the chemical, and the duration and frequency of the exposure (Sheehan et al., 1991). The 'rule of nines' may be used for estimating the skin surface areas of certain anatomical regions (Snyder, 1975): head and neck, 9%; upper limbs, each 9%; lower limbs, each 18%; and front or back of trunk, 18%. **Table 5** gives the skin surface areas commonly used when conducting exposure assessments.

There are two common exposure scenarios to consider in calculating percutaneous absorption. One is that of a thin film of chemical on the skin. For this finite mass scenario:

$$\text{percutaneous uptake} = C \cdot J \cdot A \cdot x \cdot t$$

where C = concentration of the chemical, J = percutaneous absorption rate, A = skin surface area, x = thickness of the film layer and t = duration of exposure. The other scenario is where there is an excess amount of a chemical on the skin. In this case, the thickness of the chemical layer is not calculated and steady-state kinetics are assumed:

$$\text{percutaneous uptake} = C \cdot K_p \cdot A \cdot t$$

where K_p = permeability coefficient.

Table 5 Representative skin surface areas of a male human adult

Anatomical region	Area (cm^2)
Whole body	18000
Head and neck	1620
Head	1260
Back of head	320
Neck	360
Back of neck	90
Torso	6480
Back	2520
Chest	2520
Sides	1440
Upper limbs	3240
Upper arms (elbow to shoulder)	1440
Lower arms (elbow to wrist)	1080
Hands	720
Hands (one side)	360
Upper arms (back of)	360
Lower arms (back of)	270
Lower limbs	6480
Thighs	3240
Lower legs (knee to ankle)	2160
Feet	1080
Soles of feet	540
Thighs (back of)	810
Lower legs (back of)	540
Perineum	180

Percutaneous Absorption of Chemicals in Aqueous Solution

Beech (1980) estimated the amount of chloroform absorbed by a child swimming for 3 h in water containing 0.5 μg of chloroform per cm^3. The average 6-year-old boy is assumed to have a skin surface area of 8800 cm^2. The permeability constant (K_p) for chloroform in aqueous solution was 0.125 cm h^{-1}. The percutaneous absorption is then given by

$$
\begin{aligned}
\text{percutaneous uptake} &= C \cdot K_p \cdot A \cdot t \\
&= 0.5 \mu\text{g cm}^{-3} \times 0.125 \text{cm h}^{-1} \times 8800 \text{ cm}^2 \\
&\quad \times 3\text{h} = 1650 \mu\text{g}
\end{aligned}
$$

Percutaneous Absorption of Liquid Chemicals

Paustenbach (1988) estimated the amount of 2-methoxyethanol absorbed by a worker wearing a heavily contaminated glove on one hand for about 30 min:

$$
\begin{aligned}
\text{percutaneous uptake} &= J \cdot A \cdot t \\
&= 2.82 \text{ mg cm}^{-2}\text{h}^{-1} \times 400 \text{ cm}^2 \times \\
&\quad 0.5\text{h} = 564 \text{ mg}
\end{aligned}
$$

For comparison, the amount taken up via inhalation by the same worker exposed for 8 h ($10 \, \text{m}^3$ of air inhaled) at the occupational exposure limit of $16 \, \text{mg m}^{-3}$ was also estimated. The efficiency of inhalation uptake is assumed to be 80%:

$$\text{inhalation uptake} = 16 \, \text{mg m}^{-3} \times 10 \, \text{m}^3 \times 0.8 = 128 \, \text{mg}$$

These calculations indicate that the uptake of 2-methoxyethanol following 30 min of skin exposure (one hand) is over four times that from inhalation for 8 h. From this example, it is clear that the cutaneous route of entry can contribute significantly to the total absorbed dose.

Percutaneous Absorption of Chemical Vapours

The absorption of chemical vapours through the skin has been studied. **Table 6** shows the permeability constants measured in these studies. McDougal *et al.* (1990) observed that in general rat skin appears to be 2–4 times more permeable than human skin to chemical vapours. From a mixed percutaneous and inhalation exposure to chemical vapours, skin absorption accounts for about 10–30% of the total dose, with the inhalation route accounting for 70–90%. Furthermore, whereas the uptake of chemical vapours by inhalation is linearly proportional to the vapour concentration, absorption through skin exposure becomes saturated as the vapour concentration increases. In most workplaces, the airborne concentration of chemicals is too low for the uptake of vapours through the skin to be significant. In environments where the airborne concentrations are high, e.g. 10- or 1000-fold higher than the occupational exposure limit, respirators are worn to control inhalation exposure. Consider a worker who wears an airline respirator for 30 min in a room containing $250 \, \text{mg m}^{-3}$ of nitrobenzene (50 times the occupational exposure limit). For the purposes of this assessment, the head and arms of the worker were assumed to be exposed (surface area $= 5000 \, \text{cm}^2$), while the rest of the body (surface area $= 13\,000 \, \text{cm}^2$) was covered with clothing. The available data (Piotrowski, 1977) suggest that clothing reduces the percutaneous uptake rate of vapours by about 20%, i.e. the inhibition factor. The amount of nitrobenzene vapour absorbed through the skin would be

$$\text{percutaneous uptake} = C \cdot K_p \cdot A \cdot i \cdot t$$
$$= 250 \, \text{mg m}^{-3} \times 11.1 \, \text{cm h}^{-1} \times$$
$$(5000 + 13000 \times 0.8) \, \text{cm}^2 \times 0.5 \, h \times 10^{-6} \, \text{m}^3 \, \text{cm}^{-3} = 21.37 \text{mg}$$

where $i =$ inhibition factor for clothing.

From this example, it is clear that if one enters an environment which contains high concentrations of airborne contaminants, even if a supplied-air respirator is worn to limit inhalation exposure, percutaneous uptake of the chemical vapour may be significant.

Table 6 Percutaneous absorption of chemical vapours *in vivo*

Chemical	Permeability coefficient (cm h^{-1})	
	Rat	Human
Benzene	0.15	0.08
2-Butoxyethanol		2.1–28.8
Bromochloromethane	0.79	
Dibromomethane	1.32	
Halothane	0.05	
Hexane	0.03	
Isoflurane	0.03	
Methylene chloride	0.28	
Nitrobenzene		11.1–25.00
Perchloroethylene	0.67	0.17
Phenol		15.74–17.59
Styrene	1.75	0.35–1.42
Toluene	0.72	0.18
1,1,1-Trichloroethane		0.01
m-Xylene	0.72	0.24–0.26

CONCLUSION

Although cutaneous contact with chemicals is a common occurrence in industrial settings, for decades the human health hazard has seldom been quantified. This has been partly due to a lack of knowledge about the percutaneous absorption rates and a lack of available methods to determine them. The other reason is that many occupational hygienists and physicians assumed that gloves and protective clothing probably prevented exposure. However, there is now good evidence that many chemicals can penetrate most barriers at a low but measurable rate.

As a result of the emerging interest in exposure and health risk assessments, relatively reliable techniques for estimating the percutaneous absorption of chemicals are now available. In those instances where precise estimates are needed, chemical-and media-specific tests can be performed using either human skin *in vitro* or animal skin *in vivo*. If animal data are generated, the differences between the animal and human skin must be accounted for. While specific experimental data on percutaneous absorption will be most valuable, mathematical models may provide a useful tool to make estimations of percutaneous absorption rates. They can also be used to evaluate exposure conditions beyond those feasible in *in vivo* experiments and to examine the impact of various parameters controlling percutaneous absorption.

A review of the information discussed in this chapter suggests the following generalizations concerning percutaneous absorption:

(1) The cutaneous bioavailability of chemicals bound to soil can range over five order of magnitude. Consequently, it is crucial to understand and account for the various factors governing the matrix effects.

(2) The rate of percutaneous absorption can be appreciable for those chemicals with a high *n*-octanol–water partition coefficients. For example, studies of nitrobenzene, phenol, dimethylformamide, dimethylacetamide, carbon tetrachloride and several glycol ethers suggest that even when good hygienic practices are in place, the dose due to percutaneous absorption can often be as much as half of that due to inhalation. Although for many chemicals such an increase in dose may pose no significant hazard, for those chemicals where the margin of safety between the occupational exposure limit and toxicity is small, such an incremental contribution to dose should not be overlooked.

(3) The percutaneous absorption of chemical vapours is particularly worthy of consideration when the atmospheric concentration of the chemical is 10–1000-fold higher than the occupational exposure limit, even when the worker is using adequate respiratory protection.

REFERENCES

Andersen, M. E. and Keller, W. C. (1984). Toxicokinetic principles in relation to percutaneous absorption and cutaneous toxicity. In Drill, V. A. and Lazar, P. (Eds), *Cutaneous Toxicity*. Raven Press, New York, pp. 9–27.

Beech, J. A. (1980). Estimated worst-case trihalomethane body burden of a child using a swimming pool. *Med. Hypothesis*, **6**, 303–307.

Berner, B. and Cooper, E. R. (1987). Models of skin permeability. In Kydonieu, A. F. and Berner, B. (Eds), *Transdermal Delivery of Drugs*, Vol. II. CRC Press, Boca Raton, FL, pp. 107–130.

Borsadia, S., Ghanem, A. H., Seta, Y., Higuchi, W. I., Flynn, G. L., Behl, C. R. and Shah, V. P. (1992). Factors to be considered in the evaluation of bioavailability and bioequivalence of topical formulations. *Skin Pharmacol.*, **5**, 129–145.

Bronaugh, R. L., Stewart, R. F., Congdon, E. R. and Giles, A. L., Jr. (1982). Methods for *in vitro* percutaneous absorption studies. I. Comparison with *in vitro* results. *Toxicol. Appl. Pharmacol.*, **62**, 474–480.

Dugard, P. H. (1983). Skin permeability theory in relation to measurements of percutaneous absorption in toxicology. In Marzulli, F. N. and Maibach, H. I. (Eds), *Dermatotoxicology*. Hemisphere, Washington, DC, p. 102.

Fiserova-Bergerova, V., Pierce, J. T. and Droz, P. O. (1990). Dermal absorption potential of industrial chemicals: criteria for skin notation. *Am. J. Ind. Med.*, **17**, 617–635.

Flynn, G. L. (1990). Physicochemical determinants of skin absorption. In Gerrity, T. R. and Henry, C. J. (Eds), *Principles of Route-to-Route Extrapolation for Risk Assessment*. Elsevier, New York, pp. 93–127.

Guy, R. H. and Potts, R. O. (1993). Penetration of industrial chemicals across the skin: a predictive model. *Am. J. Ind. Med.*, **23**, 711–719.

Guy, R. H., Hadgraft, J. and Maibach, H. I. (1982). A pharmacokinetic model for percutaneous absorption. *Int. J. Pharm.*, **11**, 119–129.

Guy, R. H., Hadgraft, J. and Maibach, H. I. (1983). Percutaneous absorption: multidose pharmacokinetics. *Int. J. Pharm.*, **17**, 23–28.

Kao, J., Hall, J. and Helman, G. (1988). *In vitro* percutaneous absorption in mouse skin: influence of skin appendages. *Toxicol. Appl. Pharmacol.*, **94**, 93–103.

Marzulli, F. N., Brown, D. W. C., and Maibach, H. I. (1969). Techniques for studying skin penetration. *Toxicol. Appl. Pharmacol.*, **3**, 79–83.

McDougal, J. N., Jepson, G. W., Clewell, H. J., III, Gargas, M. L. and Andersen, M. E. (1990). Dermal absorption of organic chemical vapours in rats and humans. *Fundam. Appl. Toxicol.*, **14**, 299–308.

McKone, J. E. (1990). Dermal uptake of organic chemicals from a soil matrix. *Risk Anal.*, **10**, 407–419.

Menon, G. K. and Elias, P. M. (1997) Morphologic basis for a pore-pathway in mammalian stratum corneum. *Skin Pharmacol.*, **10**, 235–246.

Pannatier, A., Jenner, B., Testa, B., and Etter, J. C. (1978). The skin as a drug-metabolizing organ. *Drug Metab. Rev.*, **8**, 319–343.

Paustenbach, D. J. (1988). Assessment of the developmental risks resulting from occupational exposure to select glycol ethers within the semiconductor industry. *J. Toxicol. Environ. Health*, **23**, 29–75.

Piotrowski, J. (1977). *Exposure Tests for Organic Compounds in Industrial Toxicology*. Publication No. 77–144. National Institute for Occupational Safety and Health, Cincinnati, OH.

Raykar, P. V., Fung, M., and Anderson, B. D. (1988). The role of protein and lipid domains in the uptake of solutes by human stratum corneum. *Pharm. Res.*, **5** 140–150.

Reifenrath, W. G., Chellquist, E. M., Shipwash, E. A., Jederberg, W. W., and Krueger, G. G. (1984). Percutaneous penetration in the hairless dog, weanling pig and grafted athymic nude mouse: evaluation of models for predicting skin penetration in man. *Br. J. Dermatol.*, **111**, 123–135.

Rougier, A. D., Dupuis, D., Lotte, C. and Roguet, R. (1985). The measurement of the stratum corneum reservoir. A predictive method for *in vivo* percutaneous absorption studies: influence of application time. *J. Invest. Dermatol.*, **84**, 66–68.

Scheuplein, R. J. (1967). Mechanism of percutaneous absorption. II. Transient diffusion and the relative importance of various routes of skin penetration. *J. Invest. Dermatol.*, **48**, 79–88.

Scheuplein, R. J. and Blank, I. H. (1985). Permeability of the skin. *Physiol. Rev.*, **51**, 702–747.

Shatkin, J. A. and Brown, H. S. (1991). Pharmacokinetics of the dermal route of exposure to volatile organic chemicals in water: a computer simulation model. *Environ. Res.*, **56**, 90–108.

Sheehan, P., Meyer, D. M., Sauer, M. M. and Paustenbach, D. J. (1991). Assessment of the human health risks posed by exposure to chromium contaminated soils at residential sites. *J. Toxicol. Environ. Health*, **32**, 161–201.

Simon, G. A., and Maibach, H. I. (1998). Relevance of hairless mouse as an experimental model of percutaneous penetration in man. *Skin Pharmacol. Appl. Skin Physiol.*, **11**, 80–86.

Snyder, W. S. (1975). *Report of the Task Group on Reference Man*. International Commission of Radiological Protection Publication No. 23. Pergamon Press, New York.

Surber, C., Wilhelm, K. P., Maibach, H. I., Hall, L. L. and Guy, R. L. (1990). Partitioning of chemicals into human stratum corneum: implications for risk assessment following dermal exposure. *Fundam. Appl. Toxicol.*, **15**, 99–107.

Vickers, C. F. H. (1963). Existence of reservoir in the stratum corneum. *Arch. Dermatol.*, **88**, 20–23.

Wester, R. C. and Maibach, H. I. (1985). *In vivo* methods for percutaneous absorption measurements. In Bronaugh, R. L. and Maibach, H. I. (Eds), *Percutaneous Absorption. Mechanisms, Methodology, Drug Delivery*. Dermatology Series, Vol. 6. Marcel Dekker, New York, pp. 245–266.

Wester, R. C. and Noonan, P. K. (1980). Relevance of animal models for percutaneous absorption. *Int. J. Pharm.*, **7**, 99–110.

Wester, R. C., Noonan, P. K. and Maibach, H. I. (1980). Percutaneous absorption of hydrocortisone increases with long-term administration. *Arch. Dermatol.*, **116**, 186–188.

Zatz, J. L. (1985). Computer simulation using multi-compartmented membrane models. In Bronaugh, R. L. and Maibach, H. I. (Eds), *Percutaneous Absorption, Mechanisms, Methodology, Drug Delivery*. Dermatology Series, Vol. 6. Marcel Dekker, New York, pp. 165–181.

FURTHER READING

Exposure Assessment Group (1992). *Dermal Exposure Assessment: Principles and Applications*. EPA/600/8-91/011B, Interim Report. US Environmental Protection Agency Office of Health and Environmental Assessment, Washington, DC.

Leung, H.-W. and Paustenbach, D. J. (1994). Techniques for estimating the percutaneous absorption of chemicals due to occupational and environmental exposure. *Appl. Occup. Environ. Hyg.*, **9**, 187–197.

Chapter 30
Inhalation Toxicology

Paul M. Hext

C O N T E N T S

INTRODUCTION

Inhalation represents one of the major routes by which the body can be exposed by accident or design to foreign materials. This is well recognized in the context of human occupational exposures since it may result in the development of respiratory or systemic diseases. In this context, legislation has been developed over many years that requires monitoring of the workplace and application of adequate control procedures to prevent excessive exposure. However, there is often the need to understand further the mechanisms involved in the development of diseases induced by existing materials and additionally there is a need to established the toxicity profile of new materials entering the workplace or general environment. Experimental studies, often in animals, represents the only way to fulfil these needs. Hence this chapter is confined predominantly to the design and conduct of inhalation studies in experimental species with reference to man where appropriate.

When conducting experimental investigations on the fate or effects of airborne materials, a number of problems are encountered which are unique to the inhalation route of exposure. In the first instance it is necessary to ensure that the material under investigation can reach the target site or sites within the respiratory tract at concentrations appropriate to the needs of the study. The experimentalist must therefore have an understanding of the anatomy of the respiratory tract, mechanisms of deposition, particularly in the case of aerosols, and species differences with respect to these points, since in most cases studies are performed in species other than man. Second, in conducting inhalation studies the exposure and generation systems must be appropriate to the requirements of the study. The latter is particularly important in the case of studies performed for regulatory purposes where very high atmospheric concentrations are advocated if the material under test has a low toxic potential. Atmospheres, once generated, must also be monitored or analysed at regular intervals to demonstrate stability and, if an aerosol, that the particle size characteristics are acceptable. The foregoing indicates that inhalation toxicity studies involve a considerable technological input which may vary extensively according to the physical and chemical characteristics of the material being investigated. The inhalation toxicologist must therefore understand a number of disciplines, such as aerosol physics, that are not normally encountered in general toxicology.

The aim of this chapter is to provide the reader with a review of the basic principles and practices involved in conducting inhalation studies, but the principles of deposition and dosimetry can be applied also when assessing occupational or environmental exposure to man. It is not possible here to cover in detail the theoretical backgrounds to technology and study design, or the structure of the respiratory tract, its functions and responses to exposure, all of which are essential for a full understanding of the science of inhalation toxicology. These topics are extensively covered in textbooks dedicated to this topic and the reader should refer to these if a greater depth of knowledge is required (see References and Bibliography).

DOSIMETRY

The most important parameter in the majority of toxicity tests is the dose administered to the experimental animal or system. In virtually all modes of administration apart from inhalation it is easy to determine the dose since this is usually administered on an easily controlled weight per kilogram body weight basis. In inhalation studies it is clearly more difficult to assess the dose received by the animal since this is dependent on several factors, the major ones being (1) atmospheric concentration, (2) duration of exposure, (3) pulmonary physiological characteristics of the test species during the exposure period(s) and (4) deposition/absorption patterns of the test material. It is readily apparent that the dose will be related to the product of concentration (C) and time (T) for any given exposure provided that (3) and (4) above remain constant. This $C \times T$ product is commonly used to relate exposure to the magnitude of a toxic response and is frequently referred to as 'Haber's law', following from notes in the work of Haber (1924), who investigated the comparative lethalities of potential war gases. Further background on this important contribution to the laws governing inhalation toxicology can be found in Witschi (1997). In many cases, particularly those involving relatively short-duration exposures to materials such as phosgene which have a predominantly direct action on the pulmonary system, the observed toxicity follows Haber's law fairly closely, i.e. the response is directly proportional to the product $C \times T$. However, with the growing interest in relationships between concentration and exposure time, and in mechanisms of toxicity, it is becoming increasingly apparent that many materials do not follow Haber's law. This is frequently seen with those exhibiting systemic toxicity. Such toxicity depends upon the combined processes of uptake by the respiratory tract, tissue distribution, metabolism in potential target organs and elimination. Since many of these processes may be highly efficient at low concentrations but saturable at higher concentrations, a basis for non-linear relationships between concentration, time and toxic phenomena becomes apparent. A more detailed appraisal of the toxicokinetics of inhaled materials is beyond the scope of this chapter but is addressed in more detail in the general texts referred to in the References and Bibliography

The respiratory parameters of an animal will dictate the volume of air inhaled and hence the quantity of test material entering the respiratory system. Commonly used parameters for a number of experimental species and man are given in **Table 1** to illustrate this point and include alveolar surface area because this represents the target tissue for most inhaled materials. It can be seen

that by taking the ratios of these parameters and comparing the two extremes, i.e. the mouse and man, that (1) a mouse inhales approximately 30 times its lung volume in 1 min whereas a man at rest inhales approximately the same volume as that of his lung. This can increase with heavy work up to the same ratio as the mouse, but is not sustained for long periods. This means that the dose per unit lung volume is up to 30 times higher in the mouse than man at the same inhaled atmospheric concentration. (2) The minute volume of the mouse is in contact with five times less alveolar surface area than man, hence the dose per unit area is up to five times greater in the mouse. (3) The lung volume in comparison with the alveolar surface area in experimental animals is less than in humans, meaning that the extent of contact of inhaled gases with the alveolar surface is greater in experimental animals.

While it is possible, and frequent practice, to refer to standard respiratory parameters for different species in order to calculate inhaled dose and deposited dose with time, it is common for inhaled materials to influence the breathing patterns of test animals. The most common examples of this are irritant vapours, which can reduce the respiratory rate by up to 80%. This phenomenon results from a reflexive pause during the breathing cycle due to stimulation by the inhaled material of the trigeminal nerve endings situated in the nasal passages. The duration of the pause and hence the reduction in the respiratory rate are concentration related, permitting concentration–response relationships to be plotted. This has been investigated extensively by Alarie (1981) and forms the basis of a test screen for comparing quantitatively the irritancy of different materials, and has found application in assessing appropriate exposure limits for human exposure when respiratory irritancy is the predominant cause for concern.

While irritancy resulting from the above reflex reaction is one cause of altered respiratory parameters during exposure, there are many others. These include other types of reflex response, such as bronchoconstriction, the narcotic effects of many solvents, the development of toxic signs as exposure progresses, or simply a voluntary reduction in respiratory rate by the test animal due to the unpleasant nature of the inhaled atmosphere. The extent to which these affect breathing patterns and hence inhaled dose can only be assessed by actual

Table 1 Respiratory parameters for common experimental species and man (from Altman and Dittmer, 1974)

Species	Body weight (kg)	Lung volume (ml)	Minute volume (ml min^{-1})	Alveolar surface area (m^2)	Lung volume% / surface area	Minute volume% / lung volume	Minute volume% / surface area
Mouse	0.023	0.74	24	0.068	10.9	32.4	353
Rat	0.14	6.3	84	0.39	16.2	13.3	215
Monkey	3.7	184	694	13	14.2	3.77	53
Dog	22.8	1501	2923	90	16.7	1.95	33
Human	75	7000	6000	82	85.4	0.86	73

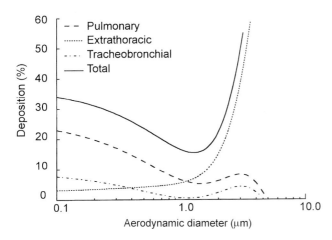

Figure 1 Deposition pattern of particles in the respiratory tract of the rat. From Raabe *et al.* (1977, 1988).

measurements made during the exposure. Such measurements are being incorporated increasingly into routine toxicity tests in order to estimate more accurately the inhaled dose. The methodology is relatively simple and has been adapted to small experimental animals from the standard plethysmographic techniques used on human subjects. From these parameters it is possible to assess the quantities of test atmosphere breathed in by the animal. It must be remembered that these techniques do not give the quantity of the inhaled material that is absorbed by, or deposited in, the respiratory tract.

In the case of aerosols, the particle size dictates the quantities and regional deposition of the particles. An approximation of dose can therefore be obtained by reference to plots of deposition efficiency as a function of particle size. **Figure 1** is an example, based on the studies of Raabe *et al.* (1977, 1988), of such a plot and shows the total and regional deposition curves for various particle sizes in the rat. Factors governing such deposition are considered later in this chapter. For more accurate assessment or determination of dose for both particulate and vapour atmospheres chemical analysis of tissues or exposure to radioisotopically labelled materials may be required in conjunction with measurement of respiratory physiology parameters.

PHYSICAL CHARACTERISTICS AND REGIONAL ABSORPTION/DEPOSITION

The fate of inhaled materials depends on both physical and chemical characteristics and the physical and biological characteristics of the respiratory tract. All atmospheres to which man or animals may be exposed may be divided initially according to the physical form of the test material and then aspects of the respiratory tract considered with respect to this division. Thus atmospheres are divided into those which are vapours or

gases and those which are aerosols. The latter term refers to both liquids and solids suspended in the air and encompasses other terms used for solid aerosols such as 'particulates' and 'dusts'.

Gases and Vapours

An initial assumption that is frequently made regarding a vapour or gas is that, because of its physical form, it will penetrate and be absorbed uniformly throughout the respiratory tract. This assumption is generally incorrect. The chemical characteristics and concentration of the material and conditions or characteristics of the respiratory tract all influence the sites to which the material may penetrate and the proportion absorbed. When an atmosphere is inhaled, it mixes with air-saturated water vapour and comes into contact with the tissue lining the various regions of the tract. Many gases or vapours, e.g. ammonia, formaldehyde and sulphur dioxide, are extremely soluble in water and therefore will be absorbed rapidly in the upper respiratory tract. At lower concentrations, and indeed at concentrations as high as hundreds or thousands of parts per million (ppm), there may be total absorption in these regions with none of the atmosphere penetrating to the lower respiratory tract. Therefore, any direct toxic effects of this class of material will be confined generally to these regions, particularly the nasal passages, where the pattern and type of lesion are characteristic of exposure to this class of material (Buckley *et al.*, 1984). With increasing inspired concentration, a gradient of concentration will develop from the nose to the alveolus, toxic effects occurring at each level in proportion to the local concentration of material and defence mechanisms of particular tissues. With materials which have low solubility in water, the humidity in the respiratory system has little effect on upper respiratory tract absorption and these materials penetrate readily to the pulmonary regions, even at relatively low concentrations, where, if they are direct tissue toxicants, they may exert toxicity. Well known examples of this class are ozone and nitrogen dioxide.

That, the site of deposition of vapours according to their solubility in water is only a general rule. Other factors may have a considerable influence on where vapours may deposit or become absorbed. In mixed atmospheres where both a vapour and particulate are present, the vapour may adsorb on the particle and the deposition pattern then is governed by the influence of particle deposition, a fact which is addressed later in this section.

The marked capacity of different areas of the respiratory tract to metabolize inhaled materials (Dahl and Lewis, 1993) may also influence the regional uptake of vapours. For example, the nasal passages are known to be rich in cytochrome P450 monooxygenase enzymes (Hadley and Dahl, 1982, 1983), by virtue of which they have a considerable capacity to metabolize inhaled vapours or gases. If the metabolite proves to be toxic then the observed tissue effects may be site-specific. This accounts for the effects of some compounds, e.g. 3-trifluoromethyl-pyridine (Hext and Lock, 1992) and methyl bromide (Hurtt *et al.*, 1987), to induce upper respiratory tract lesions that are specific to the olfactory epithelium and may also exhibit marked species differences with respect to effects (Hext *et al.*, 1994). Another result of the metabolic capacity of the upper respiratory regions is that not only may the inhaled vapour be absorbed totally in this region, but also the compound that subsequently enters the bloodstream may be a metabolite rather than the parent compound. The bronchiolar regions also have cells, Clara cells, that are capable of metabolizing inhaled xenobiotics with the potential of cell-, site- or species-specific toxicity (Hook *et al.*, 1990). There are important interspecies differences in the distribution of Clara cells; these cells being limited to the distal airways in humans but being found throughout the respiratory system of mice.

Gases and vapours whose absorbtion is not influenced by respiratory tract metabolism, which do not exert substantial direct toxicity and which penetrate to the alveolar region, will be absorbed into the blood across the alveolar air–blood interface. Their rate of uptake is dependent upon the blood–air partition coefficient. This is defined as the equilibrium that develops between the gas or vapour in the blood and that in the alveolar air. As this coefficient increases, the rate of uptake into blood increases and hence increasingly greater amounts of the inhaled gas or vapour are absorbed into the blood. Conversely, for vapours of low partition coefficient, such as those of very low water solubility, only a small proportion will be absorbed and hence the main part will be exhaled. If these absorption characteristics are applied to inhalation studies where a constant concentration is maintained in both the atmosphere and the lung, during the early phases of exposure when the blood concentration is low there will be a steady uptake until the equilibrium point is reached, at which stage the blood concentration remains constant. Once exposure ceases, the equilibrium shifts in the opposite direction and absorbed vapour will diffuse back into the alveolar air and be exhaled; a good example is provided by the uptake and subsequent release of carbon monoxide. The above represents an idealized illustration; the toxicokinetics of the chemical once it has entered the blood and hence body may influence these processes and a detailed appraisal of toxicokinetics is provided elsewhere in this book (Chapter 4).

Aerosols

An aerosol can be considered as a suspension of particles in a gas, air being the gas in the majority of cases dealt with in inhalation toxicology. When such an atmosphere is inhaled the particles may deposit anywhere within the respiratory tract, the actual deposition site being dictated by their size. Before understanding the relationship between size, deposition mechanism and site, it is necessary to realise that it is not the physical size of the particle that is important here but the aerodynamic size, which will vary according to a number of variables, the most important of which is density. Shape, for instance of a fibre, will also have an influence, but this is generally less than might be expected.

The aerodynamic size or diameter of a particle is determined using specialized instrumentation and is defined as the diameter of a sphere of unit density having the same settling velocity as the particle in question. The relationship between the aerodynamic diameter and physical diameter is broadly covered by the following equation:

$$\text{aerodynamic diameter} = \text{physical diameter} \times (\text{density})^{1/2}$$

Thus, a particle of 1 μm physical diameter and density of 4 g cm^{-3} will behave aerodynamically in air in a similar manner to a particle of unit density and diameter of 2 μm.

Depending on the particle size, especially for those of < 1 μm, additional correction factors have to be added to the above equation and more detailed treatises on the physical aspects of aerosols may be found in Hidy (1984), Hinds (1982) and Vincent (1989, 1995) and also those texts referred to in the Introduction. Instrumentation used most commonly for assessing aerodynamic size and particle size distribution in inhalation chamber atmospheres will be covered later.

Deposition in the Respiratory Tract

Deposition of particles within the respiratory tract is governed by three main factors: (1) the anatomical structure of the respiratory tract, (2) the airflow patterns and (3) the aerodynamic size of the particle.

Anatomical Structure
The physiological role of the lung is to enable oxygen to be absorbed into the blood to provide the needs of biological respiration and to remove carbon dioxide. In order to achieve this there must be a very large surface area available to facilitate this process efficiently. In man, the surface area of the gas-exchange region (the alveoli) is of the order of 80 m^2. To enable air to enter the respiratory tract through one initial conducting airway but to then provide 80 m^2 surface area of gas-exchange tissue, the initial airway, which has a cross-sectional area of approximately 2 cm^2, must divide repeatedly, each division or branch resulting in two airways, both of smaller diameter but with a concomitant increase in total cross-sectional area. Thus the structure of the lungs can be considered simplistically as a series of dividing tubes, the number of new tubes doubling at each division and the total cross-sectional area increasing **(Figure 2)**.

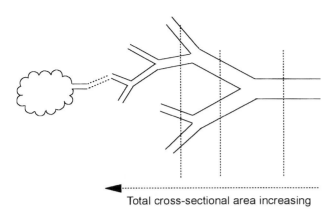

Total cross-sectional area increasing

Figure 2 Diagrammatic representation of the branching of the respiratory tract to illustrate increasing cross-sectional area and hence decreasing velocity of inhaled air.

Airflow Patterns

Air entering the respiratory tract has a velocity related to the volume and cross-sectional area of the airway. Any particle suspended in the inhaled air will have the same velocity. At the first airway branch the velocity will decrease since the same volume is passing through an increased surface area. Further reductions in velocity occur at each subsequent branch such that within the deeper regions of the lung the velocity is virtually zero and gaseous diffusion becomes the mechanism of oxygen and carbon dioxide transport. In parallel with velocity changes, the inhaled air undergoes changes of direction due to the structure of the upper respiratory tract (nasal and laryngeal regions) and then as a consequence of the branching of the airways. In the upper unbranched regions and the upper part of the branched airways, the directional change is relatively abrupt whereas further along the airways, the directional change is slight. Combining these two factors, inhaled air undergoes a continued reduction in velocity together with a range of directional changes when passing from the nose or mouth to the deep regions of the lung. Any particle suspended in the inhaled air will potentially be subject to the same changes in behaviour.

Particle Size

The aerodynamic size of a particle dictates how it will behave in air and is related to the settling rate of the particle in air. Hence large particles will settle quickly and will be influenced less by turbulence in the air. Taking this in conjunction with the structure of the respiratory tract and the airflow patterns, larger particles that are inhaled within the airstream can remain suspended at high velocity but will begin to 'settle out' as the velocity decreases. In addition, the kinetics of larger particles which have initial high velocities are such that when an abrupt change in direction occurs they are less likely to follow the change in direction of the gas stream and will deposit in the region of the directional change. Smaller particles will follow the directional change of the air stream and remain suspended, especially if the branching becomes less abrupt. However, as the velocity reduces they will be more influenced by gravity and will start to settle out according to their settling velocity. Those of very fine size and therefore very low settling velocity act more like gas molecules and undergo Brownian diffusion.

The above factors in combination lead to four principle mechanisms by which inhaled particles deposit within the respiratory tract: inertial impaction, gravitational sedimentation, Brownian diffusion and interception, together with the additional mechanism of electrostatic precipitation. These are defined as follows.

Impaction

Impaction occurs where the airstream undergoes a directional change **(Figure 3A)**. The momentum of the particle is such that it is unable to change course and deposits on the wall of the airway. Particles of aerodynamic size of greater than 0.5 μm may deposit by this mechanism. This mechanism can operate only where there is a combination of both velocity and directional change and is confined predominantly to the upper respiratory tract and higher branching points in the tracheobronchial system of man but can operate down to the alveolar duct region of smaller experimental animals. Factors influencing deposition by this mechanism include the physical size and density of a particle and breathing pattern.

Gravitational Sedimentation

All particles are subjected to gravity and when this force exceeds other forces to which the particle is subjected, such as velocity and buoyancy, the particle will deposit on the wall of the respiratory tract **(Figure 3B)**. This mechanism predominates in the lower regions of the respiratory tract where velocities are low. Factors influencing deposition by this mechanism are those mentioned above for impaction with the addition of residence time within the respiratory tract.

Brownian diffusion

Very fine particles, i.e. those smaller than approximately 0.5 μm, are subject to bombardment by gas molecules and thus acquire random movement in air, termed Brownian motion. Within the respiratory tract particles moving in such a manner may contact the wall of the airway and deposit **(Figure 3C)**. Deposition by this mechanism is favoured by air velocities being low or absent and therefore predominates in the bronchiolar and alveolar regions.

Interception

Where there is a change in direction of the airflow, irregularly shaped particles such as fibres or fume aggregates may make partial contact with the wall of the airway and become deposited **(Figure 3D)**.

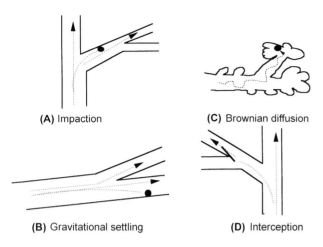

Figure 3 Diagrammatic representations of the mechanisms influencing the deposition of particles in the respiratory tract.

Electrostatic Charge

Aerosols generated for inhalation experiments frequently carry substantial electrostatic charge as a result of the methods of generation employed. Such charges can enhance the fraction and site of deposition of the inhaled aerosol by both particle–particle charge interaction and particle–respiratory tract charge interaction.

Regional Deposition of Particles

When conducting inhalation studies with aerosols, it is important to understand the relationship between particle size and regional deposition. In man, this relationship is well defined. The fraction of an atmosphere that is capable of entering the respiratory tract via the nose or mouth is defined as the 'inhalable' fraction. This is now a standardized definition for this fraction used by the International Standards Organization (ISO, 1995) and is considered to represent the fraction of the atmosphere, and hence any particle, with an aerodynamic diameter of < 100 μm. Particles of this size will deposit in the nose or mouth and penetrate no further into the respiratory tract. With decreasing size, particles will penetrate further into the respiratory tract and those capable of reaching the alveolar regions, which are perceived to represent the greatest risk to health, are defined as 'respirable'. In man the upper size range for this respirable fraction is considered to be 10 μm. This apparent size cut-off is used for defining the sampling characteristics of instruments for measuring airborne particles (detailed later). Hence for measuring the respirable fraction of an atmosphere, a sampler should collect specifically particles of this size or less. This fraction has become well known as PM_{10} and is defined more accurately as the mass concentration of a particulate aerosol as determined with sampling instruments having a 50% cut-off point of size-sampling of 10 μm. It should be recognized that this fraction contains particles that will deposit in regions of the respiratory tract other than the alveolar region and also that the coarser part of this fraction will penetrate to a limited extent only to this region. The finer part will indeed penetrate efficiently to the alveoli and for many years the fraction of 2.5 μm or less has been used to identify this 'higher risk' proportion of particles. The concern in recent years that this fraction in the environment may represent an even greater health hazard than the classical 10 μm respirable fraction has led to the development of instruments for measuring this fraction specifically, termed $PM_{2.5}$, using a 50% cut-off at 2.5 μm as the instrument sampling characteristics. Both PM_{10} and $PM_{2.5}$ are used by a number of regulatory agencies in conjunction with regulations designed to measure and control environmental particles that arise from the activities of man.

Taking the above considerations and definitions in the context of inhalation studies conducted in experimental animals, allowance will need to be made for differences in particle deposition patterns compared with man. A comparison of respiratory tract deposition in different species can be found in the review paper by Schlesinger (1985). The rat, for example, the most commonly used species for toxicity testing, is an obligate nose breather and has a complex nasal turbinate structure which will filter out many of the relatively fine particles which would be expected normally to penetrate to the alveoli in man. Thus, whereas 15 μm is considered to represent the upper size limit for particles that can reach the alveolar regions in man, the limit is more likely to be in the region of 5–6 μm in the rat, as shown in **Figure 1**.

EXPOSURE SYSTEMS

Exposure systems for short- or long-term inhalation studies fall into three main categories: whole body, nose/head only and masks. Masks are used predominantly for larger experimental species and will not be dealt with here. The remaining two categories can be divided further into those operating in the dynamic or static modes. In dynamic systems, the test atmosphere passes through the exposure chamber and is renewed continuously. This ensures atmospheric stability and no reduction in oxygen concentration as a result of the respiration of the test animals. It is the mode in which the great majority of inhalation studies are conducted and is the only mode in which reasonable numbers of test animals can be exposed to materials for appreciable periods of time. Static systems are sealed and generally depend upon the air within the chamber to maintain any exposed animals. The exposure time is therefore relatively short, although some systems, in order to extend the exposure time, are designed to replace the consumed oxygen and remove exhaled carbon dioxide. The atmospheric concentration generally will not remain stable in these systems. If the atmosphere is generated continuously then it will increase in concentration, whereas if generated only at the initiation of a study it will decrease owing to absorption by the test animal and also adsorption on the walls of the exposure system. The advantage of static systems is that they are relatively simple to operate and consume only a fraction of the material required to generate a dynamic atmosphere at equivalent concentrations. Hence they are used predominantly in research studies, particularly if the test material is isotopically labelled, or for other specialized applications, such as assessing the toxicity of products evolved during the combustion of materials.

Dynamic systems, of whatever size or design, must involve a considerable amount of ancillary equipment to maintain appropriate conditions of airflow, temperature and relative humidity. There is a wide range of designs currently in use, some being commercially available whereas others have been designed and built by individual laboratories. **Figure 4A** shows the general design for a chamber of approximately 250 l capacity in which small experimental species may be exposed, whole body, to experimental atmospheres and **Figure 4B** shows a typical nose-only exposure chamber. The latter mode of exposure is used frequently for exposure to particulates since it reduces to an absolute minimum the deposition of test atmosphere on the pelt of the test animal. This is an important factor to take into account when exposure is to aerosols, which may exert systemic toxicity since with whole body exposure the quantities depositing in the fur and subsequently ingested during grooming can exceed considerably the quantity depositing in the respiratory tract (Langard and Nordhagen, 1980; Iwasaki *et al.*, 1988).

The main criteria for the design and operation of any dynamic system are as follows:

■ The concentration of the test atmosphere must be reasonably uniform throughout the chamber and should increase and decrease at a rate close to theoretical at the start or end of the exposure. Silver (1946) showed that the time taken for a chamber to reach a point of equilibrium was proportional to the flow rate of atmosphere passing through the chamber and the chamber volume. From this, the concentration–time relationship during the 'run-up' and 'run-down' phase could be expressed by the equation

$$t_x = k\frac{V}{F}$$

where t_x = time required to reach $x\%$ of the equilibrium concentration, k = a constant of value determined by the value of x, V = chamber volume and F = chamber flow rate. The t_{99} value is frequently quoted for exposure chambers, representing the time required to reach 99% of the equilibrium concentration and providing an estimate of chamber efficiency. Thus, at maximum efficiency, the theoretical value of k at t_{99} is 4.605, and the closer to this that the results of evaluation of actual chamber performance fall, the greater is the efficiency and the better the design of the chamber.

■ Flow rates must be controlled in such a way that they are not excessive, which might cause streaming effects within the chamber, but must be adequate to maintain normal oxygen levels, temperature and humidity in relation to the number of animals being exposed. A minimum of 10 air changes per hour is frequently advocated and is appropriate in most cases. However, the chamber design and housing density also need to be taken into account and some designs, such as that of Doe and Tinston (1981), function effectively at lower air change rates.

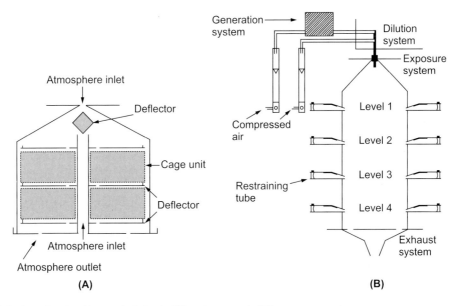

Figure 4 Typical designs for short-term whole-body **(A)** and nose-only **(B)** exposure systems.

■ The chamber materials should not affect the chemical or physical nature of the test atmosphere

In addition, it is desirable, and frequently a regulatory necessity, to monitor and record air flow, temperature and humidity within the chamber.

The above criteria apply equally to those chambers already illustrated (Figure 4) which are designed predominantly for short-term studies (days to months) and to those built on a larger scale to accommodate large numbers of experimental animals for durations of up to several years. The latter can vary from a relatively simple design of 2 m³ capacity (similar to Figure 4A) to the more complex design described by Doe and Tinston (1981), where the cages are suspended on carriers which rotate within the chamber. More detailed considerations of theoretical and practical design and operation of inhalation chambers may be found in Drew (1978), Leong (1981) and MacFarland (1983).

ATMOSPHERE GENERATION

Atmosphere generation systems fall into two classes: those concerned with particulate atmospheres, such as aerosols of solids or liquids, and those concerned with non-particulate atmospheres, such as gases or vapours. In all cases there should be sufficient control over the generation system to provide reasonably stable atmospheres. Gases and vapours should normally be controlled to within 5–10% of target concentration with little difficulty, whereas particulates, which present invariably the greater difficulties of control, may vary acceptably to within 20% of target.

Gases and Vapours

Gases and vapours may be generated in several ways, including direct dilution of a gas with clean air and vaporization of a liquid, either by the addition of heat and/or by increasing the surface area of the liquid. The latter is achieved frequently by either atomization into a reservoir chamber such that the aerosol droplets volatilize before passing into the main exposure chamber or by passing the liquid over heated glass beads (as described by Miller *et al.*, 1988) or similar apparatus designed to increase the surface area of the liquid. Other common methods include bubbling air through the heated liquid or simply taking vapour from the headspace of a cylinder containing a readily volatile material such as a compressed gas. The advantage with generation methods based on atomization or passage over a heated surface is that generally total volatilization of a mixture of volatile materials can be achieved to give an atmosphere composed of the individual components in similar proportions to that found in the liquid mixture. Bubblers

or headspace generation may result in differential volatilization if components of a mixture have different vapour pressures, i.e. the most volatile component will vaporize predominantly first followed by components of lower volatilities. This can result in variations not only in concentration but also in the composition of the test atmosphere. Similar problems of differential volatilization using these methods should be taken into consideration when generating vapour from a relatively pure liquid containing traces of less volatile but toxic impurities. The majority of the liquid can be generated with adequate control of concentration but the less volatile component will concentrate within the container and may be generated subsequently at toxic concentrations. This potential problem does not arise when generating by continuous total volatilization.

Particulates

The generation of particulate atmospheres is more complicated owing to the physical characteristics of the material and of the generated aerosol. The latter, for inhalation studies, must be capable generally of penetrating to all regions of the respiratory tract. Aerosol generation systems must therefore be capable of producing particles of a suitable size. It is convenient to consider liquid and solid aerosol generation systems separately.

Aerosol Generation From Liquids

There are two commonly used processes by which an aerosol can be generated under laboratory-controlled conditions: condensation from saturated vapours or dispersion of solutions or suspensions by aerosolization or nebulization. Condensation generators produce only relatively low concentration aerosols, but can be used to produce aerosols containing a very narrow range of particle sizes. Aerosols of materials with only moderate volatility at ambient temperature and pressure may be generated as condensation aerosols. This involves heating the test material and passing air over, or through it, to carry away the vapour phase created by the raised temperature. The air then passes through a flue where it is cooled to room temperature. This causes the vapour phase to become supersaturated and to condense on to any nuclei present in the air stream. The nuclei grow until the vapour phase of the test material reaches a new point of saturation. An aerosol produced in this way is usually monodisperse, i.e. all the particles have a very similar size. The mass concentration of the aerosol will be limited by the change in saturated vapour concentration caused by the increase in temperature. Only aerosols of essentially pure materials should be generated in this way as the removal of the vapour phase from above the heated material may cause a fractional distillation from mixtures of chemicals with different vapour pressures.

Atomization and Nebulization

Atomization and nebulization are two methods of liquid atomization which use compressed air as a motive force. Atomizers are very simple devices which use a high-velocity air jet to disrupt a stream of the test liquid as it leaves a narrow orifice. There are many designs based on this principle. An example of a commercially available atomizer that may be used to produce test atmospheres is the Schlick atomiser (**Figure 5A**; Gustav Schlick GmbH, Germany). This is made from stainless steel and is therefore suitable for use with a wide range of liquids, including organic solvents. This atomizer is representative of the most common type of atomizer where the air jet forms an annulus around the inner liquid jet as shown. The Schlick atomizer is designed as an industrial device used, for example, in drying, spray drying, spray painting or glue spreading, but it is suited equally to the generation of atmospheres in inhalation toxicity. The extended inner jet prevents volatile materials evaporating within the jet throat, which could result in precipitated solute blocking the jet and causing either stoppages or irregular operation.

Atomizers produce a broad-spectrum aerosol containing a wide range of particle sizes. However, although the mean diameter of the aerosol can vary substantially, many commercially available atomizers generate aerosols with large mean diameters and as such their use may be limited for inhalation toxicology, so more suitable devices such as the nebulizer have been developed.

Nebulizers are more sophisticated than atomizers. The main difference between the two types of aerosol generator is the inclusion of some form of size selection device in the nebulizer. This is usually a baffle placed in the path of the air–liquid mixture. The Wright nebulizer, (Wright 1958; **Figure 5B**) is an example and is constructed generally from polyacrylic resin. This does, however, preclude the use of this device with materials containing many organic solvents. Several other nebulizers have been designed to provide aerosol therapy via the respiratory tract and are equally applicable to inhalation toxicology. One example, the Acorn nebulizer (Medic-aid, Chichester, Sussex, UK), is shown diagrammatically in **Figure 5C**. The performance of this and a number of similar devices has been characterized extensively by Clay *et al.* (1983), Newman *et al.* (1985) and Bretz *et al.* (1984). Such devices are usually very compact. Since they are generally injection moulded from polyacrylic resins or similar materials, they may similarly be unsuitable for materials which contain organic solvents. However, they do offer the most consistent output between different generators owing to their closely controlled method of manufacture.

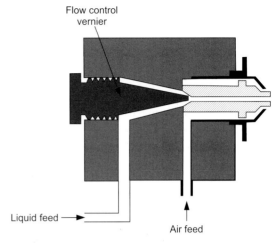

(A) The Schlick atomizer

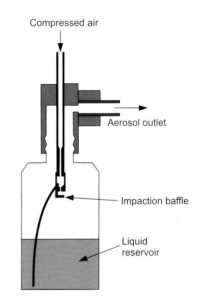

(B) The Wright nebulizer

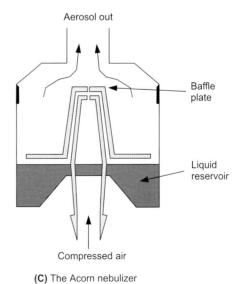

(C) The Acorn nebulizer

Figure 5 Commonly used liquid aerosol generation systems.

Aerosol generation from solids

There are two main forms of dry particle dispersion system: those that disperse from a compressed sample of the test material and those that disperse from the free-flowing material. Both types are in common use.

Dust generation systems based on the Wright Dust Feed Mechanism (Wright, 1950; **Figure 6A**) are used widely and are available in a number of different commercial forms. The material to be generated is first packed and compressed into a hard cake and during aerosol production a thin layer is scraped off into the air stream. The scraper is driven into the cake by a series of gears powered by a constant-speed motor. The gears can be adjusted to achieve a range of scraper advancement speeds and hence dust generation rates. More sophisticated systems use electronically controlled motors or similar devices to provide improved control over feed rates.

Systems based on compressing material into a hard cake are not suitable for materials which are near to their melting point at room temperature. If such materials were used, the pressure could cause the melting point of the material to be exceeded, resulting in fusion into a solid or wax. Systems based on Wright's generation methodology may not always provide the fine control over dust dispersion and hence concentration that is now required in many studies, especially when developing automatic feed-back control using a combination of dust monitor and generator to control concentration and stability.

An alternative approach to Wright's generation system is the use of rotating brush generators to disperse test material packed into a barrel **(Figure 6B)**. These systems, which are now used routinely in many laboratories, employ a piston to push the lightly packed material on to a rotating brush made from stainless steel or plastic. The design of the brush chamber and associated airflow exerts considerable shear forces on the generated materials, breaking up aggregates and improving dispersion. Rotating brush generators are capable of fine control of atmospheric concentration and, unlike many other designs of generator, they can be used for generation of atmospheres of fibrous materials.

The other major group of dust generation systems disperse material directly from the freely flowing bulk sample without any compaction into a cake. The Rotating Table Dust Generator (RTDG) was described by Mark *et al.* (1985) and represents an inexpensive system of this type. The device is shown in **Figure 6C**. The bulk material is placed in a hopper and a stirrer blade is passed down the centre. The hopper exhaust is positioned over a groove in the rotating table. Several concentric grooves of different depths may be cut into each table to extend the range of concentrations available without changing the table. Dust from the hopper fills the groove as it rotates beneath the hopper exhaust. After the dust has

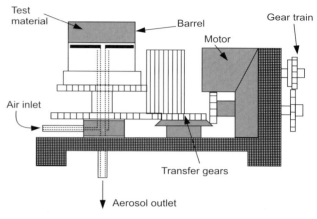

(A) Wright's dust feed mechanism

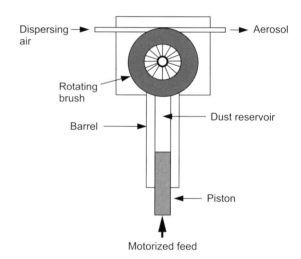

(B) Rotating brush generator

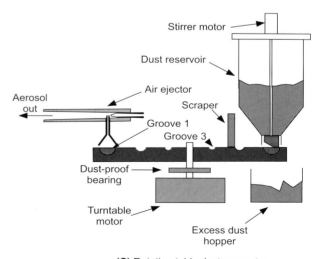

(C) Rotating table dust generator

Figure 6 Commonly used solid aerosol generators.

been levelled, it is transferred beneath the inlet of an air ejector, which lifts it from the groove. The air velocity and turbulence within the air ejector dissociate the test material into individual particles. The concentration of the test aerosol can be adjusted and controlled by altering the rate at which the table rotates, by using a different groove or by adjusting the air flow through the air ejector. Other systems using free-flowing powders include those based on air jet mills (Bernstein *et al.*, 1984), fluidized beds (Carpenter and Yerkes, 1980) or simply screw-feed devices supplying the material directly to an air ejector.

The atmosphere generation systems described above are provided as examples of the wide range of systems, based on an equally wide range of principles, that can be used to generate experimental atmospheres over a range of concentrations. Although many generators will produce atmospheres from a range of different materials, there are also many specialized generation systems that have been developed to create a specific atmosphere from one material or, at the most, a narrow class of materials. For more detail of the principles and practices of atmosphere generation, the reader is referred to books in the general reference list which describe these more fully.

ATMOSPHERE ANALYSIS

An atmosphere having been generated, it is necessary to confirm that it is chemically and physically suitable to provide a valid assessment of the inhalation toxicity of the test material. This is a two-stage process; the first stage involves the collection of a representative sample of the atmosphere, generally from the breathing zone of the test animals, and the second is concerned with the determination of the physical and chemical nature of the atmosphere. The frequency of sampling for analysis is dependent on a number of factors, including the stability of the test atmosphere, the method of sampling or analysis and the concentration of test material. All these factors need to be considered for each new material but, as a general rule, sampling should be performed at least hourly during exposure. Instruments are now available to give continuous qualitative, semi-quantitative or quantitative assessments of both particulate or non-particulate atmosphere concentrations. These help to assess continuously the stability of test atmospheres and to reduce the frequency of manual sampling and analysis, and are becoming integral parts of fully automated atmosphere control systems.

Vapours and Gases

When considering vapours and gases, the first stage generally represents few problems. However, the possible reactivity of the atmosphere with components of the sampling system and the volume taken for analysis must be considered in every case. The latter is important since the flow rate through and atmosphere distribution within the inhalation chamber must be unaffected by the volume removed for sampling. In general, the sampling rate should not represent greater than 5–10% of the total chamber flow rate.

Atmospheres of vapours or gases can be considered as homogeneous mixtures and, as such, would be unaffected by the physical nature of the sampling process. In this instance, the process becomes a matter of collecting sufficient material to allow a meaningful chemical analysis. The amount needed can vary enormously, depending on the type of analysis to be performed. Gas chromatography (GC), high-performance liquid chromatography (HPLC), gas chromatography–mass spectrometry (GC–MS) and infrared gas analysis (IRGA) are all commonly used to measure non-particulate atmosphere concentrations, as are 'wet' chemistry and spectrophotometry. Many of these methods may be automated in order to take and analyse samples repeatedly from a range of inhalation and exposure chambers. The results may be collated using a microcomputer in addition to being used to trigger alarms should the measured concentration fall outside a pre-set range.

Gas and vapour concentrations can be expressed in terms of either mass-per-volume or volume-per-volume units, the latter usually as parts per million (ppm). Conversion between mass-per-volume and volume-per-volume units for gases and vapours requires incorporation of the molecular weight of the substance into the necessary calculation together with the molecular volume of the gas or vapour (the molecular volume is the volume occupied by 1 gram molecule of a gas or vapour at a specified temperature and pressure). The resultant relationship is expressed as

$$\text{mg m}^{-3} = \text{ppm} \times \frac{\text{molecular weight}}{\text{molecular volume}}$$

Since the molecular volume varies according to temperature, the molecular volume at normal atmospheric pressure will vary according to the equation

$$\begin{array}{l}\text{Volume occupied by 1 gram} \\ \text{molecule at temperature } t(^{\circ}\text{Kelvin})\end{array} = \frac{t(K)}{273} \times 22.414$$

Therefore, when converting between ppm volume-per-volume units and weight-per-volume units, the molecular volume must first be corrected for temperature.

Particulates

Particulate atmospheres are more complicated to analyse than non-particulate atmospheres. Gases and vapours can be transferred through sample lines to a remote analyser with normally little or no degradation or surface adsorption of the sample in many cases. This is not true of an aerosol. The particles within an aerosol will have a tendency to settle out by gravity even within a dynamically mixed atmosphere. This can cause changes in both the mass concentration and the aerodynamic size distribution of an aerosol. In addition, the inertial forces acting on an aerosol as it passes through a sample line may cause similar changes as larger particles are removed selectively by impaction at curves and bends in the line. Because of these considerations, it is generally advocated that samples are taken in the breathing zone of the test animals. Further discussion on the complexities of aerosol sampling can be found in Vincent (1989).

Two fundamental aspects of an aerosol must be measured: mass concentration and aerodynamic size distribution. The first aspect can be measured easily by drawing a known volume of test atmosphere, at a known flow rate, through a filter. A basic sampling system is shown schematically in **Figure 7A**. A wide range of aèrosol samplers are available, each with a slightly different sampling inlet efficiency, and those concerned or interested in detailed sampling criteria should consult Vincent (1989) or similar texts. The filter mass is weighed before and after sampling to provide a gravimetric estimate of mass collected, or the filter may be analysed chemically for one or more components in order to provide a more detailed description of the chemical nature of the aerosol. The atmospheric concentration of the particulate is calculated simply from the mass collected divided by the volume of air sampled and is expressed most commonly as mg m^{-3} or mg l^{-1}.

The aerodynamic size distribution of an aerosol is determined generally using a cascade impactor (see **Figure 7B**). In such a device, the aerosol is accelerated repeatedly through a series of increasingly finer jets that play upon a flat collection surface. As the particles are accelerated they achieve sufficient momentum to prevent them following the change in direction of the airflow and they are deposited by impaction on the collection plate. In this way particles with increasingly smaller aerodynamic diameters are collected on the successive stages. The impactor is designed such that under defined operating conditions the particle size of material collecting on each stage is known, hence the quantity of material depositing on each stage can be assigned a specific 'cut-point'. This information is then converted to cumulative percentage, as shown in **Table 2**, and then linearized by plotting 'cut-point' particle size against cumulative percentage on log-probability paper, as shown in **Figure 8**. From such a plot, the particle size distribution is demonstrated graphically and the mean aerodynamic diameter (often referred to as the D_{50}) can be found. The distribution of particle size can be expressed as the geometric standard deviation (GSD), which is calculated from the particle sizes at the 16% or 84% points (these represent one standard deviation from the mean) according to the following equations:

$$\text{GSD} \quad \frac{D_{84}}{D_{50}} \text{ or } \frac{D_{50}}{D_{16}} \text{ or } \frac{D_{84}}{D_{16}}$$

Where specific size fractions of an atmosphere are required to be analysed, usually in the context of occupational and environmental exposure, samplers are available that have been designed to have sampling characteristics that collect only those fractions. Thus,

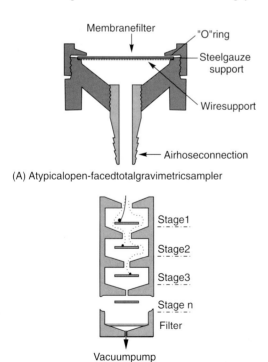

(A) A typical open-faced total gravimetric sampler

(B) A typical cascade impactor

Figure 7 Typical designs of (A) a sampler for measuring the total particulate present in an aerosol and (B) a cascade impactor for determination of the particle size distribution of an aerosol.

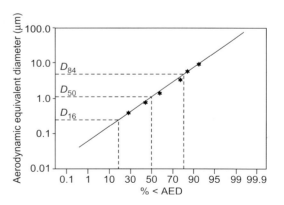

Figure 8 Logarithmic-probability plot of data (Table 2) derived from atmosphere sampling using a six-stage cascade impactor. Plotting cumulative percentage of deposited material against aerodynamic cut-off for each stage allows graphical derivation of mass median aerodynamic diameter (D_{50}) and geometric standard deviation (GSD).

Table 2 Cascade impactor data for plotting particle size distribution

Aerodynamic diameter cut-off (μm)	Weight on stage (mg)	% of total	Cumulative % (less than previous cut-off)
9.8	0.65	13	
6.0	0.45	9	87
3.5	0.80	16	78
1.55	1.40	28	62
0.93	0.75	15	34
0.52	0.50	10	19
Filter	0.45	9	9
Total	5.0	100	

as mentioned earlier, the PM_{10} and $PM_{2.5}$ fractions of environmental aerosols are defined as such owing both to the design characteristics of the samplers used to collect these fractions and the relevance to human respiratory tract deposition patterns of particles falling into these categories.

Sampling an aerosol using filter or impaction techniques as described provides accurate gravimetric data on atmospheric concentrations and also samples which can be analysed chemically if required. However, they all require finite sampling and processing times, often in minutes or hours, to provide such data, i.e. they do not provide real-time information. A range of direct-reading instruments capable of providing information on aerosol stability, concentration and particle size are now available commercially. Those used most commonly in inhalation toxicity studies can be considered as aerosol spectrometers, using light scattering to provide information on the aerosol of interest. Since the light-scattering properties of different aerosolized materials and particles sizes differ, in their simplest form the output of these instruments provides data only on the real-time stability of the atmosphere. By appropriate calibration, the instrument output can be modified to provide a measure of the gravimetric concentration of the aerosol. At the high concentrations used in many inhalation studies, the number of particles and instrument limitations allow only continuous concentration measurements to be made, but such instruments can be used to monitor stability and can be used in automated feed-back systems to adjust the atmospheric concentration automatically. More complex laser-based systems are capable of measuring also the physical or aerodynamic size of particles. To facilitate this, the atmospheric concentration is usually required to be low or may require one or more dilution stages to be included between the test atmosphere and the instrument, leading to possible problems of larger particle losses within the dilution systems.

Other instruments that are available to provide real-time aerosol information include piezobalances and β-attenuation samplers. The former contains a quartz crystal (or crystals if particle sizing versions are used) that oscillates at a stable frequency. When particles deposit on the crystal there is a change in frequency that is proportional to the deposited mass. The latter sampler contains a radioactive source that emits β-radiation. Particles depositing on a film situated between the source and detector will attenuate the amount of radiation that reaches the detector and this change is converted into a measure of aerosol concentration. Since different materials attenuate radiation to differing extents, the instrument requires calibration, such as against a gravimetric filter sampler, if the instrument output is to be converted to the aerosol mass concentration.

CONCLUSION

This chapter provides a basic introduction to the principles and practice of inhalation toxicology. It should be apparent that this discipline is very technically oriented, requiring knowledge and experience of a wide range of technical equipment in addition to general toxicology. While more detailed theoretical information on the aspects covered can be found in the textbooks recommended, the difficulties frequently encountered when generating different classes of materials as experimental atmospheres can only be understood and overcome by actual experimentation and experience.

REFERENCES AND BIBLIOGRAPHY

General Reading

Crapo, J. D., Smolko, E. D., Miller, F. J., Graham, J. A. and Hayes, A. W. (Eds) (1989). *Extrapolation of Dosimetric Relationships for Inhaled Particles and Gases.* Academic Press, San Diego.

Fiserova-Bergorova, V. (Ed.) (1983). *Modelling of Inhalation Exposure to Vapours: Uptake, Distribution and Elimination,* Vols 1 and 2. CRC Press, Boca Raton, FL.

McClellan, R. O. and Henderson, R. F. (Eds) (1995). *Concepts in Inhalation Toxicology.* Taylor and Francis, London.

Mohr, U. (Ed.) (1989). *Inhalation Toxicology, the Design and Interpretation of Inhalation Studies and Their Use in Risk Assessment.* Springer, New York.

Phalen, R. F. (1984). *Inhalation Studies: Foundations and Techniques*. CRC Press, Boca Raton, FL

Phalen, R. F. (1996). *Methods in Inhalation Toxicology*. CRC Press, Boca Raton, FL.

Salem, H. (Ed.) (1987). *Inhalation Toxicology*. Marcel Dekker, New York.

Witschi, H. P. and Brain, J. D. (Eds) (1985). *Toxicology of Inhaled Materials*. Springer Berlin.

Specific Topics

Alarie, Y. (1981). Toxicological evaluation of airborne chemical irritants and allergens using respiratory reflex reactions. In Leong, B. K. G. (Ed.), *Inhalation Toxicology and Technology*. Ann Arbor Science, Ann Arbor, MI, pp. 207–231.

Altman, P. L. and Dittmer D. S. (1974). *Biological Data Book*, Vol. III. Federation of American Societies for Experimental Biology, Bethesda, MD.

Bernstein, D. M., Moss, O., Fleissner, H. and Bretz, R. (1984). A brush feed micronising jet mill powder aerosol generator for producing a wide range of concentrations of respirable particles. In Liu, B. Y. H., Pui, D. Y. H. and Fissan, H. J. (Eds), *Aerosols*. Elsevier, New York, pp. 721–724.

Bretz, R., Hess, R. and Bernstein, D. M. (1984). Aerosol generation from a viscous liquid: characterisation of a medication nebuliser. In Liu B. Y. H., Pui, D. Y. H. and Fissan, H. J. (Eds), *Aerosols*. Elsevier, New York, pp. 717–720.

Buckley, L. A., Jiang, X. Z., Morgan, K. T. and Barrow, C. S. (1984). Respiratory tract lesions induced by sensory irritants at the RD50 concentration. *Toxicol. Appl. Pharmacol.*, **74**, 417–429.

Carpenter, R. L. and Yerkes, K. (1980). Relationship between fluid bed aerosol generator operation and the aerosol produced. *Am. Ind. Hyg. Assoc. J.*, **41**, 888–894.

Clay, M. M., Pavia, D., Newman, S. P., Lennard-Jones, T. and Clarke, S. W. (1983). Assessment of jet nebulisers for lung aerosol therapy. *Lancet*, **ii**, 592–594.

Dahl, A. R. and Lewis, J. L. (1993). Respiratory tract uptake of inhalants and metabolism of xenobiotics. *Annu. Rev. Pharmacol. Toxicol.*, **33**, 383–407.

Doe, J. E. and Tinston, D. J. (1981). Novel chambers for long term inhalation studies. In Leong, K. J. (Ed.), *Inhalation Toxicology and Technology*. Ann Arbor Science, Ann Arbor, MI, pp. 77–88.

Drew, R. T. (Ed.) (1978). *Proceedings of a Workshop on Inhalation Chamber Technology*. Brookhaven National Laboratory, New York. Report No. BNL 51318.

Haber, F. R. (1924). *Funf Vorträge aus den Jahren 1920–1924*. Springer, Berlin.

Hadley, W. H. and Dahl, A. R. (1982). Cytochrome P-450 dependent monooxygenase activity in rat nasal epithelial membranes. *Toxicol. Lett.*, **10**, 417–422.

Hadley, W. H. and Dahl, A. R. (1983). Cytochrome P-450 dependent monooxygenase activity in nasal membranes of six species. *Drug Metab. Dispos.*, **11**, 275–276.

Hext, P. M. and Lock, E. A. (1992). The accumulation and metabolism of 3-trifluoromethylpyridine by rat olfactory and hepatic tissues. *Toxicology*, **72**, 61–75.

Hext, P. M., Gaskell, B. A., Lock, E. A. and Pigott, G. H. (1994). Species differences in the toxicity and metabolism of 3-trifluoromethylpyridine (3-FMP) in olfactory tissue. *Inhal. Toxicol.*, **6** (Suppl.), 366–368.

Hidy, G. M. (1984). *Aerosols—An Industrial and Environmental Science*. Academic Press, Orlando, FL.

Hinds, W. C. (1982). *Aerosol Technology—Properties, Behavior and Measurement of Airborne Particles*. Wiley, New York.

Hook, G. E. R., Gilmore, L. B., Gupta, R. P., Patton, S. E., Jetten, A. M. and Nettesheim, P. (1990). The function of pulmonary Clara cells. In Thomasson, D. G. and Nettesheim, P. (Eds), *Biology, Toxicology and Carcinogenicity of Respiratory Epithelium*. Hemisphere, New York, pp. 38–59.

Hurtt, M. E., Morgan, K. T. and Working, P. K. (1987). Histopathology of acute toxic responses in selected tissues from rats exposed to methyl bromide. *Fundam. Appl. Toxicol.*, **9**, 352–365.

ISO (1995). *Air Quality—Particle Size Fraction Definitions for Health-related Sampling*. ISO Report No. ISO 7708: 1995(E). International Standards Organization, Geneva.

Iwasaki, M., Yoshida, M., Ikeda, T. and Tsuda, S. (1988). Comparison of whole-body versus snout-only exposure in inhalation toxicity of fenthion. *Jpn. J. Vet. Sci.*, **50**, 23–30.

Langard, S. and Nordhagen, A. L. (1980). Small animal inhalation chambers and the significance of dust ingestion from the contaminated coat when exposing rats to zinc chromate. *Acta Pharmacol. Toxicol.*, **46**, 43–46.

Leong, B. K. J. (Ed.) (1981). *Inhalation Toxicology and Technology*. Ann Arbor Science, Ann Arbor, MI.

MacFarland, H. N. (1983). Designs and operational characteristics of inhalation exposure equipment—a review. *Fundam. Appl. Toxicol.*, **3**, 603–613.

Mark D., Vincent J. H., Gibson H. and Witherspoon W. A. (1985) Application of closely graded powders of fused alumina as tests dusts for aerosol studies. *J. Aerosol Sci.*, **16**, 125–131.

Miller, R. R., Letts, R. L., Potts, W. J. and McKenna, M. J. (1988). Improved methodology for generating controlled test atmospheres. *Am. J. Ind. Hyg. Assoc. J.*, **41**, 844–846.

Newman S. P., Pellow P., Clay M., and Clarke S. W. (1985). Evaluation of jet nebulisers for use with gentamycin solutions. *Thorax*, **40**, 671–676.

Raabe, O. G., Yeh H., Newton G. J., Phalen R. F. and Velasquez, D. J. (1977). Deposition of inhaled monodisperse aerosols in small rodents. In Walton W. H. (Ed.), *Inhaled Particles IV*. Pergamon Press, Oxford, pp. 3–21.

Raabe, O. G., Al-Bayati M. A., Teague S. V. and Rasolt A. (1988). Regional deposition of inhaled monodisperse coarse and fine aerosol particles in small laboratory rodents. In Dodgson J., McCallum R. I., Bailey M. R. and Fisher D. R. (Eds), *Inhaled Particles VI*. Pergamon Press, Oxford, pp. 53–63.

Schlesinger, R. B. (1985). Comparative deposition of inhaled aerosols in experimental animals and humans: a review. *J. Toxicol Environ. Health*, **15**, 197–214.

Silver, S. D. (1946). Constant flow gassing chambers: principles influencing design and operation. *J. Lab. Clin. Med.*, **31**, 1153–1161.

Vincent, J. H. (1989). *Aerosol Sampling—Science and Practice*. Wiley, Chichester.

Vincent, J. H. (1995). *Aerosol Science for Industrial Hygienists*. Pergamon Press, Oxford.

Witschi, H. (1997). The story of the man who gave us 'Haber's Law'. *Inhal. Toxicol.*, **9**, 201–209.

Wright B. M. (1950). A new dust feed mechanism. *J. Sci. Instrum.*, **27**, 12–15.

Wright B. M. (1958). A new nebuliser. *Lancet*, **ii**, 24–25.

Chapter 31

Mixed Routes of Exposure

John J. Clary

CONTENTS

INTRODUCTION

Mixed routes of exposure to chemicals are very common in both occupational and environmental settings. While many human exposures are by multiple exposure routes, one route usually predominates. There may be a tendency to think of the predominant route as the only route of major concern. For example, in an occupational setting inhalation exposure may be the primary concern. This leads to the establishment of acceptable workplace exposure levels, i.e. threshold limit values (TLVs) and permitted exposure levels (PELs) by the American Conference of Governmental Industrial Hygienists (ACGIH) and OSHA, respectively. Airborne material, especially vapours, can result in pulmonary, oral and dermal exposure in the workplace. In some cases a skin notation is added to a TLV or PEL due to a concern for severe irritation from the chemical in question. Concern about assessing total exposure is addressed by the ACGIH TLV Committee in some cases where adequate data exist (obtained by the use of biological monitoring). The ACGIH TLV Committee has established a biological exposure index (BEI) for some chemicals where biological monitoring is feasible. Adequate data must exist to use this approach and analytical data may be more difficult to collect, but it is clear that this is the best method to assess total exposure in the workplace.

Environmental exposures are often from several routes of exposure. A toxic material may be in the air and/or drinking water. In addition to oral exposure, dermal exposure is possible if water is used for bathing. If the toxic material is volatile and in the water, heating of the water could result in pulmonary exposure. Although one route of exposure is the major one, the other routes may be a factor in determining both total exposure and metabolite production.

Many regulatory agencies and industries rely on risk assessment in making risk management decisions. Risk assessments usually examine several routes of exposure, each independently, and add the exposures together to define the total exposure and risk. While this approach has limitations, total exposure data usually do not exist in human or animal experiments used in the risk assessment. Many times very conservative default assumptions are used.

Differences in absorption rate and metabolic breakdown by different routes of exposure may result in changes in the metabolite blood level or key tissue, and affect toxicity. The ultimate toxic agent may be formed as a result of metabolism by the liver. Portal circulation following oral exposure will result in the production of metabolites more rapidly than systemic circulation (pulmonary). Distribution to the target organ is also a factor to consider. In addition, species difference in absorption and metabolism may further complicate the issue.

The route of exposure(s) is a factor both in the design of toxicity studies and in the evaluation of a chemical's effect in humans. When testing a chemical for toxicity in animals, the route of primary concern should be the route of exposure(s) during human use. Various factors have to be incorporated into experimental design. If pulmonary exposure is the primary concern, then an inhalation study should be conducted. A whole body exposure study has been used in evaluating many chemicals, but a nose-only exposure might give a better indication of just the effect of pulmonary exposure. Aerosol, vapour or dust exposure in a whole body inhalation exposure will result in test material being deposited on the fur of experimental animals. Dermal and oral exposure (as a result of grooming) may result in a significant exposure under these conditions.

If the oral route is the primary route of concern, then the questions of incorporating the test material in drinking water or feed or using a gavage technique should depend on the most likely human exposure. If the material is a pesticide, in addition to inhalation and dermal workplace exposure, oral exposure, on or in food, is also possible.

The length of exposure period, short time, such as intravenous (instantaneous) or oral (bolus), compared with longer exposures such as in drinking water, inhalation exposure over a 6 h period or continuous dermal exposure, may also be important for the response if multiple routes of exposure are of concern. A workplace exposure could result in both inhalation and dermal exposure. Dermal exposure would most likely continue until the exposed individual changed clothes and washed the affected areas. Absorption and metabolism most likely will proceed at different rates, and this possibly could affect the course and nature of the toxic response.

This chapter will discuss the question of multiple exposure routes in both experimental animals and humans. Multiple routes of exposure could have a significant effect on the toxic response in animal experimentation and in human experience.

MIXED EXPOSURE IN ANIMALS

Inhalation

Nose Only Versus Whole Body

Nose-only inhalation exposure is selected over whole-body exposure many times because of cost or availability of test material or other concerns such as contamination of the chamber by radiolabelled material. Handling of the animals in a nose-only study is more labour intensive and the exposure is more likely to be stressful than a whole-body exposure. In a nose-only exposure no test agent is likely to be found on the fur or skin. Dermal and oral exposures are minimized under these conditions. Grooming in whole-body exposure studies could result in significant ingestion of test materials, especially dusts, mist or aerosol, or by experimental animals or their offspring in multi-generation studies. Oral exposure also results from vapour or particle exposure as a result of being trapped or dissolved in the mucus fluid in the respiratory tract and being removed by the mucociliary escalator and then swallowed.

There have been very few studies that have compared nose-only with whole-body exposure in terms of response. In an inhalation study in mice comparing water aerosol exposure with nose-only or whole-body inhalation, a small increase in maternal toxicity, foetal malformations and variations were observed in the nose-only exposed mice, suggesting that stress of the exposure method was a factor (Tyl *et al.*, 1994).

In a rat inhalation study of respirable chromium, rats were housed in conventional cages or fibre-glass tubes that allowed exposure to the nose only (Langard and Nordhagen, 1980). The rats in conventional cages excreted 8.4 times more faecal and 5.5 times more urinary chromium than the rats in the fibre-glass tubes. This suggests that significant additional exposure is primarily by the oral route (grooming).

An argument for whole-body inhalation exposure in animal experiments may be that this type of inhalation exposure results in some dermal exposure, more like the normal exposure scenario in humans for workplace chemicals (although there may be greater oral exposure due to grooming). For example, it is common for occupationally exposed workers to receive both inhalation and dermal exposure to airborne chemicals during the normal workday if adequate protective measures are lacking.

Oral

In early nutrition experiments to establish nutrient requirements for trace elements and vitamins, the problem of ingestion of the faeces by the rat was an experimental detail that had to be considered to prevent underestimating the requirement. Ingestion of faeces could still be a source of continuous oral exposure if the test agent or its metabolite (given by inhalation or the dermal or oral route) is excreted in the faeces. The resulting total exposure might be higher and the duration of exposure might be a factor in the production of toxic effects no matter what the route of exposure is.

The effect of duration of the exposure can be a factor in the response. This was demonstrated when a 1 week gavage dosing was compared with administration of the same concentration of test chemical in the drinking water for 1 week (La *et al.*, 1996). Formation of DNA adducts and cell proliferation were measured. The gavage dosing resulted in 2–4 times the adduct formation and up to three times the cell proliferation, demonstrating the effect of a bolus dose versus continuous dosing also by the oral route.

Dermal

In dermal studies, exposure by the oral route is possible through grooming. This may be prevented by the use of a collar, placement of the test material on the animal and individual housing. If the test agent is volatile and care is not taken to prevent volatilization, inhalation exposure is possible.

Group Versus Individual Housing

Group housing versus individual housing may be a factor in multiple routes of exposure. Individual housing may be useful in preventing or reducing exposure from a coprophagy, grooming or off-gassings by fur of test materials.

Multiple Routes of Exposure

Toxicity studies, in general, normally use a single route of exposure. This makes the calculation of dose and the interpretation of results easier. Very few studies make an attempt to determine, calculate or estimate the effect of exposure from all routes simultaneously on the toxic response. This is understandable, as the contribution by exposure from other routes is most likely very small in comparison with the main route of exposure.

In a 1983 study, an attempt was made to study the effects of total exposure to shale (inhalation, ingestion and dermal) in hairless mice (Bernfeld and Homberger 1983). The exposure was carried out by mixing the test material (shale) with the bedding for 68 weeks. Five groups of 200 hairless female mice were used: one group on conventional bedding material (dried and ground corncob as a negative control group), one group on processed shale (termed 100% processed shale), one group on a 1:1 mixture of processed shale and conventional bedding material (termed 50% processed shale), one group on a 1:9 mixture of processed shale and conventional bedding material (termed 10% processed shale) and one group on natural shale (termed 100% natural shale). Half of the animals in each group (100 mice) received about 25 μg of lanolin per mouse per week, over approximately 1 in^2 area of the lower back, to simulate possible synergistic effects of ointments or skin lotions applied simultaneously with the shale. The other half received five weekly portions of 0.1 ml of acetone, as a negative control group to the lanolin treatment. The particle size distribution of processed shale ranged from particles of 0.1 μm diameter to a mesh size of 60 or more. About 2% of the weight of the shale consisted of particles of 1 μm or less, about 23% of particles of 10 μm or less and about 36% of particles of 44 μm or less. This suggests that up to approximately 20% was respirable.

A dose-related coat of black powder was observed during the experimental period covering the surface area of the skin of the hairless mice. In addition, visual evidence at necropsy supported an observation that dose-related amounts of shale had been ingested and inhaled as estimated by lung, trachea and larynx colour.

Histopathological evaluation of all sites of abnormal gross appearance and selected sections of skin, large and small intestines, caecum, lungs, trachea and larynx of all animals revealed no deleterious effects due to the exposure of the mice to processed or natural shale. The only major pathological findings were a significant number of lymphomas in all groups, including the controls. The prevalence of lymphoma was unrelated to the bedding materials and a high incidence was found in historical controls.

This study is an example of an investigation of potentially chronic and carcinogenic effects evaluated simultaneously as a result of dermal, ingestion and dust inhalation exposure in a single study.

This study might be criticized today because of good laboratory practice issues and the use of an unacceptable protocol from a regulatory point of view; but it is still a rational attempt to evaluate the combined toxic effects of three routes of exposure. It might be considered today as an interesting screening study. The same approach could be used for screening pigments or other coloured non-volatile materials.

HUMANS

Exposure of humans (occupationally or from environmental sources) is usually mixed, from both the route point of view and perhaps the agents involved. In a single day we are all exposed to environmental airborne chemicals from many ambient sources, low-level contaminants in food and dermal exposure to other chemicals in material we handle. Occupational exposure can also be significant in chemical production and use.

Occupational Exposure

Occupationally exposed workers can have dermal, inhalation and possible oral exposure when working with many chemicals. The evaluation of agricultural workers exposed to pesticides is a good example of mixed exposure from the inhalation, dermal and oral routes. Inhalation and dermal exposure would be expected during normal use. Oral exposure could result from vapour or particles being trapped or dissolved in the mucus fluid in the respiratory tract and being removed by the mucociliary escalator and then swallowed. Ingestion of food from pesticide-treated crops may contain a pesticide residue; or a low level of pesticide may be found in the drinking water.

Dermal exposure to chemicals can result in significant inputs to the total dose in many workplace situations. Dermal exposure may increase in relative importance when airborne occupational exposures are reduced. Dermal exposure normally occurs by one of three pathways: (i) immersion (direct contact with a liquid or solid chemical substance); (ii) deposition of aerosol or vapour and uptake through the skin; or (iii) surface contact (transfer from contaminated surfaces such as clothes).

Even the eye may be an important route of exposure for some chemicals such as nerve agents. Airborne nerve agents, in addition to pulmonary exposure, have been reported to penetrate the conjunctiva rapidly and stimulate the muscarinc receptors. Individuals exposed to nerve gas (such as the sarin released in the Tokyo subway) experience lacrimation and rapid miosis. Miosis is not normally seen or is delayed following dermal exposure (Holstege *et al.*, 1997).

The most common method for the measuring exposure in occupationally exposed workers is the air level of the chemical in question. The occupational exposure limits most commonly used are the TLV and PEL, which are normally based on air levels. Biological monitoring, where possible, is recommended as the most precise means of estimating the total absorbed dose of a chemical or pesticide by multiple routes. Dermal exposure is difficult to measure routinely, but estimates can be derived for the measurement of dermal exposure. Personal air sampling is the preferred method for the measurement of inhalation exposure, including the measurement of the respirable fraction and/or any vapour component of a chemical. Airborne exposure monitoring conducted simultaneously with biological monitoring is useful in determining the sources of exposure. If biological monitoring indicates a much greater exposure than predicted by just airborne exposure, then dermal exposure or even dietary exposure may be a problem.

Environmental Exposure

Inhalation, dermal and oral exposure are all potential routes of exposure in the environment. Environmental exposures are often mixed. The sources of the exposure are more varied than that found in the workplace. Inhalation exposure can come from factory emissions, incineration, spills of volatile chemicals, volatilization from bodies of water and automobile exhaust, to name only a few. Dermal exposure can come from the air, water, soil and direct contact. Oral exposure can come from food, soil and water. All these exposures may be occurring at the same time and contributing to the total exposure of the individual.

An example of this multiple exposure is a study concerned with the risks to humans and wildlife posed by dioxin-contaminated soil (Paustenbach, 1989). Exposure was by dermal contact (soil), inhalation (dust) and ingestion (soil by children and food and water by adults). Environmental exposure to plants, fish, birds, wildlife and grazing livestock can result in contamination of food in addition to potential toxic effects to these environmental species. Other factors that influenced the exposure were absorption by the various routes, bioaccumulation (soil–wildlife, fish food chain, soil sampling, residential vs industrial sites), uptake by plants, run-off, biological half-life, leaching into ground water, weather and others.

Other Exposures

Multiple exposure may occur from other sources such as cosmetics, food and drugs. The use of cosmetics results in primary dermal exposure, but oral exposure may also take place from lipstick. Other cosmetic ingredients may be added to food or be present as a natural component (e.g. lactic acid). Both dermal and oral exposure will occur. Many drugs may be administered by several routes. The rate of absorption of drugs may be a key factor in determining the route(s) selected by a physician. Ideally, the correct concentration of a drug or active ingredient at the target site is desired. Differences in absorption, distribution and metabolism considerations could lead to multiple routes of administration (exposure) in some cases.

Biological Markers of Exposure

Biological monitoring uses primarily human data and animal experimentation only indirectly. Biological monitoring may be used as an identification of total exposure, a marker of a toxic effect, or a marker of susceptibility to a toxic agent. The biological marker can be the chemical itself or a metabolite. It can be measured in human blood, urine, hair, fingernails or other biological fluid or samples. Depending on the nature of the biological marker, either short- or long-term exposure may be estimated. Currently the ACGIH TLV Committee has set acceptable BEI values based on biological monitoring for approximately 35 chemicals found in the workplace (American Conference of Governmental Industrial Hygienists, 1994). These values are established by determining the level of the biological marker in individuals exposed just to inhalation exposure of the chemical of concern. The use of biological markers allows total exposure from all routes to be compared with inhalation-only exposure.

Blood lead is a good example of biological monitoring, measuring total exposure from inhalation and ingestion in a workplace situation. Inorganic blood lead has been used as background for occupational exposure limits for lead (Skerfving, 1993). A two-compartment model is used to describe lead metabolism. There is a rapid compartment (reflecting soft tissues), with a lead half-time of about 1 month, and a slow lead half-time (reflecting the bone lead pool), with a half-time of approximately a decade. There are significant interindividual variations in lead metabolism. The whole-blood lead level is useful for biological monitoring for recent absorption. The relationship between exposure and blood lead concentration is curvilinear, with a decreasing impact of rising exposure. Blood lead level may be affected by the slow release of lead from the bone lead pool. The average blood lead level in individuals exposed only to 'background' lead exposure varies considerably. Blood lead levels in workers are roughly related to air lead levels in the workplace. These air levels may underestimate exposure as they do not take into account additional exposure from other routes through food, drink and tobacco. Total exposure can be estimated by biological monitoring.

Biomarkers based on metabolites have also been used. For example, benzene exposure results in muconic acid in urine, resulting from the ring opening of a benzene metabolite. *S*-Phenylcysteine resulting from the addition of benzene oxide to a cysteine sulphydryl group in albumin and in haemoglobin is another biomarker for benzene exposure (Bechtold and Henderson, 1993).

Biological monitoring can be used as an estimate of the absorbed dose of a chemical, especially if animal and human metabolism and pharmacokinetic data are available. An example of this approach is a study of atrazine applicators (Lucas *et al.*, 1993). Enzyme-linked immunosorbent assays (ELISAs) were used to detect atrazine and its metabolites in the urine. The primary urinary metabolite was the mercapturic acid conjugate of atrazine. This study demonstrated a correlation between cumulative dermal and inhalation exposure and total atrazine equivalents excreted over a 10 day period.

Most biomarkers are correlated with air concentrations. Once this correlation has been established it can be used to determine the different sources of exposure and the amount that each route of exposure contributes to the total exposure. Air concentrations and biological monitoring have been used to evaluate the exposure of occupationally exposed factory workers to the solvent methylene chloride (Ghittori *et al.*, 1993). The air concentrations were determined by personal passive dosimeters. The biological monitoring of workers was performed by determining the concentration of carbon monoxide in alveolar air and methylene chloride in urine. A correlation between the methylene chloride concentration in air and the carbon monoxide concentration in alveolar air was found when workers who smoked were removed from the analysis. Smokers who worked with methylene chloride had elevated carbon monoxide levels compared with non-smoking workers, thus demonstrating the impact of smoking as another source of exposure that elevates carbon monoxide levels. In this case, a significant linear correlation was found between the air concentration of methylene chloride in the breathing zone and the methylene chloride concentration in urine.

RISK ASSESSMENT

Risk assessment is widely used to make risk management decisions. All sources of exposure are considered in risk assessment. Exposure results in potential inhalation, dermal and oral exposure if the chemical of concern is airborne and respirable. In addition to direct inhalation and dermal exposure, airborne fallout can enter the water supply and be deposited on growing food crops, resulting in additional dermal and oral exposure. Leachate from landfill or contamination of surface water from surface run-off or airborne deposition can result in contamination of the water used for drinking and personal hygiene.

In most cases, risk assessment is based on data from each source that come from different experiments and possibly different species. Physiologically based pharmacokinetic (PBPK) modelling is used to integrate all exposures and other factors such as absorption, distribution, metabolism and elimination by the different routes and also species difference (Medinsky and Klaassen, 1996). PBPK modelling can be used to examine toxicity resulting from separate exposure routes and the influence of the time separating two routes of chemical exposure. PBPK modelling provides a basis for extrapolation across species, routes and doses and is a useful tool for risk assessment.

Risk assessment as practised has built-in conservative default assumptions such as water consumption, absorption by various routes and animal to human extrapolation. The resulting risk assessment is most likely predicting a risk greater than the real risk because of the conservative approach used. This in itself is acceptable, but determining the actual risk would require that a realistic exposure scenario is established and the effect on the total toxic response is determined. Any synergistic or inhibiting effects of one route versus another should also be determined.

Many of these exposure estimates are derived from modelling. For example, a modelling approach has been used to demonstrate the effects of gasoline-contaminated drinking water (Shehata, 1985). The model estimated ambient and indoor air quality from volatilization from drinking water. Oral and dermal burdens were estimated using benzene, toluene and xylene as surrogates for gasoline. Exposure to vapours during showering in the confined area of a bathroom was estimated to be possibly high enough to cause acute mucous irritation. While this type of information is useful for risk assessment, it is based on exposure modelling of several routes of exposure and not actual data. The use of risk assessment is widespread and these types of exposure estimates from multi-route exposure can be a source of concern. Exposure assessments can have a large impact on the risk assessment process. More sound experimental data in both animal and humans are needed to evaluate how good these estimates really are.

Another example of modelling is illustrated by an assessment of total exposure from trichloroethane (TCA)-contaminated water during showering (Byard, 1989). Exposure from three sources and two routes was estimated (inhalation, dermal water and dermal vapour). It is interesting that in this assessment, the predicted exposures during showering by the inhalation and dermal water routes were similar. The exposure to the skin by dermal vapour exposure was estimated to be 1% of the inhalation or dermal water dose.

SUMMARY

While risk management decisions are based on risk assessments that estimate total exposure from all sources, the design of toxicological experiments in animals is usually route specific. **Figure 1** illustrates a hypothetical case where multiple exposure data from both animal and humans are used to model exposure and carry out a risk assessment. A comparison of acute lethal doses by different routes points out how the difference in the route of exposure can affect the toxic response. There are very few cases where experiments in animals were designed to assess total exposure from several routes such as may be found in the human experience and derived from risk assessment. Thought should be given to conducting mixed exposure studies in animals to evaluate how predictive the PBPK and risk assessment modelling are in estimating the actual response.

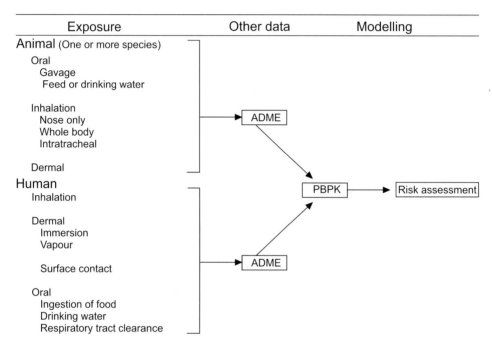

Figure 1 Multiple exposures and risk assessment. ADME = adsorption, distribution metabolism and excretion; PBPK = physiologically based pharmacokinetics.

REFERENCES

American Conference of Governmental Industrial Hygienists (ACGIH) (1994). *The Threshold Limit Values and Biological Exposure Limits*. (ACGIH, Cincinnati, OH).

Bechtold, W. E. and Henderson, R. F. (1993). Biomarkers of human exposure to benzene. *J. Toxicol. Environ. Health*, **40**, 377–386.

Bernfeld, P. and Homberger, F. (1983). Total exposure of mice to powdered test substance (e.g., shale). *Prog. Exp. Tumor Res.*, **26**, 110–127.

Byard, J. L. (1989). Hazard assessment of 1,1,1-trichloroethane in ground water. In Paustenbach, D. J. (Ed.), *The Risk Assessment of Environmental and Human Health Hazards: a Textbook of Case Studies*. Wiley, New York, pp. 331–344.

Ghittori, S., Marraccini, P., Franco, G. and Imbriani, M. (1993). Methylene chloride exposure in industrial workers. *Am. Ind. Hyg. Assoc. J.*, **54**, 27–31.

Holstege, G. P., Kirk, M. and Sidell, F. R. (1997). Chemical warfare nerve agent poisoning. *Med. Toxicol.*, **13**, 923–933.

La, D. K., Schoonhoven, R., Ito, N. and Swenberg, J. A. (1996). The effect of exposure route on DNA adduct formation and cellular proliferation by 1,2,3-trichloropropane. *Toxicol. Appl. Pharmacol.*, **140**, 108–144.

Langard, S. and Nordhagen, A. L. (1980). Small animal inhalation chambers and the significance of dust ingestion from the contaminated coats when exposing rats to zinc chromate. *Acta Pharmacol. Toxicol.*, **46**, 43–46.

Lucas, A. D., Jones, A. D., Goodrow, M. H., Saiz, S. G., Blewett, C. Seiber, J. N. and Hammock, B. D. (1993). Determination of atrazine metabolites in human urine: development of a biomarker of exposure. *Chem. Res. Toxicol.*, **6**, 107–116.

Medinsky, M. A. and Klaassen, C. D. (1996). Toxicokinetics In Klaassen, C. D. (Ed.), *Casarett & Doull's Toxicology. The Basic Science of Poisons*, 5th edn. McGraw-Hill, New York, pp. 187–198.

Paustenbach, D. J. (1989). A survey of health risk assessment. In Paustenbach, D. J. (Ed.), *The Risk Assessment of Environmental and Human Health Hazards: a Textbook of Case Studies*. Wiley, New York, pp. 27–124.

Shehata, A. T. (1985) A multi-route exposure assessment of chemically contaminated drinking water. *Toxicol. Ind. Health*, **1**, 277–298.

Skerfving, S. (1993). Inorganic lead. *Arbete och Halsa*, **1**, 125–238.

Tyl, R. W., Ballantyne, B., Fisher, L. C., Fait, D. L., Savine, T. A., Pritts, I. M. and Dodd, D. E. (1994). Evaluation of exposure to water aerosol or air by nose only or whole-body inhalation procedures for CD-1 mice in developmental toxicity studies. *Fundam. Appl. Toxicol.*, **23**, 251–260.

INDICES

SUBJECT INDEX

This Index contains topics, biological terms and normal endogenous biological materials.

A

A1, and apoptosis 193

A431 human epidermal cell line 413

A-esterase activity, birds and mammals 1334

Aα-fibres 612

A/D ratio *see* adult/developmental toxicity ratio

AAALAC *see* Association for Assessment and Accreditation of Laboratory Animal Care International

AALAS *see* American Association for Laboratory Animal Science

abdominal aorta 357

abdominal skin, percutaneous absorption *in vitro* studies 580

abdominal vena cava, for large blood samples 386

aberrant splicing 226

abortion
  in laboratory workers 510
  in pigs 2145
  spontaneous 1038, 1203, 1204, 1205, 1464, 1465, 1530

ABR *see* auditory brainstem responses

abridged application procedure, EU 1629

abscess, sterile 530

absorbed dose 9, 18, 1772

absorption 17, 67, 68–70
  dose-dependent kinetics and 83
  estimation 523
  extent 69–70, 76
  factor (AF) 1765–6
  half-life 69
  mechanisms 547–9
  in multiple route exposure 606, 607
  rate 69, 75–6
    constant 69, 75, 146
    organic solvents 2029
  saturation 1620

toxins 604
uptake models 1460

abstract publishing 1940

abuse of drugs *see* drug abusers; drugs of misuse

accelerators, rubber industry 2014, 2016

acceptable daily intake (ADI)
  determining 1646
  dietary components 1984, 2065
  food chemicals 1560, 1603, 1656
  MRLs 1643
  pesticides 1611, 1993
  plant protection products 1605, 1609
  repeated exposure studies 57, 60
  risk assessment 1574
  as safe dose in humans 91
  study design 322
  veterinary drugs 1635

acceptable operator exposure level (AOEL) 322, 1605, 1608, 1609

accident conditions 1450

accidental exposure, to PCBs 642

accreditation processes 1452, 1491

accumulation, biomonitoring 1485

acetaldehyde breakdown, herbicides 2006

acetate, as biomarker 1862

acetyl coenzyme A 108, 273

acetylation 18, 98, 108–9, 115, 285, 564

acetylator status 28, 108, 111, 119, 120, 461, 1549, 1850

acetylcholine 6, 365, 429, 430, 546-7, 632, 808, 812, 823, 1256, 1257

acetylcholinesterase 368,
  cardiac toxicity 824

acetylcholinesterase
  antidotal studies 426, 429–30
  biomarkers 1461, 1462, 1848, 1866–7, 1906
  clinical chemistry 368
  inhibition 12, 950–5, 1242–3, 1510, 2091

reactivation 430

N-acetylcysteine conjugate 107

N-acetylglucosamine, and apoptosis 183

N-acetyl-β-D-glucosaminidase (NAG) 356, 363, 678, 1462, 1862

acetyltransferases 108, 272-3
  O-acetyltransferase 109, 273
  N-acetyltransferase (NAT) 108, 109, 111–12, 216, 1457, 1891–2

ACGIH *see* American Conference of Governmental and Industrial Hygienists

achlorhydria, nitrite formation 2120, 2122

acid(s)
  –base reactions 1366
  absorption 69
  neutral drug screen (ANS) 1502, 1503–4
  phosphatase 343, 345, 1495
  precipitation 1365, 1366, 1371, 1376–81

acidification, and aluminium mobilization 1379

acidity regulators 1984–5

acidophilic bodies 175

acinar cells 546, 895–7, 2018

aconitase, inhibition 6

aconitidase 644

Aconitum napellus see monkshood

Acorn nebulizer 595

acoustic distortion product (ADP) 781, 806–7

acoustic startle response 654, *655, 656,* 661

acquired behaviour 658

acquired immunodeficiency syndrome *see* AIDS

acrodermatitis enteropathica, zinc deficiency syndrome 1565

acroosteolysis, in plastics industry 2019

acrosome 338

actin 160, 195, 776, 782, 894

actin-binding proteins, as calpain substrate 189–90
actinic elastosis 836
α-actinin 894
actinomyces 562
actinomyosin 939
actinomyosin adenosinetri-phosphatase 818, 950
activated partial thromboplastin time 361, 389
activation *see* enzymes
activators, rubber industry 2014, 2016
active energy dependent transport 547
'active metabolites' 870–2
active oxygen species 240
active transport 548
actual received dose 149
actuarial tables 1749
acute dermal toxicity *see* skin
acute dietary testing, LC$_{50}$ 1344–5
acute exposure *see* acute toxicity studies
acute lethality testing 35
acute myeloid leukaemia, oncogene activation 1457
acute overdose, commonly encoutered substances 1496
acute phase proteins 367
acute reference dose (ARfD) 1603, 1609, 1993
acute renal failure 685
acute toxicity studies
    advantages 55–6
    animal species choice 325
    animal welfare 493
    classification 5
    data interpretation 327–8, 331–2
    definitions 34–5, 1446, 1772
    dermal *see* skin
    development of assessment 35–8
    dose level selection 325–6
    factors affecting 45
    factors affecting metabolism and toxicity *326*
    Good Laboratory Practice (GLP) 440
    inhalation 46, 327
    intepretation 1337–8
    interspecies extrapolation 1447
    LD$_{50}$ values 13, 16, 39, 326, 425, 1593
    lethal injury to heart 821
    long-term effects 55

metabolic consequences *325*
new substances 1591, 1622
non-rodent 44–5
oral tests *324*, 326–7, 1329, 1343–4
parameters studies 39–40
parenteral 47
pesticides 1609
pharmaceuticals 1616
principles and procedures 38–50
protocol design 40–2, 325–8
rationale, design and use 1331–4
refinement 495–9
replacement 499
screening 35
statistical design 495
testing for effects 33–54
wildlife toxicology 1329–34
acyl-CoA:amino acid *N*-acyltransferases *216*
adaptation, rate 651
adaptive DNA repair pathway 1023–4
adaptive enzyme induction 6
adder, common (*Vipera berus*) 2181
addictive behaviours, management 1444
addictive substances 1151, 1443
addition reactions 613
additive effects 20, 50, 1416, 1787
    see also mixtures of chemicals
additives *see under* food; plastics; rubber
adducts 161–2, 1026–7, 1636
    see also macromolecular adducts
adenohypophysis 372, 980–1
adenoma, biomarker 1856
adenosine 806
adenosine diphosphate (ADP), and apoptosis 191, 192
adenosine monophosphate *see* cyclic adenosine monophosphate
adenosine triphosphatase (ATPase) 341, 343, 366, 631, 642
    actinomyosin 818
    Ca^{2+} 156, 806, 809
    Mg^{2+} 341
    Na$^+$/K$^+$ *see* sodium/potassium
    ouabain-sensitive 812
adenosine triphosphate (ATP)
    and apoptosis 185
    cardiac toxicology 806–7
    clinical chemistry 366
    depletion 190

hepatotoxicity 868
levels, as biomarker 1848
neurotoxicity 631, 642
pathology 341, 343
pulmonary toxicology 185, 722
reduced synthesis 681
skeletal muscle toxicity 938
sulphation 105
synthesis 127
weigh-master role 166
S-adenosylmethionine 109
adenovirus, and apoptosis 194
adenylate cyclase 779, 785, 819, 820, 982
adenylate kinase 357
adhesion molecules 168, 189–90
adhesions 532
adhesives 1295
ADI *see* acceptable daily intake
adipose tissue 810–11
    accumulates pesticide residues 1343
    adrenal hormone action 370
    biomarker 1589, 1858
    biomonitoring 1844, 1905, 1906
    dioxin levels 88
    distribution in 70, 71
    interspecies 88
    nitrate and nitrite levels 2116, 2117
    organic solvents 2038
    PBPK studies 89–90, 144
    PCBs 810–11
    PCBs in 642
    pharmacokinetic analysis 284
    as protective against dioxin 283–4
    as storage site 17
    styrene levels 2020
ADME (absorption/distribution/metabolism/excretion) studies 67–8
Administration of Radioactive Substances Advisory Committee 466
administration route
    see also exposure route
    drug(s) 21
    synthetic materials 1739
    toxicants 1504
    in toxicity testing 1616, 1622
ADP *see* acoustic distortion product; adenosine diphosphate
adrenal cortex 179, 346, 984–6

adrenal gland
  clinical chemistry 370
  drug toxicity *369*
  hypertrophy, nitrites 2135, 2136–7
  in vitro test *418*
  radiation-induced changes 1691
  susceptibility to drug-induced lesions 369
  tumours in plastics industry 2022
  weight 346
adrenal medulla *986*
adrenaline (epinephrine) 262, 547, 808, 2184
α-adrenergic receptors 808, 813
β-adrenergic receptors 808, 813, 896
adrenocorticotrophic hormone (ACTH) 369–70, 980
adsorption on storage 1909
adult respiratory distress syndrome (ARDS) 732, 2179–80
adult/developmental toxicity (A/D) ratio 1187–8
adverse effects 21–2, 34
  acute toxicity studies 38
  biomarker 1842
  definition 4, 34, 1394
  distasters 1427, 1437, 1450
  factors affecting 21–2
  from fires 1924–5
  human studies 456
  predictability 1438
  risk assessment 1754
  and safety of medicine 1426, 1429
  synthetic materials 1738, 1739, 1740
  types 21
advisory committees (UK) 1578, 1594, 1595, 1637
aerial spraying 1339, 1341, 1355, 1727
aerodynamic diameter formula 590
aerosols
  aerodynamic size distribution 598
  chemical 315
  concentration 598
  deposition mechanisms 588, 590
  dose–response assessment 1762
  electrostatic charge 592
  environmental 599
  exposure 603
  eye irritation tests 740

generation from liquids 594–5
generation from solids 596–7
generator diagrams *596*
inhalational toxicity 590–2
mixtures 315–16
particle size 16, 595
particulate sampler *598*
physics 588
repeated exposure studies 60
respiratory tract potency *625*
skin deposition 605
spectrometry 599
toxicity 46
toxicity testing 316
water inhalation study 604
aerospace workers and idiopathic environmental illness 1705, 1708–9, 1710
affinity chromatography 372, 2152, 2153
affinity constant 84
Afghanistan, chemical warfare 2080
aflatoxicosis 1994
African scorpions 640
African swine fever virus, and apoptosis 194
agarose gel electrophoresis 187, *188*
agave (*Agave lecheguilla*) 1519, 1523
Agave lechaguilla see agave
age effects
  and clearance 84
  drug safety 1439
  on metabolism 115, 1417
  on microbial metabolism 572
  PBPK modelling 89
  on radiation toxicology 1683, 1692, 1693
  and response to toxic agents 15, 21, 1416, 1417
  steady state concentration and 83
ageing, role of genetic mutations in 1037
Agelaius phoeniceus see blackbird, red-winged
Agelenopsis see spiders
Agency for Toxic Substances and Disease Registry (USA) 669, 1749
agonal signs 41
agonosis 43
agoraphobia, toxic 1709

agranulocytosis 394–5, 1426, 1427
Agreement on Sanitary and Phytosanitary Measures (WTO) 1569, 1649
Agreement on Technical Barriers to Trade (WTO) 1569
Agricola, Georgius 1474
agricultural biotechnology 1454, 1459
agricultural chemicals
  see also herbicides; insecticides; pesticides *and Chemical Index*
  cartilage and bone toxicity 965
  combustion products 1919
  human studies 453
  industry 438
  pharmacogenetics 215
  plant-protection products 1548
  regulatory aspects 1548, 1960
  reproductive toxicity 1143
  and wildlife toxicology 1328, 1343, 1347
Agricultural Chemicals Regulation Law (Japan) 37
Agricultural Compound Unit (New Zealand) 1611
agricultural effluents 1340, 1343, 1351, 1354–5, 1514
Agricultural Pests Control Act 1927 (Canada) 1600
agricultural soils 1377, 1383
agricultural waste, disposal 2114
agricultural workers
  pesticide exposure 605, 1548, 1993
  reproductive risks 463
  risks of death 1825, 1830
agrochemicals *see* agricultural chemicals; pesticides
Agrostemma gigatho see corn cockle
AHH *see* arylhydrocarbon hydroxylase
AhR *see* aromatic hydrocarbon receptor
α-AIB *see* α-aminoisobutyric acid
AIDS 229, 1003–4
air
  see also indoor air
  expired *see* breath
  filtration 488, 512, 514
  patterns of exposure to 603
air conditioning systems *see* heating, ventilation and air conditioning systems
air jet mills 597

American Academy of Forensic
Sciences 1491
American Antivivisection Society
486
American Association for the
Accreditation of Laboratory
Animal Care 487
American Association of Clinical
Chemists 1491
American Association for
Laboratory Animal Science 492
American Association of Poison
Control Centers 459
American Association of Poisons
Control Centers, National Data
Collection System 38
American Board of Forensic
Toxicology (ABFT) 1489, 1491
American College of Toxicology
493
American Conference of
Governmental Industrial
Hygienists (ACGIH)
  behavioural toxicity studies 668
  biological monitoring 1485,
    1910
  mixed route of exposure 603,
    606
  occupational toxicity studies
    1458, 1475, 1477
  origins 1482
  peripheral sensory iritation
    studies 625
  threshold limit values 1483,
    1594
American Crop Protection
Association (ACPA) 1602
American Medical Association
(AMA) *402*, 486
American National Standards
Institute (ANSI) 1458, 1662
American Society for Testing and
Materials (ASTM), and wildlife
toxicology 1328
American Veterinary Medical
Association 487, 497
Ames test 279, *403*, 499, 565, 567,
1045–6, 1383, 1434, 1448, 1479,
1756
  see also mutation tests;
    Salmonella triphimurium
amidases, hydrolysis 105
amide hydrolysis 105
amine group oxidation 102
amine oxidase (AO) 238–9

amino acid transferase 372
amino acids
  as biomarker 1849, 1861
  conjugation 98, 109
  metabolism 105, 568
  modification 159
  necessary for bone growth 971–2
  substitution 231
  transport system *681*
aminoaciduria 679, 1862
γ-aminobutyric (GABA) receptors
  632, 634, *641*, 651, 1244
γ-aminobutyric (GABA) synapse
  640
aminoglycoside nephrotoxicity
  cascade *687*
α-aminoisobutyric acid (α-AIB)
  1255, 1256
δ-aminolaevulinic acid (ALA)
  392, 1343, 1461
δ-aminolaevulinic acid dehydrase
  (ALAD)
  as biomarker 1848, 1864, 1867
  biomonitoring 1906
  haematotoxicity 392
  lead inhibition 1345, 2056
  nephrotoxicity 683
  wildlife toxicity 1344
δ-aminolaevulinic acid synthetase,
  as biomarker 1863–4
aminophospholipid translocase, and
  apoptosis 183
ammoniation of cereals 2147, 2153
amnesia, predictability in animal
  tests 1438
amphibians 111, 178, 1327, 1330,
  1353
amphiphilic agents 730, 945
Amsinkia intermedia see fiddleneck
amylase *356*, 365, 547, 572, 897
amyloid 296, 367
amyloidosis 943
amyotrophic lateral sclerosis (ALS)
  239, 636
Anabaena, blue–green algae toxicity
  1516
anaemia
  and arsenic 2051
  and benzene 100
  clinical chemistry 366
  erythropoietin therapy 1971
  and fungicides 2003
  haematotoxicity studies 389, 390
  and lead 2056
  megaloblastic 389–90, 391

microcytic 389–90, 391
  and organic solvents 2037
  parenteral toxicity studies 535
  pernicious 562, 1125
anaemic hypoxia, from fires 1920,
  1921
anaerobic bacteria, in large intestine
  562–3
anaerobic cabinets 563
anaerobic pyrolysis 1916
anaesthesia/anaesthetic agents
  for blood sampling 386–7
  cardiac toxicity 817–18
  clinical chemistry 357, 362
  forensic analysis 1491, 1495
  inhalation *498*, 2030
  for injections 527
  local 522, 741, 816, 817, 946–7,
    955–6
  neurotoxicity 641
  occupational exposures 1463
  pancreatic toxicity 898
  potency 2030
  regulatory aspects 1548
  reproductive toxicity 1145, 1156,
    1465
  as sign of toxicity 40, 41
  and spontaneous abortion 1464
analgesia/analgesics 40, 41, 219,
  386, 460, 536
analysis of variance (ANOVA)
  1177
  see also statistical analysis
analytical chemistry 1941–2
analytical measures of exposure
  1461
analytical methods 358, 1446–7,
  1646–7
anaphylactoid reactions
  adverse drug reaction 1427,
    1438
  food additives and 1986–7
  insect stings and 2183
  laboratory occupational hazard
    511
  parenteral toxicity 522, 535
  regulations 1549
Anas americana see wigeon,
  American
Anas platyrhynchos see mallard
Anas rubripes see black duck
anatomical site concentration
  differences 1495
Androctonus see scorpion
androgen 984, 1394–5, 1400, 1403

androgen receptor (AR) 689, 983–4
androgen receptor antagonists 1328
androgenic binding protein 372
androgenic hormone-related
  processes 1401
anemone, Bermuda 820
Anemonia sulcata 820
aneuploidy 1081, 1141
angina 394, 460, 527, 805, 822
angio-oedema, LAA 512
angiogenesis 282
angiography 756
angiosarcoma, and vinyl chloride
  1771
angiotensin 675, 684
aniline 4-hydroxylase 217
animal carcinogenesis, and human
  risk 1536–9
animal care *see* animal welfare
Animal Cruelty Act 1876 (UK) 486
animal feeds 444, 1514, 1515,
  1518, 1648, 2158–9
  see also cattle, *etc.*
animal grooming, exposure 603,
  604
animal hair, LAA 511
animal housing 489–90, 740
animal husbandry 323–4, 490–1
animal– plant warfare 215
Animal Remedies Act 1956
  (Ireland) 1558
animal rights 36, 485, 493
Animal (Scientific Procedures) Act
  (UK) 36, 1960
animal stings and bites
  cardiotoxicity 2179, 2189, 2190
  neurotoxicity 2179, 2188, 2190
  pancreatic toxicity 2180, 2188
  respiratory toxicity 2179–80,
    2189
  skin damage 2178, 2182, 2183,
    2185, 2187, 2189
animal studies
  see also inter/intraspecies *and*
    also specific types of animals,
    e.g. rat; species; strains
  acute toxicity 38–50, 1741
  antidotal assessment *431*–2
  behaviour, ethological analyses
    653–4
  cardiotoxicity 815
  combustion 1925–6
  comparability of groups 57
  cytogenetic assays 1083, 1086–7

dietary restriction 323
drugs 527, 1430–1
endangered species, biomarker
  1845
endogenous synthesis of nitrates
  2118–19
ethics 1957, 1958, 1959
factors influencing toxicity
  15–16
gastro-intestinal flora 561–4
harmonization 37–8
hazard bioassays 28, 1754–5,
  1763
health status 57
immunotoxicology 1005, 1006–9
intraocular pressure (IOP) values
  749
legal limitations 1591, 1664
long-term 1618–20
methodology 1536
mixed exposure to toxins 604–5
MRLs 1643
multi-generation 604
nitrate/nitrite/*N*-nitroso toxicity
  2123–5, 2135–6
number of animals needed 25
pancreatic cancer 922–6
particulates ingestion 1772
of pharmaceuticals 1616
placental toxicity 1243, 1247–8,
  1250–4
protocol design 22–5, 40–2,
  1964
Redbook protocols 1635, 1659
reduction/replacement 52, 53,
  148, 402, 499–500, 1622
repeated exposure protocols 57
reproductive toxicity 1137–40,
  1142–3
research programmes 1940, 1941
safe dose 91
skin irritation tests 832, 843–4
skin sensitization tests 841–3
species choice 1039, 1314
synthetic materials 1739, 1741,
  1742
teratogenicity 1169–79, 1181–8,
  1189, 1222, 1245–6
tightly specified 1535
toxicity testing 2
use of laboratory animals 402
variables 431
weight gain 323
animal technician, antineoplastic
  drugs exposure 515

animal toxins 820–1, 1444,
  2177–99
animal welfare 485–507
  humane treatment 401
  humane treatment diagram *502*
  information resources 471
  legislation/policy 36, 486–7
  quality assurance 444
  regulations 61, 64, 1734, 1740
  responsibility 500–1
  severe pain or distress signs *497*
Animal Welfare Act 1970 (US) 486
Animal Welfare Act 1995 (US) 487,
  501
Animal Welfare Act (USA) 36, 486,
  1664
anisocytosis 391
ankylosing spondylitis, radiation-
  induced 1692
annular furnace 1926
anogenital distance 1406
Anolis carolinenis see lizard, green
  anole
Anopheles albimanus see mosquito
anophthalmia 758
anorexia 283, 814, 815–16, 1351–2,
  1724
  see also feeding behaviour;
    starvation
anosmia 21
ANOVA *see* analysis of variance;
  statistics
anoxia 785, 1510–11, 1848, 1869
Anser anser see goose, greylag
ANSI *see* American National
  Standards Insitute
antagonistic interactions 20, 50,
  305, 306, *313*, *426*, 1395, 1416
antagonists 33, 35, 126
Antarctica *see* polar regions
anthelmintics 527, 634, 641, 1999
Anthosa 2190
anthrax disease 1726
anthropogenic origins, chemical
  hazard 1328, 1330
anthropogenic pollution 1329, 1370
  see also pollution
anthroposophic medicines 1550
antiabortefacient 1392
antiallergy drugs 262–3
antianginal drugs *220*
antiarrhythmics *219*, 817–18
antibiotic resistance genes 1024–5

antibiotics *522*, 532, 819–20, 1146
  see also specific antibiotics, e.g.
    penicillin (*in Chemical Index*)
  anaphylactic reactions 1549
anticancer drugs 261–2
  and female reproductive disorders
    1465
  and gut microflora 572
  molecular interactions 163
  for phosgene toxicity 2099
  supplies in CB attack 1729
antibodies
  for adduct analysis 1885
  antiCD₃, and apoptosis 188
  antiheroin 942
  anti-latex IgE 510
  antinuclear 682
  as biomarker 1848
  biotinated 338
  for ochratoxin analysis 2158
anticaking agents 1985
anticarcinogens 157
anticholinesterase properties 29,
  429, 636, 1475, 1554, 1996
anticholinesterases
  behavioural effects 1348–9,
    1351, 1352
  and brain cholinesterase levels
    1344
  clinical chemistry 368
  design of studies 328
  differential toxicity 1335
  intermittent exposure 1351
  natural exposure 1351
  as pesticides 1994, 1995–8
  and predation behaviour 1348
  reproductive effects 1352
  safety studies 1444
  secondary toxicity 1341–2
  for snakebites 2181
  sporadic lethality 1328
  wildlife toxicology 1329, 1343
Anticipated Residue Contribution
  1602
anticoagulants 229, 230, 357, 387,
  756, 989, 1345, 1455, 1510–11
antidegradants 2014
antidiuretic hormone *see* arginine
  vasopressin
antidotes 425–51
  additive 433
  antagonism 430
  comparison 432–3
  detoxifying *426*
  direct *426*

dose assessment 432
efficacy 430–3
enzyme-catalysed reaction 428–9
enzyme-poison complex reaction
  429–30
evaluation 1452
experimental assessment 431–2,
  431
forming detoxifying substance
  429
mechanism of action *426*–30
new 426
pharmacological *426*, 430
phenobarbital index 460
prophylactic administration 432
related mechanisms 430
studies 25
synergistic 433
in toxicology laboratory 516
antifertility 523
antifreeze 1510
  see also ethylene glycol *in
    Chemical Index*
antigen-presenting cells (APCs)
  1000
antigenic determinants 338, 997
antigens 549
antimetabolites 261
antimicrobials
  see also antibiotics
  microbiological endpoints 1645
antioxidant(s)
  and apoptosis 191
  biochemistry 127
  as biomarkers 1847, 1867, *1868*
  defence systems 158, 168,
    1867–9
  dietary role 1978–9, 1982–3,
    1984, 1985–6
  function of cells 160
  in IEI 1705
  neurotoxicity 634
  nitrite intake and 2132, 2137
  regulations 1552, 1653
  response element 277
  in rubber industry 2017
antiozonants 2017
antisense oligonucleotides 196
antisera 428
antistatics 2023
antitack agents 2014, 2017
antitoxins, in CB attack 1729
α₁-antitrypsin deficiency 29
Antivenom Index 2177

antivivisection *see* animal rights
ants 2184–5
anuria 40, 41
anus
  mucosal radiation-induced
    changes 1689
  and peroral toxicity 545
anutrient chemicals 216–17
anxiety, in idiopathic environmental
  illness 1708, 1709, 1710,
  1714
AOELs *see* acceptable operator
  exposure levels
aortic anatomy 805
aortic aneurysm, in firefighters
  1928, 1929
AP *see* alkaline phosphatase
AP-1 transcription factor 168
Apaf *see* apoptotic protease
  activating factors
APCs *see* antigen-presenting cells
apical junctions 548
Apidae 2182
aplastic anaemia *389–90*, 1438,
  1634
apnoea 40, 41, 615
APO1, and apoptosis 193
Apocynum spp. *see* dogbane
apolipoproteins 367
apoptogens 197
apoptosis 175–202
  biochemistry 126, 187–90
  definition 175
  distinguishing features 177
  drug- and chemical-induced
    197–200
  from radiation 1690
  genetic regulation 192–7
  induction phase 192
  inhibition 1127–8
  initiation 192
  liver remodelling by 880–1
  molecular and cellular concepts
    157, 163–9
  morphological features 176,
    183–7
  mycotoxins and 2149
  occurrence 178–9
  ototoxicity 792
  and p53 1031
  pathology 338, 340, 344
  pathophysiology 178
  response levels 177–8
apoptotic bodies, formation 183

azo reductase enzymes 564
azo reduction 104
azo structures 1041, 1079, 1090

B

B lymphocytes 341, 998
baboon, sequenced CYP genes *216*
Bacillus anthracis 1726, 1727
Bacillus brevis 2149
background levels of toxins 1781,
  1792, 1893–4
background pathology 295
bacon, nitrate and nitrite levels
  2113
bacteria
    as CB weapon 1726
    as chemical warfare agents *2082*
    foodborne hazard 2145
    for *in vitro* testing 52
    metabolism 72
    Microtox 1319, 1320
    mutagenic 128
    Mutatox 1320
    nitric oxide production 2119
bacterial mutation tests 1041–50,
  1756
bacterial reductases 565
bactericides 34
Bacteroides 562, 563
baculovirus, and apoptosis 195
bad, and apoptosis 193, 194
bak, and apoptosis 193
BAL *see* biomonitoring action levels
balance disorders 787–95
Balb/c 3T3 cells *410*
BALF *see* broncheoalveolar lavage
  fluid
Balkan endemic nephropathy 2154,
  2159
banana 222
bandaging for snakebite area 2180
banded krait 2179
Banisteriopsis caapi 222
banned and restricted substances,
  OECD inititatives 1571
barbiturate-type inducer 113
bark scorpion *see* scorprion
barracuda 2191
barrier cream 511
Bartlett test 300
basal cell carcinomas 837
basal cells 779
basal lamina 340
base-pair transformation 7–8

base-set data requirements 1479,
  1480, 1590–1
basement membrane 383
basic drug screen (BDS) 1500,
  1502, 1504
basic fucsin-picric acid method 343
basilar membrane 776, 778, 780,
  781, 786
basilar papilla 791
basophilic granules 175
basophils 263, 384
Basque separatists 1727
BAT *see* best available technology;
    Biologische Arbeitsstoff-Toleranz-
    Wert
bathmotropic effects 43
bats, susceptibility to pesticides
  1339
battery manufacture workers 668
BAX 168, 191, 194, 197
BAX protein up-regulation, NSAIDs
    and 132
BCF *see* bioconcentration factor
BCL_2 168, 189, 200
bcl-2, and apoptosis 192, 193, 194,
  195, 197, 199
bcl-w, and apoptosis 194
bcl-XL, and apoptosis 191, 193
bcl-Xs, and apoptosis 193
BCL/D1 cells *410*
BEAM *see* brain electrical activity
  mapping
beans
    nitrate and nitrite levels
      2112–13, 2115
    ochratoxin analysis 2158
    toxicity 1983
bedding 58, 356, 512, 514
beef
    ingestion, standard assumptions
      1773, 1775
    nitrate and nitrite levels 2113
beer
    and degreasers' flush 1415
    nitrate, nitrite and NDMA levels
      2113–14, 2115, 2118
    ochratoxin analysis 2158
bees 1646, 1647, 2181
beet (*Beta vulgaris*)
    nephrotoxicity 1522
    nitrate and nitrite levels 2112–13
beetle, grandis 259
behavioural aberrations
    adverse drug reaction 1430
    as biomarker 1846, 1855–61

field studies 1354
from fires 1920, 1921
quantification 1353
wildlife species 1327, 1328,
  1345–7
behavioural approaches, in IEI
  treatment 1714, 1716
behavioural assessments 39, 45,
  657–8
behavioural conditioning, in IEI
  1707–8
behavioural response audiometry
  780
behavioural thermoregulation
  664–5
behavioural toxicity 23
    aggression induction 653
    assessment 650–73
    athletic performance 652
    cognitive tests 656–7
    complex schedules 660–1
    discrimination performance
      661–2
    endocrine disruption 653
    EPA guidelines 665
    EU guidelines 665
    functional observation batteries
      (FOB) *651*
    habituation phenomenon 651
    human testing 666–9
    lead 2056
    motor function 651–3, 654,
      662–4
    naturalistic behaviour 653
    neonatal testing 665–9
    organic solvents 2036, 2041–2
    organophosphates 1997
    reinforcer types 664–5
    risk assessment 670
    safety studies 1443
    schedule-controlled operant
      behaviour *658–9*
    schizophrenia 665
    sensory function 654–6
    sensory testing 661–2
    sexual behaviour 653
    simple schedules 659–60
    tests for children 669
BEI *see* biological exposure indices
Beirut bombing 1721
Belgium, nitrate levels 2112
bench mechanics biomonitoring
  1904
bench-scale extraction experiments
  1777–8

bone marrow (*Contd.*)
nephrotoxicity 675
nitrate toxicity 2125
organic solvent toxicity 2037
peroxidases 103
radiation-induced changes 1685, 1686, 1690
sampling 388
suppression, cytokines for 1971
Bonferroni *t* test 1332
bonito 2193
Boolean operators 479
boomslang (*Dispholidus typus*) 2178
borderline products, regulatory aspects 1553
Borgias 35
Bothotus see under scorpion
Bothrops spp. *see* snakes, crotaline
botulism 428, 549, 633, 640, 1340, 1513, 1726, 1989, 2104
Bouin's stain 336, 345
bound residues, guidelines 1636
bounding information 1766–7, 1786
bowel *see* large intestine
Bowman's membrane *410*
box jellyfish (*Chironex fleckeri*) 2189
Box–Behnken designs 314
bracken fern, toxicity to horses 1519
bradycardia 40, 41, 43, 614, 615, 811, 823, 824
bradykinin, NOS and 2119
bradypnoea 40
Braer disaster 1826–7
brain
biomarkers 1866
cholinesterase 1338, 1343, 1344, 1351, 1354, 1523, 1996
drug damage 103
electrical activity mapping (BEAM) 1713, 1716
enzyme distribution 1857
fog 1709
free radical damage 634
haemorrhage 1217
hypoglycaemia 636
imaging 1707
immersion fixation 347
iron levels 634
ischaemia 636
lead damage 2055–6
mercury concentration 570
morphometry 339

MPTP oxidized 132
NQO2 in 240
organic solvent damage 2029, 2030, 2035, 2036, 2040
perfusion fixation 347
pesticide residues 1343
pharmacogenetics 232
radiation damage 1690–1
tumours 1928, 1929, 2015, 2019, 2132
weight 64, 1856
brainstem, in ALS 239
Branta canadensis see goose, Canada
Brassica spp. *see* broccoli; brussels sprouts; cabbage; kale
Brazil, fumonisin contamination of cereals 2165
BRCA1, as biomarker 1850
bread, contamination 1824, 1825, 2116, 2117
breakfast cereals
see also cereals
fortification 1552
breast
cloned enzymes 242
irradiation 1691, 1693
breast cancer
cyclic induction 266
and dietary fat 1980, 1981
endocrine related 1399
environmental effects 1392, 1399–400
hormone treatment 1392
interspecies variation 278, 279
MCF-7 cells 1402
and organochlorine compounds 1400, 1995
and PCBs 163
in plastics industry 2020, 2021
rarer in Asian women 1398
risk 572
in rubber industry 2015
and selenium 1983
surgery, and fertility cycle 266
tamoxifen treatment 284
breast–ovary cancer genes, biomarker 1850
breast-feeding 1224–7
breath
apparatus in PBPK *146*
biomarker 1845, 1848, 1855, 1867
biomonitoring 1907
elimination in 72

source of cP450-generated metabolism 1865
tests 365
breathing
laboured 497
patterns 262, 1713, 1920
rate *see* respiratory rate
zone 607
breathing apparatus, for firefighters 1938
breeding colonies 357
BRI *see* building-related illness
brine shrimp 414
brine shrimp (*Artemia* spp.) 1187
Brinvilliers, Marquise de 35
British Library 477
British Pharmacopeia 536, 537
British Toxicology Society 326, 425
broccoli
see also kale
nitrate and nitrite levels 2112
broncheoalveolar lavage 704, 722, 729
broncheoalveolar lavage fluid (BALF) 1762
bronchi 20, 46, 262, 343, 510
bronchiolar cells 722, 726, 732
bronchioles, inhalation effects 20
bronchitis 1269–70, 1961
bronchodilators *220*, 262–3, 810
bronchospasm 252
Bronsted acidity 614
broom, toxic ingredients 1552
broomweed (*Gutierrezia microcephala*), reproductive toxicity 1521
Brownian diffusion 591
Brunner's glands 545
brush borders 345, 363, 678, 680, 681, 683, 688, 690
brussels sprouts, nitrate and nitrite levels 2112–13
BS *see* Bloom's Syndrome
BTB *see* blood–testes barrier
bubblers 594
bubonic plague bacteria 1727
buccal
see also oral
absorption 545
cavity 545
microflora 561–2
mucosa, radiation-induced changes 1689

buckwheat (*Fagopyrum esculantum*), photosensitization effects 1523
Buehler technique 841, 1005
Buenos Aires, car bombing 1722
buffers, biomonitoring 1904
bufuralol 1′-hydroxylase 217
building materials 1295, *1296*, 1298, 1304
building-related illness (BRI) 1292
Bulgarian agents and CB weapons 1727
bulking agents 1552, 1653, 1985
bullfrog (*Rana catesbeiana*) 1330–1, 1353
bumblebee 2182
bundle of His 805
Bureau of Biologists (USA) 1973
Bureau of Chemistry (USA) 1534
Bureau of Medical Devices and Diagnostic Products (USA) 1662
burns 833, 1724, 1818, 1916, 1917, 1927, 2087
Bursa of Fabricius 385
Buteo jamaicensis see hawk, red-tailed
Buthidae 2189
Buthus see scorpion
buttercup (*Ranunculus* spp.), toxicity 1518, 1520
butyrylcholinesterase 368, 429, 824, 1730, 1866
butylhydroperoxide, as biomarker 1868
by-products in rubber manufacture 2014
bystander risk *see* occupational risk

C

c-fibres 612, 1705
c-fos 16, 168, 190, 193, 195
c-jun 168, 190, 193, 195
c-myc 167, 189, 193, 196
C-reactive protein (CRP) 366–7
C-S lyase 568
cabbage, nitrate and nitrite levels 2112–13
CAC *see* Codex Alimentarius Commission
cacosmia 1708
CADDY project 1609
cadherin, as calpain substrate 189–90

caecum 521, 545, 556, 605, 1985, 1986, 1987, 1990
Caenorhabditis elegans 177, 190, 194, 1092, 1189
caeruloplasmin binding to copper 2064
caffeine *N*-3 demethylase *217*
caged field trials 1349–50
caging 58, 356, 512, 514
calcineurin, as calpain substrate 190
calcitonin 968
calcium
  –calmodulin–calcineurin signalling 684
  –phosphate balance 1987
  -dependent and papain-like proteases *see* calpains
  adenosine triphosphatase *see* adenenosine triphosphatase, Ca^{2+}
  and apoptosis 187, 188, 189, 192
  as calpain substrate 190
  cardiac toxicology 809, 811, 812
  CO_2 effects 61
  compartmentation changes 167
  dysregulation 198
  extra-skeletal binding 973
  homeostasis 127, 156, 163–4, 1859, 2036, 2059, 2162
  intracellular *164*, 168, 194, 807–8, 813, 982
  and lead uptake 2055
  in outer hair cells, organ of Corti 787
  in pancreatic juice 897
  skeletal muscle toxicology 939
calcium channel(s) 639, 806, 817, 818, 2066
calcium channels blockers 956
calcium phosphate, in tooth enamel 967
calcium pumps 156, 938
calmodulin, interaction with lead 2055
calmodulin-dependent kinase 190
calpain 164, 189, 191, 193
calreticullin induction 168
Calycanthus spp. *see* sweet shrub
CAM *see* chorioallantoic membrane assay
camel, lens 242
Cameroons lake disaster 38, 1817
cAMP *see* cyclic adenosine monophosphate

Canada
  classification and labelling requirements 1477, 1603–4
  food additives regulation 1659
  food contact materials regulation 1659
  nitrite levels 2132
  pesticide regulation 1600, 1601
  risk assessment 1602–3
Canadian Council on Animal Care 486
cancer
  see also carcinogenesis *and individually named organs*
  and acetylation status 112
  and apoptosis 163
  bioassays, dose selection 148
  chemotherapy *see* chemotherapy
  chronotherapy 266
  circadian radiosensitivity 260
  determination of cause 1952
  development stages 1875
  diet and 1980–3
  DNA degradation pattern 187
  endocrine-related 1391
  following Seveso disaster 1818
  genetic aspects 1538, 1847, 1891
  incidence, USA 1787
  potency factors (CPF) 1751, 1764–6, 1771, 1782, 1786
  prevention programmes 1940, 1942
  radiation-induced 1695, 1821
  registration records 1532, 1533
  research history 1944
  risk assessment 148, 1782, 1784, 1790, 1830, 2050
Cancerline 1947
Candida albicans 413
cannibalism in animals 58
CAP *see* compound action potential
capillaries, dermis 829
capsules, dosing procedures 60
car
  see also automobile(s)
  accidents *see* road traffic accidents
  bombs 1722
carbohydrate 115, 1966
carbonating agents 1985
carbonic anhydrase 159, 160
carbonyl reductase 104, *216*, 241, *242*, 243
carboxyhaemoglobin (COHb) 150, 1843, 1920, 1921, 1924, 1927

carboxyhaemoglobinaemia *392*
carboxylators 238
carboxylesterases 105, 1866
carboxylic acid ionophores 821
carcass searches 1354
carcinoembryonic antigen (CEA), as
   biomarker 1849
carcinogen(s)
   see also specific types, e.g.
      aflatoxin (*in Chemical Index*)
   –protein adducts 225
   acceptable risk level 1787, 1788
   added risk 1786
   antagonistic interactions 314
   apoptosis 198
   binding 571
   classification 1537, 1593, 1766
   determining safe exposures 1484
   dose-response assessments 1759,
      1763–5, 1766
   epigenetic 7, 128, 314
   exposure to 225
   in fires 1821
   in food 1981–2
   genotoxic 8
   mixtures 314–15
   naturally occurring 1981
   PBPK modelling 1770
   primary 7
   promoters 314
   risk assessment 1751, 1753,
      1754, 1755
   scaling factors 1769
   synergism 314–15
   synthesis 566–7
   toxicokinetics 85
   trace quantities 1574–6
   ultimate 7
Carcinogen Assessment Group
   (USA) 147
Carcinogen guidelines (EPA) 1766
Carcinogen Potency Database
   (CPDB) 1105, 1111
carcinogenesis/carcinogenicity
   see also genetic carcinogens;
      genetic toxicology; *individually
      named organs*
   acetylaminofluoroene 110
   acrylamide 1455
   as adverse drug reaction 1427
   aflatoxins 1537, 2154
   4-aminobiphenyl 1537
   anabolic steroids 1549
   animal studies 1536–8
   aromatic amines 120

arsenic 1382, 2051
asbestos 1537
benzene 1455, 1537
benzidine 1537, 1587
beryllium 2061
bioassays 2, 336
biochemistry 126
biomarker 1845, 1849–50, 1856,
   1866, 1867, 1875, 1886
biomonitoring 1904–5, 1906–7,
   1911
bis(chloromethyl) ether 1537
cadmium 2053–4
chlorambucil 1537
chlorination byproducts 1383–4
chloroform 1455
chromium 1539, 2062
coal tars 1537
cutaneous 836, 837
cyclophosphamide 1537
definition 7
dichloromethane 1537
dietary factors 58, 1980–1
diethylstilbeostrol 1537
dioxins 87
epidemiology 1537
erionite 1537
erythrosine (FD&C Red 3, E127)
   1553
ethylene oxide 1455
in firefighters 1929
food products 1563
formaldehyde 1455, 1456, 1537
fumonisins 2165
and gastro-intestinal microflora
   561
genetic factors 1027–35,
   1099–101
herbicides 2005
heterocyclic amines 274
hydrazine 1455
initiation 314
interspecies extrapolation 1536
liver enlargement and
   remodelling by 880–1
medical devices 1734, 1735,
   1742
melphalan 1537
methotrexate 1455
methoxsalen + UV-A 1537
mineral oil 1537
multistage model 314
2-naphthylamine 1537
nickel 1537, 1539, 2063

nitrates 1382, 2124, 2130–1,
   2137
nitrites 1383, 2128
nitrobenzene 104
N-nitroso compounds 1383,
   2132
non-genotoxic 1034–5, 1101–2,
   1119–20, 1121
organic solvents 2036, 2037,
   2039
organophosphates 1998
and parenteral toxicity 525–6
phenol 1455
piperidine 1455
plastics industry 2019–23
promotion 314
radiation-induced 1692–3, 1697
radon 1538
rubber industry 2014–19
saccharin 1537, 1553
selenium 2065
shale oils 1537
species differences 59
testing
   alternative tests 64, 401
   guidelines 1434–5
   long-term 356, 1618–19
   new substances 1591,
      1618–19, 1628
   and parenteral toxicity 64,
      401, 521
   repeated-dose 64, 330
   replacement tests 499
   veterinary drugs 1643
tobacco smoke 1537, 1538
transplacental 1207–9
TSG and 1892
urea 1455
vinyl chloride 1417, 1537, 1551
wastes 1827–8
wood dust 1475
carcinoma *see* cancer
Carcinus aestuarii, biomarker 1852
cardiac, *see also* heart
cardiac action potential 805
cardiac anomalies 1465
cardiac arrest 50
cardiac arrhythmias 806, 807, 808,
   810, 814, 816, 823
   acute toxicity 40, 41, 43, 50
   and adverse drug reactions 1427,
      1429, 1430
   and barium 1757
   clinical chemistry 366
   ECG 806

cardiac arrhythmias (*Contd.*)
  and fires 1921, 1923
  and halogenated hydrocarbons
    461, 1505
  and organic solvents 2036, 2037
  and organophosphates 1997
  and terfenadine 125–6
  'torsade de pointes' 824
cardiac chrono-pathology 264
cardiac conduction pathway 343,
  805
cardiac contraction 805–6
cardiac myocytes 807
cardiac myopathy 43, 2064
cardiac output 83, 92, 364, 366
cardiac puncture 357
cardiac stimulants 220
cardiac toxicity *see* cardiotoxicity
cardiac toxicology 803–26
cardiac tumours, in rubber industry
  2015
cardiac weight 343
cardinal, northern (*Cardinalis
  cardinalis*), subacute feeding trials
  1338
Cardinalis cardinalis see cardinal,
  northern
cardiomyopathy 807, 813, 942,
  1430
cardiopathy, selenium deficiency
  2065
cardiotoxic agents 807–16
cardiotoxicity
  adverse drug reactions 1427,
    1438
  animal stings 2179, 2189, 2190
  biochemical basis 806–7
  clinical chemistry 366
  fluoroacetate 6
  mechanisms 816–24
  nitrites 2126
  organophosphates 1998
  pathological basis 807
  pharmacogenetics 240
  signs 40, 43
  terfenadine 38
cardiovascular agents 25, 1439
cardiovascular effects
  collapse 15, 1984
  and drinking water hardness
    1381
  in firefighters 1928–9
  of Gila monster bite 2182
  in vitro test systems *417*

organic solvents 2041
plant toxins 1522
radiation-induced 1691
Seveso disaster 1818–19
cardiovascular system 343
carnitine acyltransferase 1866, 1868
Carolina jessamine (*Gelsemium*
  spp.), neurotoxicity 1520, 1521
carpenter ant 2184
carpet, IEI and 1708
carrier proteins 371
carrion-eating species *see* predatory
  species
carrot, nitrate and nitrite levels
  2112–13
Carson, Rachel 1599
cartilage
  articular 342
  embryology 966
  physiological aspects 968
  radiation-induced changes
    1691–2
  structure and function 966–7
  toxic damage 968–75
cartridge respirators 516
CAS *see* Chemical Abstracts
  Service
cascade impactor 598, *599*
CASE *see* computer-automated
  structure evaluation
case-control studies 1456, 1466,
  1529, 1532–3, 1539, 1755
case-referent studies *see* case-
  control studies
caspases 164–5, 191, 194–5
cassava 900, 918, 920, 1553, 1984
cassia, toxic to domestic animals
  1513
castor oil plant (*Ricinus communis*),
  toxicity 345, 1518, 1519, 1727
cat
  see also domestic animals
  acetaminophen (paracetamol)
    susceptibility 1509
  aflatoxin LD_{50} 2154
  allergenic sebaceous glands 512
  allergens 511–12
  aminophenol hydroxylation 11
  benzoic acid lethality 535
  blood pressure response to
    depressors 535
  chlorate herbicides susceptibility
    1512
  common toxicoses 1510–13

ethylene glycol toxicity 110
food contamination 1825
garbage toxicity 1512
human contact 490
LAA 511
phenol metabolism 111
pyrethrin/pyrethroid toxicity
  1510
stratum corneum skin
  permeability *579*
vomiting reflex 546
cat scratch disease 514
catalase 158, 344, 809, 1866, 1868,
  2161
catalepsy 40, 41
cataract 20, 160, 758, 762–4, 1430,
  1687–8, 2003, 2004
catechol *O*-methyltransferase *216,*
  813
catecholaminergic systems 641, 808
catecholamines 346, 806, 813
catfish 2191
cations
  complexing 1368, 1369
  soil storage 1369
cattle
  see also ruminants
  blue–green algae toxicity 1516
  cornea *410*
  CYP 216
  CYP genes 216
  ginger neuropathy 1824
  lead toxicity 1515
  methionine salt 532
  molybdenum toxicity 1515
  nitrate toxicity 1509, 2123, 2124
  ochratoxin toxicity 2161, 2164
  salt toxicity 1517
  selenium toxicity 1515
  T_3 and T_4 concentration 371
cattle feed, contamination 1554,
  2153
caudal vein lesions 529
cauliflower, nitrate and nitrite levels
  2112–13
causal factors in legal matters 1952
cause of death, inaccuracies on
  death certficates 1529
cause–effect relationship 1354
CB *see* terrorism, chemical and
  biological
CBN *see* contraction band necrosis
CC10 *see* Clara cell protein
CCK *see* cholecystokinin;
  cholecystokinin-pancreozymin

chicken (*Gallus domesticus*)
(*Contd.*)
  and apoptosis 178
  arsenic in feed 1951–2
  biliary excretion 555
  contaminated drinking water
    1340
  eggs 233
  eye tests 751
  fumonisin toxicity 2165
  heterocyclic amines 271
  intravenous injection site 526
  liver 234
  malathion sensitivity 1342
  neurological tests 23
  neurotoxicity 638, 1824
  nitrate and nitrite levels 2113
  ochratoxin toxicity 2160, 2161
  organophosphate studies 1997
  studies 792
chicory, nitrate levels 2113
chief cells 545
child-resistant packaging 1603,
  1604
childhood syndromes, associated
  with tumour suppressor genes
  1032
children
  see also neonates
  air pollution studies 1270–1,
    1273–4
  allergic reaction to insect stings
    2183
  cancer 1464, 1465, 1820
  in clinical trials 1618
  CNS defects from plastics
    industry 2020
  copper toxicity 2064
  drug therapy 1227–9
  exposure assessment 1776, 1782,
    1783
  eye injuries 737
  informed consent 455
  iron levels 2065
  lead toxicity 639, 973, 1205,
    1227, 1769, 2055, 2056, 2057
  mass poisoning 460
  mercuric toxicity 2058, 2059,
    2060
  nitrate levels 2116–17, 2118,
    2122, 2129, 2132, 2133, 2136
  nitrite intakes 2134, 2136
  ochratoxin regulations 2158–9
  over-the-counter (OTC) drugs
    1228–9

passive smoking 1267, 1273
poisoning statistics 38
radiation injury 1691, 1694,
  1695, 1697
risk assessment 1754
screening, biomarkers 1845
selenium deficiency 2065
skin reactivity of 831
snakebites 2178
testing initiative 1587
thyroid cancer 1820
Chile, deliberate food poisoning
  1724
chimeric animals 1964
chimney sweeps, scrotal cancer 2,
  1474
chimpanzee *579*, 1971, 2050
China
  fumonisin contamination of
    cereals 2165
  nitrate levels 2114, 2131
  N-nitroso compounds levels
    2133
Chinese cabbage, nitrate levels
  2113
Chinese hamster ovary (CHO) cells
  24, 752, 753
  and apoptosis 196, 198
  cytogenetic assays 1081, 1082,
    1083, 1084, 1434
  β-hexosaminidase *412*
  Hgprt gene 1051, 1053
  mutant UV-1 1023
  and nitrates/nitrites 2124–5,
    2128
  recombinant human
    erythropoietin cloning 1971
  V79 system 1051–3, 1083
Chinese restaurant syndrome 1988
CHIP *see* Chemicals (Hazard
  Identification and Packaging)
  Regulations
chiral factors in metabolism 115
Chironex fleckeri see box jellyfish
chitin synthesis inhibitors 2000
chlor-alkali workers 663
chloracne 284, 838, 1444, 1554,
  1818
chloride channels 641, 764, 897
chloride ion 104
chlorination 1381, 1383–4
chlorine-containing wastes 281
chlorofluorocarbons, natural 1366
chloroquine myopathy 944

chlorzoxazone 6-hydroxylase *217*
choking agents 1724
cholecystokinin (CCK) 880, 897,
  992
cholecystokinin-pancreozymin 895
cholelithiasis 883
cholera 820, 1310
cholestasis 132, 356, 359, 361,
  883–4, 1843, 1849, 1858, 1859,
  1860
cholesterol 370, 823, 860, 862, 938,
  1978
cholesterol ester hydrolase 897
cholesterol lowering agents 946
cholesterol stones 898
cholostrum 549
cholic acid, as biomarker 1858
cholinergic agonists 897
cholinergic cells, damage 642
cholinergic fibres 615
cholinergic muscarinic system,
  radiation-induced changes 1689
cholinergic reflex mechanisms 256
cholinergic symptoms from
  anticholinesterases 1995
cholinergic synapses 6
cholinergics 808
cholinesterase *216*, *356*, 359,
  368–9, 466, 760, 1342, 1485,
  1906
cholinesterase inhibitors 369, 823,
  1337, 1345, 1906, 1996, 2006
Chondodendron toxicity 34
chondritis, radiation 1691
chondrocytes 342
chondrodystrophies 965, 969
chondrogenesis 966, 968
choreiform movements 638
choreoathetosis/salivation (CS)
  syndrome 1244
chorioallantoic membrane *411*, 499,
  752
chorionic gonadotrophin 538
Christison, Robert 1490
chromaffin reaction 346
chromatid damage, biomarker 1848
chromatin 161, 164, 183, 187, 189,
  2054
chromatographic methods
  see also specific methods
  in forensic testing 1497–500
chromodacryorrhoea 40, 41
chromophores 337, 836–7

Committee on Scientific Dishonesty (Denmark) 1958
Committee on Toxicology (USA) 1935
Committee for Veterinary Medicinal Products (CVMP) (EU) 1638, 1639, 1641
common chemical sense 612
Common Sense Initiative, US EPA 1587–8
communication
    amongst peers 1940
    by expert witness 1948
    for risk management 1814, 1829, 1911
communications industries, radiofrequency radiation 1418–19
companion animals *see* domestic animals
comparative toxicology of birds and mammmals 1334–5
    see also extrapolation, inter-species
comparison subjects 1531–2, 1533
compartment syndromes 940
compartment system for distribution 77, 78, 79, 1768
compartmentalization 141
compensation 1716, 1959
Competent Authorities 1557, 1578, 1590, 1591
competitive agonism 305, 626
competitive binding assays 1402
competitive inhibition 305
complete negative correlation 304–5
complete positive correlation 304
complexation reactions 1366
component interaction analysis 305
compound action potential (CAP) 781, 783, 785, 786, 787
compound effect summation 303
Comprehensive Environmental Response, Compensation and Liability Act (USA) 1750
computers and computer-aided systems 39
    programs for fraud 1958
    quantitative structure-activity response (QSAR) models 52, 53
    standard operating procedure (SOP) 448

structure evaluation (CASE) 713, 1103
    in tests 667, 668, 754
concentration–dose addition 304
concentration–effect curve 748
concentration–time curve 1834, 1835
    see also plasma
Concise International Chemical Assessment Documents (CICADs) 1592, 1612
concussion 636
condensation generators 594
Condylactis gigantea see anemone, Bermuda
confidence limits, in PBPK modelling 150
confidentiality of data 1894, 1911, 1957
confocal microscopy 339, 347
    through focusing (CMTF) 748
confounders, multiple 1447
confoundings 1531, 1535
confusion 1758
congenital malformations 510, 1219–22, 1419, 1697, 2041
Conium maculatum see hemlock
conjugation reactions 17, 18, 105–9, 216, 359, 1334
conjunctival chemoreceptors 755
conjunctival damage 605, *741*
conjunctival fibroblasts 757
conjunctival haemorrhage 742
conjunctival hyperaemia 614, 738, *741*–2, 742–*3*
conjunctival redness 622
conjunctivitis 40, 41, 510, 512, 738, 756
connective tissue 343, 530
consent for testing 1957
conservatisms, compounding 1782
constant relative density 1908
constants 1834–5
constipation 40, 2061
construction industry, risk of death 1830
consultations by IEI patients 1712, 1716
Consumer Labelling Initiative (CLI) (US) 1589, 1603
Consumer Product Safety Act (USA) 37, 1589
Consumer Product Safety Commission (CPSC) (USA) 37, *413*, 1589, 1750

consumer products 303, 1550, 1595
Consumer Protection Act (UK) 1550
consumer safety 471
contact dermatitis *see* dermatitis
contact lenses 1667
container closure systems 1603, 1604, 1737
contraceptive steroids, environmental oestrogen effects 1565
contraceptives, regulatory aspects 1548, 1549
contraction band necrosis (CBN) 813–14, 819, 820
contrived field tests 1352
control animals 59, 61, 64–5
Control Limits, Health and Safety Executive (UK) 1594
Control of Pesticides Regulations (UK) 1546
control substances, for validation of endocrine activity screens 1403
Control of Substances Hazardous to Health (COSHH) (UK) 37, 463, 1481, 1594, 1596
Controlled Ecosystem Pollution Experiment (CEPEX) 1318
controlled field studies 1327, 1328
    aquatic toxicology 1318, 1319
controls, in IEI 1705
Convalaria spp. *see* lily-of-the-valley
convulsants 640–1
convulsion *see* seizure
Conway microdiffusion dish *1497*
cooking methods *see* food
Coombs test 391
Cooper Committee, Study Group in Medical Devices 1662
coordination tests 654
copper smelting industry 1246
copperhead 2178
coprophagy prevention 604
coproporphyria 1705, 1864
coproporphyrinogen as biomarker 1864
coral (*Goniopora* spp.) 819, 820
cormorant, double-crested (*Phalacrocorax auritus*) 1329, 1355
corn
    see also cereals
    nitrate and nitrite levels 2112

corn cockle (*Agrostemma gigatho*),
toxicity to food-producing animals
1518
cornea
ALDH3 activity 237
changes 40, 41, 44
chemoreceptors 755
ciliary nerve PSI stimulation 619
dehydration 747
deposits 757
epithelium 741, 746, 751
injury 738, *741*, *745*, 746, 747,
748, 750
isolated tissue tests 751–2
neovascularization 742
oedema 738, 747
opacity 741–2, 745, 748, 751
pathology 347
permeability 741, 746, 753
protein *410*, 752
re-epithelialization 746
revascularization, grading system
742–3
swelling 748
thickness 496, 738, 746, 747–8,
748
transplants, growth factor therapy
1972
ulceration, FDA grading 745
corned beef, nitrate and nitrite levels
2113
coronary arteries 264, 343, 523,
805, 812, 1929, 2126
coronary heart disease (CHD) 1978,
1979–80
coronary thrombosis, diet and 1978
corpus luteum 372
correlation coefficients 89
correlation spectroscopy, biomarkers
1862
corrosion, local effect 19
corrosive effects 1455
corticotrophic releasing hormone
(CRH) *369*
Corydalis spp. *see* fitweed
Corynebacterium diphtheriae 639
COSHH *see* Control of Substances
Hazardous to Health; Control of
Substances Hazardous to Health
Regulations
Cosmetic Products (Safety)
Regulations 1989 (UK) 1550
Cosmetic, Toiletry and Fragrance
Association 503

cosmetics
air pollution 1298
cutaneous toxicity 828, 835
definition 1550
EU regulations 1559–60
and gastro-intestinal microflora
564
human testing 464
hypersensivity reactions 1550
mixtures 606
N-nitroso compounds 2115
neonatal toxicity 1226
permitted/prohibited lists 1557,
1559–60
phamacogenetics 215, 230
regulatory aspects 1544, 1550
cost-benefit analyses 28, 1789,
1792
cost-effectiveness, approximate
methods 1331
co-substrates 429
cottonmouth 2178
Coturnix japonica see quail,
Japanese
cough 512, 614
coumarin 7-hydroxylase *217*
Council for the Defense of Medical
Research 486
Council of Europe 37, 1571
Committee of Experts on
Flavouring Substances 1657
Committee of Experts on
Materials and Articles Coming
into Contact with Food 1657
Council of the European
Communities 486
Council for International
Organizations of Medical Science
454, 486
councilman bodies 175
counselling for test results 1957
counterterrorism forces 1721
courtroom, expert witness in
1950–1
covalent binding 6, 127–8, 230
coverings or coating, for foods
1654
cow *see* cattle
cowbird, brown-headed (*Molothus
ather*) 1347
cowpox virus, and apoptosis 195
CPDB *see* Carcinogen Potency
Database
CPF *see* cancer potency factors
CPK *see* creatine phosphokinase

CPSC *see* Consumer Product Safety
Commission
crab
biomarker 1852
horseshoe 402, 537
cranial nerve paresis 757
craniorachischisis 969
crayfish 820
CRC Critical Reviews in Toxicology
1676
creatine, as biomarker 1859, 1861,
1862
creatine kinase (CK)
as biomarker 1848, 1857, 1858,
1861, 2031
clinical chemistry 355–6, 357,
366
half-life 1858
levels following CO_2 in rats 61
pathology 343
and skeletal muscle toxicity 939,
940, 941, 943, 944, 951
as substrate 160
creatine phosphate 807
creatine phosphokinase (CPK) 531,
534, 1860
creatinine 43, 1859, 1860, 1861
creatinine-corrected units 1908
credibility 25, 1557, 1579
Creutzfeld–Jacob disease 1964
criminal poisoning *see* poisoning
cristate 778
criterion of judgment in legal
matters 1952
critical illness myopathy 947
Critical Incident Stress management
1729
CrmA, and apoptosis 193, 195
cross-sectional studies 1456, 1534
cross-tachyphylaxis 612
Crotolaria spp. *see* rattlebox
Cruelty to Animals Act (UK) 36
crustaceans 1311, 1314, 1318,
1319–20, 2052
see also individual species
cryomicrotome 751
cryopreservation techniques 271
crypt assay reports on radiation
1689, 1690
cryptorchidism 1248
Crystal Ball software 1782
p-crystallin *242*
crystalluria 363
crystal violet staining 753
CS-syndrome 1998

cytoplasmic vacuolization 551
cytoskeletal active compounds 638
cytoskeletal effects of metal toxins 2067–8
cytoskeletal proteins 631
cytosolic binding proteins 126
cytosolic enzymes 98, 105, 108, 109
cytosolic glutathione transferase 118
cytosolic receptors 126
cytosolic reductase 104
cytosolic SOD activity biomarker 1868
cytostatic drugs 515
cytotoxic agents 258, 522, 536, 1463, 1766
cytotoxic hypoxia from fires 1920
cytotoxic T lymphocyte assay (CTL) 1007
cytotoxic/suppressor T cells 341
cytotoxicity 126
  assays 752–5
  index 52
  mechanism 136
  medical devices 1734, 1735, 1740, 1743

D

D$_{50}$ *see* mean aerodynamic diameter
dab, North Sea (*Limanda limanda*) 1870
Dad-1, and apoptosis 193
DADs *see* delayed after-polarizations
dairy foods 1773, 2113, 2115, 2117
damage *see* DNA, damage
damage inducible (*din*) genes 1022
dander 511, 1300
  see also hair
danger symbols 1477, 1603
Dangerous Chemical Substances and Proposals Concerning Their Labeling (USA) 37
dangerous dose 1831
Dangerous Properties of Industrial Materials 1476
Dangerous Substances Directive *see* EU, Directive 67/548/EEC; EU, Directive 79/831/EEC
dangerous substances and preparations, EU regulations 1590, 1593–4, 1609–10
Danish, *see also* Denmark

Danish painters' disease *see* organic solvent syndrome
Danish porcine nephropathy 2145, 2154, 2160
Daphnia spp. 1318, 1320
  D. magnus 408
data
  interpretation 1941
  monitoring 1958
  requirement, regulatory procedures 1572–3, 1601
  transformation, in exposure reconstruction 1458
databanks 481
databases 477–81
  chemical substances 1456
  chromium exposures 1457–8
  clinical chemistry 358
  control 59
  for expert witness 1947
  indexing 480
  limitations 1461
  pesticides 1603
  toxicity criteria 1759, 1766
  in toxicology 39, 53, 1676, 1939, 1943
Datura stramonium see jimsonweed
Daubert decisions 1947, 1948–50
Davidson's fixative 336, 347
DBA *see Dolichos biflorus* agglutinin
De Materia Medica 35
De Venenis 35
deacetylation, acetaminophen 117
deafness *see* hearing loss
dealkylation 101–2
deamination 101–2
death
  causes 1502, 1529
  certificates 1529, 1535
  following testing in animals 8–9
  from poisoning 38, 1353, 1444, 1489–90
  from whole-body irradiation 1686
  genes 194
  medicolegal investigation 1489
  as quantal response 13
  receptors 196
  records, use in epidemiology 1532
  risk of 1830
  see also lethality
death camas, *Zygadenus* spp., cardiovascular effects 1522

debrisoquine 4-hydroxylase *217*
debrisoquine hydroxylation defect 218
decalcification 342, 782
decapitation 497, *498–9*
dechlorination 104, 566
decision-making tools 1787, 1791, 1829
Declaration of Helsinki 454
decomposed remains 1495, 1496, 1503
decontamination procedures 1511, 1729
deconvolution 655
Dedrick plots 89
default assumptions 603, 1784–5, 1787
definitive tests, field studies 1353–4
degeneration 340
degradation 1734, 1779–80
degreasers' flush 1415
dehalogenation 98, 104
dehydration 367, 1687
dehydration constant 613
7-α-dehydroxylation 567
Delaney Clause, Food, Drug and Cosmetics Act 1938 (USA) 1552–3, 1561, 1563, 1658, 1749
delayed after-polarizations (DADs) 812
delayed hypersensitivity response (DHR) 1007
delayed polyneuropathy 329
demethylation 115, 222, 225–6, 569–70, 572
demographic expansion 1443
demyelination 347, 638, 639, 822, 944
dendrites 631, 703
Denmark
  Committee on Scientific Dishonesty 1958
  nitrate and nitrite levels 2112, 2118, 2130
dental amalgam 1204, 1227, 1249
dental caries 1381
dental exposure, mercury 643
dental workers, latex allergy 510
dentifice 967
dentine 967, 1735, 1736, 2057
dentists, female 1204
dentition 343
  see also teeth
deoxyadenosine *1878*
deoxycytosine *1878*

deoxyguanosine 1878, *1881*
deoxynucleotidyl transferase 340
deoxypyridinoline, as biomarker 1859
deoxyribonucleic acid *see* DNA
Department of Agriculture (USA)
  acute toxicity studies 36
  and agricultural biotechnology 1459
  animal test reduction 494
  animal welfare 486, 496
  Food Safety Inspection Service 1563
  National Food Consumption Survey 1602
  obligations 1599
  regulatory efforts 1561
  veterinary drug regulation 1633–8
  wildlife protection 1347
Department of Defense (USA) 824
Department of the Environment (USA) 1090
Department of Health (UK) 439, 450, 454
Department of Trade and Industry (UK) 459
Department of Transportation (USA) 496, 1588–9
dephosphorylation 429
depolarization 639, 640, 938
depolarizing after-potentials 824
depression
  chronotherapy 266
  in IEI 1707, 1708, 1709, 1710, 1714, 1715
  organic solvents 2030, 2033, 2035, 2036, 2037, 2038, 2039, 2040, 2041
  pharmacogenetics 234
  plastics industry 2020, 2021
  potatoes 1984
  rubber industry 2015
dermal/dermis *see mainly* skin
dermal bioavailability 581, 584
dermal exposures 604, 1339
dermal to inhalation extrapolation 148
dermal toxicity test, in hairless mice 605
dermatitis
  contact 7, 23, 510, 511, 711, 830, 834–6, 838–40, 1779, 1985, 2062–3

  see also allergic contact dermatitis
  cumulative 833
  from rotenone 1999
  in IEI 1715
  occupational 1415
dermatological effects, predictability in animal tests 1438
Derris spp.
  D. eliptica 1999
  D. mallaccensis 1999
Descartes, R,n, 36
descriptive studies, methodology 1533
desensitization 626, 1714
desiccants 2006
design of studies 22–5, 148, 1964
  see also individual study types
designer drugs 1392, 1491
designer species 135
detection methods, specific and non-specific 67
deterministic effects of radiation 1684, 1685–92
dethiolase enzyme 160
detoxification 17, 18, 19, 56, 228, 357, 427, 545
  antidotal studies 427
  and biohandling 17, 18
  by enzymes *224*
  clinical chemistry 357
  endogenous 431
  in liver 19, 1329
  ovarian, impaired 1150
  and pancreatic disease 911–12
  pathways 272
  peroral toxicity 545
  pharmacogenetics 228
  repeated-dose toxicity studies 56, 328
  treatment for IEI 1715
  vs toxication 116–21
Deutsche Forschungsgemeinschaft 1910
developing countries
  chlorinated hydrocarbon toxicity 1510
  mycotoxin toxicity 1524
  paraquat 1512
  pesticide morbidity and mortality 1548
  pollutant emissions 1371
  regulation less stringent 1544
  WTO membership 1570
developmental delay 239

developmental toxicity 8, 1167–201
  see also congenital malformations; embryo toxicity; foetal toxicity; reproductive toxicity
  alternative testing 415
  development stage and type of effects 1218–22, 1234–6
  endocrine-related 1399
  and environmental endocrines 1406–7
  interspecies variation 283
  lead 2056
  male-mediated 1185
  mechanisms 1188–91
  neurotoxicity 642, 655, 669, 1467
  organic solvents 2041
  postnatal evaluations 1181–5
  radiofrequency radiation 1419
  regulatory health assessment 1179–81
  screening protocols 1185–8
  Segment II study 1169, 1176–9
developmentally relevant genes 1190–1
device master file 1679
dextran-coated activity charcoal technique 982
dextromethorphan *O*-demethylase *217*
DHEA *see* dihydroepiandrosterone
DHR *see* delayed hypersensitivity response
diabetes 132, 263, 1427, 1969, 2132
diabetes mellitus 1037, 1216
diabetic cataract 160, 764
diabetogenic substances 991–3
diacylglycerol, and apoptosis 190, 191
diagnostic equipment 1661
diagnostic pharmaceuticals, regulatory aspects 1548
diagnostic recombinant products 1966
diagnostic tests, biotechnological 1454
diagonal radioactive zone 1890
dialkylphosphoryl-enzyme complexes 429, 1996
Dialog 1947
dialysis 363, 425, 523, 535, 724, 1379, 2060
diamine oxidase, oxidation 103

DNA (*Contd.*)
lung 723
mapping and sequencing
see human genome project
metabolism 391
microinjections into pronucleus 1964
as molecular target 160–2
mustard gas binding 2084
mutation and cancer 1027–35, 1099–101
PCR amplification 218
plasmids 1024–5
point mutations 1025–7
probes 239, 563
proteins 1966–8
recombinant technology 1723, 1963, 1964, 1965, 1966
repair
adaptive pathway 1023–4
and apoptosis 195
arsenic 2052
cadmium 2054
carcinogen effect 314
chromium 2062
enzymes 8, 1892
error-prone and post-replication 1022–3
excision 1020–2
inhibition 261
mechanism 6, 164, 1882
mismatch 1023
and mutagenicity 1019–24
ootocytes 1150–1
and plasmids 1025
replication 195
response elements 722
sequencing 218, 229
size and stereochemical properties of interacting molecule 162
strand breakage 390, 567, 634
structure 1017–19
synthesis
and apoptosis 198
cardiac toxicity 808–9
circadian 256, 258
fertility cycle variation 266
inhibition 261
reproductive toxicity 1142, 1145
skin 258, 833
unscheduled (UDS) 271, 567, 1104
thymus 284

transcription 1019
translation 1019
DNA acetyltransferase 273
DNA polymerase 340
DNA sulphotransferase 273
DNA-derived therapeutic products 1966
DNAse 189, 897
Doctor of Philosophy requirements 1938, 1939
dog
acute toxicity studies 45
aflatoxin LD_{50} 2154
allergens 512
ALP isoenzyme 359
alternative tests to 402
aminophenol hydroxylation 110
anaesthesia 387
atrioventricular node 343
biceps femoris absorption 531
biliary excretion 555
bilirubin 360
blood collection and sampling 357, 386, *386*
body weight/surface area difference 92
breathing rate 46
cancer studies in plastics industry 2021
carbamate herbicide toxicity 1512
ceftizoxime clearance 89
chlorphenoxy herbicide toxicity 1512
cholecalciferol toxicity 1511
cholinesterase inhibition 369
combustion toxicity studies 1924
common toxicoses 1510–13
CYP genes 216, *216*
dander allergen 512
developmental period 1696
exercise pens 490
fungicide toxicity 2002, 2003
garbage toxicity 1512
hair allergen 512
HDL fraction 367
herbicide toxicity 2005
hexobarbitone toxicity 111
hydrogen cyanide toxicity 2102
intravenous injections 526, 529
intubation 544, 549
ischaemic damage 336
islet cell 346
left ventricle papillary muscles damage 336

liver amine oxidase (AO) 238
long bone haematopoiesis 383
longissimus dorsi absorption 531
mab markers 338
methaemoglobin model 393
neurotrophic factor pharmacokinetics 1972
nitrite toxicity studies 2123
ochratoxin toxicity 2159
osmotic minipump 528
phosgene 2097
pulmonary oil microembolism 534
repeated exposure studies 59
reproductive cycle 372
saliva allergen 512
secondary toxicity 1510
sinuatrial node 343
stratum corneum skin permeability *579*
tPA safety evaluation 1970
treatment groups 358
troponin measurement 366
tumorigenicity of medical devices 1742
vomiting reflex 546
zinc intoxication 1513
dogbane (*Apocynum* spp.), cardiovascular effects 1522
Dolichos biflorus agglutinin (DBA) 1061
Doll, Richard 1529, 1536, 1539
Domagk, Gerhard 34
domestic animal toxicity 1510–13
Domestic Preparedness Program (USA) 1729
dominant lethal mutation 523, 1038, 1060–1, 1143, 1144
dominant oncogenes
see proto-oncogenes
doomsday cults 1728
dopamine 16, 642–3, 1348, 2039
dopamine agonists and antagonists 1328
dopamine oxidase, inhibition by disulfiram 2016
dorsal root ganglia 347
dose
-dependent kinetics 21, 83–5
additivity 303, 309, *313*
administered 79
in animal bioassay 1750
calculation 1774–5
definition 9

driving under the influence of
alcohol (DUI) 1491
see also alcohol (*in Chemical Index*)
driving under the influence of drugs
other than alcohol (DUID) 1491
dromotropic effects 43
Drosophila melanogaster 216, 414,
1050, 1056–8, 1092, 1189, 1190,
1869
drowning 814
drowsiness 43, 460
drug(s)
absorption categories 552
abuse/misuse
behavioural toxicity 664
cardiotoxicity 813–15
cross-reactivity 1501
eye toxicity 757
forensic analysis 1491, 1495
immunotoxicity 1003
medicinal use 1550
occupational toxicity 1416
regulatory aspects 1550
reproductive toxicity 1143,
1146, 1151, 1154, 1224,
1254–7
safety aspects 1444
screening (DAS) 1502, 1503
administration route 21
adverse effects *see* adverse drug
reactions
anti-inflammatory 263
anticancer 261–2
biomaterials and 1745–6
carcinogenicity testing 1618–19
and chemical toxicity 460–1,
1417
circadian toxicology 252–4
clinical trials 457
combinations 1504
controlled and scheduled (UK)
1545
delivery system development
1966
dependence, adverse drug
reaction 1430
development and toxicity testing
265–6, 1436–7, 1974
dietary inclusion 523
disasters 1426–9, 1439–40, 1634
efficacy 1425, 1426, 1429, 1562
evaluation and approval 1425
forensic analysis 1495, 1501
gastro-intestinal absorption 521

gut microflora metabolism 572
human testing 453
interactions 21
acute toxicity 38, 50
drug–chemical interaction,
pregnant women 1216,
1217
drug–drug interactions 125–6
drug–food interactions 125–6
FDA guidance 1438–9
and metabolism 113
occupational toxicity 1415–16
prediction 1437–9
regulation 1426
studies 1565
liver detoxification 344
manufacturers *see* pharmaceutical
companies
metabolic effects 109–10
metabolism 216–18, 863, 866,
910
and myopathies 942–7
neuroleptic 264–5
over-the-counter *see* over-the-
counter drug(s)
oxidation consequences 215–18
and pancreatitis 915–20, 991–3
processing 1968
prohibited list 1550
pulmonary excretion 256
receptor theory of drug action 34
reduction 215–18
regulatory aspects
and clinical research 1439
EU 1557–9, 1621–30
history 1634
Japan 1544, 1565–7
Norway 1544, 1568–9
patterns 1543
processing 1972–3
USA 1544, 1615–20, 1662,
1665
safety
and efficacy 1549
margin calculations 91
regulatory aspects 1425,
1429–34, 1622, 1634
requirements, UK 1425
seasonal exposure 267
side-effects *see* adverse effects
specialized uses 1548
substrates for CYP2D6
polymorphism *219–21*
surveillance schemes 457–8
targeting 1966

testing
forensic 1495, 1501
guidelines 2, 40
on healthy human volunteers
1546
and thrombocytopenia 395
toxic-therapeutic ratio 260
toxicity 21–2, 1425–41, 1549
Type A and B action 21
veterinary *see* veterinary drug(s)
Drug Safety Research Trust 458
Drugs, Cosmetics and Medical
Instruments Law (Japan) 37
dry cleaning industry *678*, 2037
see also service industries
dry eye syndrome 755
DT diaphorase *see* quinone
reductase
dually perfused human placental
cotyledon 1236–7
Duboscq colorimeter 1490
ducks *see* poultry
duct of Santorini 894
duct of Wirsung 894
ductal cells, pancreas 897
Dunlop Committee *see* Committee
on Safety of Drugs
duodenal absorption 69
duodenal chyme 545
duodenal mucosa 545
duodenal ulcer 227, 236
duodenum 545, 546, 556
Durham–Humphrey amendment,
Food, Drug and Cosmetics Act
1938 (USA) 1562
dust
acute toxicity 46
aflatoxin determination 2152
cereals, respiratory effects 1475
chemical contaminants absorbed
on 1299
effects 20
emissions 1815, 2015
exposure 603
generation systems 596–7
inhalation dose calculation 1774,
1775
organic and inorganic 1299
resuspension 1300
as source of contamination of
samples 1909
Dutchman's breeches (*Dicentra
cucullaria*), neuroxicity 1520
dyaphyseal dysgenesis 972
dyes 39, 163, 918, 2014

dyschromatopsia 756
dyskinesia, predictability in animal tests 1438
dysphasia from peroral exposure 19
dyspnoea 40, 41, 512, 728, 731
dystrophic calcification 727

E

E1B19K, and apoptosis 194
E_{50} values 752, 753
E-numbers 1655
eagle, bald (*Haliaeetus leucocephalus*) 1329, 1341
Eagle River Flats, Alsaka 1341
ear
    canal, parathion percutaneous absorption 578
    inner 347, 775–83, 784–96
    melanin in 129
early warning systems 457, 1729–30
Earth Summit *see* United Nations Conference on Environment and Development
earthworms
    as biomarkers 1866
    contact lethality test *408*
    Eisenia foetida 408, 409
    Lumbricus rubellus 408, 409
    toxicity rating 408, *409*
Ebers papyrus 35, 472, 1527
Ebstein's anomaly of tricuspid valve 1205
EC_{50} (median effective concentration) 1312, 1313, 1315
    for blepharospasm 620
    choosing 48
    data for modelling 1834
    sensory irritants *624*
    subchonic toxicity testing 1345
ecdysone agonists 2000
ECG *see* electrocardiogram
Echinaceae purpurea, MRLs 1642
Echis ocellatus see viper, saw-scaled/carpet
Echium plantagineum see viper's bugloss
echothiophate, eye absorption systemic toxicity 762
ecoepidemiology 1407
ECOFRAM *see* Ecological Committee on FIFRA Risk Assessment Methods

Ecological Committee on FIFRA Risk Assessment Methods (ECOFRAM) 1328, 1352
ecological fallacy 1755
ecological health and integrity 1314–15
ecological toxicology, definition 1328
ecotoxicology *see* environmental toxicology
ectoderm 828
ectoparasiticides 1633, 1636–7, 1649, 1993, 1995
eczema 510, 1430, 2145, 2148
ED_{50} (median effective dose) 301
ED (exposure dose) 4, 9, 13, 18
    ED_{01} 48
    ED_{50} 9–10, 11, 36, 39, 48, 2030
    ED_{99} 11
    ED_{100} 48
edge associations, critical 1353
editorial review 457
Edman degradation 1883–4
EDSTAC *see* Endocrine Disrupter Screening and Testing Advisory Committee
Edward syndrome 1081
EEG *see* electroencephalogram
effect addition 304
effective dose 323, 1842, 1843, 1844–5, 1848
efficacy
    antidotes 430–3
    and drug safety 1549
    pesticides 1601
    testing 1573
    veterinary drugs 1634
EGF *see* epidermal growth factor
eggs
    bioassay 1334
    nitrate, nitrite and *N*-nitroso levels 2115, 2116, 2117, 2120
    single-dose acute tests 1330
    suceptibility to xenobiotics 1330
    tainted 234
eggshell thinning
    brown pelican 1351
    and chlorinated hydrocarbons 1329, 1343, 1345, 1548
    poultry 1520
    raptorial birds 1351, 1354
    waterfowl 1354
egr-1, and apoptosis 193

Egypt
    ancient writings 1489, 1527
    chemical warfare 2080
EINECS *see* European Inventory of Existing Commercial Chemical Substances
ejaculatory function 1142
EKA *see* exposure equivalents for carcinogenic chemicals
EKG *see* electrocardiogram
elastic fibres 829
elastic stain 336
elastomers 2013
elderly people
    adverse drug reactions 1427, 1428, 1439
    skin reactivity 831
    statistical artefacts 1529
electric shock, aggression 653
electricity, sensitivity 1714
electrocardiogram (ECG/EKG) 39, 805–6
    abnormalities *see* cardiac arrhythmias
    changes 809, 811, 817, *818*, 819, 822, 823
    P wave 805, 806, 807
    P–R interval 822
    Q–T interval *806*, 817, 819, 823
    QRS complex 805, 817
    recording 45
    S–T segment 805, *806*, 809, 811, 819, 823
    T-wave 805, 806, 809, 823
    U-wave 823
electrochemical conductance, for DNA adduct analysis 1889
electrode paste production workers, exposure risks 1886
electroencephalogram (EEG)
    activity 251
    following organic solvents 2032
    in IEI 1707, 1713
    radiation-induced changes 1691
electrolyte(s)
    balance 363–4, 366–7
    disturbances, ethanol myopathy 938, 940
    forensic analysis 1495, 1498
    imbalance 1757
    transport, radiation-induced changes 1689, 1690
electromagnetic flowmeter 679
electromagnetic radiation 1418–19

electromyocardiogram (EMG) 943, 944
electron(s)
  -withdrawing group 221–2
  donor 238
  ejection 1683
  impact (EI) 1499
  secondary 1683
  transfer 1985
  transport chain 635
electron microscopy 338–9, 764, 781, 782, 787, 790, 867–8
  ethanol myopathy 938
  soft tissue tumours 340
electron spin resonance 619
electronic bibliographic databases 474
electronic literature sources 477–81
electronics industries, radiofrequncy radiation 1418–19
electro-oculography 756
electrophiles 100, 130, 156, 161, 162, 167–8
electrophoresis 187, 188, 366, 367
electroplaters, biomonitoring 1904
electroretinography 756, 764
Elementa Medicinae et Chirurgiae Forensis 36
elements, speciation 1365
elephant, weight 51
elimination *see* excretion
ELISA *see* enzyme-linked immunosorbent assay
elixirs, toxic 1426–8
E_m *see* resting membrane potential
emaciation 41
embolization, arterial 814
embryo, parenteral toxicology 528
embryogenesis 178, 1464, 1684
embryolethality 528, 1243
embryonic stem cells, gene transfer 1964
embryotoxicity
  see also congential malformations; developmental toxicity; placenta; skeletal abnormalities
  cadmium 2053
  circadian toxicology 258
  dioxin 284
  disulphide formation and 159–60
  fungicides 2002
  organic solvents 2040, 2041
  placental toxicity 1243

in pregnant rat 534
  radiation 1696, 1697
emergency planning 1728, 1729, 1814, 1832, 1836–7
Emergency Planning and Community Right-to-know Act 1589–90
emesis *see* vomiting
EMG *see* electromyocardiogram
EMIT *see* enzyme-multiplied immunoassay technique (EMIT)
emphysema 29, 722, 732, 1928
employees, education and training 1463
employers, responsibilities 1481
emulsifiers 1552, 1653, 1985, 1987–8
enantioselective metabolism 226
encapsulation dosing procedures 60
encephalomalacia, horses 2145, 2163
encephalopathy 235, 1430, 2031
endive, nitrate and nitrite levels 2112–13
endocarditis 814
endocardium, pathology 343
endocochlear potential (EP) 777, 781, 785, 787
endocrine
  -active compounds, definition 1394
  disruption 664, 980–1, 1316, 1392–3, 1394, 1400, 1534
  feedback axis 369
  function 369–73, 1395–6, 1400–1
  glands, definition 1395
  homeostasis 1391
  hormone assays 981–3
  hyperplasia 346
  mimic, definition 1394
  modulation *see* endocrine, disruption
  myopathies 947–50
  receptors 983–4, 1402
  system 979–95
    male, toxins affecting 1146–7
    pathology 346
    radiation-induced changes 1691
    signs of toxicity 40, 1391–414
    target organ toxicity 984–93
    tissues 1395

Endocrine Disrupter Screening and Testing Advisory Committee 1393–5, 1400, 1401, 1402, 1403, 1408
endocytosis 680, 682, 685, 693
endocytotic vesicles 791
endolymph, cochlea 775, 776, 777, 779, 780, 784, 789, 795
endometrial cancer 135, 458, 1392, 1399, 1400
endometrial glands, premenstrual, basophilic bodies in 175
endometrial ischaemic death 177
endometrium, pathology 346
endoneural capillary system 633
endonucleases 127, 187, 1963
endoperoxides in diet 1980
endoplasmic reticulum
  see also rough or smooth endoplasmic reticulum
  circadian toxicology 254
  cytochrome P450 in 99
  distribution 71
  enzymes 98, 156
  hepatotoxicity 861, 868
  outer hair cells 786
  pathology 338, 344
  peroral toxicity 548
  pharmacogenetics 232
  stress components 168
endorphins, in human placenta 1256
endothelial bone 966
endothelial cells 632, 633, 2119
endothelium 383
endotoxins
  in animal husbandry 1516–17
  cardiotoxicity 819–20
  concentration 537
  parenteral toxicity 536
  and TNF, toxicology 259
endotracheal route of exposure 59
energy
  deposition 1683
  in experimental carcinogenesis 1980–1
  intake 92
  requirements of body 127
  stressors 1329
Enforcable Consent Agreements (ECAs) 1585
engineering controls 461, 514
enhancement of toxicity 21
enkephalins, in human placenta 1256

enterochromaffin cells 343–4

enterococci 562

enterohepatic circulation 18, 555–6, 557, 568–9, 570, 689

enterooxyntin 546

enterotoxaemia, domestic animals 1512

enterotoxicosis, domestic animals 1512

environmental carcinogens, biomarker 1849

Environmental Chemicals Data and Information Network 481

environmental conditions
  and chemical toxicity 1419
  improvements in quality 1370–1
  PBPK modelling 147–8
  repeated exposure studies 57–8

environmental contaminants
  see environmental pollutants

environmental costs 1752–3

environmental disasters 1443
  see also disasters

environmental endocrines
  see also environmental oestrogens
  debate 1400, 1404
  developmental effects 1406–7
  dosage 1396–7
  effects on wildlife populations 1407
  and human disease 1399–400
  low-level exposure 1395
  regulatory issues 1393–4
  screening and testing 1401–4, 1407–8
  toxicology 1391–414

environmental epidemiology 1529

environmental exposure 19, 606
  regulatory aspects 1415
  renal dysfunction markers 678
  safety margins 91
  to dioxin 87
  to organic solvents 2037

environmental factors
  affecting metabolism 109–10, 112–14
  interactions 1415–24
  pesticide residue effects 1548
  and toxicity 16, 21, 45

environmental field sampling 1781

environmental groups 1945

environmental guidelines
  see guidelines

Environmental Health Criteria (IPCS publications) 476, 1571, 1592, 1612, 1759

environmental health effects 1534

environmental illness see idiopathic environmental illness

environmental influences, on response to toxic agents 1418–19

environmental monitoring 1460

Environmental Mutagen Information Center 478

Environmental Mutagen Society 1038

environmental neurotoxins, abnormal tremor 663

environmental oestrogens
  see also environmental endocrines
  breast cancer 1392
  effects on fish 1565
  EPA (USA) investigations 1393–4
  epidemiological and toxicological co-operation 1534
  exposure 1398
  human health effects 1392
  hypothesis 1399
  regulatory focus 1529
  reproductive effects 1565
  unreproducible experiments 1404–5

environmental pollutants 524, 1464, 1564
  persistent 1553–4

environmental pollution
  biomarkers 1531, 1841, 1842, 1866, 1870
  by industrial chemicals, in Japan 1547
  human health effects 1530–1
  IEI and 1711
  mercury 1826, 2057

Environmental Protection Agency (EPA) (USA)
  acute toxicity studies 37, 45
  and agricultural biotechnology 1459
  air pollution studies 1269, 1292
  attitude to epidemiology 1528
  ban on chorinated hydrocarbons 1329
  biopharmaceutics regulations 1973
  Carcinogen Assessment Group 147, 1763–4, 1770

  Common Sense Initiative 1587–8
  developmental neurotoxicity guidelines 1467
  education 1936
  environmental oestrogen investigation 1393–4
  Existing Chemicals Program 1586–90
  exposure calculations 1775
  field studies requirements 1327, 1328, 1353
  formation 1599
  guidelines 1637
  industrial chemicals regulation 1545, 1581–6
  master testing List (MTA) 1585
  multigeneration testing protocol 1406
  Office of Pollution Prevention and Toxics (US) 1581
  pathology 347
  PBPK modelling 1769
  'pen-in-field' protocol 1349
  peroral toxicity 550
  pesticide MRLs 1563
  Pollution Prevention Recognition Program 1583
  powers 1459, 1480–1
  pre-manufacturing notice 1557
  quality assurance 437
  reference guidelines 1352
  registration of end-use product 1350, 1352, 1353
  regulatory function 1328
  reproductive risk assessment guidelines 1467
  risk assessment 1749, 1751, 1752, 1756, 1784, 1788–9
  subchronic toxicity test 1344
  surface area scaling factors 1769
  threshold margin of safety for wildlife 1331
  veterinary drug regulation 1633–8
  Worker Protection Standard 1603

environmental regulations
  see regulatory aspects

environmental risk assessment
  see under risk assessment

environmental somatization 1709, 1715

environmental sources of toxic exposure 1444

environmental stressors 1353, 1407, 1848

Environmental Teratology Information Center 478

environmental toxicology 2, 3, 27, 642–3, 1319–20, 1328, 1450–1

enzymatic detoxicants *426*

enzymatic testing, in field studies 1354

enzyme(s)
  abbreviations *356*
  and absorption 70
  activation 121, 224, 564–6
  activities, PBPK modelling 89
  and acute toxicity 35
  aflatoxin metabolism 2150
  assays 45
  biomonitoring 1906
  catalysis 98
  cDNA cloning 135
  changes, as biomarker 1848, 1856–8, 1860, 1867
  detoxification activities, cellular sensing 157
  dialkyl phosphorylated 429
  digestive 88
  distribution in tissues 1857
  EC numbers 356
  engineering 1454
    see also biotechnology industries
  exogenous 429
  as food additives 1552
  gastrointestinal function 365
  half-life 1857, 1858
  hydrolysis 18, 1883
  inactivation 127, 130
  inducibility 100
  induction 113
    adaptive 6
    as biomarker 1847, 1848, 1856, 1865–6
    in chronic intake 83, 90
    consequences 114
    as double-edged tool 911
    extrahepatic 911
    from organic solvents 2032–3
    hepatic 866–7, 910–12
    non-cP450 1866
    pancreatic 911–12
  inhibition 6, 8, 114, 159, 1847, 1848, 1866–7
  inhibitors 1455
  localization 1857
  metabolic 73

in nucleic acid manipulation 1965
  oxidative 102–3
  Phase I and II 216
  plasma 359–60
  polymorphisms, biomarker 1850
  preparations 1985
  restriction, history of 1963
  stabilization 113
  synthesis, pancreatic 895
  urinary 363, 367
  xenobiotic metabolism 1890–2

enzyme immunoassay (EIA) 370, 1501–2, 1503

enzyme–substrate theory 34

enzyme-linked immunosorbent assay (ELISA)
  adducts 1885, 1887, 1889
  aflatoxin 2152–3
  biotechnology products 1972
  in clinical chemistry 360
  in endocrine toxicology 983
  in forensic testing 1502
  laboratory ocupational hazard 510
  ochratoxin 2158
  in respiratory toxicology 706, 710
  snake venom 2180

enzyme-multiplied immunoassay technique (EMIT) 983, 1501

enzymuria 685, 687

eosin staining 345

eosinophilia 384, 389, 728

eosinophilia–myalgia syndrome (EMS) 395, 946, 1463, 1553, 1568

eosinophilic pneumonitis *727*

eosinophils 702, 729

EP *see* endocochlear potential

EPA *see* Environmental Protection Agency

epicardium 804

epichlorohydrin 1035

epicutaneous techniques, sensitization studies in animals 841–2

epidemic, definition 1527

epidemiological studies 454, 457
  biomarkers 1538
  breast cancer 571
  definition 1527
  end-points 1529–30
  environmental 1529, 1534

health and chemical exposure 461

hepatocellular cancer 274

historical aspects 1527–9

and idiopathic environmental intolerance 1716

laboratory workers 515

methodology 1529, 1535

nitrates, nitrites and *N*-nitroso compounds 2129–33

observational 1456

organic solvent toxicity 2041–2

prognostic criteria 1450

protein and colonic cancer 568

reproductive outcomes 1463

risk assessment 1755–6, 1770

study designs 1531–4

techniques 22, 25

teratogenic eye toxicity 758–9

and toxicology 1449, 1455–7, 1527–42

workforce health status 464

epidermal growth factor (EGF) 729, 1972

epidermal growth factor (EGF) receptor 189–90

epidermis 828
  back-diffusion 582
  circadian toxicology 258
  diffusion 46
  keratinocytes 411–*12*, 413
  lichenification 835
  pathology 340
  thickness 583

epididymides 371

epigenetic *see* non-genotoxic

epiglottis 544

epilation radiation-induced 1688

epilepsy 166, 2030

epinephrine *see* adrenaline

epineurum 633

epithelial cells
  and apoptosis 199
  lining 548
  proliferation 126
  radiation-induced damage 1690

epithelium, passage across 70

epoxide hydrolase
  as biomarker 1866
  biotransformation 115
  bromobenzene toxicity and 118
  catalysis 130–1
  induction 1866
  interspecies extrapolation 279

epoxide hydrolase (*Contd.*)
  in liver microsomes 280
  pharmacogenetics 216
epoxygenase *217*
Epping jaundice 1825
Epstein–Barr virus 194
equine leukoencephalomalacia
  1520, 2163
equipartition of energy principle
  1683
equipment, standard operating
  procedures (SOP) 447, 448
ergonomic costs of fires 1927
ergosterol synthesis inhibition 2004
ergotism 1994, 2145, 2148
EROD *see* ethoxyresorufin *O*-
  deethoxylase
erosion 340
erthyrocytes
  aplasia 391
  recycling 864
eruptions 40
Ervatarnina orientalis 820
erythema 21, 40, 41, 340, 510, 832,
  835, 836, 840, 1688, 1741
erythroblast, radiation-induced
  changes 1694
erythrocyte(s) 384, 387–8
  binding 254
  biomonitoring 1906
  catalase activity 1868
  cellular membrane 413
  cholinesterase activity 368, 466,
    1996
  clinical chemistry 357, 362
  coproporphyrinogen oxidase
    1705
  count 387, 2002, 2006
  enzymes 105
  fragility test, synthetic materials
    1741
  haemolysis *418*, 529
  in vitro assays 415
  lifespan 1879, 1893
  pharmacogenetics 238, 243
  radiolabelled 365
  regulation 1971
  sedimentation rate (ESR) 535
erythropoiesis 384
erythropoietin 185, 265, 361, 384,
  391, 1966, 1971
erythropoietin, transgene models
  1964
escape from fire, hindrances 1916

Escherichia coli
  cardiotoxicity 819
  cytogenicity 1092
  DNA repair 1020–2, 1024, 1025
  and gastro-intestinal microflora
    568
  hepatotoxicity 883
  lac Z system 1062–3, 1064
  lipopolysaccharide, NOS and
    2119
  nitrates and 2124
  nitrites and 2128
  nitrogen oxide study 1278
  and parenteral toxicity 536
  pharmacogenetics 235, 241
  tester strains 1044, 1045
Establishment License Application
  (USA) 1974
esterases, inhibition 114
Estimation and Assessment of
  Substance Exposure (EASE),
  knowledge-based system 1479
estuary pollution 1866
ET_{50} (median effective time) 1314
ETA (Basque separatist
  organization) 1727
ethanol myopathy 938–42
ethanol-metabolizing system 103
ethical issues
  animal studies 1535, 1536
  guidelines 453, 454
  human studies 453, 1447, 1535,
    1536
  medical ethics 1955–6
  prospective studies 1435
  in toxicology 1893–4, 1955–6,
    1957–8
ethnic factors 236, 1567
  clinical testing 1573
  dietary habits 1646
  effects on metabolism 112
  null genotype 1891
ethnic–nationalist conflicts 1723
17β-ethoxycoumarin 4-hydroxylase
  217
7-ethoxycoumarin *O*-deethylase
  217
ethoxyresorufin *O*-deethoxylase
  (EROD) as biomarker 1865
Eubacterium spp. 563, 568
euchromatin 160
eukaryotes 216, 1019–20, 1051–61
Eupatropium rugosum
  see snakeroot, white

Euphausiids 1314
Euphorbia spp. *see* spurge
European Association of Poison
  Control Centres 459
European Centre for Ecotoxicology
  and Toxicology of Chemicals
  (ECETOC) 746
European Centre for the Validation
  of Alternative Methods 504
European Coal and Steel
  Commmunity 1555
European Commission 459, 1556
European Community *see* European
  Union
European Community Coordination
  (ECCO) 1607, 1608
European Court of Human Rights
  1572
European Court of Justice 1572
European daily food factors 1646
European Economic Community 37
European Environmental Mutagen
  Society 1038
European experts, list 1639
European Inventory of Existing
  Commercial Chemical Substances
  (EINECS) 1556–7, 1590, 1592
European law, takes precedence
  over domestic statutes 1555
European Licensing Authority 1429
European Medicines Evaluation
  Agency (EMEA) 1559, 1621,
    1623, 1625, 1627, 1639
European Monetary System 1555
European Pharmacopeia 536, 1571
European predictive operator
  exposure model (EUROPOEM)
    1609
European Public Assessment Report
  (EPAR) 1625
European Space Agency 477
European Union (EU)
  see also Committee on
    Proprietary Medicinal Products
    (CPMP)
  abridged application procedure
    1629
  animal testing harmonization
    501
  binding values 1595
  biotechnology products
    regulation 1558
  Chemical Agents Directive 1481

European Union (EU) (*Contd.*)

  classification and labelling
      requirements 1476–7, 1479,
      1486, 1557, 1609–10, 1627,
      1628
  clinical trials requirements
      1622–3
  Commission and Council
      Directives 1556
  cosmetics regulation 1550,
      1559–60
  Council of Ministers 503
  dangerous preparations
      regulations 1593–4
  drug safety requirements 1425
  existing industrial chemicals
      regulation 1592–6
  existing substances regulation
      1480, 1590, 1608
  expert report requirements 1627
  food additives regulation 1653–7
  food chemical regulation 1560
  foods, novel 1546
  Good Laboratory Practice (GLP)
      standards 438, 1609, 1621–2
  hazard criteria 1557
  historical development 1555–6,
      1621
  human studies 462
  indicative limits 1595
  industrial chemicals regulation
      1556–7, 1590–6
  institutions and structure 1621
  laws and other instruments 1556,
      1621
  marketing authorization
      procedures 1622, 1623,
      1625–6, 1627–9
  medical devices regulation
      1671–2
  member states 1556
  minimum pre-marketing data set
      1583, 1584
  MRL 1641–3
  multi-state authorization
      procedure 1557
  mutual recognition
      (decentralized) procedures
      1625–6, 1640–1
  national marketing authorization
      procedures 1626–7
  new pesticides regulation
      1605–8
  new substances programme
      1478–9

nitrate levels 2112, 2114
Notification of New Substances
    (NONS) Regulations 1478
novel foods regulation 1560
occupational exposure levels
    (OELs) 1483, 1594–5
*Official Journal of the European
    Communities* 1592, 1621, 1643
pesticide regulation 1557,
    1604–10
pharmaceuticals regulation 1544,
    1557, 1621–30
post-marketing authorization
    procedures 1629–30
pre-marketing authorization
    procedures 1551, 1553,
    1623–7
pre-marketing notification 1557
regulations 2
    see also European Union
      Regulations
    development 1555–60
    harmonization 1557, 1572,
      1590, 1638, 1649, 1654
    pharmaceutical regulations
      1557–9
Risk Assessment Directive 1479
Risk Assessment Regulation
    1480
Scientific Committee on
    Cosmetology 1560
Scientific Committee for Food
    1560
seventh amendment 1590
toxological hazard classification
    1486
Transparency Directive 1545
veterinary drug regulation 1558,
    1637–48
Working Group on the Safety of
    Residues 1643
European Union (EU) Directives
  65/65/EEC 1557, 1621, 1623,
      1629, 1638
  67/548/EEC (Dangerous
      Substances Directive) 37,
      1139, 1545, 1556, 1557, 1590,
      1592–3, 1596, 1605, 1609–10
  70/524/EEC 1648
  75/318/EEC (pharmaceutical
      testing) 1557, 1621
  75/319/EC (expert reports) 1627,
      1629
  75/319/EEC (CPMP) 1557, 1621

76/768/EEC (Cosmetics) 1560
76/769/EEC 1595
78/631/EEC (annulled) 1610
79/117/EEC 1557
79/831/EEC (sixth amendment)
    1545, 1556, 1564, 1590, 1591
80/117/EEC 1594–5
80/778/EEC (drinking water
    quality) 1609
81/851/EEC 1558, 1638, 1639,
    1648
81/852/EEC 1558, 1638, 1639
83/570/EEC 1558
86/362/EEC 1610
86/363/EEC 1610
86/469/EEC (residue
    surveillance) 1647
86/609/EEC (animal protection)
    486, 1622
87/18/EEC 1564, 1621
87/22/EEC 1558, 1638
88/320/EEC (Good Laboratory
    Practice) 1564, 1621, 1622
88/379/EEC (classification and
    labelling) 1478, 1610
88/388/EEC 1655
88/642/EEC 1595
89/105/EEC (Transparency
    Directive) 1569
89/107/EEC 1653, 1656
89/109/EEC 1654, 1655
90/18/EEC 1564
90/128/EEC 1655
90/385/EEC (medical devices)
    1672
90/394/EEC 1595
90/642/EEC 1610
91/414/EEC 1557, 1605, 1608,
    1609
91/414/EEC (plant protection
    products) 1605
91/507/EEC 1621
93/39/EEC 1621, 1629
93/42/EEC (medical devices)
    1671
96/22/EEC (residue surveillance)
    1647
96/23/EEC (residue surveillance)
    1647
96/51/EC 1648
97/41/EC 1610
97/57/EEC 1605
98/8/EC (Biocidal Products
    Directive) 1611

European Union (EU) Regulations
258/97 (Novel Foods) 1560
541/95 1629
542/95 1629, 1640
1069/98 1629
1146/95 1629
2232/96 1655
2309/93 1621, 1623, 1625, 1629, 1639
2377/90 1638, 1643, 1644
euthanasia 61, 496–7, 497–8, *498*
evaporation on storage 1909
evaporimeter 845
evoked potentials 661, 1713
evolution 215
ex vivo studies 52
examination for toxicology 1938–9
Excerpta Medica 473
excipient solvents 533–4
excision repair of DNA 1020–2
excitable membrane function 126–7
excitotoxicity 166, 631, 634, *635*, 644
excitotoxins *634–6*
excretion 18, 67, 72–3, 74–5, 78–80
see also metabolism
dose-dependent kinetics and 83
extent 73
first-order 73
half-life, concentration 86
interspecies 88
rate 72–3, 79
rate constant 77, 80, 86
saturation 83, 84
sigma minus method 85
excretory products, as biomarkers 1849
exemption, from routine testing 1601
exencephaly 528
exercise
avoidance 665
variables 356
exhaled air 552, 581
EXICHEM database 1571
Existing Chemicals Program, EPA (USA) 1586–90
existing drugs, MRLs 1647
existing industrial chemicals, EU regulation 1592–6
existing plant protection products 1608–9
existing products, dossiers 1608

Existing Substances Regulation, EU 1480, 1590, 1608
exocrine cells 545
exogenous dyes 360–1
exogenous enzymes 429
exophthalmos 40, 41
experimental design 293–5, 299–300, 455
see also study design
experimental errors 294
experimental hypo-responders 294
experimental myopathies 950–5
Experimental Use permits (EUPs) 1600
expert advice 1449, 1639
expert report, EU requirements 1627
expert systems 1449
Expert in Toxicology, DGPT 1943
expert witness 1946–51
export and import of chemicals, US 1588
exposure
acute toxicity 34–5
assessment 1460, 1752, 1772–86
biomarkers 1461, 1538
in occupational setting 1456
retrospective 1770
temporal relevance 1893
-based finding 1583
biomonitoring 1899–906
chamber 593
characteristics, effects on toxicity 16
chemical 1328, 1474
control, in IEI 1716
data 1530
definition 1750
dose *see* ED
–effect relationship 1313, 1315
environmental 606
equivalents for carcinogenic chemicals (EKA) 1911
estimates, statistical and analytical issues 1781–2
expression 147
groups, choosing 60–1
history in IEI 1711
index 128
intermittent 1351
limits, occupational, PBPK modelling 149
measurement 1530–1
misclassification risk 1755
nose-only 604

parameters 45
pathways 1772, 1787
patterns 1474, 1535–6
potency index 91
reconstruction, data transformation 1458
repeated *see* repeated exposure toxicity
retrospective measurement 1530
route 5, 17, 18–20
effects 45
mixed/multiple 603–9, 1904–5
and nephrotoxicity 704–5
occupational toxicity 1464, 1485
of organic solvents 2029
PBPK modelling 147–8
pesiticides 1993
in protocols 40
regulatory aspects 1548, 1619
in repeated exposure studies 59
risk assessment 1754
-to-route extrapolation 1766, 1769
secondary 60
soil and groundwater 1366
-specific toxicity criteria 1765–6
and total body burden 149
scenario construction 1772–3
single (acute) 55
sources, wildlife toxicology 1339–42
studies 23
systems 592–3
time (duration) 13, 20, 1739, 1745, 1772, 1786
whole body 604, 623
withdrawal 1715
Exposure factors handbook 1775
exsanguination *498–9*
extenders in rubber 2017
external chain of custody 1491
external dose *see* exposure dose
extracellular fluid 549, 675
extraction
procedure 1369, 1739
ratio 74
extrahepatic enzyme induction 911
extrahepatic toxins 133
extramedullary haemopoiesis, spleen 341
extraocular muscles 614, 757

extrapolation
  see also interspecies
    extrapolation
  disaster studies 1833, 1834
exudates 41, 342
exudation 539
eye
  see also ophth- *and parts and*
    diseases of the eye
  acute inflammatory reaction 755
  adverse drug reactions 1427
  allergic response 512
  arsenic retention 2051
  blinking 739
  chemical injuries 737–8
  concentration-response for
    threshold sensation *616*
  contact of substance with 19, 20
  cosmetics 759
  cytotoxicity assays 752–5
  enucleated methods 751–2
  episceral venous complex 614
  exposure to toxins 605
  fixation 336, 347
  hypertension 614, 757
  hypoplasia 758
  inferior conjunctival sac for
    material testing 739, 740
  inflammation signs 738
  injury 8
    disasters 1814, 1819
    fires 1920, 1925, 1928
    fungicides 2003
    jellyfish venom 2189
    Lewisite 2089
    methanol 2040
    mustard gas 2084, 2087
    nerve agents 2091
    phosgene 2098
    radiation 1684, 1687–8, 1696
    riot control agents 2104
    scoring system *741*
    scorpion venom 2188
    snake venom 2179
    volcanoes 1816
  intraocular pressure (IOP)
    measurements 748–50
  irrigation 741, 2013, 2016, 2020,
    2021, 2032, 2181
  irritation 622–3, 737–55
    see also eye irritation tests
  itching as allergic response 512
  local anaesthesia effects 747
  malformations 757
  metabolism 756

peripheral sensory irritation 614,
  755
signs of toxicity 44
slit-lamp biomicroscopy 746
and systemic toxicity *755–9,*
  759–64
tests in repeated exposure 63
toxicology 737–74
toxin absorption sites 759–60
triparanol toxicity 1634
eye drops, vasoconstrictor effects
  1550
eye irritation tests 23, 25, 738–46
  alternative methods 410, 747–55
  animal welfare 494, 499
  computer-based modelling 754
  Draize scoring 496, 740–1,
    744–6, 752
  human studies 466
  immunotoxicology 1005
  in vitro 739
  modification 466
  rabbit studies 745, 841, 843–4
  results 742, 744–6

F

FA *see* Fanconi's anaemia
fabrics, biocompatibility testing
  1738
facial parasthesia 524
facial warming 236
FACScan flow cytometer *680*
factor IX 1965
factor VIII 1965, 1966, 1970
factor VII
  and diet 1980
factorial designs 313
Factories Inspectorate (UK) 1960
factory
  see also occupational toxicology;
    workplace
  biomonitoring 1904
  emissions, inhalation exposure
    606
facts, real vs junk science 1946–7
factsheets 1448–9
FAD *see* flavin
faecal excretion 18
  dioxin 90
  elimination rate constant
    calculation 86
  mecury 2059
  sigma minus method 85
  toxicokinetics 69, 70, 72

faeces
  absence 40
  bacterial flora *563*
  bolus weight 1645
  chemical excretion 581
  clinical chemistry 362
  mutagenic activity 566
  N-nitroso compounds 567
  stained 40
FAEES *see* fatty acid ethyl esters
Fagopyrum esculantum
  see buckwheat
FAK *see* focal adhesion kinase
Falco peregrinus see peregrine
  falcon
fallopian tubes *see* oviducts
false positives 404, 1501
familial motor neuron disease 239
family environment *see* home
  environment
Fanconi's anaemia (FA) 1033–4
FAO *see* Food and Agriculture
  Organization
farm animal studies 45
farm animals, *see also* food-
  producing animals *and specific*
    animals
farmers *see* agricultural workers
Farr, William 1527, 1528, 1529
Fas 190, 191, 193, 195–6, 199
fasciculations 40, 41, 430, 950, 951
Fasciola hepatica see liver fluke
fasciotomies 941
fast twitch fibres 342
fasting *see* feeding behaviour
fat
  see also adipose tissue
  dietary 58, 1980
  heated, as source of oxygen free
    radicals 1979
  partition coefficients of organic
    solvents 2029
  in tissues, interspecies 88
fat cells 829
fat storage cells *see* Ito cells
fatigue 1686, 1687, 1703, 1706,
  1724
fatty acids
  composition changes with
    organic solvents 2036, 2037
  essential 1979–81
  metabolism 99, 1868
  monounsaturated 1978
  non-esterified 367
  oxidation 869

fatty acids (*Contd.*)
  pharmacogenetics 216
  polyunsaturated 1980
  saturated, blood cholesterol and 1978
  storage pool, fumonisins and 2165
fatty liver-haemorrhagic syndrome (FLHS) 233–4
fault indemnity 1959
fault tree analysis 1832
FBI forensic laboratories 1942
FCA test *see* Freund's Complete Adjuvant test
FDA *see* Food and Drug Administration (FDA) (USA)
FDCs *see* follicular dendritic cells
fecundity 1465, 1846
Federal Insecticide, Fungicide and Rodenticide Act (FIFRA) (USA) 37, 487, 1328, 1350, 1459, 1467, 1563, 1599, 1600, 1636, 1750
feedback mechanisms 546, 980–1, 986–7
feeding behaviour 1328, 1347, 1351
feeding studies, chemical effect on renal function 678
feedstock chemicals, occupational exposures 1463
feedstuffs *see* animal feeds
feet *see* foot
female reproductive system 1147–56
  see also pregnancy
  drug and chemical effects 1155–6
  exercise effects 1156
  health evaluation 1465–6
  occupational hazards 1465–6
  physiology 1147–9
  toxic mechanisms 1149–55
feminization 654, 862, 1226–7
femoral blood concentrations 1495, 1504
femur 341
Fenton reaction 633, 641
feral animals *see* wildlife species
fermentation
  peroral toxicity 545
  plants, source of biological hazards 1459
  process, biopharmaceutics regulations 1973

ferret
  black-footed ferret (*Mustela nigripes*) 1347
  Siberian (*Mustela evermanni*) 1346
  studies 45, 110, 2199
ferritin 2065
ferrochelatase 392, 1864, 1906, 2056
fertility 465
  see also reproductive system
  cycle, toxicology 266
  female 1465
  and fungicides 2002
  male 62, 1464
    see also sperm quality
  and organic solvents 2041
  and radiation 1688, 1696
  reduced 1463
  study, Japanese requirements 1567
  toxic effects on 23–4
fertilization, regulation 1464
fertilizers 1371–2, 1383, 1514, 2114
fescue, tall (*Festuca arundinaceae*), reproductive system toxicity 1521
Festuca arundinacea see tall fescue
FETAX system *see* frog embryo teratogenesis assay: *Xenopus*
FEV *see* forced expiratory volume
fever 169, 235, 265
fibre inhalation 20
fibrinogen 264, 366, 2179
fibrinolysis 264, 385
fibroblasts 196, 315, *412*, 530, 567, 728, 810, 829
fibromyalgia 1703, 1710, 1714
fibronectin 342
fibrosis 6, 19, 807, 873–4
Fick's law 46, 143, 578, 582
fiddleback spider 2186
fiddleneck (*Amsinkia intermedia*), hepatoxicity 1519
field studies
  animal behaviour 1346
  definitive tests 1353–4
  ecology 1327
  EPA guidelines 1353
  granular formulations 1350
  non-destructive sampling 1345
  population estimation 1353
  screening tests 1353–4
  statistical analysis 1353
  test design 1354

FIFRA *see* Federal Insecticide, Fungicide and Rodenticide Act
figure-of-eight mazes 651
filamin, as calpain substrate 189–90
fillers 2014, 2022
filter cages 514
fine needle aspiration 344
finger-prick blood samples 19
fingernails *see* nails
Finland
  BALs 1910, 1911
  nitrate, nitrite and *N*-nitroso levels 2114, 2118, 2132
Finnish Institute of Occupational Health 666
fire ants (*Solenopsis* spp.) 2184
fire coral jellyfish 2190
fire extinguishers 460
firefighters
  risks 1821, 2033
  toxicity studies 1916, 1920, 1926–9
fires
  see also combustion
  airport 1821–2
  atmosphere in 1916–17, 1920–4
  combustion products 1915–16, 1924
  deaths in 1494–5, 1917
  disasters 1821–3
  exposure tests 24–5
  hazard investigation 1924–7
  incapacitating factors 1920
  nature and toxicity of atmospheres 1917–19
fireworks 1524
first-aid management 22
first-order reactions 69, 73, 74, 75, 79–80, 84
first-pass metabolism 22, 56, 69–70, 545, 548, 552
fish
  acute toxicity studies 38
  alternative testing 407
  aluminium toxicity 1379
  and apoptosis 178
  arsenic levels 2052
  biomarker 1852, 1866, 1867, 1869
  CHD and 1980
  dioxin 281
  environmental endocrine effects 1407
  environmental oestrogen effects 1565

fish (*Contd.*)
  farming 1548, 1648
  gonadal recrudescence assay
    1403, 1408
  heterocyclic amines 271
  ingestion, risk assessments 1780,
    1785
  liver oils 1552
  mercury toxicity 1249, 1310,
    1826, 2057–8
  MRLS 1646, 1647
  nitrate, nitrite and *N*-nitroso
    levels 2114, 2115, 2116, 2117,
    2118, 2120, 2132
  oil spillage and 1826–7
  phenol metabolism 111
  poisonous 2191–4
  pollutants in 1870
  predatory 1378, 1379
  scombrotoxic 1554
  stinging 2191–2
  toxicology studies 45, 790, 1311,
    1314, 1316, 1318, 1319–20
  vitellogenin 1407, 1408
Fish and Wildlife Service (USA)
  1331, 1332
fish-eating human populations,
  methylmercury exposure 1379
fish-eating wildlife species 1329,
  1339–440
fish-odour syndrome 233–4
Fisheries Act (Canada, 1971) 1311
fishermen, risk assessment 1775,
  1780, 1826, 1830
Fisher's exact test 300, 301
fit *see* seizure
fitweed (*Corydalis* spp.),
  neurotoxicity 1520
five-day dietary tests 1335–6
fixation 336, 338, 339
fixed dose procedures 44, 326
flame, trauma from 1916
flame photometry 367
flame retardants 2014, 2022
flaming, combustion 1916
flashover 1822
flatulence 40
flavin (FAD), reduction 104
flavin monooxygenase (FMO) 102,
  216, 232–3, 725
flavoprotein cofactors 103
Flavor and Extract Manufacturers'
  Association 1658
flavours and flavour enhancers
  1985, 1988

regulatory aspects 1552, 1653,
  1654, 1655, 1656–7
flea and tick control products,
  toxicity 1510
flip-flop kinetics 75
floating necrosis 872
floor and furniture waxes 1295
flounder, European (*Platichthys
  flesus*) 1870
flour *see* cereals
fluctuation tests 1048
fluidized beds 597
fluorescein
  flare 746
  fundus angiography 764
  permeability 751
  retention 752
  staining 746, 751, 752
fluorescence microscopy 346,
  781–2
fluorescence spectrometry *680*,
  1882, 1889
fluorescent polarization
  immunoassay (FPIA) 1502
fluoridation, water 1534
fluoroacetyl coenzyme A 6
fluorochromes 1848
fluorometer 750
fluorophotometry 746
flushing 114, 460
flux 578, 582
fly
  see also Drosophila
  house 259
FMO polymorphisms 233–5
foaming agents 1985
FOB *see* functional observational
  battery
focal adhesion kinase (FAK2), and
  apoptosis 195
focal granulomatous plaques 532
focal hyperplasia, incidence 296
focal myopathies 946–7
focal necrosis 539
fodrin 189–90, 195
foetal alcohol syndrome 660, 757,
  758, 2040
foetal development 1465
  biomarkers 1465
  and lead 1487
  PCBs damage 642
  regulation 1464
  stages and types of effects
    1218–22
foetal distress syndrome 1427

foetal exposure and eye toxicity
  758–9
foetal heart rate 1216
foetal loss 1465, 1466, 1530
  see also abortion, spontaneous
foetal malformation, in mouse
  inhalational study 604
foetal metabolism 1240
foetal metallothionein gene
  expression 2067
foetal Minamata disease 1249
foetal toxicity *see* foetotoxicity
foetotoxicity
  arsenic 2051
  CO 1921–2
  dioxin 282, 1818
  firefighters 1929
  food contamination 1825
  fumonisins 2164
  fungicides 2002, 2003
  interspecies variation 281
  lead 1205, 2055, 2057
  lithium 1205–6
  mercury 2057, 2058, 2059
  methylmercury 1204
  nitrites 2128, 2135
  non-lethal 8
  organic solvents 2041
  placental toxicity 1243
  radiation 1696, 1697
  reproductive studies 23
foliage, herbicide/pesticide residues
  1341, 1349, 1518
follicle stimulating hormone (FSH)
  986–7
  as biomarker 1858
  breast cancer surgery 266
  dioxin effects 163
  female 1147, 1148, 1151, 1155
  male 1141, 1143
follicular cell tumours in plastics
  industry 2022
follicular dendritic cells (FDC)
  1000
follow-up period, cohort studies
  1531
food 316–17
  see also nutrition
  allergies 1706, 1986
  cardiotoxic materials in 823
  consumption 39, 61, 63, 83, 84,
    1846, 1855, 1859
  contamination
    accidental 1824–5
    adulteration 1823–4

food

Fusarium spp. (*Contd.*)
  mycotoxins 1516
   F. nygamai 2163
   F. solani 726
   F. subglutinans 2163
Fusobacterium 563
FVC *see* forced vital capacity

G

G1-S phase 260
G2-M phase 260
GABA *see* γ-aminobutyric acid
GADD 153, 167, 168
gait abnormality 40, 41, 1997
galactorrhoea, adverse drug reaction
  1430
galactose, and apoptosis 183
galactosidase, as biomarker 1862
galactosylhydroxylysine, as
  biomarker 1859
Galen 35, 460
gallbladder
  passage of drugs and chemicals
   557
  tumours 2018
gallstones 898, 899, 1843
Gallus domesticus see chicken
Gambierdiscus toxicus 819, 2191
game species
  cadmium levels 1375, 1378
  feeding trials 1330
  mercury concentration 1355
  xenobiotic tolerance 1337–8
gametogenesis, regulation 1464
gangrene 1382, 1516
  see also necrosis
gap junctions 779, 806, 810, 854
garbage toxicity, domestic animals
  1512–13
Gardener's syndrome 1034
gardening, biomonitoring 1780
Gardner hypothesis 1695
garlic as antioxidant 1984
gas chromatography 597, 1491
gas chromatography–mass
  spectrometry (GC–MS) 597,
  1499–500, 1503, 1504
gas masks for CB attack 1729
gas stoves 1278, 1279, 1296
gas–liquid chromatography (GLC)
  367, 1499, 1500, 1502–3
gases
  see also war gases
  absorption 589–90

aliphatic 2034
atmosphere analysis 597
atmosphere generation 594
biomonitoring 1907
exposure 20
incidents, risk of death 1830
indoor air pollutants 1296–8,
  1303
inorganic 1296
lake emissions 181
mixtures 315–16
mortality data 1834–5, 1917
in repeated exposure studies 60
rubber industry emissions 2015
sampling 597
toxicity 46
uptake, PBPK modelling *146,
  148–9*
volcanic 1815
gasping 41
Gasserian ganglia 347
gastric, *see also* gastro-intestinal
gastric acid secretion 227
gastric cancer *see* stomach cancer
gastric contents 1495, 1504
gastric fluids, bench-scale extraction
  experiments 1777–8
gastric mucosa 108, 547
gastric parietal cells 365
gastric secretion 546
gastric ulcer 227, 236, 2061
gastrin 365, 546, 547
gastro-enteric target 524–6
gastro-intestinal tract
  see also specific areas, e.g.
   stomach
  absorption 19
   aluminium 2060
   cadmium 2052–3
   lead 2055
   mercury 2058
   parenteral toxicity 521, 523
   peroral toxicity 552
   tin 523
   toxicokinetics 67, 69, 75
   zinc 2066
  atresia 1348
  cancer 235, 2002
  clinical chemistry 364–7
  epithelium 338, 343
  flora 561–76
   detoxification 569–71
   factors affecting metabolism
    and toxicity 571–3
   human 1645

and parenteral toxicity 521,
  522
and peroral toxicity 555, 556
protective effects 569–71
species differences and
  metabolism 572
haemorrhage 132, 282, 458
and idiopathic environmental
  intolerance 1704
and metabolism 98
mucosa 105, 339, 551
nitrobenzene reduction 104
and parenteral toxicity 522, 530,
  532
pathology 343
PBPK studies 89–90
pH 252
toxicity
  adverse drug reactions 1427,
   1438
  arsenic 1515, 2051
  copper 1380
  domoic acid 2193
  fish poisoning 2192
  food additives 1986
  food contamination 1825
  garbage poisoning 1512–13
  herbicides 2004, 2006
  horses 1519
  houshold product ingestion
   1512
  iron 2065
  lead 1475
  mushrooms 1513
  mycotoxins 1516
  nitrates 2119
  nitrites 2120
  nitrogen 1514
  potatoes 1984
  radiation 1684, 1685, 1686,
   1687, 1689
trace element uptake deficiency
  2049
ulceration 363, 365, 524, 525,
  1430
gastro-oesophageal junction, in
  peroral toxicity test 553
gatekeepers, trial judges 1949
gaussian distribution 11, 12, 322,
  1785
gavage 55, 59, 549, 550, 551
  acute toxic response 555
  dosing 67, 75, 554, 604
  oesophageal injury to treated rats
   553–4

geeldikkop 2148
GEES *see* generalized estimating equations
gel electrophoresis *219*, 1845
gel filtration 363
gelatin capsules 549
gelling agents 1985
Gelsemium spp. *see* Carolina jessamine
gelsolin, and apoptosis 195
gender differences
    AITC 134
    and behaviour 664
    cadmium toxicity 1374, 2053
    enzyme induction 2033
    in idiopathic environmental intolerance 1707
    metabolism 111
    nephropathy 129
    nitrate intakes 2116
    nucleus of the preoptic area 1406
    pesticide sensitivity 1338
    radiation toxicology 1683, 1692
    and response to toxic agents 1343, 1416
gene–environment interactions 215
General Agreement on Tariffs and Trade (GATT) 1569, 1611, 1649
general drug screen (GDS) 1502, 1503
general population *see* population
generalized estimating equations (GEES) 1178
generally recognized as safe (GRAS) 725, 1563, 1658
genes
    see also specific genes
    amplification 339, 1967
    developmentally relevant 1190–1
    dosage 162
    expression 53, 169
    families 99
    loci 236
    mapping 1091
    mutation *see* mutagenicity
    new variants 215
    phenotypes and genotypes 218
    rearrangements 340
    and regulation of apoptosis 193
    sequencing 1548
    stress-related 167
    superfamily 216–18
    transcription activation 126, 2067

genetic abnormalities
    biochemistry 126, 128
    as biomarker 1848, 1849
    from radiation 1683, 1693, 1695
    molecular concepts 157, 162, 163, 168
genetic code 1017, *1018*
genetic engineering 1963
genetic factors
    in acetylation 108
    affecting drug effects 110
    and metabolism 111–12
    and response to toxic agents 1338, 1416
genetic manipulation 135
genetic modification 1454, 1553
    see also genetic enginering
genetic polymorphisms
    see polymorphisms
genetic predisposition 461
genetic risks, in radiation studies 1694
genetic screening 235
genetic toxicology
    guidelines 1038–9, 1061
    in vitro test systems 1039–58
    interpretation of data 1064–5
    mammalian mutation tests 1051–6, 1058–61
    restriction site mutation analysis 1062
    tissue-specific genetic polymorphisms 1061–2
    transgenic models 1062–4, 1111–14
genetic variants 238
genetically engineered products, testing 1463
genetically modified organisms (GMOs) 1459, 1548, 1560, 1584, 1628, 1629
genetically susceptible subpopulations 28–9
genetics, applied 1963
Geneva Protocol 2080
genito-urinary cancer in firefighters 1928, 1929
genomic instability radiation-induced 1695–6
genotoxic carcinogens 8, 874, 1101–6, 1114, 1434
    see also rodent carcinogenicity tests
genotoxic chemicals 7, 1484

genotoxic initiators 7
genotoxicity 8
    2-naphthylamine 134
    arsenic 2051
    bioassays 1460
    biochemistry 128
    biomarker 1845
    biomonitoring 1906–7
    dose extrapolation 1766
    firefighters 1929
    fumonisins 2165
    human studies 465
    Japanese test battery 1567
    medical devices 1734, 1735, 1742
    nitrites 2128
    ochratoxins 2160
    organic solvents 2040
    PBPK modelling 1770
    plastics industry 2020
    risk assessment 1750
    rubber industry 2015
    testing 24, 1435, 1448
        EU requirements 1622
        extrapolation 1435, 1448
        harmonization 1573
        new pharmaceuticals 1617, 1618–19
        new substances 1591
        replacement tests 499
    toluene exposure 1456
genotype 218, 1850
GENSTAT statistical program 301
geographic distribution 1527
geographical location 1910
geometric mean 1781, 1782
George III, King 1849
gerbil, aminophenol hydroxylation 110
Gerbillinae, interspecies differences 283
germ cells
    acrosome 345
    assays 1086, 1088
    chromosomes 1145
    damage from radiation 1684, 1688, 1692
    pathology 336
germ layer differentiation 8
German Society of Experimental and Clinical Pharmacology and Toxicology 1943
germander (*Teucrium* spp.), adverse effects 1427

Germany
  BALs 1910, 1911
  Biologische Bundesanstalt für
    Land- und Forstwirtschaft
    (BBA) 1607
  CB agent threat 1724
  chemical warfare 2079, 2080,
    2100
  classification and labelling 1477
  MAK values 1483–4, 1594
  nitrate and nitrite levels 2112,
    2114, 2116, 2117, 2118, 2131,
    2132
  Technische Richtkonzentrationen
    (TRK) values 1484, 1594
  toxicology education 1943
germinal follicles 341
GESAMP (Working Group on the
  Evaluation of Harmful Substances
  Carried by Ships) 1310–11
gestation 23, 758–9, 1696
Gettler, Alexander O. 1490–1
GFR *see* glomerular filtration rate
GGTP *see* γ-glutamyl transpetidase
GH *see* growth hormone
Giemsa stain 341
Gila monster (*Heloderma horridum*;
  H. suspectum) 2181–2
ginger paralysis 1824
glabrous skin 829, 830
glandular stomach 546, 556
glass fibre emissions 1293
glass for samples, contamination
  from 1909
glaucoma 20, 757
glaucopsia 738
glazing agents 1653, 1985
glial cells 347, 631, 632, 634, 643
glial fibrillary acid protein 347
GLIM statistical program 301
glioma, *N*-nitroso compounds 2132
gliosis 631
GLOBAL dose–response computer
  programs 1764, 1771
global revolutionary group 1728
globulins 253, 367, 368, 897
  see also microglobulins
glomerular basement membrane
  336
glomerular filtration 255–6, 257,
  362, 428, 684, 686, 1462
glomerular function 72, 362
glomerular mesangial cells 183
glomerular permeability 363

glomerulonephritis, mercury-
  induced 682
glomerulus 345, 363
*Glossary for Chemists of Terms used
  in Toxicology* 1811–12
glove powder 510
gloves 510, 583
GLP *see* good laboratory practice
D-glucaric acid as biomarker 1865
glucocorticoid receptor-binding
  protein 2066
glucocorticoids 187, 188, 1869
glucogenesis 283, 939
glucose
  as biomarker 1861
  conjugation 107
  homeostasis 283
  levels following CO_2 in rats 61
  necrosis prevention 166
  plasma measurements 365
  uptake, organ of Corti 790
  urine levels *see* glycosuria
glucose transporters 779
glucose-1-phosphate,
  glucuronidation 106
glucose-6-phosphatase 383, 391,
  868, 872
glucose-6-phosphate dehydrogenase
  28, 159, 337, 344, 384, 2187
β-glucosidase 566, 571–2
glucosuria 683
  see also glycosuria
glucuronic acid 18, 106, *107*, 111,
  116, 132, 236, 371, 862, 1866
β-glucuronidase 272, 556, 568–9,
  572, 1228
glucuronidation 98, 106–7, 114,
  115, 255, 568
glucuronosyl-*S*-transferases (GST)
  markers 135, 1866, 1891
glues 1961, 2029, 2036
glutamate 166, *1878*
glutamate dehydrogenase 356, 359,
  1857
glutamate receptors 634
glutamine 106, *107*, 109
γ-glutamyl transferase (GGT) 107,
  363, 1849, 1862, 2059
γ-glutamyl transpeptidase (GGTP)
  43, 337, 344, 1255–6
γ-glutamylcysteinylglycine 107,
  130
glutaredoxin (GRX) 160

glutathione
  activities 255
  and apoptosis 191
  as biomarker 1842, 1848,
    1862–3
  biomarker 1842, 1843, 1891
  circadian toxicology 257
  conjugation 18, 98, 107, 116–17,
    121, 130, 131, *134*, 1865
  depletion 28, 158
  metabolism and 104, 105
  oxidative stress and 158
glutathione peroxidase 127, 158,
  793, 1276, 1870
glutathione reductase 104, 729,
  793, 1857, 1868–9, 1870
glutathione *S*-transferase
  biomarker 1850, 1865, 1868,
    1870
  biotransformation 107, 115, 118
  catalysis 130
  clinical chemistry 359, 363
  in epidemiology 1537–8
  hepatotoxicity 871
  interspecies extrapolation 279
  pathology 344
  pharmacogenetics 281
glutathione-protein mixed
  disulphides 159
glutathione/GSSG ratio 191, 255,
  1868–9
S-glutathionylation reactions 160
gluten-free products 1553
glyceraldehyde-3-phosphate
  dehydrogenase 160, 1843
glycine 18, 109, 111
glycocholic acid, as biomarker
  1858
glycogen 862, 1861
glycogen phosphorylase b 160
glycolysis 357, 939
glycoproteins, as biomarker 1856
glycosaminoglycan metabolism 758
glycosuria 332, 362, 679, 686, 689,
  690, 1862
GM-CSF *see* granulocyte–
  macrophage colony-stimulating
  factor
GMOs *see* geneticaly modified
  organisms
gnotobiotic animal studies 1645
goat *216*, 371, 579, 1515
Gobius criniger see goby, Pacific
goblet cells 545, 755, 1690

goby, Pacific (*Gobius criniger*) 2193
goitre 1430, 1983
goitrogens 1121–3
golden hamster *see* hamster
goldenrod, rayless (*Haplopappus heterophylus*) neurotoxicity 1520
goldfish, monochromatic stimuli 661
Goldner trichrome 342
golf courses 1329, 1523
Golgi apparatus 860, *861*, *862*, 864
Gomori's stain 341
gonadosomatic index 1408, 1870
gonadotoxins *989*
gonadotrophic hormones 371, 980, 982
   see also follicle stimulating hormone (FSH); luteinizing hormone (LH)
gonads 23, 1684, 1696
Goniopora spp. *see* coral
Gonyaulax spp. 2192
Good Agricultural Practice 1548, 1574, 1610
Good Clinical Practice 465, 1562, 1622, 1623
Good Laboratory Practice (GLP)
   advisory leaflets (UK) 439
   applications to computer systems 450
   appropriate clothing 443
   archives 449–50
   clinical chemistry 358, 373
   current standards 438–40
   and EPA 1561, 1563–4, 1591
   epidemiology 1528, 1536
   EU requirements 1609, 1621–2
   extrapolation studies 1436
   facility management 440
   human studies 465
   laboratory areas 444
   medical devices 1663, 1664
   mouse dermal toxicity test 605
   occupational toxicology 1406
   OECD 1570, 1591, 1601
   pathology techniques 337
   peroral studies 550
   personnel education and training 443
   principal investigation 442
   principles 440–50
   quality assurance 437, 1664
   regulations 437, 448, 487, 1561

scope 440
standard operating procedures (SOPs) 440
statistics 293
study report 448–9
testing facility 444
toxicological studies 323–4
training records 448
Good Laboratory Practice Monitoring Authority (UK) 439
Good Manufacturing Practice 1622, 1649, 1655
good scientific practice 293
goose
   Canada (*Branta canadensis*) 1328, 1349
   greylag (*Anser anser*) 1341
gout 942, 943
government hearings 1945
GPT *see* γ-glutamyl transpeptidase
graded response 9
grading, skin irritation tests 844
grain *see* cereals
Gram-negative bacteria 1292, 1301, 1302
Gram-positive bacteria 1301
granular formulations of pesticides 1338, 1339, 1340, 1341, 1350
granulocyte–macrophage colony-stimulating factor (GM-CSF) 703, 999, 1000, *1002*, 1971, 2087
granulocytes 384–5, 1686, 1882, 1964
granulocytopenia 389, 394–5
granulocytopoiesis 385
granuloma, foreign-body 532
granzyme B, and apoptosis 193
grapefruit juice 21–2, 1427, 1429, 1865
graphical methods 49, 1941, 1951
grass *see* cereals
Graunt, John 1527, 1528
Gray PBPK model 1249
gray unit 1684
Greek ancient writings 1489, 1527
Greek Fire 2079
greenhouse effect 1451
Greenland *see* polar regions
grey literature 476–7
Griffonia simplicifolia isolectin B4 338
grinders, biomonitoring 1904
grip strength 41

gross indices 1846, 1855
groundcherry (*Physalis* spp.), neurotoxicity 1521
groundnut *see* peanut
groundsel (*Senecio* spp.)
   alkaloids 133
   hepatoxicity 1519
groundwater
   arsenic 1382
   cadmium 1377
   contamination, modelling 1772, 1773
   dispersion of toxicants 1832, 1833
   heavy metals 1369
   near waste disposal sites 1372
   nitrate 1382
   vinyl chloride 1770–1
grouper 2191
grouse
   sage (*Centrocercus urophasianus*), dimethoate toxicity 1343
   sharp-tailed (*Tympanuchus phasianellus*), aberrational behaviour 1348
grouting workers, acrylamide exposures 1587
growth, nutrients for 317
growth factor receptors, as calpain substrate 189–90
growth hormone (GH) 950, 970, 980, 1455, 1463
growth hormone deficiencies 1964
growth promoters 1524, 1549, 1554, 1648, 1649
growth retardation 1691, 1692, 1696, 1697, 2066
grp78 chaperone molecule 167
grp94 chaperone molecule 167
Grunwald/Giemsa stain 1087
GRX *see* glutaredoxin
GSH *see* glutathione
GST *see* glucuronosyl-*S*-transferases
GSTT1, as biomarker 1850
GTTI human gene 1538
Guam disease 635
guanine 128, 2084
guanylate cyclase 159
Guidance for Exposure Assessment 1781
Guidance for Industry on Single Dose Acute Toxicity Testing for Pharmaceuticals 40

guidelines
  endocrine disrupting effects 1400
  environmental 1763–4, 1770, 1775
  harmonization 1636
  in vitro cytogenetic assays (UK) 1081, 1083, 1084
  for testing 31, 1434–6
Guidelines for Testing of Chemicals 37
guinea pig
  aflatoxin LD_{50} 2154
  allergens 511
  aminophenol hydroxylation 110
  anaphylaxis 535
  arsenic metabolism 2050
  β-glucuronidase and β-glucosidase 572
  biliary excretion 555
  blepharospasm test *612, 613, 619, 620, 621, 623–4*
  brain FMO 232
  breathing rate 46
  cancer studies in rubber industry 2018
  chemical respiratory sensitization assessment 705–6
  cortisol as plasma maker 356
  CYP genes 216
  dermal studies 46
  developmental period 1696
  dioxin toxicity 85, 87, 282
  famciclovir conversion 239
  gastro-intestinal tract 544
  HDL fraction 367
  hepatocyte LD_{50} for dioxin 284
  hepatotoxicity marker 359
  hypersensitivity reactions 340
  interspecies differences 274–5, 283
  intravenous injection site 526
  LAA 511
  LD_{50} intravenous dosing 525
  lens 242
  liver 872
  model for interferon testing 1971
  nerve agents 2091, 2093
  nitrate toxicity 2124
  nitrite toxicity 2127–8, 2135
  organic solvents 2041
  ototoxicity studies 776, *778, 783, 789, 792, 794*
  pseudoeosinophils 385

repeated-dose studies 329
respiratory effects of sulphuric acid 1281
respiratory hypersensitivity 705
safety of biologicals 535
skin sensitization tests *841*, 842, 1005
stratum corneum skin permeability *579*
T_3 and T_4 concentration 371
Gulf War 2081
Gulf War syndrome 28, 2096
Gulf War Veteran's Illness, Presidential Advisory Committee 1729
gulls
  environmental endocrine effects 1407
  herring 654
  laughing (*Latrus atricilla*), aberrational behaviour 1348
  PCBs in 642
gut *see* gastro-intestinal tract
Gutierrezia microcephala
  see broomweed

H

h-gate 639, 640
Ha-ras, and apoptosis 189
Haber rule 327, 1834–5
Haber–Weiss reaction 633
habitat 1328, 1407
habituation, in motor activity *652*
haem
  iron absorption 2065
  metabolism 2068
  synthesis 1863–4, 2056
haem oxygenase isozyme-1 2066
haemabsorbents 1734–5
haemagglutination 338
haemangiomas 1248
haemangiosarcoma 1533, 2015
haemapoietic system tumours 2019
haematochromatosis 869
haematocrit 364, 387
haematology 39, 62
  acute toxicity 39
  insecticide studies 2000
  in long-term toxicity studies 331–2
  in repeated exposure studies 61, 62, 63
  test abnormalities 389–96

haematopoiesis
  and apotosis 179, 191
  haematology 383–4, 391
  and hepatotoxicity 865
  pathology 336, 341
  pharmacogenetics 240
  radiation-induced changes 1684, 1685, 1686, 1696
  signs of toxicity 43–4
haematopoietic stimulating factors 1971
haematotoxicity
  adverse drug reactions 1427, 1438
  benzene 1475
  lead 1475, 1513
  nitrobenzene 104
  organic solvents 2033, 2041
  pharmacogenetics 241
  rodenticide toxicity 1511
  snake venom 2179
haematoxylin staining 345
haematuria 43
haemochromatosis 902, 2065
haemocompatibility of medical devices 1735, 1741
haemoconcentration 357
haemodyalysis 941
haemoglobin (Hb)
  abnormal 384
  adducts, as indicators of exposure 1457
  in antidotal studies 429
  biomarker 1845, 1879–80, 1883–4, 1890, 1892–3
  carbon monoxide binding 430, 1282, 1921
  and cardiotoxicity 821
  clinical chenistry 358, 364
  foetal 394
  genotyping 1890–1
  glycosylated 365
  in haematology 384, 387
  physiology 392
  Soret band 368
  synthesis, biomonitoring 1906
haemoglobinuria 367
haemolysis
  and alternative testing 410, 413
  clinical chemistry 357
  in haematology 383
  nitrobenzene effects 104
  oxidant effects 28
  test for synthetic materials 1741
haemolytic anaemia 384, *390*, 391

haemolytic jaundice 360
haemoperfusion 425, 724
haemorrhage
  alveolar 728
  brain 1217
  clinical chemistry 367
  conjunctival 742
  gastro-intestinal tract 132, 282, 458
  kidney 344
  pericardial 807
  radiation-induced 1686, 1688
  subendocardial 814
  traumatic 539
haemorrhagic cystitis 1430
haemorrhagic pancreatic necrosis 899
haemosiderosis 535
haemostasis 385
Hague Convention 2079
Hahnemann, Samuel 2
hair
  analysis 1496
  autopsy samples 1495
  biomonitoring 606, 1907
  contaminated 1355
  depigmented 1515
  elimination via 18, 72
  follicles 46, 256, 577, 830, 847
  and indoor air pollution 1300
  LAA 511
  loss 1511, 1515, 1519
  mercury levels 2059, 2060
  removal 46
hair cells, organ of Corti (HCs) 776–8, 780, 782–7, 788–95
hair dyes and products 230, 1550
hair/beauty establishements
  see service industries
Halabja chemical war effects 2080
Haldane coefficient 393
half-life
  absorption 69
  as biomarker 1879
  biomonitoring 1905–6
  data in risk assessment 1780, 1792
  elimination, calculation 86
  human studies 462
  interspecies 51
  reducing 97
  relationship to clearance 79–80
  scaling factors 1769
  short-range toxins 131
  terminal 77, 84

toxicokinetics 73–4
  using MRT 85
Haliaeetus leucocephalus see eagle, bald
Halichondria spp. *see* sponges, marine
Halley, Edward 1528
hallucinations from solvent abuse 2029, 2036
halogen atoms, oxidation 101
Halotegon spp., nephrotoxicity 1522
ham, nitrate and nitrite levels 2113
hamster
  see also Chinese hamster ovary (CHO) cells
  acetaminophen toxicity 110
  aflatoxin toxicity 2154
  aminophenol hydroxylation 110
  arsenic toxicity 2050, 2051
  brain FMO 232
  cadmium toxicity 2054
  cancer studies in plastics industry 2019
  CYP genes 216
  developmental period 1696
  dioxin toxicity 85, 282
  gallium toxicity 2063
  gene mutation assay 24
  β-glucuronidase and β-glucosidase 572
  hepatotoxicity testing *417*
  indium toxicity 2063
  interspecies differences 274–5, 283
  LAA 511
  laryngeal tumours 525
  lung culture *417*
  NAT enzymes 108
  nitrate toxicity 2126
  nitrite toxicity 2127
  NOS 2119
  ochratoxin toxicity 2160
  oestrogen effect on liver 284
  tamoxifen protection against hepatocarcinogenesis 284
hand
  percutaneous 577, 578, 583
  washing, and response to toxic agents 1417
Haplopappus heterophylus
  see goldenrod, rayless
haptens 705, 835–6
haptoglobin 254
hard metal 1904, 2063, 2064

hardeners, in plastics industry 2022
harm criterion 1812, 1829, 1830, 1831
harmonization
  see also International Conference on Harmonization
  of classification systems 1478
  Council of Europe 1571
  of drug safety regulations 1426, 1430, 1431–4, 1622
  European 1572, 1590, 1654
  guidelines 1636
  international 37–8, 55, 1611, 1662
  Nordic Community 1572
  OECD 1572, 1612
  of pesticide regulations 1605, 1611
  of regulatory issues 1546–7, 1604, 1648–9
  of toxicological testing requirements 1567
Harmonized Electronic Dataset 1480
harrassment, peripheral sensory irritant effects 615
hawk, red-tailed (*Buteo jamaicensis*) 1342, 1355
HAZARD 1 Fire Hazard Assessment Method 1927
Hazard Communication Standard 37, 1477
hazard index 312–13, *313*, 1787
hazard quotient 312, 1786–7
hazardous exposures, routes and nature 509–10
Hazardous Materials Transportation Act (USA) 37
Hazardous Substances Act (USA) 37
Hazardous Substances Data Bank 481, 1677
hazardous wastes, sites 669
hazards 1811–12
  acute 1338–44
  affected by physical agents 1418–19
  analysis 27–9, 38, 1927
  anthropogenic 1328–30
  assessment 475
  classification and labelling 36–7, 1476–8, 1610, 1675
  definition 34, 1449, 1811
  EU criteria 1486, 1557

hazards (*Contd.*)
  evaluation 554–7, 1318, 1332,
    1415–24, 1449–50
  identification 314, 456, 1460,
    1461, 1476–8, 1536–8, 1753–8
  impact severity 1960
  prediction, probabilistic methods
    1328
  relationship to risk 1812
  risk assessment *1829*
Hb *see* haemoglobin
HBV *see* hepatitis B virus
HCs *see* hair cells, organ of Corti
HDL *see* high-density lipoprotein
  cholesterol
head
  male adult skin surface area *583*
  trauma 636
head-only exposure 46
headache 43, 454, 460, 515
headlice 460, 1995
headspace generation 594
health, vs survival 1961
health care workers
  biological hazards 1459
  cytotoxic material studies 515
  exposure to medical devices
    1679
  laboratory hazards 510
  reproductive risks 463
health effects, planning 1832
Health Effects Assessment Summary
  Tables 1759
health guidance values, UK 1486
Health Industry Manufacturers
  Association (HIMA) 1743
health information systems 1661–2
health insurance, permitted/
  proscribed lists 1544–5
health products, toxicological effects
  1552
Health Protection Branch, Health
  Canada 1659
Health Research Extension Act 487
health risk
  assessment 147–8, 1461–2
  assessment *see mainly* risk
    assessment
Health and Safety at Work Etc. Act
  1974 (UK) 1481, 1545, 1547,
  1595–6
Health and Safety Commission
  (UK) 1481, 1594, 1595

Health and Safety Executive (UK)
  459, 1486, 1545, 1590, 1594,
  1595, 1695, 1812
Health and Safety Guides (IPCS
  publications) 1571
Health and Safety Laboratory (UK)
  1910
health and safety regulations 36–7
health status 1416, 1504–5,
  1509–10, 1531
health supplements 1550, 1551,
  1552, 1567
health surveillance 467, 1485–6
health surveys 461–4
healthy human volunteers 1546,
  1547
healthy worker effect 1532, 1535
hearing loss 643, 655, 784, 785,
  786, 787–95
hearing problems 130
heart 343
  see also cardiac; cardio-;
    coronary heart disease;
    myocardial; myocardium
  anatomy *804*, 805
  block 43
  blood, forensic sampling 1495,
    1496, 1504
  clinical chemistry 365–7
  disease 1427, 1456, 1928
  embryology 803–4
  enzyme distribution 1857–8
  failure, congestive 285, 366,
    808, 812
  left atrium 805
  left ventricle 343, 805
  muscle, biomarker 1848
  normal contraction 805–6
  NQO2 in 240
  oxidation in 103
  radiation-induced changes 1691
  rate, as biomarker 1855
  right atrium 805
  right ventricle 805, 814
  and taurine 361
  weights 336, 343
heat 1343, 1418–19
heat inducible genes 2066
heat shock 169, 196
  cognate protein 2066
  elements 2066–7
  factors (HSFs) 167, 2066
  proteins (hsp)
    and apoptosis 193

  as biomarkers 1842, 1848,
    1869
  environmental enzyme toxicity
    1395
  interspecies variation 281
  metal toxicity 2066–7
  molecular concepts 163, 167,
    168, 169
heating appliances 1278, 1300
heating, ventilation and air
  conditioning (HVAC) systems
  515, 1293–5, 1300
heavy metals 3, 58, 1712, 1848,
  1868
  see also metals
HEDSET *see* Harmonized
  Electronic Dataset
Heinz bodies 384, 391, 393
HeLa cells 410, 2157
Helenium spp. *see* sneezeweeds
Helicobacter pylori infection 562
heliotrope (*Heliotropum* spp.) 133,
  1519
hellebore
  false (*Veratrum*) 818
  false (*Veratrum californicum*),
    reproductive system toxicity
    1521
Helly's fluid 345
Heloderma see Gila monster
helper T cells 341, 1704
Helsinki declaration on human
  experiment 1958
HEMASTIX reagent strip 495, 496
hemlock (*Conium maculatum*) 34,
  1521
hen *see* chicken
henbane (*Hyoscyamus niger*),
  neurotoxicity 1521
Hep-G$_2$ cells, and apoptosis 191
hepatectomy, partial 284
hepatic, *see also* liver
hepatic angiosarcoma, adverse drug
  reaction 1430
hepatic circulation *see* liver,
  circulatory system
hepatic cytochrome P450 255, 272
hepatic injury *see* hepatotoxicity
hepatic microsomal oxidase 255
hepatic mixed function oxidase
  activity 58
hepatic monoesterase 1337, 1339,
  1342, 1345
hepatic monooxygenase 1329, 1334
hepatitis 132, 236, 1427, 2064

hepatitis B (HBV) 274, 1100
hepatocarcinogenesis
see also specific carcinogens, e.g.
aflatoxins in the Chemicals
Index
aflatoxin B1 278
biomarkers 1869
circadian toxicology 259
interspecies variation 271, 275
oestrogen induced 284
and parenteral toxicity 526
protective clinical trials 278
hepatocarcinoma
and aflatoxins 1538, 1982, 2145,
2153–4
aromatic amines 120
benzopyrene 130
diet effects 58
epidemiological studies 274
and mycotoxins 1883
nitrites 2127
and peroral toxicity 551
pharmacogenetics 235, 240
in plastics industry 2022
rat and mouse 1127–9
in rubber industry 2018
in Thailand 278
and vinyl chloride 1456, 1475,
1538
hepatocellular hypertrophy 338
hepatocellular necrosis from snake
venom 2180
hepatocytes
in alternative testing 416, 418
apoptosis *179, 180, 181–2,* 198
biliary dysfunction *417*
biomarkers 1843, 1862, 1880
cadmium binding 2053
calcium homeostasis and 156
carbonic anhydrase III 160
clinical chemistry 359
damage marker 359
DNA 275
embryonic 865
enzyme induction and 113
functions 860–5
gap junctions 854
GST A1 induction 274
hypertrophy 344
incubation with tamoxifen 285
and laboratory occupational
toxicity 551
modelling 306
NOS and 2119
organocytosis 183

peroxisome proliferation *417*
relationship to sinusoid and
Kupffer cells *857*
structure 860, *861*
test system 407
in toxicological tests 271
hepatosomatic index 1870
hepatotoxicity
see also liver
acetaminophen (paracetamol)
110, 113, 116–17, 1427
activation of toxins 868–73
acute 868
adverse drug reactions 1427
aflatoxins 274, 1516
alkaloids 133
biomarker 1842, 1843, 1845,
1849, 1858, 1859, 1860, 1862,
1887
blue–green algae toxicity 1516
bromobenzene 100, 118, 133
carbon tetrachloride 16, 117–18
and cardiotoxicity 810
chloroform 111
chronic, agents causing 877
circadian toxicology 257
clinical chemistry 358
copper 2064
death from 15
dioxin 1818
dose–response relationship 56
ethanol 28, 199
evaluation 1462
food contamination 1825
fumonisins 2164–6
fungicides 2002
haloalkanes 121
hepatic enzyme inducers 135
herbicides 2005
in horses 1519
in vitro test systems *417*
isoniazid 119
marker 359
metabolism 133
methanol 119
neomycin 1455
and nephrotoxicity 691
nitrites 2126
NSAIDs 132, 136
nutrition effects on metabolism
115
OCs 1995
oestrogen-induced 284
organic solvents 2029, 2033,
2035–6, 2037, 2039, 2041

PCBs 1554
and peroral toxicity 551, 552
pharmacogenetics 230–1, 239
phenacetin 103
phomopsins 2148
plasma enzyme assessment 355,
361
predictability in animal tests
1438
protection from *201*
radiation 1684, 1685, 1690, 1696
repeated exposure studies 56
signs 43
solvents 133–4
sporidesmins 2148
and time of dosing 16
toluene 1456
toxic changes 867–84
toxic plants 1519
white phosphorus 1511
herbicides
aquatic toxicity 1313
circadian toxicity 259
domestic animal toxicity 1510,
1511–12
endocrine toxicity 990
groups 1998, 2003, 2004–6
and habitat quality 1328
interspecies variation 281
nestling studies 1349
neurotoxicity 638
pancreatic toxicity 927
pulmonary toxicity 43
in warfare 2105
hereditary effects from radiation
1684, 1692, 1693–6
hereditary thymine-uraciluria 235
heritable chromosome assays 1086
heritable defects and genetic
damage 1035–8, 1101
heritable translocation tests 1143
heron
black-crowned night-herons
(*Nycticorax nycricorax*) 1340
great blue (*Ardea herodias*) 1329
Herpes simplex 836
herring gull 654
Hershberger assay 1403
heterochomatin 160
heterophils 385, 539
heterozygosity 234
HGMP *see* Human Genome
Mapping Project (HGMP)
high-density lipoproteins (HDL)
367, 1978

high-dose effects *see* maximum tolerated dose (MTD), evaluation of
high-dose testing 1434
high-explosive (HE) shells 2102
high-molecular-weight substances, characteristics 1966
high-pressure liquid chromatography (HPLC) 597, 712, 1455, 1491, 1500, 1862, 1882, 2158
high-production-volume (HPV) chemicals 1480, 1585, 1587, 1592
high-throughput screens 1401, 1402
high-toxicity laboratory 515
Hill criteria 1755–6
HIMA *see* Health Industry Manufacturers Association
hippocampal granule cells 638
hippocampal responses to ischaemia 168
Hippocrates 35, 460, 472, 1841, 1849
Hiroshima 1692, 1693, 1697
his genes 1042
histamine decarboxylase 344
histamine-like substances, release radiation-induced 1688
histidine 24, 764, *1878*, 1882, 1883
histidine genes *see his* genes
histiocytes 532
histochemistry 337–8
histology 39, 61, 64
histology technicians, exposure to chemicals 515
histones 160–1, 190, 1880
histopathology 331, 335–7, 531, 539, 1846, 1847, 1856
   eye irritation tests 746
historical aspects
   biotechnology 1963–4
   chemical exposures 1474
   occupational exposure limits 1482
   toxicology 1–4, 35–6, 1489–91, 1731–2, 1935–6, 1944
   warfare agents 2079–81
history (patient), risk assessment development 1750
HIV *see* human immunodeficiency virus
hives 510
HL-60 cells, and apoptosis 199
HLA *see* human leukocyte antigen

HLA-DPB1 as biomarker 2061
Hodgkin's disease 395, 1692
Hohenheim, P.A.T.B. von 36
holding rooms for animals 58
hole in the head disease 2163
holocytochrome *c* 165
Holy Fire 2148
home environment, effect on toxicity 1415, 1416, 1417–18
Home Office (UK) animal studies statistics 38, 53
homeopathy 2, 1451, 1550
homeostasis 34, 159, 192, 370, 1397–8
homicide 543
   see also poisoning, homicidal
homocysteine, CHD and 1979
homogeneity tests, standard operating procedure (SOP) 446
honey 1646, 1647, 1984
honeybee 2182
hoof abnormalities, selenium toxicity 1519
hormesis 1397, 1445, 1451–2, 1951–2
hormone assays 981–3
hormone replacement therapy 458, 1398
hormones 879, *981*, 1395
   see also individual hormones
hornet 2182
horse
   arsenic toxicity 1518
   common toxicoses 1517–20
   CYP genes 216
   encephalomalacia 2145
   fumonisin toxicity 2164
   gastro-intestinal problems 1519
   lead toxicity 1518
   leukoencephalomalacia 1520, 2163
   liver failure 1519
   mycotoxin toxicity 1516, 1520
   nervous system disorders 1519
   nitrate/nitrites 1519, 2122, 2123
   plant toxicity 1518–19
   snake bites 1517
   stratum corneum skin permeability *579*
   sudden death 1519
   T_3 and T_4 concentration 371
horseradish 134
horseradish peroxidases 103
horsetail, neurotoxic to horses 1519

hospital
   admissions due to toxic exposures 1444
   needs in CB attack 1729
host-cell derived proteins, as impurities 1968
house dust mites 1302
household products
   see also cleaning products *in Chemical Index*
   adverse effects 1450
   allergy 1704
   classification and labelling 1589, 1603–4
   domestic animal toxicity 1510, 1512
   human studies 464
   N-nitroso compounds 2115
   potentially hazardous 1443
   regulatory aspects 37
   risk assessment 1444
housing
   conditions 58
   as exposure factor 604
Howell–Jolly bodies 391
HPLC *see* high-pressure liquid chromatography (HPLC)
HPV *see* human papilloma virus
HSF *see* heat shock factors
hsp *see* heatshock proteins
human activity, and soil composition 1329
human chorionic gonadotophin assays 1465
Human Fertilisation and Embryology Act 1990 454
Human Genome Mapping Project (HGMP) 1090–2
human immunodeficiency virus (HIV) 159, 636, 814, 1957
human leukocyte antigen (HLA) 1037
human papilloma virus (HPV) 1100
human populations, immunotoxicity 1005–6
human studies 25, 453–70
   see also interspecies extrapolation
   acute toxicity testing 33, 38, 55
   aluminium toxicity 1379, 2060
   anaesthesia 104
   antidotal assessment 433
   and apoptosis 178
   aquatic toxicology 1310
   barbiturate metabolism 111

human studies (*Contd.*)
  behavioural toxicity testing 666–9
  breathing rate 46
  bufarolol toxicity 115
  cadmium toxicity 2053–4
  carcinogenicity, prediction from animal testing 1536–8
  case surveillance 458
  case–control studies 455, 458
  ceftizoxime clearance 89
  cohort studies 455
  combustion studies 1926–7
  cyanide toxicity 1923
  cytochrome P450 enzymes 99
  data evaluation 455–6
  data sources 456–7
  developmental period 1696
  dioxin toxicity 87, 88, 90
  DNA repair deficiency syndromes 1033–4, 1101
  dose–response relationship 1534
  dosimetric scaling in 147
  effect studies 465–7
  environmental endocrine toxicity 1399–400
  environmental toxicity 1328, 1376–81, 1530–1, 1534
  epidemiological studies 455
  epithelial cells, apoptosis 199
  ethics 1535
  ethylene glycol toxicity 55
  exposure assessment case study 1778
  exposure to toxicity test 605–7
  eye toxicity 759
  factors affecting metabolism 109–10
  food chain contamination 1373, 1375, 1376
  furan toxicity 90
  genetic factors 110, 111–12
  genome mapping 216–17, 1090–2
  harmonization problems 1567
  hazard evaluation 28–9
  hepatic enzyme inducers 135
  hydrogen cyanide toxicity 2101
  hypothesis testing 455
  indoor air contaminants 1292–3, 1294
  irritant or allergic dermatitis 838–40
  isoniazid toxicity 119–20
  justification 464–5

  kinetic behaviour prediction 147
  latency period 456
  Lewsite effect 2088–9
  male adult skin surface area 583
  mercury levels 2058
  metabolism 146, 466–7
  methanol toxicity 119
  methodology 1536
  monitoring of environmental mutagens 1090
  MPTP toxicity 132
  NAT enzymes 108
  nephropathy 2154, 2159
  nerve agents toxicity values 2091
  nitrate, nitrite and *N*-nitroso compounds 2115–18, 2121, 2122, 2123, 2129–31, 2133–5, 2136
  nitrates, endogenous synthesis 2119–20
  nitrogen dioxide exposure 51
  organic solvents toxicity 2033–4, 2037
  organophosphate toxicity 955
  organophosphates 955
  percutaneous absorption 580
  pharmacokinetic studies 466–7
  pharmacology clinical trials 1616
  protein content 1869
  PSI studies 622–3
  quantitative evaluation 456
  radiation toxicity 1686, 1693, 1696
  relevant data 572
  riot control agents 2013
  risk assessment 1449–50, 1755
  safety margin calculations 91
  stratum corneum skin permeability 579
  sulphur mustard vapour effects 2084
  surveillance schemes 456–7
  synthetic materials sensitization tests 1740
  tissue preparations for safety evaluations 135
  toxicity data 453–70
  weight 51
humane animal research 493–501
humectants 1985
humidity 16, 58, 1419
humus 1367, 1368
Huntington's disease 166, 634, 636

Huskvarna, chronic renal disease 1428
Hussein, Sadam 1723, 1726
HVAC systems *see* heating, ventilation and air conditioning systems
hyaline droplets 63, 64, 691
hyberbaric oxygen therapy 1921
hybrid site-specific proteins 1966
hybridoma technology 1454, 1966
  see also biotechnology industries
Hydra attenuata 414, 1187
hydration 98, 105
hydrocarbon nuclear translocator protein 163
hydrocephalus 1217
hydrocortisone *see* cortisol
hydrogen bonds 613–14, 1369
hydrogen peroxidase 633
hydrogen peroxide 127, 1867, 1868
hydrological cycle 1370
hydrolysis 17, 98, 105, 110, 216, 254, 255, 523, 550
hydrophilic and hydrophobic species 547
hydroxybutyrate dehydrogenase, as biomarker 1860
17-hydroxycorticosteroid, as biomarker 1865
6β-hydroxycortisol, as biomarker 1865, 1867
hydroxyl radical 127
hydroxylation 100–2, 110, 112, 115, 221, 225, 226, 229, 230, 231, 240, 272, 273, 277
hydroxyproline, as biomarker 1859
20β-hydroxysteroid dehydrogenase 241
5-hydroxytryptamine 222, 236, 547, 632, 641, 706, 730, 815, 834, 956-7, 1960, 2039
Hydrozoa 2190
hygienic research 2013
hymenoptera 2182–5
Hymenoxys spp. *see* bitterweed
Hyoscamus niger see henbane
hyothalamic–pituitary–gonadal axis, assay 1403
hyper-responders 294
hyperactivity 41, 1986
  see also attention disorders
hyperaemia, in human subject PSI 623
hypercalcaemia, ECG/EKG profile *806*

hypercarbia 765
hypercholesterolaemia 823, 1978
hyperestrogeneism 2145
hypergastrinaemia 1125, 1126
hyperglycaemia, and adverse drug
    reactions 142
Hypericum perforatum see St John's
    wort
hyperinsulinaemia 815
hyperkalaemia 532
hyperlipidaemia 358, 364, 815,
    1427
hypernatraemia 364
hyperosmia in IEI 1708
hyperoxia 724, 728, 764, 765
hyperparathyroidism 900, 949–50
hyperplasia 556
hyperpnoea 41
hyperproteinaemia 367
hypersensitivity reactions
    acute toxicity 41
    in eye 20
    immunotoxicity 1004–5
    myocarditis 807
    systemic pulmonary toxicity
        726, 729
    to cosmetics 1550
    to drugs 21
    to snake venom 2180–1
    type I 510
    type IV 510
hypersusceptible (hyperreactive)
    groups 9, 12, 14, 1831, 1833,
    1835
hypertension 21, 264, 822, 823,
    1216
hyperthermia 6, 40, *522*
    see also heat
hyperthyroidism 948–9
hypertonia 40, 41
hypertrophy 685
hyperventilation 1709, 1713, 1714
hypervitaminosis A 969, 972
hypnotics *536*, 1491, 1495
hypoactivity 41
hypocalcaemia 365, 530
hypocarbia 1709
hypochlorhydria 562
hypochondria 1709, 1711
hypogammaglobulinaemia 562
hypoglossus nucleus 642
hypoglycaemia 283, 365, 458, *806*,
    982
hypoglycaemic drugs *220*, 228, 365
hypokalaemia 1430

hypokalaemic myopathy 940, 941,
    945
hypolipidaemic agents 367, 368,
    920, 922, 1978
hypomagnesaemia 683, 940
hyponatraemia 364
hypophosphataemia 940
hypopnoea 40
hypoproteinaemias 367
hyposusceptible (hyporeactive)
    groups 9
hypotension 944
hypothalamic–pituitary–endocrine
    axis *369*, 1400
hypothalamic–pituitary–ovarian axis
    372, 1147–8, 1151
hypothalamic–pituitary–testicular
    axis 371, 1140–1
hypothalamic-releasing hormones
    981
hypothalamus 251, 346, 347, *369*
hypothermia 40, *522*
    see also heat
hypotheses in toxicology 1939
hypothyroidism 949, 950
hypotonia 40, 41
hypovolaemic shock 822
hypoxaemia 26, 56, 1920
hypoxanthine-guanine
    phosphoribosyl transferase
    (HGPRT) 24
hypoxia 6, 168, 808, 969, 1216,
    1920

I

I-bands 938
Ia antigen 340
IAP, and apoptosis 195
IARC *see* International Agency for
    Research on Cancer
IATA *see* International Air Transport
    Association
iatrogenic disease 938, 1446
ICAD, and apoptosis 195
ICAO *see* International Civil
    Aviation Organization
ICE *see* interleukin-1-converting
    enzyme
ICH *see* International Conference on
    Harmonization
ichthyootoxic fish 2191
ichthypsarcotoxic fish 2191
ICRP *see* International Commission
    on Radiological Protection

ICSH *see* interstital cell stimulating
    hormone
icterus 360
ID_{50} 34–5, 52, 1876–7
idiopathic environmental illness
    (IEI) 1703–20
    aetiological theories 1704–7
    as behavioural phenomenon
        1707–9
    evaluation and diagnosis
        1711–13
    as illness belief system 1710–11
    as misdiagnosed illness 1709–10
    prevalence 1704
    research recommendations
        1715–16
    social and political implications
        1716–17
    treatment 1713–15
idiosyncratic reactions 4, 21, 1416,
    1549
IEI *see* idiopathic environmental
    illness
IFN *see* interferon
Ig *see* immunoglobulin
IH *see* inhibition concentration
Iito (fat storing/stellate) cells 864–5
IL *see* interleukin
IL-2 gene expression 191
ileum 562
illness belief system, IEI as
    1710–11
ILO *see* International Labour
    Organization
ILSI *see* International Life Sciences
    Institute
imaging systems 1661
imidazole *N*-methyltransferase *216*
immediate-type allergic reactions
    704
immersion fixation 339
immune haemolytic anaemia 1438
immune sensitization test for
    synthetic materials 1740
immune system 997, *998*
    cell mechanisms 998–1001
    cell-mediated responses 126
    compromised 1416
    cytokines 1001–3
    detecting changes 1969
    disorders, 5-HT inhibitors 1960
    functions, biomarker 1849
    immature 1337
    long-term effects 1446
    modulation 409

immune system (*Contd.*)
  related parameters 1008, 1009
  type 2 responses 710
immune-complex-type
  glomerulonephritis 682
immune-mediated reactions 6–7,
  19, 23, 178
immuno-allergic reactions 1444
immunoassays 367, 371, 514, 1491,
  1500–2
  see also enzyme-linked
    immunosorbent assay; enzyme-
    multiplied immunoassay
    technique
immunobiology, respiratory
  sensitization to chemicals 702–13
immunochemical analysis,
  macromolecular adduct 1885–7
immunocytochemistry 336, 338,
  339, 340, 342
immunoelectrophoresis 368
immunoenzymometric methods 365
immunogenicity 1964, 1967
immunogens 1302
immunoglobulins
  biomarker 1848
  Ig 999
  IgA 868
  IgE 510, 512, 682, 702–4, 705,
    999, 1004
  IgG 682, 1004
  IgM 1004
  and neonatal immunity 549
immunohistochemistry 237, 239,
  342
immunoinhibition methods 366
immunological testing, in IEI 1713
immunological theories, of
  idiopathic environmental
  intolerance
    aetiology 1704–5
immunoradiometric assays (IRMAs)
  983
immunosuppression 7, 85, 389,
  1003–4
  biomarkers 1862
  and carcinogenesis 1130, 1131
  fumonisins 2165
  haematotoxicity 389
  mycotoxins 1516
  myopathies 946, 948
  nephrotoxicity 684–5
  repercussions 7
  toxicokinetics 85
immunosurveillance 8

immunotherapy 428, 1967–8, 2184
immunotoxicology 997–1016
  animal studies 1005, 1006–9
  biomarkers 1875
  dioxin 87
  in human populations 1005–6
  hypersensitivity 1004–5
  immunosuppression 1003–4
  in vitro studies 1009–10, 1012
  molecular 1011–12
  ochratoxins 2160
  organometallic compounds 2001
  procedures 1967–8, 1974
  risk assessment 1756
  testing 1448
  wastes 1827–8
implant 60, 530, 1731, 1741
  see also medical device
implantation 539, 1464
imposex, molluscs 1407
impurities, importance in toxicology
  1445–6
in situ hybridization 239, 345
in vitro diagnostic devices 1661,
  1667
in vitro fertilization, legal
  restrictions 1547
in vitro studies 52–3, 401–24, 453,
  1449
  acute toxicity 52–3
  developmental toxicity 1184,
    1186–7, 1188, 1247
  genetic toxicology 1039–58
  haemolysis test for synthetic
    materials 1741
  human studies 453
  immunotoxicology 1009–10,
    1012
  in vivo correlations 1438
  metabolic activation 1039–41
  ototoxic effect of salicylates 786
  percutaneous absorption 580
  skin irritation and sensitization
    845–7
  toxokinetics 67
  UK guidelines 1081, 1083, 1084
in vivo studies
  design 44–5
  in vitro correlations 1438
  limitations *404*
  percutaneous absorption 579–80
  rationale *404*
inborn errors 234, 2049
incinerator emissions 606, 1776,
  1780

increased capillary fragility 385
indentation tonometry 749
independent effects of mixed
  chemicals 20
independent expert advice 1544,
  1562, 1578, 1638, 1658
independent joint action 304
index of exposure 128
Index Medicus 473, 478
indexing 474
India
  ancient writings 1489
  childhood cirrhosis 2064
  fumonisin contamination of
    cereals 2165
Indian cobra venom 820
indicative limits, EU 1595
indigenous compounds 1890
indigestion, in laboratory workers
  515
individual response 8, 135–6, 1708
indoor air, pollution 626
indoor air contaminants 1291–307
  building improvement plans
    1304
  gases 1296–8, 1303
  human health 1292–3, *1294*
  microbial 1303
  and outdoor (I/O) concentrations
    1291–2, 1295
  outdoor sources 1293
  particulates 1298–302, 1303
  sampling and characterization
    1302–3
  sick building syndrome (SBS)
    1292, 1299
  sources 1293–6
induction pathway 189
induction pathway *see mainly*
  enzyme induction
inductive period, skin sensitivity
  835
industrial accidents 737, 1547,
  1818–21, 1830
Industrial Bio-Test 437
industrial chemicals
  classification and labelling 1545,
    1551
  notification 1545
  occupational hazards 1550
  OECD inititatives 1571
  product information 1456
  as raw materials 1549, 1550
  regulatory aspects 1550–1,
    1581–90

industrial chemicals (*Contd.*)
EU 1556–7, 1590–6
Japan 1545, 1564
UK 1595–6
USA 1545
reproductive toxicity 1111,
1139–40, 1146, 1156, 1465
risk assessment and management
1460–1
safe working practices 1545,
1551
sperm evaluation studies 1467
spillages 1551
toxicological testing 1545, 1551
workplace exposure limits 1545,
1551
industrial effluents/emissions
environmental oestrogen effects
1565
field study evaluation 1352
and habitat quality 1328
Japanese experience 1564
treatment processes 1565
wildlife toxicity 1339, 1343
industrial hygiene data, IEI 1712
industrial hygienist 1458, 1530
industrial products, risk assessment
1444
industrial safety regulations 1960
industrial site evaluation 1772,
1792
industrial toxicology
see occupational toxicology
industrialized areas, pollution 316
industry, environmental effects
1328, 1373–4
Industry Health and Safety Law
1972 (Japan) 1565
infared thermography 844
infections 814, 2133
inferior olive nucleus 642
infinite dose situation 582
inflammatory agents, NOS induction
2120
inflammatory bowel disease 900
inflammatory mediators 1705,
1715–16
inflammatory response
and apoptosis 196
avoidance 176
as biomarker 1843, 1855
cellular effects 126
chronopathology 263
circadian toxicology 263
definition 6

dose–response relationship 9
eye 20
and idiopathic environmental
intolerance 1705–6
local effect 19
molecular concepts 169
and necrosis 164, 177
pathology 340, 343
peripheral sensory irritation 611
skin 837
to Lewisite 2089
to sulphur mustard 2085
influenza virus, biomarker 1849
influenza-like syndrome from PTFE
1915
information resources 471–83
see also databases
information sharing 1959
information sources, safety
assessment 1675–7
infradian frequency 251
infrared spectroscopy 597, 712
infusion techniques 522, 527–8
ingestion
see also peroral
of contaminated food and water
1339
standard assumptions 1773
workplace exposures 1474
inhalable fraction 461, 592
inhalant abuse 2029, 2038
inhalation 20
acute toxicity 46
aerosol container closure systems
1737
cadmium 2052, 2053
CB agents 1724
chamber 46
dosing 432, 523
exposure route 59, 60, 604,
1474, 1504
extrapolation from oral data 148,
1832
gases, mortality data 1834–5
hydrogen cyanide *2101*
lead 2055
mercury 2058
metabolites formed during
exposure 148
of mixtures 21
nickel 2063
nitrogen dioxide 51
organic solvents 2029
PBPK modelling 145, 1768

and peripheral sensory irritation
623
risk assessment 461
risks 1773, 1780
testing
determination of LC_{50} 49
interpretation of results 26
toxicology 20, 46, 588–601
vs percutaneous route 19
xenobiotics 1339
inherited cancer genes 1101
inherited somatic mutations 1538
inhibin B, as biomarker 1858
inhibition 305
concentration (IH) 1312
factor 584
initiator(s) 566, 2023
initiator, -promoter scheme 7
injection
fever 537
site, carcinogenesis 1130–1
subcutaneous 523
technique 526–7
injury without warning, peripheral
sensory irritation 615–16
innervation 545–6
innovatory products, definition
1623
inotropic effects 805, 808, 816, 818
Insecticide Act 1910 (USA) 1599
insecticides 2, 259, 460, 524, 641,
824, 1994–2000
*see also individual compounds in
Chemical Index*
biological origin 1999–2000
biomonitoring 1902
cardiotoxicity 824
circadian toxicology 259
domestic animal toxicity 1510
effects 651
and environmental toxicology 2
in food chain 1826
forensic analysis 1491
human studies 460
and invertebrate food base 1328
mammalian selectivity ratio
(MSR) 1547
metabolism 101
molecular interactions 163
neurotoxicity 43, 641
parenteral toxicity 524
placental toxicity 1242–5
poultry toxicity 1523

insecticides (*Contd.*)
  species sensitivity differences 110
  time course of effects 1956
  wildlife toxicity 1341
insects 38, 111, 178, 462, 1994, 1999–2000, 2182–4
insertion sequences 1027
Institute of Occupational Health (Finland) 1910
Institution of Chemical Engineers, hazard definition 1811
institutional animal care and use committee 487, 501–3
institutional review board 454
instrumentation, forensic toxicology 1491
insulin 346, 458, 522, 527, 530, 982, 991, 1455, 1965, 1966, 1969-70
  see also diabetogenic substances
insurance risk tables 1749
integrated field and laboratory studies 1354–5
Integrated Risk Information System (IRIS) 1759
Integrated Uptake and Exposure Biokinetic Model 1769
integrin, as calpain substrate 189–90
integumentary signs of toxicity 40
intellectual property rights 1569
interaction factor 313
interactive effects
  chemicals within cells 158
  drugs *see* under drugs
  mixed chemicals 20, 305, 306–13
  PBPK modelling 148–9
  toxic 1342–3
  zero response surfaces *310*
Interagency Coordinating Committee on the Validation of Alternative Methods 411
intercalcated discs 804, 813
interferons (IFN) 115, 703, 710–*11*, 999, 1002, 1455
intergeneric microorganisms 1584
Intergovernmental Forum on Chemical Safety 1592
interindividual *see* intraspecies
interlaboratory testing 16, 49, 626
interleukin-1 converting enzyme (ICE), and apoptosis 194, 195

interleukins 185, 1972
  after exposure to TMA *711*
  as biomarkers 1869
  in IEI 1704, 1706
  IL-1 265, 533, 722, 729, 864, 1000, 1001, 1002, 1012
  IL-2 265, 266, 341, 999, 1002, 1012
  IL-3 999, *1002*
  IL-4 682, 703, 999, 1000, 1002
  IL-5 703, 999, 1002, 1012
  IL-6 703, 864, 999, 1002, 1276
  IL-7 1002
  IL-8 1002
  IL-10 703, 999
  IL-12 999
  IL-13 703, 999
intermediate cells, cochlea 779
intermediate syndrome 426, 1996, 1997
internal dose *see* ID_{50}
Internation Chemical Safety Cards 1571
International Agency for Research on Cancer (IARC) 1104–6, 1383, 1434, 1537, 1571
International Air Transport Association (IATA) Restricted Articles Regulations 37
International Association of Forensic Toxicologists 1491
International Civil Aviation Organization (ICAO) 37
International Commission on Radiological Protection (ICRP) 1684
International Conference on Harmonization (ICH)
  data collection 1436
  genotoxicity testing 1039
  guidelines 1138, 1169, 1430, 1434–5, 1436, 1439, 1627, 1630
  medical devices 1662, 1667
  pharmaceutical safety testing 2, 1426, 1430, 1622
  registration 1546–7
  Safety Working Group Consensus Regarding New Drug Applications 40
international copyright law 475
International Council for Laboratory Animal Science 486

International Court of Justice 1572
International Covenant on Civil and Political Rights 453–4
International Environmental Information System (INFOTERRA) 1571–2
international estimated daily intake for the European diet (IEDI) 1609
International Federation of Pharmaceutical Manufacturers Associations (IFPMA) 1431
International Labour Organization (ILO) 476, 482
International Life Sciences Institute (ILSI) 1106
international normalized ratio (INR) 229
International Organization for Standardization (ISO) 461, 536, 538, 592
  exposure assessment 461
  extracts of solids 538
  inhalable fraction 592
  ISO 10993 testing standards 1670
  medical device testing 1668–71
  medical devices guidelines 536, 1662, 1733–7, 1738, 1742, 1743, 1744
international organizations, regulatory powers 1569–72
international periodicals directories 475
International Programme on Chemical Safety (IPCS) 459, 1452, 1570, 1571, 1592, 1612, 1659, 1703, 1759
  see also Environmental Health Criteria
International Register of Potentially Toxic Chemicals (IRPTC) 1571
international regulation 1648–9
International System for Human Cytogenetic Nomenclature (ISCN) 1083
International Uniform Chemicals Information Database 481
International Workshop on Immunotoxicology and Immunotoxicity of Metals 1009
Internet 53, 477, 482, 1723, 1759, 1947
internodal pathways 850

interspecies extrapolation 147,
271–90, 1435–7, 1447–8, 1449,
1461, 1754–5, 1763, 1769
see also interspecies variability
acute toxicity 28, 51, 55
agrochemical toxicity 25
allometric scaling 51
appropriateness 1754–5
arsenic toxicity 2052
carcinogenicity 1536
chronic high dose studies 80–90
dioxin body burden 88
dose–response assessments
1758–9, 1760, 1763
dosimetric scaling 147
environmental endocrine toxicity
1391, 1392–3
in vitro tests 53
inter-route 147–8, 1766
legal matters 1952
low-dose risk 90–1
mathematical modelling 1941
mycotoxin data 2148
nitrate/nitrite toxicity data 2136
occupational toxicity 1461
organic solvents 2041–2
PBPK modelling 51–2, 607,
1767–9, 1771
and prediction 1534
problems 430
radiation data 1694, 1695
regulatory aspects 1430–1, 1574,
1575
repeated exposure studies 59
risk assessment 1447–8, 1449
role of toxicokinetics 67
safety evaluations and 135
therapeutic protein testing 1967
interspecies variability
see also interspecies
extrapolation
acute toxicity 45, 50–2
adducts *275*
AITC 134
cadmium toxicity 2054
clinical chemistry 371
dioxin toxicity 282
disaster studies 1834
domestic animals 1509
dose adjustment 147, 1758
erythrocyte fragility test 1741
haematology 385
immunogenicity 1964
metabolism and 110–11
in metabolism of tamoxifen 285

MPTP susceptibility 132
negligible risk and 90
prenatal toxicity 282
peripheral sensory irritation 626
safety margin calculations 91, 92
study design 135, 322
testicular atrophy 82–3
uncertainty factors 1760
interstital cell stimulating hormone
(ICSH) 987
interstitial fibrosis *727*, 807
interstitial oedema 722
interstitial pneumonitis *727*
interstitial pulmonary fibrosis 315
intertest comparability 1352
intervention studies, methodology
1534
intestine
see also gastro-intestinal
absorption 69, 88
bacterial metabolism, dietary
modification *573*
biomarkers *1879*
blood flow 252
crypt cells, apoptosis 179
epithelium 197, 337, 524, 548,
1684
half-life extension 556
hydrolysis 523
mouse dermal toxicity test 605
mucins 561
mucosa 368, 547, 568
peroxidases 103
segments, interspecies
extrapolation 555
toxicity 556
villi 545, 554, 1687, 1689, 1690
intolerance 4, 21
INTOX system 459
intoxication, definition 1445–6
Intra-agency Regulatory
Alternatives Group 411
intra-alveolar oedema 732
intra-arterial route 527
intracellular fluid 70
intracerebral route 47, 524, 527,
641, 644
intracerebroventricular route 527,
528
intracranial pressure, raised 1427
intracutaneous route, local reaction
538–9
intracutaneous testing, synthetic
materials 1741
intradermal techniques 841, 842

intragastric route, varying LD$_{50}$ 525
intraluminal instillation 525
intramembranal bone 966
intramuscular myodegeneration 522
intramuscular route 523, 526–7,
531–2
intramuscular route of exposure 19,
47, 55
intramuscular toxicity 412
intramyelinic oedema *638*, 639
intraocular pressure 496, 614,
748–9, *749*, *750*
intraocular tissue, medical devices
toxicity testing 1741
intraperitoneal route
activity promotion 532
acute toxicity 47
animal dechlorination reactions
566
bioavailability 533
in carcinogenicity studies 525
LD$_{50}$ 525, 534
liver change 533
neonatal mouse 525–6
neurotoxicity 642
parenteral toxicity 523, 526,
532–3
synthetic materials 1739–40
visceral penetration risk 526
intrapleural route 525, 527
intrapulmonary injection, lung
squamous cell carcinoma 525
intraspecies variability
acute toxicity 45
AhR differences 1892
biochemical 1509
disaster studies 1834
DNA repair 1892
dose–response assessments 1760
extrapolation by *in vitro* testing
53
genetic polymorphism 1890
similarities and differences in
acute testing 50–2
tools to examine 135
intrathecal route 527
intratracheal route 432
intrauterine contraceptive devices
1674
intrauterine development 8
intrauterine growth retardation
(IUGR) 1219, 1254–7, 1696
intrauterine position effects 1406
intravascular injection, distribution
and 70

intravenous route
  acute toxicity 47
  alternative testing 412
  artefacts and alterations 529–30
  by injection 526
  by osmotic minipump 528
  in carcinogenicity studies 525
  comparison with oral data 75
  distribution and 70, 78
  guidelines 523
  nausea and vomiting 524
  and plasma clearance calculation 79
  repeated exposure 55, 59
  solution bags 1737
  statistical moment analysis 85
intravitreal route 644
intrinsic toxicity 523–4
inulin as marker 1972
invertebrates 38, 1327, 1328, 1349, 1355
  see also specific invertebrates
investigation brochure (IB) 1623
investigational device exemption (IDE) 1662, 1663
Investigational New Animal Drugs Application (INAD) (USA) 1634
Investigational New Drug Application (IND) 1546, 1615
iodotyrosine 1868
ions
  exchange–adsorption reactions 1366
  transport 754, 779, 784–7, 790, 807, 938–9, 1843
  transporters 189–90
ion channels 777
  neurotoxins 639–40
ionization 1683
ionized molecules, absorption 69
ionizing radiation 464, 1154, 1464, 1465
ionotropic effects 43
IORT treatment for radiation injury 1689
IPCS *see* International Programme on Chemical Safety
IQ 566
Iran–Iraq chemical warfare 2080
Iraq 1249, 1726–7, 1825–6, 2080
iris, injury 741, 745
Irish Republican Army 1727, 1730
iritis 40, 41, 742–3
IRMAs *see* immunoradiometric assays

irradiation *see* radiation
irrigation, and soil salinization 1371
irritant dermatitis 832–4, 838–40
irritants 40, 1455, 1475
  see also eye; lung; mucous membrane; peripheral sensory; respiratory tract; skin
  acute toxicity 40
  airborne toxicants 1487, 1828
  chemical warfare 2080
  effects 56
  fires 1821
  medical devices 1734, 1735, 1740–1
  occupational toxicity 1455, 1475
  testing 839
    see also eye irritation testing
  vapours 589–90
irritation
  see also eye; lung; mucous membrane; peripheral sensory; respiratory tract; skin
  cumulative 60
  definition 611
  lung or skin 1474
  peripheral sensory (PSI) 23, 611–30
  primary 23
  testing 25
irritative/corrosive effects 1475
ischaemia
  clinical chemistry 364
  hippocampal responses 168
  myocardial 805, 815
  nephrotoxicity 681, 684
  NMDA 166
  pathology 343
  reperfusion 158
  stria vascularis 785, 786
ISCN *see* International System for Human Cytogenetic Nomenclature
Islamic extremists 1722
ISO *see* International Organization for Standardization
isoboles 307–11, *309*
isobolograms 311, 312
isocitrate dehydrogenase *356*, 939
isoelectric focusing 752
isoenzymes 355, 363
isoleukotrienes 896
isomers 115
isoniazid-type inducer 113
isopleths 1833, *1835*, 1836

isoprostanes 896
Israel, deliberate food poisoning 1724
itai-itai disease 1373, 1564, 2053
Italy
  fumonisin contamination of cereals 2165
  nitrate and nitrite levels 2112, 2114, 2116, 2130, 2131
Iva augatifolia see sumpweed

J

J-receptor 615
Japan
  see also Matsumoto; Minamata; Tokyo
  cosmetics regulation 1550
  deliberate food poisoning 1724
  drug regulation 1428, 1430, 1544, 1565–7
  environmental pollution by industrial chemicals 1547
  food production regulation 1567–8
  foreign manufacturing approvals 1566
  functional foods regulation 1552, 1567–8
  government ministries 438
  industrial chemicals regulation 1545, 1564
  marketing authorization 1566
  mercury-exposed pregnant women 1249
  nitrate levels 2114
  N-nitroso compounds levels 2133
  post-war radiation exposure 1035
  pre-manufacturing notification 1565
  regulatory processes 1554–5, 1564–8, 1649
  reproductive toxicological testing 1567
  sarin gas attack *see under* sarin
  Tokyo subway sarin gas attack 955
jaundice
  acute toxicity 41
  from food contamination 1825
  from NSAIDs 132
  and hepatic necrosis 1426, 1427

knowledge-based system,
  Estimation and Assessment of
  Substance Exposure (EASE)
  1479
Kochia scoporia, hepatoxicity 1519
Koch's postulates 1952
kohlrabi, nitrate levels 2113
Kosteve, Vladimir 1727
Koupparis, Panos 1724–5
Krebs cycle *see* tricarboxylic acid
  cycle
krill *see Euphausiids*
Kruskal–Wallis one-way ANOVA
  300
Kupffer cells 200, 274, 385, *857*,
  858, 862, 864, 873, 881
Kurbegovic, Muharem 1725
Kussmaul sign 40
kwashiorkor 823, 897, 903, 910
  see also protein deficiency
kyphosis 41

L

L929 cells *410*
L5178Y mutation test 1434
LAA *see* laboratory animal allergy
labelling *see* classification and
  labelling
laboratory
  accreditation 492–3
  animals *see* animal welfare and
    animal studies
  animals, allergy to 511–14, 516
  practice
    see also interlaboratory
    ethical aspects 1958
    reproducibility of results 1893
    samples, sources of error 1911
    toxicology 3
  studies
    animal behavioour 1346
    forensic 1489
    reproductive behaviour
      1347–8
  workers
    and congenital malformation
      510
    latex allergy 510
Laboratory Animal Technician
  certification (US) 492
Laboratory Animal Welfare Act
  (US) 1966 486
lachrymation
  and accidents 8

acute toxicity 40, 41
  as allergic response 512
  from nerve gas 605
  grading 742–3
  peripheral sensory irritation 614
  reflexes 755
lactate dehydrogenase (LDH)
  acute toxicity 43
  assays 1462
  in BALF, dose–response
    assessment 1762
  biomarker 1848, 1858, 1859,
    1860, 1861, 1862
  cardiotoxicity 806
  clinical chemistry 355–6, 359,
    366
  isoenzymes 366, 372
  pathology 343
  and wildlife toxicity 1345
lactation 23, 340, 1548, 1549
lactic acid producing bacteria (LAB)
  571–2
lactic acidosis 126, 1430, 1438
lactic aciduria 679, 1862
Lactobacillus 562
lactoferrin 897
lactoperoxidase 103
lactotrophic hormone (prolactin)
  980
Lactrodectus mactans see black
  widow spider
lag phase prior to absorption 69, 75
Lake Nyos disaster 1817
LAL test 537
lamb's lettuce, nitrate levels 2113
lambsquarters (*Chenopodium* spp.),
  nephrotoxicity 1522
laminar flow cabinets 515
laminin, mustard gas and 2085
lamins, and apoptosis 190, 195
land-use planning 1831, 1832, 1836
Langerhans cells 340, 828, 830,
  835, 991
lanolin 835, 836
Lantata camara, hepatotoxicity
  1519
lapilli 1815, 1816
large intestine
  microflora 562–4, *564*
  modelling 556
  mucosal oxidases 571
  predominant organism
    identification 563
  rate of transfer 69

Larus argentatus 654
laryngeal nerve, peripheral sensory
  iritation stimulation 619
larynx
  cancer 1456, 1982, 2132
  granulomas 27
  mouse dermal toxicity test 605
laser Doppler flowmetry 845
last measured concentration 79
late asthmatic response 510
latency period 1531
latency to toxicity 5, 6
  before tumour appearance 64
  and LD_{50} 15
  phosgene-induced 2098
  radiation-induced 1692
  repeated exposures 56, 63
  risk assessment and 1755
  skin absorption 1778
lateral cisternae system, outer hair
  cells 786, 787
lateral plasma menbrane, outer hair
  cells 786
lateralization technique, in human
  subject PSI 623
latex industry 2018
lathyrism 634
Lathyrus sativas 634
Latrus atricilla see gull, laughing
laundromats 1216, 1226
lauric acid 12-hydroxylase *217*
lava 1815, 1816
Law 44, Chemical Substances
  Control Law, (Japan) 1565
law, *see also* legal aspects of
  toxicology
law enforcement, use of toxic
  chemicals 1547
LC *see* Langerhans cells
LC_{50} (median lethal concentration)
  13
  acute toxicity 36
  age effects 1337
  alternative testing 407
  aquatic toxicity 1312, 1313,
    1315
  caution/reproducibilty 1337
  choosing 48
  combustion studies 1926, 1927
  data for modelling 1834
  defining 46, 49
  determination 49
  mixtures 317
  nitrogen dioxide 51
  repeated exposure toxicity 55

leukaemia (*Contd.*)
   nitrates 2124
   organic solvents 2037
   and parental occupational
      exposure 1465
   plastics industry 2020
   radiation 1464, 1692, 1693,
      1695, 1697
   rubber industry 2015, 2018
   toxicology 395
leukaemogenesis 395
leukocytes 384–5, 833
   acetylation enzymes 108
   biomarkers 1845, 1880, 1892
   clinical chemistry 362–3
   count 61, 387, 388
   and cutaneous toxicity 833
   DNA 1882, 1885, 1886, 1891
   parameters 388
   and parenteral toxicity 533
   pathology 341
leukocytosis 389
leukoencephalopathy, radiation-
   induced 1691
leukopenia 235, 389, 394, 2089
leukotrienes 702, 845, 1981
   role in respiratory damage from
      fires 1917
Leydig cells 371, 987–8, 1464,
   1859
LH *see* luteinizing hormone
Li–Fraumeni syndrome 1031–2
liability 1948, 1959
libido 1142, 1146, 1154–5
Libya, chemical warfare 2080–1
licences 1543
licensing, UK 1546
Licensing Authority (UK) 1559,
   1627
lichen planus, civatte bodies 175
lichenification of epidermis 835
life span 1769, 1773
ligand exchange 1369
ligand-protein theory 34
light microscopy 781, 782, 951,
   952
light-induced cutaneous toxicity
   836–7
lightning, risk of death 1830
lily-of-the-valley (*Convalaria* spp.),
   cardiovascular effects 1522
lima beans, toxicity 1984
Limanda limanda see dab, North
   Sea
limb explants 967

limbic kindling in IEI 1706
limit of detection (LOD) 1781–2
limit tests 44, 45
Limited Announcements, New
   Substances Notification Scheme
   1590
limits of detection 1563
Limulus spp.
   amoebocyte lysate test 53, 413,
      537
   L. polyphemus 537
line transect sampling 1353
linoleic acid deficiency, effect on
   metabolism 115
lionfish 2191
lipaemia 357
lipases 156, 347, 356, 365, 897
lipid(s)
   barrier 69
   clinical chemistry 361, 365, 367,
      370
   damage 104, 128
   deficiency, effect on metabolism
      115
   lowering drugs 1124
   metabolism 868–9, 939
   pathology 355
   peroxidation 6
      biochemistry 127, 136
      as biomarker 1848, 1867
      and carbon tetrachloride
         toxicity 118
      in cardiotoxicity 807, 808,
         809
      in cartilage and bone toxicity
         872
      in cutaneous toxicity 837
      in eye toxicity 757
      and gastro-intestinal
         microflora 570
      human placenta 1246
      induction 167
      in nephrotoxicity 687
      ochratoxin and 2162
      pharmacogenetics 158, 237,
         240
   solubility 69, 71, 143
   as targets 34
   tests 359
   theory of inhalation anaesthetics
      2030
lipid hydroperoxides 6, 158, 1866
lipid peroxidase 764
lipofuscin 867
lipophilic pathway 581

lipophilicity 131, 581
lipoproteins 815, 868–9
liposomes 570
lipoxygenases 158, 159
lipstick 606
liquid chromatography 1500
liquid formulations, toxicity 1338
liquid scintillation counting 534
liquids, assessing chemicals in
   1777–8
Lisa ramada 1870
Listeria monocytogenes 1007
literature for expert witness 1947
literature review, tier testing *403*
litter, non-contact absorbent 514
liver
   see also hepatic, hepato-
   acetylation enzymes 108
   adrenal hormone action 370
   alcohol dehydrogenase 242
   alcoholic disease 236
   amine oxidase (AO) 238
   anatomy and physiology 853–9,
      860–5
   apoptosis 132, 198
   autopsy specimens 1495, 1496
   azoreduction 564
   bile acids 567
   bioavailability alteration 555
   biomarkers *1879*
   biomonitoring 1905
   blood flow 254, 2033
   cancer *see* hepatocarcinoma
   carbonyl reductase 242
   cell, *see also* hepatocyte
   cell nuclei
      accumulation of Ca^{2+} 187–8
      peroxisome proliferator 2022
      regeneration 126
   cholinesterase 368
   circadian blood flow 254
   circulatory system 545, 548,
      552, 556, 853–4, *855*, 856, *858*,
      859
   cirrhosis *see* cirrhosis
   clearance/excretion assays 1462
   clinical chemistry 358–61
   cytochrome P450 99, 218, 274,
      277
   cytosol enzyme reduction 104
   damage *see* hepatoxicity
   dechlorination reactions 566
   detoxification 19, 344
   development 865–6
   dioxin accumulation 88

liver (*Contd.*)
  disease
    apoptosis in 175
    effect on metabolism 114–15
    and forensic testing 1504–5
    porphyria 29
  ducts 545
  dysfunction and injury 1462
  enlargement 880–1, 1986
  enzyme induction 135, 910–11
  enzymes 98
    biomarker 1843
    biotransformation 98
    distribution 1857
    excereion 21, 1462
    following carbon tetrachloride
      1857, *1858*
    hydration 105
    induction 135, 910–11
    reduction 104
    sulphation 105
    systems 550
  erythropoietin 384
  failure 943
  fatty 1862, 1863
  FMO expression 232
  forensic toxicology 1504
  function tests 359
  gene product excretion 217–18
  glucuronide conjugate formation
    556
  glutathione conjugation 107
  haemopoiesis 383
  half-life extension 556
  innervation 854
  Kupffer cells 103, 385
  mercury uptake 2058
  metabolic function 70, 148, 254,
    272
  microsomes 107, 111, 274, 285
  mitochondrial enzymes 103
  mitoinhibitory pathways 126
  morphometry 339
  necrosis 6, 102, 281, 360, 361,
    1430
  nodules 565
  normal adaptive changes 866–7
  NQO 240
  oxidative stress 912
  parenchymaal organization
    855–9
  PBPK studies 89–90
  perfusion, furan 90

pesticide residue accumulation
  1343
pharmacokinetic analysis 284
portal exposure 603
remodelling 880–1
substance activation in 19
as target organ 43, 131
taurine 1862
as tissue compartment in PBPK
  144
tissue in mutagenicity tests
  1039–41
toxicity *see* hepatotoxicity
for toxicokinetic modelling 307
transplant 884
tumours
    see also hepatocarcinoma
    diet effects 58
    dioxin 88
    food additives and 1986
    fungicides 2002
    ochratoxins 2159
    and peroxisome proliferators
      7
    plastics industry 2019,
      2020–1, 2022, 2023
    rubber industry 2015, 2016,
      2018
    vinyl chloride 1771
  vulnerable to xenobiotics 1462
  weight 336, 344, 1859
  xenobiotic metabolism 1339
liver fluke (*Fasciola hepatica*) 882,
  2119
liver pate, nitrate and nitrite levels
  2113
liver sausage, nitrate and nitrite
  levels 2113
lizards
    acute testing 1353
    green anole (*Anolis carolinenis*)
      1330–1
    venomous 2181–2
LLNA *see* local lymph node assay
LMS *see* multistage model,
  linearized version
LMW5-HL, and apoptosis 194
Loa loa control 1999
loading dose 88
LOAEL *see* lowest observed
  adverse effect level
lobbies for anti-vivisection 36
Lobelia spp. *see* wild tobacco
lobster studies 820

local anaesthetics *see* anaesthesia/
  anaesthesia/anaesthetic agents,
  local
local effects 5
local lymph node assay (LLNA)
  708, 842–3, 1005, 1009, 1010
local tolerance studies 1616–17,
  1628
lock and key receptor–ligand model
  1397
locoweed, neurotoxic to horses
  1519
LOD *see* limit of detection
Loewe additivity 304
log-normal distribution 47
log-probit plot 10, 12, 13, 48, 431
logistic function 49
logit analysis 49, 1331–2
Lonchocarpus utilis 1999
London principles report 1756
London smog 1265, 1268–9
long-term carcinogenicity studies
  1618–19
long-term effects 1446, 1451
long-term toxicity studies, Good
  Laboratory Practice (GLP) 440
loop of Henle 345, 363, 675, 785
Los Angeles
  CB agent threat 1724, 1725
  smog 1265–6, 1275, 1278
Lotus corniculatus see birdsfoot
  trefoil
Lotus tetragonolobus 345
Louis-Bar syndrome *see* ataxia
  telangiectasia
Love Canal (USA) disaster 1372,
  1827–8
low birth weight 1464, 1465
low linear energy transfer 1683
low volume eye test (LVET) 739
low-density lipoproteins (LDL)
  367, 1978
low-dose effects 1397, 1404,
  1451–2, 1460, 1563
  see also hormesis
lowest observed adverse effect level
  (LOAEL) 57, 60, 1180, 1181,
  1483, 1759–60, 1787
Loxosceles spiders 2186–7
LS cells *410*
LT$_{50}$ 13, 1314
luncheon meat, nitrate, nitrite and
  N-nitroso levels 2113, 2120

marketing authorization
 EU procedures 1544, 1622,
   1623–7
 Japan 1566
 'need' clause 1568–9
 renewals and variations 1629–30
 responsibilities of holder 1625,
   1629
 UK procedures 1627
marketing of toxicologist 1947
Markov, Georgi 1727
marmoset monkey
 see under monkey
Marsh test, arsenic 1490
masculinization in women 862
mass intoxication 1445
mass median aerodynamic diameter
 (MMAD) 20, 1762
mass median diameter (MMD)
 1281
mass spectrometry 1500, 1501
 in forensic toxicology 1491
 of macromolecular adducts
   1882, 1883, 1885, 1889
mass transfer 582
mass-transfer coefficients 582
mast cells
 in alternative testing 412
 in cutaneous toxicity 829, 830,
   833
 function, nitrites and 2128
 hyperplasia radiation-induced
   1690
 in immunotoxicity 997, 1000
 in nephrotoxicity 702, 706
 in respiratory sensitization 707
Master of Science requirements
 1938, 1939
Master testing List (MTA), US EPA
 1585
MAT *see* mean absorption time
matching, comparison group 1533
MATCs *see* maximum acceptable
 toxicant concentrations
Material Safety Data Sheet (MSDS)
 37, 516, 833, 1448–9, 1459, 1478,
 1712
maternal acidosis 1189
maternal toxicity
 and childhood tumours 1465
 developmental effects 758–9
 drug levels in breast milk
   1225–6
 factors influencing transplacental
   transfer 1241–2

in mouse inhalation study 604
 risk assessment 1754
mathematical modelling 581, 1451,
 1461, 1563, 1575
matrimony vine (*Lycium* spp.),
 neurotoxicity 1521
matrix attachment regions 189
Matsumoto, sarin incident 1721,
 1723, 1726, 1729
Maximale Arbeitskonzentrationen
 Commission (MAK) 1477, 1482,
 1483–4, 1485, 1594
maximally exposed individual
 (MEI) 1775
maximally tolerated does (MTD)
 1619
maximization patch method,
 synthetic materials testing 1740
maximum acceptable toxicant
 oncentrations (MATCs) 1316
maximum allowable concentrations
 (MAC) 1482
maximum contamination limits
 (MCL) 1784, 1790
maximum exposure limit (MEL)
 (UK) 1484, 1594
maximum feasible dose, in dose
 selection 1620
maximum lifespan potential (MLP)
 89
maximum likelihood method 44
maximum residue level (MRL) 3,
 1563, 1570, 1574, 1603, 1609,
 1610, 1611, 1639–40
 animal testing 1643
 establishing 1647–8
 EU regulation 1641–3
 existing drugs 164
 fish 1646, 1647
 pesticides 1993
 pollutants 3
 practicability 1646
 regulatory aspects 1563, 1570,
   1574, 1603, 1609, 1610, 1611,
   1639–40
 toxicity testing 1643, 1644
maximum safe concentration,
 residues 1635
maximum tolerated dose (MTD)
 carcinogenicity 1106–7
 chronic studies 65
 definition 1755
 epidemiology 1535
 evaluation of 1110–11
 PBPK modelling 148

repeated exposure 60
 subchronic studies 62
Mayo Clinic 815
maze techniques 657
MCF-7 breast cancer cell assay
 1402
McKone's model 582
MCL *see* maximum contamination
 limits
mcl-1, and apoptosis 193
McNemar's test 301
MCV *see* mean corpuscular volume
McVeigh, Timothy 1722
MDCK cells *410*
mean absorption time (MAT) 75
mean cell volume 387
mean corpuscular haemoglobin
 content (MCHC) 387
mean corpuscular volume (MCV)
 389
mean residence time (MRT) 75,
 84–5
meat
 and cancer 1981, 1982
 cooked 274
 cured/processed 2113, 2114,
   2116, 2118, 2132
 dioxin 281
 fried 566
 ingestion, risk from 1772
 nitrate and nitrite levels 2113,
   2114, 2115, 2116, 2117, 2118,
   2127, 2132
 PAHs 1791
 radioactivity 1821
 raw, inspection 1637
 red, drug residues 1647
Meat Inspection Act (USA) 1563
meat wrapper allergy 1915
mechanoreceptors 661
mechanotransduction 776
media involvement 1576
median effective concentration
 see EC$_{50}$
median effective dose *see* ED$_{50}$
median effective time *see* ET$_{50}$
median eminence 347
median lethal concentration
 see LC$_{50}$
median lethal dose *see* LD$_{50}$
median lethal molar concentration
 49
median lethal time *see* LT$_{50}$
median response 12

mediastinitis from peroral exposure 19

Medicaid 458

Medical and Biologic Effects of Environmental Pollutants 1676

Medical Device Amendment 1976 (USA) 1662, 1663, 1733

medical devices
American National Standards Insitute (ANSI) 1662
biocompatibility 1666, 1670, 1672, 1738–42
biological testing 1668
chemical characterization 1742–3
classification 1666, 1667–8, 1671–2, 1734–7
combination product 1733
definition 1661, 1732–3
direct contact 1732–3
duration of contact 1734
external 1735
finished product 1733
fraudulent 1662
Good Laboratory Practice 1664
guidelines 1733–7
historical aspects 1662, 1733–4
implantable 1732, 1735
implantation tests 539
indirect contact 1733
International Commission on Harmonization 1662, 1667
materials and components 1672–3, 1731
non-implantable 1732
parenteral toxicity 523, 538
potential toxicity 1643
premarketing procedures 1663–4, 1737–8
public perception 1674
raw materials 1672–3
regulatory aspects 1548–9, 1562, 1661–81
EU 1671–2
US 1662–5
risk assessment 1743–6
sterilization 1667, 1668, 1679–80, 1740
surface 1735
target organ toxicity 1734
testing 1672–80
International Standards Organizations (ISO) 1662
ISO 1668–71
needs 1734–8

United States Pharmacopeia 1668, 1669
toxicity testing 1665–72
toxicology 1731–47
uses and abuses 1672
vs drug 1733

medical ethics *see* ethical issues

medical evaluation, postplacement periodic 513–14

medical examinations 462

Medical Examiner's Office, New York 1490

medical industries, radiofrequency radiation 1418–19

Medical Literature Analysis and Retrieval System (MEDLARS) 478

medical planning 1837

medical practice, cultural factors 1558, 1567

medical products 522

Medical Research Council (UK) 454

Medical Research Council Ethics Series 1958

medical screening, in the workplace 1460

medical and surgical supplies 1661, 1667

medical surveillance 462, 1460

medical toxicology 1443, 1444–5, 1447, 1452

Medicines Act 1968 (UK) 1425, 1546, 1627, 1637, 1638

Medicines Act Leaflet, MAL 4 1622

Medicines Commission (UK) 1425

Medicines Control Agency (UK) 458, 1425, 1436, 1578, 1627, 1638

MediConf 473

MEDLARS *see* Medical Literature Analysis and Retrieval System

Medline 1676–7, 1943, 1947

medulla 546

medulla oblongata 347

megakaryocytes 385, 395

'megalin' receptor 791

mehrotoxicity, lead 2056

MEI *see* maximally exposed individual

meiosis 40, 41, 605

MEL *see* maximum exposure limit

melanin 129

melanocytes 779, 830

melanogenesis 779

melanomas 837

melanosome 830

melatonin 163

melon, nitrate and nitrite levels 2112–13

membrane
ion pumps 126–7
permeability 252
phospholipids, methylation 896
receptors 163

membranous labyrinth 775

Memorandum of Understanding, Dow Corning Corporation 1585

memory disturbances in IEI 1707

memory search 667

Menière's disease 787

meningitis, and adverse drug reactions 1427

Menkes disease 2064

menstrual function 234, 251, 340, 830, 1148–9, 1463, 1464, 1465

mental health needs in CB attack 1729

mental retardation radiation-induced 1696, 1697

mentors in toxicology 1937, 1939, 1942

mephenytoin 4′-hydroxylase *217*

mephenytoin, metabolic pathways *225–6*

β-mercaptopyruvate sulphur transferase 428

Merck Index 222, 1677

MERL *see* Marine Environment Research Laboratory

Merrell Dow Pharmaceuticals 1948–9

mescal beans (*Sophora* spp.), neurotoxicity 1520, 1521

mesenchymal cells 340, 804

mesenchymal induction 968–9

MeSH (Medical Subject Heading) 480

Mesobuthus tamulus see scorpion, red

mesocosm *see* controlled field study

mesoscale models 1781

mesothelioma 1131, 2017

MEST *see* mouse ear swelling test

meta-analysis 1456–7

metabolic acidosis 2040

metabolic activation 17, 18, 52, 56, 130–5, 545, 1039–41, 1056

metabolic clearance calculation 80

metabolic constants 145–6

metabolic inhibitors 870
metabolic phenotyping 112, 265
metabolic poisons 604, 807
metabolic polymorphisms, and
  cancer 1538
metabolic rates 72–3, 357
metabolic retroversion 234
metabolic theory of idiopathic
  environmental intolerance
  aetiology 1705
metabolism 67, 74–5
  see also biotransformation;
    inborn errors of metabolism;
    kinetics; toxicokinetics
  affecting biological activity 97
  bacterial 72
  biomarkers of susceptibility
    1850, 1877
  in biomonitoring 461
  BPK modelling and 148
  definition 72
  dose-dependent kinetics and 83
  of drugs 21, 22
  effects 21, 65
  enzyme-catalysed 73
  extent 73
  factors affecting 109–15
  first-pass 22, 69–70, 73, 523
  incomplete absorption and 70
  inhibition 114
  intermediary 92, 98, 159
  interspecies differences 85
  major reactions 98
  mixed routes of exposure 606,
    607
  molecular concepts 157–8
  in multiple route exposure 606
  pharmacogenetics 215
  phase 1 reactions 98–105, 110,
    115
  phase 2 reaction 105–9, 110–11,
    115
  and plasma clearance 79
  products 97
  reducing excretion 98
  in repeated exposure studies 56
  saturation 85
  scaling factors 1769
  studies 24
metabolites
  as biomarkers 607
  biomonitoring 1906, 1907
  relationship with macromolecular
    adducts 1878, 1879
  sigma minus method and 86

toxic 429, 1329
  ethical issues 1956–7
  toxicokinetics 72
metal smelters, and plant metal
  concentrations 1373
metal storage diseases 902
metal workers, risks 1463, 1474
metal-based compounds, toxic-
  therapeutic ratio 260–1
metallothionein 1848, 1869, 1870,
  2053, 2054, 2059, 2067
metals
  see also heavy metals
  biocompatibility testing 1738
  cardiotoxicity 822
  chelation 1985
  fume fever 2066
  fungal extraction from soil 1369
  hepatotoxicity 822, 870
  immunotoxicity 1004
  indestructibility 1366
  medical devices 1734
  occupational exposures 1463
  placental toxicity 1245–6
  teratogenicity and embryotoxicity
    1203–9
metamorphosis, and apoptosis 178
metaphase analysis 1085, 1088
metaphysis 342, 966
metastatic mineralization 969
methaemoglobin 15, 384, 392–3,
  428, 432, 565, 572, 2120, 2123,
  2125–6, 2129, 2131, 2135, 2136
methaemoglobin reductase 392
methaemoglobinaemia
  in acute toxicity 28
  adverse drug reaction 1430
  antidotal studies 429
  biochemistry 127
  compounds producing 393
  drinking water toxicity 1383
  effect 392
  and fire intoxication 1920
  and gastro-intestinal microflora
    565, 572
  haematotoxicity 391, 392
  herbicide toxicity 2005
  hydrogen cyanide toxicity 2102
  insecticide toxicity 2000
  in neonates, food additives and
    1989
  and nitrate-accumulating plants
    1522
  nitrobenzene toxicity 104
  spectrophotometry 393

methaemoglobinuria 384
5-methyl hydroxylation 227
methylation 18, 98, 109, 896, 2050
methyltransferases 109
MFO system see mixed function
  oxidase system
Mg^{2+}-ATPase 341
MHC see major histocompatibility
  complex
MIC_{50} 1645
mic, biomarker 1849
Michaelis constant 146
Michaelis–Menten kinetics 84, 90,
  145, 305
micro-organisms, pathogenic, in
  sewage sludge 1372
microalgae 1310, 1314, 1318,
  1319–20
  see also micro-organisms
microbial, see also micro-organisms
Microbial Commercial Activity
  Notice (MCAN) 1584
microcapsule, liver kidney and
  spleen weight decrease 551
microcephaly, radiation-induced
  1696, 1697
micrococci 562
microcosms, aquatic toxicology
  1318, 1319
microdensitometry, integrating 338
microdialysis 644
microdiffusion 1497
microencapsulation 60, 550
micro-exposure techniques 1775
microglia 338, 632, 633
microglobulins
  biomonitoring 1906, 1910
  and cadmium toxicity 2053
  clinical chemistry 363
  labioratory occupationa risks 511
  measurement 63
  nephropathy marker 129, 271,
    678, 692, 1374
micrognathia 972
micronuclei 1848
  assays 1085, 1087–8, 1460
micronutrient deficiencies 913–14,
  1551–2
micro-organisms
  and building/interiors materials
    1295
  catalytic propeties 1368
  as CB weapon 1723, 1726
  emitted volative organic
    compounds 1298

mitosis 340, 544
mitotic index, fertility cycle
    variation 266
mitotic rate 256
mixed function oxidase 725, 732,
    1317
mixed leukocyte reaction (MLR)
    1000, 1007
mixed routes of exposure 603–9
mixtures
    acute effects assessment 49–50
    additivity 50, 312
    analysis 305
    antagonism 50, 309, 312
    binary 312
    biomarkers 1841
    chemical 303–19
    complex 314
    effects 20–1, *308*
    factorial designs 313
    interaction 148–9, 309, 313–14
    occupational toxicity hazard
        1418
    organic solvents 2033, 2042
    risk assessment 1751
    simple 314
    study methods 305–14
    synergy 309, 312
    toxicity studies 303
    whole 306
mixtures of chemicals, occupational
    toxic hazard 1418
MKV *see* Moolgavkar–Knudson–
    Venzon
MLD *see* LD₁
MLP *see* maximum lifespan
    potential
MLR *see* mixed leukocyte reaction
MMAD *see* mass median
    aerodynamic diameter
MMD *see* mass median diameter
mode of action, risk assessment
    1754
model species
    see also species
    for drug testing 1431
    human genome project 1092
    reproductive studies 1328
    wildlife 1327
modelling
    see also mathematical modelling
    chronic ocular hypertensive
        rabbit 749
    computer-based eye irritation
        tests 754

gastro-intestinal parameters
    556–7
mathematical for percutaneous
    toxicity 581
physicochemical properties based
    581–2
physiologically based
    pharmacokinetic 607
risk assessment 1575
skin absorption 578
two-compartment for
    biomonitoring 606
modified reproduction tests 1351–2
modified starches 1552, 1653
modifying factor 1759–60
modulus 776
molar units in biomonitoring 1907
molarity, definition 1446–7
molecular biology
    definition 1965
    technology 336, 339–40
    and toxicology 136
    use 1966
molecular epidemiology 1457,
    1534, 1538
molecular immunotoxicology
    1010–12
molecular orbital energies 713
molecular probes 339
molecular targets 158–63
molecular toxicology 155–74
molecular volume, definition 597
molecular weight (MW) of toxic
    agent 1217
molluscicides 1998, 2006
molluscs 1407, 1866, 2192
Molothus ather see cowbird, brown-
    headed
molybdenum cofactor deficiency
    239
molybdenum hydroxylase 239
Mon Voisin, Madame 35
monitored release schemes 1960
monitoring
    see also screening
    ambient 461
    ambient and biological 1602
    biological 461, 464
    personal 461
    pollutants 1460
    to prevent CB incidents 1728
    for toxicity 61–2
monkey studies
    acute toxicity 45
    aflatoxin LD₅₀ 2154

ceftizoxime clearance 89
circadian variation 254
CYP genes 216
delayed spatial alternation 660–1
dioxin exposure 87
fumonisin toxicity 2165
hepatic microsomes 273
interferon testing model 1971
intubation 544, 549
IQ 272
LDL fraction 367
liver 274, 872
marmoset
    arsenic metabolism 2050
    β-glucuronidase and β-
        glucosidase 572
    intravenous injection site 526
mercury toxicity 2058, 2059
MPTP toxicity 132
nerve agent toxicity 2095
ochratoxin pharmacokinetics
    2161
ototoxicity 787
patas monkey 787
pharmacodynamic and
    pharmacokinetic toxicity 329
phosgene 2097
progesterone level 372
reproductive cycle 372
rhesus monkey
    biliary excretion 555
    dioxin susceptibility 282
    experimental toxicity 429
    internal carotid artery infusion
        530
spatial contrast ssensitivity 661
squirrel monkey 663
stratum corneum skin
    permeability *579*
vomiting reflex 546
monkey virus B, infection
    transmission 514
monkshood (*Aconitum napellus*)
    34, 818
monoamine oxidases (MAO) 103,
    114, 222, 814, 939
Monoclonal Amphetamine/
    Metamphetamine Assay (EM)
    EMIT immunoassay 1501
monoclonal antibodies
    see also biotechnology products
    in antidotal studies 426
    development 1964, 1965, 1967,
        1973–4
    endocrine toxicology 983

monoclonal antibodies (*Contd.*)
  IgE 707
    measurement 366
    in occupational toxicology 1454
    in pathology 341, 344
    pharmacogenetics 230
    poisoning antidotes 428
monocytes 385
monodealkylation 429
monogastric species 1509, 1513
Monographs on the Evaluation of
  the Carcinogenic Risk (of
  Chemicals) to Humans 476
mononuclear blood cells 277
mononuclear phagocytes 533
monooxygenases 115, 343
Monte Carlo analysis 1758,
  1782–5, 1789–90, 1791
mood 222, 1714
Moolgavkar–Knudson–Venzon
  (MKV) model 1770
morbidity
  in acute toxicity testing 39
  statistics, interpretation 1533
Morinaga incident 2051
morphine placental opioid system
  1256–7
morphological teratogenic effects 8
morphometric analysis 339, 342,
  722
Morris water maze 657
MORT-1, and apoptosis 193
mortality
  see also death; lethality
  rates, regional 1531–2
  statistics, availability 1533
  and survival, field testing 1354
mosquito
  Anopheles albimanus 216
  control 1998
  larva 259
most likely estimate scenarios 1775
motion sickness 527
motor activity changes 41
motor end plates,
  acetylcholinesterase 368
motor neurone disease (ALS) 239,
  635
motor system impairment 655
mould-release agents, rubber
  industry 2014, 2017
Mount St Helens 1816–17
mouse
  activity promotion 532
  acute lethality studies 428

adrenal medulla 346
aflatoxin LD_{50} 2154
age effects on metabolism 115
aggressive behaviour 653
AITC toxicity 134
allergens 511
amine oxidase (AO) 239
apoptosis 178, 193, 197
arsenic metabolism 2050
aryl hydrocarbon receptor-
  deficient 281
barbiturate metabolism 111
bite infection transmission 514
blood sampling site *386*
body weight
  and LD_{50} 51
  /surface area difference 92
bone marrow 385
brain FMO 232
breast cancer surgery timing 266
breathing rate 46
bromobenzene toxicity 118
cadmium toxicity 2054
cancer studies 262, 278, 291
  non-genotoxic 1120, 1131–2
  in plastics industry 2019,
    2021, 2022, 2023
  in rubber industry 2015, 2016,
    2018
  skin 315
cardiac puncture 387
ceftizoxime clearance 89
circadian variations 252–3, 255,
  256
cleft palate effect of dioxin 282
combustion toxicity studies
  1924, 1926
cornea, permeability procedure
  750
CYP genes 216
dechlorination reactions 566
deer (*Peromyscus maniculatus*)
  1335
dermal studies 46, 554, 1944
designer 1964
developmental period 1696
dietary studies 58, 1982, 1985,
  1986
dioxin toxicity 85, 282
dominant lethal test 1060–1
ear, model for skin 340
ear swelling test (MEST) 842
embryo limb bud testing 414
eye/permeability test *410*
FMO expression 232

fungicide toxicity studies 2004
furan toxicity 90
gastro-intestinal microflora 563
germ cell cytogenetic assays
  1088
β-glucuronidase and β-
  glucosidase 572
hair follicle allergen 511
hairless, in dermal contact test
  605
HDL fraction 367
hepatic enzyme inducers 135
hepatocarcinogenesis 271
hepatocytes, apoptosis from
  acetaminophen *179*
herbicide toxicity studies 2004,
  2005, 2006
heterocyclic amines 272
hexobarbitone toxicity 111
hydration and renal clearance
  533
hypersensitivity reactions 1005,
  1007
IgE test 704, 707–10
interleukin-2 343
interspecies difference 274–5,
  283
intestinal studies 260
intravenous injection sites 526
irradiation toxicity 1951
isotonic saline LD_{50} 533
killer cells 341
L929 fibroblasts *410*
LAA see Laboratory animal
  allergy
LD_{50} 407–8, 525
^{14}C-leucine label *412*
liver
  apoptosis 199
  electrophoretic variants 239
  microsomes 279
  tamoxifen metabolites 285
  toxicity 257, 551, 853, 866,
    872, 1825
  tumours 526, 1127–9
lymphoma
  cell cultures 407–8
  L5178Y TKS+/-s assay
    1053–4
macrophage, and apoptosis 199
medullary space 383
mercury toxicity 2059
metallothionein role studies 2067
methaemoglobinaemia,
  insecticide 2000

mouse (*Contd.*)

  methylmercury 570
  microcapsule dosage 551
  motor activity 651
  nasal passages 342
  nerve agents toxicity 2091
  neurotoxicity test *417*
  NIH 3T3 fibroblasts 1099–100
  nitrate toxicity 2123, 2124, 2125, 2135
  nitrite toxicity 2123, 2125, 2126, 2127, 2128
  nitroreduction and liver and lung tumours 565
  ochratoxin toxicity 2160, 2161, 2162
  orbital sinus blood sample 387
  organic solvents toxicity 2041
  organophosphate toxicity 638, 1997
  osmotic minipump 528
  ototoxicity 791, 795
  parathion toxicity 1342
  PCB toxicity 131
  percutaneous absorption 577, 579
  phosgene toxicity 2097
  plethysmography 623–4, 625
  pregnant, subcutaneous dosing 528
  PSI plethysmography *621*
  PSI respiratory rate depression *620*
  radiation studies 260, 1694, 1695, 1696
  repeated exposure studies 59
  reproductive cycle 372
  respiratory rate depression *613*
  respiratory sensitization assessment 706–7
  skin *see* mouse, dermal studies
  somatic spot test 1058–9
  specific locus test 1059–60
  sperm analysis 1142
  spinal cord amine oxidase (AO) 239
  stratum corneum skin permeability *579*
  sulphur mustard toxicity 2084
  teratogenicity study 258
  testicular atrophy 82–3
  ³H-thymidine label *412*
  toxicity rating scheme 408
  transgenic 1062–4
  tumorigenicity
    of high-fat diet 1980
    of medical devices 1742
    of radiation 260
  upper GI tract 544
  urinary allergens 511, 514
  white-footed (*Peromyscus leucopus*) 1345
  wood, biomarkers 1866
mouth *see* buccal; oral; peroral
moving average method 49
MRI *see* magnetic resonance imaging
MRL *see* maximum residue level
mRNA *see* RNA, messenger
mrp *see* multidrug resistance-associated proteins
MRT *see* mean residence time
MSDS *see* Material Safety Data Sheet
Msp1, lung cancer and 1891
MTD *see* maximum tolerated dose
MTT assay 752
mucin 338, 343
mucociliary escalator 604, 605
mucofilaments 340
mucopolysaccharides 829, 966, 967, 969
mucoprotein 897
mucosal epithelium 549
mucous membranes
  contact with medical devices 1735, 1736
  irritation 2006, 2032
  radiation-induced changes 1689, 1690
mucus
  ductal cells 897
  in oral exposure 604
muffle furnace 1926
Muller cells 644
Mullerian duct regression 179
mullet, grey *see Lisa ramada; Oedalechilus labeo*
multidrug resistance-associated proteins (mrp) 864
multigeneration tests 1143, 1185, 1406
multimedia applications 475
multinuclear giant cell 539
multiple chemical sensitivity syndrome 1416, 1450
  see also idiopathic environmental illness
multiple dosing combinations 433
multiple myeloma from organic solvents 2037
multiple route exposure 606, *608*
multi-species toxicity studies 1430–1
multistage models 1537, 1764, 1766, 1771
Musca domestica 216
muscarinic cholinergic receptors 430
muscarinic receptor-associated effects 1242
muscarinic receptors, stimulation by airborne agents 605
muscle
  adrenal hormone action 370
  cell damage, biomarker 1848, 1860
  damage 342
  distribution in 70
  enzyme distribution 1857
  fibres 539, 938, 939, 941, 942, 944
  function 126–7
  ginger toxicity 1824
  implant testing 1741
  injury
    biomarkers 1861
    signs 40
  irritancy 413
  iso-enzymes, as biomarker 1861
  metabolism radiation-induced changes 1689
  necrosis 951–5
  PBPK studies *90*, 144
musculoskeletal system 341–2, 1691–2
mushrooms
  Amanita spp.
    acute toxicity 34
    neurotoxicity 634
    A. phalloides 34
  as carcinogens 1981
  nitrate and nitrite levels 2112
  toxic metal concentrations 1369
  veterinary toxicology 1513
mussels
  biomarkers in 1866
  Mytilus edulis 1870
  toxicity 634, 2192–3
mustard, AITC in 134

Mustela spp.
  M. evermanni see ferret, Siberian
  M. nigripes see ferret, black-
    footed
  M. vison see mink
mutagenic, *see also* carcinogenesis;
  genetic damage; genetic
  toxicology
mutagenic carcinogens 873
mutagenic hepatocarcinogens
  874–6
mutagenicity 7–8, 24, 523, 567,
  571
  aflatoxin 2154
  arsenic 2052
  biomarker 1867
  definition 7–8
  ethidium bromide 1455
  fungicides 2002
  and gastro-intestinal microflora
    571
  herbicides 2005
  nitrates 2124–5
  nitrites 2128
  OCs 1995
  organophosphates 1997–8
  and parenteral toxicity 523
  and peroral toxicity 567
  in plastics industry 2019, 2020,
    2021
  in rubber industry 2015
  site-directed 1966
  testing 2, 24, 401, 1434–5, 1567,
    1573, 1628
mutagens *see mainly specific types,
  e.g. benzo[a]pyrene in Chemical
  Index*
mutagens
  determining 'safe' exposures
    1484
  literature on 1038
  risk assessment 1751, 1756
'MutaMouse' *see* transgenic models
mutation
  assay 24
  biochemistry 126, 128
  lung or skin 1474
  from medical devices 1742
  PBPD model 1770
  pharmacogenetics 226
  from radiation 1684, 1688, 1692,
    1693, 1694, 1695
mutual acceptance of data (MAD)
  (OECD) 1564, 1570, 1591

Mutual Recognition (decentralized)
  Procedure, EU 1625–6, 1640–1
Mutual Recognition Facilitation
  Group (MRFG) 1625
myasthenia gravis, treatment 1995
Mycobacterium tuberculosis 841
mycotoxicoses 2145, 2147, 2154
mycotoxins 2145–76
  *see also specific mycotoxins,
    e.g.* aflatoxin
  as CB weapon 1726
  food contamination 1994
  human studies 462
  indoor air pollution 1301–2
  metal extraction from soil 1369
mydriasis 40, 41, 759
myelin 64, 347, 2037
myelin cells 631
myelinopathies 638–9
myeloid cell types 383
myeloid inclusion bodies 818
myeloperoxidase 103, 112, 240
myelotoxicity 241, 265, 2037
myocardial damage 366
myocardial fibrosis 814–15
myocardial hypertrophy 815
myocardial infarction 229, 264,
  367, 814, 823
myocardial ischaemic necrosis, diet
  and 1978
myocardial necrosis 808, 814, 818,
  821
myocardial scar tissue 343
myocardium 336, 343, 804, 805,
  821
myocytes 804
myocytolysis 807
myoepithelial cells 340, 341
myofibrillar alteration 807
myofibrillar degeneration *see*
  contraction band necrosis (CBN)
myofibrillar lysis 807
myoglobin 340, 342, 360, 384, 941
myoglobinaemia 941
myoglobinuria 942, 1861
myopathies 366, 1997
  drug(s)-induced 942–7
myosin 341, 343, 894
myosin ATPase 342
myotactic reflex 42
Myrothecium spp. 2149
Mytilus edulis see mussels
myxoedema, radiation-induced
  1691

N

Na+/K+ *see* sodium/potassium
NAD 190, 191, 237–8, 240
NADH2 diaphorase 344
NADH 103, 104, 753
NADH dehydrogenase flavin 809
NAD(P)H: quinone oxidoreductase
  216, 240
NADP/NADPH ratio 191
NADPH
  cP450 reductase induction 1866
  generation 28
  in haematology 384
  oxidation 99, 102–3
  pharmacogenetics 232, 240–1
  redox cycling and 127
  reduction 104
  in systemic pulmonary toxicity
    724, 730
NAFTA *see* North Atlantic Free
  Trade Areas
Nagasaki bombing 1692, 1693,
  1697
nails 18, 606, 1495, 1907
Naja nigricollis see cobra
narcosis 8, 25, 2034
narcotics 2030
nasal congestion, as allergic
  response 512
nasal discharge 40
nasal epithelium, histopathology
  315
nasal mucosa
  cytotoxicity from formaldehyde
    16
  epithelium, glutaraldehyde effects
    62
  eye effects and 20
  irritation 315
  nerve PSI stimulation 619
  site of eye drug absorption
    759–60
  toxicity 56
nasal particle disposition 46
nasal PSI 614
nasal resistance, IEI and 1705
nasal sinuses 342
nasal tumours 16, 2018, 2020, 2063
nasal turbinates 704
nasal washings in IEI 1715–16
nasolacrimal ductules 755
nasolacrimal occlusion 760
nasopharyngeal region inhalation
  toxicity 46

NAT *see* *N*-acetyltransferase

national approaches, regulatory aspects 1547

National Cancer Institute (USA) 551, 765, 1434

National Estimated Daily Intake (NEDI) 1602

National Fire Protection Assocation (NFPA) (US) 1458

National Food Consumption Survey (USA) 1602

National Health Services Central Register (UK) 1531

National Institute of Building Sciences (USA) 1927

National Institute of Environmental Health Sciences (USA) 1935, 1936, 1942

National Institute for Occupational Safety and Health (NIOSH) (USA) 481, 650, 1458, 1588–9, 1677, 1936

National Institutes of Health (NIH) (USA), guidelines 1459

National Library of Medicine (USA) 478, 1676–7

National Pollutant Discharge Elimination System (NPDES) 1311

national population
  see also population
  as comparison subjects 1531

National Research Council (USA) 1752
  biomarker paradigm 1464, 1875

National Residue Program, Food Safety and Inspection Service 1637

National Theoretical Maximum Daily Intake (NTMDI) 1602

National Toxicology Program (NTP) (USA)
  carcinogenicity 1102, 1106, 1108, 1434
  cutaneous toxicity 835
  education 1940
  immunotoxicity 1006–7
  pathology 341, 344, 346
  reproductive toxicity test protocol 1140
  safety aspects 1968

natriuretic hormone 364

natural disasters, toxic effects 1444

natural flavours 1654

natural killer (NK) cells 188, 343, 865, 999, 1001

natural selection 215

natural toxicants 1366, 1371, 1534, 1554, 1977

naturally occurring toxicity 1366, 1371, 1534, 1554, 1977

nature-identical flavours 1654

nausea 43, 524, 811

Nazi physicians 453

nbk, and apoptosis 193

NCEs *see* normochromatic erythrocytes

NDMA, false conclusion 298

near-maximum lethal toxicity 13

near-threshold lethal toxicity 13

nebulization 595

neck
  male adult skin surface area *583*
  radiation-induced tumours 1691

necrogens 197

necropsy
  see also autopsy; post-mortem
  acute toxicity 39
  dermal toxicity test 605
  gross 42, 45
  procedures 62
  in repeated exposure studies 61, 64

necrosis
  and acute toxicity 40, 42
  arachnidism 2186–7
  biochemical changes 126, 187, 188
  cause 6, 126
  characterization 176
  and circadian toxicology 255
  definition 6, 175
  distinguishing features 177
  ergot toxicity 1516
  molecular concepts 163–9
  morphology 183
  nitric oxide 199
  secondary 187
  zonal 6

necrotizing myopathies 942
  see also muscle necrosis

necrotizing vasculitis 822

'need' clause, marketing authorizations 1568–9

needles, stainless steel, for sampling 1909

negative control substances 340

negative effects 1450–1

negligence 1450

Neisseria spp. 562

nematocysts 787
  on jellyfish 2189, 2190

nematodes 177, 178, 1999

neo-Nazis 1728

neon ions, radiation-induced changes 1690

neonatal mouse test 525

neonates
  blood flow 83
  development 8
  dioxin exposure 88
  exposure via milk 72
  food additives consumption 83–4, 1985, 1989
  hGH safety 1970
  metabolism 115
  mortality 1203
  neoplasia 7
  nitrite levels 2120
  peroral toxicity 549
  prenatal treatment effects 651
  toxicology 1224–9

neoplasia *see* mainly cancer; tumours

neoplasia
  aberrant crypt foci 571
  and peroxisome proliferation 1124

NEP *see* neutral endopeptidase

nephritis-like reaction, radiation-induced 1691

nephro-, *see also* kidney; renal

nephrocalcinosis 357, 1430

nephron 345, 676

nephropathy *522*, 685
  adverse drug reaction 1430
  analgesic 679, 688
  humans 2154, 2159
  and parenteral toxicity 522
  pigs 2145, 2154, 2159
  poultry 2145
  predictability in animal tests 1438
  urinary markers *678*

nephrosclerosis, food additives and 1986

nephrotic syndrome 682

nephrotoxicity
  adverse drug reactions 1427, 1430
  bismuth 2061
  bromobenzene 118
  cadmium 1373–4, 1475, 2053, 2054

nephrotoxicity (*Contd.*)
  cholecalciferol 1511
  and circadian toxicity 256
  clinical chemistry 355, 361, 362,
    367
  copper 1514–15
  ethylene glycol 1426, 1428,
    1512
  evaluation 1462
  furosemide 198
  gallium 2063
  haloalkanes 121
  herbicides 2004, 2005, 2006
  indium 2063
  lead 1475, 1515
  metal-based compounds 260–1
  mycotoxin 1516
  nitrite 2126
  organic solvents 2029, 2035,
    2036, 2038, 2041
  organophosphates 1998
  and parenteral toxicity 523
  PCBs 131
  pesticide residues 1343
  phenacetin 1428
  plants 1522
  radiation 1685, 1691, 1696
  reactive intermediates 131
  responses 675–700
  signs 43
  snake venom 2179
  sulphonamides 98
  test systems *417*
  uranium 1475
  white phosphorus 1511
nephrotoxins 305, *417*, 680, 1862
Nerium oleander *see* oleander
Nero 35
nerve agents 1721–30, 1996–7,
  2089–96
  absorption 2090–1
  clinical effects 2091
  clinical investigations 2091–2
  half-lives 2091
  history 2080, 2081
  long-term effects 2095–6
  mechanism of action 2091
  military use 2090
  pesticides 1996–7
  physicochemical agents 2090
  prognosis for casualties 2095
  terrorist use 1721–30, 2090
  toxicity 2090
    management 2092–5
  types 2082

nerve cells 179, 195, 631–2, 643
  see also neurons
nerve growth factors 178
nervous system
  see also neural, neuro-
  and apoptosis 178
  cells *see* nerve cells; neurons
  demyelination, organophosphorus
    pesticides 1333
  development, in tadpoles 1956
  function 126–7
  immature 1337
  nerve terminals 631, 640–1
  OC effects 1995
  organophosphate toxicity 1997
  pathology 346–7
  radiation-induced changes
    1690–1
  sprouting 631
  toxicity *see* neurotoxicity
nesting behaviour 1352, 1353
'net acid gas' 1266
net affinity 427
Netherlands
  nitrate and nitrite levels 2112,
    2114, 2115, 2116, 2118, 2132,
    2133
  novel food controls 1546
  occupational exposure levels
    1594
Netherlands Animal Welfare Society
  486
network theory of molecular
  mechanisms *157*
neural crest, test system 414
neural membranes, and organic
  solvents 2030, 2038
neural pathway methods for PSI
  recording 619–21
neural tube defects *see* spina bifida
neurasthenia 1710
neurobehavioural effects
  fires 1920
  lead 2055, 2056
  malformations 8
  organic solvent syndrome 1529
  organic solvents 2032
  protein deficiency and 16
  screening 495
neuroblast cell, radiation-induced
  changes 1697
neurocognitive function in
  idiopathic environmental
  intolerance 1707

neurodegenerative disorders,
  mechanisms 636
neuroendocrine activity
  assay 1328
  radiation-induced changes 1690
neurofibrillary degeneration,
  aluminium 1379
neurofilaments 631, 637, 638
neurogenic inflammation in IEI
  1715–16
neuroleptanalgesic 539
neuroleptic drugs 264–5, 1430
neurological disease, and apoptosis
  178
neuromuscular junctions 6, 790
neuromuscular symptoms, radiation-
  induced 1686
neuromuscular transmission 950–1
neuron(s) 631
  chemical lesions 641–2
  cholinergic 638
  degeneration 631
  inability to regenerate 126
  NOS and 2119
  radiation-induced changes 1690
  -specific enolase 344, 2031
neuropathy
  delayed-onset peripheral 55
  from ginger 1824
  from honey 1984
  skeletal muscle toxicity 944
  from solvents 131
  target esterase (NTE) 638, 2095
  from toxic oil syndrome 1824
neurophysiological effects in
  idiopathic environmental
  intolerance 1716
neuropsychological testing in
  idiopathic environmental
  intolerance 1713
neuroretina 756
neurosensory epithelia *see* organ of
  Corti
neurotoxic esterase, biomarker
  1345
neurotoxic theories of idiopathic
  environmental intolerance
  aetiology 1706–7
neurotoxicity 631–47
  adverse drug reactions 1427,
    1430
  aluminium 1380, 2060
  animal stings and bites 2179,
    2188, 2190
  avermectins 1999

neurotoxicity (*Contd.*)
  and behavioural toxicity 651
  biochemistry 126–7
  biomarkers 1875
  bismuth 2061
  blue–green algae toxicity 1516
  dose–response assessment 1758
  ethylene oxide 1455
  fires 1920, 1921
  FOB screen 63
  food contamination 1825
  horses 1519
  in vitro test systems *417*
  lead 1518, 2055
  and lethal synthesis 6
  mercury 1564–5, 2058
  methylmercury 569–70
  MPTP 132
  NMDA 166
  organic solvents 2030–2, 2034
  placental toxicity 1244, 1246
  predictability in animal tests
    1438
  pyrethroids 1998
  radiation 1686, 1687
  risk assessment 1756
  shellfish 2192
  signs 40, 43
  sodium chloride 1517
  tests 23
  transport mechanism 632
  vincristine 1455
  vitamin B$_6$ 1552
neurotransmitters 632, 640, 642,
  643
neurotrophic factors 788
neutral endopeptidase (NEP), IEI
  and 1705
Neutral Red uptake assay 753–4
neutrons 1683
  activation measurement
    biomonitoring of cadmium
    1905
  radiation-induced changes 1690,
    1693
neutropenia 394–5, 1549
neutrophil leukocytosis 535
neutrophils 103, 200, 384, 1686,
  1843, 2119
New Animal Drugs Application
  (NADA) (USA) 1634
new chemical substances
  see also novel foods and food
    ingredients
  dossier 1601, 1605, 1606

regulatory aspects
    EU 1478–9, 1627–9
    USA 1582–6
  toxicological studies 1557, 1565,
    1581, 1606
New Chemicals Program (USA)
  1583
New Drug Application (NDA)
  (USA) 1562, 1615, 1974
New Drug Approval (USA) 1544
New Zealand
    Agricultural Compound Unit
    1611
    fumonisin contamination of
    cereals 2165
newborn *see* neonate
newt, Californian (*Taricha torosa*)
  818, 2193
NF$_{kb}$-dependent genes 168
NFPA *see* National Fire Protection
  Association
nicotine adenosine dinucleotide
  phosphate *see* NADHP
nicotinic receptor-associated effects
  1242
nictitating membrane changes 42
nifedipine dehydrogenase *217*
nigericin, and apoptosis 192
Nightingale, Florence 1529
nightshades (*Solanum* spp.),
  neurotoxicity 1521
NIH *see* National Institutes of
  Health
Niigata disaster 1826, 1828, 2057
NIOSH *see* National Institute for
  Occupational Safety and Health
nitrate reductase 562, 567, 572,
  2122
nitrate-accumulating plants, and
  methaemoglobinaemia 1522
nitric oxide synthases (NOS) 812,
  2119–20
nitrite reductase 567
nitro reduction 104
nitroreductase *216*
nitrosation reactions 567
Nitzschia pungens 634, 2193
NK cells *see* natural killer cells
NMR *see* nuclear magnetic
  resonance
no correlation 304–5
no observed adverse effect level
  (NOAEL)
    behavioural toxicity 657

developmental toxicity 1172,
    1179, 1180
  disadvantages 1761
  human studies 462
  mixtures 314
  occupational toxicity 1483
  regulations 1574, 1612
  repeated exposure studies 56, 57,
    60
  in risk assessment 1757,
    1759–61, 1787
  as safe dose in animals 91
  study design 322
no observed effect concentration
  (NOEC) 1312, 1316, 1318
no observed effect level (NOEL) 12
  air pollutants 316
  antidotal studies 433
  regulations 1448, 1449, 1451,
    1602, 1635, 1643
  repeated exposure studies 56, 60,
    64
NOAEL *see* no observed adverse
  effect level
Nobel, Alfred 460
nodes of Ranvier 631, 637
NOEC *see* no observed effect
  concentration
NOEL *see* no observed effect level
noise *see* ototoxic interactions
non-bacterial thrombotic
  endocarditis 814
non-carcinogens
    dose–response assessments
    1759–62
    risk expression 1786–7
non-clinical safety studies 1616–18
non-competitive inhibition 305
non-genotoxic (epigenetic)
    carcinogens 7, 126, 1119–20,
    1131–2
non-Hodgkin's lymphoma 1995,
    2005
non-invasive procedures 62
non-linear kinetics *see* dose-
    dependent kinetics
non-mutagenic hepatocarcinogens
    876–81
non-necrotizing arteritis 1551
non-protein nitrogen compounds,
    toxicity 1514
non-reproducible results 1445
non-sensory epithelia 778–9
non-specific cholinesterase 368
non-specific effects 35

non-threshold effects 1758
noradrenaline 808, 812, 813, 2039
Nordic countries, regulatory
procedures 1568–9, 1572
Nordic Working Group on Food
Toxicology 1568
norepinephrine *see* noradrenaline
normal equivalent deviant ranges
48
normit chi-squared-squared method
49
normoblasts 384
normochromatic erythrocytes
(NCEs) 1087
Norsk Medisinaldepot 1568
North American Free Trade
Agreement (NAFTA) 2, 1604,
1649
northern bobwhite (*Colinus
virginianus*)
anticholinesterase exposure 1351
avian embryo bioassay 1334
behaviour 1346, 1348, 1352
chronic testing 1350
dose–response anomalies 1330
fenthion toxicity 1338
inhalation and oral toxicity
studies 1331
as model species 1329
parathion toxicity 1351
reproduction tests 1350, 1351
subacute testing 1332, 1333–4,
1338
subchronic toxicity testing 1344
Norway
nitrate and nitrite levels 2116,
2117, 2118, 2133
pharmaceuticals regulation 1544,
1568–9
NOS *see* nitric oxide synthases
nose
-only exposure 60
see mainly nasal
Notice of Commencement of
Manufacture 1583
Notice to Applicants 1621
notification, meaning 1546
Notification of New Substances
(NONS) Regulations (EU) 1478
Notification of New Substances
Regulations (UK) 37, 1590
notification schemes 1543, 1545
novel foods and food ingredients
1551, 1553, 1560

NPDES *see* National Pollutant
Discharge Elimination System
nQUERY ADVISOR statistical
program 301
NTP *see* National Toxicology
Program
NUC, and apoptosis 189
nuclear, fear of word 1959
nuclear aberrations 571
nuclear chromatin 681
nuclear condensation 183
nuclear disaster 1443, 1820–1
nuclear industry, and radiation
damage 1692
nuclear magnetic resonance (NMR)
spectroscopy 234, 364, 678–9,
1849, 1850–1, 1862
nuclear proteins, ribosylation 190
nuclear receptor genes,
polymorphism 1892
nuclear scaffold structures 163
nuclear transport, *bcl-2* gene and
194
nuclear waste 1313
nuclear weapons 1444, 1723
37 kDa nuclease, and apoptosis 189
nuclease P_1 treatment method 1887,
1888–90
nucleic acid
damage by free radicals 1683
interactions with toxins 163
modification, endogenous
1878–9
replication interference 8
study 1965
as targets 34, 160–2
nucleophiles 684, 689, 835
nucleophilic sites in genome 161
5-nucleotidase 337, 344–5, *356*,
359
nucleotide monophosphate 261
nu,e ardente 1815
null genotype 1891
Nuremberg Code 453
nutrition
see also food
antioxidants 158
balanced 317
as biomarker 1845
biomonitoring 1780, 1907
bone and cartilage growth needs
969–70
deficiencies 8, 317, 792, 823,
969–74, 1977, 2064–5
and diet 1551, 1980–3

dosing procedures 59–60
drug inclusion 523
and drug metabolism 113
exposure 19
risk assessment 1602–3
fibre 561, 572
gut microflora metabolism
572–3
habits
inter-ethnic variations 1646
poor 1552
hazard evaluation 28
imbalance 316–17
and indoor air contaminant
effects 1292
ingestion, standard assumptions
1773
maternal diet and foetal growth
1217
and metabolism 109–10, 115
and radiation effects 1690
repeated exposure studies 58
restriction 323
science development 1977
selenium requirements 2065
in standard operating procedure
(SOP) 446
status 15–16, 366, 938, 939,
1690
and toxicity 15–16, 21, 1415,
1416, 1417, 1977–83
toxicokinetics studies via 75
tumour-promoting activity 568
variables 356
vascular disease and 1978–80
Nutrition Canada Survey 1602
nuts
aflatoxin contamination 2153
nitrate levels 2115
toxicity and 1983–4
Nycticorax nycricorax see heron,
black-crowned night-
nystagmus 40, 42, 757, 788

O

OAEs *see* otoacoustic emissions
oak (*Quercus* spp.), toxicity 1513,
1518, 1522
obesity *see* size factors
obsessive-compulsive disorder, IEI
and 1709
obstructive nephropathy, adverse
drug reaction 1430
Occam's razor, ethics 1957

occult blood 364–5
occupational disease 701
occupational epidemiology,
  definition 1456
occupational exposure
  see also idiopathic environmental
  illness; occupational hazards
  acute toxicity 46
  aluminium 2060
  arsenic 1246
  asbestos 1006
  beryllium 2061
  biomarkers 1877, 1886
  biomonitoring 1899–914
  cadmium 2053–4
  carbon monoxide *1283*
  chromium 2062
  dioxin 88
  guidelines 57, 618
  human studies 466
  lead 2055, 2056
  mercury 643
  metals, during pregnancy 1203,
    1204, 1205, 1206
  nickel 2063
  nitrogen oxide 1278
  organic solvents 2031, 2033,
    2037, 2039
  paternal 1464
  PBPK modelling 148, 149
  PEL 606
  pesticides 1548, 1993
  peripheral sensory irritation
    effects 616
  regulatory aspects 1415, 1752
  reproductive system toxins 1138,
    1150, 1156
  rubber industry 2015
  safety margins 91
  tetrachloroethelene, perinatal
    exposure 1216–17, 1226
  TLV 606
  to toxins 266, 605, 1444
  veterinary drugs 1637
occupational exposure limit (OEL)
  1481–5
  airborne 1481
  biological monitoring 1910
  definition 1481–2
  EU 1483, 1594–5
  health-based 1483–4
  historical aspects 1482
  in-house 1486
  lists 1482–3, 1484–5, 1486

Maximale Arbeitskonzentrationen
    Commission 1482
  PBPK modelling 149
  percutaneous toxicity 584
  peripheral sensory irritation
    625–6
  regulations 1459, 1594
  toxicological background
    1483–5
  USSR (former) 1482
occupational exposure standard
  (OES), UK 1483–4
occupational factors 1415–24
occupational hazards 509–20, 828
  see also occupational exposure
  allergic reactions 509
  cancer risk prediction 1770
  disturbance of mood and sleep
    515
  evaluation 27
  exhaust hoods 510
  gloves 510
  industrial chemicals 1550
  infection 509
  lymphocyte cytogenetics 515
  mixing operations 510
  physical injury 509
  protective clothing 510
  reproductive effects 510, 1465–7
  sister chromatic exchanges 515
  socially acceptable 1474
  target tissues 1753
  test diets 510
  urine mutagenicity 515
  zoonoses 514–15
occupational history 1531
occupational hygiene 584, 1473,
  1487
occupational industrial exposures,
  and metabolism 112–13
occupational legislation 1458–9
occupational medicine 456, 1458
occupational mortality 1529
occupational risks 1476, 1602,
  1830
Occupational Safety and Health Act
  1970 (USA) 37, 1453, 1458,
  1467, 1481, 1482, 1588
Occupational Safety and Health
  Administration (OSHA) (USA)
  acute toxicity 37
  laboratory occupational toxicity
    515
  mixed routes of exposure 603
  multistage risk models 1537

permissible exposure limits
    (PELs) 660, 1482
  regulations 1435, 1453, 1477,
    1481, 1588
  risk assessment 1749
occupational safety
  recommendations 1648
occupational sensitization, chemical
  route 705
occupational surveillance
  programme 464
occupational toxicology 1453–71,
  1473–88
  definition 3
  history 2
ochratoxicosis 2159–60, 2161
octanol–water partition coefficient
  145, 581–2, 613, 810, 1312, 1315,
  1317, 1318, 2030
ocular *see* eye
oculomucocutaneous syndrome
  1427, 1438, 1549
odds ratio (OR) 1533
odour intolerance in idiopathic
  environmental intolerance 1704,
  1705, 1706, 1707–9, 1714, 1716
OECD *see* Organization for
  Economic Cooperation and
  Developemt
Oedalechilus labeo 1870
oedema
  acute alcoholic rhabdomyolysis
    940
  acute toxicity 40, 42
  cellular 815, 822
  dermatitis 832, 835
  dioxin toxicity 282
  pathology 342
  stria vascularis 785
  synthetic materials testing 1741
oedematous pancreatitis 898, 906–7
OEL *see* occupational exposure
  limit
oesophagus
  blood supply 545
  cancer
    in firefighters 1929
    from fumonisins 2163
    and mycotoxin toxicity 1516
    from nitrates 2131
    from *N*-nitroso compounds
      2132, 2133
    in rubber industry 2015
  drug transport 555
  epithelium 544, 554

oesophagus (*Contd.*)
  innervation 545
  mucosa, radiation-induced
    changes 1689
  peroral toxicity 544, 553
  submucosa 544
oestradiol, effects on chloroform
  metabolism 111
oestrogen(s)
  agonists 1395, 1401
  antagonists 1395, 1401
  carcinogenicity 1131
  clinical chemistry 370
  conjugates 568
  definition 1394–5
  effects on liver 284
  endocrine toxicology 983, 988
  evaluation of effects 1400
  natural 1392, 1396
    see also 17β-oestradiol
  neonatal toxicity 1226–7
  pancreatic toxicity 911, 917
  response elements 1395
  structure 1396
  synthetic 1396
  therapeutic use 1398
oestrogen receptor
  affinities 1397
  binding 1395–6, 1401
  endocrine toxicology 984
  and gastro-intestinal microflora
    570
  interspecific variation 1407
  multiple forms 1397
oestrogenic activity 163, 1153–4,
  1244, 1315–16
  see also environmental
    oestrogens
  DDT 1841
oestrogenic hormone-related
  processes 1400–1
oestrogenicity, assay 1328
oestrone hydroxylases *217*
oestrous cycle 340, 1148
oestrus-related activity patterns 653
Office of Device Evaluation *1665*
Office of Hazardous Materials
  Safety 1589
Office of Pollution Prevention and
  Toxics, US EPA 1581
Office of Population Censuses and
  Surveys publication, occupational
  morality 1529
Office of Research Integrity (USA)
  1958

Office of Technology Assessment
  (USA) 1462
office workers, risk of death 1830
*Official Journal of the European
  Communities* 1592, 1621, 1643
offspring effects, predictability in
  animal tests 1438
OHSA Communication Standard
  1459
oil contamination 1824, 1826–7
oil red O stain 336
oils, nitrate and nitrite levels 2116
Oklahoma bombing 1721, 1722
okra, nitrate and nitrite levels 2112
old people *see* elderly people
oleander
    common pink (*Nerium oleander*),
      cardiovascular effects 1522
    toxicity to horses 1519
olfaction, in human subject PSI 623
olfactory epithelium 315, 590
olfactory threshold in IEI 1706
olfactory warning 21, 1707–8
oligodendria 631
oliguria 43, 362, 682
olive oil–water partition coefficient
  of organic solvents 2030
Olympic Committee's Medical
  Commission 1958
omeprazole 5-hydroxylase *217*
Onchocerca volvulus control 1999
oncholysis 1427, 1428, 1438
oncogene(s)
    and apoptosis 192, 196
    biomarker 1847, 1849, 1892
    carcinogenicity 1099–100
    expression 339
    mutagenicity 1028
    pathology 340
    proteins, altered 1460
    transition mutations 162
oncogenesis, definition 7
oncogenicity, chronic studies 57
Oncorhynchus mykiss see trout,
  rainbow
onion
    as antioxidant 1984
    cardiovascular effects 1522
    nitrate and nitrite levels 2112
online searching 479
oocyte, radiation-induced changes
  1685, 1688–9
open-field enclosures 651
operant behaviour 1345, 1346
ophthalmic *see* mainly eye

ophthalmic decongestion
  preparations 738
ophthalmoscopy 331, 764
Opisthorchis viverrini see liver fluke
opisthotonos 42
optic nerve 119, 757, 765
optical brighteners in plastics
  industry 2023
optical pachymeters 747
oral cancer 1892, 1929, 1982, 2132,
  2133
oral clearance 79
oral contraceptives
  adverse effects 1427, 1428–9,
    1438
  carcinogenicity 1129
  combined 1155
  ethinyloestradiol 1392
  hepatotoxicity 879
  human studies 458
  manufacture, toxic hazards 1455
  neonatal toxicity 1226
  and oestrogen 1392, 1398
  progesterone-only (POPs)
    1155–6
  reproductive toxicity 1150,
    1154–5
  and venous thromboembolism
    1428–9
oral dosing 465, 522, 523
oral drainage 545
oral examination for toxicology
  1938–9
oral exposure to toxins 604
oral LD_{50} 407
oral microflora 561–2
oral mucous membranes 1516,
  1686, 1689
oral ulceration from radiation 1686,
  1689
oral-to-dermal extrapolation 148
Orange Book 37
ore-crushing workers 668
Orfelia 472
Orfila, J.B. 36, 1490, 1935
organ(s)
  blood flow 74
  burden assessment, occupational
    1905
  fixation 64, 336
  pathology 62, 336
  perfusion 85, 416
  potential target 373
  signs of toxicity 44
  transplant recipients 215

organ(s) (*Contd.*)
  transplantation 684
  weight
    analysis, PBPK modelling 145
    as biomarker 1846, 1855–6
    checks 45
    in long-term toxicity studies 331
    pathology 336
    in repeated exposure studies 61, 64
organ of Corti 347, 776–8, 780, 781–3, 787, 790
organic matter, in soil 1368, 1369
organic solvent syndrome (Danish painters' disease) 1527, 1529, 1539
Organization for Economic Cooperation and Development (OECD) 2
  acute toxicity studies 36, 37
  animal testing harmonization 501
  aquatic toxicology initiatives 1311, 1314
  banned and restricted substances 1571
  existing substances, risk assessment programme 1480
  guidelines 326, 439, 465, 1139, 1400, 1404, 1436, 1612
  harmonization 1478, 1572, 1612
  high production volume (HPV) chemicals program 1480, 1585
  industrial chemicals 1571
  information resources 482, 487
  mutual acceptance of data (MAD) 1564, 1591
  Principles of Good Laboratory Practice 439, 442, 445, 1591
  regulatory procedures 1570–1
  and wildlife toxicology 1328
  Working Group on Endocrine Disrupters 1393, 1401
organizational information resources 482
organogenesis 23
organophosphate anticholinesterases 6, 12, 25, 329
ornithine carbamyltransferase 356, 359, 1345
ornithine conjugation 109, 111
ornithine decarboxylase gene 167
orosomucoid 254

orotate phosphoribosyltransferase 261
Orphan Drug Act 1984 (USA) 1662
orphan drug procedure 2
Osaka, CB incident 1726
OSHA *see* Occupational Safety and Health
osmolality 332, 362, 364, 365, 366
osmotic load, high 521
osmotic minipump 60, 528–9
osprey (*Pandion haliatus*) 1329, 1341
osteitis, radiation 1691
osteoblasts 968, 1858
osteocalcin 1859
osteoclasts 1858
osteogenesis 968
osteomalacia 1427
osteopathy, adverse drug reaction 1430
osteoporosis 973, 1859
osteosarcommas 1081
OTC *see* 'over-the-counter' drugs
otoacoustic emissions (OAEs) 781, 783, 786
ototoxic interactions 795–6, 1418–19, 1430
outer root sheath, hair follicles 830
ovarian cancer 278, 1400
ovarian cells, apoptosis 179, 196, 198
ovarian receptors 372
ovary
  clinical chemistry 372–3
  cloned enzymes 242
  cycles 1148–9
  development 1148
  drug toxicity 369, *369*, 987, 1152–3
  hypothalamic–pituitary pathway 1148
  pathology 346
  physiological considerations 986–7
  radiation-induced injury 1685, 1688
  weight 336
over-the-counter (OTC) drugs 1562
  availability 1550
  children 1228–9
  cross-reactivity in testing 1501
  demand for 1549–50
  in pregnancy 1215, 1222–4, 1226
overdosage 4, 21, 116

overexposure 22
oviducts 1149
ovulation 372, 1148–9
owl, barn (*Tyto alba*) 1355
Oxford Childhood Cancer Study 1697
oxidants 28, 158, 192
oxidase, mixed function 373
oxidation 17, 98–103
  β-oxidation 109, 939
  circadian toxicology 254
  cytochrome P450-dependent 221, *227*, 228, 232
  drugs 114–15
  FMO substrates *233*
  genetic polymorphisms 218–43
  non-cytochrome P450-dependent 102–3
  N-oxidation 102–3, 233, 234, 272
  pharmacogenetics 216, 226, 232
  S-oxidation 101–2, 233
  species differences 110
oxidation state 1365
  see also speciation
oxidation–reduction P450 systems 254–5
oxidation–reduction reactions 1366
oxidative haemolysis 391
oxidative metabolism 218, 280, 315, 785
  see also oxidation
oxidative phosphorylation 127, 794, 806, 811, 813, 821, 822, 939, 969
oxidative pyrolysis 1916
oxidative reactions 564
oxidative stress
  and apoptosis 191–2, 199
  as biomarker 1845, 1848, 1866, 1867, 1869
  cell killing 166
  DNA adducts from 1881
  in eye toxicity 762–3
  in haematology 391
  in liver 912
  molecular concepts 158, 159–60, 168–9
  and nephrotoxicity 681
  in other pancreatic diseases 909–10
  in pancreatic disease 904–14
  pharmacogenetics 240
  role 163
oxirane ring 100
oxireductase 238

oxygen
  availability 127, 1919
  blood gas level, in fires 1920
  depletion from fire 1916
  free radicals, sources 1979
  metabolites 158
  oxidation reactions and 99
  reduction 104
  as target 34
oxyhaemoglobin dissociation curve
  384, 393, 1921, 1922
oxyradicals, as biomarker 1867
oyster, toxicity 2192

P

P13 kinase, and apoptosis 191
p53
  and apoptosis 189, 193, 195, 196
  as biomarker 1849
  expression, nitric oxide synthesis
    and 200
  induction, radiation-induced
    1690
  molecular concepts 168
  mutations 1427, 1429, 1457,
    1538
  suppressor gene 1030–1, 1101
  in testing 1448
  transcription factor 168
  and tumorigenesis 1892
P450 *see under* cytochromes
pachymetry 738
packaging
  see also classification and
    labelling; food contact
    materials
  CB agents threats 1724
  requirements 36–7
  synthetic materials 1736–7
packed cell volume (PCV) 387
paclitaxel 6-hydrogenase *217*
paedatric *see* child/ren
paints and varnishes 1417, 1418,
  1419, 1704, 1708, 2055
palate 179, 191
  see also cleft lip and palate
Palestinians, deliberate food
  poisoning 1724
palm, permeability 577, *578*
palpation 45
palpitation 236
Palythoa 820

pancreas
  acinar cells 895–7
  anatomy and physiology 894–5,
    991
  cancer 132–3, 235, 898, 901–2,
    920–6, 2015
  diseases and definitions 897–8
  drug and chemical toxicity 369,
    910–27
  ducts 545, 897
  evolution 893, 894
  in vitro test system *418*
  in miscellaneous systemic
    diseases 902–3
  peroral toxicity 547
  secretion 364, 546, 894, 897
  toxicity, oxygen free radical
    903–10, 912–14
pancreastasis 908–9
pancreatitis
  acute 897, 898–900, 906–10,
    915–17, 991–3
  chronic 900–1, *902*, 917–20
  drug(s)-induced pancreatitis
    915–20, 991–3
  from animal stings and bites
    2180, 2188
  recurrent (non-gallstone) 909
  tests 365
pancytopenia 389–90, 394
Pandion haliatus see osprey
panic attacks in IEI 1708, 1709,
  1710, 1714
pannus 742
Paoli Railroad Yard PCB litigation
  1949
Papanicolaou stain 344
papillary muscles 343
papillotoxic agents 363
paprika, nitrate levels 2113
PAPS *see* 3′-phosphoadenosine-5′-
  phosphosulphate
papules 835
para-acute dosing 39
Parabuthus see scorpion
Paracelsus 36, 47, 472, 1474, 1547,
  1937
paracrine effects 981
paradigm shift, in environmental
  toxicology 1749–50
paraesthesia 465, 1999
paraffin wax embedding 338
paralysis 42, 1824, 1997, 2192
paraparesis 634
parasitic infections 365, 367

parasthesia, facial 524
parathyroid gland 369, 1691
parathyroid hormone (PTH)
  949–50, 968
paravertebral muscles, implantation
  into 539
parenchymal cells of liver, radiation-
  induced changes 1684, 1685
parenteral infusions 522, 533–5
parenteral routes 60, 526–9
  see also specific route, e.g.
    intravenous
parenteral toxicity 521–42
  acute 46
  alternative testing 412–13
  indications 522–6
  long-term studies 521
parietal cells 545, 546
parkinsonism
  adverse drug reaction 1430
  free radicals 634
  genetic suscepibility 29
  MPTP and 132
  neurotoxicity 635, 636, 641
  pharmacogenetics 29, 223, 225,
    232
Parkinson's disease
  see parkinsonism
paroxysmal atrial tachycardia (PAT)
  811
parsley, nitrate and nitrite levels
  2112–13
partial addition, mixture effect *313*
partial hepatectomy as promoter
  566
particle accelerators 1683
α-particles 1683
particles *see* particulates
particulates
  see also winter smog/particulates
    complex
  atmosphere analysis 597–9
  atmosphere generation 594
  breathing zone samples 598
  characterization and sources
    1299
  deposition 46, 592
  dispersion system 596
  dose–response assessment 1762
  effects on human populations
    1281–2
  from volcanoes 1815
  gravitational sedimentation 591
  high-energy 1683
  'higher risk' 592

PET scan in idiopathic
environmental intolerance 1707,
1713, 1716
Peter of Albanos 35
petrous bone, decalcification 347
pets *see* domestic animal
Peyer's patches 344, 549, 557
PGF synthase, ox lung cloned *242*
pH
effects on absorption 547
factors affecting 546–7
of formulation 46
modifiers, prevention of
ochratoxicosis 2161
urine in long-term toxicity studies
332
phagocytes 200, 731, 908–9
phagocytosis 6, 176, 183, 384, 534,
997
Phalacrocorax auritus
see cormorant, double-crested
Phalaris 222
Pharmaceutical Affairs Bureau
(Japan) 1566
Pharmaceutical Affairs Law (Japan)
1544, 1566
pharmaceutical industry
development 2
responsibilities 1426, 1438
restrospective data 1435
safety standards 1439
pharmaceutical use, biotechnology
products 1548, 1558
pharmaceuticals *see* drugs
pharmacodynamics
in acute toxicity testing 34, 39
differences, uncertainty factors
and 1762
in dose selection 1620
extrapolation studies 1438
interactions 1416
peroral 543
testing, in marketing
authorization applications
1628
pharmacogenetics 215–18
pharmacogenotyping 222
pharmacokinetics
aberrant 125–6
acute toxicity testing 39
basic concepts 73–5
biomonitoring 461, 607
chronic studies 65
circadian 252–6
definition 67

derivation 73–80
differences, RDDRs and 1762
dose–response assessments 1758
end-points, in carcinogenicity
testing 1620
of ethanol 552
interactions 1416
models 19–20, 582–3
order of reaction 73
parameters and constants 68–73
peroral toxicity 543
regulations 1436, 1438, 1443
in repeated exposure studies 56
scaling, physiologically based
51–2
studies 24, 1616, 1646
testing, in marketing
authorization applications
1628
'worst-case' scenario 19–20
pharmacological effects 8
pharmacological toxicology 3
pharmacology 125, 1547
pharmacovigilance 1629, 1640
pharyngeal cancer in firefighters
1929
pharyngeal mucosa,
radiation-induced changes 1689
pharyngeal particle deposition 46
pharynx 544
Phase I and II enzymes and
reactions 17–18, 216, 254, 273,
568
phase-contrast microscopy 781
Phaseolus vulgaris 345
Phasianus colchius see pheasant,
ring-necked
pheasant, ring-necked (*Phasianus
colchius*) 1332, 1333–4, 1340,
1341
phenotypes
ADH 236
ALDH 237
as biomarker 1847, 1890–1
and biotransformation 112
debrisoquine 223
ethnic differences 236
functional 218
metabolic 265
pharmacogenetics 231
studies 224
tests 222
phenyalanine-free amino acid
mixtures 1553

phenylalanine-tRNA formation
inhibition 2161–2
S-phenylcysteine adduct analysis
1882
phenylketonuria, food additives and
1990
Philadelphia chromosome 1080,
1099
PhIP$_2$ *see* phosphatidylinositol
4′,5′-bisphosphate; phospholipid
phlebitis 529
phobic disturbance in IEI 1709
phocomelia 1430, 1956
see also thalidomide *in Chemical
Index*
Phomopsis spp. 2146
P. leptostromiformis 2148
Phoradendron spp. *see* mistletoe
phosphatases, as calpain substrate
190
phosphate molecule synthesis
interference 6
phosphatidylchlorine 896
phosphatidylserine 187
phosphatidylserine receptors 183
3′-phosphoadenosine-5′-
phosphosulphate (PAPS) 105, *106*
phosphodiester alkylation 162
phosphodiesterase, inhibition 817
phosphoenolpyruvate carboxykinase
283
phosphoglycerate kinase 372
phospholipases 127, 129, 190
A 195
A$_2$ 897, 899, 938
C (PLC) 896
phospholipidosis 338, 344, *730–1*,
756, 1430
phospholipids 191, 254, 255, 367,
548, 685, 807, 809, 860, 938
phospholipids, attack 1867
phosphorus-32 postlabelling 279,
280, 284, 1845, 1846, 1849,
1888–90
photoallergy 837
Photobacterium phosphoreum 753
photocell arrays 651
photochemical air pollution
see summer smog/photochemical
complex
photoimmunotoxicity 836
photoperiod effects on toxicity 16,
58
photophobia 756, 757
photoreceptors 757

photosensitivity 1427, 1428, 1430, 1438

photosensitization 413, 415, 836–7, 1523, 2148

phototoxic retinopathy 490

phototoxicity 340, 413, 415, 837

Phyllobates aurotaenia see frog, Columbian

Physalia physalis see Portuguese man-o'-war

Physalis spp. *see* groundcherry

physical abuse, IEI and 1710

physical agents, effect on chemical hazards 1418–19

physical examination
  in acute toxicity 45
  in idiopathic environmental intolerance 1711, 1712

physical mechanisms of IEI aetiology 1704–7

physical and mental development, and environmental endocrines 1392

physical stress effects 167

physical trauma from fire 1916

physician, approach to toxicology 1447–8

physiological function in acute toxicity testing 39

physiological indicators of health, wildlife species 1327, 1328

physiological parameters, allometric scaling 51

physiological variation in biomonitoring 1908

physiologically based pharmaco-dynamic (PBPD) model 1770

physiologically based pharmacokinetic (PBPK) modelling 141–50
  acute toxicity studies 51–2, 53
  applications in toxicology 147–9
  case study 1770–1
  chronic high-dose studies 88, 89–90
  classical vs 141–2
  clearance studies 74
  definition 141
  determining parameter values 145–7
  development 143–7
  dose–response assessment 1767–9
  environmental health risk assessment 1792

establishing an adjusting occupational exposure limit (OEL) 149

formulation of mathematical relationship 144–5

inhalation model *1768*

metabolic interactions in chemical mixtures 148–9

mixed routes 607, 608

occupational toxicity 1416, 1460

parameters 1768

peroral toxicity 543, 556

personal protective equipment evaluation 149

refining experimental design in toxicity testing 148

and reformulation 147

route-to-route extrapolation 1766

safety margins 91

scaling 51–2

theory and principle 143

tissue compartments selection 144

uncertainties and limitations 149–50

validation 1780

phyto-oestrogens 570–1, 1392, 1398, 1403, 1404, 1407

Phytolacca dodecandra see pokeweed

phytometabolism, organophosphorus insecticides 1341

phytoplankton 1310

phytoremediation 1373

Pica pica see magpie, black-billed

piezobalances 599

pig
  aflatoxin toxicity 2145, 2153, 2163, 2164
  arsenic toxicity 1515
  CYP genes 216
  fetal eye *in vitro* cornea, preparation 752
  FMO expression 232
  intraperitoneal dosing necrosis 534
  monogastric 1513
  mustard gas 2085
  mycotoxin toxicity 1516
  nerve agents 2094
  nitrite levels 2123
  ochratoxin toxicity 2158, 2159, 2161, 2164
  phenol metabolism 111
  salt toxicity 1517

sciatic nerve injection damage 531

selenium toxicity 1515

stratum corneum skin permeability *579*

sulphonilamide residues 1637

T_3 and T_4 concentration 371

testicular cloned aldo-keto reductase *242*

trichlorfon toxicity 636

pig farming, toxic gases 1516–17

pigeon
  arsenic metabolism 2050
  domestic (*Columba livia*), behavioural testing 1346
  performance after carbon disulphide exposure *660*

pigmentation 830, 836, 837, 2190

pigweed, rough (*Amaranthus* spp.), nephrotoxicity 1522

pike *see* fish, predatory

piloerection 40, 42

pineapple 222

pink disease 2058

pinna 780
  reflex 42

pinocytosis 547, 549

pinprick tests, in LAA 512

Pinus ponderosa see ponderosa

pit cells 865

Pithomyces 2146
  P. chartarum 2148

pituitary gland 298, 346, 369, 1691

pituitary hormones 369, 371, 950

pituitary–target organ feedback systems 980–1

pituitary–thyroid axis 371

pK of formulation 46

pK_a 546

PKC *see* protein kinase C

placebo 425, 1715

placenta
  as barrier 17
  blood vessels 1237–8
  chemical toxicity 1241–2
  clinical chemistry 372
  cloned enzymes 242
  and drugs of abuse 1254–7
  metabolism 1240
  pathology 344
  structure and function 1233–9
  tissue evaluation 1236–9
  trophoblasts 1255–6
  villus tissue and cells 1238–9

polyamine transport mechanism 128

polychotomous response 47

polychromatic erythrocytes (PCEs) 1087

polyclonal antibodies 982

polyclonal antisera 338

polycythaemia 389, 391–2

polyethylene tubing 526

polyfume fever 1915

polygenic mutations in multifactorial conditions 1037

polygraph tests 1948

polyhydramnios 1206

polymer industry 1734, 1915, 1917, 2013–28

polymerase chain reaction (PCR)
  ADH 236, 237
  CYP2D6 218, 219
  in pharmacogenetics 218, 229, 234, 235
  safety technology 1966

polymeric matrix testing 1742

polymodal nociceptor 612

polymorphisms 21, 38, 112, 135, 217–43, 274, 1549, 1890

polymorphonuclear leukocytes 384, 533

polymorphs 384

polymyositis 943

polyneuropathy, organophosphate-induced delayed 1996, 1997

polyuria 40, 42, 43, 362, 682

ponderosa (*Pinus ponderosa*), reproductive toxicity 1521

pons 347

pony *see* horse

POPs *see* progesterone-only oral contraception

population
  -based studies, male reproductive health 1466
  composition ratios 1353
  dynamics 1327
  estimation, in field testing 1353
  exposures 1535
  risk 1813
  size, as biomarker 1846, 1847

porcelain factory biomonitoring 1904

pork
  heterocyclic amines 271
  nitrate and nitrite levels 2113

porphobilinogen, as biomarker 1864

porphyria 383, 392, 1705, 1713

porphyria cutanea tarda 29, 1226

porphyrin
  biomarker 1849, 1863–5
  as biomarker 1461
  clinical chemistry 362
  complex 99
  dioxin-induced 1818
  excretion, arsenic and 2051
  hepatic 29
  metabolism 2068
  synthesis 1863–4

porphyrinuria 2063

portal vein 545, 555, 556

Portuguese man-o'-war (*Physalia physalis*) 2189

positive control substances 340

positive/negative lists *see* permitted/proscribed lists

post-drug potentiation (PDP) 950–1

post-drug repetition (PDR) 950

poster presentations 1941

post-marketing authorization procedures, EU 1629–30

post-marketing surveillance (PMS) 22, 457, 1960

post-mortem drug testing 1501

post-mortem interval 1495

post-natal evaluations, teratogenicity 1181–5

post-natal growth 969–70

post-registration observations 1435

post-traumatic stress disorder 1707

post-traumatic syndrome 1825, 1828

posture 252

potassium changes, as biomarker 1861

potassium channels 639, 805, 806, 822, 897

potato
  see also Solanum spp.
  nitrate and nitrite levels 2112–13, 2115, 2116
  toxicity 1984

potency 39

Potential Daily Intake (PDI) 1602

potentiation 20, 50, 305, 306, *313*

Pott, Percival 472, 1474

potters 456

poultry
  see also specific types, e.g. chicken
  aflatoxin toxicity 2145, 2149, 2154

cardiotoxicity 819
  common toxicoses 1520–4
  fumonisin toxicity 2163
  mycotoxin toxicity 1524
  ochratoxin regulations 2158
  salt toxicity 1522–3

Poultry Products Inspection Act (USA) 1563

PPARα *see* peroxisome proliferation associated receptor

prairie dog (*Cynomys* spp.), poisoned 1347

prandial state 552–3, 557

prealbumin 254, 371, 511

precipitation on storage 1909

preconceptual irradiation 1695

precursors for *in vitro* testing 52

predation
  see also feeding patterns; secondary toxicity
  pesticide effects 1348

predator species
  eggshell thinning 1351, 1354, 1548
  secondary/tertiary toxicity 1341, 1346–7

pre-derived cancer values 1758

pre-derived non-cancer values 1758

pre-employment medical screens 513

pre-existing disease 461

pregnancy
  chemical and drug exposure 1216–24
  detection 1465
  diethylstilboestrol effects 1406
  and drug toxicity 21
  exposure to metal compounds 1203–6
  and increased susceptibility to toxicants 1464
  17β-oestradiol levels 1398
  outcome abormalities radiation-induced 1694
  pathology 340
  studies of chemicals and 23
  viral infections and neurotoxicity 665

Pregnancy Discrimination Act 1467

pregnant women, in clinical trials 1618

pre-historic toxicology 1527

pre-incubation tests 1047–8

pre-keratins 828

pre-leptone spermatocyte radiation-induced changes 1688
preliminary safety data 464–6
pre-manufacture notice (PMN) 1459, 1545, 1581
  exemption 1581
  Japan 1565
  USA 1557
pre-marketing approval, medical devices 1663–4
pre-marketing authorization
  drugs 1543, 1544
  EU 1551, 1552, 1557
  food additives, USA 1658
  novel foods, EU 1551, 1553
  pesticides 1543, 1557
  terminology 1543
  veterinary medicines 1558
pre-marketing notification 37, 1545, 1557
pre-Marketing Notification of New Chemicals Act (USA), amendment 37
premature ventricular contraction (PVC) 811, 818
prematurity 1464, 1465
prenatal irradiation effects 1696–7
pre-neoplastic foci 692
preputial separation, in juvenile male rats 1406
prescribers see clinicians
prescription medications, cross-reactivity in drug testing 1501
presentation, effects on toxicity 16
preservatives 1552, 1560, 1611, 1653, 1985, 1988–9
pre-synaptic terminal 813, 814
prey base, removal by anticholinesterase 1352
Preyer's reflex 42, 780
PRIMA see Pollutant Responses in Marine Animals
primary effects 26
'primary irritation' see chemical burns; irritation
primary literature 475
primates
  see also humans
  combustion toxicity studies 1923
  human contact 490
  metanol toxicity 119
  model for interferon testing 1971
prime toxicant 307

printing industry
  noise and chemical hazards 1418
  reproductive risks 1463
prions, as impurities 1968
probabilistic analysis 1328, 1449, 1782–4, 1785, 1792
probability
  density functions 1784
  distribution 1782
  quantifying 1573, 1574
  of response 48
probe, labelled DNA 239
probit analysis 48, 49, 493, 1331–2, 1334, 1344–5, 1763
procarboxypeptidase 897
procarcinogens 7
procaspases 164, 191
process flavourings 1654
proctitis 524
prodromal syndrome, radiation-induced 1686
product(s)
  databases 1448–9
  factsheets 1448–9
  formulation, differential hazard 1338–9
  licence 1425
  and process validation 1678
  safety 402, 403, 738, 755
  toxicology 3
Product Licence (UK) 1544, 1627
Product License Application (USA) 1974
Product Stewardship agreements 1585
proelastase 897
professional organizations, forensic toxicology 1491
Professors in Toxicology 1937
progesterone 266, 372, 534–5, 1149, 1155–6, 1403
prognostic criteria and factors 1450
programmed cell death
  see apoptosis
'prohaptens' 836
prokaryotes 216, 1019, 1966, 1969
prolactin 372
prolactin effects, assay 1328
prolapsus 42
proliferating cell nuclear antigen 338
proline nitrosation 2121
promoters 7, 88, 126, 566
pronase in adduct analysis 1883
pro-oxidants 168

Propionibacterium 563
proportional mortality ratio (PMR) 1532
prospective cohort studies 1456, 1532
prospective studies, ethical issues 1435
prostaglandin synthases 103, 241, 678, 729, 732
prostanoids, concentration in lung 128
prostate
  cancer 1983, 2015, 2054
  cells, apoptosis 179, 196
  -specific antigen (PSA), biomarker 1849
prostatic acid phosphatase DNA adduct analysis 1890
prostheses 523
  see also medical devices
prostration 40, 42
protease inhibitors, adverse effects 1427
proteases 127, 156, 194, 1883
proteasomes 164
protection ratio 433
protective clothing see personal protective equipment
protective proteins, as biomarker 1847
protein(s)
  see also specific types, e.g. heat-shock proteins
  adducts 1843, 1844, 1845, 1847, 1877–80, 1887
  antibodies 1885
  attack 1867
  binding 51, 71, 73, 126, 128
  C, activation by snake venom 2179
  catabolism 159
  cell cycle involvement 168
  changes, as biomarker 1858–9
  damage, metal toxicology 2066
  deficiency 16, 115, 970–1
    see also kwashiorkor
  degradation 1883–4
  dietary 58, 2120
  engineering 1454
    see also biotechnology industries
  as impurities 1969
  inhibition 189
  interactions with chemicals 85
  interactions with toxins 163

protein(s) (*Contd.*)

levels in BALF, in dose–response assessment 1762

modification, endogenous 1878

phosphatase inhibitor 199

post-translation modification 1878

synthesis 113, 114, 188, 1843, 1848–9, 1862–3, 1869

as targets 34, 159–60

therapeutic 1964–74

thiols 128

tissue content, interspecies 88

visualization, as biomarker 1856

protein kinases 190

C (PKC) 190, 195, 808, 896, 2055

proteinase-K, in adduct analysis 1883

proteinuria 43, 363, 367, 678, 682, 685, 687, 689, 690

proteolysis 819

proteolytic enzymes 701

proteomics 169

prothrombin 361, 389, 2179

prothrombinase 2179

protista for *in vitro* testing 52

proto-oncogenes 364, 395, 1028–30, 1099–100

protocol design 40–2, 64–5

protoporphyrin 1864, 1906

provisional tolerable weekly intake (PTWI) 91

provocation-neutralization in IEI 1713, 1714

proximal tubule 345, 362, 363, 676

pruritis 510

PSA *see* prostate-specific antigen

pseudoallergic reactions 1986–7

pseudocholinesterase 29, 1906

see also butyrylcholinesterase

pseudoeosinophils 385

pseudogene *216*, 230, 237

pseudohypoparathyroidism 950

pseudomembranatous colitis 1438

Pseudomonas 536, 1301

pseudoperoxidase activity 364

psychedelic drugs *220*

psychedelic effects 222

psychiatric disorders in IEI 1707, 1709, 1710, 1714, 1716

psychiatric evaluation in IEI 1712, 1715

psychoactive drugs, forensic analysis 1491

psychogenic asthma attacks 1708

psychological disturbance, adverse drug reactions 1427

psychological stress 1708, 1710, 1729, 1927

psychomotor retardation 235

psychosomatic symptoms, idiopathic environmental intolerance and 1711

psychotomimetic agents 2082

psychotropic drugs 264–5, 1443

psychotropic effects 223

PTH *see* parathyroid hormone

ptosis 40, 42, 757

PTWI *see* provisional tolerable weekly intake

Ptychodiscus brevis 2192

public health

pests, pesticide efficacy 1601

protection 1426

Public Health Service 487

public hygiene insecticides, EU regulation 1611

public perception

of medical devices 1674

of risk 1576–8, 1959

of science 1959

public relations 1576

public risk 1812–13

public safety, regulatory aspects 1439

PUFA *see* polyunsaturated fatty acids

puffer fish 34, 639, 816, 2193

pugilist brain 636

pulmonary, *see also* lung

pulmonary alveolar proteinoses *727*

pulmonary arterial hypertension 730

pulmonary cadmium absorption 2052

pulmonary capillaries 724, 728

pulmonary damage, from riot control compounds 2013

pulmonary drug excretion 256

pulmonary endothelial cells 730

pulmonary epithelium, target tissue 128

pulmonary exposure to chemicals 603

pulmonary fibrosis 725, 728, 731, 1430, 2060

pulmonary function tests in idiopathic environmental intolerance 1709

pulmonary hyperplasia 728

pulmonary hypersensitivity 702

pulmonary hypertension 730, 815

pulmonary lipid embolism *727*

pulmonary lipidosis 730–1

pulmonary oedema 724, *727*, 732

acute 809

from fires 1917

from organic solvents 2036–7

from phosgene toxicity 2099

interstititial 728

in pigs 2145, 2163, 2164

pulmonary ossification *727*

pulmonary phospholipidosis *730*–1

pulmonary pneumocytic dysplasia 728

pulmonary surfactant 731

pulmonary system 342

pulmonary toxicity, systemic 721–36

pulmonary uptake of organic solvents 2029

pulmonary vascular leak syndrome 343

pulmonary vasculitis *727*

pulse exposures 1535, 1536

pulse rate 264

pulsed field gel electrophoresis 563

pumpkin, nitrate and nitrite levels 2112

pupillary reflex 42, 45, 764

Pure Food and Drug Act (USA) 36

Purkinje cells 637, 643

Purkinje fibres 805, 816, 818

see also ventricular ectopic pacemaker activity

purslane, nitrate levels 2113

purulent exudate 530

PVC *see* premature ventricular contraction

pyknosis 821

pyloric sphincter 545

Pyrethrum cinariaefolium 34

pyrexia 127

Pyridinium spp. 2192

pyridinoline, as biomarker 1859

pyroclastic debris 1815

pyrogen test 535–6

pyrogenicity 522, 535

pyrogens, as impurities 1968

pyrolysis 315, 1916, 1919–20

Q

Q fever, infection transmission 514
QA *see* quality assurance
QEEG *see under* electro-
encephalogram
QRA *see* risk assessment,
quantitative
QSAR *see* quantitative structure-
activity relationship
quadriceps, risk in intramuscular
dosing 527
quail *see* northern bobwhite
quail
Japanese (*Coturnix japonica*)
age effect on LC_{50} 1337
carbofuran sensitivity 1342
dose–response anomalies
1330
as model species 1344
parathion sensitivity 1342
subacute toxicity testing 1332,
1333–4
quality assurance 293, 437–51,
1563–4, 1664
quality control 45, 535–9, 1628,
1973
quantal response 9, 10–11, 13
quantified risk analysis 1829
quantitative structure–activity
relationship (QSAR) 317, 613,
1449
see also strcture–activity
relationship
quantity of absorbed dose per unit
mass 1684
quarrying, risk of death 1830
quasi-folded proteins 167
Quercus spp. *see* oak
questionnaires 1450, 1529–30
quinone oxidoreductase 104, 240–1
quinone reductase, DT diaphorase
104

R

R-*ras*, and apoptosis 193
rabbit
acute toxicity 45
adrenaline 529
aflatoxin LD_{50} 2154
aluminium toxicity 427
amphetamine metabolism 102
arsenic metabolism 2050
baseline temperature 536

biliary excretion 555
blood sampling 386
cardiotoxicology 811, 813, 818
cornea, epithelial cells and
plasminogen activator 753
coronary artery test systems *417*
cyanide toxicity *760*
cyotchrome P450 antibodies 218
CYP genes 216
dermal and oral 46
developmental period 1696
dioxin susceptibility 282
endotoxin sensitivity 536
ethylene glycol toxicity 110
eye irritation tests 739
eye toxicity 409, 410
FMO expression 232, 233
gastric pH 555
β-glucuronidase and β-
glucosidase 572
HDL fraction 367
hepatotoxicity marker 359
hexobarbitone toxicity 110, 111
immature 536
in vitro lung tests *417*
interferon testing model 1971
intra-arterial dosing 527
intravenous injection site 526
kidney ketone reductase 242
LAA 511
long bone haematopoiesis 383
muscle implantation 535
NAT enzymes 108
neuropathy from ginger 1824
nitrate toxicity 2123, 2124
nitrite toxicity 2123, 2125
ochratoxin pharmacokinetics
2161
oral drug administration 522
N-oxidation inhibition 232
parenteral techniques 526
phosgene 2097
pulmonary oil microembolism
534
pyrogen test 522, 526, 535, 536
replacement 402
sacrospinal muscle 342
skin irritation studies 843
sperm analysis 1142
stomach pH 555
stratum corneum skin
permeability *579*
synthetic materials testing 1741
tPA safety evaluation 1970
upper GI tract 544

water injections 533
weight 51
wild 1350
race *see* ethnic factors
rad (unit) 1684
radial arm maze 657
radiant furnace 1926
radiation
see also ultraviolet light
absorption 1683
and apoptosis 188, 1690
β-radiation 599
biomarker 1849
dose–response model 1766
exposure 1035
γ-radiation 1683, 1693
hormesis and 1951
-induced lethality 260
ionizing
and apoptosis 177, 191, 199
carcinogenesis 1692–3
cellular stage 1684
densely ionizing 1683
deterministic effects 1685–92
hereditary effects 1693–6
nature of action 1683–4
partial body 1685, 1687–92
physical and chemical stages
1683
prenatal 1696–7
reproductive toxicity 1154
stochastic effects 1692–7
tissue 1684
toxicology 1683–701
whole-body 1685, 1686–7
lung toxicity 728
and menstrual disorders 1465
occupational exposures 1463
radiofrequency, toxicity 1418–19
sickness, acute 1820
toxicology 260
radicals, reactions 161
radioactive zone, diagonal 1890
radioactivity
accidental release 1820, 1828,
1833
bioavailability 581
radioallergosorbent test (RAST)
510, 513, 514
radiofrequency radiation
see radiation, radiofrequency
radioimmunoassay (RIA) 371,
982–3, 1502, 1885, 1889, 1967,
2158

rat (*Contd.*)

  intromission latency 653

  islet cell 346

  jejunum length 554–5

  LAA 511

  LDH activity 355

  liver

    apoptosis 199

    carcinogenesis 259, 271

    enzyme inducers 135

    hepatotoxicity 230–1, 359, 417, 853, 866, 872

    interspecies differences 279

    necrosis 361

    pathology 344

    thyroxine excretion 1123

  male, testosterone 511

  mammary gland 278, 571

  medullary space 383

  MeHg in faeces 570

  mercury 2058

  metallothionein gene expression 2067

  methionine salt, intramuscular dosing 532

  methotrexate, circadian response 261

  microflora 563, 565

  microsomes 279

  milk allergen studies 1005

  mitochondria 810

  as model species 1335

  motor activity 651

  muscle necrosis 951–5

  myelosuppression 527

  nasal passages 342

  nasal turbinate structure 592

  nephritis 511

  nerve agents 2091

  nitrate, nitrite and *N*-nitroso toxicity 2120, 2122, 2123–4, 2125–8, 2135, 2199

  NMR of urine *679*

  nutrient requirements for trace elements and vitamins 604

  nutrition effects on metabolism 115

  ochratoxin pharmacokinetics 2161, 2162

  ocular teratogenesis 758

  olfactory bulb of brain 232

  orbital sinus blood sample 387

  organic solvents 2041

  organophosphate studies 1997

  oropharynx bacterial infection 514

  ototoxicity 794

  ozone toxicity studies 1275, 1276

  parenteral techniques 526

  PCB toxicity 131

  peritoneal cells *411*

  peritonitis 532

  pesticide sensitivity 1338

  phosgene 2097

  phrenic nerve test *417*

  plasma ALP 359

  poisons 2006

  prandial state bioavailability 552

  preferred intraperitoneal dosing 526

  pregnant, osmotic minipump use 528

  proteinuria 511

  proximal tubule 345, 417

  pulmonary fibrinogenesis 527

  pulmonary oil microembolism 534

  renal tubule 680, 1862

  repeated acquisition task 661

  repeated exposure studies 59

  reproductive cycle 372

  reproductive system *see* rat, female/male

  respiratory tract deposition pattern of particles *589*

  riot control agents 2013

  running wheel 652, 664

  skin permeability 584

  splanchnic artery necrosis 527

  stomach

    absorption 546

    section 544

  strain, survival 323

  strain differences 239

  subcutaneous sarcoma 530

  sulphur mustard 2084, 2086

  T_3 and T_4 concentration 371

  tamoxifen 285

  target tissues for non-mutagenic carcinogens *1120*

  testis

    ABP 372

    atrophy 82–3

    toxicity 372

  thromboarteritis 529

  troponin measurement 366

  tumorigenicity of medical devices 1742

  upper GI tract 544

  urinary aeroallergens 514

  urinary biomarkers *1864*, 1885

rat bite fever 514

rate constant 70, 73, 77, 79, 86

rattlebox

  (*Crotolaria* spp.) 133, 730, 1519

  (*Sesbiana* spp.) 1518

rattlesnake 2178

  Mojave (*Crotalus scutulatus*) 2178, 2179, 2180

  Sistrurus 2178

  western diamondback 2178

raw materials, medical devices 1672–3

ray designs 306

Raynaud's phenomenon 2019

Rb see retinoblastoma gene

RD_{50} (respiratory depression) 612–13, 620, 621–2

RDA *see* recommended daily allowance

RDDR *see* regional deposited dose ratios

reactions

  see also first-order reactions

  order 73–5

reactivation 429, 430

reactive airways dysfunction syndrome 1915

reactive effects 35

reactive intermediates 130–2, 133–5, 157–63

reactive metabolite 223

reactive oxygen species (ROS) 34, 127, 128, 192, 199, 635, 643, 684, 691

reactive radical metabolites 104

reality checks on model results 1781

reanl cells, regeneration 126

Reaper, and apoptosis 193, 195

reasonable man, legal concept 1677–8

reasonably maximal exposure scenarios 1775

receptor

  agonists 631

  antagonism 430

  binding assays 1402–3

  definition 1395

  interaction 6

  ligand binding, transcriptional activity 1402

  -mediated events 126

regulatory procedures (*Contd.*)
Nordic Council 1568–9
patterns 1543–7
reinforcing agents in rubber industry 2017, 20114
Reissner's membrane 776, 780, 782
relative potency factor 311
relative risk (RR) 1533
release pathways 189
release testing 1678
relevance of expert witness report 1949
reliability of expert witness report 1949
religious conflicts 1723
religious cults 1728
REM *see* rapid eye movements
Remote Access to Marketing Authorizations (RAMA) 1436
renal, *see also* kidney; nephro-
renal blood flow 254, 255
renal cells
apoptosis 179
damage, extrapolation studies 1754
epithelial 362
renal clearance assessment 1861
renal insufficiency 943
renal papilla 345
renal tubules 256, 257, 337, 338, 345, 685
renal vascular resistance 678, 684
renin 345, 364
–angiotensin system 370, 684
repeated application irritation testing 844
repeated dose toxicity studies 328–31, 1591, 1616, 1618, 1622
repeated exposure toxicity 22, 55–66
repeated insult patch testing (RIPT) 839–40
replication factor C, and apoptosis 195
reporter gene assays 1402
reports from students 1940–1
Reports of the Scientific Committee for Food, EU 1656
reproducibility of results 45
reproductive efficiency, epidemiological measurement 1529–30

reproductive system
see also female reproductive system; male reproductive system
cell changes 179
clinical chemistry 372
genetic mutations 1038
male 1140–7
environmental effect *see* sperm count
environmental endocrine effects 1391, 1399, 1400
occupational hazards 1466–7
physiology 1140–2
toxic agents 1142–7
workplace semen samples 1529
pathology 345–6
plant toxicity 1521
screening tests in animals 1137–40, 1142–3
weight 1395, 1400, 1402–3, 1407
reproductive toxicity
biomarkers 1858–9
carbamate pesticides 1351
classification 1593
diethylstilboestrol 1392
dioxin 87
environmental oestrogens 1565
fungicides 2002, 2003
laboratory studies 1347–8
mechanisms 1464
medical devices 1734, 1735
model species 1328
mycotoxin 1516
new drugs 1617–18
nitrates 2124, 2129–30
nitrites 2127
occupational hazards 1463–7, 1929
organic solvents 2041
organophosphorus pesticides 1351
prednisone 1455
radiation 1684, 1688–9
rifampin 1455
risk assessment 1467, 1751, 1756
streptomycin 1455
studies 8, 23–4, 1137–8, 1168–9
testing 499, 1329, 1567, 1628
toxicology laboratory 510

wildlife species 1327, 1328, 1339–440
xenobiotic effects 1347–8
reptiles
phenol metabolism 111
studies 790
wildlife toxicology 1327, 1330, 1353
RER *see* rough endoplasmic reticulum (RER)
research
ethics committees 1960
experience for toxicology 1939–40
laboratories, source of biological hazards 1459
and risk assessment 1753
reservoir effect 577, 579
residence time, standard assumptions 1773
residual capacity, inhalation toxicity 46
residuals 75, 77
residue file, EU Regulation 2377/90 1643, 1644
residues
analysis 1354
cut-off assessment 1635
depletion studies 1646
maximum safe concentration 1635
monitoring 1637
surveillance, UK 1647–8
wildlife species 1327
resin
embedded sections 339
manufacture, formaldehyde exposure 1456
resistant starch 561
resorption phase, chemical 578
Resource Conservation and Recovery Act (USA) 1749–50
resources 1957, 1961
respirable fraction 461, 512, 592
respirators 149–50, 584, 1714
respiratory allergens 702, 706, 712
respiratory allergy 701
respiratory depression *see* RD_{50}
respiratory homeostasis maintenance drugs 25
respiratory irregularities 42
respiratory protective equipment 514, 516

rodenticides (*Contd.*)
  and parenteral toxicity 523
  poultry toxicity 1524
  testing 45
  wildlife toxicity 1345
  yellow phosphorus 1523–4
ROELEE 84 statistical program 301
Romanowsky stain 336, 341, 385, 1087
roofing workers, exposure risks 1886, 1887
rooting powders 2005
rope of death 222
ROS *see* reactive oxygen species
rose allergy 1708
rotarod techniques 654
rotating brush generators 596
Rotating Table Dust Generator *596*
rough endoplasmic reticulum (RER) 860, *861*, 864, 894, 895
route of administration
  see administration route
route of exposure *see* exposure route
Royal College of Physicians of London 433, 454
Royal Society (UK), Study Group of Risk Assessment 1811
Rp-2/Rp-8, and apoptosis 193
RTECS *see* Registry of Toxic Effects of Chemical Substances
rubber industry 564, 1667, 1738, 2013–18
Rules governing medicinal products in the European Union 1621, 1627
rumen
  see also forestomach
  microflora, in nitrogen toxicity 1514
Rumex spp. *see* curlydock
ruminants 527, 544, 1509, 2122
  see also cattle; forestomach
  wild 1375, 1378
running memory 667
running wheels 651
Russia *see* USSR (former)
rye *see* cereals

S

S9 fraction preparation 1040–1
β-S100 biomarker 2031
S phase 256
S-PLUS statistical program 301

SA node *see* sinoatrial node
Saccharomyces cerevisiae see yeast
saccule 778
sacrifice animals 61, 65
safe dose 91
Safe Drinking Water Act (USA) 1393, 1750
Safe Medical Devices Act 1990 (USA) 1662
safe working practices, industrial chemicals 1545
safety
  see also apparent safety margin
  assessment 35, 36, 135, 1941
    acute toxicity 35, 36
    biochemistry 135
    biodrugs 1967–9
    biomaterials 1738–9, 1746
    education 1941
    information sources 1675–7
    medical devices 1675–7
    packaging materials 1737
    pre-clinical 1968
    reference sources 1676–7
    transgene models 1964
  assurance procedures 91–2
  definition 34
  demonstration in acute toxicity studies 38–9
  factors (coefficients)
    factsheets 1448
    food 316
    Food and Drug Administration (FDA) (USA) 1635
    indoor air pollution 316
    new chemicals 1448
    occupational toxicity 1461
    regulations 1575, 1643
    study design 322
  file, EU Regulation 2377/90 1643, 1644
  margin in risk assessment 91
  needs in CB attack 1728
  parameters, medical devices 1737–8
  pharmacology 125, 1616
  phrases (S-phrases) 1477
  ratios *11*
  regulations 1960
  symbols 1594
  testing 1621, 1628–9
Safety Association of Marketed Medicine 458
sago palm *seeds* 635
Saimiri sciureus 663

St Anthony's Fire 2145, 2148
St Johns wort (*Hypericum perforatum*), photosensitization effects 1523
saline, percutaneous absorption *in vitro* studies 580
salinity changes as biomarker 1842, 1848, 1869
saliva 18, 72, 562, 1845, 2120, 2122, 2134
salivary glands 237, 343, 1689
salivation 42, 497
salmon lice control 636
Salmonella spp.
  in garbage toxicity 1512
  and gastro-intestinal microflora 561, 565, 572
  /microsome assay 566
  S. typhimurium 272, 279, 499, 566
    mutagenic DNA repair 1022, 1025
    mutation tests 1042, 1043–6, 1049, 1050, 1102, 1103–4, 1185–6
    toxicity studies 24, 2124, 2128
  S. typhosa 536
salmonids (fish) 1311, 1314
SALT *see* skin-associated lymphoid tissue
sampling
  contamination 1909
  misuse 1911
  pollutants, in samples 1909
  procedures, validation 1893
  sources of error 1908–9
  standardization 1908
  strategies 1530, 1905
San Francisco Bay Area Region Poison Control Center 737
sandwich enzyme immunoassay 514, 983
sanitary and phytosanitary measures 3
SAR *see* structure–activity relationships
sarcolemma 539, 808
sarcomas 837
  herbicides 2005
  induction 530–1
  spleen 565
  subcutaneous 522, 529, 530
sarcoplasmic calcium 938

sarcoplasmic reticulum 808, 809, 812, 813, 816, 820, 821, 938, 939
Sarobatus vermiculatus see black grease-wood
SAS statistical program 301
sassafras 1552, 1981
saury 2193
sausage, nitrate and nitrite levels 2113
SBS *see* sick building syndrome
scabby grain intoxication 2149
scabies 460
scala media 776, 779, 789
scala tympani 776, 779
scala vestibuli 776, 779
scalds, deaths from 1917
scale containment 1960
scaling factors in risk assessment 1769
scalp 577, 578
scanning calorimetry 619
scanning electron microscopy (SEM) 339, 347, 756, 782
scanning lens monitoring 756
scanning synchronous fluorescence spectrophotometry 1882, 1889
scar formation 177
scatter diagrams 1836
scavenger systems 515
SCE *see* sister chromatid exchange
Schiff's reaction 344
Schistosomas haematobium 636
schistosomiasis treatment 1995
schizophrenia as neurotoxic process 665
Schlick atomiser 595
Schmiedeberg 1935
Schmorl's stain 867
Schwann cells 631, 639
sciatic nerve 527, 531
Science and judgments in risk assessment 1752
Scientific Committee on Animal Nutrition (EU) 1648
Scientific Committee on Cosmetology (EU) 1560
Scientific Committee on Food (EU) 91, 1560, 1655–6, 1657
Scientific Committee for Occupational Exposure Limits to Chemical Agents (SCOEL) 1595
scleroderma 944, 2019
scombroid fish 2193–4
scorpion fish 2191

scorpions 2187–8
Androctonus 820, 2188
Bothotus 2188
Buthus 2188
Centruroides 820, 2187–8, 2189
Mesobuthus tamulus 2188
Parabuthus 2188
Tityus 820, 2188
scramblase 187
screening
see also monitoring; testing
definition 1394
information data set (SIDS) 1480, 1585, 1587
level assessments 1586
objectives 1400
protocols, developmental toxicity 1185–8
tests
environmental endocrines 1407–8
field studies 1353–4
forensic toxicology 1497
standardized 1328
scrotum 577, 578
cancer 2, 456, 1474
sea anemones 640, 2190
sea bass 2191
sea nettle (*Chrysaora quinquecirrha*) 2189
sea snake 2178, 2179
sea urchin *414*
aquatic toxicology 1319, 1320
seafood
see also shellfish *and individual foods, e.g.* mussels
arsenic 1382
histamine 823
methylmercury 1564–5
seagulls, PCBs in 642
seals, PCBs in 642
seasonality, and xenobiotic toxicity 1342–3, 1419
sebaceous glands 46, 829–30
sebum 830
Second World War *see* Word War II
second-hand smoke *see* passive smoking
secondary effects 4, 21, 26, 125
secondary/tertiary toxicity
anticholinesterases 1341–2
birds 1524
carrion-eating species 1341
dogs 1510
famphur 1342

laboratory testing 1353
predator species 1341, 1346–7
secrecy 1961
Secretary of Agriculture (US) 486
secretin 895
security against terrorism 1721
sediments
field sampling 1781
toxicant dispersal 1832
toxicity, aquatic toxicology 1319
seed dressings, toxicity 1825–6
seeds
chemically treated 1341, 1343
contaminated 1339
mercury toxicity 2057
segmental necrosis 944
seizure-related deaths 1494, 1504
seizures
in acute toxicity 40, 41
in animals 497, 644
diazepam for 430
herbicide toxicity 2006
neurotoxicology 641
pharmacogenetics 235, 239
solvent abuse 2029
strychine toxicity 1510
selective ion monitoring (SIM) 1500
selective ion monitoring (SIM), GC mass spectrometry (SIM-GCMS) 231
seleniferous plants 1519
self-medication 1549
self-poisoning (acute overdose), commonly encoutered substances 1496
Sellafield 1695
SEM *see* scanning electron microscopy
semen
see also sperm
analysis 1467
quality 1145–6, 1463, 1466
samples 1529
semi-automated digital image analysis 339
semi-quantitative prognostic criteria 1450
seminal fluid 372
seminiferous epithelium 345
seminiferous tubules 346, 371–2
Senecio spp. *see* groundsel
sensation changes 40
sensitive population, response to toxic agents 1416

sensitivity 47, 150, 1785–6, 1833–4
sensitization
    contact 340
    effects, OEL notation 1485
    lung or skin 1474
    medical devices 1734, 1740
    patch testing 838–9
sensory irritation 21
    see also peripheral sensory
        irritation
    biological models 619–22
    chemical models 618–19
    concentration-response data 616
    cutaneous toxicity 832–3
    determination methods 618–23
    effective concentration (EC) 616
    exposure dosage *617*
    incapacitating concentration (IC)
        617
    mixtures 307
    peripheral 611–29
    response 616–18
    significance 615–16
    in warfare 2082
sensory nerve fibres, IEI and 1706
sensory nerve receptors 612, 623
sensory thresholds 655
sentinel animals 58, 1870
sepiapterin reductase *242*
sequential dosing procedures 44
serine *1878*
serotinergic system 222, 223
serotonin *see* 5-hydroxytryptamine
    (5HT)
Sertoli cells 346, 371–2, 418, 1141,
    1142, 1404, 1464
serum
    biochemistry as biomarker
        1858–9, 1929
    horse butyrylcholinesterase 429
    lipid, dioxin levels 282
    parameters 43
    sickness 1549, 2181
    tests 355
service industries, toxic exposures
    1453
Sesbania spp. *see* rattlebox
set dose procedures 44
SETAC *see* Society of
    Environmental Toxicology and
    Chemistry
seventh amendment, EU 1590
Seveso disaster 2, 38, 1443, 1444,
    1724, 1818–19

sewage
    aquatic toxicity 1310
    environmental oestrogen efffects
        1565
    sludge 1371–2
    treatment plants, hormone levels
        1407
sex
    see also gender differences
    chromosome, abnormalities
        1081, 1694
    hormone binding globulin
        (SHBG) 372, 1398
    hormones and agonists 1129
    -linked conditions 1036, 1056–7
    ratios, altered 1392
sexual abuse, idiopathic
    environmental intolerance and
    1710
sexual assault, and acid phosphatase
    1495
sexual behaviour 664
    see also libido
sexual changes, as biomarker 1855
sexual differentiation 179
Sgp-2, and apoptosis 193
sheep
    aflatoxin toxicity 2154
    copper toxicity 1514
    CYP genes 216
    facial eczema 2145, 2148
    herbicide toxicity 2006
    lupinosis 2145, 2148
    methionine salt 532
    nitrate toxicity 2124
    nitrite levels 2123
    pharmacogenetics 223
    selenium toxicity 1515
    T_3 and T_4 concentration 371
Sheffield (Brightside) disaster 1821
shellfish
    see also seafood
    biomarkers 1852
    cadmium concentrations 822
    contamination 1825
    diarrhoeic 2194
    neurotoxicity 639, 2192
    oil contamination 1826–7
    paralytic 2192
    poisonous 2177, 2191
    saxitonin toxicity 1554
    toxin 816
shift work 1419
Shigella spp. 561

shipping
    and aquatic toxicity 1310–11
    disasters 1826–7
ships, anti-fouling 1548
shock-associated odour 666
shop workers, risk of death 1830
short-chain fatty acids 561
short-range toxins 131
short-term exposure limit 625
short-term mutagenicity tests 1434
short-term repeated dose studies 5,
    39, 57
showering exposure 1773, 1780,
    1786
shrew 51, 1866
shrimp *see* brine shrimp
sialic acid biomonitoring 1910
sick building syndrome (SBS)
    1292, 1299, 1530, 1703
sickle cell anaemia 384
side-effects 4, 21, 1435
sideroblastic anaemia 389, 391
siderophagocytosis 532
Sidman avoidance 657
SIDS *see* screening information data
    set
sigma minus method 80, 85
signal transduction 159, 163–4,
    169, 190, 194
signalling 190, 202
significant new use notice (SNUN)
    1583
significant new use rule (SNUR)
    1581, 1583, 1587
Silent Spring 2
silicon microphysiometer 753, 847
silicone biocompatibility testing
    1738
silicosis 1475
silk combustion products 1923
silo filler's disease, nitrogen dioxide
    1517
simian virus 40 415
simple dissimilar action 304–5
simple independent action 304
simple joint action 304
simulated field trials *see* caged field
    trials
single application irritation testing
    see Draize test
Single European Act 1987 1555
single-dose toxicity studies
    see also acute toxicity testing
    embryotoxicity 1334
    LD_{50} test 1328

single-dose toxicity studies (*Contd.*)
  oral 1330, 1332–3, 1335–6
  regulations 1616
single-generation reproduction
  studies 1328
singlet oxygen $^1O_2$ 127
sink effects
  indoor air particles 1299–300
  ozone and nitric oxide 1274–5
sinoatrial (SA) node 805, 808, 811,
  817
sinus arrest 811
sinus tachycardia 819
sinusitis 1703, 1711
sinusoid epithelial cells 855, 856,
  857, 858, 864, 881
sinusoids 545
SIRC cells 410
sister chromatid exchange assays
  (SCE) 276, 515, 567, 1088–90,
  1460
Sistrurus see rattlesnake
site-of-contact effects 1474
sixth amendment *see* EU Directives,
  79/831/EEC
size factors
  obesity 366, 1981
  and response to toxic agents
  1416
SK *see* ethyl bromoacetate
skeletal, *see also* bone; cartilage
skeletal abnormalities 40, 951, *952,
  966,* 968–70, 972, 1217, 1245–6
skeletal fluorosis 1381
skeletal muscle
  autopsy samples 1495
  biomarker 1848
  enzyme distribution 1858
  fibre simplification 342
  necrosis 366
  NQO2 in 240
  nuclei ATPase activity 187
  toxicity 938–64, 1512
skeletal remains, forensic
  examination 1495, 1496
skin
  see also cutaneous; dermal;
    percutaneous; subcutaneous
  abrasions 46, 363
  absorption
    human studies 463, 465
    of lead 2055
    modelling 578
    of organic solvents 2029–30

as source of error in
    biomonitoring 1908
  time factors 1778
  toxicokinetics 69, 70, 75
adipose layers reached by soil
  chemical 582
allergic response 512
animal and human 584
and apoptosis 197
assessment 340
barrier function 577
cancer 836, 837
  arsenic 1382, 2051
  biomarkers 1892
  and dietary fat 1980
  interspecies variation 278
  mixtures 315
  occupational toxicity 1474
  in plastics industry 2019,
    2020
  in rubber industry 2015
  and ultraviolet light 1538
cells *see* keratinocytes
condition, as biomarker 1855
contact studies 60, 1735, 1736,
  1740–1, 1765
damage
  animal stings and bites 2178,
    2182, 2183, 2185, 2187,
    2189
  in disasters 1814
  fungicides 2002
  lake gas 1817
  Lewisite 2088, 2089
  radiation 1684, 1685, 1688
  rubber chemicals 2014, 2016
  sulphur mustard 2084, 2085,
    2087
  toxic oil syndrome 1824
disorders
  adverse drug reactions 1427
  predictability in animal tests
    1438
dosing 523
exposure 19–20
  see also percutaneous;
    subcutaneous
  assessing 1777–8, 1780
  dose calculation 1774, 1775
  sensitivity analysis 1786
  soil 1776–7, 1778
  standard assumptions 1773
  to chemicals 605
functions 830–1
in humans 623

hydration 46
irritation
  alternative tests 411–12
  analogy 754
  characterization of 834
  cumulative 60
  nickel 2062–3
  organic solvents 2032
  primary 23
  repeated exposure 56
  results evaluation 844–5
  selected microscopic changes
    833
  tests 494
lotions 605
mouse dermal toxicity test 605
notation 603
oncogenicity bioassay 58
painting study 554
penetration studies 499, 578, 580
permeability 579
pigmentation, arsenic 2051
prick tests 510, 513
sensitization 413
structure 577–8, 828–30
surface areas, 'rule of nines'
  estimation 583
tags and papillae 1248
as tissue compartment in PBPK
  144
toxicity
  acute 46
  diisocyanates 1475
  effects 829, 831–8
  in vitro assays 845–7
  in vivo results 844–5
  OEL notation 1484–5
  signs 44
  testing 327, 838–44
  xylenes 1475
skin-associated lymphoid tissue
  (SALT) 830–1
skipjack 2193
SLE *see* systemic lupus
  erythmatosus
sleeping
  problems in IEI 1714
  sickness 1994
  time, as biomarker 1855
slimming aids 1551
slit-lamp biomicroscopy 496, 738,
  746, 747, 751, 756
slow acetylators 273
slow twitch fibres 342

small business sector 1453, 1481, 1487

small intestine 552, 562

small mammals
  feeding trials 1330
  subacute dietary toxicity test 1333–4

SMART *see* somatic mutation and recombination test

smelter factory 1904, 2051

smog, *see also* London smog

smoke from fires 46, 1821–3, 1916, 1917, 2128
  see also tobacco smoke

smoked foods 1982

smokers/ing
  adducts in 1883, 1885, 1890
  biomarkers 1845
  biomonitoring 1904, 1905
  cadmium 2052
  and cancer 1538, 1981
  carbon monoxide levels 607
  β-carotene and 1983
  CHD and 1978
  contamination 1915
  drug metabolism 113
  effect on COHb levels 1921
  ethylene oxide 1784
  hazards 28, 1439
  Hb adducts 1883
  idiopathic environmental intolerance and 1705
  interaction
    with asbestos exposure 1417
    with chemicals, in firefighters 1929
    with lead exposure 1417
  laboratory ban 516
  and lung function tests in firefighters 1928
  nitrate metabolism 2122
  nitrosamine adducts 1885
  N-nitroso compounds 2115
  PAHs 1886
  passive *see* passive smoking
  and phenotypes 1891
  polycythaemia 391
  and reference limits 1910
  risks 223, 274, 279, 513, 1529, 1751
  as source of error 1908
  vitamin E and 1983

smokestacks 1376

smooth endoplasmic reticulum 105, 113

smooth muscle 460

snails, aquatic toxicity 1316

snakebites
  acute toxicity 38
  horses 1517
  management 2180–1
  phosphodiesterase DNA adduct analysis 1890
  statistics 2178
  toxic manifestations 2178–80

snakeroot, white (*Eupatropium rugosum*), neurotoxicity 1519, 1520

snakes 2177–81
  cobra (*Hemachatus haemachatus*; *Naja nigricollis*) 820, 2178, 2179, 2180
  coral snake (*Micrurus fulvius*) 2178, 2180, 2181
  crotaline
    (*Bothrops* spp.) 957
    rattlesnake (*Crotalus scutulatus*) 2178, 2179, 2180
  pit viper 2180
  saw-scaled/carpet viper (*Echis ocellatus*) 2181
  sea snake 2178, 2179
  viper 2178

snapper 2191

sneezeweeds (*Helenium* spp.), hepatoxicity 1519

sneezing 512, 614, 2102

Snow, John 1528

snuff 2115, 2132

Soap and Detergent Association 503

soaps, allergy 1704

social and regulatory toxicology 1447

Social Security Act 1975 511

societal differences and risk acceptance 1961

Society of Environmental Toxicology and Chemistry (SETAC) 1316, 1328

Society of Forensic Toxicologists 1491

Society of Toxicology (SOT) (USA) 39, 326, 402, 425, 472, 493, 1770, 1935–6

socioeconomic factors in air pollution studies 1272, 1274

Socrates 1489

SOD *see* superoxide dismutase– catalase system

sodium changes, as biomarker 1861

sodium channel blockers 1510

sodium channels 639, 640

sodium/potassium (Na^+/K^+) ATPase
  and cardiotoxicity 807, 808, 809, 811, 812, 816, 818, 821, 823
  and ototoxicity 779, 785
  pathology 341
  species differences 286
  pump 812, 818, 822

soil(s) 577
  absorption, in disasters 1828
  agricultural 1376
  buffering capacity 1376
  cation storage 1369
  chemical bioavailability 1777, 1778
  chromium contamination 1778–9, 1780
  composition 1329, 1367
  definition 1366
  dioxin contamination 281, 606, 1818
  field sampling 1781
  forming factors 1367
  horizons 1367
  ingestion 1773, 1774, 1775–7, 1782–3, 1788
  lead contamination 1780
  loading 582
  material binding, cycling and transformation 1368–70
  matrix, movement to skin 582
  mineralogical and chemical composition 1367–8
  mining activities contamination 1373
  natural 1375–6
  nature and properties 1366–8
  near waste disposal sites 1372
  nitrate contamination 2112
  organic contaminants 1369
  organic matter 1368, 1369
  PAH contamination 1791
  parent material 1367
  particles, surface area 1367
  pH 1368
  profiles 1367
  reference values for metal contamination 1373
  salinization 1371

soil(s) (*Contd.*)
  self-purification 1370
  solution 1367, 1368
  texture 1367
  toxicant dispersal 1832
  wildlife hazard 1340–1
soil(s)–water systems
  acidification 1376
  interrelated 1365
  pollution 1370–81
  selenium 1380
Solanum spp. *see* nightshades
solder flux, respiratory effects 1475
soldering, lead neurotoxicity 639
Solenopsis spp. *see* fire ants
solid–water interface 1365, 1368
solvent(s)
  see also organic solvents (*in
    Chemical Index*)
  abuse 2029
  extraction 367
  in food 1985
  idiopathic environmental
    intolerance and 1708
  intoxication 1715
  in plastics industry 2023
  in rubber industry 2014,
    2017–18
somatic cell assays 1085–6
somatic effects of radiation 1684,
  1692
somatic mutation and recombination
  test (SMART) 1057
somatization, IEI and 1709, 1715
somatosensory discrimination 661
somatotrophs *see* growth hormone
  (GH)
somnolence 42
Sophora spp. *see* mescal beans
SOPs *see* standard operating
  procedures
sorbitol dehydrogenase 356, 359,
  1462
sorghum, cyanide-containing plant
  1519
SOT *see* Society of Toxicology
soybean fumonisins 2165
SP-1 transcription factor 168
space of Disse 855, *858*, 864
Spain
  nitrate levels 2112
  toxic oil syndrome 38, 1444,
    1551, 1554, 1568, 1824

sparrow
  house, subacute feeding trials
    1338
  white-throated (*Zonotrichia
    albicollis*), migratory behaviour
    1348
spasticity 42, 1983
spatial processing 667
special sense organs 346–7
speciality medical devices 1661,
  1667–8
speciation
  arsenic 1382, 1515
  chromium 1458
  elements 1365
  mercury 1378
  terminology 1445
species
  see also model species
  affecting toxicity 2, 15
  differences *see* interspecies
    variability
  diversity 1327
  overcrowding 1842
  selection 59, 293, 739, 1967
  sensitivity in repeated exposure
    studies 59
specific effects 35
specific gravity 362
specific ion electrodes 367
specific locus test 24, 1143
specimen sampling *see* sampling
SPECT in idiopathic environmental
  intolerance 1707, 1713, 1716
spectrofluorimetry 1498
spectrometry *see* specific techniques
spectrophotometry 597, 982, 1491,
  1498, 1882, 1889
  see also specific techniques
spectroscopic methods
  see also specific techniques
  in forensic testing 1497
speech problems, and PCBs 642
sperm
  see also semen
  analysis 1142, 1143
  clinical chemistry 362
  count
    as biomarker 1858
    environmental encrocine
      effects 1391, 1392
    reduced 1392, 1399, 1404,
      1464
    variability 1399

morphology, glutaraldehyde
  effects 62
quality 1464, 1466–7
spermatids 346
spermatocyte 372
spermatogenesis 371, 1141–2
  clinical chemistry 371
  dibromochloropropane (DBCP)
    effects 1466
  nitrate effects 2125
  organic solvent effects 2041
  radiation effects 1688–9
  semen analysis 1467
  toxins affecting 1145–6
sphincter of Oddi 894
sphinganine inhibition, fumonisins
  2165
sphingomyelin pathway, and
  apoptosis 191
sphingomyelinase D, in spider
  venom 2186
sphingosine inhibition, fumonisins
  2165
spiders 2185–7
  Agelenopsis 820
  Argiope spp. 820
  black widow spider 640, 2185–6
  brown spider 2186
  necrotic effects 2186–7
spillages, chemical 606, 1339–440,
  1545, 1551
spina bifida 969, 1216, 1696
spinach, nitrate and nitrite levels
  2112–13
spinal cord
  amyotrophic lateral scoliosis
    (ALS) 239, 1983
  glycine receptor antagonist 641
  neurotoxic action 640
  organic solvent toxicity 2031
  pathology 347
  peroral toxicity 546
  radiation-induced damage 1690
spinal reflex check 45
spiral ligaments 779, 785, 795
spirits, nitrate levels 2115
spleen 103, 341, 383, 565, 1762,
  2126
spleen colony formation (CFU-S)
  260
splenomegaly 391
SPM *see* particulates, suspended
spongiform encephalopathy, adverse
  drug reaction 1430
spongiotrophoblast 282

spontaneous abortion *see* abortion

spraying, metabolic excretion 460

spring greens, nitrate and nitrite levels 2113

spring parsley (*Cymopterus watsonii*), photosensitization effects 1523

SPSS statistical program 301

spurge (*Euphorbia* spp.), toxicity 1518

squamous cell carcinomas 837, 1692

squamous epithelium, mitosis 340

squamous metaplasia from formaldehyde 16

squirrel monkey 663

Sri Lanka, deliberate food poisoning 1724

Stabe, Casina 1528

stability data, in marketing authorization application 1628

stability tests, standard operating procedure (SOP) 446

stabilizers 1552, 1653, 1985, 2022

Stachybotris spp. 2149

stacks *see* incinerators

staggers 223

staining techniques 64, 342

stakeholders in risk assessment 1829

Standard Operating Procedures (SOPs) 293, 444, 445, 446, 447–8

standard texts 475–6

standardized mortality ratio (SMR) 1532

Standing Committee on Plant Health (EU) 1605, 1607–8, 1610

Stanford–Binet intelligence test 669

stapes 776

Staphylococcus spp.
  enterotoxin B 1690
  in garbage toxicity 1512
  in intestine 562

starling, European (*Sturnus vulgaris*) 1348, 1349, 1352

startle reflex 42

starvation
  see also anorexia; feeding behaviour
  effect on metabolism 115

Stas–Otto method 1490

static monitoring, exposure data 1530

statistics 291–302
  acute toxicity testing 45, 47–50, 1331–2
  age adjustment 298
  analysis of variance (ANOVA) 1177
  bias 291
  bioassay 1331–2
  chance 291
  clinical trials 1439
  combination 296, 297
  comparison methods 292, 300–1
  confidence interval 292
  confounding variables 301
  continuous data 301
  control groups 297, 298
  correlation coefficients 301
  developmental toxicology 1177–8
  dose-related trend 300
  false conclusion 298
  false positive 291
  field studies 1353
  formal models 296
  heterogeneity 300
  hypothesis testing 292
  LD_{50} 301
  low-dose extrapolation 297–8
  meta-analysis 1456–7
  misuse 1533
  multivariate methods 301
  NOEL estimation 297–8
  non-parametric methods 297
  null hypothesis 300
  observation context 298
  paired data 301
  pairwise comparison 300
  pooled data 297
  probability 292
  ranked data 301
  response variable 300
  software 301
  stratification 297
  subchronic toxicity testing 1344–5
  survival differences 298
  tests 292, 300–1, 1332
  time-to-tumour models 296
  trend analysis 297
  variables 295–6, 301
  wildlife toxicology 1330, 1331

statum granulosum 828

STATXACT statistical program 301

steady state 80–2, 83, 87, 582

steam distillation 1497

stellate cells *see* Ito cells

stem cells 383, 1684, 1686, 1687

stercobilinogen 360

stereocilia 776–7, 782, 790–1

stereospecificity 614

stereotactic injections 641

sterility, radiation-induced 1688

sterilization 1454, 1455, 1667, 1668, 1679–80

sternum, bone marrow 341

sternutators 2102

steroid binding proteins 1892

steroid hormone assays 1317

steroid receptors 126, 984

steroid-type inducer 113

steroidogenesis, *in vitro* assay 1402

Stevens–Johnson syndrome 755

stillbirths 1203, 1205

stinging *see* sensory irritation

stingrays 2190–1

stochastic reinforcement of waiting 660

stochastic response to radiation 1684, 1685

stomach
  see also forestomach; gastric; gastro-
  absorption 69
  ALDH3 in 237
  cancer
    gastric carcinoma 240
    nitrates 2130–1
    nitrites 2132
    N-nitroso compounds 567, 2132
    in plastics industry 2022
    in rubber industry 2015
    vitamin C and 1982
  carcinoid tumours 1124–7
  dosing into 549
  modelling 556
  mucosal radiation-induced changes 1689
  occlusion 11
  secretions 546

stomatitis 235

stonefish 2191

storage sites 17

strain
  differences, and metabolism 111
  and sensitivity in repeated exposure studies 59
  and toxicity 15, 2054

stratum corneum
  absorption 69
  chemical crossing estimation
    model 582
  cutaneous toxicity 828, 830, 831,
    833, 843, 845, 847
  diffusion 46, 582
  fat content 583
  penetration phase 578
  percutaneous toxicity 577
  and transfer rate 578
stratum germinativum (basal layer)
  828
stratum lucidium 828
stratum spinosum 828
Straub tail 42
strawberry, nitrate levels 2113
Streptobacillus meliniformis 514
Streptococcus 562
streptokinase 366, 538
Streptomyces spp.
  S. avermitilis 1999
  S. cinnamonensis 819
  S. cuspidosporus 765
  S. sparsogenes 765
Streptopelia risoria see dove, ringed
  turtle-
stress
  -activated protein kinase, and
    apoptosis 195
  cellular responses 166–9
  and chemical toxicity 1419
  clinical chemistry 357
  and cocaine toxicity 1419
  detection with polygraph 1948
  following disasters 1828
  effect on toxicity 1417
  in firefighters 1928–9
  following food contamination
    1825
  in mouse inhalational study 604
  reduction techniques 1714, 1729
  -related autonomic reaction in IEI
    1708
  as source of error in
    biomonitoring 1908
  variables 356
  following volcanic eruption 1817
stress proteins 168, 1461, 1847,
  1869, 2066–7
stressors
  endogenous and exogenous
    1337–8
  and reproductive failure 1465

stria vascularis
  amnioglycosides effects on
    792–3
  cis-Platinum effects on 793–4
  in ototoxicity 779, 780, 782,
    784–5
  trimethylin effects on 794, 795
structure–activity relationships
  (SAR)
  and alternative testing 407, 411
  and animal welfare 499
  and aquatic toxicity 1315
  and cutaneous toxicity 846
  in environmental health 1756
  and eye toxicity 754
  genotoxic carcinogens 1102–4
  and hepatotoxicity 876
  and nephrotoxicity 701, 706
  new chemical substances 1581
  in new product testing 1635
  oestrogen agonists and
    antagonists 1401
  and parenteral toxicity 524
  regulatory aspects 1583–4, 1618,
    1635
  and repeated exposures 61
  and respiratory toxicity ·712–13
  in risk assessment 1449 ·
student presentations in toxicology
  1940–1
student–mentor relationship 1937,
  1939
Student's *t*-test 300
study design and conduct 22–5
Study Director 386, 439, 440,
  441–2, 444, 449
Study Group on Combination
  Effects 304
Study Group on Medical Devices
  (Cooper Committee) 1662
stupor 42
Sturnus vulgaris see starling,
  European
styrene, vapour and colour vision
  impairment 756
styrene epoxygenase *217*
subacute intoxication, definition
  1446
subacute myelo-opticoneuropathy
  (SMON), and clioquinol 1427,
  1428, 1566
subacute toxicity studies 39
  design 328–31, 1534
  dietary tests 1333–4
  feeding trials, in captivity 1338

LD$_{50}$ protocol 1330
  repeated exposure 57
  reproducibility 1332, 1448
subadditivity 305, 1416
subarachnoid space 779
subchronic toxicity studies 39
  design 328–31
  environmental health risk
    assessment 1772
  Good Laboratory Practice (GLP)
    440
  medical device testing 1742
  oral tests 324
  repeated exposures 57, 62–4
  wildlife toxicity 1344–5
subcutaneous, *see also* skin
subcutaneous exposure 19, 47,
  525–6, 530–1
subcutaneous implantation 528
subcutaneous infection 530
subcutaneous injection 525
subcutaneous sarcoma 530
subdural haematoma 636
subendocardial haemorrhage 814
sublethal toxicity 15, 1333, 1353,
  1831
sublingual neutralization for
  idiopathic environmental
  intolerance 1715
subspecialities of toxicology 3
substance P, idiopathic
  environmental intolerance and
  1705
substantia nigra 103, 223, 232, 641
substrate specificity 233, 241
succinate, as biomarker 1862
succinate dehydrogenase 342
succinyl-coenzyme A 392
sudden death, horses 1519
sugar
  and lectins 183
  nitrate and nitrite levels 2115,
    2116, 2117
suggestive responses in idiopathic
  environmental intolerance 1708
suicide 38, 234, 543, 1443, 1444
suicide substrates enzyme
  inactivators 130
suing expert witness 1948
sulphaemoglobinaemia 391
sulphatase 568
sulphate 16, 18, 105
sulphation 98, 105–6, 115, 255
sulphomucin 897
sulphonation 528

sulphones 101
sulphotransferases 105–6, 216, 272–3, 285
Summary of Product Characteristics (SmPC) 1438, 1623, 1627
summer smog/photochemical complex 1265–6, 1267, 1273–80
sumpweed (*Iva augatafolia*), reproductive system toxicity 1521
suntan, artificial 1550
superfusion chamber 751
superoxide anion radical O_2^- 127, 1867
superoxide dismutase (SOD) 127, 158, 239, 636, 809, 1867–8, 2161
superoxide dismutase (SOD)–catalase system 1276
supervised trials median residue (STMR) 1609
suppliers, responsibilities 1476, 1480, 1481
supply-side testing programs 1478–81
suppressor genes 162
suppressor mutations 1026
supra-additive interactions *see* synergistic interactions
sural nerve 637
surface area
    and body weight 51, 92
    scaling factors 1769
    sensitivity analysis 1786
    soil and groundwater toxicity 1367, 1369
    soil particles 1367
surface exposures, in the workplace 1474
surrogate data 1602
surrogate models, for human exposures 1534
surrogate species *see* model species
Surveillance of Work Related Occupational Respiratory Disease (SWORD) (UK) 701
survival
    factors, and apoptosis 193
    genes 194
    vs health 1961
Susrata 1731
sutures, bioabsorbable 1744–5
sweat
    bench-scale extraction experiments 1777–8
    chromium toxicity 1779

diffusion 46
excretion 18
radioactivity excretion 581
sweat glands 577, 829, 847
Sweden, nitrate and nitrite levels 2114, 2118
Swedish National Food Administration 1379
Swedish National Institute of Occupational Health 668
sweet potatoes 726
sweet shrub (*Calycanthus* spp.), neurotoxicity 1520
swine *see* pigs
Swiss roll techniques 343
Switzerland
    BALs 1910
    fumonisin contamination of cereals 2165
    nitrate and nitrite levels 2116, 2117, 2118
symbols, in classification and labelling 1477, 1557, 1594, 1603
sympathetic nervous system 368, 1142
sympathomimetic drugs 219, 1438
symposium format progress reports 1940–1
symptom diary 1712
symptom questionnaires 1530
synaptic clefts 640
synaptic vesicles 632
Synechocystis spp. 1092
synergistic interactions 20, 28, 50, 305, 306, 313, 1395, 1405–6, 1416
synthetic hormones 1455, 1465
synthetic materials 1731, 1739
synthetic protein membranes 754
synthetic reactions 216
Syrian golden hamster *see* hamster
SYSTAT statistical program 301
systemic absorption 523
systemic circulation 555, 603
systemic lupus erythematosus (SLE) 764, 944
systemic toxicity
    acute 35, 56
    aflatoxins 1516
    definition 5
    fires 1917
    medical devices 1735
    synthetic materials testing 1741
    testing 40

T

T_3 *see* triidothyronine, thyroid hormones
T_4 *see* tetraiodothyronine (thyroxine), thyroid hormones
T cell(s)
    and apoptosis 188
    functional subpopulations 703–4
    helper (Th cells) 703, 729, 998–9
    hybridomas, and apoptosis 190
    and immunotoxicity 998–1000, 1012
    in latex allergy 510
    lifespan 1882
    mitogen 710
    pathology 341, 343
    response 682
    skin-infiltrating 830, 835
    subset alterations in IEI 1704
    Swiss mouse fibroblast cell line 413
    thymocytes 341
    zones 341
T cell receptor (TCR) complex 998
T syndrome 1244, 1998
tables for computation 49
tachycardia 40, 42, 43, 460, 811, 824
tachyphylaxis 612, 619, 725
tachypnoea 40, 42
tacrolimus, diabetogenic effect 764
tadpole tail regression 178
talin, as calpain substrate 189–90
Tamil guerillas 1724
Tamm–Horsfall glycoprotein 362, 678
tampons 1667
tandem mass spectrometry 225
Tantramar copper swamp 1368
tapwater *see* drinking water
tardive dyskinaesia 663
target organ(s)
    accumulation testing 1967
    acute toxicity 15, 39, 43
    biochemistry 128–30
    for cell apoptosis by toxins 184–6
    dose 9, 91, 147
    identification in acute toxicity testing 39
    medical devices toxicity 1734, 1741
    regulatory aspects 1676

testis (*Contd.*)
    lead toxicity 1475
    organic solvents toxicity 2041
    physiological considerations 987
    radiation-induced damage 1688
    reproductive toxicity 1141
    size 336
    solvent toxicity 131
    and taurine 361
    toxicity 336
    toxicological effects 987–8
    tumours 1392, 1399, 2002, 2015, 2018, 2022, 2054
    weights 336
testosterone 815, 984, 988, 1143
    as biomarker 1858–9, 1861
    effects on liver microsomal enzyme activity 111
    6β-hydroxylation 286
testosterone–oestradiol binding globulin 372
testosterone 6p-dehydroxylase 217
tetanus toxin, biomarker 1849
Tetrahymena/motility, alternative test 411
Tetraodan 639
Tetraodontiformes 2193
tetrapyrole ring system 384
Teucrium spp. *see* germander
textile industry 564
TGF-β 864, 873
Th cell *see* T cell(s), helper
Thackray, Charles 1474
thalassaemia 29
Thames (river) 1370
theca cells 372
Thelotornis capensis see vine snake
Theophrastus 35, 472, 1489
theoretical maximum daily intake (TMDI) 1609
theoretical maximum residue contribution (TMRC) 1602
therapeutic adjuvant 460–1
therapeutic confirmatory studies, phase III clinical trials 1616
therapeutic drugs, toxic–therapeutic ratio 260–5
therapeutic exploratory studies, phase II clinical trials 1616
therapeutic index (TI$_{50}$) 11, 39, 323, 426
therapeutic potential 460
therapeutic range of drug blood concentration 527

therapeutic sources, toxic exposure 1444
Thermactinomycetes 1301
thermal decomposition 1916, 1917–18
thermal injury in fires 1927
thermal process flavourings 1654, 1655, 1657
thermister probe thermometer 536
thermoastics 2018
thermography, contact 844
thermolysis 1916, 1925
thermoreceptor 612
thermosets 2018
thesis
    defence committee 1939–40
    writing 1941
thickeners in food 1985
thighs, male adult skin surface area *583*
thin-layer chromatography (TLC)
    in drug screening 1503
    in forensic toxicology 1491, 1498–9
    ochratoxin 2157–8
    in pharmacogenetics 235
thiols
    conjugate 108
    -disulphide interchange reactions 159
    oxidation 167
    protein 159
    and stress component expression 168
thiomethyl shunt 131
thiopurine methyltransferase *216*
thioredoxin (TRX)-thioredoxin reductase 160
The Third Principle 47
thorn apple *see* jimsonweed
Three Mile Island accident 1959
threshold
    carcinogens 1763
    concentration (TC$_{50}$) 616
    definition 1483, 1759
    dosage 12
    dose–response 34
    effects 1758
    levels 34, 64, 1354
    limit value (TLV) 2
        ACGIH 1483, 1594
        biological monitoring 1911
        chemical exposure and motor activity 651
        history 1482

        mixed routes of exposure 603
        occupational exposures 606, 1458–9
        PSI 625–6
        repeated exposures 60
        vinyl chloride 1475
    margin of safety for wildlife, US EPA 1331
    of regulation 1659
    to induce toxicity 56
Threshold Limits Committee 603, 1482
throat, peripheral sensory irritation 614
thrombin inhibition by snake venom 2179
thrombocyte count 387
thrombocytopenia 235, 385, 389–90, 395, 2179, 2182
thrombocytosis 535
thromboembolism 458, 1438
thrombosis 529, 809, 1979–80
thrombospondin, and apoptosis 187
thromboxane A2, diet and 1980
thromboxane synthetase inhibitors 684
thymic lymphomas in rubber industry 2015
thymidine 235, 338, 722, *1878*
thymidine kinase 256, 261
thymidine phosphorylase 261
thymidylate synthase 261
thymocytes 178, 179, 183, 188, 197, 198, 200, *410*
thymus 282, 283, 341, 385, 1693
thyroglobulin 370, 1122, 1123
thyroid function
    assay 1403
    clinical chemistry 366
    evaluation 1400
    nitrate toxicity 1514
thyroid gland
    arsenic retention 2051
    C cells 346
    carcinogenesis 1120–3, 1820, 2015, 2016, 2021, 2022
    clinical chemistry 370–1
    disorders 948–50
        food additives 1987
        from ENB 62
        fungicides 2001, 2002, 2003
        herbicides 2006
        nitrates 2125, 2130
        radiation 1691
    hypertrophy 234

thyroid gland (*Contd.*)
 in vitro test *418*
 pathology 346
 physiological considerations
  988–9
 toxic conjugate effect 569
 toxicological effects 369, 989–91
 weights 336
thyroid hormone(s)
 clinical chemistry 365, 369, 371
 dioxin effects 163
 and nervous system development
  642
 -related processes 1401
 thyroxine (T$_4$) 369–70, 984, 989,
  990, 1122
 triiodothyronine (T$_3$) *369–70*,
  989
thyroid receptors 984
thyroid stimulating hormone (TSH)
 980, 990–1, 1121, 1123
thyrotrophic 4-methylhydroxylase
 217
TI$_{50}$ *see* therapeutic index
tibial nerve 637
tidal volume 46, 615
Tier I screens (TIS) 1184–5
tight junctions 777, 779
timber *see* wood
time
 above tissue concentration,
  scaling factors 1769
 of death, investigation 1495
 -dependent sensitization in IEI
  1706–7
 effects, repeated exposure studies
  58
 factors, models incorporating
  1778
 –response relationship of
  pollutants 1870
 to toxic effect 15
 -weighted average (TWA) 1459,
  1484, 1588
timing of sampling 1908, 1910
tinea capitis, irradiation 1693
tingible bodies 175
tinnitus 130, 785, 786
tissue(s)
 see also target organ(s)
 affinity for substance 77
 –air partition coefficients 145
 –blood partition coefficient 145,
  146

compartment choice in PBPK
 144
contact with medical devices
 1735, 1736
cytokinetics 256
distribution 88, 128–30
enzyme levels, as biomarkers
 1865–7
fibrosis from radiation 1686
fixation 64, 336
forensic toxicology
 measurements 1941–2
inflammation or damage, lung or
 skin 1474
levels 45, 53
pathology 62, 1855
permeability 17
protein binding 71
rejection, HPLC 1862
response to implants 1731, 1732,
 1736
sensitivity in chronic studies 65
solubility 143
-specific genetic polymorphisms
 1061–2
specificity 128–38, 178
susceptibility patterns 256
Tityus see scorpion
TLC *see* thin layer chromatography
TLV *see* threshold limit value
TNF *see* tumour necrosis factor
TNF-R-associated death domain
 (TRADD) 193, 196
TNF-related apoptosis-inducing
 ligand (TRAIL) 196
tobacco
 chewing 2132
 replacement 220
 smoking *see* smokers/ing
 wild (*Lobelia* spp.), neurotoxicity
  1521
toenails *see* nails
Toffana, Mme 1490
Tokyo sarin incident 1721, 1723,
 1726, 1728, 1729, 1730, 1827
tolerable daily intake (TDI) 91,
 1574
tolerance, repeated-dose toxicity
 studies 328
tomato
 fumonisins 2165
 nitrate and nitrite levels 2112–13
tongue 343, 545
tongue (food), nitrate and nitrite
 levels 2113

tonometry 756
tooth *see* teeth
toothpaste 230
top dose 60
topoisomerases, and apoptosis 190
torsade de pointes see cardiac
 arrhythmias
torsion 42
torso, male adult skin surface area
 583
torts, toxic 1946
torture, use of toxic chemicals 1547
total body dose, biodegradable
 biomaterials 1745
total suspended particulates (TSP)
 1269, 1270, 1271, 1272
total volatile organic compounds
 (TVOCs) 1297–8, 1302
tourniquet as source of error in
 biomonitoring 1908
TOXBACK 1947
toxic cardiopathy 821–4
Toxic and Deleterious Regulation
 Law (Japan) 37
toxic dose 323
toxic equivalency factor 304, 1416
Toxic Exposure Surveillance System
 459
toxic gases, in animal husbandry
 1516–17
toxic interactions *see* interactive
 effects, toxic
toxic metabolites *see* metabolites,
 toxic
toxic myocarditis 807
toxic oil syndrome 38, 1444, 1551,
 1554, 1568, 1824
Toxic Release Inventory 1587,
 1589–90
toxic shock syndrome 1674
toxic stress 807
Toxic Substances Control Act 1976
 (TSCA) (USA)
 acute toxicity 37
 animal welfare 487
 behavioural toxicity 650
 chemical testing program
  1584–5
 environmental health risk
  assessment 1750
 industrial chemicals 1557
 information gathering authorities
  1586
 notification schemes 1545

Toxic Substances Control Act 1976
(TSCA) (USA) (*Contd.*)
  occupational toxicity 1459,
    1467, 1480–1
  pathology 347
  peroral toxicity 550
  wildlife toxicity 1328, 1334
toxic torts 1946
toxic wastes *see* waste disposal sites
toxic–therapeutic ratio 252, 260
toxication 116–21, 1329
toxicity (*general only*)
  action 34
  administration routes 1504
  biochemical basis 125–36
  circadian 257–65
  classification and labelling 5,
    1610
  data
    New Substances Notification
      Scheme 1590
    regulatory uses 1648
  in dead animals 23
  definition 4, 34, 1750
  description and terminology 4–6
  elimination by genetic
    manipulation 1553
  end-points, in carcinogenicity
    testing 1620
  equivalence factors (TEF) 1756,
    1757
  information sources 1759
  mechanisms 125–6
  monitoring 61–2
  nature of 6–8
  overt signs 1354
  ranking 36–7
  recommended procedures 63
  seasonal exposure 267
  species-specific 405
  subchronic 465
  testing *see* test(ing)
  types 328
toxicodynamics 34, 67, 92, 305,
  1444, 1446
toxicokinetics 67–95
  see also pharmacokinetics
  and biomonitoring 1485
  bird studies 1347
  clinical trials 1616
  definition 67
  extrapolation studies 1436
  human 1446
  medical devices 1742
  parameter selection 92

physiologically based studies
  306
  safety studies 1443, 1444
  separation from toxicodynamic
    aspects 92
  steady-state 1835
  wildlife studies 1353
toxicological disasters *see* disasters
Toxicological Excellence in Risk
  Assessment 1759
toxicological hazards *see* hazards
toxicological risk *see* risk
toxicologist
  co-operation with epidemiologists
    1538
  duties 1955–7
  education 1935–44, 1951
toxicology (*general only*)
  see also specific subjects, e.g.
    legal aspects of toxicology, *etc.*
  applied 1941–2
  chemical and analytical methods
    1447
  databases 1676
  definition 155, 1443
  education 1935–44
  endpoints 1529
  and epidemiology 1527–42
  etymology 1547
  experimental 1534
  historical aspects 1474–6,
    1489–91, 1527
  laboratory 509–20
  methodological differences from
    epidemiology 1535
  pathological techniques 335–53
  studies
    design 22–5, 322–34
    review 25–7
Toxicology Training Program
  (USA) 1935
Toxicology Data Bank 1677
toxicovigilance 458–60
toxinology 3
TOXKITS 1320
Toxline 478, 1676, 1943, 1947
Toxnet 1677, 1759
trachea 20, 46, 342, 544, 605
tracheobronchial system 591, 1814,
  1859, 1885
tracing, vital status 1531
TRADD *see* TNFR-associated death
  domain
trade barriers and disputes 1648–9

Trade-related Aspects of Intellectual
  Property Rights 1569
TRAIL *see* TNF-related apoptosis-
  inducing ligand
training programme, for respirator
  use 516
Trait, de toxicologie 36
trans-species *see* interspecies
N,O-transacetylation 108–9
transaminases 43, 868, 1462
transcriptase-polymerase chain
  reaction (PCR) 712
transcription
  activation 113
  activity 1402
  factors 190
  and hepatotoxicity 866–7
  interspecies variation 281
  mutagenicity 1019
  pharmacogenetics 232, 235, 240
  proteins 168
transdermal *see* skin
transducer radiotelemetry system
  749
transduction channel of hair cells
  790, 791
transduction pathways, and
  apoptosis 190
transfection, endocrine receptors
  1402
transferrin 1910, 2065
transforming growth factor (TGF)-β
  193, 729, 1690, 1972, 1929
transgene technologies 1964
transgenic animals 135, 682,
  1062–4, 1111–14
transglutaminases 177, 189
transient effects 5, 6, 1179
transition kinetics 1890
transition mutations 162
translation of mRNA 1019
translocator protein 281
transmission electron microscopy
  338–9, 756
Transparency Directive, EU 1545
transparency in risk estimates 1788
transplacental transport 1464, 1465
transport
  active 73
  atmospheric 1371, 1374–5
  mechanisms 1367, 1371
  requirements 37
  in soil 1367, 1370
  transplacental 1464, 1465
transulphuration 428

trapezoidal rule 79, 84–5
trauma
    see also stress
    in fires 1927
    from NMDA 166
    from parenteral injections 60
    injuries 1503
    linked to alcohol and drug use
        1444
treat and plate tests 1048–9
Treatise on Poisons 1490
treatment, toxic exposures 1444
Treaty of Maastricht 1992 1555,
    1556
Treaty of Rome 1555, 1621
tree nuts, as carcinogen 1982
tremor 40, 42, 497, 663
Treponema pallidum 1092
Trevan approach 36, 40
Tribulis terrestris 883, 2148
tricarboxylic acid cycle (Krebs
    cycle, TCA) 6, 337, 634, 643,
    822
Trichinella spiralis 1008
Trichoderma spp. 2149
Trichodesma europeum,
    hepatotoxicity 1519
trichothiodystrophy (TTD) 1034
trichrome stain 336
Trifolium hybridum see clover,
    alsike
trigeminal chemoreceptors 626
trigeminal nerve, peripheral sensory
    irritation effects 615
triglycerides, as biomarker 1848,
    1858, 1859, 1860, 1863
trimethylamine *N*-oxide, as
    biomarker 1862
trimethylaminuria 234
Tripartite Agreement 1662, 1733
TRK *see* Technische
    Richtkonzentrationen
tRNA *see* RNA, transfer
trophic factor withdrawal 178
trophoblastic tissue, human placenta
    1238
tropics 566
tropomyosin 343, 366, 894
trout
    rainbow (*Oncorhynchus mykiss*)
        409, 1311
    test system *414*
TRPM-2, and apoptosis 193
TRX *see* thioredoxin
trypsin protein catabolism 159

trypsinogen 899
tryptophan *1878*
tryptophan fluorescence
    spectroscopy 756
TSCA *see* Toxic Substances Control
    Act
TSCA Experimental Release
    Application (TERA) 1584
TSG *see* tumour suppressor genes
TSH *see* thyroid stimulating
    hormone
TSP *see* total suspended particulates
TTD *see* trichothiodystrophy
tuberculosis 514, 757
tubulin proteins 2067
tumorigenicity
    adriamycin 1455
    benzo[*a*]pyrene 115
    biomarkers 1848, 1892
    definition 7
    in environmental health risk
        assessment 1766
    fat in diet and 1980
    and gastro-intestinal microflora
        565
    medical devices 1742
    OCs 1995
tumour(s)
    see also carcino-; neoplasm *and*
        specific types of tumour, e.g.
        sarcoma
    apoptosis machinery 202
    blood flow 256
    cells 238, 1080–1
    dose reducing tumour incidence
        50% (TD$_{50}$) 274
    genes, biomarker 1849–50
    incidence
        and diet 16, 58
        latency to 64
        nitrates 2124
        nitrites 2126, 2127, 2128,
            2135
        random differences in controls
            65
    initiating activity 567
    markers 1849–50
    PBPK modelling 1770
    production, LMS 1764
    promoters, synthesis 567–9
    promoting activity, FC 567
    risk assessment 1754, 1755
    suppressor genes (TSG) 192,
        1030, 1032, 1100–1, 1849,
        1892

tumour necrosis factor(s) (TNF)
    and apoptosis 192, 193, 195, 196
    circadian toxicity 259, 265
    immunotoxicity 1001, 1002
    nephrotoxicity 703
    systemic pulmonary toxicity
        722, 729
    TNF-α 191, 199, 864, 873, 999,
        1000, 1001
    TNF-β 864
    TNF-L 195
tumour necrosis factor receptor
    (TNF-R) 163, 193, 196
tuna 2193
tunnel disasters 1827
Turdus migratorius see robin,
    American
turf farms 1329, 1348
turkey
    see also poultry
    nitrate and nitrite levels 2113
    X disease 2145
turnip, nitrate and nitrite levels
    2112–13
TVOCs *see* total volatile organic
    compounds (TVOCs)
TWA *see* time-weighted average
twins, cancer study radiation-
    induced 1697
two-generation studies 83, 1404,
    1405
Tympanuchus phasianellus
    see grouse, sharp-tailed
typhus 2
tyre
    curing fumes 2014
    workers, risks in rubber industry
        2015, 2017
tyrosine residues 370
Tyto alba see barn owl

U

U1-70 kDa, and apoptosis 190, 195
ubiquitin, as biomarker 1848, 1869
UCR *see* unit cancer risks
UDP-glucosyltransferases *216*
UDP-glucuronyltransferase 285,
    1403
UDS *see* unscheduled DNA
    synthesis
UF *see* uncertainty factor
ulceration 340, 343, 363, 365, 524,
    525, 553, 745, 1430, 1686, 1689
ulcerative colitis 565

ulcerogenic drugs 364
ultradian frequency 251
ultrafiltration 363
ultra-rapid metabolizers 224
ultrasound techniques 747, 951, 1216
ultraviolet
  filters, in cosmetics 1560
  light
    absorbers in plastics industry 2022
    and apoptosis 199
    arsenic interaction with 2052
    circadian toxicity 252
    cutaneous toxicity 836, 837
    DNA damage 1892
    in epidemiology 1538
    gene expression alterations 167
    mutagenic DNA repair 1019–20, 1023, 1025, 1034
umbilical cord, blood lead levels 2057
*umu*DC genes 1022
uncertainty factor (UF) 13, *91*, 313, 1759–60, 1787
unconditioned response to odour 1707–8
underground storage tanks 1372
uniform resource locator (URL) 482
unit cancer risks (UCR) 1764–5
United Kingdom (UK)
  BALs 1910, 1911
  benchmark value 1486
  chemical warfare 2080
  nitrate and nitrite levels 2112, 2114, 2116, 2117–18, 2130, 2133, 2134
  toxicology education 1942–3
United Nations
  Committee of Experts on the Transport of Dangerous Goods 37
  Conference on Environment and Development 1478
  Conference on Environment and Health 1592
  Environment Programme 476
    see also International Program on Chemical Safety
  human studies 453
United States of America (USA)
  Army 824
  BALs 1910

biotechnology products regulation 1584
chemical warfare 2080
chemicals export and import 1588
classification and labelling requirements 1477, 1603–4
Congress 438, 486
consumer protection 1589
cosmetics regulation 1550
dietary exposure, risk assessment 1602–3
drug regulation 1544, 1615–20
food additives regulation 1658–9
fumonisin contamination of cereals 2165
harmonization of regulation 1649
industrial chemicals regulation 1581–90
medical devices regulation 1662–5
new chemicals, regulatory program 1582–6
nitrate, nitrite and *N*-nitroso levels 2113, 2116, 2117, 2118, 2131, 2132
occupational and bystander risk assessment 1602
pesticide regulation 1599, 1600, 1601
supply-side testing and risk assessment 1480–1
toxicology education 1935–42
veterinary drug regulation 1633–8
worker protection 1588–9
United States Department of Agriculture (USDA)
  see Department of Agriculture (USA)
United States Pharmacopeia
  medical device testing 1668, 1669
  parenteral toxicity studies 536
  plastics classification 1733
University of Pittsburgh combustion device 1926
University of Surrey toxicology curriculum 1942–3
unscheduled DNA synthesis (UDS) 271, 567, 1104
up-and-down procedure 326

uracil NDA glycosulase 1892
urea 43
  see also blood urea nitrogen
ureter 1691, 1928
uricase 344
uridine diphosphate glucuronic acid
  see UDP
uridine kinase 261
uridine phosphorylase 261
urinalysis 61, 62, 63, 332, 362, 1460, 1466
urinary bladder
  AITC toxicity 134
  cancer
    acetylator status and 28, 1891
    adverse drug reaction 1430
    aromatic amines 120
    circadian studies 258
    in firefighters 1928
    food additives and 1990
    isoniazid 112
    nitrates 2131
    N-nitroso compounds 2132
    and phenotypes 1457, 1891
    in plastics industry 2021
    ras genes 1029–30
    in rubber industry 2015
    and smoking 1538
  carcinogenesis 258, 566, 1129–30
  epithelium 339
  mucosa 345
  pH 135
  radiation-induced changes 1691
  stones, and food additives 1987
urinary excretion 18
  arsenic 2052
  and bioavailability calculation 76
  biomarkers 1844, 1845, 1846, 1847, 1848, 1849, 1855, 1859, 1861–5, 1876–7, *1879*, 1885
  cadmium 2054
  clearance rate calculation 80
  elimination rate constant calculation 86
  radioactivity elimination 72
  sigma minus method 85
urinary protein
  as biomarker 1861, 1906
  clincal chemistry 363
  LAA 511
urinary tract 344–5, 1691, 2154

urine
  aflatoxin determination 2152
  autopsy samples 1495
  biomonitoring 606, 1899, 1904,
    1905, 1906, 1908, 1909, 1910
  chemical excretion 581
  clinical chemistry 357
  enzymes 363
  ethanol levels in fire victims
    1916
  mercury levels 2060
  metabolite excretion 466
  metabolite measurement,
    temporal relevance 1893
  nitrate levels 2122
  N-nitroso proline levels 2120
  ochratoxin analysis 2158
  pharmacogenetics 231
  samples
    in firefighters 1927
    for toxokinetic studies 67
  sediment 362
  volume 362
urobilin 360
urobilinogen 360, 362
urogenital signs of toxicity 40
urokinase 538
urological cancer 241
uroporphyrin 1864, 2051
uroporphyrinogen 29, 1864
urticaria 512, 516
Uruguay round 1569, 1611, 1649
user-side risk assessment/
  management 1481–6
users, responsibilities 1476
USSR (former)
  chemical warfare 2080
  MACs 1484
  nitrate levels 2114
  OELS 1482
uterotrophic assay 1395, 1402–3,
  1407
uterus
  apoptosis of cells 179
  cancer and related diseases 1400
  hypotonus, and adverse drug
    reactions 1427
  peroxidases 103
  and reproductive toxicity 1149
  tumours in rubber industry 2015
  weight 1395, 1402–3, 1407
utricles 778, 788
UV *see* ultraviolet

V

vaccines
  development and production
    1454, 1964
  genetically engineered, protection
    against CB weapons 1723
  regulatory aspects 1633–4, 1641
vacuolar myopathies 942
vacuolation 340
vacuum cleaning 1299, 1300
vaginal cancer 1215, 1228
vaginal cytology, glutaraldehyde
  effects 62
vaginal mucosa 346
vaginal opening, in juvenile female
  rat 1406
vaginosis 234
vagus nerve 546, 547
Val/Val, and lung cancer 1891
validation
  of new chemical products 1448
  of toxicological techniques 846
valve
  cusp 343
  disease, carcinoid and
    ergotamine-induced 815
van der Waals bonds 1369
Van Slyke monometric gas analysis
  apparatus 1490
vapour(s)
  absorption 584, 589–90, 605
  atmosphere analysis 597
  atmosphere generation 594
  emissions
    CB agents 1724
    completed pathways 1772
  exposure 19, 20, 21, 56, 59, 60,
    603, 607
  inhalation studies 26
  pressure 145, 543, 2029
  sampling 597
  toxicity 46
vasa recta 675
vascular disease 1382, 1978–80
vasculitis 938
vasoactive action 429
vasoconstriction 40, 42, 681
vasoconstrictors, in local
  anaesthetics 530
vasodilatation 40, 42, 1475
vasodilators, for scorpion bite 2188
Vedas 35
vegetable oils, carcinogenic 1980

vegetables
  green 230
  ingestion, standard assumptions
    1773
  nitrate, nitrite and *N*-nitroso
    levels 2111, 2112–13, 2115,
    2116, 2117, 2118, 2120, 2130,
    2136, 2137
vehicle control 549
Veillonella spp. 562
vein, clearance 74
venomous animals 2177–91
venoms *see* animal toxins
venoms, properties 2177, 2178
venous sinuses 383
venous thromboembolism, and oral
  contraceptives 1427, 1428
*Ventilation for Buildings: Design
  Criteria for the Indoor
  Environment* 1304
ventilation systems *see* heating,
  ventilation and air conditioning
  systems
ventilatory capacity 1270–1, 1273,
  1276–8, 1279, 1928
ventricular arrhythmias 806, 816,
  824
ventricular depolarization 805–6
ventricular ectopic pacemaker
  activity (Purkinje fibres) 811, 812
ventricular extrasystoles 817
ventricular fibrillation 43, 808, 811,
  819, 821
ventricular repolarization 805
ventricular tachycardia 811, 817
ventromedial hypothalamic nuclei
  815
verapamil *O*-demethylase *217*
Veratrum see hellebore, false
vertebral bodies, bone marrow 341
vertebrates, sexual differentiation
  179
Verticimonisporium spp. 2149
vertigo 788
very low density lipoproteins
  (VLDL) 367, 861, 869
vesicant agents 2082, 2083–8
vesiculation of skin 832
Vespidae 2182
vestibular dark cells 779, 784, 785
vestibular dysfunction 794
vestibular membrane *see* Reissner's
  membrane
vestibular system 775, 778

vestibular toxicity, caloric or
  rotational stimulation 788
Vesuvius 1815–16
veterinary drugs
  abuse potential 1637
  classification and labelling 1637
  efficacy studies 1634
  food safety assessment 1634–5
  legal violations 1637, 1647,
    1648
  MRLs 1642
  non-therapeutic 1549
  occupational exposures 1637
  pesticidal ingredients 1548
  pre-marketing authorization
    1558
  regulations 1549, 1633–52
  residues 1563, 1574
  socioeconomic aspects 1649
  toxicological testing 1635
  variation in use 1640
  withdrawal period 1636, 1647
veterinary facilities, source of
  biological hazards 1459
Veterinary International Conference
  on Harmonization (VICH) 2,
  1649
veterinary medicine 491, 522, 531
Veterinary Medicines Directorate
  (UK) 1638
Veterinary Pharmaceutical
  Committee 1639
Veterinary Products Committee
  (UK) 1637
veterinary toxicology 3, 1509–26
vial equilibrium technique 145
vibration 662, 1418–19
Vibrio cholera 820
VICH see Veterinary International
  Conference on Harmonization
video tape in courtroom 1951
Vietnam, chemical warfare 2080,
  2105
vimentin, and apoptosis 195
vine snake (Thelotornis capensis)
  2178
vinyl chloride workers,
  haemangiosarcoma 1533
violence, risk of death 1830
violin spider 2186
viper 2178
  pit 2180
  saw-scaled/carpet (Echis
    ocellatus) 2181
Vipera berus see adder, common

Viperidae 2178
viper's bugloss (Echium
  plantagineum), hepatoxicity 1519
viral hepatitis 868
virtually safe doses (VSD) 1764–5
Virus Act (USA) 36
viruses
  carcinogenicity 1100
  as CB weapon 1726
  as chemical warfare agents 2082
  as impurities 1968
  regulation see micro-organisms
viscosity of formulation 46
visual cortex, methyl mercury
  damage 643
visual dysfunction/impairment 129,
  614, 615, 738, 757, 765
visual evoked potentials 756
vital fluorescent labels 342
vital status, tracing 1531
vitreous humour, forensic testing
  1495, 1503, 1504
vitronectin 187
vitronectin receptors 183
VLDL see very low density
  lipoproteins (VLDL)
VOCs see volatile organic
  compounds
volatile screen (VS) 1502
volatile toxins 1491, 1495
volcanoes 1815–17
voles (Microtus spp.) 1335
voltage activated channels 639
volume
  effects on absorption 547
  factors affecting 546–7
voluntary consent 453
voluntary regulation schemes 1543,
  1545–6, 1586, 1589, 1637
volunteer testing 567, 1960
Volvariella volvacea 820
volvulus 364
vomiting
  in acute toxicity 40, 41
  agents in warfare 2028
  cardiac toxicity 811
  centre 546
  clinical chemistry 364
  human studies 460
  induction 1511
  peroral toxicity 549
  protective reaction 1347
  response 553
vomiting (emesis) 40, 41, 364, 549

von Kossa stain 342
VSD see virtually safe doses
vulcanization 2016
vulcanizers 2015
Vulpes macrotis see kit fox
vulvovaginitis 2145

W

Wallerian degeneration 347
waltzing syndrome 638
warble fly control 1342, 1355
warfare
  agents see chemical warfare
    agents; nerve agents
  radiation effects in 1692, 1693
S-warfarin 7-hydroxylase 217
wartime, development of toxicology
  during 2
wasps 2182
waste disposal
  disasters 1827–8
  from farms 2114
  regulations 1960
  sites 314, 669, 1372–3
wasting syndrome 283
water
  see also drinking water;
    groundwater
  acidification 1376
  aerosol 604
  aluminium levels 2060
  consumption in studies 61, 63
  contaminated 1339, 1340, 1828
  field sampling 1781
  fluoridation 1534
  hardness see drinking water
  increased consumption in
    poisoning 1523, 1524
  intake variables 356
  mixed routes of exposure 607
  natural chemical composition
    1370
  pH
    and methylmercury 1379,
      1380
    and selenium 1380
  pollution 1870
    see also aquatic toxicology
  quality 1340, 1673
  self-purification 1370
  solubility 71
  trace metals anthropogenic inputs
    1370

water distribution systems
  asbestos content 1380
  CB agents and 1727
  copper content 1380
  corrosion 1377
  lead content 1378
  pesticide exposure 1993
water hemlock (*Cicuta* spp.),
  neurotoxicity 1519, 1520
water-soluble formulations,
  availability and toxicity 1340
waterborne diseases 1383, 1384
waterfowl
  eggshell thinning 1354
  lead toxicity 1340–1, 1343, 1523
  nest and brood abandonment
    1348
  nesting grounds 1355
  susceptibility to diazinon 1328
watermelon, aldicarb contamination
  1548
waxes 1295
weakness 460
weaver ant 2184
weavers 456
*Webster's New Collegiate
  Dictionary* 425
Wechsler Intelligence Scale for
  Children 669
weedkillers *see* herbicides
weeds 462
weever fish 2191
weigh-masters 164, 166
weight
  see also size factors
  loss 235
weight-of-evidence (WOE)
  classification 313, 1757
welding fumes 314
Western blot methods 235, 273, 510
wetlands, drainage 1355
whale
  blue, weight 51
  mercury toxicity 2057
wheat *see* cereals
wheezing, as allergic response 512
white blood cells *see* leukocytes
white supremacist groups 1728
WHO *see* World Health
  Organization
whole-body concentration,
  dosimetric scaling 147
widgeon, American 1328, 1350
Wilcoxon matched-pair signed-ranks
  test 301

wild tobacco (*Lobelia* spp.),
  neurotoxicity 1521
wildlife species
  acute toxicity 1329–34, 1338–44
  and agricultural chemicals 1328,
    1343, 1347
  behavioural aberrations 1327,
    1328, 1345–7
  biomarkers 1345, 1407–8, 1866
  in captivity 1338, 1343, 1345,
    1349
  chemical screening 1327, 1329
  endocrine disruption 1392–3
  energy stressors 1329
  environmental endocrine effects
    1407
  exposure effects 1328
  exposure sources 1339–42
  feeding habits 1328
  feeding patterns 1347
  fish-eating 1329, 1355
  laboratory tests 1345
  lack of chemical avoidance 1347
  lead toxicity 1340–1
  physiological indicators of health
    1327, 1328
  reproductive impairment 1327,
    1328
  residue burders 1327
  soil hazards 1340–1
  species studies 45
  sublethal exposures 1333,
    1344–54
  susceptibility to toxic chemicals
    1328–9
  test protocols 1330–4
  toxicology 1327–64
  water requirements 1440
  white phosphorus toxicity
    1340–1
  xenobiotic tolerance 1344
Wiley, Harvey 1534
Wilms' tumour 262, 1032, 1464
Wilson's disease 427, 869, 897,
  902, 910, 2064, 2068
wine, nitrate levels 2115
winter smog 1265, 1266, 1268–73,
  1272, 1273
withdrawal or deficiency syndromes
  1451
  see also negative effects
withdrawal periods, veterinary drugs
  1636, 1647
Withering, William 2
witness *see* expert witness

Wolffian duct differentiation 179
wood
  burning 1917–18, 1935
  dust, respiratory effects and
    carcinogenicity 1475
  preservation 1790, 1995, 1998,
    2001, 2002, 2004
  protection 1548
woodworkers, respiratory function
  1456
wool, combustion products 1923
Worker Protection Standard (US)
  1588–9, 1603
workers
  exposure studies 467, 1755
  older 46
  protection 604, 1588–9
working groups, EU 1643, 1656,
  1657
workplace
  see also occupational toxicology
  atmosphere 314
  exposure guidelines 755, 1545,
    1551
  exposures 1474
  eye safety 755
  improvement, ethics and 1911
  management, and LAA 513–14
  monitoring 1460, 1463
  reproductive hazards 1463–7
  standards 1459
Workplace Hazardous Material
  Information System (WHMIS)
  (Canada) 1477
World Health Organization (WHO)
  see also International Programme
    on Chemical Safety
  air pollution studies 1268, 1271,
    1272, 1273, 1274, 1280, 1292
  Air Quality Guidelines for
    Europe 1271, 1279, 1282
  Cell Products Safety Commission
    1463
  Codex Alimentarius Commission
    1570
  Expert Group of pesticide
    residues 1960
  –FAO Joint Expert Committee on
    Food Additives 91
  Food Additives Series 1659
  human studies 454, 458, 462
  information 476, 482
  parenteral toxicity studies 531
  pathology studies 341

World Health Organization (WHO)
acute toxicity studies 37
World Medical Association 454
World Trade Center bombing
1722–3
World Trade Organization (WTO)
1569–70, 1649
World War I, chemical warfare
2079–80, 2083, 2089, 2096, 2098,
2100, 2102
World War II 453, 460, 472, 2080,
2100, 2102, 2145
worst-case scenario 19–20, 1775
wound-healing properties of growth
factors 1972
Wright Dust Feed Mechanism 596
Wright nebulizer 595
Wright's stain 1087

X

X-linked conditions *see* sex-linked
conditions
X-ray diffraction 619
X-ray fluorescence spectrometry for
biomonitoring 1905
X-rays 634, 1683, 1693
xanthine dehydrogenase 238
xanthine oxidases 101, 103, 238–9
Xanthium spp. *see* cocklebur
xenobiotics
additive effects 1342
dermal exposure 1339, 1349
dietary presentation 1337
endocrine active

see environmental oestrogens
exposure routes 1339
exposure sources 1339–42
hepatic monoesterase (HMO)
metabolism 1339
ingestion 1339
inhalation 1339, 1349
interactions with natural stressors
1342–3
metabolism 215, 216, 1337
monooxygenase metabolism
1329
pharmacogenetics 215
recovery from exposure to 1346
reproductive toxicity 1347–8
secondary effects 1444
susceptibility 1338, 1343
tolerance 1337–8, 1344
toxicity determinants 1329
wildlife toxicity 1327, 1344
Xenopus laevis see frog, African
clawed
xeroderma pigmentosa 1033, 1892

Y

yeast (*Saccharomyces cerevisiae*)
52, 1019, 1022, 1092
Yellow Book 37
Yellow Card scheme 458
yellow jacket 2181
yellow rice disease 2145
yellow scorpion (*Leirus
quinquestriatus*) 820, 2188
yellow thick head disease 2148

Yersinnia pestis 1727
yew (*Taxus* spp.), cardiovascular
effects 1522
yoghurt
live 1552
starter cultures 1645
'Yokkaichi asthma' 1280
yolk sac 383
Yousef, Ramzi 1722–3
youth culture 222
Yun Chi Ch'i Ch'ien 35

Z

Z-band 813, 819
Z-discs 938
Zenker's stain 345
zero-order absorption 69
zero-order reaction 73, 84
zinc deficiency syndrome,
acrodermatitis enteropathica 1565
zinc proteases, in snake venom
2179
zinc protoporphyrin 392, 1485
zoanthids *see Palythoa*
Zollinger–Ellison syndrome 1125
Zonotrichia albicollis see white-
throated sparrow
zoonoses 514–15
Zopyrus 35
Zygadenus spp. *see* death camas
zygote 8, 1684
zymbal gland tumours 2015, 2021

CHEMICAL INDEX

This Index contains xenobiotics (industrial chemicals, drugs and foreign environmental materials) and their metabolites. Naturally occuring and biological substances are to be found in the Subject Index.

actinomycin 163, 184, 188, 199, 262, 727, 974, 1145, 1455
Adamsite *see* chlorodihydro-phenarsazine
adenosylcobalamin 2064
adipates 2017, 2022
adiponitrile 1922
adrenaline/lidocaine combination 947
adrenergic agonists and antagonists 16, 430, 433
adriamycin (doxorubicin)
  and apoptosis 184, 185, 192, 1430, 1861
  biomarker 1861, 1867
  cardiac toxicity 808–9, 821
  circadian toxicology 255, 262
  hepatotoxicity 872
  mechanism of action 127
  orrupational toxicology 1455
  pancreatic toxicity 904, 926
  parenteral toxicity 524, 527
  pharmacogenetics 240
  skeletal muscle toxicity 945
  systemic pulmonary toxicity 727
  toxic reactions 1430
AF-2 *see* furylfuramide
AF64A 642
AFB1 oxides 276
aflatoxicol 2149
aflatoxins 2145, 2149–54
  A$_1$ 882
  B$_1$ 231, 271, 274–8, 569, 571, 1042, 1044, 1251–2
    adducts 1883, 1885, 1886–7
    8,9-epoxygenase 217
    hepatocarcinogenesis 278
    -2,3-oxide, hepatotoxicity 130
    phase I and II metabolism 276, 277
    stereochemical factors and 162
  B, in diet 1982
  biomarkers 1845, 1848, 1880, 1881, 1882
  G$_1$ 1251–2
  hepatotoxicity 58, 877, 1537, 1538
  N^7-guanine, DNA adducts 1885
  and *p53* mutation 1457
  toxicity to food-producing animals 1515–16, 1524
  veterinary toxicology 1516, 1520
8-AG *see* 8-azaguanine (8-AG)
agarose 368

Agent Orange *see* 2,3,7,8-tetra chlorodibenzodioxin (TCDD)
aglycone 556
β-agonists
  ban 1647–8
  testing 1554
AITC *see* allyl isothiocyanate
ajmaline 219, 222, 223
alachlor 2003, 2005
β-alanine 235
Alar 1790
alclofenac 1960
alcohol
  see also ethanol and other specific alcohols
  abuse 2040–1
  acute overdose 1496
  aggressive behaviour after 653
  consumption, hazard evaluation 28
  intoxication hindering escape from fire 1916
  metabolism 113, 114, 235
  teratogenicity 258
aldehydes 307, 315, 530, 1275, 1298, 1868
  air pollution 1298
  biomarker 1867, 1868
  chlorination byproduct 1383
  irritant properties 2032
  metabolism 103, 104
  mixtures 307, 315
  parenteral toxicity 530
  reduction 104
aldesleukin 1965
aldicarb 101, 102, 1006, 1336, 1341, 1347, 1548, 1994, 1998
aldomet *see* α-methyldopa
aldosterone 364, 369–70, 675
aldrin 641, 879, 1243–4, 1329, 1994
alfoxolone 641
alginic acid 1985
alicyclic solvents 2037
aliphatic alcohols 757–8, 2023
aliphatic hydrocarbons 1504, 2034–7
aliphatic nitriles, unsaturated 551
aliphatic solvents 2034–7
alkali compounds 1987
alkali elements 1381
alkaline earth elements 1381
alkaloids
  indole 222–3
  nicotinic 1520, 1521

  pyrrolizidine 133, 730, 872, 873, 881, 882, 1981
  veterinary toxicology 1519, 1520, 1521
  vinca 638, 942, 943, 992, 1152, 1153
alkanes 1868, 2034–5
alkanolamines 2115
n-alkenals 1867
alkenes 104, 161, 1879, 2034–5
N^3-alkyladenine 1885
n-alkylamines 612
alkylating agents 527, 1104, 1144, 1146, 1465, 1882, 1883
alkylbenzenes 149, 2032
alkylene epoxides 7
N^l-alkylgaunine, DNA adducts 1885
O^6-alkylguanine
  biological activity 2146, 2153–4
  biomarker 1865
  biosynthesis 2150–2, 2151
  characteristics 2035
  chemical structure 2146, 2150
  competing pathways 115–17
  control and decontamination 2153
  determination 2152
  DNA adducts 115, 1881, 1883, 1885, 1917, 1918, 1919, 2151
  enzyme induction 1866
  equine-derived 2186
  fish poisoning 2193
  from polymers 1917, 1919
  Hb adduct levels 1880
  immunological screening 2152–3
  LD$_{50}$ 2150, 2154
  metabolism 71, 105, 110, 113, 114, 1883, 2149, 2155
  occurrence 2153
  physical and spectroscopic data 2150
  production 2152
  renal clearance 97
  scorpion sting 2188–9
  spider bite 2187
alkyl-lead 2054–5
alkyloctyl phosphorofluoridates 638
alkylsulphonic esters 2022
alkynes 2034
allergens 53, 262, 511–12, 702, 1299, 1300–1, 1302
allethrin 824, 1244
alloxan 881, 991, 992
alloys 2049, 2064

allyl alcohol 103, 255, 810, 872, 873, 882, 920
allylaldehyde 103, 119
allylamine 103, 809–10
allyl formate 881, 882, 883
allylglycine 641
allylisopropylacetamide 114
allylisothiocyanate 126
allyl isothiocyanate (AITC) 134
ALO1576 763
L-alosine 634
alphaxalone 1427, 1438
alprazolam 1495
alprenolol 219, 760
alteplase 1965, 1966
alum 1824
aluminium 2060
 and acid precipitation 1377
 and Alzheimer's disease 1379–80
 in antacids 1380
 antidotes 427
 biomonitoring 1900, 1904, 1905, 1907
 biovailability 1380, 1381
 cartilage and bone toxicity 973
 in drinking water 1379, 1381
 as environmental pollutant 1379–80
 ligands 1365–6, 1369
 mobilization 1379
 neurotoxicity 1379, 1380
 placental toxicity 1245–6
 solubilization 1371
 speciation 1365–6
 toxicity 1379
aluminium hydroxide 2022
aluminium phosphide 2006
aluminium sulphate 1824
amalgams 2049
amanitines 34, 870, 1513
amantidine 1495
amethocaine hydrochloride 2087
amidarone (Cordarone X) 1427
amidephrine 15
amidopyrine 1426
amiflamine 219
amikacin 685, 787, 788
amines 305, 2014, 2023, 2032
amino acid pyrolysates 1038
amino acids 548, 1983
aminoacridines 163
D,L-aminoadaptic acid 644
aminoalkyltrialkoxydisilane 11
2-aminoanthracine 1046, 1047

p-aminoazobenzene 2023
3-aminobenzamide 190, 200, 201
aminobenzene 1146
p-aminobenzoic acid 105
aminobenzotriazole 872, 1865
4-aminobiphenyl (ABP) 225, 1537, 1845, 1880, 1891
γ-aminobutyric acid (GABA) antagonist 641
aminocyclohexanols 71–2
2-amino-3,6-dihydro-3-methyl-7H-imidazo[4,5-f]quinoline-7-one 566
4-aminodimethyaniline 565
2-amino-3,8-dimethylimidazo [4,5-f]quinoxaline 272, 274, 1061
3-amino-1,4-dimethyl-5H-pyrido [4, 3-b]indole(Trp-P-1) 571
aminofluorene 120
aminoglutethimide 1121
aminogluthemide 1395
aminoglycosides 129, 130, 522, 685–6, 784, 787–93, 795–6, 819
p-aminohippurate 129, 364, 679, 1462
2-amino-3-methyl-3H-imidazo [4,5-f]quinoline 272, 274, 566
2-amino-1-methyl-6-phenylimidazo [4,5-b]pyridine 272, 274, 1881
3-amino-1-methyl-5H-pyrido [4, 3-b]indole 571
1-amino-2-naphthol 565
6-aminonicotinamide 972
aminonitriles 1983
aminophenols 110, 113, 117, 390, 393, 680, 688–9, 1907
aminophylline 816
aminoplasts 2018
β-aminopropionitrile 974
4-aminopropiophenone 393, 429
p-aminopropiophenone, for hydrogen cyanide poisoning 2102
aminopyridines 817, 822
aminopyrine 113, 2121
aminosalicylic acid (5-ASA, PAS) see aspirin; salicylates
amiodarone 219, 730, 755, 757, 818, 943–4, 945, 989, 1428
amitraz 1994, 2000
amitriptyline 51, 219, 264, 807, 819, 1495
amitrole 990, 2006
amitryptyline 1495

ammonia 117, 362, 568, 589, 751, 1297, 1516–17, 2018, 2119
ammonia compounds, in food 1514, 1987
ammonium bisulphate 1281
ammonium bisulphite 1281
ammonium hexachloroplatinate 711
ammonium hydroxide 752
ammonium metabisulphate 1281
ammonium phosphate 1514
[S]15[s]N-ammonium acetate 2119
[S]15[s]N-ammonium chloride 2119
ammonium sulphate 1266, 1281
ammonium sulphite 1281, 1987
ammonium tetrachloroplatinite 711
amoscanate 764
amoxapine 945, 1495
amoxycillin 2099
amphenidone 1634
amphetamines
 cardiac toxicity 808, 814
 controlled drug 1545
 derivatives 218
 forensic analysis 1491, 1503
 immunoassays 1501
 metabolism 102
 misuse 1550
 pharmacogenetics 219
 reproductive toxicity 1146
 risk acceptance 1960
 site-dependent blood concentrations 1495
 skeletal muscle toxicity 942
 steam distillation 1497
amphiphilic drugs 385, 730–1, 945
amphotericin B 536, 819, 945
ampicillin 756, 807, 1025
amygdalin 566
amyl nitrate 1550
amyl nitrite 3, 393, 426, 429, 460
anabolic steroids 815, 948, 1146, 1549, 1554
anastrozole 1403
anatoxin A 1516
androgen 370–1
andromedol 1984
angiotensin converting enzyme inhibitors 2188
anilines
 and anaemia 390
 biomonitoring 1900, 1907
 and gastro-intestinal microflora 565
 haemoglobin toxicity 393

anilines (*Contd.*)
  herbicides 2003, 2005
  metabolism 104, 110
  in oils 1824
  toxic reactions 1430
annatto, in food 1987
Antabuse *see* disulfiram
antacids 1380, 2060–1
anthracyclines 127, 807, 808–9
anthrax 1726–7
anthrocyanins 1987
α_1-antichymotrypsin 340
anticancer drugs 240, *240*, 258,
  262, 683–4, 727–9, 756–7, 1866
anticholinergic drugs 429, 430,
  1430
anticoccicidal drugs 1648
anticonvulsants 225, 258, 2092
antidepressants 218, *219*, 232, 819,
  1146, 1491, 1496, 1504, 1714
antidiabetic drugs 241
antiemetic drugs 229
antiepileptic drugs 1494
antifoaming agents 1985
antifouling compounds 1548, 1611,
  2001
antifreeze 1512
  see also ethylene glycol
antigenic agents 536
antihaemophilic factor 1965, 1970
antihistamines *219*, 262, 1127,
  1223, 1427, 1429, 1550, 2184,
  2190
antihypertensive drugs *219*
anti-inflammatory drugs 263, 1438
  see also non-steroidal anti-
    inflammatory drugs
antimalarial drugs 227
antimony 1451, 1489, 1491, 1496,
  1907
antimony trioxide 2018, 2022
anti-oestrogens *220*, 1392, 1403
  see also tamoxifen
antiperistaltic drugs *220*
antipsychotic drugs *219*
antipyretics *536*, 688
antipyrine 114–15, 253, 395
antirheumatic agents 1439
antisecretory drugs 1124, 1125–7
α_1-antitrypsin 254
antituberculosis drugs 119, 391
antitussive drugs *220*
antiulcer drugs 16
antivenin 2180
anxiolytics 641, 819

apamin 820
aphidicolin 185
apocynamarin 1522
apomorphine 1403, 1511, 1520,
  1547
appetite suppressants *220*
aprindine 219
1-(β-D-arabinofuranosyl)cytosine
  (Ara-C) 185, 195, 199
Ara-C *see* 1-(β-D-arabinofuranosyl)
  cytosine
arene oxides 130
arginine 229, 2119
aristolochic acid 554
Arochlor 24, 1254, 1343, 1348,
  1866
  see also polychlorinated
    biphenyls
aromatase inhibitors 1395
aromatic acids 109
aromatic amines 7, 28, 456, 874–6,
  1039, 1041, 1056, 1057, 1079,
  1104
  adducts 162
  biomarkers 1880, 1882, 1885,
    1886
  biomonitoring 1904
  carcinogenesis 7, 1104, 2015
  cytogenicity 1079
  human studies 456
  metabolism 112, 120
  mutagenicity 1039, 1041, 1056,
    1057
  reaction with DNA 161
  susceptibility 28
aromatic amino acids 568
aromatic hydrocarbons 2037–40
  acute overdose 1496
  and blood–testis barrier 1463
  forensic testing 1504
  inducing GSTs 1866
  toxicity 2030
aromatic hydroxylamines 1867
arsenates 2050
arsenic 2050–2, 2066
  acute overdose 1496
  animal toxicity 1513, 1518,
    1951–2
  anthropogenic emissions 1370
  antidotes 427
  biomarker 1864
  biomonitoring 1900, 1904, 1907
  carcinogenic 1382
  cardiac toxicity 822
  in drinking water 1382

forensic testing 1491, 1504
gastro-intestinal toxicity 1515
general symptoms 1513
in groundwater 1382
hepatotoxicity 870, 881, 882
in humus layer 1375
as impurity in fertilizer 1371
marketing controls 1595
Marsh test 1490
in mining areas 1382
as natural poison 34
nephrotoxicity 6
ototoxicity 784
PBPK modelling 142
poisoning 1382, 1490
reproductive toxicity 1156
and skin cancer 1382
in soils 1329, 1373
solubilization 1371
speciation 1382, 1515
teratogenicity 1206, 1246–7
and vascular disease 1382
arsenic compounds
  organic *see* organoarsenicals
  peripheral neuropathy 1515
  rodenticides 1510–11
  toxicity to animals 1512, 1515
arsenic oxide 2014
arsenic sulphide 2050
arsenic trioxide 1900, 2050, 2051
arsenic trisulphide 2050
arsenilic acid 1515
arsenite 2066
arsenobetaine 2052
arsenopyrite 2050
arsine 390, 2082
artificial sweeteners 1431, 1552
arylamides 101
arylamines 28, 101, 108–9
arylesterase 216
aryl hydrocarbons 867
arylhydroxamic acid 109
arylphosphates 2022
AS *see* ascorbic acid (AS)
5-ASA *see* aminosalicylic acid
asbestos
  binding values (EU) 1595
  carcinogenicity 1131, 1537
  as combustion product 1927,
    1929
  environmental source 1380
  health hazard 1380
  human studies 456, 463
  immunotoxicity 1006
  inhalation 1446

asbestos (*Contd.*)
  lung disease 1475
  occupational exposure 1456, 1487
  parenteral toxicity 525
  in plastics industry 2022
  release in fires 1821
  and smoking 28, 1417, 1445
  in water distribution systems 1377
  workplace exposure 1475
ascorbic acid (AS) 1130, 2121, 2137
  see also vitamin C
aspartame 1653, 1989, 2161
L-aspartate 634
asphalt 922
aspirin
  see also salicylates
  acute toxicity 51
  cardiac toxicity 807
  cartilage and bone toxicity 969
  circadian toxicity 263
  endocrine toxicology 991
  and gastro-intestinal microflora 565
  haematotoxicity 390, 391
  neonatal toxicity 1223
  nephrotoxicity 688
  ototoxicity 786
  pancreatic toxicity 908
  parenteral toxicity 525
  peroral toxicity 549, 552
atrazine 607, 2003, 2006
atropine
  antidotal studies 429, 430, 1355, 1510, 1998
  for carbamate poisoning 1998
  cardiac toxicity 824
  for fish poisoning 2192
  laboratory occupational hazard 516
  for OP poisoning 1998
  peroral toxicity 548
  placental toxicity 1256
  skeletal muscle toxicity 955
  in toxic plants 1521
  toxic reactions 1430
  treatment of nerve agent poisoning 2090, 2092, 2093–4
atropine sulphate, for scorpion bite 2188
ATX-II 820
auramine 463
auritricarboxylic acid 188, 198

averantin 2151
avermectins 641, 1999
averufin 2151
AY-9944 730
8-azaguanine (8-AG) 1052
azaserine 58, 924, 925
azathioprine 915, 917, 945, 1010, 1153
azides 392
azinophos methyl 1335
5-(aziridin-1-yl)-2,4-dinitro-benzamide 241
azobisformamide 2014, 2017, 2023
azobisisobutyronitrile 2023
azo compounds 564–5, 2022, 2023
azodicarbonamide 2022
azo dyes 7, 240, 1986
azoles 2001, 2003
azothioprine 727, 764
azoxymethane 571
azoxystrobin 1608
AZT *see* zidovudine

B

bacitracin 1648
bacitracin zinc 538
baking soda 2190
BAL *see* dimercaprol
banamine hydrochloride 1518
BAPP *see* 2,2-bis(4-amino phenoxyphenyl) propane
barbital 553
barbiturates
  acute overdose 34, 1496
  behavioural toxicity 651
  clinical chemistry 357
  controlled drug 1545
  in drug combinations 1504
  drugs of abuse screen (DAS) 1503
  forensic analysis 1491
  haematology 390–1
  induction 113, 114
  injection 498
  metabolism 111, 113, 114, 115
  neurotoxicity 641
  pharmacogenetics 226
  reproductive toxicity 1151
  skeletal muscle toxicity 944
  toxicity study design 325
barium 805, 822, 1757
barium chloride 1757
barium oxide 2022
barium sulphate 1757

bases, absorption 69
batrachotoxins (BXT) 639, 816, 818, 821, 824, 2104
Baytex 4 *see* fenthion
BBN *see* N-butyl-N-(4-hydroxy-butyl)-nitrosamine
BCLE *see* butyryl cholinesterase
BCNU *see* 1,3-bis(2-chloroethyl)-1-nitrosourea
beetroot red 1987
belladonna 2
Bendictin 1948–9
benomyl 758, 2000, 2002
benoxaprofen (Opren) 132, 1427, 1428, 1438, 1439
bentazon 259
benzaldehyde 237, 239, 613, 2038
benz[*a*]anthracene 280, 1791, 2017
benzene 2037
  air pollution 1267, 1298
  and alcohol 2033
  and apoptosis 184
  biomarkers 1867, 1882, 1884
  biomonitoring 1900, 1904, 1907, 1908, 1910
  carcinogenicity 1455, 1537, 2015
  characteristics 2035
  chromosomal abnormalities 395
  circadian toxicity 257
  as combustion product 1927
  in diet 1981
  early research 1482
  epidemiology 2042
  excretion 98
  exposure routes 607
  haematology 390, 395, 1475
  human studies data 463
  immunotoxicity 1004
  impurity in toluene 1445–6
  interactions 2034
  marketing controls 1595
  metabolism 100, 103, 2032, 2038
  ototoxicity 795
  PBPK modelling 142, 150
  pharmacogenetics 240–1
  risk assessment 1770
  rubber additive 2014, 2017, 2018
  in styrene 2039–40
  with toluene, PBPK modelling 149
  toxic reactions 1430
  vapour 16, 56
benzene-*trans*-1,2-dihydrodiol 105

benzene epoxide 2037
benzene hexachloride 1995
benzene oxide 105, 395
benzidine 112, 120, 569, 569, 1041, 1537, 2021, 2023
benzidine-based dyes 564, 1587
benzimidazole carbamate fungicides 2002
benzine oxide 607
benzoates 1653
benzodiazepine antagonist 433575
benzodiazepines
  acute overdose 1496
  antidotal studies 426, 433
  behavioural toxicity 651
  circadian toxicology 254
  drugs of abuse screen (DAS) 1503
  forensic analysis 1491
  HPLC 1500
  neurotoxicology 641
  pancreatic toxicity 895
  pharmacogenetics 228
  reproductive toxicity 1146
  withdrawal symptoms 1549
benzofurans 1982, 1986
benzoic acid 107, 109, 142, 535, 1989, 2017, 2038
benzol 463
benzonitrile 1919, 1922
benzophenes 2022
benzo[a]pyrene
  absorption data 1778
  biomarker 1852, 1870
  chiral factors and 115
  DNA adducts from 1881, 1886
  as electrophile 130
  and gastro-intestinal microflora 569, 571
  interspecies extrapolation 278–81
  metabolism 113
  mutagenicity 1042, 1044, 1047
  pancreatic toxicity 920
  PBPK modelling 142
  pharmacogenetics 217
  risk assessment 1791
  stereochemical factors and 162
benzo[a]pyrene 217, 278–81, 569, 571, 920, 1042, 1044, 1047
benzo[o]pyrene 569
benzo[a]pyrene-4,5-oxide 279
benzo[p]pyrene 1905, 2004, 2017
4-benzoquinoneimine 688–9

benzotriazoles 2022
benzoyl peroxide 2020, 2022, 2023
benzoylphenylureas 2000
4-benzoylpyridine 243
N-benzoyl-1-tyrosyl-p-aminobenzoic acid 365
benzphetamine 113
benzpyrene 395, 549
benzpyrene-7,8-dihydrodiol 105
benzydamine 232
benzyl alcohol 2038
benzylamine 103
benzylamine oxidase (BzAO) inhibitors 810
benzyl bromide 2102
N-benzylimidazole 232
benzylpenicillin 522
beryllium 870, 881, 973, 2061
beta-blockers 219, 228, 426, 430, 2188
betamethasone 2087
bethanidine 818
BHA see butylated hydroxyanisole
BHT see butylated hydroxytoluene
bicuculline 641
bicyclophosphate esters 641
biphenyl ethers 990
bipyridyls 1867, 2003, 2004
2,2-bis(4-aminophenoxyphenyl) propane (BAPP) 15, 26
biscarbamates 990
bischloroether 1952
1,3-bis(2-chloroethyl)-1-nitrosourea (BCNU) 728, 729, 756
bis(2-chloroethyl) sulphate 755
bis(chloromethyl) ether 1484, 1536, 1537
bis[2-(dimethylamino)ethyl] ether 738
2,2,-bis(p-2,3-epoxypropxyl)-phenylpropane 2020
1,1´-bisethylidene (tryptophan) (EBT) 946
4,4´-bis(methylsulphonyl)-2,2´,5,5´-tetrachlorobiphenyl 131
bismuth 870, 2061
bismuth subcitrate 2061
bismuth subgallate 2061
bismuth subnitrate 2061
bismuth subsalicylate 2061
bisphenol A 1396, 1565, 2020
4,5-bisphosphate (PIP$_2$) 896
bispyridinium 2093
biuret 1514

BL-6341 1124
bleach 737, 2092
bleomycin 127, 184, 185, 727, 728, 762, 1042, 1430, 1455
BOP see N-nitrosobis(2-hydroxypropyl)amine
borate 1496
Bordeaux mixture 2000, 2001
boric acid 1467
boron compounds 2001
botulinus toxin 428, 549, 633, 640, 1340, 1513, 2104
bovine somatotropin 1649, 1970
BPDE see 8α-dihydroxy-9α,10α-epoxy-7,8,9,10-tetrahydrobenzo [a]pyrene
brass, source of lead 1378
BrDU see bromodeoxyuridine; 5-bromo-2´-deoxyuridine (BrDU)
bretylium 818
brevitoxins 2192
Brij-78759
brimonidine 239
British antiLewisite (BAL) see dimercaprol
brodifacoum 1510–11, 1524, 2006
bromadialoneo 2006
bromhexine 730
bromide 1496
bromine 1328
bromobenzene 100, 118–19, 125, 133, 142, 691
bromobenzene-3,4-oxide 133, 691
bromobenzyl cyanide 2102
2-bromo-bis(glutathion-S-yl) hydroquinone 691
bromocriptine 1548
5-bromo-2´-deoxyuridine (BrDU) 338, 344, 722, 1089
bromodichloromethane 142
bromoethylamine 2-hydrobromide 184
bromoform 1784
2-bromohydroquinone 119, 691
4-bromophenol 118, 691
2-bromoquinone 691
2-bromosemiquinone 691
bromosulphalein (BSP) 361
5-bromouracil 548
bromoxynil 2003, 2005
brompheniramine 1495
BTP see butylated triphenyl phosphate
bufodienolides 821

cantharidin 1518
canthoxanthin 1987
caproic acid 1989
caprolactam 1537
capsaicin 612
captan 2001, 2002
captofol 2001, 2002
caramel 1987
carbadox 1648
carbamates 951–5
  age/maturation effects 1337
  behavioural effects 1348
  and brain cholinesterase levels
    1343
  cholinesterase inhibition 1345
  contamination of food 1548
  deactivation by HMOs 1334
  dog toxicity 1512
  enzyme inhibition 1866
  equine poisoning 1518
  fungicides 2000, 2001–2
  immunotoxicity 1006
  insecticides 1995, 1998
  lability 1329
  metabolism 105
  placental toxicity 1242–3
  reproduction testing 1351
  secondary poisoning 1341
  in wildlife diet 1347
carbamazepine 10,11-oxide 130
carbamazine 253–4
carbapenems 686
carbaryl 24, 227–8, 1243, 1342,
  1523, 1548, 1994
carbendazim 2000, 2002
carbenoloxone 945
carbimazole 1549
carbinolamine 102
carbocations, reaction with DNA
  161
carbofuran 1331, 1336, 1339, 1341,
  1342, 1347, 1348, 1350
carbohydrates 359, 370, 1981
carbolines 222, 223, 641
carbon, from wood burning 1917
carbonates 2014, 2017
carbon black 1282, 2014, 2017
carbon dioxide
  acute toxicity 38
  air pollution 1296
  Bhopal disaster 1819
  blood analysis 61
  with CO 1924–7
  as combustion product 1928
  fires 1821
  formate oxidation 2040

  from lake water 1817
  from volcanoes 1815
  from wood burning 1917–18
  and gastro-intestinal microfloral
    563
  inhalational toxicity 590
  metabolism 2036, 2041
  in plastics industry 2021
  removal in inhalational studies
    592
  tests 357
carbon disulphide
  acute toxicity 43
  behavioural toxicity 660
  biomonitoring 1900
  eye toxicity 756
  and heart disease 1456
  human studies 463
  as inhibitor 114
  neurotoxicity 637
  ototoxicity 784
  sperm evaluation studies 1467
  toxicity 637, 1430
carbon monoxide (CO)
  acute overdose 1496
  air pollution 1267, 1268
  analysis in tissues 1491
  in animal husbandry 1516–17
  antidotes 426, 430
  biomarkers 1842
  biomonitoring 1485, 1900, 1905,
    1908, 1910
  with carbon dioxide 1924–7
  cardiac toxicity 821
  and cardiovascular disease 34
  in combustion products
    1917–18, 1920–2, 1927, 1928,
    1929
  dose–response assessment 1758
  early OEL 1482
  effects on humans 1282–3
  in fires 1821, 1822
  foetal half-life 1922
  forensic analysis 1491, 1495
  from lake water 1817
  from volcanoes 1815
  and haemotoxicity 384, 391–4
  with HCN 1924
  indoor sources 1296
  microdiffusion 1497
  mixed routes of exposure 607
  neonatal toxicity 1218
  quantitative analysis 1490
  in smoke 1446
  in tobacco smoke 28

  toxicity, elevated temperature and
    1919–20
  toxicokinetics 1282
carbon steel 2064
carbon tetrachloride 2035–6
  activation 6
  alcohol and 2033
  biomarker 1857, 1858, 1859,
    1861, 1862, 1867
  biomonitoring 1900, 1907
  cardiac toxicity 810, 821
  characteristics 2035
  with chlordecone 149
  circadian toxicology 257, 259
  epidemiology 2042
  genotoxicity 200
  hepatotoxicity 16, 56, 132, 869,
    872, 873, 877, 881
  human studies 463
  as impurity in trichloroethylene
    1445
  as inhibitor 114
  interactions 2033
  metabolism 104, 115, 117–18
  with methanol 149
  pancreatic toxicity 900, 914,
    916, 920, 927
  PBPK modelling 142, 150, 1767
  percutaneous toxicity 585
  peroroal toxicity 551
  systemic pulmonary toxicity 731
  toxicity enhanced by ketones
    1418
  toxic reactions 1430
carbonyl fluoride 1915, 1918
carboplatin 260–1, 784
carboxyatractyloside 1518, 1520
carboxyhaemoglobin 393–4, 1267,
  1282, 1283, 1494–5, 1504, 1905
carboxylic acids 131
carboxyphosphamide 238
cardenolides 1520
cardiac glycosides 237, 285, 428,
  808, 811–12, 818, 821, 1549
carisprodol 1495–6, 1503
carmustine *see* 1,3-bis
  (2-chloroethyl)-1-nitosourea
carotenes/carotenoids
  as antioxidants 158, 1978, 1982,
    1983, 2137
  in foods 1653, 1987, 2131
carprofen 1642
catecholamines 256, 346, 357, 632
catechols 100, 990
Cau p 1 allergen 511

Cau p II allergen 511
ceftazidime 687
ceftizoxime 89
cellulose 1552, 1985, 2022
cellulose acetate 368
Centruroides toxin 820
cephaloglycin 686, 687
cephaloridine 686–8
cephalosporins 127, 128, 129, 390, 552, 686, 687
CFCs *see* chlorofluorocarbons
chaconines 1521, 1984
channel black 2017
charcoal 425, 2153
chenodeoxycholic acid 360, 567
chlomipramine 219
2-chloracetophenone 2102
α-chloralose 2006
chlorambucil 191, 727, 1537
1-chloramitriptyline 730
chloramphenicol
　adverse drug reactions 1438, 1439
　cardiac toxicity 807
　drops for mustard gas eye damage 2087
　eye absorption and aplastic anaemia 761
　and gastro-intestinal microflora 569
　haematotoxicity 390–1, 395, 1634
　maximum residue limits (MRLs) 1642
　parenteral toxicity 533–4
　therapy for phosgene poisoning 2099
chlorate herbicides 1512
chlordane 879, 1226, 1243–4, 1342, 1343, 1523
chlordecane 637
chlordecone (Kepone) 142, 149, 879, 1146, 1154, 1244, 1418, 1475
chlordiazepoxide 1495
chlorendic acid 2022–3
chlorfenvinphos 142
chlorhexidine 1642
chloride 355, 364, 428, 1504, 2102
chlorinated cyclodienes 1243–4
chlorinated hydrocarbons
　acute overdose 1496
　banned by US EPA 1329
　behavioural effects 1346
　brain residues 1343

cardiac toxicity 804
　and CNS 1510, 1518
　domestic animal poisoing 1510
　and eggshell thinning 1343, 1345
　equine poisoning 1518
　forensic analysis 1491, 1504
　and hepatic monoesterase (HMO) activity 1342, 1345
　human studies 461
　indoor sources 1295
　and menstrual disorders 1465
　microdiffusion 1497
　persistence in environment 1510
　poisoning, developing countries 1510
　poultry poisoning 1523
　reproductive effects 1339–40, 1350
　secondary poisoning 1341
　in soil and groundwater 1372
　stability 1329, 1341
chlorinated phenols 1310, 1366, 1373, 1383
chlorinated solvents 39
chlorine
　as chemical warfare agent 2082, 2096
　dangerous dose 1831
　in fires 1821
　gas 1724
　peripheral sensory irritation 626
　risk assessment 1832–3
　in rubber 2018
　soil content 1328
chlorine dioxide 989
chloroacetaldehyde 100–1
chloroacetone 2102
chloroacetophenone (CN) 623, 744, 745, 748, 750, 751, 2103
chloroalkanes 142, 2022
chloroalkyl thio compounds 2001, 2002
chlorobenzenes 1372, 1900
2-chlorobenzylidene malononitrile (CS) 623, 745, 2080, 2082, 2103, 2104
2-chlorobuta-1,3-diene
　see chloroprene
chlorocatechols 1907
chlorocresol 535
chlorocyclizine 730
chlorodihydrophenarsazine (DM) 2081–2, 2082, 2102, 2103
2-chloroethylnitrosoureas 2132
chlorofluorocarbons 460

chloroform 2036
　anaesthesia 2, 2030
　biologically based model 1770
　bounding information 1767
　carcinogenicity 1455
　cardiac toxicity 810
　chlorination byproduct 1383
　circadian toxicity 255, 257
　cytotoxicity 126
　dose–response model 1764
　genotoxicity 200
　hepatotoxicty 877
　injection 498
　kidney response 689–90
　maximum residue limits (MRLs) 1642
　metabolism 104, 111, 2036
　Monte Carlo analysis 1784
　natural 1366
　PBPK modelling 142
　percutaneous toxicity 583
　peroral toxicity 551
　risk assessment 1757, 1766
α-chlorohydrin 1147
chloromethyl methyl ether 1537
chloropentafluorobenzene 142
chlorophacinone 2006
chlorophenols 21, 38, 1900, 1907
chlorophenoxy acids 1900
p-chlorophenylalanine 763
chlorophyll 384, 1987, 2148
chloroprene 1464, 2015
2-chloropropionate 634
chloroquine 128, 129, 393, 730, 755, 756, 942, 944, 945, 1861
3-chlorostyrene 612
chlorothalonil 2001, 2004
chlorothiazide 548
chlorotrifluoroethylene 691
chlorozotocin 727
chlorpheniramine 219, 1495
chlorphenoxy herbicides 1512
chlorphentermine 730
chlorpromazine
　apoptosis and 188, 198
　cardiac toxicity 816, 819
　hepatotoxicty 859
　maximum residue limits (MRLs) 1642
　mg/kg 264
　peroral toxicity 553
　pharmacogenetics 219, 233
　systemic pulmonary toxicity 730
　tests 366
　tissue specificity 129

cytisine 1520
cytisol 277
cytokeratins 341
cytokines 364, 722
cytosine arabinoside 184, 258, 261, 527, 727
cytosol 359, 691
cytoxan 1144

D

D&C Red No 9 565
D&C Yellow 1430
2,4-D 1512, 1907, 2003, 2005, 2104
dacarbazine 524, 727
dactinomycin 199
daidzein 570
daidzin 570
dantrolene sodium 2186
dapsone 390, 393, 1642, 2187
DAS *see* diacetoxyscirpenol
daunorubicin 243, 262, 808
daunorubicinol 243
DCE *see* dichloroethane
DCVA *see* trans-3-(2,2-dichlorovinyl)-2,2-dimethylcyclo-propane carboxylic acid
DCVC *see* dichlorovinylcysteine
DDD *see* 1,1-dichloro-2,2-bis (p-chlorophenyl)ethane
DDE *see* dichlorodiphenyl-dichloroethylene
DDM *see* 4,4′-diaminodiphenyl-methane
DDT *see* dichlorodiphenyl-trichloroethane
debrisoquine 112, 218, 219, 222, 225
decabromodiphenyl oxide 2014, 2018, 2022
n-decane 623
decanoyl peroxide 2023
decosahexaeonic acids 1981
DEF *see* S,S,S-tributyl phosphoro-trithoate
deferoxamine 427, 792, 2068
defoliants 2006, 2080
degreasing agents 918, 922
degreasing solvents 460, 1419
dehydromonocrotaline 133
DEHP *see* di(2-ethylhexyl)phthalate
deltamethrin 1244, 1998, 1999
demeton 1336
deoxycholic acid 360, 567

11-deoxycortisol 370
N-(deoxyguanosin-8-yl)-2-aminofluoroene 120
deoxynivalenol (DON) 823, 1254, 1515–16, 2149
6-deoxypenciclovir 239
derris 1999
desacetylpieristoxin 1984
desferioxamine *see* deferoxamine
desipramine 1495, 1497
O-desmethylangolensin 570
desmethylimipramine 219, 325
desmin 342
desogestrel 1427, 1428
detergents 230, 905, 1297
dexamethasone 285, 758, 969, 1010
dexfenfluramine 815, 1427
dextran sulphate 881
dextromethorphan 219
DFP *see* diisopropyl phospho-fluoridate
N-(5,5-diacetoxypentyl)doxorubicin 199
diacetoxyscirpenol (DAS) 1254, 1515–16, 2149
diacylglycerol 808
dialkylhydrazines 876, 877
dialkylnitrosoamine 2123
dialkyl phosphorofluoridates 638
dialkyltin salts 882
diallyl sulphones 1984
2,4-diaminoanisole 1038
4,4′-diaminodiphenylmethane (DDM; MDA) 220, 882, 1824, 1825, 1902, 1907, *1910*, 2017, 2021
diaminodiphenyl sulfone 2020
diaminopropidium iodide 163
diaminotoluenes 876
diamorphine 1545, 1550
o-dianisidine 463, 1587, 2102
diazepam
    antidotal studies 426, 430
    cardiac toxicity 817
    circadian toxicity 254, 264–5
    clinical chemistry 366
    for OP poisoning 1998
    pharmacogenetics 228
    skeletal mucle toxicity 944
    for spider bite 2186
    therapy for nerve agent poisoning 2093, 2095
    toxicity 265
diazinon 898, 955, 1328, 1329, 1339, 1350, 1351, 1523, 1994

diaziquone 240
diazomethane 225, 635
6-diazo-5-oxo-L-norleucine (DON) 924
diazoxide 992
dibenz[*a,h*]anthracene 280, 2017
dibenzofurans 1827
dibenzo[*a,i*]pyrene 280, 2017
dibenz[*b,f*]-1,4-oxazepine (CR) 623, 745, 748, 750, 751, 2082, 2103, 2104
1,2-dibromobenzene 872
dibromochloropropane (DBCP) 1144, 1146, 1399, 1464, 1466
1,2-dibromoethane 121
dibromosulphthalein 255
di-*n*-butylamine 2016
3,5-di-*t*-butyl-4-hydroxytoluene 725
dibutylnitrosamine 2016
dibutylphthalate 2017, 2022
dibutyltin 200, 882
dibutyryl cyclic AMP 2099
dicamba 2003, 2005
dichlorbenzidine 463
dichloroacetic acid 566
dichloroacetylene 691
dichlorobenzenes 142, 692
dichlorobiphenyl 114
1,1-dichloro-2,2-bis (p-chlorophenyl)ethane (p,p-TDE; DDD) 566, 1343, 1345
dichloro(2-chlorovinyl)arsine *see* lewisite
dichlorodifluoromethane 461, 2022
dichlorodiphenyldichloroethane (DDD) *see* 1,1-dichloro-2,2-bis (p-chlorophenyl)ethane
dichlorodiphenyldichloroethylene (DDE) 1329, 1343, 1345, 1346, 1348, 1354, 1844
dichlorodiphenyltrichloroethane (DDT)
    biomarkers 1841, 1844
    cardiac toxicology 824
    diagnostic brain residues 1343
    domestic animal toxicity 1510
    eggshell thinning 1345, 1354, 1548
    endocrine toxicology 985, 1407
    environmental oestrogen efffects 1565
    and gastro-intestinal microflora 566
    human studies 460

ethanol (*Contd.*)
    treatment for ethylene glycol
       toxicity 1512
    volatile screen 1502
ethanolamine 1455
ethchlorvynol 1496, 1497
ethene *see* ethylene
ether 357, 498
    see also diethyl ether
ethidium bromide 163, 1455
ethinyloestradiol 22, 284, 569, 879,
    1129, 1392, 1397
ethion 1335
ethionine 882, 883, 971–2, 1862
ethoprop 1336
ethoxyacetic acid 1907, 2041
6-ethoxy-1,2-dihydro-2,2,4-
    trimethylquinolone 2017
2-ethoxyethanol 1901, 2030, 2033,
    2041
2-ethoxyethyl acetate 1901
ethoxyquine 130
ethyl acetate 142, 2034
ethyl acrylate 142, 148, 547, 554
ethyl aminobenzoate 413
ethylbenzene 612, 1901, 2033,
    2035
ethyl bromoacetate (SK) 2102
ethyl chlorosulphonate 2102
ethyldeshydroxysparsomycin 765
1,1′-ethylene-2,2′bipyridylium 724
4′-ethylenebis(2-chloroaniline),
    biomonitoring 1902, 1907, 1910
ethylene-bisdithiocarbamates 1123,
    2000, 2001
ethylene bis(tetrabromo)
    isophthalimide 2022
ethylenediamine (EDA) 59, 1475
ethylenediamine tetra-acetic acid
    (EDTA) 357, 384, 388, 535, 622,
    973
ethylene dibromide 880, 1038,
    1145, 1146, 1377, 1467, 1557,
    1770
ethylene dichloride 142, 1557
ethylene (ethene) 259, 1880, 1881,
    1883, 1901, 2019
ethylene glycol
    antidotes 15, 426, 429
    dinitrate biomonitoring 1901,
       1907
    in elixirs 1634
    LD$_{50}$ 15, 55
    metabolism 97, 110, 2032
    mixtures 49

    peroral toxicity 553, 555
    pharmacogenetics 237
    toxic reactions 1430
ethylene glycol monoethers 553
ethylene glycol–xylene, Seveso
    disaster 1818
ethylene oxide
    biomarkers 1845, 1865, 1879,
       1882
    biomonitoring 1901
    DNA adducts 1881, 1885, 1886
    exposure levels 1484
    Hb adducts 1880, 1883–4
    interspecies variations in toxicity
       274
    mixtures 21
    mutagenicity 1035
    PBPK modelling 142
    in plastics industry 2019
    prohibited 1557
    reroductive toxicity 1156
    and spontaneous abortion 1464
    toxic hazard 1455
ethylene–propylene rubber 2013
ethylenethiourea (ETU) 2001,
    2002, 2014, 2016
ethyleneurea 1766
ethyl glycol (EG) 1189
2-ethylhexanoic acid 466
2-ethylhexanol 550
5-ethylidene-2-norbornene (ENB)
    61–2
N-ethylmaleimide 816
ethylmaltol 1988
ethyl mercury 681
ethylmethane sulphonate 200, 1023,
    1052, 1145
ethylmethylphenyl glycidate 1988
ethylmorphine 111, 113, 219, 255
N-ethylmorpholine 738
o-ethyl-o,p-nitrophenyl phenyl-
    phosphothioate 1335, 1342, 1345,
    1997
N-ethyl-*N*-nitrosourea 1030
ethylnodiol diacetate 879
ethyl octyl phosphorofluoridates
    638
4-ethyl-1-phospha-2,6,7-
    trioabicyclol[2.2.2]octane-1-oxide
    1925
N-ethylpiperidine 738
p-ethyl phenol 570
ethylvanillin 1988
etidocaine 529
etoposide 185, 199, 200, 262, 727

etretinate 946
ETU *see* ethylenethiourea
eugenol 708
euphorbin 1518
euphoron 1518
exhaust fumes *see* diesel
    combustion products;petrol/diesel
    fumes

F

Fab fragments 426, 428, 1447,
    2181
fagopyrin 1523
famciclovir 239
famphur 1341, 1342, 1355
fatty acid ethyl esters (FAEEs) 813
FC-11 *see* trichlorofluoromethane
FC-12 *see* dichlorodifluoromethane
FC-14 *see* dichlorotetrafluoroethane
fecapentaenes 567–8
Fed d 1 allergen 512
felodipine 22
fenabutatin oxide 2001
fenbuconazole 2001, 2003
fenclofenac (Flenac) 569, 1427,
    1428
fenfluramine 220, 730, 804, 815,
    1155, 1427
fenitrothion 1335, 1994
fenofibrate 859
fenoldopam mesylate 527, 821
fenoprop 2003, 2005
fenoxycarb 2000
fenpropimorph 2001, 2004
fensulfothion 1336, 1337
fentanyl citrate 527, 539
fenthion 1338, 1340, 1341, 1346,
    1352
fentin 2000, 2001
fenvalerate 1244, 1245
feprazone (Methrazone) 1427
ferbam 2000, 2001
ferric compounds *see* iron(II)
ferritin 822
ferrocyanides 1985
ferro-manganese alloy production
    668
ferrous compounds *see* iron(II)
fertilizers 305
fexofenadine 1429
fibreglass 2019
fibroblast growth factor 1972
fibronectin 342
filgrastim 1965

finasteride 1403
fipronil 1994, 2000
flavonoids 566, 1429, 1984, 2131, 2137
flax*seed* flour 570
flecainide 220, 222
flectol H 882
fluanisone 527, 539
fluazifop 142, 259
fludarabine 727
flumazanil 426, 430, 433
flumethrin 1994, 1998
flunisolide 758
fluoran 1987
fluorescein 746, 751, 752, 753, 760
fluoride
  acute overdose 1496
  analysis in tissues 1491
  biomonitoring 1901, 1907, 1910
  bound by ligand exchange 1369
  cartilage and bone toxicity 967, 973
  in drinking water 1381
  PBPK modelling 142
  storage sites 17
fluorocarbons 1455
fluorocene 338
fluorochrome penetration 750
fluorocitrate 643
fluorodeoxyuridine 185, 261
fluoroelasomers 2013
fluoropyrimidines 261
5-fluoropyrimidin-2-one 238
fluoroscein dyes 1987
fluorotrichloromethane 1901, 1907
5-fluorouracil
  causing apoptosis 184
  circadian toxicology 261, 266
  interaction with sorivudine 1565
  neurotoxicology 643
  pancreatic toxicity 926
  parenteral toxicity 524
  peroral toxicology 548
  pharmacogenetics 235, 238
  systemic pulmonary toxicity 727
fluoxetine 220, 232, 730, 1495
flupentixol 220
fluphenazine 220
flurandrenolide 758
flutamide 1403
[tau]-fluvalinate 1642
folate 257, 391, 972, 2040, 2131
folcodine 220
follicle stimulating hormone (FSH) 369, 371, 1965

folpet 2001, 2002
food colourings 530, 564, 1123, 1653
formaldehyde
  antidotal studies 429
  carcinogenicity 1456, 1537
  chemical mixtures toxicity 315
  as combustion product 1929
  in diet 1981
  dose profiling 16, 56
  eye toxicity 765
  idiopathic environmental illness 1705, 1706, 1709, 1713
  indoor sources 1295, 1298
  inhalation toxicity 20, 589
  irritant effects 16, 1475
  lung cancer 1456
  metabolism 119
  methanol oxidation 2040
  mixtures 21
  mutagenicity 1038
  occupational hazards 510, 515
  pancreatic toxicity 902
  peripheral sensory irritation 623, 626
  pharmacogenetics 237
  from polyethylene 1918–19
  reproductive toxicity 1156
  respiratory sensitization 16, 707–11
  risk assessment 1757, 1766
  in rubber 2016, 2018
  toxic hazard 1455
  from wood burning 1918
formalin 510
formate 119, 429, 765, 1455, 1901, 1907, 2040, 2041
2-formyl-3,4-dihydro-2*H*-pyran 738
Fos protein 240
fostriecin 199
fotemustine 727
Fowler's solution 460
FPL 52757 863–4, 881, 882
frusemide *see* furosemide
FTY 720 184
5-FU *see* 5-fluorouracil
fuel oil 922
Fuller's earth, decontaminant 2083, 2087, 2092
fulvic acids 1368
fumaric acid 549, 1985
fumonisins 1252–3, 2145, 2146, 2162–6
  A_1 2163
  A_2 2163

  B_1 1515–16, 1520, 2146
  B_2 2163
  B_3 2163
  B_4 2163
furan-2-al *see* furfural
furans 90, 132, 142, 726–7, 1756, 1757
furazolidone 819, 1642
furfural 237, 1901
furnace black 2017
furoic acid 1907
furosemide (frusemide) 184, 198, 253, 785, 795, 915, 1010, 1430
furylfuramide (AF-2) 1038

G

GA *see* tabun
gadolinium chloride 873, 881
galactoflavine 972
galactosamine 6, 184, 1860, 1861
galena *see* lead sulphide
gallic acid 1518, 1522
gallic acid esters 1985
gallium 2063
gallium arsenide 2050, 2063
ganglio-*n*-tetrosylceramide *see* asialo GM1
gas, bottled 920
gasoline *see* petroleum products
GB *see* sarin
GD *see* pinacolyl methylphosphono-fluoridate
GE *see* isopropyl ethylphosphono-fluoridate
gelsemine 1520
genestein 1396
genistin 197, 570
gentamicin
  cardiotoxicity 819
  circadian toxicology 16, 265
  nephrotoxicity 685
  ototoxicity 789, 792, 795
  parenteral toxicity 531, 537
  tissue take-up 128, 129
  toxic reactions 1430
gentian violet 738
germanium 1567–8
germanium compounds 1552
gestodene 1427, 1428–9
GF *see* cyclohexyl methyl-phosphonofluoridate
gigathenin 1518
ginerol 806
ginseng 1552

gitoxin 237
glass 2022
gliotoxin 197
glucagon 346, 547, 759, 991
D-glucaric acid 1848
glucocorticoids 757, 758
    antidotal studies 428
    and apoptosis 197
    endocrine toxicology 984, 985,
        990–1
    for insect stings 2184
    manufacture, toxic hazards 1455
    for mustard gas respiratory tract
        lesions 2087
    skeletal muscle toxicity 947
    therapy for phosgene poisoning
        2099
gluconate 428
glucono-δ-lactone 2127
glucose 355–6, 358, 362, 684,
    1495, 1496, 1504
glucosinolates 1983, 1984
glucuronides 107, 537
glufosinate 2003, 2006
glutamate 115, 632, 634, 1988
glutamate antagonists 635
glutamine 236
glutaraldehyde 26, 62, 548, 701,
    711
glutathione
    circadian toxicology 257
    haematotoxicity 384, 393
    interspecies variation in toxicity
        277
    metabolism 100
    mixtures 315
    nephrotoxicity 681
    neurotoxicity 634
    pathological changes 344
    systemic pulmonary toxicity 724
    tests 361
glutathionine 262
glutethimide 1122, 1496, 1503,
    1545
glycerol 2022
glycerol formal 534
glyceryl dinitrates 1907
glyceryl triacetate 740, 750
glycidyl ethers 1884, 2023
glycine 236, 392, 632
glycoconjugates 343
glycogen 336
glycol ethers 585, 804, 1156, 1467,
    2023, 2032, 2041
glycolic acid 2032

glycols 2014, 2020
glycoproteins 338, 364
glycosaminoglycans 342
glycosides
    cardiac 237, 285, 428, 808,
        811–12, 818, 821, 1549
    cytogenicity 1090
    in toxic plants 1522
glycosides food toxicology 1983–4
glyphosate 1512, 2003, 2006
gold 390, 395, 870, 1003, 1004,
    1130, 1489
gossypol 185, 1553
grain dusts 701
gramicidin D 819
granisetron 220
grayanotoxins (GTX) 639, 818,
    821, 824
griseofulvin 552, 569, 867, 870
growth factors 1972
GTX see grayanotoxins
guanethidine 1427
guanoxan 220
N7-guanyl-aflatoxin B1 1845
S-[2-(N-guanyl)ethyl]glutathione
    121
guanylic salts 1988
guianidine derivatives 2016

H

H1-blockers 738
H2 antagonists see histamine H2
    antagonists
H7 191, 199
H16 426
haematoporphyrin 762
haemocyanin 384
haemophilus B, conjugate vaccine
    1965
haemoprotein 254
haemorrhagins 2179
haemosiderin 2065
Hagedorn oximes 429, 2094, 2095
haloacetonitriles 1383
haloalkanes/haloalkenes 121, 161,
    690–1, 871, 2032
haloethylglutathione 121
halogenated compounds, forensic
    screening tests 1497
halogenated hydrocarbons
    abusive use 1505
    aliphatic 313
    aromatic 810–11, 872, 911, 917,
        922, 1004

chlorination byproducts 1383
    metabolism 104
    nephrotoxicity 689–91
    protein adducts 1887
    steam distillation 1497
halogens, bioavailability in drinking
    water 1381
haloperidol 220, 243, 264, 553,
    663, 1403
halothane
    activation 132
    adverse drug reactions 1438,
        1439
    anaesthesia 2030
    animal euthanasia 498
    biomarker 1849
    biomonitoring 1901
    cardiac toxicity 810, 818
    cartilage and bone toxicity 966
    metabolism 101, 102, 104
    reproductive toxicity 1145
    tests 357
haloxyfop 2003, 2005
harmaline 222, 223
harmalol 222
harman 222
harmine 222
hashish see cannabis
HCH see hexachlorocyclohexane
heavy metals 2049
    and acid precipitation 1377
    animal toxicoses 1513, 1523
    cartilage and bone toxicity 965
    combustion products 1919
    as contaminants in food crops
        1369
    endocrine toxicity 987–8
    environmental contamination
        1564
    forensic analysis 1491, 1495,
        1497
    groundwater contamination 1369
    human studies 461
    and menstrual disorders 1465
    natural high concentrations 1366
    neonatal toxicity 1217, 1218
    plant root uptake 1369
    renal injury 680–1
    reproductive effects 1146, 1350
    screening methods 1497, 1554
    in soils 1329
    toxicology 257
helanine 1519
helenaline 1519
heleurine 1519

hydroxocobalamin 428
hydroxquinone 990
3α-hydroxy bile acids 360
N-hydroxy-2-acetylaminofluorene
    metabolism 102
hydroxyalkenals 158, 1868
hydroxyamines 393, 556
1-hydroxyaminonaphthalene 876
4-hydroxyamphetamine 220
p-hydroxybenzoic acid 1989
3-hydroxybutyrate 365
hydroxychloroquine 764, 945
hydroxycobalamin *see* vitamin B12
hydroxycoumarins 231, 231
4-hydroxycyclophosphamide 729
4-hydroxydebrisoquine 112, 222
8-hydroxydeoxyguanosine 1845,
    1867, 1868, 2015
6-hydroxydopamine 641
β-hydroxyethoxyacetic acid 84
2-hydroxyethyl mercaptoethanol
    1865
N_3-(2-hydroxyethyl)adenine 1885
hydroxyethyl amines 2115
N-(2-hydroxyethyl)valine 1845,
    1884
2-hydroxy-5-hexanone 2035
hydroxyhippuric acid 1989
5-hydroxyindol-3-ylanic acid 236
hydroxylamines 104, 109, 161, 413,
    426, 429, 1883, 2094, 2119
11β-hydroxylase 370
4-hydroxymethamphetamine 220
N-(3′-hydroxy-4i-methoxyphenyl)-
    2-chloroamides 612
R-4′-hydroxy-*N*-methylphenytoin
    226
5-hydroxymethyluracil 235, 1845
N-hydroxy-2-naphthylamine 134
4-hydroxynonenal 184, 764, 896
hydroxyochratoxin 2156
4-hydroxyphenoxy)benzoic acid
    466
2-hydroxyphenylacetaldehyde 231,
    231
2-hydroxyphenylacetic acid 231
2-hydroxyphenylethanol 231
hydroxyproline 722
4-hydroxypropranolol metabolism
    100
2-(hydroxypropyl)amine 2115
3-hydroxypropylmercaptouric acid
    1865
1-hydroxypyrene 1905, 1927

4-hydroxy-1-(3-pyridyl)butan-1-one
    1883
8-hydroxyqunilines 1565–6
3β-hydroxy-5β-steroids 236
hydroxytamoxifen 284–5
5-hydroxytryptamine antagonists
    763
hydroxyurea 258
1′-hydroxyversicolorone 2151
hymenoxon 1519
hyoscyamine 1521
hyoscyamus 1489
hypericin 1523
hypochlorite 737, 905
hypoxanthine 103

I

ibotenate 634, 641, 1513
ibufenac 132
ibuprofen 263, 1550
ICI 162 1124
ICI 164,384 1395
ICI 182,780 764, 1403
ifosfamide 262, 727, 1862
imazalil 2001, 2003
imidazoles 1147, 1429
3,3′-iminodipropionitrile 637, 638
imipenem 686
imipramine
    acute toxicity 325
    cardiac toxicity 805
    eye toxicity 756
    forensic screening tests 1497
    pharmacogenetics 222, 232, 233
    post-mortem changes 1495
    site-dependent blood
        concentrations 1495
    systemic pulmonary toxicity 730
indigo dyes 1987
indinavir (Crixivan) 1427
indium 2063
indium arsenide 2063
indocyanine green 361
indolcarbazoles 163
indol-3-carboxylic acid scopine
    ester 763
indoles 132, 222–3, 2131
indol-3-ylmethanal 238
indomethacin 184, 253, 254, 807,
    1427, 1428, 1917
indoprofen (Flosint) 1427
indoramin 220
inosinic acid 1988

inositol triphosphate (PIP3) 808,
    896
insulin-like growth factor 1972
interferons 1964, 1965, 1966,
    1971–2
intermidine 1519
inulin 362, 1462
iodide 2102
iodine 1328, 1329, 1365, 1551,
    1552, 1969
iodoacetamide 167
iodochlorohydroxy quinoline 413
iodoquinol (Yodoxin, Moebiquin),
    adverse effects 1566
iodothalamate 362
2-iodo-3,7,8-trichlorodibenzo-*p*-
    dioxin 90, 142
ioxynil 2003, 2005
ipecacuanha 2, 546
4-ipomeanol 132, 726–8, 727
iprindole 730
iprodione 2000, 2002
iproniazid 114
irinotecan 262
iron 2064–5, 2066
    in ancient Indian writings 1489
    bioavailablity in drinking water
        1381
    biomonitoring 1905
    cardiac toxicity 822
    cartilage and bone toxicity 973
    chelation 634, 2068
    deficiency 1551, 2053
    ferric *see* iron(III)
    fortification 1223, 1552
    haematotoxicity 384
    hepatotoxicity 870
    ligand exchange 1369
    metabolism 1863
    neonatal toxicity 1217
    stains for 867
    transport, as biomarker 1864
iron(II) sulphide 2050
iron(III) 2065
iron(III) mitoxantrone 184
iron(III) oxide 2017
isobutanol 1298
isocyanates 701, 1004, 1475, 1927,
    2014, 2021
isoeugenol 708, 711
isofenphos 142
isoflavonoids 570, 1398, 1984
isofluorophate 760
isoflurane 2030
isoleucine 229

isolinoleic esters 1428
isomyl alcohol 142
isoniazid 28, 105, 108, 112, 113, 119–20, 325, 390, 756, 1430
isonicotinic acid 119
isopentane 1867
isophorone 692
isophthalic anhydride 2020
isoprenaline (isoproterenol) 58, 430, 808, 810, 814, 1430
isoprene rubber 2013, 2015
isopropanol 237, 2041
isopropyl alcohol *see* isopropanol
isoprpyly ethylphosphonofluoridate (GE) 2089
isoprostanes 1867, 1868
isoproterenol *see* isoprenaline
isoquinolones 191
isoretinoin 1430
isosasafrole 1866
isosorbide dinitrate 460
isosorbide mononitrate 460
isothiocyanates 234, 1430
isotretinoin *see* 13-*cis*-retinoic acid
itraconazole 1429
ivermectin 1648, 1994, 1999

J

jacobine 1519
jacodine 1519
jervin 1521

K

kainate 634, 634, 641
kallikreinogen 897
kanamycin 128, 129–30, 685, 787, 789, 792, 795, 1430
kaolin 1475, 2022
Kepone *see* chlordecone
kerosene 315, 920, 922, 2087
ketoconazole 38, 50, 1147, 1403, 1427, 1429
ketones 103, 104, 362, 911, 1383, 1418, 2023, 2032
 see also individual chemicals
ketoprofen 263
kinesin 631
King's yellow 2050
kohl 759

L

β-lactam antibiotics 686–8, 1049
lactate 563, 806, 939, 969

LAL *see* limulus amoebocyte lysate
laminin 342–3
landrin 1347
lanolin 605
lantadine 1519
lanthanides 870
lanthanum 805, 822
lasiocarpine 883, 1519
latex 510–11, 828, 1667, 1674
lathyrogens 1983
α-latrotoxin 640
lauric acid 101
lazaroid U-78517F 954
lead 2054–7, 2066
 age effects 1417
 animal toxicoses 1343, 1513, 1515, 1518, 1523–4
 anthropogenic emissions 1370
 antidotal studies 426, 433
 behavioural toxicity 650, 654, 658, 661, 665–6
 binding values (EU) 1595
 biomarker 1844, 1848, 1864
 biomonitoring 1485, 1780, 1899, 1901, 1904, 1905, 1907, 1909, 1910, 1911
 cardiac toxicity 821, 822
 cartilage and bone toxicity 973, 974, 2068
 central neurotoxicity 1378, 1523
 chelation therapy 2068
 CNS symptoms 1523
 in contaminated cattle feed 1554
 and DALAD 1343, 1345
 developmental toxicity 1487
 in drinking water 1377, 1378, 1382
 exposure routes 606
 eye toxicity 759
 forensic analysis 1491
 in gull feathers 654
 haematology 390–2
 haematotoxicity 1513
 hepatotoxicity 880
 historical aspects 1482, 1489
 in home environment 1417
 human studies data 463
 and idiopathic environmental illness 1711, 1712
 industrial exposure 683
 ingestion 1340
 interaction with smoking 1417
 and lung disease 1474
 mitochondria sensitivity 683
 neonatal toxicity 1227, 1248

nephrotoxicity 683
nestling studies 1349
neurotoxicity 633, 638–9, 639, 1518
 not taken up by plant roots 1369
 ototoxicity 784
 PBPK modelling 142
 in precipitation 1370, 1377
 reproductive toxicity 1145, 1146, 1156, 1464, 1465, 1466, 1467
 risk assessment 1777
 in river Rhine 1370
 in sewage sludge 1372
 in soil 1329, 1371, 1373, 1375
 storage sites 17
 susceptibility 29
 systemic effects 1475
 teratogenicity 1205
 threshold levels 1378
 and Wilms' tumour 1464
lead arsenate 2050, 2055
lead compounds
 binding values (EU) 1595
 in leaded petrol 1266, 1267
 marketing controls 1595
 in plastics industry 2022, 2023
 rubber additive 2014, 2017
 therapeutic use 1451
lead nitrate 184
lead oxide 1446, 2055
lead shot, waterfowl poisoning 1523
lead sulphide (galena) 252, 1366, 2054, 2056
leather 564
lecithin 619
lecithin/sphingomyelin ratio 1216
lectin 338, 343
leptophos 1345, 1997
levamisole 692
lewisite 427, 1724, 2068, 2081, 2082, 2088–9
licorice 945
lidocaine *see* lignocaine
light hydrocarbons 691
lignans 570, 1984
lignocaine (lidocaine) 254, 265, 366, 522, 529, 555, 640, 817, 947, 956
 toxicity 265
lime salts 972
d-limonene 136, 692, 1757
linamarin 918, 1984
lincomycin 1438

mercury (*Contd.*)
  gastro-intestinal microflora 570
  hepatotoxicity 870
  history 2
  in home environment 1418
  human data studies 460
  immunotoxicity 1003, 1004
  inorganic 681, 1355, 2058, 2066
  interactions with selenium 1351
  ion binding 128
  kidney response 681, 683
  marketing controls 1595
  metallothionein and 2067
  in mine tailings 1355
  neonate toxicity 1226
  neurotoxicity 633, 643, 1564–5
  not taken up by plant roots 1369
  organic 1343, 1355, 1994
  ototoxicity 784
  peripheral neuropathy 1475
  reproductive toxicity 1156
  in sewage sludge 1372
  in soils 1329, 1373
  speciation 1365–6, 1378
  sperm evaluation studies 1467
  and spontaneous abortion 1465
  subchronic testing 1344
  toxicity 1344–5
  transplacental transport 1464
mercury(I) chloride 2000, 2001,
  2057
mercury(II) chloride (corrosive
  sublimate) 257, 267, 681, 682,
  822, 1490, 1528, 1861, 2001,
  2057, 2059
mercury(II) sulphide 2057
merphos 1512, 2006
mesna 809
mestranol 568
metala 2049–78
metal chelates 1867
metaldehyde 2006
metal ions, binding 128
metalloids 2049
metallothioneins 367, 533, 682,
  684, 1317, 1461
metals 104, 1952, 2000, 2001,
  2014, 2016, 2023, 2049–78
  *see also heavy metals and
    individual elements*
metam 2000, 2001
metamizol (novaminosulfon) 1427,
  1428
metamphetamine 1491
metapramine 805

metaprolol 760
metaraminol 220
methacarbamol 2186
methacholine 512
2-methacryloxypropyltrimethoxy-
  silane 27
methadone 114–15, 220, 1145,
  1154, 1497, 1503, 1504
methaemoglobin-generating
  substances 28, 426
methaemoglobin inhibitors 1902
methamidophos 1997
methamphetamine 184, 220, 814,
  1495
methanamine hexamethylene
  tetramine
methandrostenolone 815
methane 1516–17, 1917, 1927,
  2034
methanediol 2040
methanol 2040
  antidotes 425–6, 429
  biomonitoring 1902, 1907
  with carbon tetrachloride 149
  as combustion product 1927
  eye toxicity 755, 765
  forensic analysis 1491
  from wood burning 1918
  GLC 1503
  inhalation 1419
  LD_{50} 15
  metabolism 103, 119, 2032
  microdiffusion 1497
  PBPK modelling 142
  pharmacogenetics 237
  steam distillation 1497
  toxic reactions 1430
methapyriline 878, 1127, 1128
β-methasone 758
methenyl trichloride 2036
methimazole 232
3-methindole 731–2
methiocarb 1336, 1347, 1998, 2006
methionine 426, 430, 644, 793,
  972, 1970, 1973
methoprene 1999–2000
methotrexate
  and apoptosis 185
  carcinogenicity 1455
  circadian toxicology 261
  cytotoxicity 1454–5
  eye toxicity 755
  haematotoxicity 390, 391
  metabolism 16
  mutagenicity 1053, 1054

neonatal toxicity 1219
  systemic pulmonary toxicity
    727, 728, 729
methoxsalen 1537
methoxyacetic acid 142, 2041
methoxyamphetamines 220
methoxychlor 1145, 1153–4,
  1243–4, 1329, 1396
methoxydihydropyran (MDP) 26
5-methoxy-*N,N*-dimethyltryptamine
  222–3
2-methoxyethanol 142, 583–4,
  2030, 2033, 2041
  and radiofrequency radiation
    1419
methoxyethylmercury 2058
methoxyfluorane 357, 387, 498,
  818, 1430
methoxyphenamine 100, 220
8-methoxypsoralen 415, 762, 1430
2-methylacrolein 1919
methylacrylamidoglycolate methyl
  ether 554
N-methylamino-L-alanine 634
methylarsenic compounds 267,
  1907
methylating agents 1881
methylazooxymethane 876
methylazoxymethanol 184, 566,
  569, 635–6, 876, 877
methylbenzene *see* toluene
methylbenzoic acid 793, 2039
methylbromide 615, 755
methyl-1-(butylcarbamoyl)
  benzimidazol-2-ylcarbamate 758
methyl *iso*-butyl ketone 1907, 2018
methyl butyl ketone *see* 2-hexanone
methyl *tert*-butyl ether, PBPK
  modelling 142
N-methylcarbamoylmercaptouric
  acid 1865
methylchloroform *see* 1,1,1-
  trichloroethane
methyl chlorosulphonate 2102
3-methylcholanthracene 258, 279,
  280, 283, 395, 525, 549, 763
3-methylcholanthrene (3-MC) 113,
  114, 118, 866, 910
methylcobalamin 2064
S-methylcysteine sulphoxide 1522
methylcysteine sulfoxide 234
7-methyl-2′-deoxyguanosine-3′-
  monophosphate 225
2-methyl-4-chlorophenoxyacetic
  acid (MCPA) 1907

morphine 114, 184, 198, 556, 568, 569, 1430, 1491
   see also opiates
morpholines 2001, 2004
morsodren 1336, 1337
motilin 547
moulds *see* mycotoxins
moxidectin 1642
4-MP *see* 4-methylpyrazole
6-MP *see* 6-mercaptopurine
MPDP$^+$ 132, 133
MPP$^+$ 132, 133, 224
MPTP *see* methylphenyltetra-hydropyridine
muconic acid 607
mumps vaccines (Pluserix-MMR, Immravax) 1427
β-muricholate 360
muromonab 1965
muscimol 1513
musk ambrette 1430
Mus m 1 allergen 511
Mus m 2 allergen 511
mustard gases 1035, 1444
   see also nitrogen *or* sulphur mustard
MX mutagen 1383
MXT *see* maitotoxin
mycophenolate 1130
mycotoxins 2145–76
   biological activity 2146
   in biological warfare 2082
   characterization 2148
   as chemical warfare agent 2104
   in diet 58, 1982
   in mouldy food 1554
   placental toxicity 1251–4
   produced by non-storage fungi 2148–9
   structures 2145, 2146
   toxicity 1339, 1340, 1515–16, 1520, 1524
mydriatics 1548
myelin 636–7
myricetin 571

N

nabam 990
NABQI *see* N-acetyl-*p*-benzoquinoneimine
NAC *see* N-acetylcysteine
nafenopin 1127
nafoxidine 762
naloxone 426, 430, 433

2-naphthalene sulphonate 2018
naphthalene 108, 731, 763, 1455
naphthalene dihydrodiol 763
naphthalene diisocyanate 2021
naphthaquinones 358
naphthazoline 738
naphthoflavones 113, 763, 918, 925, 990
naphthotriazoles 2023
naphthoxylacetic acid 100, 228
α-naphthyl isothiocyanate (ANIT) 882, 1860, 1861
naphthylamines
   biochemistry 134
   carcinogenicity 1537, 2015, 2017
   extrapolation studies 1952
   in humans 463
   metabolism 120
   rubber additive 2014
   toxic reactions 1430
α-naphthylthiourea (ANTU) 724, 1511
NAPQI *see* N-acetyl-*p*-benzoquinoneimine
naringenin 22
natamycin 1642
neamine 792
neocarzinostatin 527
neomycin 129–30, 685, 787, 788, 791–2, 795, 819, 1455
neoprontosil 565
neostigmine bromide 2181
neostygmine 951
neriine 821
netilmicin 685
netropsin 163
neurotrophic factors 1972
Neutral Red 753, 753
ngaione 872, 877
niacin 972
nicarbazine 1521
nickel 2062–3, 2066
   anthropogenic emissions 1370
   and apoptosis 188–9
   biomarker 1849
   biomonitoring 1902, 1904, 1907, 1909, 1910
   carcinogenicity 1537, 1539
   cardiac toxicity 808
   cutaneous toxicity 835
   genotoxicity 200
   PBPK modelling 142
   placental toxicity 1249–50
   in sewage sludge 1372

   in soils 1329, 1373
   teratogenicity 127–9, 1206–9
nickel carbonyl 758
nickel chloride 664
nickel sulphate 413
nicotinamide 190, 200
nicotine
   biomonitoring 1905
   circadian toxicity 265
   extraction from tissues 1490
   favourable effects 1452
   metabolism 238, 239
   PBPK modelling 142
   peroral toxicity 548
   as pesticide 1994, 1999
   pharmacogenetics 220–1, 231, 233, 238–9
   risk acceptance 1960
   steam distillation 1497
   toxicity 265
nicotinic alkaloids 1520, 1521
nifedipine 188, 817
nimodipine 22
nitrates 2111–43
   air pollution 1266
   animal toxicoses 1509, 1514, 1519, 2135
   carcinogenic 1382
   conversion to nitrite 1383
   dose levels expression 2111
   endogenous synthesis 2118–21, 2133
   epidemiological studies 2129–31
   fertilizer, in soil 1960
   human body burdens 2133–4
   human dietary intakes 2115–18
   interspecies differences 1509, 1519
   leaching 1371
   levels in food and beverages 2112–14
   reduction 566–7
   RfD 1760
   toxicokinetics and metabolism 2121–3
nitrenium ions 161
nitric acid 1275, 1376, 1477
nitric oxide 104, 158, 199, 634, 808, 1266, 1274–5, 2119, 2121
nitric oxide radical 896, 903
nitrile rubber 2013
nitriles 2003, 2005
nitrites 2111–43
   carcinogenic 1383
   dose levels expression 2111

nitrites (*Contd.*)
  endogenous synthesis 2120,
    2134
  epidemiological studies 2131–2
  haematotoxicity 390
  human body burdens 2134
  human dietary intakes 2115–18
  levels in food and beverages
    2112–14
  susceptibility 28
  toxicokinetics and metabolism
    2121–2, 2123, 2125–8
  toxicological data in animals
    2135
4-nitroacetophenone 243
nitroalkanes 2023
nitroamines 1883
nitroarenes 1883
nitroaromatics 238, 1867
nitroarsenilic acid 1515
nitrobenzaldehyde 243
nitrobenzenes 104, 565, 572, 585,
  1902
6-nitrochrysene 565
nitro compounds 565
nitrofen 990, 1557
nitrofurans 1642
nitrofurantoin 726, 1430
nitrogen 563, 1372
  see also urea
nitrogen/argon inhalation 498
nitrogen-based fertilizers, toxicity
  1514
nitrogen dioxide
  acute toxicity 50, 51
  air pollution 1266
  ambient concentration effects on
    humans 1279
  biochemical and histopatho-
    logical effects 1278–6
  in fires 1821
  mixtures 314
  in plastics industry 2021
  respiratory effects 1279
  and response to allergens
    1279–80
  silo filler's disease 1517
  toxicokinetics 1278
  transport 158
nitrogen mustard 199, 258, 2083,
  2085
nitrogen oxides 1266, 1267, 1297,
  1376, 1927
nitrogen poisoning, rumen
  microflora 1514

nitrogen trichloride 626
nitroglutethimide 1122
nitroglycerine 460, 527, 545, 1475,
  1722–3, 1902, 2187
nitroimidazoles 1090
3-nitromalonate 635
1-nitronaphthalene 731, 876
nitrophenazide 1521
p-nitrophenol, biomonitoring 1907
3-nitropropionate 634, 635, 636
nitropyrene 130, 565, 569, 1038
nitroquinoline oxide 104, 240, 1047
nitrosamides 1982, 1989
nitrosamines
  biomarkers 1880, 1882
  carcinogenicity 2128–9
  cytogenicity 1079
  in diet 1981, 1982, 1989
  DNA adducts 1885, 1886
  genotoxicity 7
  in German food and drink 2118
  hepatotoxicity 876, 877
  mixtures 305, 314
  mutagenicity 1039
  pancreatic toxicity 902, 911,
    920, 924, 925, 926
  rubber additives 2014, 2016–17
  in tobacco smoke 2115
nitroschloramphenicol 390
N^1-nitrosoanabasin 2115
N^1-nitrosoanatabine 2115
nitrosobenzene 565
N-nitrosobis(2-hydroxypropyl)
  amine (BOP) 922, 923–4, 927
nitroso compounds
  carcinogenic 1383
  in chemical warfare 2111
  endogenous synthesis 2120–1,
    2134
  epidemiological studies 2132–3
  and gastro-intestinal microflora
    562, 566
  human studies 2115–18, 2134–5,
    2137
  rubber additives 2014
  toxicokinetics and metabolism
    2121–2, 2123, 2128–9
  toxicological data in animals
    2135–6
nitrosodiethanolamine 274, 2115,
  2121, 2123
nitrosodimethylamine 232, 234,
  2115, 2118, 2121, 2123, 2132
nitrosodiphenylamine 2016, 2017
nitrosohydroethylglycine 2121

nitrosomethylurea (NMU) 1030,
  1100
nitrosomorpholine 2121
N′-nitrosonornicotine *see* 4-(*N*-
  methylnitrosoamino)-1-
  (3-pyridyl)butan-1-one (NNK)
nitrosopiperidine 2120, 2123
nitrosoproline (NPRO) 2120, 2123
nitrosopyrrolidine 2115, 2120, 2123
nitrosothiioproline 2123
nitrosoureas 7, 1885
β-nitrostyrene 612
nitrous oxide 390, 1151
nivalenol 2104, 2149
NMU *see* nitrosomethylurea
NNK *see* 4-(*N*-methylnitrosoamino)
  -1-(3-pyridyl)butan-1-one
nocodazole 199
nomifensine (Merital) 1427, 1438
nonane 2034
non-steroidal anti-inflammatory
  drugs (NSAIDs) 51, 132, 136,
  167, 229–30, 458, 940, 1427,
  1428, 1550
nonylphenol 1396, 1397
nordoxepin 1495
norephedrine *see* phenylpropanolamine
norepinephrine (noradrenaline) 730,
  1348
norethisterone 879, 1127
norethynodrel 879
norfluoxetine 1495
norgestimate 1428
normeperidine 1495
norpropoxyphene .1495, 1504
norsolorinic acid 2151
nortriptyline 220, 819, 1495
noscapine 220
NO_x *see* nitrogen oxides
NSAIDs *see* non-steroidal
  anti-inflammatory drugs
nucleic acid
  extractants 1454, 1455
  identification chemicals 1454
  sequencing reagents 1454, 1455
nux vomica *see* strychnine
nylon 1922, 2022

O

obidoxime 426, 429, 2094
OCDD *see* 2,3,7,8-tetrachloro-*p*-
  dibenzodioxin octochloroanalog

ochratoxins 2145
  analogues 2155–7
  analysis 2157–8
  animal toxicoses 1515–16, 1524
  A (OTA) 197, 1253, 2156, 2157
  B 2155, 2156
  biological activity 2146,
    2154–62
  C 2156
  chemical characteristics and
    biosynthesis 2154–5
  chemical structures 2146, 2156
  genotoxicity 2160
  immunotoxicity 2160
  isolation and purification 2157
  mechanisms of action 2161–2
  pharmacokinetics 2160–1
  production, isolation and
    purification 2157
  toxicity 1516, 2157
OC see organochlorines
octadecysilane 1455
octane 2034
octanoic acid 1298
octanol 199
octylphenol 1404–5
17β-oestradiol
  assay 1402
  clearance rates 1408
  developmental effects 1406
  and gastro-intestinal microflora
    568, 569, 570
  grapefruit interaction 22
  natural oestrogen 1392
  normal levels 1398
  as reference substance 1397
  structure 1396
  testosterone metabolite 1395,
    1406
  toxicity and reproduction studies
    1404, 1405
  use in assay 1403
oestrogens see Subject Index
oestrogens, synthetic
  see dithethystilboestrol
oestrogen sulphate 568
oil, detection by histology 534
oil of Bergamot 413
oil spill control agents 1313
OK-432 184
okadaic acid 186, 199, 817, 2193
olanzapine 220
olaquindox 1648
oleandrin 821
oleates 534, 731–2, 2022

olefins 2034
oligomycin 816
olive oil 58
oltipraz 278, 1887
omeprazole 227–8, 1124
ondansetron 220
OP see organophosphates
opiates
  acute overdose 1496
  controlled drug 1545
  forensic analysis 1491, 1495,
    1503, 1504
  heroin injection 814–15, 942,
    944, 946
  maternal addiction 1224, 1256–7
  pancreatic toxicity 901
  reproductive toxicity 1145
  skeletal muscle toxicity 942
opium 1489, 1490
OPP see 2-phenylphenol
Orange II 565
orcinol 990
organic acids see acids
organic solvents 2029-47
  aliphatic 2034-7
  aromatic hydrocarbons 2037-40
  biological monitoring 1906
  chlorinated aliphatic 2035-7
  combustion toxicology 1919,
    1928
  enzyme induction 2032-3
  metabolism 2032, 2033-4
  mixtures 2033, 2042
  toxicity 2030-3
    behavioural 651
    narcosis 8
    occupational 1418, 1487
    ototoxicity 794-5
organoarsenicals 3, 56, 1426, 1427
organochlorines (OC)
  biomarker 1848
  biomonitoring 1902
  and breast cancer 1400
  chronic intake 82
  environmental 1370, 1553–4
  human studies 460
  as mixtures 2007
  molecular interactions 163
  oestrogenic effects 1398
  persistence 1392, 1548, 1553–4,
    1599
  as pesticides 2, 1994, 1995,
    1996–8
  placental toxicity 1243–4
  prohibited 1557

organohalides 1366, 1457
organomercurials 681–2, 1824–5,
  2000
  see also mercurials;
    methylmercury
organometallic compounds,
  fungicide 2001
organophosphates (OP)
  see also nerve agents in Subject
    Index
  acute poisoning 34
  additive effects 50
  age/maturation effects 1337
  antidotes 431
  behavioural effects 662, 1348
  biochemical disturbances 63
  biological effect monitoring
    1485
  biomarker 1848
  biomonitoring 1900, 1906
  and brain cholinesterase levels
    1343, 1523
  cardiac toxicity 807, 823–4
  cholinesterase inhibition 114,
    951–5, 1345, 1475, 1554, 1866,
    1900
  differential toxicity 1328, 1335
  domestic animal toxicity 1510,
    1512
  effect of formulation 1339
  equine toxicity 1518
  extrapolation of acute effects 51
  fungicides 2001, 2003
  herbicides 1512, 2003, 2006
  history 2, 3
  immunotoxicity 1004, 1006,
    1010
  insecticides 466, 1996–8
  lability 1329
  long-term exposure 1487
  metabolism by HMOs 1334
  as mixtures 2007
  neurotoxicology 23, 43, 55,
    637–8, 1333
  pancreatic toxicity 917
  pesticides 578
  phytometabolism 1341
  placental toxicity 1242–3
  in plastics industry 2023
  poultry toxicity 1523
  repeated exposure 1418
  reproduction testing 1351
  rubber additive 2014
  species sensitivity differences
    110

organophosphates (OP) (*Contd.*)
  sulphoxide and sulphone
    metabolites 1341
  toxicity 426, 429, 432
  varied uses 1548
  wildlife toxicity 1337, 1338,
    1341
organophosphonate 635
organosilicones 751
organotins 523, 1004, 1006, 2000,
  2001, 2022
orpiment 2050
osmosin 1427, 1428
OTA *see* ochratoxin A
ouabain 265, 807, 821
oxalates 97, 973, 1518, 1522, 2032
oxaliplatin 260–1
oxamniquine 882
β-*N*-oxatylamino-L-alanine 634
oxazepam 114
oxazolone 707, 711
oxides of nitrogen *see* nitrogen
  oxides (NO$_x$)
oximes 3, 426, 429–30, 516, 1998,
  2093, 2094–5
oxiranes 130
oxmetidine 1124
8-oxo-dG adducts 1890
2-oxothiazolidine-4-carboxylic acid
  689
oxprenolol 220
oxybisbenzenesulphonyl hydrazides
  2023
oxybuprocaine 741
oxychlordane 1343
oxycodone 1491, 1504
oxygen 238, 429, 430, 516, 590,
  1417, 2099
oxygen free radical(s) 792, 793,
  807, 809
  biology 903–4
  oxidation products (FROPS) 896
  pathology *see* oxidative stress
oxyphenbutazone 807, 1427
oxytetracycline 534, 537
oxytocin 537
oxytotic drugs 220
ozone
  air pollution 1267, 1268, 1273–4
  behavioural toxicity 653, 665
  biochemical and histopatho-
    logical effects 1276
  causing apoptosis 184
  effects on human health 1276–8,
    1283

ethics 1960
mixtures 314, 315, 316
and nitric oxide 1274–5
occurrence and production 1275
pancreatic toxicity 922
and sulphuric acid, comparison of
  factors 1280
toxicokinetics 1275
transport 158

P

PAF *see* lysophospholipid
PAHs *see* polycyclic aromatic
  hydrocarbons
paint(s) 918, 1295
paint thinners 918, 922
palladian catalysts 563
palmitic acid 813
palytoxin 820, 2104
2-PAM *see* pyridine-2-aldoxime
  methyl chloride
PAN *see* peroxyacetyl nitrate
pancuronium 947
papaverine 817
paper products 1298
PAPP *see* 4-aminopropiophenone
paraffins 2034
paraoxon 50, 102, 656, 1996
paraquat 2003, 2004
  action 127
  acute toxicity 34
  antidotes 428
  behavioural effects 1346
  biomarker 1867
  cardiac toxicity 821
  cationic 1369
  developing countries 1512
  inducing enzymes 1866
  LD$_{50}$ 51
  mechanism of toxicity 125
  pancreatic toxicity 904
  systemic pulmonary toxicity
    723–4
  tissue take-up 128
  toxic reactions 1430
parathion 1994
  biomonitoring 1902
  birds, toxicity 1336, 1337, 1342,
    1523
  cardiac toxicity 824
  effect on invertebrate food source
    1355
  metabolism 101, 102
  oxidative desulphuration 1329

PBPK modelling 142
percutaneous absorption 578
and predation behaviour 1348
reduced sensitivity 1342
regional differences in
  percutaneous absorption 578
reproductive effects 1351
secondary poisoning 1342
parathion-methyl
  behavioural effects 1348–9, 1352
  birds, toxicity 1336, 1337
  effect on invertebrate food source
    1355
  human studies 466
  placental toxicity 1243
paroxetine 220
PAS *see* p-aminosalicylic acid
patulin 2146
PBBs *see* polybrominated biphenyls
PCBs *see* polychlorinated biphenyls
PCP *see* phencyclidine
peanut oil 911
peanuts, roasted 1005
pectin 572
pegaspargase 1965
pemoline (Volital) 1427
penchloromethane 2035–6
penciclovir 239
penconazole 2001, 2003
penethamate 1642
D-penicillamine 427, 552, 755,
  942, 1430, 1513, 1514–15, 2068
penicillins
  biomarker 1849
  cardiac toxicity 807
  in chemical warfare 2099
  eye toxicity 756
  haematotoxicity 390
  immunotoxicity 1004
  irritation 413
  nephrotoxicity 686
  neurotoxicology 641
  parenteral toxicity 532
  peroral toxicity 547
penitrem A 2146, 2147
pennyroyal oil 731
S-(1,2,3,4,4-pentachloro-1,3-
  butadienyl) glutathione 690
pentachloroethane 142
pentachlorophenol 6, 917, 1902,
  1907, 2001, 2002
pentaerythritol 460
pentagastrin 1548
pentamidine 915, 992
pentane 2022, 2034

2,4-pentanedione 15, 26
pentanol 199
pentazocine 942
pentobarbital *see* phenobarbitone
pepleomycin 727
peptides 265, 1964, 2082
peptidoglycans 571
perbenzoates 2022
perchloric acid 1455
perchloroethylene
 see tetrachloroethylene
perfluorodecanoic acid 869
perfluorophenyl isothiocyanate
 1883, 1884
perfluorophenylthiohydantoin 1884
perfluoropropene 1915
perfumes 230
perhexiline 220, 221
periciazine 220
perlolidine 1521
perloline 1521
Perls' Prussian Blue 867
permethrin 460, 651, 1244, 1245,
 1994, 1998, 1999
peroxides 160, 2014, 2023, 2106
peroxisomes 344, 680
peroxyacetyl nitrate (PAN) 1278
peroxyacyl nitrates 1275
peroxynitrite 160, 199, 633, 634
perphenazine 220
perthane 1243–4
pertussis toxin 819
PE *see* polyethylene
pethidine 366, 1491, 1497, 1504
petroleum ether 920
petroleum hydrocarbons 691–2,
 1310, 1313
petroleum jelly, for mustard gas eye
 damage 2087
petroleum pollutants, avian embryo
 bioassay 1334
petroleum products
 car exhaust 606
 contamination 1373
 fractionation 920–2
 gasoline 607, 658, 2034
 groundwater contamination 1772
 interactions 2034
 lead additive 2054–5
 methanol in 2040
 paternal workplace exposure
  1464
 petrol/diesel fumes 917, 918,
  919, 1215
 in plastics industry 2023

underground storage tanks 1372
 unleaded petrol 692
phalloidin 782, 870, 1513
phasin 1518
phenacetin 103, 105, 390, 569, 569,
 1427, 1428, 1438
phenanthridine 239
o-phenanthroline 200
phencyclidine (PCP, angel dust)
 89, 942, 1491, 1495, 1503, 1545,
 1550
phenelzine 112
phenformin 112, 125, 220, 1430,
 1438
phenindione 241, 807
p-phenitidine 103
phenitrothion 259
phenobarbital *see* phenobarbitone
phenobarbitone
 bromobenzene toxicity and 118
 carcinogenicity 1127
 cardiac toxicity 818
 circadian toxicology 267
 DNA damage and 126
 endocrine toxicology 990
 and gastro-intestinal microflora
  566, 569
 hepatotoxicity 866, 867, 872,
  880
 increased 117
 inducing GSTs 1866
 LD$_{50}$ 51
 metabolism 106, 113, 114, 119
 pancreatic toxicity 910, 918, 925
 peroral toxicity 548
 use in assay 1403
phenol–formaldehyde composite
 1709, 2018
phenolphthalein 1427, 1429
phenols
 biomonitoring 1902, 1903, 1907
 fungicides 2001, 2002
 and gastro-intestinal microflora
  568–9
 haematotoxicity 395
 human studies 463
 metabolism 98, 100, 107, 111
 microdiffusion 1497
 parenteral toxicity 535
 percutaneous toxicity 585
 rubber additive 2014, 2016
 steam distillation 1497
 toxic hazard 1455
phenolsulphonphthalein 546

phenothiazines
 cardiac toxicity 819
 forensic analysis 1491, 1497
 haematotoxicity 395
 hepatotoxicity 884
 mutagenicity 1042
 parenteral toxicity 536
 reproductive toxicity 1146
 tissue specificity 129
 toxic reactions 1430, 1438
phenoxyacetates 2104
phenoxybenzamine 684
3-phenoxybenzoic acid 466, 569
phenoxy herbicides 2004–5
phentermine 730, 815, 1427, 1501
phenylacetone 102
phenylacetone oxime 102
phenylalanine 1518, 1989
phenylalanine mustard 527
phenylarsonic aresenicals 1515
phenylbutazone 253, 390, 756, 807,
 1438
S-phenylcysteine 607
phenyldiamines 413, 1861
phenylenediamines 1849, 2014,
 2020
phenylephrine 738
R-5-phenyl-5-ethylhadantoin 226
phenylglyoxylic acid 1907, 1910,
 2040
phenylhydroxylamine 393, 565
phenylimidazopyridine 1881, 1886
phenylisopropylamine 1501
phenyl isothiocyanate (PITC) 1883,
 1884
phenylmercapturic acid 2037
phenylmercury 2058
phenylnaphthylamine 2014, 2017
2-phenylphenol 2001
 sodium salts (OPP/SOPP)
  1129–30
3-phenylpropan-1-ol 101
phenylpropanolamine (PPA) 814,
 1501
phenyl sulphate 98
phenylthiohydantoin 1883, 1884
phenylthiourea 724
phenylureas 990
phenytoin
 cardiac toxicity 807, 817
 circadian toxicity 252, 254, 265
 disaster 1427
 endocrine toxicology 989, 991,
  992
 eye toxicity 760

polychlorinated biphenyls (PCBs)
(*Contd.*)
  PBPK modelling 142
  peroral toxicity 549
  persistence 1370, 1392, 1553–4
  placental toxicology 1251
  risk assessment 1756, 1770,
    1777, 1778
  risk management 1588
  in sewage sludge 1372
  sorbed to humus 1369
  toxicity 1554
  transplacental transport 1464
polychloroprenes 2013
polycyclic aromatic hydrocarbons
  (PAHs)
  adducts 162, 1880, 1887
  air pollutants 1267, 1300
  analysis 1883
  and apoptosis 197, 198
  aquatic toxicity 1316, 1317
  atmospheric deposition 1376
  biomarkers 1848, 1870, 1880,
    1882, 1886
  biomonitoring 1904–5
  bioremediation 1373
  circadian toxicology 271
  as combustion product 1927,
    1929
  cutaneous toxicity 27
  in diet 1982
  genotoxicity 7
  hepatic monoesterase (HMO)
    induction 1345
  hepatotoxicity 876, 879
  induction 113
  interspecies variation in toxicity
    278
  metabolism 1883
  mixtures 315
  mutagenicity 1026–7
  neonatal toxicity 1226
  oil spillages 1826–7
  pancreatic toxicity 917, 920
  persistence 1370, 1376
  reaction with DNA 161
  reproductive toxicity 1142, 1144,
    1145, 1146, 1150, 1153
  risk assessment 1756, 1791
  in rubber 2017
  in sewage sludge 1372
  and smoking 28
  in soils 1369, 1370, 1376
polycyclic aromatic hydrocarbon-
  type inducer 113

polydimethylsiloxane 1985
polyesters 1922, 2018, 2020
polyether 1922
polyethylene (PE) 1130, 1918,
  1919, 2018, 2019
polyethylene glycols 533–4, 740,
  744, 748, 750, 908, 2023
polyfluorocarbons 2018
polyglycols 2022
polyhalogenated biphenyls 1956,
  1982
    see also polybrominated
      biphenyls; polychlorinated
      biphenyls
polyhydric alcohols 1989
polyhydroxyphenols 990
polymers, combustion products
  1922–3
poly(methyl methacrylate) 2018,
  2019
polymyxin B 537, 538
polyols 1989
  brominated 2022
polyphenolics 1984
polypropylene 1918–19, 2018,
  2019
polypropylene glycol 552
polypropylene homopolymer 626
polypropylene-polyethylene
  copolymer 626
polysaccharides 571, 1981
polystyrene 2018
polytetrafluoroethylene (PTFE)
  1282, 1915, 1918
polythene *see* polyethylene
polyunsaturated fats 807
polyunsaturated fatty acids (PUFA)
  634, 904–5
polyurethanes (PU) 1918, 1919,
  1922, 1923, 1925, 2013, 2018,
  2021
poly(vinyl chloride) (PVC) 2018,
  2019
    see also vinyl chloride
    combustion products 1918, 1925,
      1928
    film, allergy 1915
    hot wire cutting 1915
    human studies 466
    PBPK modelling 1770–1
    peripheral sensory irritation 626
    waste from chimneys 1960
poly(vinylidine chloride) 2018
Ponceau MX 879, 1127
Pondimin *see* fenfluramine

potassium 355, 357, 364, 366, 370,
  463, 1430, 1979
potassium arsenite 460
potassium ascorbate 2087
potassium cyanide 635, 1724
potassium (KS+s) 808, 940, 941
    see also sodium/potassium
PPA *see* phenylpropanolamine
practolol 1427, 1428, 1438, 1439,
  1549
pralidoxime *see* pyridine-2-
  aldoxime methyl chloride
praseodymium 870
pravastatin 946
praziquantel 1642
prazocin 2188
prednisolone 758, 969
prednisone 22, 552, 758, 1455
5-pregnenolone 370
pregnenolone-16α-carbonitrile 113,
  285
prenalterol 426, 430
prenylamine 809
primaquine 391, 393
primidone 390, 391
printing inks 564
probenecid 691
procainamide 103, 105, 108, 112,
  218, 220, 221, 265, 817
procaine 105
procarbazine 727, 1145
procarcinogens 231
prochlorperazine 220
proflavine sulphate 415
proglycem *see* diazoxide
proguanil 227
promazine 730
promethazine 188, 220
prontosil 104, 325, 565
propachlor 569, 2003, 2005
propafenone 220
propandiol 237, 1438
propane 1867
propane thiosulphonate 428
propanil 390, 393, 1845, 2003,
  2005
propanol 553, 612, 626, 1298,
  1417, 1491, 1503, 1706, 1902
propanolol 1495
proparacaine 762
propellants 460, 1985
propionaldehyde 237, 613
propionic acid 554, 1989
propionitrile 1922

propofol (Diprivan) 234, 1427
propoxyphene 1495–6, 1500, 1503, 1504
propranolol 100, 228, 252, 254, 265, 555, 760
N-propylamine 220, 222
propylbenzene 101
propylene 2019
propylene glycol 460, 533, 740, 1426, 1427, 1428, 2020
propyleneimine 680
propylene oxide 21, 1880, 1884
propyl gallate 1985
propyl methanesulphonate 1145
n-propyl disulphide 1522
2-*n*-propylpent-4-enoic acid 121
propylthiouracil (PTU) 941, 989, 1121, 1403
prostaglandins 241, 243, 361, 525, 657, 741, 786, 845, 1981, 2161
prostigmine 951
proteins
    see also mycotoxins
    allergens 702
    in animal poisons 2184, 2186
    binding 253–4
    catalytic activities 217
    in food toxicology 1983
    hepatic metabolism tests 359
    metabolites 568
    nephropathy marker 678
    neuronal synthesis 631
    phosphorylation 982
    tests 355, 362, 370
    toxicities 265
proteoglycans 364
protoanemonin 1518
proton-pump inhibitor 227
Prussian blue 391
pseudoephedrine 1501
psoralens 22, 1043, 1523
PTFE *see* polytetrafluoroethylene
PTU *see* propylthiouracil
pulegone 1655
puromycin 184, 869
PU *see* polyurethane
putrescine 103, 128, 2193
PVC resin manufacturing company 457
pyrazole 429
pyrazophos 2001, 2003
pyrene 1886, 1907
pyrenol (1-hydroxypyrene) 1905, 1907

pyrethrins 34, 524, 534, 1510, 1994, 1998–9
pyrethroids
    behavioural toxicity 651
    domestic animal poisoning 1510
    human studies 460
    hydrolysis 524
    insecticides 465
    neurotoxicology 639
    parenteral toxicity 524, 534
    placental 1244–5
    sodium channel action 639
    synthetic 465, 1994, 1998–9
pyrethrum 259, 1642, 1994
pyridazinones 990
pyridine 109, 221, 1455, 1919, 1922
pyridine-2-aldoxime methyl chloride (2-PAM) 429, 955, 1510, 1998, 2094
pyridinium oximes 429
pyridostigmine 1995, 2081, 2093
pyridoxine *see* vitamin B_6
pyromellitic dianhydride 2020
pyrrole, oxidation 637
pyrrolidine dithiocarbamate 926
pyrrolizidine alkaloids 133, 730, 872, 873, 881, 882, 1981
pyruvate 806
pyruvate decarboxylase 427

Q

quartz *see* silica
quaternary amines 69
quaternary ammonium salts 2023
quercetin 241, 566, 571
quercetin-*O*-rutinoside *see* rutin
quinacridones 2023
quinalphos 1243
quinidine 22, 395, 817–18
quinine 395, 784, 785, 787
quinolinate 641
quinolines 2014, 2017
quinols 100
quinoneimine 71
quinone methides 725
quinones 240, 835, 1043
    and apoptosis 199
    biomarker 1867
    and calcium homeostasis 156
    cell prolferation stimulation 165
    metabolism 104
    and oxidative stress 160
    redox cycling 127, 691

Quintox *see* cholecalciferol
quintozene 2001
3-quinuclidinyl benzoate 1082

R

radium 974
radon 28, 252, 259, 260, 1293, 1538, 1827, 1959
raloxifene 1392
ranitidine 572
Rat n 1A allergen 511
Rat n 1B allergen 511
realgar 2050
recombinant-methionyl human brain-derived neurotrophic factor 1972
red squill 1511
Redux *see* dexfenfluramine
refrigerants 460
reserpine 1403
resins, absorbent 2161
resmethrin 1244, 1998
resorcinol 100, 990, 2014
respiridone 220
retarders, rubber industry 2014, 2016–17
13-*cis*-retinoic acid 236, 867, 946, 1188, 1189, 1218
retinoids 197, 755, 972, 1549
retinol 236, 642
retrorsine 872
RG12195 763
rhodanese 426, 428–9
riboflavins 972, 1987
ribonucleic acid (RNA) 1988
ribostamycin 789
rice oil 1005–6, 1226
ricin 184, 1518, 1726, 1727, 2082, 2104
rickettsia 2082
rifampicin 273, 1455
ristocetin 395
ritodrine 1216
ritonavir (Norvir) 1427
road oil 922
robin 1518
robitin 1518
ronidazole 1642
rotenone 807, 1994, 1999
rubber *see* Subject Index
rubidium 805
rubratoxins 1253
rubril 565

rutin 566
ryanodine 806, 808

S

S100 protein 347
SA *see* sodium ascorbate (SA)
SAC *see* acid saccharin
D-saccharic acid-1,4-lactone 568
saccharin 81, 1537, 1553, 1653, 1658, 1989
safrole 526, 569, 879, 1981
salazopyrin 390
salicylates 524, 553, 756, 969, 989, 991, 992
   see also aspirin
   acute overdose 1496
   ATP synthesis and 127
   cartilage and bone toxicity 969
   endocrine toxicology 989, 991, 992
   eye toxicity 756
   forensic screening tests 1497
   metabolism 115
   ototoxic effects 784, 785–7
   parenteral toxicity 524
   peroral toxicity 553
   in plastics industry 2022
   rubber additive 2014, 2016
   teratological effects 971, 1223
salicylazosulphapyridine 565
salt *see* sodium chloride
salvarsan 1426
saponins 759, 1519, 1521
saquinavir (Invirase) 22, 1427
sarafotoxin 812
sargramostim 1965
sarin (GB)
   ageing 2092
   cardiac toxicity 824
   L(Ct)$_{50}$ 2091
   management 2094
   military use 2089, 2090
   mixed routes of exposure 605
   physicochemical properties 2090
   regulations 1555
   safety 1444
   skeletal muscle toxicity 955
   terrorist use 1721, 1723, 1725–6, 1728, 1729, 1730, 1827, 2092
   toxicity 2091
satumomab 1965
saxitoxins 639, 816, 818, 1554, 2082, 2104, 2192
SBP *see* sulphobromophthalein

scaritoxin 2191
scombrotoxins 1554, 2193
scopolamine 527, 1430, 1521
scorpion toxins 818, 820, 898
SDZICT 322 763
sea anemone toxins 816, 818, 820
sebacates 549, 2017, 2022
secalonic acid D 1253–4
secoisolariciresinol 570
secretin 547
Seldane *see* terfenadine
selenites 870
selenium 2065, 2066
   accumulation in plants 1515
   in agricultural drainwater 1351
   as antioxidant 158, 1983
   biomarker 1868
   biomonitoring 1902, 1907
   cardiac toxicity 823
   in drinking water 1382
   hepatotoxicity 877
   pancreatic toxicity 908, 911
   poisoning in food-producing animals 1515
   rubber additive 2014, 2016
   in soils 1328, 1329, 1371, 1380
   toxicity to horses 1518–19
selenomethionine 1351, 1354
semustine 727
sequestrene *see* ethylene diamine tetra-acetic acid
sertraline 220
sesbanine 1518
sevoflurane 2030
shale 605
shale oils 1537
shellfish toxin 816
SHI *see* sodium hippurate
sialomucin 897
sialoproteins 974
silica
   causing apoptosis 184
   early research 1482
   from volcanoes 1815, 1817
   irritant effects 1455
   and lung cancer 1457
   in mines 1827
   in plastics industry 2022
   in rubber 2017
   silicosis 1475
silicates 1985
silicon 1382, 1905
silicones 1662, 1674, 2013, 2014
siloxanes 1585
silver 1489, 1765, 2087, 2089

silybin 870
simazine 2003, 2006
simvastatin 946
sincamidine 1519
sinigrin 234
sirolimus 1130
SKF93479 1124
smoke 919–20, 1266, 1446
   see also tobacco smoke
smoke flavourings 1654, 1655, 1657
snake venoms 428, 812, 820, 956, 957–8
sodium
   cardiac action potential 805, 816
   food toxicology 1979, 1990
   forensic toxicology 1504
   mineralocorticoid action 370
   in soils 1367
   in tests 355, 358, 364, 366
sodium aluminosilicate 2153
sodium ascorbate (SA) 1130
sodium azide 1046, 1047
sodium bentonite 2153
sodium bicarbonate 546
sodium birate 618
sodium chlorate 51, 390, 393, 2003, 2004
sodium chloride 528, 537, 685, 1517, 1522–3
sodium chromate 463
sodium chromoglycate 513
sodium citrate 2087
sodium cyanide 50, 760, 1331, 1725, 1726
sodium 2,3-dimercaptopropane-sulphonate *see* dimercaprol
sodium edetate 427, 1513
sodium ethane thiosulphonate 428
sodium fluoride 357, 1994
sodium fluoroacetate (compound 1080) 6, 34, 325, 643, 1510–11
sodium hippurate (SHI) 1130
sodium iodoacetate 821
sodium lactate 1709
sodium lauryl sulphate 842, 844
sodium β-mecaptopyruvate 428
sodium metabisulphite 535
sodium monofluorate 1524
sodium nitrate 428
sodium nitrite 393, 426, 429, 433, 1519
   for hydrogen cyanide poisoning 2102
sodium nitroprusside 185, 2188

THC *see* cannabis

Δ9-THC *see* cannabis

theobromine 823

theophylline 200, 252, 256, 433, 552, 816, 823, 911, 917

thermoplastic resins 626

thiabendazole 2000, 2001, 2002

thiazoles 2016

thiazopyr 990

thioacetamide 184, 233, 257, 881, 882, 883, 1860, 1861, 1862

thioacetic acid 134

thioamides 990

thiobarbituric acid 757

thiobenzamide 184

thiocyanate 566, 1822, 1905, 1907, 1927, 2100

thioglycollic acid 134

6-thioguanine (6-TG) 24, 261, 985, 1052

thiols 2014, 2052, 2054

thiomersal 1642

thiopentone sodium 522

thiophanate 2000, 2002

thiophanate-methyl 2000, 2002

thiophosphorus insecticides, oxidative desulphuration 1329

thioredoxin 199, 200

thioridazine 129–30, 220, 819, 1146, 1495

thiotepa 231

2-thiothaizolidine-4-carboxylic acid 1907

thiouracil 1121

thioureas 233, 724–5, 1121, 2003, 2005

thiram 1415, 2001, 2002, 2014, 2016

thorium 974

thorium dioxide 881

thorotrast *see* thorium dioxide

thromboxanes, carcinogenesis and 1981

thymidine glycol 1867, 1868

thyrocalcitonin 968

ticrynafen *see* tienillic acid

tienillic acid 229, 1439

tilidine fumarate 882

tilmicosin 1645

timolol 220, 760–1, 760–1, 761

tin 1489

tiotidine 1124

TIQ *see* 1,2,3,4-tetrahydroiso-quinoline

tissue plasminogen activator 1970

titanium dioxide 1280, 1282, 2014, 2017, 2023

TMA *see* trimethylamine

TMT *see* trimethyltin

tobacco smoke
    carcinogenicity 1538
    chemical constituents 224, 1278, 1296, 1297, 1298
    epidemiology 1537
    and gastro-intestinal microflora 565
    indoor source 1293
    in vitro tests 417
    mixtures 305, 314
    neonatal toxicity 1215, 1218, 1224
    pancreatic toxicity 911, 917, 919, 920, 926
    particulate matter 1299
    passive smoking 1267, 1293
    placental function and amino acid transport 1255–6
    reproducitve toxicity 1151, 1153
    source of cadmium 1377

tobramycin 685

toclofos-methyl 2001, 2003

tocopherols *see* vitamin E

tolbutamide 228–9

o-tolidine 463, 565, 1587

tolrestat 763

toluene 2038–9
    abuse 2029
    behavioural toxicity 651, 657, 660
    with benzene 149, 1445–6
    biomonitoring 1903, 1904, 1907
    characteristics 2035
    CNS effects 1455, 2030, 2031
    as combustion product 1927
    and *o*-cresol excretion 1417
    enzyme induction 2033
    ethanol interaction 2033, 2034
    exposure routes 607, 613
    from PU 1918
    genotoxicity 1456
    hepatotoxicity 1456
    neurotoxicity 634
    and noise 1419
    occupational hazards 510, 515
    ototoxicity 784, 794, 795, 1418
    PBPK modelling 142, 149
    reproductive toxicity 1156
    rubber additive 2014, 2018
    with *m*-xylene 149

toluene diisocyanate (TDI) 413, 616, 705, 707, 709, 711, 1456, 1712, 2021

toluidine blue 344, 393

o-toluidine 1484

o-tolyl diguanidine 2016

torsemide 229

toxaphene 879, 1244, 1316, 1336, 1346, 1995

TPA *see* 12-*O*-tetradecanoʏ lphorbol 13-acetate

trace elements 1370, 2049, 2062, 2063–6

traclimus 1130

tramadol 220

transferrin 254, 363, 367, 634, 678

trematoxin 877

tremetol 1520

triacetyloleandomycin 114

trialkyl phosphorothioate 21

trialkyltin salts 882

triamcinolone 758, 969

triaryl phosphates 986

triazines 990, 1042, 1369, 1511–12, 2003, 2006

triazolam (Halcion) 22, 252, 1427, 1428, 1438

triazoles 1123, 2003, 2006

tributylin 186, 188–9, 197

S,S,S-tributyl phosphorotrithoate (DEF) 2006

tributyltin oxide (TBTO) 1007–8, 2000, 2001

tributyltins 200, 1407

tricaine/benzocaine injection 498

tricarboxylic acid 632

trichlorethylene 917

trichlorfon 635, 636, 824, 1341, 1352

trichloroacetic acid 566, 1383, 1485, 1908, 2037

1,1,1-trichloroethane 206, 2035, 2037
    biomonitoring 1903, 1908
    cardiac toxicity 810
    eye toxicity 750
    genotoxicity 24
    mixed routes of exposure 607
    PBPK modelling 142
    in rubber 2017

trichloroethanol 1908, 2036, 2042

trichloroethanol glucuronide 2037

trichloroethylene 2036–7
    anaesthesia 2030
    biomonitoring 1903

trichloroethylene (*Contd.*)
  cardiac toxicity 810
  CNS effects 1475
  and degreasers' flush 1415
  with dichloroethylene 148
  enzyme induction 2033
  with ethanol 149, 2033
  and gastro-intestinal microflora 566
  human studies 463
  impurities 1445
  nephrotoxicity 691
  ototoxicity 784, 794, 795
  PBPK modelling 142, 1770–1
  peroral toxicity 551
  protein adducts 1887
  rubber additive 2014, 2018
  systemic pulmonary irritation 731
  with vinyl chloride 149
trichlorofluoroethane 1908
trichlorofluoromethane 461, 2023
trichloromethane 2036
trichloromethyl, free radical 2036
trichloronat 1997
2,4,5-trichlorophenol 281, 1818
2,4,5-trichlorophenoxyacetic acid (2,4,5-T) 879, 1222, 2003, 2005, 2104
1,1,1-trichloropropene-2,3-oxide 279
1,1,2-trichloro-1,2,2-trifluoroethane 142
trichothecenes 390, 391, 394, 525, 1254, 2104, 2145, 2146, 2149
  see also T-2 mycotoxins
tri-*o*-cresyl phosphate (TOCP) 637–8, 1554, 1824, 1997
tricresyl phosphate (TCP) 986, 2014, 2017
tricyclic antidepressants 1495, 1504
tridemorph 2001, 2004
triethanolamine 2014
triethylamine 738, 1903, 1908, 2020
triethylenemelamine 1145
tri(2-ethylhexyl)phosphate 750
triethyltin 638–9, 639, 2001
triethyltin bromide 274
trifluoperazine 819
3-trifluormethylpyridine 590
trifluoroacetic acid 101, 102, 1908
trifluoroacetyl chloride 102, 104
triglycerides 361, 367, 548, 939
1,2,3-trihydroxybenzene 100

3,4,5-trihydroxybenzoic acid 109
Triludan *see* terfenadine
trimellitic anhydride (TMA) 706, 709, 1004, 2022
trimethoprim 390, 391, 532
trimethoxysilane 15, 16
trimethylamine 102, 103, 220, 233–4
trimethylamine oxide 679, 2127
1,2,4-trimethylbenzene, interactions 2033
2,2,4-trimethyl-2-dihydroquinolone 2017
trimethylolpropane 1925
2,2,4-trimethylpentane 692
3-[2(2,4,6-trimethylphenyl)thiothyl]-4-methylsydnone 870
trimethyltin 642, 784, 794, 2001
trimipramine 221, 1495, 1497
triparanol 730, 1430, 1634
triphenylmethane 531, 1987
triphenylmethane triisocyanate 2021
triphenyltin chloride 274
tris(chloroalkyl) phosphate esters 2022
tris(2,3-dibromopropyl) phosphate 2022
tris(dimethylamino)silane (TDMAS) 26–7
trolitazone 992
tropicamide 759
tropisetron 221
troponins 366, 812
tryptamine 222, 223, 225
Tryptan Blue 565
tryptophan 22, 283, 395, 942, 946, 1552, 1553, 1568
tryptophol 222, 236
tubocurarine 34, 954, 955
Tween 80 1086
Tween 20 551
Tylenol *see* acetaminophen
tylosin 1648
tyramine 21, 103, 114, 823, 1518

U

unsaturated fats 823
uracil 235, 990
uranium 1475, 1866
uranium oxide 1820
urates 363
urea 355–6, 362, 1455, 1514, 2003, 2005

urea–formaldehyde 1922
urethane 881, 1035, 1922
uric acid 1983

V

valeric acid 1125
valinomycin 819
valium *see* diazepam
valproic acid 121, 254, 258, 869, 993, 1189, 1216
vanadate 822
vanadium 823, 1370, 1382, 1908
vanadium pentoxide 1903
vedaprofen 1642
vegetable oils 534, 551, 823, 2014
vehicle emissions 1265–6, 1267, 1268, 1273, 1274
  see also petrol/diesel fumes
verapamil 22, 188, 198, 809, 817, 1495, 2190
veratridine 639, 816, 818
veratrosin 1521
veratrum 821
vermillion *see* mercury(II) sulphide
versicolorins 2151
versiconal 2151
villin 894
vinblastine 186, 199, 262, 942, 1146
vinca alkaloids 638, 942, 943, 992, 1152, 1153
vinclozolin 2001, 2002
vincristine 199, 262, 522, 637, 638, 942, 943, 1455
vinegar, for jellyfish stings 2190
vinorelbine 262
vinyl acetate 550, 2019
vinylbenzene *see* styrene
vinyl chloride 2019
  see also poly(vinyl chloride) (PVC)
  age effects 1417
  binding values (EU) 1595
  biomonitoring 1903
  carcinogenicity 1417, 1456, 1475, 1536, 1537, 1538, 1551
  as combustion product 1928
  DNA adducts from 1881
  extrapolation studies 1952
  from polymers 1917
  hepatotoxicity 881
  human studies 457, 463
  metabolism 100–1
  mixtures 21

vinyl chloride (*Contd.*)
  monomer 2019
  Monte Carlo analysis 1784
  pancreatic toxicity 922
  rat toxicity 1417
  reproductive toxicity 1145
  sperm evaluation studies 1467
  and spontaneous abortion 1464
  threshold limit value 1475
  toxic reactions 1430
  with trichloroethylene and 1,2-
    dichloroethylene 149
4-vinylcyclohexene diepoxide 184
vinylidene fluoride 142
vinylidine chloride 2019
L-5-vinyl-2-thiooxazolidone 1121
Vioform 1565
virginiamycin 1648
vitamin(s)
  see also food supplements *in
    Subject Index*
  deficiency, effect on metabolism
    115
vitamin(s) 548, 938, 972, 1217,
  1223, 1552, 1690, 1985, 2161
vitamin(s)
  A 127, 316, 864, 946, 969, 972,
    1430, 1551, 1552, 1982
  B$_6$ 1430, 1552, 1987
  B$_{12}$ 391, 428, 1548, 2064
  C 127, 158, 191, 200, 491,
    1982–3, 1985, 2131, 2132,
    2161
  D$_2$ 2068
  D$_3$ (cholecalciferol) 1511, 2068
  D 316, 949–50, 968, 972, 973,
    983, 1430, 2068
  E
    as antioxidant 158
    and apoptosis 191, 200
    cardiac toxicity 809
    food toxicology 1978, 1982,
      1983, 1985, 1986
    human studies 2132, 2137
    nephrotoxicity 681
    parenteral toxicity 532
    toxicokinetics 2121
    toxic response moderation
      127

  K 229, 1524
  K$_1$ 1511, 2006
vitellogenin 1407, 1408
V nerve agents 2090
volatile organic compounds (VOCs)
  1266–7, 1292, 1295, 1297–8,
  1299, 1300, 1302
volvatoxin A 820
vomitoxin *see* deoxynivalenol
VP-16 186, 195
VX *see* pinacolyl methylphosphono-
  fluoridate

W

Warbex 1342
warfarin 114, 229, 243, 569,
  1510–11, 2006
white oils 920
white phosphorus 1340–1, 1475,
  1511
white spirit 2018
wood dusts 701
WR 2721 792

X

xylenes 2033, 2039
  biomarker 1844
  biomonitoring 1903, 1908
  characteristics 2035
  CNS effects 1475
  enzyme induction 2033
  interactions 2033–4
  irritation 1475
  laboratory occupational hazard
    510, 515
  mixed routes of exposure 607
  ototoxicity 784, 795
  PBPK modelling 142
  rubber additive 2014, 2018
  skin effects 1475
  with toluene 149
xylitol 1653
xylose 107, 365
xylyl bromide 2102

Y

yellow phosphorus 1523–4
Yellow Rain 2080

Z

zearalenone 1515–16, 2145, 2146,
  2147
zenarestat 764
zeranol 284
zidovudine (AZT) 942, 946
zimeldine (Zelmid) 1427, 1438
zinc 2066
  anthropogenic emissions 1370
  and apoptosis 188
  apoptosis and 200
  associated cadmium 1374
  biomarker 1864, 1869
  cartilage and bone toxicity 965,
    968, 972, 973, 974, 2068
  circadian toxicology 257
  depletion 757
  in diet, cadmium toxicity and
    2054
  domestic animal toxicoses 1513
  fortification 1552
  from mining sites 1373
  fungicide 2001
  in Greenland snow cover 1370
  hepatotoxicity 870
  as impurity in fertilizer 1371
  metallothionein and 2067
  plant root uptake 1369
  in plastics 2022
  in sewage sludge 1372
  soil reference values 1373
  in soils 1329
  in water distribution systems
    1377
zinc carbonate 2052
zinc chloride 1475
zinc dimethyl dithiocarbamate
  see ziram
zinc naphthenate 917
zinc nitrate 2018
zinc oxide 2014
zinc phosphide 1346–7, 1510–11,
  2006
zineb 990, 2000, 2001
zinostatin 727
ziram 990, 2001, 2002, 2016, 2017
zoalene (3,5-dinitro-*o*-toluamide)
  1521
zomepirac (Zomax) 1427, 1428
zuclopentixol 221
zygacine 1522